Matthias
Maihoefer

Emergency

phone - 412-767-0505

Care and Transportation of the Sick and Injured

Student Workbook

JONES AND BARTLETT PUBLISHERS

Sudbury, Massachusetts

BOSTON   TORONTO   LONDON   SINGAPORE

Jones and Bartlett Publishers

World Headquarters
Jones and Bartlett Publishers
40 Tall Pine Drive, Sudbury, MA 01776
978-443-5000
info@jbpub.com
www.EMSzone.com

Jones and Bartlett Publishers Canada
6339 Ormindale Way
Mississauga, Ontario
L5V 1J2

Jones and Bartlett Publishers International
Barb House, Barb Mews
London W6 7PA
United Kingdom

Jones and Bartlett's books and products are available through most bookstores and online booksellers. To contact Jones and Bartlett Publishers directly, call 800-832-0034, fax 978-443-8000, or visit our website www.jbpub.com.

Substantial discounts on bulk quantities of Jones and Bartlett's publications are available to corporations, professional associations, and other qualified organizations. For details and specific discount information, contact the special sales department at Jones and Bartlett via the above contact information or send an email to specialsales@jbpub.com.

American Academy of Orthopaedic Surgeons

Chief Education Officer: Mark W. Wieting
Director, Department of Publications: Marilyn L. Fox, PhD
Managing Editor: Lynne Roby Shindoll
Managing Editor: Barbara A. Scotese

Production Credits

Publisher, Public Safety: Kimberly Brophy
Managing Editor: Carol Brewer
Associate Editor: Janet Morris
Production Editor: Karen Ferreira
V.P., Manufacturing and Inventory Control: Therese Connell
Interior Design: Shepherd, Inc.
Cover Design: Kristin E. Ohlin
Composition: Shepherd, Inc.
Printing and Binding: Courier Westford

Editorial Credits

Authors: Julie F. Chase, BS, BM, NREMT-P
Jay Keefauver, BS, EMT-P, CEMSI
Donald Royder, EMT-P

This student workbook is intended solely as a guide to the appropriate procedures to be employed when rendering emergency care to the sick and injured. It is not intended as a statement of the standards of care required in any particular situation, because circumstances and the patient's physical condition can vary widely from one emergency to another. Nor is it intended that this Student Workbook shall in any way advise emergency personnel concerning legal authority to perform the activities or procedures discussed. Such local determinations should be made only with the aid of legal counsel.
Note: The patients described in **Ambulance Calls** are fictitious.

Printed in the United States of America
09 08 07 06 05   10 9 8 7 6 5 4 3 2

CONTENTS

Section 5: Trauma

Section 6: Special Populations

Section 7: Operations

Section 8: ALS Techniques

Answer Key

EMT-Basic Review Manual for National Certification

ISBN: 0-7637-1829-7

The *EMT-Basic Review Manual for National Certification* is designed to prepare you to sit for the national certification exam by including the same type of skill-based and multiple-choice questions that you are likely to see on the exam. The review manual will also evaluate your mastery of the material presented in your EMT-Basic training program. The *EMT-Basic Review Manual for National Certification* includes:

- Practice questions with answers and model exam
- Step-by-step walkthrough of skills, including helpful tips, commonly made errors, and sample scenarios
- Self-scoring guide and winning test-taking tips
- Coverage of the entire 1994 DOT EMT-Basic curriculum

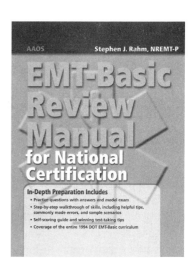

Student Review Manual

ISBN: 0-7637-2971-X (print)
ISBN: 0-7637-2970-1 (CD-ROM)
ISBN: 0-7637-2972-8 (online)

This *Review Manual* has been designed to prepare students for exams by including the same type of questions that they are likely to see on classroom and national examinations. The manual contains multiple-choice question exams with an answer key and page references. It is available in print, on CD-ROM, and online.

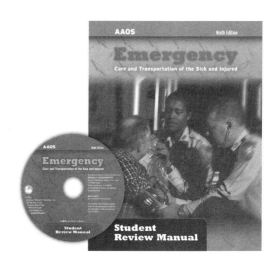

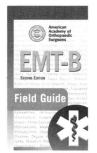

EMT-B Field Guide, Second Edition

ISBN: 0-7637-2214-6

This handy reference covers basic information from patient management tips to guidelines on helping a patient use medication. A few special features include a prescription medication reference and documentation tips. The *EMT-B Field Guide* is pocket-sized, spiral-bound, and water resistant for ready-reference in the field.

To order: Call 1-800-832-0034 or visit www.EMSzone.com

CHAPTER

1 Introduction to Emergency Medical Care

Workbook Activities

The following activities have been designed to help you. Your instructor may require you to complete some or all of these activities as a regular part of your EMT-B training program. You are encouraged to complete any activity that your instructor does not assign as a way to enhance your learning in the classroom.

Chapter Review

The following exercises provide an opportunity to refresh your knowledge of this chapter.

Matching

Match each of the items in the left column to the appropriate definition in the right column.

H	**1.** ALS	**A.** EMS professional trained in ALS
F	**2.** BLS	**B.** a system of internal reviews and audits
M	**3.** EMT-B	**C.** a system to provide prehospital care to the sick and injured
G	**4.** EMT-I	**D.** the physician who authorizes the EMT to perform in the field
A	**5.** EMT-P	**E.** responsibility of the medical director to ensure appropriate care is delivered by an EMT
K	**6.** Medical control	**F.** basic lifesaving interventions, such as CPR
S	**7.** CQI	**G.** EMS professional trained in some ALS interventions
C	**8.** EMS	**H.** advanced procedures such as drug administration
E	**9.** Continuing education	**I.** designated area in which the EMS service is responsible
E	**10.** Quality control	**J.** protects disabled individuals from discrimination
I	**11.** Primary service area	**K.** physician instruction to EMS team
	12. Medical Director	**L.** a required amount of training to maintain skills
S	**13.** Americans with Disabilities Act	**M.** EMS professional trained in BLS

Multiple Choice

Read each item carefully, and then select the best response.

 1. Control of external bleeding, provision of oxygen and CPR are included in the "scope of practice" of the:
   A. EMT-P.
   B. EMT-B.
   C. EMT-I.
   D. EMT-D.

 2. All of the following are true of medical control except:
   A. It is determined by the dispatcher.
   B. It may be written or "standing orders."
   C. It may require online radio or phone consultation.
   D. It describes the care authorized by the medical director.

_____ **3.** All of the following are components of continuous quality control except:
   A. periodic run reviews.
   B. remedial training.
   C. internal reviews and audits.
   D. public seminars and meetings.

_____ **4.** The major goal of quality improvement is to ensure that:
   A. quarterly audits of the EMS system are done.
   B. EMTs have received BLS/CPR training.
   C. the public receives the highest standard of care.
   D. the proper information is received in the billing department.

_____ **5.** Your main concern while responding to a call should be the:
   A. safety of the crew and yourself.
   B. number of potential patients.
   C. request for mutual assistance.
   D. type of call.

Questions 6-10 are derived from the following scenario: After stocking the ambulance this morning, you and your partner go out for breakfast. While entering the restaurant, you see an older gentleman clutch his chest and collapse to the floor. When you get to him, he has no pulse and is not breathing.

_____ **6.** The _____ _____ authorizes you as an EMT-B to provide emergency care to this patient.
   A. City Counsel
   B. Medical Control
   C. Medical Director
   D. Fire Chief

_____ **7.** To treat this patient, you will follow:
   A. off-line medical control
   B. on-line medical control
   C. protocols
   D. all the above

_____ **8.** The level of training that allows electrocardiogram and advanced life support to be given to this patient is:
   A. First responder
   B. EMT-B
   C. EMT-I
   D. EMT-P

_____A_____ **9.** While you checked the patient's airway, breathing, and circulation, your partner followed local protocols and called for _____ back-up.
   A. ALS
   B. CQI
   C. PSA
   D. HIPAA

_____B_____ **10.** While you performed CPR on this patient, your partner gathered the _____ that will deliver an appropriate electrical shock.
   A. EMD
   B. AED
   C. DEA
   D. GPS

Fill-in

Read each item carefully, and then complete the statement by filling in the missing word(s).

1. The training of the EMT-B should meet or exceed the guidelines of _____.

2. EMT-B training is divided into care of _____, _____, and important non-medical issues related to EMT abilities.

3. In some areas, EMT-Bs may provide selected ALS care such as automated external defibrillation, use of nonvisualized airways such as the Combitube or even endotracheal intubation, and assisting patients in taking prescription Medecines.

4. In most of the country, a communications center can be easily reached by dialing 911.

5. The appropriate care for injury or illness as described by the medical director either by radio or in written form is called Medical control.

True/False

If you believe the statement to be more true than false, write the letter "T" in the space provided. If you believe the statement to be more false than true, write the letter "F."

_____F_____ **1.** EMT-B personnel are the highest qualified members of the prehospital care team.

_____T_____ **2.** The EMT-B scope of practice may include the use of an automated or semi-automated defibrillator.

_____F_____ **3.** The purpose of continuous quality improvement (CQI) is to support discipline of personnel.

_____T_____ **4.** A professional appearance and manner by the EMT-B will help a patient build confidence.

_____F_____ **5.** Essential keys to being a good EMT-B include compassion, commitment, and desire.

_____T_____ **6.** As a health care professional and an extension of physician care, you are bound by patient confidentiality—even in your own home.

Short Answer

Complete this section with short written answers using the space provided.

1. Describe the EMT-B's role in the EMS system.

_____

_____

2. What role has the U.S. Department of Transportation played in the development of EMS?

_____

_____

3. List five roles and/or responsibilities of being an EMT-B.

_____

_____

4. Describe the two basic types of medical direction that help the EMT-B provide care.

_____

_____

Word Fun

The following crossword puzzle is an activity provided to reinforce correct spelling and understanding of medical terminology associated with emergency care and the EMT-B. Use the clues in the column to complete the puzzle.

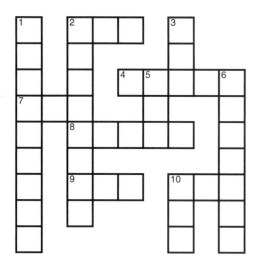

Across

2. System that provides prehospital emergency care

4. An EMT with training in BLS/CPR

7. Designed to protect individuals with disabilities

8. Section of the U.S. DOT that created programs to improve EMS

9. An individual trained to provide emergency care to the sick and injured

10. BLS intervention in cardiac arrest

Down

1. An EMT with extensive training in advanced life support

2. A type of 9-1-1 system that displays the caller's address

3. Simple lifesaving interventions, ie, CPR

5. Advanced lifesaving procedures, ie, defibrillation

6. Medical or Quality _____

10. A circular system of reviews and changes in an EMS system

Ambulance Calls

The following case scenarios provide an opportunity to explore the concerns associated with patient management. Read each scenario, and then answer each question in detail.

1. You are dispatched to a two car MVC. Upon arrival, you see minimal damage to both vehicles, as they were traveling less than 25 mph when the incident occurred. You and your partner examine all patients, and find no injuries. All patients are adults except for the driver of one vehicle. He is 16 years old, and has no complaints and no apparent injuries. He asks you if it's okay to leave.

Do you let him go?

No, he is underage and needs parent/gardian to leave

2. You are dispatched to a private residence. Several neighbors are gathered on the front lawn. There appears to be an argument taking place between two of them. A teenage boy is sitting on the doorstep, bleeding profusely from a cut above his left eye.

How would you best manage this situation?

Make your way to the patient carfuly and get local pd on scene

3. It's after midnight and you are dispatched to "laceration to the arm." You arrive to find a young man who tells you he was in a fight and his right arm was cut. You notice that his bleeding is controlled, and his vital signs are within acceptable ranges. As you apply dressings to his wound, another dispatch comes over the radio for "unconscious assault victim, police officers on the scene." You are one block away.

What do you do?

transport your patient to the hospital if you don't its neglegence

CHAPTER

2 The Well-Being of the EMT-B

Workbook Activities

The following activities have been designed to help you. Your instructor may require you to complete some or all of these activities as a regular part of your EMT-B training program. You are encouraged to complete any activity that your instructor does not assign as a way to enhance your learning in the classroom.

Chapter Review

The following exercises provide an opportunity to refresh your knowledge of this chapter.

Matching

Match each of the terms in the left column to the appropriate definition in the right column.

_____ 1. Cover
_____ 2. Burnout
_____ 3. Occupational Safety and Health Administration
_____ 4. Posttraumatic stress disorder
_____ 5. Body substance isolation
_____ 6. Pathogen
_____ 7. Transmission
_____ 8. Tuberculosis
_____ 9. Virulence
_____ 10. Hepatitis
_____ 11. Exposure
_____ 12. Infection control
_____ 13. Meningitis
_____ 14. Contamination

A. chronic fatigue and frustration
B. assuming all body fluids are potentially infected
C. regulatory compliance agency
D. concealment for protection
E. capable of causing disease in a susceptible host
F. delayed stress reaction
G. chronic bacterial disease that usually affects the lungs
H. an inflammation of the meningeal coverings of the brain
I. an infection of the liver
J. contact with blood, body fluids, tissues, or airborne particles
K. the presence of infectious organisms in or on objects, or a patient's body
L. the strength or ability of a pathogen to produce disease
M. the way in which an infectious agent is spread
N. procedures to reduce transmission of infection among patients and health care personnel

Multiple Choice

Read each item carefully, then select the best response.

_____ **1.** From the age of 1 to the age of 34, _____ is the leading cause of death.

    A. cardiac arrest

    B. congenital disease

    C. trauma

    D. AIDS

_____ **2.** The stage of the grieving process where an attempt is made to secure a prize for good behavior or promise to change lifestyle is known as:

    A. denial.

    B. acceptance.

    C. bargaining.

    D. depression.

_____ **3.** The stage of the grieving process that involves refusal to accept diagnosis or care is known as:

    A. denial.

    B. acceptance.

    C. bargaining.

    D. depression.

_____ **4.** The stage of the grieving process that involves an open expression of grief, internalized anger, hopelessness, and/or the desire to die is:

    A. denial.

    B. acceptance.

    C. bargaining.

    D. depression.

_____ **5.** The stage of grieving where the person is ready to die is known as:

    A. denial.

    B. acceptance.

    C. bargaining.

    D. depression.

_____ **6.** When providing support for a grieving person, it is okay to say:

    A. "I'm sorry."

    B. "Give it time."

    C. "I know how you feel."

    D. "You have to keep on going."

_____ **7.** When grieving, family members may express:

    A. rage.

    B. anger.

    C. despair.

    D. all of the above

_____ **8.** _____ is a response to the anticipation of danger.

    A. Rage

    B. Anger

    C. Anxiety

    D. Despair

9. Signs of anxiety include all of the following, except:

   A. diaphoresis.

   B. comfort.

   C. hyperventilation.

   D. tachycardia.

10. Fear may be expressed as:

   A. anger.

   B. bad dreams.

   C. restlessness.

   D. all of the above

11. If you find that you are the target of the patient's anger, make sure that you:

   A. are safe.

   B. do not take the anger or insults personally.

   C. are tolerant, and do not become defensive.

   D. all of the above

12. When caring for critically ill or injured patients, _____ will be decreased if you can keep the patient informed at the scene.

   A. confusion

   B. anxiety

   C. feelings of helplessness

   D. all of the above

13. When acknowledging the death of a child, reactions vary, but _____ is common.

   A. shock

   B. disbelief

   C. denial

   D. all of the above

14. Factors influencing how a patient reacts to the stress of an EMS incident include all of the following, except:

   A. family history.

   B. age.

   C. fear of medical personnel.

   D. socioeconomic background.

15. Negative forms of stress include all of the following, except:

   A. long hours.

   B. exercise.

   C. shift work.

   D. frustration of losing a patient.

16. Stressors include _____ situations or conditions that may cause a variety of physiologic, physical, and psychologic responses.

   A. emotional

   B. physical

   C. environmental

   D. all of the above

17. Prolonged or excessive stress has been proven to be a strong contributor to:

   A. heart disease.

   B. hypertension.

   C. cancer.

   D. all of the above

_____ **18.** _____ occur(s) when insignificant stressors accumulate to a larger stress-related problem.

A. Negative stress

B. Cumulative stress

C. Psychological stress

D. Severe stressors

_____ **19.** Events that can trigger critical incident stress include:

A. mass-casualty incidents.

B. serious injury or traumatic death of a child.

C. death or serious injury of a coworker in the line of duty.

D. all of the above

Questions 20-24 are derived from the following scenario: A 12-year-old boy told his grandmother he was going to collect the day's mail, located on the opposite side of the street for her. As he was returning with the mail, he was struck by a vehicle and was found lying lifeless in the middle of the street.

_____ **20.** What would be appropriate to say to the grandmother?

A. "Don't worry, I'm sure he'll be fine."

B. "What were you thinking? You will be reported!"

C. "We're placing him on a backboard to protect his back, and we'll take him to the Columbus Community Hospital. Do you know who his doctor is?"

D. It's best not to spend time talking to the grandmother.

_____ **21.** As an EMT-B, you know these types of calls are coming. How can you prepare to meet such stressful situations?

A. Eat a balanced diet.

B. Go for walks or other forms of exercise.

C. Cut down on caffeine and sugars.

D. All the above

_____ **22.** You or your partner may develop _____ after experiencing this call.

A. Critical incident stress management

B. Posttraumatic stress disorder

C. Critical stress debriefing

D. None of the above

_____ **23.** What signs of stress may you or your partner exhibit?

A. Irritability towards coworkers, family, and friends.

B. Loss of sexual activities

C. Guilt

D. All of the above

_____ **24.** When should you begin protecting yourself with BSI on this call?

A. As soon as you are dispatched.

B. As soon as you arrive.

C. After you assess the victim, and know what you need.

D. After speaking with the grandmother.

_____ **25.** The quickest source of energy is _____; however, this supply will last less than a day and is consumed in greater quantities during stress.

A. glucose

B. carbohydrate

C. protein

D. fat

_____ **26.** Stress management strategies include:

    A. changing work hours.

    B. changing your attitude.

    C. changing partners.

    D. all of the above

_____ **27.** _____ is a condition of chronic fatigue and frustration that results from mounting stress over time.

    A. Posttraumatic stress disorder

    B. Cumulative stress

    C. Critical incident stress

    D. Burnout

_____ **28.** The safest, most reliable sources for long-term energy production are:

    A. sugars.

    B. carbohydrates.

    C. fats.

    D. proteins.

_____ **29.** A _____ is any event that causes anxiety and mental stress to emergency workers.

    A. disaster

    B. mass-casualty incident

    C. critical incident

    D. stressor

_____ **30.** A CISD meeting is an opportunity to discuss your:

    A. feelings.

    B. fears.

    C. reactions to the event.

    D. all of the above

_____ **31.** Components of the CISM system include:

    A. preincident stress education.

    B. defusings.

    C. spouse and family support.

    D. all of the above

_____ **32.** Sexual harassment is defined as:

    A. any unwelcome sexual advance.

    B. unwelcome requests for sexual favors.

    C. unwelcome verbal or physical conduct of a sexual nature.

    D. all of the above

_____ **33.** Drug and alcohol use in the workplace can result in all of the following, except:

    A. absence from work more often.

    B. enhanced treatment decisions.

    C. an increase in accidents and tension among workers.

    D. lessened ability to render emergency medical care because of mental or physical impairment.

_____ **34.** You should begin protecting yourself:

    A. as soon as you arrive on the scene.

    B. before you leave the scene.

    C. as soon as you are dispatched.

    D. before any patient contact.

_____ 35. _____ is contact with blood, body fluids, tissues, or airborne droplets by direct or indirect contact.

A. Transmission

B. Exposure

C. Handling

D. all of the above

_____ 36. Modes of transmission for infectious diseases include:

A. blood or fluid splash.

B. surface contamination.

C. needle stick exposure.

D. all of the above

_____ 37. The spread of HIV and hepatitis in the health care setting can usually be traced to:

A. careless handling of sharps.

B. improper use of BSI precautions.

C. not wearing PPE.

D. sexual interaction with infected persons.

_____ 38. _____ is equipment that blocks entry of an organism into the body.

A. Vaccination

B. Body substance isolation

C. Personal protective equipment

D. Immunization

_____ 39. Recommended immunizations include:

A. MMR vaccine.

B. hepatitis B vaccine.

C. influenza vaccine.

D. all the above.

_____ 40. Why isn't tuberculosis more common?

A. Absolute protection from infection with the tubercle bacillus does not exist.

B. Everyone who breathes is at risk

C. The vaccine for tuberculosis is only rarely used in the United States.

D. Infected air is easily diluted with uninfected air.

_____ 41. You can use a bleach and water solution at a _____ dilution to clean the unit.

A. 1:1

B. 1:10

C. 1:100

D. 1:1000

_____ 42. Hazardous materials are classified according to _____, which dictate(s) the level of protection required.

A. danger zones

B. flammability

C. toxicity levels

D. all of the above

_____ 43. Factors to take into consideration for potential violence include:

A. poor impulse control.

B. substance abuse.

C. depression.

D. all of the above

Fill-in

Read each item carefully, then complete the statement by filling in the missing word.

1. The personal health, safety, and _____ of all EMT-Bs are vital to an EMS operation.

2. The struggle to remain calm in the face of horrible circumstances contributes to the _____

    _____ of the job.

3. Sixty percent of all deaths today are attributed to_____ _____.

4. Determination of the cause of death is the medical responsibility of a _____ .

5. In cases of hypothermia, the patient should not be considered dead until the patient is _____ and dead.

6. _____ is generally thought of in relation to the oncoming pain and the outcome of the damage.

7. Almost all dying patients feel some degree of _____ because of internalized anger and other factors.

8. You must also realize that the most _____ symptoms may be early signs of severe illness or injury.

9. EMS is a _____ job.

True/False

If you believe the statement to be more true than false, write the letter "T" in the space provided. If you believe the statement to be more false than true, write the letter "F."

_____ 1. Developing self-control is aided by proper training.
_____ 2. The primary mode of infection for herpes simplex is through close personal contact.
_____ 3. Denial is generally the first step in the grieving process.
_____ 4. Body fluids are generally not considered infectious substances.
_____ 5. Most EMT-Bs never suffer from stress.
_____ 6. Physical conditioning and nutrition are two factors the EMT-B can control in helping reduce stress.

Short Answer

Complete this section with short written answers using the space provided.

1. Describe the basic concept of body substance isolation (BSI).

    _____

    _____

2. List the five stages of the grieving process.

    _____

    _____

3. List five warning signs of stress.

    _____

    _____

4. List two strategies for managing stress.

    _____

    _____

5. Describe the process for proper hand washing.

_____

_____

6. Complete the following table on the toxicity of hazardous materials.

Level	Hazard	Protection Needed
0		
1		
2		
3		
4		

7. List the three layers of clothing recommended for cold weather.

_____

_____

8. List the four principal determinants of violence.

_____

_____

Word Fun

The following crossword puzzle is an activity provided to reinforce correct spelling and understanding of medical terminology associated with emergency care and the EMT-B. Use the clues in the column to complete the puzzle.

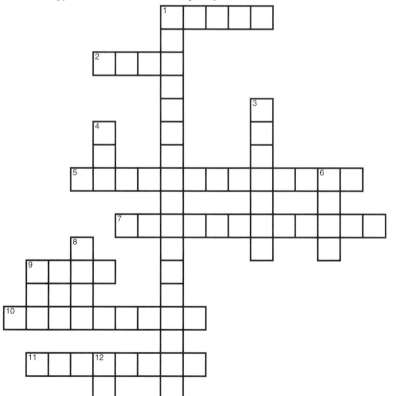

Across

1. Impenetrable barrier for tactical use
2. Confronts responses and defuses them
5. Exposure by physical touching
7. Disease of the lungs
9. Delayed reaction to past incident
10. Infection of the liver
11. Capable of causing disease

Down

1. Disease spread from person to person
3. Chronic fatigue and frustration
4. Infection control process
6. Confidential discussion group
8. Federal workplace safety agency
9. Blocks entry of an organism into the body
12. May progress to AIDS

Ambulance Calls

The following case scenarios provide an opportunity to explore the concerns associated with patient management. Read each scenario, then answer each question in detail.

1. You are dispatched to a private residence for an "unknown medical problem." You arrive to find family members gathered around the patient's bed. Your patient is breathing and has a pulse, but is not conscious. The family tells you that she's a hospice patient who has cancer. They tell you that a relative from out of state called 9-1-1, and the patient has a DNR order. They tell you to leave.

   What do you do?

   _____

   _____

   _____

2. You are dispatched to a rollover vehicle crash with three known patients. All other ambulances are out on calls; you and your partner will likely not receive assistance for at least 15 minutes. One patient has obvious head trauma, but is still breathing. Your other two patients are conscious but have significant injuries. A crowd is gathering and is watching your every move.

   What do you do?

   _____

   _____

   _____

3. In the process of working a motor vehicle crash, your arm is gashed open and you are exposed to the blood of a patient who tells you that he is HIV positive. You have no water supply in which to wash. Your patient is stable and you are able to control his bleeding with direct pressure.

   How would you best manage this situation?

   _____

   _____

   _____

Skill Drills

Skill Drill 2-1: Proper Glove Removal Technique

Test your knowledge of skill drills by placing the photos below in the correct order. Number the first step with a "1," the second step with a "2," etc.

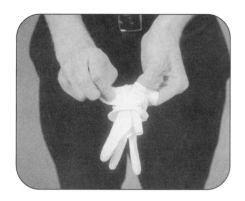

_____

Grasp both gloves with your free hand touching only the clean, interior surfaces.

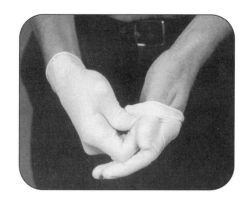

_____

Partially remove the first glove by pinching at the wrist. Be careful to touch only the outside of the glove.

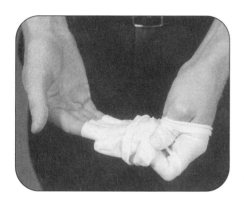

_____

Pull the second glove inside-out toward the fingertips.

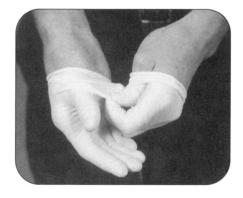

_____

Remove the second glove by pinching the exterior with the partially gloved hand.

CHAPTER

3 Medical, Legal, and Ethical Issues

Workbook Activities

The following activities have been designed to help you. Your instructor may require you to complete some or all of these activities as a regular part of your EMT-B training program. You are encouraged to complete any activity that your instructor does not assign as a way to enhance your learning in the classroom.

Chapter Review

The following exercises provide an opportunity to refresh your knowledge of this chapter.

Matching

Match each of the terms in the left column to the appropriate definition in the right column.

_____ **1.** Assault

_____ **2.** Abandonment

_____ **3.** Advance directive

_____ **4.** Battery

_____ **5.** Certification

_____ **6.** Competent

_____ **7.** Consent

_____ **8.** Duty to act

_____ **9.** Expressed consent

_____ **10.** Forcible restraint

_____ **11.** Implied consent

_____ **12.** Medicolegal

_____ **13.** Negligence

_____ **14.** Standard of care

A. able to make decisions

B. specific authorization to provide care expressed by the patient

C. confining a person from mental or physical action

D. granted permission

E. touching without consent

F. legal responsibility to provide care

G. written documentation that specifies treatment

H. unlawfully placing a patient in fear of bodily harm

I. unilateral termination of care

J. failure to provide standard of care

K. accepted level of care consistent with training

L. process that recognizes that a person has met set standards

M. legal assumption that treatment was desired

N. relating to law or forensic medicine

Multiple Choice

Read each item carefully, then select the best response.

_____ **1.** The care the EMT-B is able to provide, most commonly defined by state law, is:
  A. duty to act.
  B. competency.
  C. scope of practice.
  D. certification.

_____ **2.** How the EMT-B is required to act or behave is called the:
  A. standard of care.
  B. competency.
  C. scope of practice.
  D. certification.

_____ **3.** The process by which an individual, institution, or program is evaluated and recognized as meeting certain standards is called:
  A. standard of care.
  B. competency.
  C. scope of practice.
  D. certification.

_____ **4.** Negligence is based on the EMT-B's duty to act, cause, breach of duty, and:
  A. expressed consent.
  B. termination of care.
  C. mode of transport.
  D. real or perceived damages.

_____ **5.** While treating a patient with a suspected head injury, he becomes verbally abusive and tells you to "leave him alone." If you stop treating him you may be guilty of:
  A. neglect.
  B. battery.
  C. abandonment.
  D. slander.

_____ **6.** Good Samaritan laws generally are designed to offer protection to persons who render care in good faith. They do not offer protection from:
  A. properly performed CPR.
  B. acts of negligence.
  C. improvising splinting materials.
  D. providing supportive BLS to a DNR patient.

_____ **7.** Which of the following is generally NOT considered confidential?
  A. assessment findings
  B. patient's mental condition
  C. patient's medical history
  D. the location of the emergency

_____ **8.** An important safeguard against legal implication is:
  A. responding to every call with lights and siren.
  B. checking ambulance equipment once a month.
  C. transporting every patient to an emergency department.
  D. a complete and accurate incident report.

Questions 9-13 are derived from the following scenario: At 2 AM, a 17-year-old son accompanied by his 19-year-old girlfriend had driven to the bar to give his father (who had been drinking large amounts of alcohol) a ride home. On the way back, they were involved in a motor vehicle crash. The son has a large laceration with profuse bleeding on his forehead. His girlfriend is unconscious in the front passenger floor, and the father is standing outside the vehicle, appearing heavily intoxicated, and is refusing care.

_____ **9.** Should the father be allowed to refuse care?

    A. Yes – consent is required before care can be started.

    B. No – he is under the influence of drugs/alcohol and is therefore mentally incompetent.

    C. Yes – under implied consent.

    D. No – you would be guilty of abandonment.

_____ **10.** Why is it permissible for you to begin treatment on the girlfriend?

    A. consent is implied

    B. consent has been expressed

    C. consent was informed

    D. none of the above

_____ **11.** As you progress in your care for the patients, the father becomes unconscious. Can you begin/continue care for him now?

    A. Yes – consent in now implied.

    B. No – he made his wishes known before he fell unconscious.

    C. He just needs to sleep it off.

    D. none of the above

_____ **12.** With the son being a minor, what is the best way to gain consent to begin care, when his father has an altered mental status or is unconscious?

    A. Phone his mother for consent

    B. Call his grandparents for consent

    C. It's a true emergency, so consent is implied

    D. You're covered under the Good Samaritan Laws

_____ **13.** Your responsibility to provide patient care is called:

    A. Scope of practice

    B. Duty to act

    C. DNR

    D. Standard of care.

_____ **14.** Presumptive signs of death would not be adequate in cases of sudden death due to:

    A. hypothermia.

    B. acute poisoning.

    C. cardiac arrest.

    D. all of the above

_____ **15.** Definitive or conclusive signs of death that are obvious and clear to even nonmedical persons include all of the following, except:

    A. profound cyanosis.

    B. dependent lividity.

    C. rigor mortis.

    D. putrefaction.

_____ **16.** Medical examiner's cases include:

    A. violent death.

    B. suicide.

    C. suspicion of a criminal act.

    D. all of the above

_____ **17.** HIPAA is the acronym for the Health Insurance Portability and Accountability Act of 1996. It:

    A. makes ambulance services accountable for transporting patients in a safe manner.

    B. protects the privacy of health care information and to safeguard patient confidentiality.

    C. allows health insurers to transfer an insurance policy to another carrier if a patient does not pay his or her premium.

    D. enables emergency personnel to transfer a patient to a lower level of care when resources are scarce.

Fill-in

Read each item carefully, then complete the statement by filling in the missing word(s).

1. The _____ _____ _____ outlines the care you are able to provide.

2. The _____ _____ _____ is the manner in which the EMT must act when treating patients.

3. The legal responsibility to provide care is called the _____ _____ _____.

4. The determination of _____ is based on duty, breach of duty, damages, and cause.

5. Abandonment is _____ of care without transfer to someone of equal or higher training.

6. _____ consent is given directly by an informed patient, where _____ consent is assumed in the unconscious patient.

7. Unlawfully placing a person in fear of immediate harm is _____, while _____ is unlawfully touching a person without their consent.

8. A(n) _____ _____ is a written document that specifies authorized treatment in case a patient becomes unable to make decisions. A written document that authorizes the EMT not to attempt resuscitation efforts is a(n) _____ _____.

9. Mentally competent patients have the right to _____ _____.

10. Incidents involving child abuse, animal bites, childbirth, and assault have _____ _____ requirements in many states.

True/False

If you believe the statement to be more true than false, write the letter "T" in the space provided. If you believe the statement to be more false than true, write the letter "F."

_____ **1.** Failure to provide care to a patient once you have been called to the scene is considered negligence.

_____ **2.** For expressed consent to be valid, the patient must be a minor.

_____ **3.** If a patient is unconscious and a true emergency exists, the doctrine of implied consent applies.

_____ **4.** The EMT can legally restrain a patient against their will if the patient poses a threat to themselves or others.

_____ **5.** The best defense against legal action for the EMT is to always provide care in a manner consistent with ethical and moral standards.

Short Answer

Complete this section with short written answers using the space provided.

1. In many states, certain conditions allow a minor to be treated as an adult for the purpose of consenting to medical treatment. List three of these conditions.

_____

_____

2. When does your responsibility for patient care end?

_____

_____

3. There will be some instances when you will not be able to persuade the patient, guardian, conservator, or parent of a minor child or mentally incompetent patient to proceed with treatment. List five steps you should take to protect all parties involved.

_____

_____

4. List the two rules of thumb courts consider regarding reports and records.

_____

_____

5. List four steps to take when you are called to the scene involving a potential organ donor.

_____

_____

Word Fun

The following crossword puzzle is an activity provided to reinforce correct spelling and understanding of medical terminology associated with emergency care and the EMT-B. Use the clues in the column to complete the puzzle.

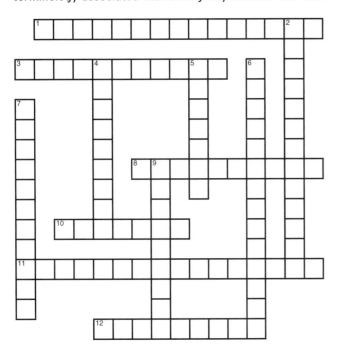

Across

1. Care that the EMT-B is authorized to provide
3. Relating to medical law
8. Failure to provide standard of care
10. Touching another person without their expressed consent
11. Direct permission to provide care
12. Responsibility to provide care

Down

2. Evaluation and recognition of meeting standards
4. Able to make rational decisions
5. Placing one in fear of bodily harm
6. Assumed permission to provide care
7. Unilateral termination of care
9. A serious situation, such as an injury or illness

Ambulance Calls

The following case scenarios provide an opportunity to explore the concerns associated with patient management. Read each scenario, then answer each question in detail.

1. You are dispatched to a woman complaining of abdominal pain. You arrive to find the 17-year-old female crying and holding her abdomen. She tells you that she fell down the stairs, and that she is pregnant. She is not sure how far along she is, but she is experiencing cramping and spotting. She asks you not to tell anyone, and says that if you tell her parents she will refuse transport to the hospital.
   What do you do?

   _____

   _____

2. You are off-duty when you see a child injured while riding his bike. You examine him and find abrasions on both knees, but no other injuries. He needs help getting to his house up the street. He tells you that his mother is not home, but his grandfather is (although he is bedridden). Looking through the window, you see the house is full of clothing, garbage, and papers.
   What do you do?

   _____

   _____

3. It is late in the night when police summon you to an auto crash. On arrival the officer directs you to the back of his patrol car. Sitting on the seat is your patient, snoring loudly with blood covering his face. The officer states that the patient was involved in a drunk driving accident in which he hit his head on the rear-view mirror. The patient initially refused care at the scene. You were called because his wound continues to bleed. Assessment reveals a sleeping 56-year-old man with a deep, gaping wound over the right eye with moderate venous bleeding. During assessment the patient wakes suddenly and pushes you away. He tells you to "leave him alone."
   What actions are necessary in the management of this situation?

   _____

   _____

   _____

CHAPTER

4 The Human Body

Workbook Activities

The following activities have been designed to help you. Your instructor may require you to complete some or all of these activities as a regular part of your EMT-B training program. You are encouraged to complete any activity that your instructor does not assign as a way to enhance your learning in the classroom.

Chapter Review

The following exercises provide an opportunity to refresh your knowledge of this chapter.

Matching

Match each of the terms in the left column to the appropriate definition in the right column.

_____ 1. Anterior

_____ 2. Capillary

_____ 3. Anatomic position

_____ 4. Superior

_____ 5. Midline

_____ 6. Carotid

_____ 7. Medial

_____ 8. Inferior

_____ 9. Femoral

_____ 10. Proximal

_____ 11. Brachial

_____ 12. Distal

_____ 13. Midaxillary

_____ 14. Radial

_____ 15. Posterior

A. closer to the midline

B. farther from the midline

C. farther from the head; lower

D. standing, facing forward, palms facing forward

E. imaginary vertical line descending from the middle of the forehead to the floor

F. front surface of the body

G. closer to the head; higher

H. imaginary vertical line descending from the middle of the armpit to the ankle

I. back or dorsal surface of the body

J. closer to the midline

K. connects arterioles to venules

L. major artery that supplies blood to the head and brain

M. major artery that supplies blood to the lower extremities

N. major artery of the lower arm

O. major artery of the upper arm

For each of the bones listed in the left column, indicate whether it is an upper extremity bone (A) or a lower extremity bone (B).

_____ **16.** Acetabulum

_____ **17.** Patella

_____ **18.** Clavicle

_____ **19.** Fibula

_____ **20.** Calcaneus

_____ **21.** Ulna

_____ **22.** Acromion

A. upper extremity bone

B. lower extremity bone

For each of the muscle characteristics described in the left column, select the type of muscle from the right column.

_____ **23.** Attaches to the bone

_____ **24.** Found in the walls of the gastrointestinal tract

_____ **25.** Carries out much of the automatic work of the body

_____ **26.** Forms the major muscle mass of the body

_____ **27.** Under the direct control of the brain

_____ **28.** Found only in the heart

_____ **29.** Responds only to primitive stimulus, such as heat

_____ **30.** Can tolerate blood supply interruption for only a very short period

_____ **31.** Responsible for all bodily movement

_____ **32.** Has its own blood supply and electrical system

A. skeletal

B. smooth

C. cardiac

For each of the parts of the nervous system in the left column, select the phrase in the right column with which it is associated.

_____ **33.** Spinal cord

_____ **34.** Central nervous system

_____ **35.** Sensory nerves

_____ **36.** Motor nerves

_____ **37.** Brain

_____ **38.** Peripheral nervous

A. exits the brain through an opening at the base of the skull

B. transmits electrical impulses to the muscles, causing them to contract

C. brain and spinal cord

D. links the central nervous system to various organs in the body

E. carries sensations of taste and touch to the brain

F. controlling organ of the body system

Multiple Choice

Read each item carefully, then select the best response.

_____ **1.** The topographic term used to describe the location of an injury that is toward the midline center of the body is:

A. lateral.

B. medial.

C. midaxillary.

D. midclavicular.

_____ **2.** Topographically, the term distal means:

A. near the trunk.

B. near a point of reference.

C. below a point of reference.

D. toward the center of the body.

_____ **3.** The leaf-shaped flap of tissue that prevents food and liquid from entering the trachea is called the:

    A. uvula.

    B. epiglottis.

    C. laryngopharynx.

    D. cricothyroid membrane.

_____ **4.** Which of the following systems is responsible for releasing chemicals that regulate body activities?

    A. nervous

    B. endocrine

    C. cardiovascular

    D. skeletal

_____ **5.** Which of the following vessels does NOT carry blood to the heart?

    A. inferior venae cavae

    B. superior venae cavae

    C. pulmonary vein

    D. pulmonary artery

Questions 6-10 are derived from the following scenario: Kory, a 16-year-old skateboarder, attempted to "gap" (jumping down a flight of stairs) with his skateboard, landing on his right side. He hit the pavement with his unprotected head, and had two bones sticking out by his right ankle.

_____ **6.** His open wound would be known as a(n):

    A. ulna/radial fracture

    B. acromion/humerus fracture

    C. tib/fib fracture

    D. patella/fibula fracture

_____ **7.** You would want to keep what part of his spinal column immobilized, so as not to move all 7 vertebrae?

    A. Cervical

    B. Thoracic

    C. Sacrum

    D. Coccyx

_____ **8.** If he were to develop pain in his upper-right quadrant, what organ may be causing the pain?

    A. liver

    B. stomach

    C. spleen

    D. appendix

_____ **9.** Kory was found in what position?

    A. prone

    B. supine

    C. shock position

    D. recovery position

_____ **10.** In order to keep his spinal column straight, in what position would you place him on the cot?

    A. prone

    B. supine

    C. Fowler's position

    D. Trendelenburg position

Labeling

Label the following diagrams with the correct terms.

1. Directional Terms

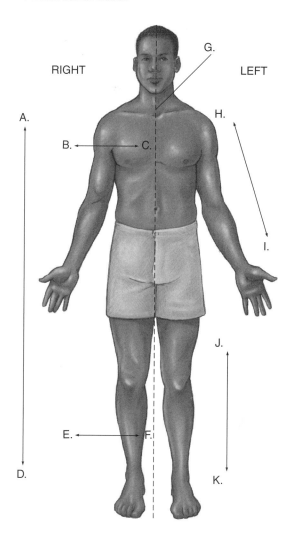

RIGHT

LEFT

A. _____

B. _____

C. _____

D. _____

E. _____

F. _____

G. _____

H. _____

I. _____

J. _____

K. _____

2. Anatomic Positions

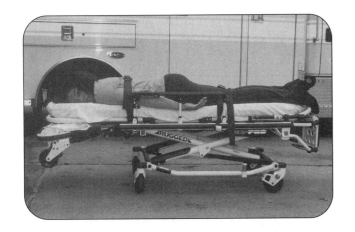

_____

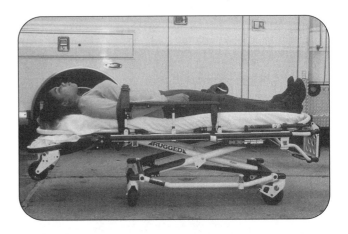

_____

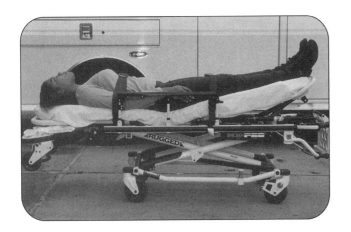

_____

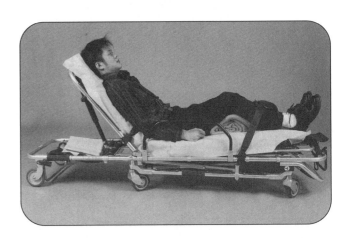

_____

3. The Skeletal System

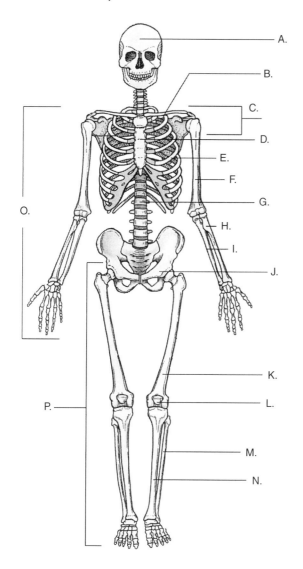

A. _____

B. _____

C. _____

D. _____

E. _____

F. _____

G. _____

H. _____

I. _____

J. _____

K. _____

L. _____

M. _____

N. _____

O. _____

P. _____

4. The Skull

A. _____

B. _____

C. _____

D. _____

E. _____

F. _____

G. _____

H. _____

I. _____

J. _____

K. _____

L. _____

M. _____

N. _____

O. _____

P. _____

Q. _____

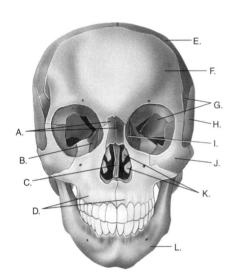

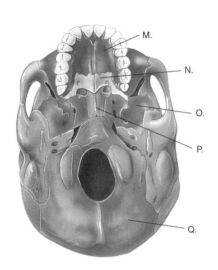

5. The Spinal Column

A. _____

B. _____

C. _____

D. _____

E. _____

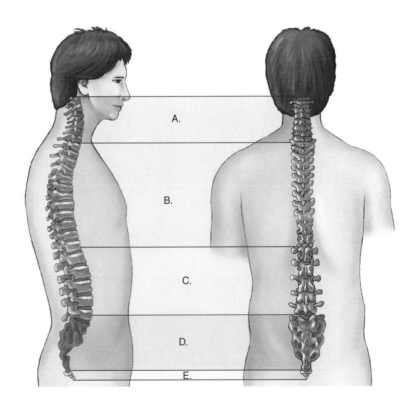

6. The Thorax

A. _____

B. _____

C. _____

D. _____

E. _____

F. _____

G. _____

H. _____

I. _____

J. _____

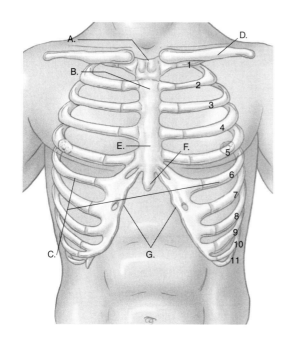

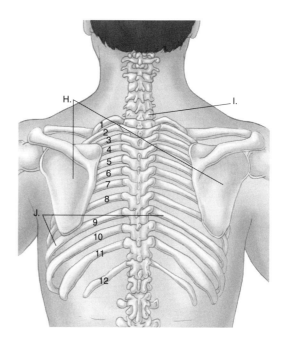

7. The Pelvis

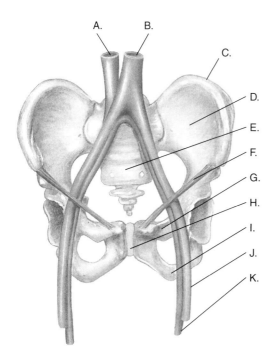

A. _____

B. _____

C. _____

D. _____

E. _____

F. _____

G. _____

H. _____

I. _____

J. _____

K. _____

8. The Lower Extremity

A. _____

B. _____

C. _____

D. _____

E. _____

F. _____

G. _____

H. _____

I. _____

J. _____

K. _____

L. _____

M. _____

N. _____

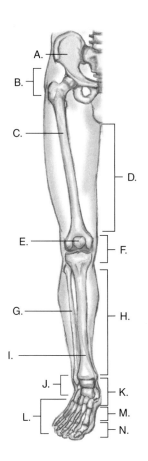

9. The Shoulder Girdle

A. _____

B. _____

C. _____

D. _____

E. _____

F. _____

G. _____

H. _____

I. _____

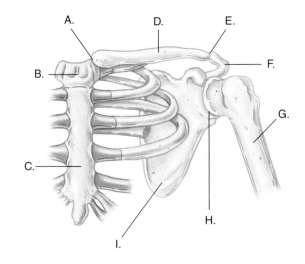

10. The Upper Extremity

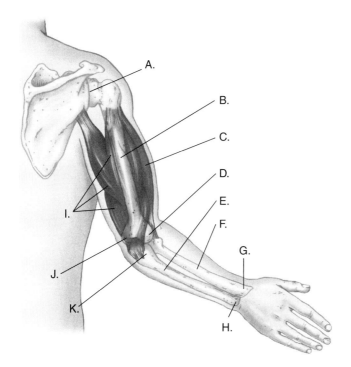

A. _____

B. _____

C. _____

D. _____

E. _____

F. _____

G. _____

H. _____

I. _____

J. _____

K. _____

11. Wrist and Hand

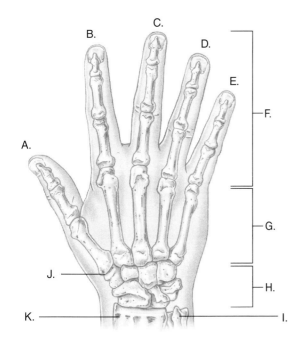

A. _____

B. _____

C. _____

D. _____

E. _____

F. _____

G. _____

H. _____

I. _____

J. _____

K. _____

12. The Respiratory System

A. _____

B. _____

C. _____

D. _____

E. _____

F. _____

G. _____

H. _____

I. _____

J. _____

K. _____

L. _____

M. _____

N. _____

O. _____

P. _____

Q. _____

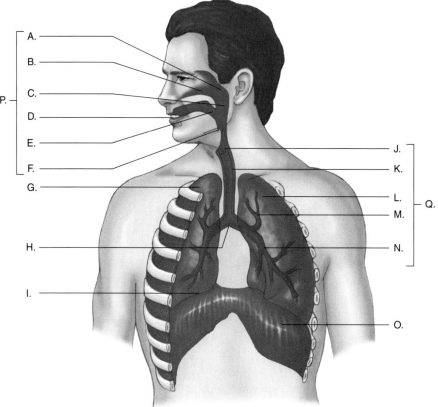

13. The Circulatory System

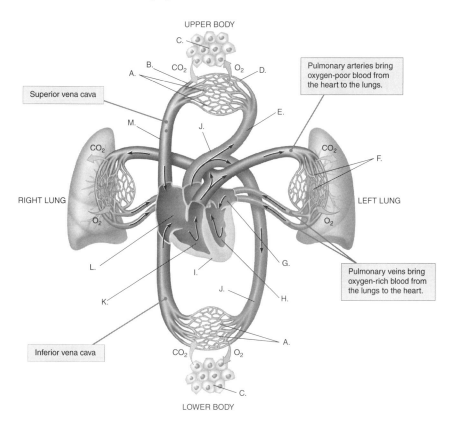

A. _____

B. _____

C. _____

D. _____

E. _____

F. _____

G. _____

H. _____

I. _____

J. _____

K. _____

L. _____

M. _____

14. Electrical Conduction

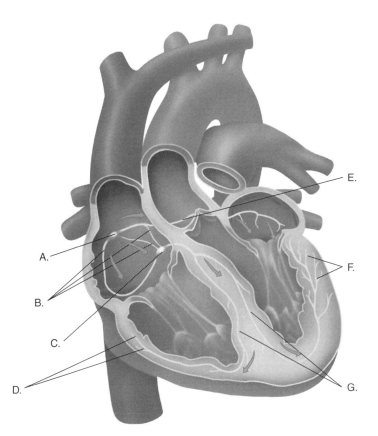

A. _____

B. _____

C. _____

D. _____

E. _____

F. _____

G. _____

15. Central and Peripheral Pulses

A. _____

B. _____

C. _____

D. _____

E. _____

F. _____

G. _____

H. _____

I. _____

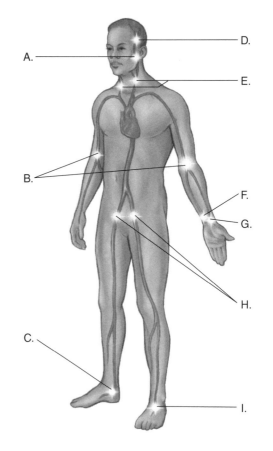

16. The Brain

A. _____

B. _____

C. _____

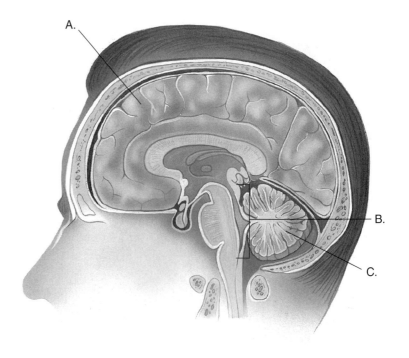

17. Anatomy of the Skin

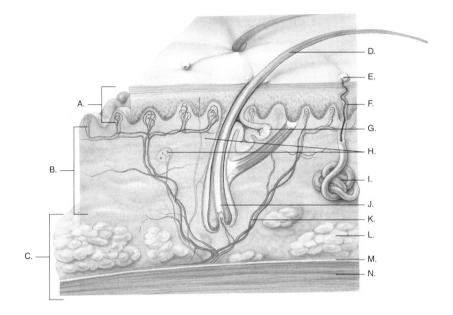

A. _____

B. _____

C. _____

D. _____

E. _____

F. _____

G. _____

H. _____

I. _____

J. _____

K. _____

L. _____

M. _____

N. _____

18. The Male Reproductive System

A. _____

B. _____

C. _____

D. _____

E. _____

F. _____

G. _____

H. _____

I. _____

J. _____

K. _____

L. _____

M. _____

N. _____

O. _____

P. _____

Q. _____

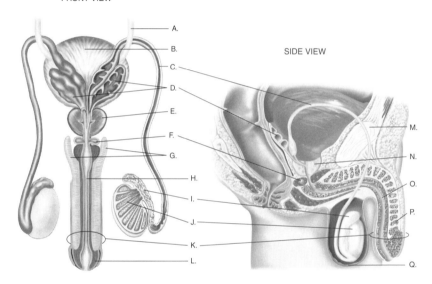

FRONT VIEW

SIDE VIEW

19. The Female Reproductive System

A. _____

B. _____

C. _____

D. _____

E. _____

FRONT VIEW   SIDE VIEW

Fill-in

Read each item carefully, then complete the statement by filling in the missing word.

1. There are _____ cervical vertebrae.

2. The movable bone in the skull is the _____ .

3. There is a total of _____ lobes in the right and left lungs.

4. There are _____ pairs of ribs that attach posteriorly to the thoracic vertebrae.

5. The spinal column has _____ vertebrae.

6. The ankle bone is known as _____ .

7. The 11th and 12th rib are called _____ _____.

True/False

If you believe the statement to be more true than false, write the letter "T" in the space provided. If you believe the statement to be more false than true, write the letter "F."

_____ 1. The aorta is the major artery that supplies the groin and lower extremities with blood.

_____ 2. The largest joint in the body is the knee.

_____ 3. The phalanges are the bones of the finger and toes.

_____ 4. The right atrium receives blood from the pulmonary veins.

_____ 5. There are 12 ribs that attach to the sternum.

Short Answer

Complete this section with short written answers using the space provided.

1. List the four components of blood and each of their functions.

_____

_____

2. List the five sections of the spinal column and indicate the number of vertebrae in each.

_____

_____

3. What organs are in each of the quadrants of the abdomen?

RUQ _____

_____

LUQ _____

_____

RLQ_____

_____

LLQ_____

_____

4. List in the proper order the parts of the heart that blood flows through.

1. _____   6. _____

2. _____   7. _____

3. _____   8. _____

4. _____   9. _____

5. _____

Word Fun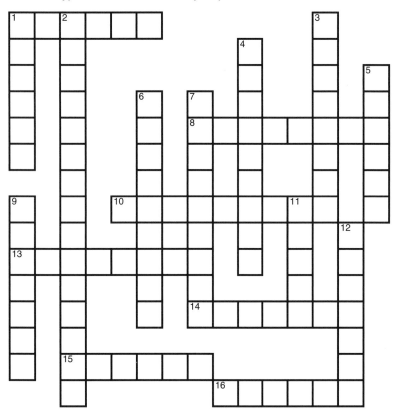

The following crossword puzzle is an activity provided to reinforce correct spelling and understanding of medical terminology associated with emergency care and the EMT-B. Use the clues in the column to complete the puzzle.

Across

  1. Inner layer of skin

  8. Nearer to the feet

10. Lower chamber of heart

13. Front surface of the body

14. Away from the midline, sides

15. Slow, dying respirations or pulse

16. Bone on thumb side of forearm

Down

  1. Nearer the end

  2. Behind the abdomen

  3. Lower jawbone

  4. Adequate circulation of blood

  5. Upper chamber of the heart

  6. Back surface of the body

  7. Appears on both sides

  9. Windpipe

11. Large solid organ in RUQ

12. Sitting up with knees bent

Ambulance Calls

The following case scenarios provide an opportunity to explore the concerns associated with patient management. Read each scenario, then answer each question in detail.

1. You are dispatched to the scene of a bar fight. A 34-year-old man has been stabbed in the right upper quadrant of the abdomen with a knife.

Using medical terminology, indicate which organ(s) might be affected. How would you describe this patient's injuries?

_____

_____

_____

2. You are dispatched to a one car MVC, car versus telephone pole. You arrive to find an unrestrained driver who is complaining of chest pain. You notice the steering wheel is deformed.

Based on the MOI and his chief complaint, what are his potential injuries?

_____

_____

_____

3. You are dispatched to a local BMX bike track just down the road from the fire station. You arrive to find 14-year-old male patient walking toward you, holding his left arm in place. He tells you that as he was turning a corner on the track, he fell off his bike and landed on his shoulder.

What possible injuries does this patient have?

_____

_____

_____

CHAPTER

5 Baseline Vital Signs and SAMPLE History

Workbook Activities

The following activities have been designed to help you. Your instructor may require you to complete some or all of these activities as a regular part of your EMT-B training program. You are encouraged to complete any activity that your instructor does not assign as a way to enhance your learning in the classroom.

Chapter Review

The following exercises provide an opportunity to refresh your knowledge of this chapter.

Matching

Match each of the terms in the left column to the appropriate definition in the right column.

_____ **1.** Pulse

_____ **2.** Auscultation

_____ **3.** Palpation

_____ **4.** Perfusion

_____ **5.** Blood pressure

_____ **6.** SAMPLE history

_____ **7.** Sphygmomanometer

_____ **8.** Capillary refill

_____ **9.** Bradycardia

_____ **10.** Cyanosis

_____ **11.** Diaphoretic

_____ **12.** Hypertension

_____ **13.** Hypotension

_____ **14.** Sclera

_____ **15.** Tachycardia

A. the pressure of the circulating blood against the walls of the arteries

B. characterized by profuse sweating

C. white portion of the eye

D. examination by touch

E. listening to sounds within the organs, usually with a stethoscope

F. the ability of the circulatory system to restore blood to the capillary blood vessels after it is squeezed out

G. blood pressure that is higher than normal range

H. a patient's history consisting of signs/symptoms, allergies, medications, pertinent past history, last oral intake, and events leading to the illness/injury

I. blood pressure that is lower than normal range

J. rapid heart rate

K. a blood pressure cuff

L. the process whereby blood enters an organ or tissue through its arteries and leaves through its veins, providing nutrients and oxygen and removing waste

M. slow heart rate

N. the pressure wave that is felt with the expansion and contraction of an artery

O. bluish-gray skin color caused by reduced blood-oxygen levels

Multiple Choice

Read each item carefully, then select the best response.

_____ **1.** The reason that a patient or other individual calls 9-1-1 is called the:
   A. signs.
   B. symptoms.
   C. chief complaint.
   D. primary problem.

_____ **2.** Signs include all of the following, except:
   A. dizziness.
   B. marked deformities.
   C. external bleeding.
   D. wounds.

_____ **3.** The first set of vital signs that you obtain is called the:
   A. original vital signs.
   B. baseline vital signs.
   C. actual vital signs.
   D. real vital signs.

_____ **4.** Besides pulse, respirations, and blood pressure, you should also include evaluation of:
   A. level of consciousness.
   B. pupillary reaction.
   C. capillary refill in children.
   D. all of the above

_____ **5.** During inspiration:
   A. the chest rises up and out.
   B. the phase is passive.
   C. carbon dioxide is released.
   D. all of the above

_____ **6** Assess breathing by:
   A. watching for chest rise and fall.
   B. feeling for air through the mouth and nose during exhalation.
   C. listening for breath sounds with a stethoscope.
   D. all of the above

_____ **7.** The normal range for adult respirations is _____ breaths/min.
   A. 8 to 20
   B. 15 to 30
   C. 25 to 50
   D. none of the above

_____ **8.** In the _____ position, the patient sits leaning forward on outstretched arms with the head and chin thrust slightly forward.

 A. Fowler's

 B. tripod

 C. sniffing

 D. lithotomy

_____ **9.** In this position, the patient sits upright with the head and chin thrust slightly forward.

 A. Fowler's

 B. tripod

 C. sniffing

 D. lithotomy

_____ **10.** Signs of labored breathing include all of the following, except:

 A. accessory muscle use.

 B. dyspnea.

 C. retractions.

 D. gasping.

_____ **11.** The _____ is the pressure wave that occurs as each heartbeat causes a surge in the blood circulating through the arteries.

 A. systolic pressure

 B. diastolic pressure

 C. pulse

 D. ventricular pressure

_____ **12.** In responsive patients who are older than 1 year, you should palpate a pulse at the _____ artery.

 A. carotid

 B. femoral

 C. radial

 D. brachial

_____ **13.** In unresponsive patients who are older than 1 year, you should palpate a pulse at the _____ artery.

 A. carotid

 B. femoral

 C. radial

 D. brachial

_____ **14.** A pulse that is weak and _____ should be palpated and counted for a full minute.

 A. difficult to palpate

 B. irregular

 C. extremely slow

 D. all of the above

_____ **15.** When assessing the skin, you should evaluate:

 A. color.

 B. temperature.

 C. moisture.

 D. all of the above

_____ **16.** Perfusion may be assessed in the:

 A. fingernail beds.

 B. lips.

 C. conjunctiva.

 D. all of the above

_____ **17.** Poor peripheral circulation will cause the skin to appear:

    A. pale.

    B. ashen.

    C. gray.

    D. all of the above

_____ **18.** Liver disease or dysfunction may cause _____, resulting in the patient's skin and sclera turning yellow.

    A. cyanosis

    B. jaundice

    C. diaphoresis

    D. lack of perfusion

_____ **19.** The skin will feel cool when the patient:

    A. is in early shock.

    B. has mild hypothermia.

    C. has inadequate perfusion.

    D. all of the above

_____ **20.** Capillary refill reflects the patient's perfusion and is often affected by the patient's:

    A. body temperature.

    B. position.

    C. medications.

    D. all of the above

_____ **21.** With adequate perfusion, the color in the nail bed should be restored to its normal pink within _____ seconds when checking capillary refill.

    A. 1½

    B. 2

    C. 2½

    D. 3

_____ **22.** A decrease in blood pressure may indicate:

    A. loss of blood.

    B. loss of vascular tone.

    C. a cardiac pumping problem.

    D. all of the above

_____ **23.** When blood pressure drops, the body compensates to maintain perfusion to the vital organs by:

    A. decreasing pulse rate.

    B. decreasing the blood flow to the skin and extremities.

    C. decreasing respiratory rate.

    D. dilating the arteries.

_____ **24.** Blood pressure is usually measured through:

    A. auscultation.

    B. palpation.

    C. visualization.

    D. rationalization.

_____ **25.** When obtaining a blood pressure by palpation, you should place your fingertips on the _____ artery.

    A. carotid

    B. brachial

    C. radial

    D. posterior tibial

_____ 26. You must assume that a patient who has a critically _____ can no longer compensate sufficiently to maintain adequate perfusion.

   A. low blood pressure

   B. high blood pressure

   C. low pulse rate

   D. high pulse rate

_____ 27. The patient's level of consciousness reflects the status of the:

   A. peripheral nervous system.

   B. central nervous system.

   C. peripheral perfusion.

   D. distal perfusion.

_____ 28. The diameter and reactivity to light of the patient's pupils reflect the status of the brain's:

   A. perfusion.

   B. oxygenation.

   C. condition.

   D. all of the above

_____ 29. You should reassess vital signs:

   A. every 15 minutes in a stable patient.

   B. every 5 minutes in an unstable patient.

   C. after every medical intervention.

   D. all of the above

_____ 30. In the mnemonic "SAMPLE," the "P" stands for:

   A. pupillary response.

   B. pulse rate.

   C. pertinent past history.

   D. pain level.

Questions 31-35 are derived from the following scenario: You've responded to a state wrestling tournament where several wrestling matches are taking place at the same time. The room is extremely noisy with fans cheering, and you are led to a 17-year-old male who appears unconscious and is surrounded by his coaches.

_____ 31. His unconsciousness is a:

   A. sign

   B. symptom

   C. both A and B

   D. none of the above

_____ 32. What method should be used to take his blood pressure?

   A. auscultation

   B. palpation

   C. by using the carotid artery

   D. by using the femoral artery

_____ 33. By using a painful stimulus, the patient moans. Which level of unconsciousness is the patient exhibiting?

   A. A

   B. V

   C. P

   D. U

_____ 34. Your patient is also exhibiting unequal pupils. This is likely caused by:

   A. internal bleeding

   B. cataracts

   C. brain injury

   D. none of the above

_____ **35.** His skin color, temperature, and moisture are signs of:
  A. level of consciousness
  B. perfusion
  C. brain injury
  D. none of the above

Fill-in

Read each item carefully, then complete the statement by filling in the missing word.

  1. _____ _____ is the amount of air that is exchanged with each breath.

  2. The _____ is the delicate membrane lining the eyelids and covering the exposed surface of the eye.

  3. By using your _____ powers, you will be able to interpret the meaning and implications of your findings

  and the information that you have gathered while assessing the patient.

  4. The severity of a _____ is subjective because it is based on the patient's interpretation and tolerance.

  5. A patient who is breathing without assistance is said to have _____ _____.

  6. _____ _____ are the key signs that are used to evaluate the patient's initial general condition.

  7. When assessing respirations, you must determine the rate, _____, and depth of the patient's breathing.

  8. When you can actually see the effort of the patient's breathing, it is described as _____ _____.

  9. If you can hear bubbling or gurgling, the patient probably has _____ in the airway.

  10. The condition of the patient's skin can tell you a lot about the patient's peripheral circulation and _____,

  blood oxygen levels, and body temperature.

True/False

If you believe the statement to be more true than false, write the letter "T" in the space provided. If you believe the statement to be more false than true, write the letter "F."

_____ **1.** A pulse is an indicator of the condition of the heart.
_____ **2.** A blood pressure determined by palpation is less accurate than if determined by auscultation.
_____ **3.** Only the diastolic pressure can be measured by the palpation method.
_____ **4.** Labored breathing can be described as increased breathing effort, grunting, and use of accessory muscles.
_____ **5.** A conscious patient is likely to alter his or her breathing if he or she is aware that you are evaluating it.
_____ **6.** The pulse is most commonly palpated at the femoral artery.
_____ **7.** The normal pulse range for a newborn is 140 to 160 beats/min.
_____ **8.** To assess skin color in an infant, you should look at the palms of the hands and soles of the feet.
_____ **9.** Cyanosis indicates a need for oxygen.
_____ **10.** BSI precautions should be followed when a patient is jaundiced.
_____ **11.** The skin will feel hot when the patient is in profound shock or has hypothermia.
_____ **12.** Normal reaction to a bright light shone in one eye is pupil constriction in only that eye.
_____ **13.** Normal respirations in an adult are 15 to 30 breaths/min.

Short Answer

Complete this section with short written answers using the space provided.

1. Name the seven basic vital signs.

_____

_____

2. List four abnormal skin colors.

_____

_____

3. Name four factors to be considered when assessing adequate or inadequate breathing.

_____

_____

4. Define systolic blood pressure.

_____

_____

5. Define diastolic blood pressure.

_____

_____

6. Name the three factors to consider when assessing a patient's pulse.

_____

_____

7. Name the three factors to consider when assessing a patient's skin.

_____

_____

8. Describe the process for assessing capillary refill.

_____

_____

9. Define the acronym PEARRL.

_____

_____

10. Explain the difference between a sign and a symptom.

_____

_____

Word Fun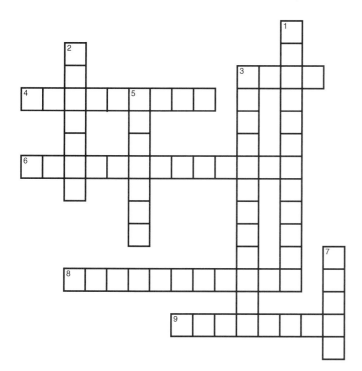

The following crossword puzzle is an activity to reinforce correct spelling and understanding of medical terminology associated with emergency care and the EMT-B. Use the clues in the column to complete the puzzle.

Across

3. Acronym used to assess LOC
4. Circulation of blood within an organ or tissue
6. Pressure against the walls of the arteries
8. BP lower than normal
9. Bluish-gray skin color

Down

1. BP that is higher than normal
2. Harsh, high-pitched inspiratory sound
3. Listening
5. Subjective finding
7. Cardiac pressure wave

Ambulance Calls

The following case scenarios provide an opportunity to explore the concerns associated with patient management. Read each scenario, then answer each question in detail.

1. It's Thanksgiving and you are dispatched to a private residence for "female choking." You arrive to find an older woman who is alert and oriented but is coughing and drooling. Family members tell you that the patient was eating a piece of strip steak when she suddenly clutched her throat and started coughing. She keeps repeating, "It's stuck in my throat!" Every time she tries to swallow, she feels that her airway becomes blocked.

How would you best manage this patient?

_____

_____

_____

2. It's the first day of a major snowfall in your area. You are dispatched to a man complaining of chest pain. You arrive to find a 50-year-old male patient sitting on the steps of his home. He tells you that he was shoveling snow from his sidewalk when suddenly he felt pain and pressure in his chest. He says that it is slightly better now, but there is still a feeling of "heaviness," and he also feels sick to his stomach.

How would you best manage this patient?

_____

_____

_____

3. You are called to a residence for a possible cardiac arrest. Family members tell you that the patient, a 57-year-old man, stopped breathing and had no pulse. They also tell you he has a cardiac history. They stopped CPR when he resumed breathing and regained a pulse, approximately 2 minutes before your arrival.

How would you best manage this patient?

_____

_____

_____

Skill Drills

Skill Drill 5-1: Obtaining a Blood Pressure by Auscultation or Palpation

Test your knowledge of this skill drill by placing the photos below in the correct order. Number the first step with a "1," the second step with a "2," etc.

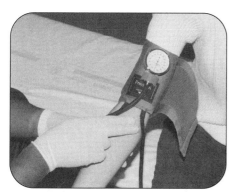

Palpate the brachial artery.

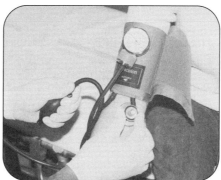

Close the valve and pump to 20 mm Hg above the point at which you stop hearing pulse sounds. Note the systolic and diastolic pressures as you let air escape slowly.

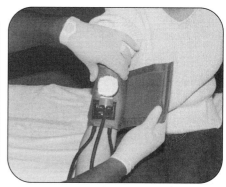

Apply the cuff snugly.

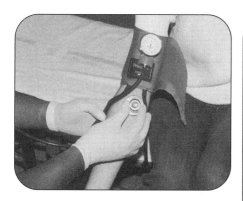

Place the stethoscope over the brachial artery and grasp the ball-pump and turn-valve.

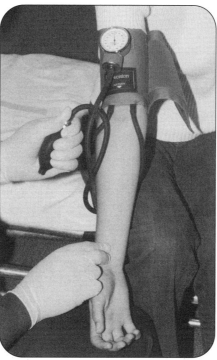

When using the palpatation method, you should place your fingertips on the radial artery so that you feel the radial pulse.

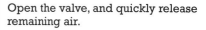

Open the valve, and quickly release remaining air.

C H A P T E R

6 Lifting and Moving Patients

Workbook Activities

The following activities have been designed to help you. Your instructor may require you to complete some or all of these activities as a regular part of your EMT-B training program. You are encouraged to complete any activity that your instructor does not assign as a way to enhance your learning in the classroom.

Chapter Review

The following exercises provide an opportunity to refresh your knowledge of this chapter.

Matching

Match each of the terms in the left column to the appropriate definition in the right column.

_____ **1.** Extremity lift

_____ **2.** Flexible stretcher

_____ **3.** Stair chair

_____ **4.** Basket stretcher

_____ **5.** Scoop stretcher

_____ **6.** Backboard

_____ **7.** Direct ground lift

_____ **8.** Portable stretcher

_____ **9.** Wheeled ambulance stretcher

A. separates into two or four pieces

B. tubular framed stretcher with rigid fabric stretched across it

C. used for patients without a spinal injury who are supine

D. specifically designed stretcher that can be rolled along the ground

E. used to carry patients across uneven terrain

F. used for patients who are found lying supine with no suspected spinal injury

G. can be folded or rolled up

H. used to carry patients up and down stairs

I. spine board or longboard

Multiple Choice

Read each item carefully, then select the best response.

_____ 1. _____ safety depends on the use of proper lifting techniques and maintaining a proper hold when lifting or carrying a patient.

   A. Your

   B. Your team's

   C. The patient's

   D. all of the above

_____ 2. You should perform an urgent move:

   A. if a patient has an altered level of consciousness.

   B. if a patient has inadequate ventilation or shock.

   C. in extreme weather conditions.

   D. all of the above

_____ 3. You may injure your back if you lift:

   A. with your back curved.

   B. with your back straight, but bent significantly forward at the hips.

   C. with the shoulder girdle anterior to the pelvis.

   D. all of the above

_____ 4. When lifting you should:

   A. spread your legs shoulder width apart.

   B. never lift a patient while reaching any significant distance in front of your torso.

   C. keep the weight that you are lifting as close to your body as possible.

   D. all of the above

_____ 5. When carrying a patient on a cot, be sure:

   A. to flex at the hips.

   B. to bend at the knees.

   C. that you do not hyperextend your back.

   D. all of the above

_____ 6. In lifting with the palm down, the weight is supported by the _____ rather than the palm.

   A. fingers

   B. forearm

   C. lower back

   D. wrist

_____ 7. When you must carry a patient up or down a flight of stairs or other significant incline, use a _____ if possible.

   A. backboard

   B. stair chair

   C. stretcher

   D. short spine board

_____ 8. If you need to lean to either side to compensate for a weight imbalance, you have probably _____ your weight limitation.

   A. met

   B. exceeded

   C. increased

   D. countered

_____ **9.** A backboard is a device that provides support to patients who you suspect have:

  A. hip injuries.

  B. pelvic injuries.

  C. spinal injuries.

  D. all of the above

_____ **10.** The team leader should do all of the following, except _____, before any lifting is initiated.

  A. give a command of execution

  B. indicate where each team member is to be located

  C. rapidly describe the sequence of steps that will be performed

  D. give a brief overview of the stages

_____ **11.** Special _____ are usually required to move any patient who weighs more than 300 lb to an ambulance.

  A. techniques

  B. equipment

  C. resources

  D. all of the above

_____ **12.** When carrying a patient in a stair chair, always remember to:

  A. keep your back in a locked-in position.

  B. flex at the hips, not at the waist.

  C. keep the patient's weight and your arms as close to your body as possible.

  D. all of the above

_____ **13.** When you use a body drag to move a patient:

  A. your back should always be locked and straight.

  B. you should avoid any twisting so that the vertebrae remain in normal alignment.

  C. avoid hyperextending.

  D. all of above

_____ **14.** When pulling a patient, you should do all of the following, except:

  A. extend your arms no more than about 15 to 20 inches.

  B. reposition your feet so that the force of pull will be balanced equally.

  C. when you can pull no farther, lean forward another 15 to 20 inches.

  D. pull the patient by slowly flexing your arms.

_____ **15.** When log rolling a patient:

  A. kneel as close to the patient's side as possible.

  B. lean solely from the hips.

  C. use your shoulder muscles to help with the roll.

  D. all of the above

_____ **16.** If the weight you are pushing is lower than your waist, you should push from:

  A. the waist.

  B. a kneeling position.

  C. the shoulder.

  D. a squatting position.

_____ **17.** If you are alone and must remove an unconscious patient from a car, you should first move the patient's:

  A. legs.

  B. head.

  C. torso.

  D. pelvis.

_____ **18.** Situations in which you should use an emergency move include those where:

   A. there is the presence of fire, explosives, or hazardous materials.

   B. you are unable to protect the patient from other hazards.

   C. you are unable to gain access to others in a vehicle who need lifesaving care.

   D. all of the above

_____ **19.** You can move a patient on his or her back along the floor or ground by using all of the following methods, except:

   A. pulling on the patient's clothing in the neck and shoulder area.

   B. placing the patient on a blanket, coat, or other item that can be pulled.

   C. pulling the patient by the legs if they are the most accessible part.

   D. placing your arms under the patient's shoulders and through the armpits, while grasping the patient's arms, drag the patient backward.

_____ **20.** An urgent move may be necessary for moving a patient with:

   A. an altered level of consciousness.

   B. inadequate ventilation.

   C. shock.

   D. all of the above

_____ **21.** Use the rapid extrication technique in the following situation(s):

   A. The vehicle on the scene is unsafe.

   B. The patient's condition cannot be properly assessed before being removed from the car.

   C. The patient blocks access to another seriously injured patient.

   D. all of the above

_____ **22.** To avoid the strain of unnecessary lifting and carrying, you should use _____ or assist an able patient to the cot whenever possible.

   A. the direct ground lift

   B. the extremity lift

   C. the draw sheet method

   D. a scoop stretcher

_____ **23.** You should use a rigid _____, often called a Stokes litter, to carry a patient across uneven terrain from a remote location that is inaccessible by ambulance or other vehicle.

   A. basket stretcher

   B. scoop stretcher

   C. molded backboard

   D. flotation device

_____ **24.** Basket stretchers can be used:

   A. for technical rope rescues and some water rescues.

   B. to carry a patient across fields on an all-terrain vehicle.

   C. to carry a patient on a toboggan.

   D. all of the above

Questions 25-29 are derived from the following scenario: You've been called to the scene of a high-speed motor-vehicle accident involving two compact cars. The first vehicle was a roll-over, ejecting the driver. The second vehicle contained both a driver and a front seat passenger who can't be reached as their door is up against a building.

_____ **25.** What device will you use to put the roll-over victim onto the wheeled ambulance stretcher?

   A. extremity lift

   B. scoop stretcher

   C. short backboard

   D. backboard

_____ **26.** For the passenger in vehicle number 2, you may need to perform a _____ on the driver in order to reach the patient.
- **A.** extremity lift
- **B.** emergency move
- **C.** short backboard
- **D.** You should do nothing different, treating each patient the same.

_____ **27.** An advantage of using the diamond carry is that:
- **A.** It uses an even number of people (less likely to drop)
- **B.** It can be done with one person, freeing up others for patient care
- **C.** They can be slid along the ground
- **D.** It provides the best means of spinal immobilization

_____ **28.** You'll likely use the _____ to transfer the patient from your cot to the hospital bed.
- **A.** diamond carry
- **B.** scoop stretcher
- **C.** portable cot
- **D.** draw sheet method

_____ **29.** After the doctor examines the patient, you are asked to transfer the patient to a specialized facility. What method will be likely used to get the patient back onto your cot?
- **A.** extremity lift
- **B.** draw sheet method
- **C.** direct ground lift
- **D.** scoop stretcher

_____ **30.** Bariatrics is:
- **A.** The branch of medicine concerned with the elderly.
- **B.** The branch of medicine concerned with the obese.
- **C.** The branch of medicine concerned with babies.
- **D.** The method used to take blood pressures.

Fill-in
Read each item carefully, then complete the statement by filling in the missing word.

1. To avoid injury to you, the patient, or your partners, you will have to learn how to lift and carry the patient properly, using proper _____ _____ and a power grip.

2. The key rule of lifting is to always keep the back in a straight, _____ position and to lift without twisting.

3. The safest and most powerful way to lift, lifting by extending the properly placed flexed legs, is called a _____ _____.

4. The arm and hand have their greatest lifting strength when facing _____ up.

5. Be sure to pick up and carry the backboard with your back in the _____ position.

6. You should not attempt to lift a patient who weighs more than _____ pounds with fewer than four rescuers, regardless of individual strength.

7. During a body drag where you and your partner are on each side of the patient, you will have to alter the usual pulling technique to prevent pulling _____ and producing adverse lateral leverage against your lower back.

8. When you are rolling the wheeled ambulance stretcher, your back should be _____, straight, and untwisted.

9. Be careful that you do not push or pull from a(n) _____ position.

10. Remember to always consider whether there is an option that will cause _____ _____ to you and the other EMT-Bs.

11. The manual support and immobilization that you provide when using the rapid extrication technique produce a greater risk of _____ _____.

12. The _____ _____ _____ is used for patients with no suspected spinal injury who are found lying supine on the ground.

13. The _____ _____ may be especially helpful when the patient is in a very narrow space or there is not enough room for the patient and a team of EMTs to stand side by side.

14. The mattress on a stretcher must be _____ _____ so that it does not absorb any type of potentially infectious material, including water, blood, or other body fluid.

15. A _____ _____ may be used for patients who have been struck by a motor vehicle.

True/False
If you believe the statement to be more true than false, write the letter "T" in the space provided. If you believe the statement to be more false than true, write the letter "F."

_____ **1.** A portable stretcher is typically a lightweight folding device that does not have the undercarriage and wheels of a true ambulance stretcher.

_____ **2.** The term "power lift" refers to a posture that is safe and helpful for EMT-Bs when they are lifting.

_____ **3.** If you find that lifting a patient is a strain, try to move to the ambulance as quickly as possible to minimize the possibility of back injury.

_____ **4.** The use of adjunct devices and equipment, such as sheets and blankets, may make the job of lifting and moving a patient more difficult.

_____ **5.** One-person techniques for moving patients should only be used when immediate patient movement is necessary due to a life-threatening hazard and only one EMT-B is available.

_____ **6.** A scoop stretcher may be used alone for a standard immobilization of a patient with a spinal injury.

_____ **7.** When carrying a patient down stairs or on an incline, make sure the stretcher is carried with the head end first.

_____ **8.** The rapid extrication technique is the preferred technique to use on all sitting patients with possible spinal injuries.

_____ **9.** It is unprofessional for you to discuss and plan a lift at the scene in front of the patient.

_____ **10.** Americans are becoming so large that a new field of medicine has been named for the care of the obese.

Short Answer
Complete this section with short written answers using the space provided.

1. List the one-rescuer drags, carries, and lifts.

_____

_____

2. List the situations where the rapid extrication technique is used.

_____

_____

3. List the three guidelines for loading the cot into the ambulance.

_____

_____

4. List the five guidelines for carrying a patient on a cot.

_____

_____

5. Describe the key rule of lifting.

_____

_____

Word Fun

The following crossword puzzle is an activity provided to reinforce correct spelling and understanding of medical terminology associated with emergency care and the EMT-B. Use the clues in the column to complete the puzzle.

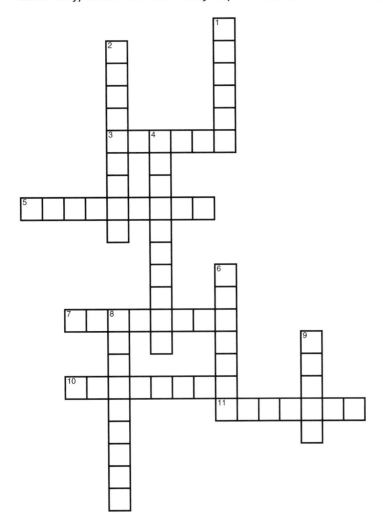

Across

3. Stretcher used with technical rescues, particularly when water is involved

5. Safest way to lift

7. Stretcher that becomes rigid when secured around patient

10. Tubular framed stretcher with fabric across

11. Four-rescuer carry with one at the head, one at the foot, and one on each side

Down

1. A ground lift used with no suspected spinal injury

2. Used to support patient with hip, pelvic, or spine injury

4. Folding device for moving seated patients up or down floors

6. Stretcher designed to roll along ground

8. Using the patient's limbs to lift

9. Stretcher that can be split into two or four sections

Ambulance Calls

The following case scenarios provide an opportunity to explore the concerns associated with patient management. Read each scenario, then answer each question in detail.

1. You are dispatched to a construction site for a 26-year-old man who fell into a ravine. He is approximately 35 feet down a rocky ledge. He is alert with an unstable pelvis and weak radial pulses. You have all the help you need from the construction crew and the volunteer fire department.

How would you best manage this patient?

_____

_____

_____

2. You are dispatched to "unknown medical problem" at a local residence. You are met at the door by the wife of the patient who tells you that her husband is in the bathroom and is not acting right. You find the 350 pound patient lying in the bathroom, stuck between the bathroom toilet and the wall. He is not breathing and has no pulse. What do you do?

_____

_____

_____

3. You are dispatched to "difficulty breathing" at a nearby apartment complex. The patient's apartment is located on the top floor of a three-story building, is accessed through an exterior entryway and no elevators are available. Your patient is morbidly obese and cannot walk.

What do you do?

_____

_____

_____

Skill Drills

Skill Drill 6-1: Performing the Power Lift
Test your knowledge of this skill drill by filling in the correct words in the photo captions.

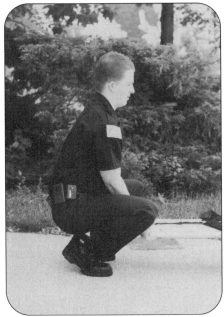
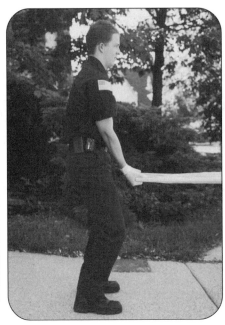
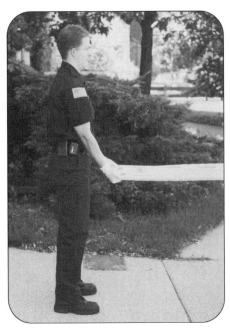

1. Lock your back into a(n) _____, inward curve. _____ and bend your legs. Grasp the backboard, palms up and just in front of you. _____ and _____ the weight between your arms.

2. Position your feet, _____ the object, and _____ weight.

3. _____ your legs and lift, keeping your back locked in.

Skill Drill 6-2: Performing the Diamond Carry
Test your knowledge of this skill drill by placing the photos below in the correct order. Number the first step with a "1," the second step with a "2," etc.

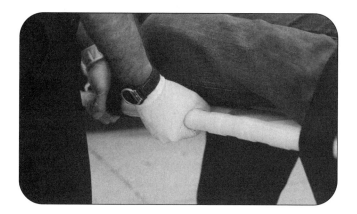

EMT-Bs at the side each turn the head-end hand palm down and release the other hand.

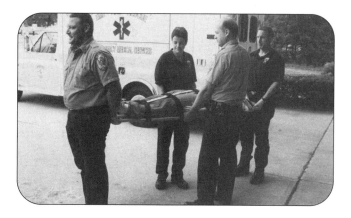

After the patient has been lifted, the EMT-B at the foot turns to face forward.

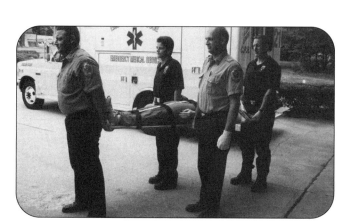

EMT-Bs at the side turn toward the foot end.

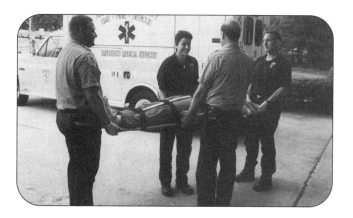

Position yourselves facing the patient.

Skill Drill 6-3: Performing the One-Handed Carrying Technique
Test your knowledge of this skill drill by filling in the correct words in the photo captions.

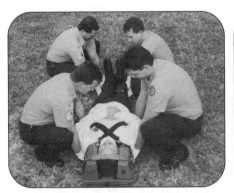

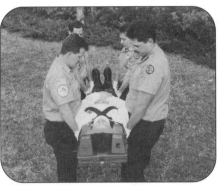

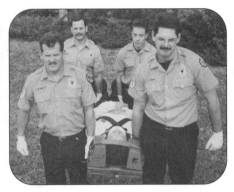

1. _____ each other and use both _____.

2. Lift the backboard to _____ _____.

3. _____ in the direction you will walk and _____ to using one hand.

Skill Drill 6-4: Carrying a Patient on Stairs
Test your knowledge of this skill drill by filling in the correct words in the photo captions.

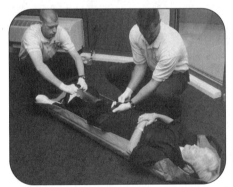

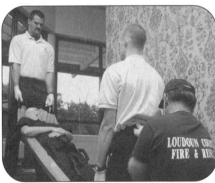

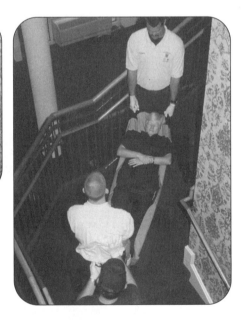

1. _____ the patient securely. Make sure one strap is tight across the _____ _____, under the arms, and secured to the handles to prevent the patient from _____.

2. Carry a patient down stairs with the _____ end first, _____ elevated.

3. Carry the _____ end first going up stairs, always keeping the head elevated.

Skill Drill 6-5: Using a Stair Chair
Test your knowledge of this skill drill by filling in the correct words in the photo captions.

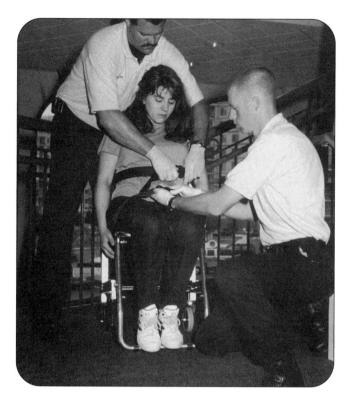

1. Position and secure the patient on the chair with
   _____ .

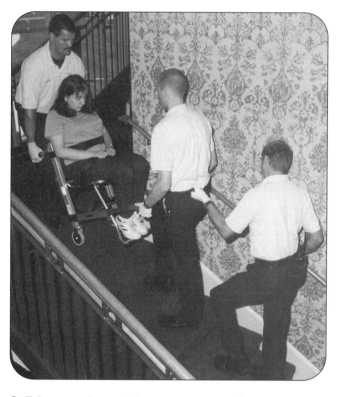

2. Take your places at the _____ and _____
   of the chair.

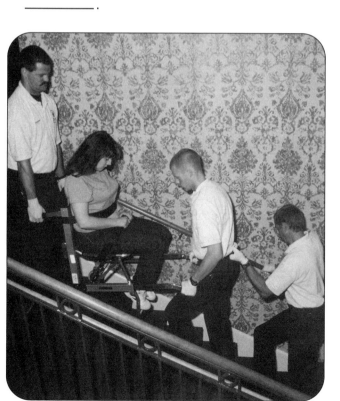

3. A third _____ "backs up" the rescuer carrying
   the _____ .

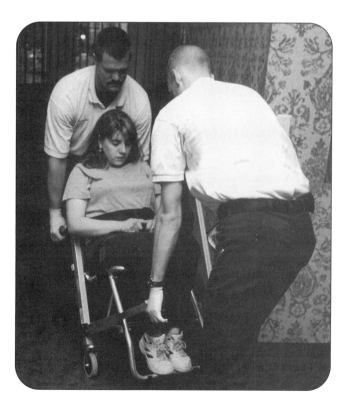

4. _____ the chair to roll on landings, or for transfer
   to the cot.

Skill Drill 6-6: Performing the Rapid Extrication Technique
Test your knowledge of this skill drill by placing the photos below in the correct order. Number the first step with a "1," the second step with a "2," etc.

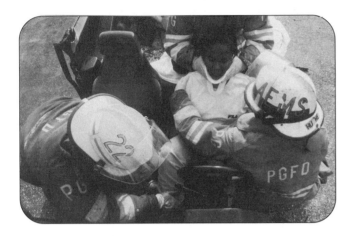

Second EMT-B supports the torso.

Third EMT-B frees the patient's legs from the pedals and moves the legs together, without moving the pelvis or spine.

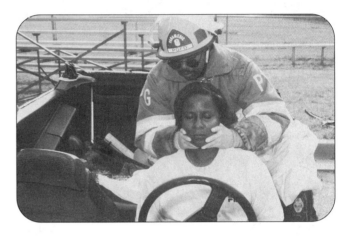

First EMT-B provides in-line manual support of the head and cervical spine.

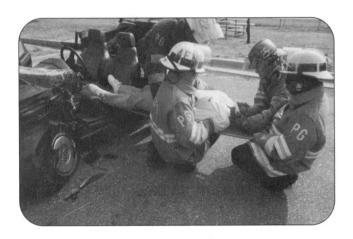

Third EMT-B exits the vehicle, moves to the backboard opposite Second EMT-B, and they continue to slide the patient until patient is fully on the board.

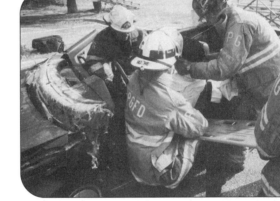

First (or Fourth) EMT-B places the backboard on the seat against patient's buttocks.

(continued)

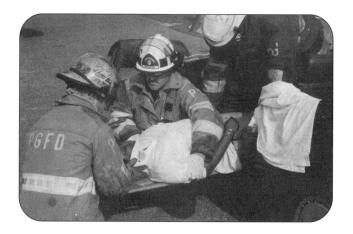

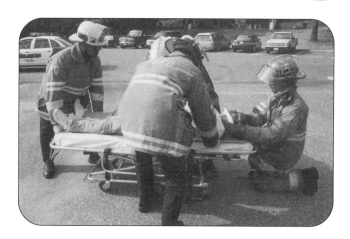

Third EMT-B moves to an effective position for sliding the patient.

Second and Third EMT-Bs slide the patient along the backboard in coordinated, 8" to 12" moves until the hips rest on the backboard.

First (or Fourth) EMT-B continues to stabilize the head and neck while Second and Third EMT-Bs carry the patient away from the vehicle.

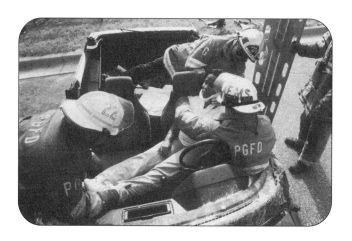

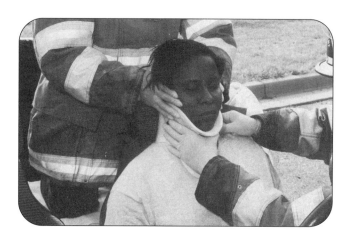

Second and Third EMT-Bs rotate the patient as a unit in several short, coordinated moves.

First EMT-B (relieved by Fourth EMT-B or bystander as needed) supports the head and neck during rotation (and later steps).

Second EMT-B gives commands, applies a cervical collar, and performs the initial assessment.

Skill Drill 6-7: Extremity Lift
Test your knowledge of this skill drill by filling in the correct words in the photo captions.

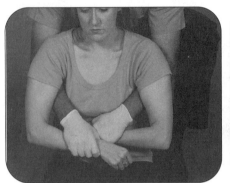 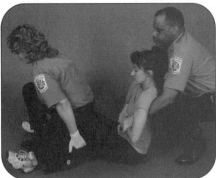 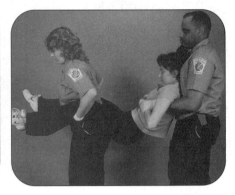

1. Patient's hands are
_____ over the chest.
First EMT-B grasps patient's wrists
or _____ and pulls
patient to a _____
position.

2. When the patient is sitting, First
EMT-B passes his or her arms through
patient's _____ and grasps the
patient's opposite (or his or her own)
_____ or _____.
Second EMT-B kneels between the
_____, facing in the same
direction as the patient, and places
his or her hands under the
_____.

3. Both EMT-Bs rise to _____.
On _____, both lift and begin
to move.

Skill Drill 6-8: Using a Scoop Stretcher
Test your knowledge of this skill drill by filling in the correct words in the photo captions.

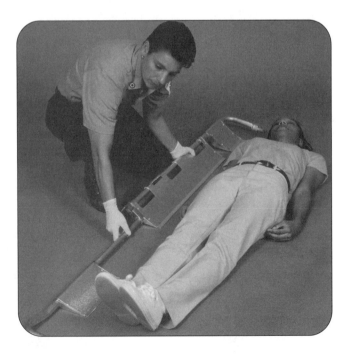 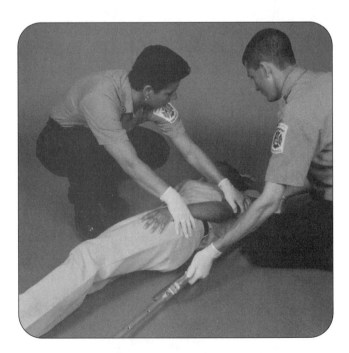

1. Adjust stretcher _____.

2. _____ the patient slightly and _____
stretcher into place, one side at a time.

(continued)

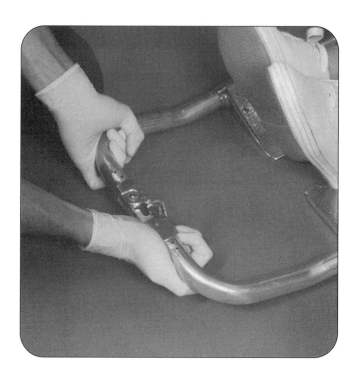

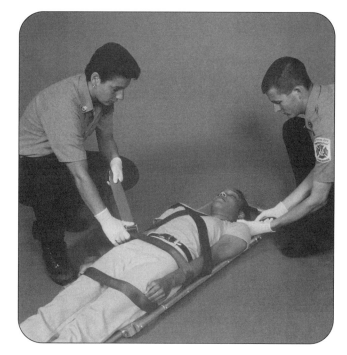

3. _____ the stretcher ends together, avoiding _____ .

4. _____ the patient to the scoop stretcher and _____ it to the cot.

Skill Drill 6-9: Loading a Cot into an Ambulance

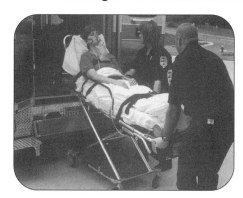

1. Tilt the head of the cot _____ , and place it into the patient compartment with the wheels on the floor.

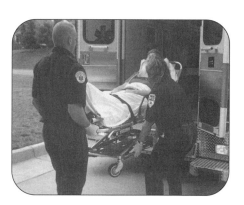

2. Second rescuer on the side of the cot releases the _____ lock and lifts the undercarriage.

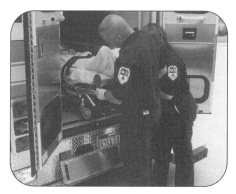

3. _____ the cot into the back of the ambulance.

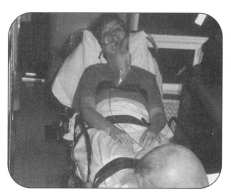

4. Secure the cot to the _____ mounted in the ambulance.

CHAPTER

7 Airway

Workbook Activities

The following activities have been designed to help you. Your instructor may require you to complete some or all of these activities as a regular part of your EMT-B training program. You are encouraged to complete any activity that your instructor does not assign as a way to enhance your learning in the classroom.

Chapter Review

The following exercises provide an opportunity to refresh your knowledge of this chapter.

Matching

Match each of the terms in the left column to the appropriate definition in the right column.

_____ 1. Inhalation	**A.** moves down slightly when it contracts
_____ 2. Exhalation	**B.** irregular breathing pattern with increased rate and depth, followed by apnea
_____ 3. Alveoli	
_____ 4. Automatic function	**C.** active part of breathing
_____ 5. Hypoxic drive	**D.** voice box
_____ 6. Tidal volume	**E.** amount of air moved during one breath
_____ 7. Diaphragm	**F.** raises ribs when it contracts
_____ 8. Intercostal muscle	**G.** controls breathing when we sleep
_____ 9. Ventilation	**H.** site of oxygen diffusion
_____ 10. Larynx	**I.** thorax size decreases
_____ 11. Hypoxia	**J.** insufficient oxygen for cells and tissues
_____ 12. Cheyne-Stokes	**K.** backup system to control respiration
	L. exchange of air between lungs and respirations environment

Multiple Choice
Read each item carefully, then select the best response.

_____ **1.** What percentage of the air we breathe is made up of oxygen?

   A. 78%

   B. 12%

   C. 16%

   D. 21%

_____ **2.** Regarding the maintenance of the airway in an unconscious adult, which of the following is false?

   A. Insertion of an oropharyngeal airway helps keep the airway open.

   B. The head tilt-chin lift maneuver should always be used to open the airway.

   C. Secretions should be suctioned from the mouth as necessary.

   D. Inserting a rigid suction catheter beyond the tongue may cause gagging.

_____ **3.** The normal respiratory rate for an adult is:

   A. about equal to the person's heart rate.

   B. 12 to 20 breaths/min.

   C. faster when the person is sleeping.

   D. the same as in infants and children.

_____ **4.** All of the following conditions are associated with hypoxia, except:

   A. heart attack.

   B. altered mental status.

   C. chest injury.

   D. hyperventilation syndrome.

_____ **5.** The brain stem normally triggers breathing by increasing respirations when:

   A. carbon dioxide levels increase.

   B. oxygen levels increase.

   C. carbon dioxide levels decrease.

   D. nitrogen levels decrease.

_____ **6.** Which of the following is not a sign of abnormal breathing?

   A. Warm, dry skin

   B. Speaking in two- or three-word sentences

   C. Unequal breath sounds

   D. Skin pulling in around the ribs during inspiration

_____ **7.** The proper technique for sizing an oropharyngeal airway before insertion is to:

   A. measure the device from the tip of the nose to the earlobe.

   B. measure the device from the bridge of the nose to the tip of the chin.

   C. measure the device from the corner of the mouth to the earlobe.

   D. measure the device from the center of the jaw to the earlobe.

_____ **8.** What is the most common problem you may encounter when using a BVM device?

   A. volume of the BVM device

   B. positioning of the patient's head

   C. environmental conditions

   D. maintaining an airtight seal

_____ **9.** When ventilating a patient with a BVM device, you should:

   A. look for inflation of the cheeks.

   B. look for signs of the patient breathing on his or her own.

   C. look for rise and fall of the chest.

   D. listen for gurgling.

_____ **10.** Suctioning the oral cavity of an adult should be accomplished within:

    A. 5 seconds.

    B. 10 seconds.

    C. 15 seconds.

    D. 20 seconds.

Questions 11-15 are derived from the following scenario: You respond to a construction site and find a worker lying supine in the dirt. He has been hit by a heavy construction vehicle and flew over 15 feet of distance before landing in this position. There is discoloration and distention of the abdomen about the RUQ. He is unconscious and his respirations are 10 breaths/min and shallow, with noisy gurgling sounds.

_____ **11.** What airway technique will you use to open his airway?

    A. Head tilt-neck lift

    B. Jaw thrust

    C. Head tilt-chin lift

    D. None of the above

_____ **12.** After opening the airway, your next priority is to:

    A. provide oxygen at 6 L/min via nonrebreathing mask.

    B. provide oxygen at 15 L/min via nasal cannula.

    C. assist respirations.

    D. suction the airway.

_____ **13.** What method will you use to keep his airway open?

    A. Nasal cannula

    B. Jaw thrust

    C. Oropharyngeal airway

    D. All of the above can be used

_____ **14.** While assisting with respirations, you note gastric distention. In order to prevent or alleviate the distention, you should:

    A. ensure the patient's airway is appropriately positioned.

    B. ventilate the patient at the appropriate rate.

    C. ventilate the patient at the appropriate volume.

    D. all of the above

_____ **15.** The correct ventilation rate for assisting this adult patient is:

    A. 1 breath per 5 seconds

    B. 1 breath per 3 seconds

    C. 1 breath per 10 seconds

    D. There is no need to assist with ventilations for this patient.

_____ **16.** Which is the preferred method of assisting ventilations?

    A. Mouth-to-mask with one-way valve

    B. Two-person BVM device with reservoir and supplemental oxygen

    C. Flow-restricted, oxygen-powered ventilation device

    D. One-person BVM device with oxygen reservoir and supplemental oxygen

_____ **17.** When a person goes _____ minutes without oxygen, brain damage is very likely.

    A. 0-4

    B. 4-6

    C. 6-10

    D. more than 10

_____ **18.** If your partner, while examining a patient, states their lungs are equal and bilateral, you would understand them to mean:

    A. both lungs have labored breathing.

    B. both lungs are equally bad.

    C. they have no lungs.

    D. clear and equal lung sounds on both sides.

_____ **19.** What are agonal respirations?

    A. Occasional gasping breaths, but adequate to maintain life

    B. Occasional gasping breaths, unable to maintain life

    C. Painful respirations due to broken ribs

    D. Another name for ataxic respirations

_____ **20.** You come upon a patient who is not injured and is breathing on their own with a normal rate and an adequate tidal volume. What would be the advantage of placing them in the recovery position?

    A. It's the preferred position of comfort for patients.

    B. It helps to protect their cervical spine when injuries are hidden.

    C. It helps prevent the aspiration of vomitus.

    D. It's easier to load them onto the cot from this position.

Labeling

Label the following diagrams with the correct terms.

    1. Upper and Lower Airways

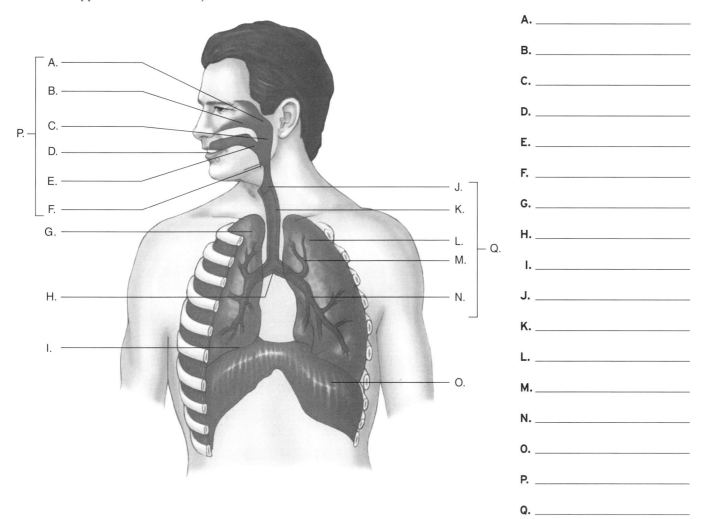

A. _____

B. _____

C. _____

D. _____

E. _____

F. _____

G. _____

H. _____

I. _____

J. _____

K. _____

L. _____

M. _____

N. _____

O. _____

P. _____

Q. _____

2. The Thoracic Cage

A. _____

B. _____

C. _____

D. _____

E. _____

F. _____

G. _____

H. _____

I. _____

J. _____

Fill-in

Read each item carefully, then complete the statement by filling in the missing word(s).

1. Air enters the body through the _____.

2. In exhalation, air pressure in the lungs is _____ than the pressure outside.

3. The air we breathe contains _____ percent oxygen and _____ percent nitrogen.

4. The primary mechanism for triggering breathing is the level of _____ _____ in the blood.

5. During inhalation, the _____ and _____ _____ contract, causing the thorax to enlarge.

6. The drive to breathe is triggered by _____ _____ or _____ _____ _____ levels in arterial blood.

7. Insufficient oxygen in the cells and tissues is called _____.

True/False

If you believe the statement to be more true than false, write the letter "T" in the space provided. If you believe the statement to be more false than true, write the letter "F."

_____ **1.** Nasal airways keep the tongue from blocking the upper airway and facilitate suctioning of the oropharynx.

_____ **2.** Nasal cannulas can deliver a maximum of 44% oxygen at 6 L/min.

_____ **3.** Oral airways should be measured from the tip of the nose to the earlobe.

_____ **4.** Compressed gas cylinders pose no unusual risk.

_____ **5.** The pin-indexing system is used to ensure compatibility between pressure regulators and oxygen flowmeters.

Short Answer

Complete this section with short written answers using the space provided.

1. List the five early signs of hypoxia.

_____

_____

2. What are the normal respiratory rates for adults, children, and infants?

_____

_____

3. How can you avoid gastric distention while performing artificial ventilation?

_____

_____

4. List the six steps for providing one-rescuer artificial ventilation with a BVM device.

_____

_____

5. List six signs of inadequate breathing.

_____

_____

6. What are accessory muscles? Name three.

_____

_____

7. When should medical control be consulted before inserting a nasal airway?

_____

_____

8. List the three steps in nasal airway insertion.

_____

_____

9. What is the best suction tip for suctioning the pharynx, and why?

_____

_____

10. What is the time limit for each episode of suctioning an adult?

_____

_____

Word Fun

The following crossword puzzle is an activity provided to reinforce correct spelling and understanding of medical terminology associated with emergency care and the EMT-B. Use the clues in the column to complete the puzzle.

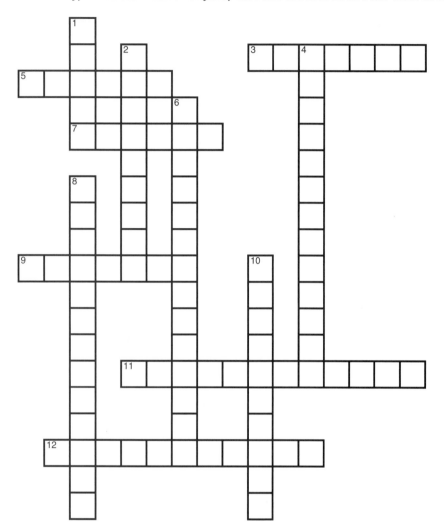

Across

3. Requires more than normal effort
5. Dying, gasping respirations
7. Larynx, nose, mouth, throat
9. Not enough O_2
11. Face piece attached to a reservoir
12. Exchange of air between lungs and outside

Down

1. Opening in neck connected to trachea
2. Mechanism that causes retching
4. Limits exposure to body fluids
6. Airway inserted in nostril
8. Airway inserted in mouth
10. Diaphragm relaxes

Ambulance Calls

The following case scenarios provide an opportunity to explore the concerns associated with patient management. Read each scenario, then answer each question in detail.

1. You are dispatched to a crash with multiple patients early one morning near the end of your shift. Your patient was the unrestrained driver of one of the vehicles. She is 38 years old and struck her face against the steering wheel and windshield. There is a large laceration on her nose and several teeth are missing. Though unconscious, she has vomited a large amount of food and blood, which is pooling in her mouth. You note gurgling noises as she attempts to breathe.

How would you best manage this patient?

_____

_____

_____

2. You are dispatched to a local restaurant for an unconscious woman. As you arrive, you are greeted by a frantic restaurant manager. She tells you that one of her staff members went into the restroom to complete the hourly cleaning routine and found a woman lying on the floor, motionless and apparently not breathing. You and your partner enter the cramped ladies' bathroom, to find an older woman who is apneic, cyanotic, and has a carotid pulse. You attempt to ventilate the patient using a BVM device, but are unsuccessful.

How should you manage this patient?

_____

_____

_____

3. You are outside doing some yard work when you hear one of your neighbors call for help. As you cross the street, you see a husband standing over his wife who is lying on the ground. He tells you that she complained of feeling lightheaded and then she suddenly passed out. He further tells you that he was able to help her to the ground without injury. When you assess her, you hear snoring sounds as she breathes.

How do you manage this patient?

_____

_____

_____

Skill Drills

Skill Drill 7-1: Positioning the Unconscious Patient

Test your knowledge of skill drills by placing the photos below in the correct order. Number the first step with a "1," the second step with a "2," etc.

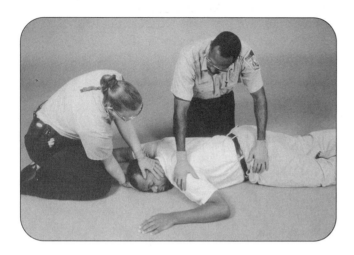

Have your partner place his or her hand on the patient's far shoulder and hip.

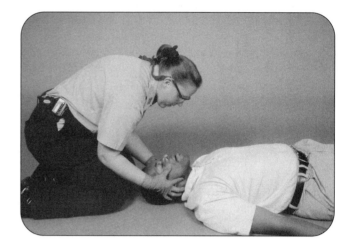

Open and assess the patient's airway and breathing status.

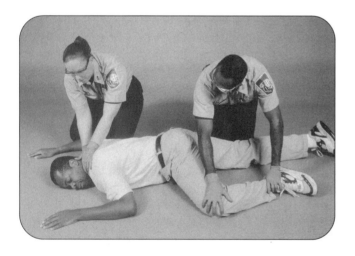

Support the head while your partner straightens the patient's legs.

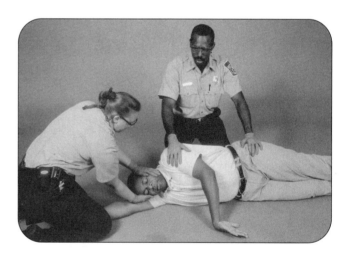

Roll the patient as a unit with the person at the head calling the count to begin the move.

CHAPTER

8 Patient Assessment

Workbook Activities

The following activities have been designed to help you. Your instructor may require you to complete some or all of these activities as a regular part of your EMT-B training program. You are encouraged to complete any activity that your instructor does not assign as a way to enhance your learning in the classroom.

Chapter Review

The following exercises provide an opportunity to refresh your knowledge of this chapter.

Matching

Match each of the terms in the left column to the appropriate definition in the right column.

_____ 1. Triage

_____ 2. Sclera

_____ 3. Subcutaneous emphysema

_____ 4. Paradoxical motion

_____ 5. Conjunctiva

_____ 6. Crepitus

_____ 7. Accessory muscles

_____ 8. Breath sounds

_____ 9. Chief complaint

_____ 10. Frostbite

_____ 11. Jaundice

_____ 12. Orientation

A. indication of air movement in the lungs

B. lining of the eyelid

C. movements in which the skin pulls in around the ribs during inspiration

D. white of the eyes

E. the mental status of a patient

F. the six pain questions

G. yellow skin color due to liver disease or dysfunction

H. a crackling sound

I. examine by touch

J. damage to tissues as the result of exposure to cold

K. the way in which a patient responds to external stimuli

L. secondary muscles of respiration

_____ **13.** OPQRST	**M.** air under the skin
_____ **14.** Palpate	**N.** motion of a segment of chest wall that is opposite the normal
_____ **15.** Responsiveness	movement during breathing
_____ **16.** Retractions	**O.** the reason a patient called for help
	P. sorting

Multiple Choice

Read each item carefully, then select the best response.

_____ **1.** The scene size-up consists of all of the following, except:
   A. determining mechanism of injury.
   B. requesting additional assistance.
   C. determining level of responsiveness.
   D. PPE/BSI.

_____ **2.** Possible dangers you may observe during the scene size-up include:
   A. oncoming traffic.
   B. unstable surfaces.
   C. downed electrical lines.
   D. all of the above

_____ **3.** With _____, the force of the injury occurs over a broad area, and the skin is usually not broken.
   A. motor vehicle crashes
   B. blunt trauma
   C. penetrating trauma
   D. gunshot wounds

_____ **4.** With _____, the force of the injury occurs at a small point of contact between the skin and the object.
   A. motor vehicle crashes
   B. blunt trauma
   C. penetrating trauma
   D. falls

_____ **5.** You can use the mechanism of injury as a kind of guide to predict the potential for a serious injury by evaluating:
   A. the amount of force applied to the body.
   B. the length of time the force was applied.
   C. the areas of the body that are involved.
   D. all of the above

_____ **6.** In penetrating trauma, the severity of injury depends on all of the following, except:
   A. the geographic location.
   B. the characteristics of the penetrating object.
   C. the amount of force or energy.
   D. the part of the body affected.

_____ **7.** In order to quickly determine the nature of illness, talk with:
   A. the patient.
   B. family members.
   C. bystanders.
   D. all of the above

_____ **8.** When considering the need for additional resources, questions to ask include all of the following, except:

   A. How many patients are there?

   B. Is it raining?

   C. Who contacted EMS?

   D. Does the scene pose a threat to you or your patient's safety?

_____ **9.** The initial assessment includes evaluation of all of the following, except:

   A. mental status.

   B. pupils.

   C. airway.

   D. circulation.

_____ **10.** The best indicator of brain function is the patient's:

   A. pulse rate.

   B. papillary response.

   C. mental status.

   D. respiratory rate and depth.

_____ **11.** An altered mental status may be caused by:

   A. head trauma.

   B. hypoxemia.

   C. hypoglycemia.

   D. all of the above

_____ **12.** All of the following are signs of inadequate breathing except:

   A. tightness in the chest.

   B. two- to three-word dyspnea.

   C. use of accessory muscles.

   D. nasal flaring.

_____ **13.** The _____ of the patient's pulse will give you a general idea of the overall status of the patient's cardiac function.

   A. rate

   B. rhythm

   C. strength

   D. all of the above

_____ **14.** The AED should be used on medical patients who are at least _____ years old and weigh more than 55 lb and who have been assessed to be unresponsive, apneic, and pulseless.

   A. 7

   B. 8

   C. 9

   D. 10

_____ **15.** In almost all instances, controlling external bleeding is accomplished by:

   A. direct pressure.

   B. elevation.

   C. pressure points.

   D. tourniquet.

_____ **16.** Assessing the _____ is one of the most important and readily accessible ways of evaluating circulation.

   A. pulse

   B. respirations

   C. skin

   D. capillary refill

_____ **17.** Skin color depends on:

    A. pigmentation.

    B. blood oxygen levels.

    C. the amount of blood circulating through the vessels of the skin.

    D. all of the above

_____ **18.** In deeply pigmented skin, you should look for changes in color in areas of the skin that have less pigment, including:

    A. the sclera.

    B. the conjunctiva.

    C. the mucous membranes of the mouth.

    D. all of the above

_____ **19.** Other conditions, not related to the body's circulation, such as _____, may slow capillary refill.

    A. local circulatory compromise

    B. hypothermia

    C. age

    D. all of the above

_____ **20.** While initial treatment is important, it is essential to remember that immediate _____ is one of the keys to the survival of any high-priority patient.

    A. airway control

    B. bleeding control

    C. transport

    D. application of oxygen

_____ **21.** Goals of the focused history and physical exam include:

    A. identifying the patient's chief complaint.

    B. understanding the specific circumstances surrounding the chief complaint.

    C. directing further physical examination.

    D. all of the above

_____ **22.** Understanding the _____ helps you to understand the severity of the patient's problem and provide invaluable information to hospital staff as well.

    A. chief complaint

    B. mechanism of injury

    C. physical exam

    D. focused history

_____ **23.** An integral part of the rapid trauma assessment is evaluation using the mnemonic:

    A. AVPU.

    B. DCAP-BTLS.

    C. OPQRST.

    D. SAMPLE.

_____ **24.** It is particularly important to evaluate the neck before:

    A. log rolling the patient.

    B. examining the chest.

    C. covering it with a cervical collar.

    D. checking for the presence of a carotid pulse.

_____ **25.** To check for motor function, you should ask the patient:

    A. to wiggle his or her fingers or toes.

    B. to identify which extremity you are touching.

    C. if they can feel you touching them.

    D. all of the above

_____ **26.** Baseline vital signs provide useful information about the:

    A. overall functions of the patient's heart.

    B. overall functions of the patient's lungs.

    C. patient's stability.

    D. all of the above

_____ **27.** When performing a detailed exam, check the neck for:

    A. subcutaneous emphysema.

    B. jugular vein distention.

    C. crepitus.

    D. all of the above

_____ **28.** The purpose of the ongoing assessment is to ask and answer the following questions, except:

    A. Is treatment improving the patient's condition?

    B. What is the patient's diagnosis?

    C. Has an already identified problem gotten better? Worse?

    D. What is the nature of any newly identified problems?

_____ **29.** When reevaluating any interventions you started, take a moment to ensure that:

    A. oxygen is still flowing.

    B. backboard straps are still tight.

    C. bleeding has been controlled.

    D. all of the above

_____ **30.** The last step of the scene size-up for the medical patient is:

    A. consider c-spine.

    B. consider additional resources.

    C. initial assessment.

    D. None of the above.

Questions 31-33 are derived from the following scenario: You've been called to a park where an 86-year-old man has fallen and can't get up. He is pale, cool to the touch, and clammy.

_____ **31.** After ensuring the scene is safe, your next step is to:

    A. provide c-spine.

    B. provide oxygen.

    C. BSI.

    D. determine the number of patients.

_____ **32.** After assessing his ABC's, your next step is to:

    A. complete a focused history and physical exam.

    B. complete a rapid trauma assessment.

    C. complete a detailed assessment.

    D. identify patient priority and make a transport decision

_____ **33.** After completing the initial assessment, your next step is to:

    A. evaluate responsiveness.

    B. reconsider the MOI.

    C. rapid trauma assessment.

    D. focused trauma assessment.

_____ **34.** After evaluating the responsiveness of the medical patient during the focused history and physical exam, your next step for the responsive patient is the:

    A. baseline vitals.

    B. history of illness.

    C. sample history.

    D. None of the above

Fill-in

Read each item carefully, then complete the statement by filling in the missing word(s).

1. From a practical point of view, prehospital emergency care is simply a series of _____ about treatment and transport.

2. The best way to reduce your risk of exposure is to follow _____ _____ _____ (BSI) precautions.

3. You cannot help your patient if you become a _____ yourself.

4. You should park your unit in a place that will offer you and your partner the greatest _____ but also rapid access to the patient and your equipment.

5. _____ is a process of identifying the severity of each patient's condition.

6. The _____ _____ is based on your immediate assessment of the environment, the presenting signs and symptoms, mechanism of injury in a trauma patient, and the patient's chief complaint.

7. The first steps in caring for any patient focus on finding and treating the most _____ _____ illnesses and injuries.

8. With an unresponsive patient or one with a decreased level of consciousness, you should immediately assess the _____ of the airway.

9. If a patient seems to have difficulty breathing, you should immediately _____ the airway.

10. Assess the skin temperature by touching the patient's skin with your _____ or the back of your hand.

11. Correct identification of high-priority patients is an essential aspect of the _____ _____ and helps to improve patient outcome.

True/False

If you believe the statement to be more true than false, write the letter "T" in the space provided. If you believe the statement to be more false than true, write the letter "F."

_____ **1.** Responsiveness is evaluated with the mnemonic DCAP-BTLS.

_____ **2.** An ongoing assessment is not necessary for stable patients.

_____ **3.** Distinguishing between medical and trauma patients is less important than identifying and treating their problems appropriately.

_____ **4.** The apparent absence of a palpable pulse in a responsive patient is not caused by cardiac arrest.

_____ **5.** A patient with a poor general impression is considered a priority patient.

Short Answer

Complete this section with short written answers using the space provided.

1. What is the single goal of initial assessment?

_____

_____

2. What is the general impression based on?

_____

_____

3. What do the letters ABC stand for in the assessment process?

_____

_____

4. What four questions are asked when assessing orientation and what purpose do these questions serve?

_____

_____

5. What are the three goals of the focused history and physical exam?

_____

_____

6. List the elements of DCAP-BTLS.

_____

_____

7. List at least five significant mechanisms of injury in an adult.

_____

_____

Word Fun

The following crossword puzzle is an activity provided to reinforce correct spelling and understanding of medical terminology associated with emergency care and the EMT-B. Use the clues in the column to complete the puzzle.

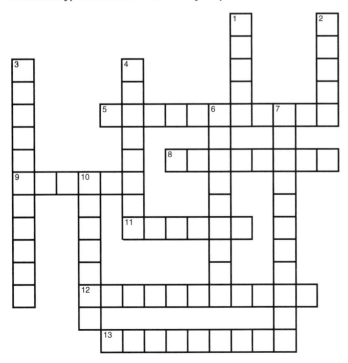

Across

5. Skin pulls in around ribs
8. Involuntary muscle contractions, to protect
9. Pain assessment acronym
11. Acronym for history
12. Below 95 degrees F
13. Distal discomfort or pain

Down

1. Broad area trauma without broken skin
2. Rattling, moist sounds
3. Motion in opposite direction
4. Grating or grinding
6. Formation of clots
7. Times four
10. Coarse breath sounds

Ambulance Calls

The following case scenarios provide an opportunity to explore the concerns associated with patient management. Read each scenario, then answer each question in detail.

1. You are dispatched to a motor vehicle collision where you find a 32-year-old man with extensive trauma to the face and gurgling in his airway. He is responsive only to pain. You also note that the windshield is spider-webbed and there is deformity to the steering wheel. He is not wearing a seat belt.

   How would you best manage this patient? What clues tell you the transport status?

   _____

   _____

   _____

2. You are dispatched to a local residence for "difficulty breathing." You find a man standing in his kitchen, leaning against a counter, and holding a metered-dose inhaler. As you question him, you see that he is working very hard to breathe, hear wheezing, and note that he can only answer you with one- or two-word responses.

   How do you manage this patient?

   _____

   _____

   _____

3. You are dispatched to "man fallen" at a private home. You arrive to find an older man who is semiconscious (response to painful stimuli) and has fallen down a flight of wooden stairs onto a cement basement floor. He has bruising and a small laceration above his left eye.

   How do you manage this patient?

   _____

   _____

   _____

Skill Drills

Skill Drill 8-1: Performing a Rapid Physical Exam

Test your knowledge of this skill drill by placing the photos below in the correct order. Number the first step with a "1," the second step with a "2," etc.

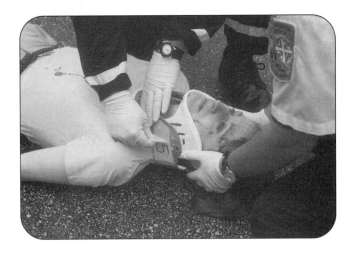

_____

Apply a cervical spinal immobilization device on trauma patients.

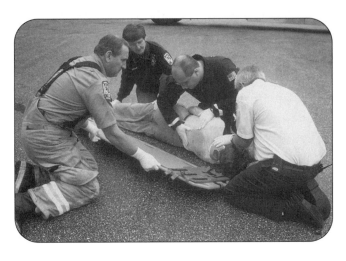

_____

Assess the back. In trauma patients, roll the patient in one motion.

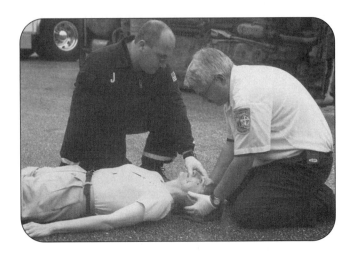

_____

Assess the head. Have your partner maintain in-line stabilization.

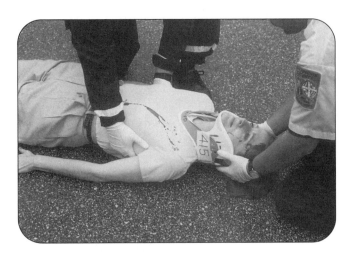

_____

Assess the chest. Listen to breath sounds on both sides of the chest.

(continued)

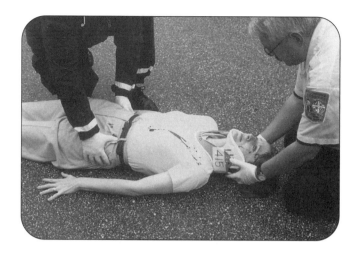

Assess the pelvis. If there is no pain, gently compress the pelvis downward and inward to look for tenderness or instability.

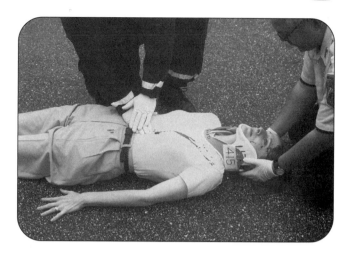

Assess the abdomen.

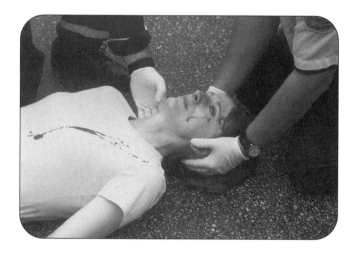

Assess the neck.

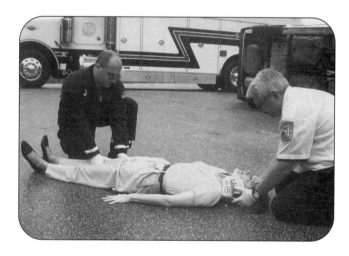

Assess all four extremities. Assess pulse, motor, and sensory function.

Skill Drill 8-3: Performing the Detailed Physical Exam

Test your knowledge of this skill drill by placing the photos below in the correct order. Number the first step with a "1," the second step with a "2," etc.

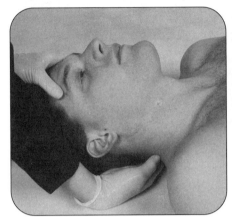

_____

Palpate the front and back of the neck.

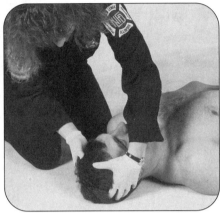

_____

Observe and palpate the head.

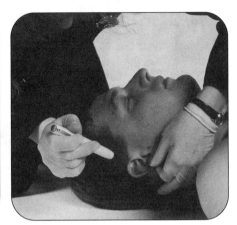

_____

Check the ears for drainage or blood.

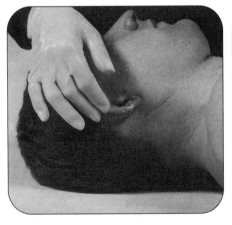

_____

Look behind the ear for Battle's sign.

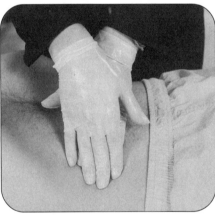

_____

Gently palpate the abdomen.

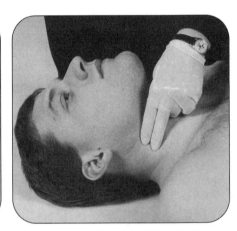

_____

Observe for jugular vein distention.

(continued)

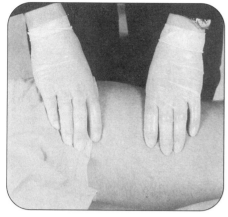

Inspect the extremities; assess distal circulation and motor sensory function.

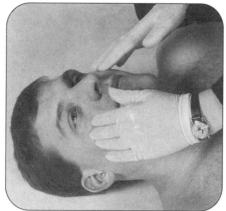

Palpate the maxillae.

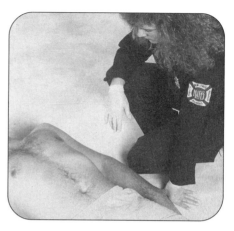

Inspect the chest and observe breathing motion.

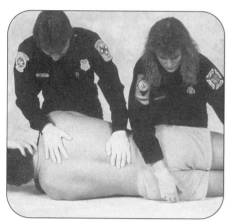

Log roll the patient and inspect the back.

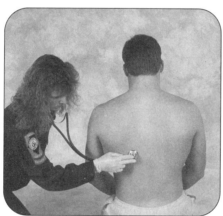

Listen to posterior breath sounds (bases, apices).

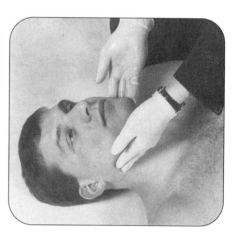

Palpate the mandible.

(continued)

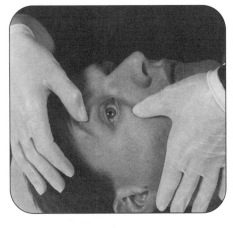

Inspect the area around the eyes and eyelids.

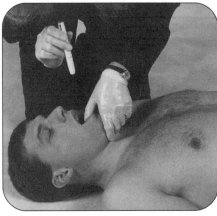

Assess the mouth and nose.

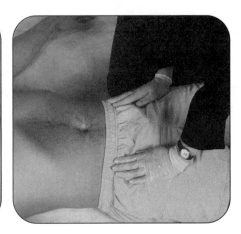

Gently press the iliac crests.

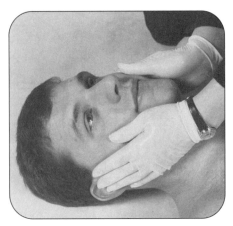

Palpate the zygomas.

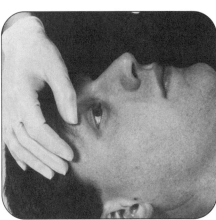

Examine the eyes for redness, contact lenses. Check pupil function.

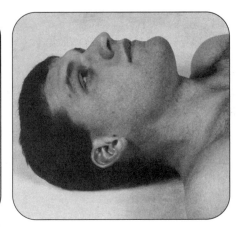

Inspect the neck.

(continued)

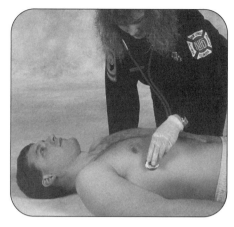

Listen to anterior breath sounds (midaxillary, midclavicular).

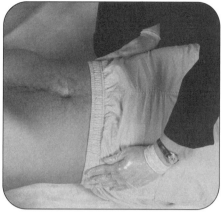

Gently compress the pelvis from the sides.

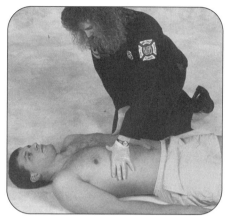

Gently palpate over the ribs.

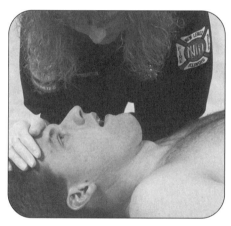

Check for unusual breath odors.

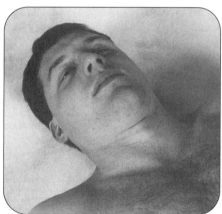

Observe the face.

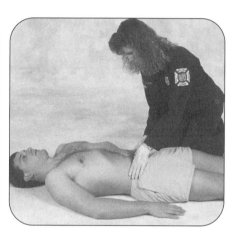

Observe the abdomen and pelvis.

CHAPTER

9 Communications and Documentation

Workbook Activities

The following activities have been designed to help you. Your instructor may require you to complete some or all of these activities as a regular part of your EMT-B training program. You are encouraged to complete any activity that your instructor does not assign as a way to enhance your learning in the classroom.

Chapter Review

The following exercises provide an opportunity to refresh your knowledge of this chapter.

Matching

Match each of the terms in the left column to the appropriate definition in the right column.

_____ **1.** Base station

_____ **2.** Mobile radio

_____ **3.** Portable radio

_____ **4.** Repeater

_____ **5.** Telemetry

_____ **6.** UHF

_____ **7.** VHF

_____ **8.** Cellular telephone

_____ **9.** Dedicated line

_____ **10.** MED channels

_____ **11.** Scanner

_____ **12.** Channel

_____ **13.** Rapport

A. "hot line"

B. a trusting relationship built with your patient

C. communication through an interconnected series of repeater stations

D. assigned frequency used to carry voice and/or data communications

E. radio receiver that searches across several frequencies until the message is completed

F. VHF and UHF channels designated exclusively for EMS use

G. vehicle-mounted device that operates at a lower frequency than a base station

H. a process in which electronic signals are converted into coded, audible signals

I. radio frequencies between 30 and 300 MHz

      J. hand-carried or hand-held devices that operate at 1 to 5 watts

      K. special base station radio that receives messages and signals on one frequency and then automatically retransmits them on a second frequency

      L. radio frequencies between 300 and 3,000 MHz

      M. radio hardware containing a transmitter and receiver that is located in a fixed location

Multiple Choice

Read each item carefully, then select the best response.

_____ **1.** The base station may be used:

    A. in a single place by an operator speaking into a microphone that is connected directly to the equipment.

    B. remotely through telephone lines.

    C. by radio from a communication center.

    D. all of the above

_____ **2.** The transmission range of a(n) _____ is more limited than that of mobile or base station radios.

    A. portable radio

    B. 800 MHz radio

    C. cellular phone

    D. UHF radio

_____ **3.** Base stations:

    A. usually have more power than mobile or portable radios.

    B. have higher, more efficient antenna systems.

    C. allow for communication with field units at much greater distances.

    D. all of the above

_____ **4.** _____ are helpful when you are away from the ambulance and need to communicate with dispatch, another unit, or medical control.

    A. Base stations

    B. Portable radios

    C. Mobile radios

    D. Cellular phones

_____ **5.** Digital signals are also used in some kinds of paging and tone alerting systems because they transmit _____ and allow more choices and flexibility.

    A. numerically

    B. faster

    C. alphanumerically

    D. encoded messages

_____ **6.** As with all repeater-based systems, a cellular telephone is useless if the equipment:

    A. fails.

    B. loses power.

    C. is damaged by severe weather or other circumstances.

    D. all of the above

_____ **7.** In the simplex mode, all of the following are true, except:

    A. when one party transmits, the other must wait to reply.

    B. you must push a button to talk.

    C. it is called a "pair of frequencies."

    D. radio transmissions can occur in either direction, but not simultaneously in both.

_____ **8.** Principle EMS-related responsibilities of the FCC include:

    A. monitoring radio operations.

    B. establishing limitations for transmitter power output.

    C. allocating specific radio frequencies for use by EMS providers.

    D. all of the above

_____ **9.** Information given to the responding unit(s) should include all of the following, except:

    A. the number of patients.

    B. the time the unit will arrive.

    C. the exact location of the incident.

    D. responses by other public safety agencies.

_____ **10.** You must consult with medical control to:

    A. notify the hospital of an incoming patient.

    B. request advice or orders from medical control.

    C. advise the hospital of special situations.

    D. all of the above

_____ **11.** The patient report commonly includes all of the following, except:

    A. a list of the patient's medications.

    B. the patient's age and gender.

    C. a brief history of the patient's current problem.

    D. your estimated time of arrival.

_____ **12.** In most areas, medical control is provided by the _____ who work at the receiving hospital.

    A. nurses

    B. physicians

    C. interns

    D. staff

_____ **13.** For _____ reasons, the delivery of sophisticated care, such as assisting patients in taking medications, must be done in association with physicians.

    A. logical

    B. ethical

    C. legal

    D. all of the above

_____ **14.** Standard radio operating procedures are designed to:

    A. reduce the number of misunderstood messages.

    B. keep transmissions brief.

    C. develop effective radio discipline.

    D. all of the above

_____ **15.** Be sure that you report all patient information in a(n) _____ manner.

    A. objective

    B. accurate

    C. professional

    D. all of the above

_____ **16.** Medical control guides the treatment of patients in the system through all of the following, except:

    A. hands-on care.

    B. protocols.

    C. direct orders.

    D. post-call review.

_____ **17.** Depending upon how the protocols are written, you may need to call medical control for direct orders to:

    A. administer certain treatments.

    B. transport a patient.

    C. request assistance from other agencies.

    D. immobilize a patient.

_____ **18.** During transport:

    A. you must periodically reassess the patient's overall condition.

    B. it is not necessary to report changes in the patient's condition.

    C. you are required to check vital signs once.

    D. once treatment is provided, it is safe to finish your paperwork, since the patient's condition will remain stable.

_____ **19.** While en route to and from the scene, you should report all of the following to the dispatcher, except:

    A. any special hazards.

    B. traffic delays.

    C. abandoned vehicles in the median.

    D. road construction.

_____ **20.** Situations that might require special preparation on the part of the hospital include:

    A. HazMat situations.

    B. mass-casualty incidents.

    C. rescues in progress.

    D. all of the above

_____ **21.** The _____ officially occurs during your oral report at the hospital, not as a result of your radio report en route.

    A. patient report

    B. transfer of care

    C. termination of services

    D. all of the above

_____ **22.** Effective communication between the EMT-B and health care professionals in the receiving facility is an essential cornerstone of _____ patient care.

    A. efficient

    B. effective

    C. appropriate

    D. all of the above

_____ **23.** Components that must be included in the oral report during transfer of care include:

    A. the patient's name.

    B. any important history.

    C. vital signs assessed.

    D. all of the above

_____ **24.** Your _____ are critically important in gaining the trust of both the patient and family.

    A. gestures

    B. body movements

    C. attitude toward the patient

    D. all of the above

_____ **25.** If the patient is hearing impaired, you should:

    A. stand on the patient's left side.

    B. shout.

    C. speak clearly and distinctly.

    D. use baby talk.

_____ **26.** The functional age relates to the person's:

    A. ability to function in daily activities.

    B. mental state.

    C. activity pattern.

    D. all of the above

_____ **27.** When caring for a visually impaired patient, you should:

    A. use sign language.

    B. touch the patient only when necessary to render care.

    C. try to avoid sudden movements.

    D. never walk them to the ambulance.

_____ **28.** When attempting to communicate with non-English-speaking patients, you should:

    A. use short, simple questions and simple words whenever possible.

    B. always use medical terms.

    C. shout.

    D. position yourself so the patient can read your lips.

_____ **29.** The patient information that is included in the minimum data set includes all of the following, except:

    A. chief complaint.

    B. the time that the EMS unit arrived at the scene.

    C. respirations and effort.

    D. skin color and temperature.

_____ **30.** Functions of the prehospital care report include:

    A. continuity of care.

    B. education.

    C. research.

    D. all of the above

_____ **31.** A good prehospital care report documents:

    A. the care that was provided.

    B. the patient's condition on arrival.

    C. any changes.

    D. all of the above

_____ **32.** When completing the narrative section, be sure to:

    A. describe what you see and what you do.

    B. only include positive findings.

    C. record your conclusions about the incident.

    D. use appropriate radio codes.

_____ **33.** Instances in which you may be required to file special reports with appropriate authorities include:

    A. gunshot wounds.

    B. dog bites.

    C. suspected physical, sexual, or substance abuse.

    D. all of the above

Questions 34-38 are derived from the following scenario: You have just finished an ambulance run where a 45-year-old man had run his SUV into a utility pole. The driver was found slumped over the steering wheel, unconscious. A large electrical wire was lying across the hood of the vehicle. After securing scene safety, you were able to approach the patient and completed a rapid physical assessment, in which you found a 6-inch laceration across his forehead. The patient regained responsiveness, was alert and oriented, and refused care.

_____ **34.** Should an EMT document this call, since the patient refused care?

    A. No – You only need to document when you have actually provided care.

    B. No – This was not a billable run.

    C. Yes – and is best signed by the patient as "Refusal of Care."

    D. Both A and B

_____ **35.** What would be important to document?

    A. That the scene needed to be made safe

    B. That ensuring scene safety delayed care

    C. That you completed a rapid physical assessment

    D. All of the above

_____ **36.** While writing the report, you made an error. How should this be corrected?

    A. Draw a single line through it.

    B. Erase the mistake.

    C. Cover up the mistake with correction fluid.

    D. All of the above

_____ **37.** What are the consequences of falsifying a report?

    A. It may result in the suspension and/or revocation of your license.

    B. It gives other health care providers a false impression of assessment/findings.

    C. It results in poor patient care.

    D. All of the above

_____ **38.** If the patient refuses to sign the refusal form:

    A. Sign it yourself and state: "Patient refused to sign."

    B. You cannot let him leave the scene until he either goes with you or signs the form.

    C. Have a credible witness sign the form testifying they witnessed the patient's refusal of care.

    D. If they refuse care, you don't have to document.

Fill-in

Read each item carefully, then complete the statement by filling in the missing word(s).

  1. Written communications, in the form of a written _____ _____ _____, provide you with an

     opportunity to communicate the patient's story to others who may participate in the patient's care in the future.

  2. A two-way radio consists of two units: a _____ and a _____.

  3. A _____ _____, also known as a hot line, is always open or under the control of the individuals at

     each end.

  4. With _____, electronic signals are converted into coded, audible signals.

  5. Low-power portable radios that communicate through a series of interconnected repeater stations called "cells" are

     known as _____ _____.

  6. _____ are commonly used in EMS operations to alert on- and off-duty personnel.

7. When the first call to 9-1-1 comes in, the dispatcher must try to judge its relative _____ to begin the appropriate EMS response using emergency medical dispatch protocols.

8. The principal reason for radio communication is to facilitate communication between you and _____ _____.

9. You could be successfully sued for _____ if you describe a patient in a way that injures his or her reputation.

10. Regardless of your system's design, your link to _____ _____ is vital to maintain the high quality of care that your patient requires and deserves.

11. To ensure complete understanding, once you receive an order from medical control, you must _____ the order back, word for word, and then receive confirmation.

12. By their very nature, _____ _____ do not require direct communication with medical control.

13. Maintaining _____ _____ with your patient builds trust and lets the patient know that he or she is your first priority.

14. Children can easily see through lies or deception, so you must always be _____ with them.

15. If the patient does not speak any English, find a family member or friend to act as a(n) _____.

16. The national EMS community has identified a _____ _____ _____ that should enable communication and comparison of EMS runs between agencies, regions, and states.

17. _____ adult patients have the right to refuse treatment.

True/False
If you believe the statement to be more true than false, write the letter "T" in the space provided. If you believe the statement to be more false than true, write the letter "F."

_____ **1.** The two-way radio is actually at least two units: a transmitter and a receiver.

_____ **2.** Base stations typically have more power and much higher and more efficient antenna systems than mobile or portable radios.

_____ **3.** A cellular telephone is just another kind of portable radio that is available for EMS use.

_____ **4.** The transmission range of a mobile radio is more limited than that of a portable radio.

_____ **5.** A dedicated line, a special telephone line used for specific point-to-point communications, is always open or under the control of the individuals at each end.

_____ **6.** The written report is a vital part of providing emergency medical care and ensuring the continuity of patient care.

_____ **7.** EMS systems that use repeaters are unable to get good signals from portable radios.

_____ **8.** Small changes in your location will not significantly affect the quality of your transmission.

_____ **9.** Your reporting responsibilities end when you arrive at the hospital.

_____ **10.** Patients deserve to know that you can provide medical care and that you are concerned about their well-being.

Short Answer

Complete this section with short written answers using the space provided.

1. List the five principal FCC responsibilities related to EMS.

_____

_____

2. List five guidelines for effective radio communications.

_____

_____

3. List the six functions of a prehospital care report.

_____

_____

4. Describe the two types of written report forms generally in use in EMS systems.

_____

_____

Word Fun

The following crossword puzzle is an activity provided to reinforce correct spelling and understanding of medical terminology associated with emergency care and the EMT-B. Use the clues in the column to complete the puzzle.

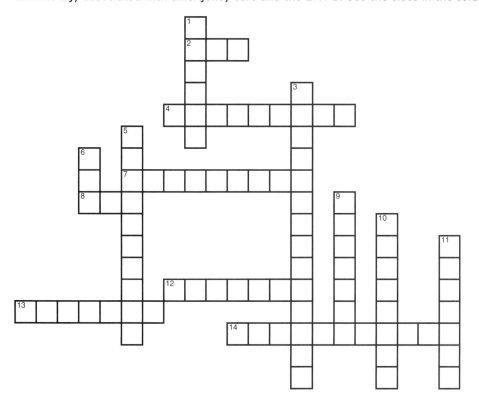

Across

2. Frequencies between 300 and 3,000 MHz

4. Electronic signals converted into coded audible signals

7. Point-to-point

8. Agency with jurisdiction over radios

12. Radio receiver that searches

13. Transmit in both ways, but not at the same time

14. Hardware in a fixed location

Down

1. Transmit and receive simultaneously

3. Outline specific directions, protocols

5. Frequencies for exclusive EMS usage

6. Frequencies between 30 and 300 MHz

9. Trusting relationship

10. Receives on one, transmits on another

11. Assigned frequency

Ambulance Calls

The following case scenarios provide an opportunity to explore the concerns associated with patient management. Read each scenario, then answer each question in detail.

1. You are in the dispatch office filling in for the EMS dispatcher who needed to use the restroom. The phone rings and you answer it to find a hysterical female screaming about a child falling in an old well. The only information she is providing is that he is 5 years old and is not making any noise. The address is on the computer display.

   How would you best manage this situation and what additional help would you call for?

   _____

   _____

   _____

2. You respond to an "unknown medical problem" in an area commonly populated by Hispanic Americans. You arrive to find several individuals speaking to a middle-aged man. They seem to be concerned about him, and motion you toward the patient. You attempt to gain information about the situation, but your patient does not speak English and you do not speak Spanish. The patient has no outward appearance of any problems.
   What should you do?

   _____

   _____

   _____

3. You are dispatched to the parking lot of a grocery store for a "confused child." You arrive to find a young boy who is developmentally disabled. He cannot communicate who he is or where he lives. He is frightened but appears otherwise unharmed.
   What should you do?

   _____

   _____

   _____

CHAPTER

10 General Pharmacology

Workbook Activities

The following activities have been designed to help you. Your instructor may require you to complete some or all of these activities as a regular part of your EMT-B training program. You are encouraged to complete any activity that your instructor does not assign as a way to enhance your learning in the classroom.

Chapter Review

The following exercises provide an opportunity to refresh your knowledge of this chapter.

Matching

Match each of the terms in the left column to the appropriate definition in the right column.

_____ 1. Absorption

_____ 2. Contraindication

_____ 3. Side effect

_____ 4. Adsorption

_____ 5. Dose

_____ 6. Indication

_____ 7. Action

_____ 8. Pharmacology

_____ 9. Capsules

_____ 10. Topical medications

A. lotions, creams, ointments

B. effect that a drug is expected to have

C. the study of the properties and effects of drugs and medications

D. amount of medication given

E. gelatin shells filled with powdered or liquid medication

F. any action of a drug other than the desired one

G. to bind or stick to a surface

H. therapeutic use for a particular medication

I. process by which medications travel through body tissues

J. situation in which a drug should not be given

Multiple Choice

Read each item carefully, then select the best response.

_____ **1.** The proper dose of a medication depends on all of the following, except:

    A. the patient's age.

    B. the patient's size.

    C. generic substitutions.

    D. the desired action.

_____ **2.** Nitroglycerin relieves the squeezing or crushing pain associated with angina by:

    A. dilating the arteries to increase the oxygen supply to the heart muscle.

    B. causing the heart to contract harder and increase cardiac output.

    C. causing the heart to beat faster to supply more oxygen to the heart.

    D. all of the above

_____ **3.** The brand name that a manufacturer gives to a medication is called the _____ name.

    A. trade

    B. generic

    C. chemical

    D. prescription

_____ **4.** The fastest way to deliver a chemical substance is by the _____ route.

    A. intravenous

    B. oral

    C. sublingual

    D. intramuscular

_____ **5.** The form the manufacturer chooses for a medication ensures:

    A. the proper route of the medication.

    B. the timing of its release into the bloodstream.

    C. its effects on target organs or body systems.

    D. all of the above

_____ **6.** Solutions may be given:

    A. orally.

    B. intramuscularly.

    C. rectally.

    D. all of the above

_____ **7.** In the prehospital setting, _____ is the preferred method of giving oxygen to patients who have sufficient tidal volume, and can provide up to 95% inspired oxygen.

    A. a nasal cannula

    B. a nonrebreathing mask

    C. a bag-valve mask

    D. any of the above

_____ **8.** Characteristics of epinephrine include:

    A. dilating passages in the lungs.

    B. constricting blood vessels.

    C. increasing the heart rate and blood pressure.

    D. all of the above

_____ **9.** Epinephrine acts as a specific antidote to:

   A. adrenaline.

   B. histamine.

   C. asthma.

   D. bronchitis.

_____ **10.** Nitroglycerin relieves pain because its purpose is to increase blood flow by relieving the spasms or causing the arteries to:

   A. dilate.

   B. constrict.

   C. thicken.

   D. contract.

_____ **11.** Nitroglycerin affects the body in the following ways (select all that apply):

   A. It decreases blood pressure.

   B. It relaxes veins throughout the body.

   C. It often causes a mild headache after administration.

   D. It increases blood return to the heart.

Questions 12-16 are derived from the following scenario: You are called to a home of a known 34-year-old man with diabetes. When you arrive, you find the patient supine and unconscious on the living room floor, snoring.

_____ **12.** Medications most EMT-Bs carry in the ambulance that would pertain to this call include:

   A. insulin, oxygen, and oral glucose.

   B. nitroglycerin, oxygen, and oral glucose.

   C. activated charcoal, oxygen, and oral glucose.

   D. none of the above

_____ **13.** Oral glucose:

   A. is a suspension.

   B. should be given to this patient.

   C. is placed between a patient's cheek and gum.

   D. is not carried by EMT-Bs.

_____ **14.** The government publication listing all drugs in the United States is called the:

   A. United States Pharmacopoeia.

   B. The Department of Transportation Reference Guide.

   C. US Pharmacology.

   D. Nursing Drug Reference.

_____ **15.** Oral glucose is _____ for this patient.

   A. indicated

   B. contraindicated

   C. not normally given

   D. none of the above

_____ **16.** Oxygen:

   A. is a drug.

   B. should be applied to this patient.

   C. does not burn.

   D. all the above

Fill-in

Read each item carefully, then complete the statement by filling in the missing word.

1. _____ is a simple sugar that is readily absorbed by the bloodstream.

2. _____ is the main hormone that controls the body's fight-or-flight response.

3. Nitroglycerin is usually taken _____.

4. In all but the _____ _____ route, the medication is absorbed into the bloodstream through various body tissues.

5. When given by mouth, _____ may be absorbed from the stomach fairly quickly because the medication is already dissolved.

6. A _____ is a chemical substance that is used to treat or prevent disease or relieve pain.

True/False

If you believe the statement to be more true than false, write the letter "T" in the space provided. If you believe the statement to be more false than true, write the letter "F."

_____ 1. Oxygen is a flammable substance.

_____ 2. Glucose may be administered to an unconscious patient in order to save his or her life.

_____ 3. Epinephrine is a hormone produced by the body to aid in digestion.

_____ 4. Nitroglycerin decreases blood pressure.

_____ 5. Sublingual medications are rapidly absorbed into the digestive tract.

_____ 6. Vital signs should be taken before and after a medication is given.

_____ 7. Even though medications can react with each other, this is not a potentially harmful condition for the patient.

_____ 8. Nitroglycerin should only be administered when the patient's systolic blood pressure is below 100 mm Hg.

Short Answer

Complete this section with short written answers using the space provided.

1. List seven routes of medication administration.

_____

_____

2. Describe the general steps of administering medication.

_____

_____

3. Describe the action of activated charcoal and the steps of administration that are specific to this medication.

_____

_____

4. List three characteristics of epinephrine.

_____

_____

5. How is an epinephrine auto-injector activated?

_____

_____

6. List five effects of nitroglycerin.

_____

_____

7. Explain why metered-dose inhalers are often used with a spacer.

_____

_____

Word Fun

The following crossword puzzle is a good way to reinforce correct spelling and understanding of medical terminology associated with emergency care and the EMT-B. Use the clues in the column to complete the puzzle.

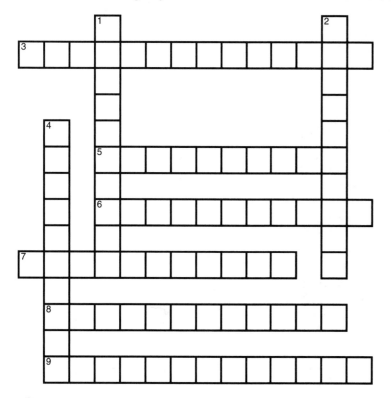

Across

3. Through the skin

5. Process for medication to travel

6. Into the vein

7. Raises heart rate and blood pressure

8. Into the bone

9. Dilates arteries in angina patients

Down

1. Therapeutic use for medication

2. Under the tongue

4. Binding to or sticking to a surface

Ambulance Calls

The following case scenarios provide an opportunity to explore the concerns associated with patient management. Read each scenario, then answer each question in detail.

1. You are dispatched to "difficulty breathing" at one of your town's many parks. As you near the park entrance, you see a crowd of people who frantically wave for you. You arrive to find a city employee who was apparently mowing the park grounds when he accidentally mowed over a yellow jacket nest. He was wearing coveralls, but he was repeatedly stung around his neck and face. He appears to be somewhat confused; you can hear stridor with each inspiration and his blood pressure is 80/40. Your local protocols allow EMT-Bs to carry EpiPens.

   How do you best manage this patient?

   _____

   _____

   _____

2. You are dispatched to an "unknown medical problem" at 1212 Main Street. You were called after police were summoned to subdue a combative male shopper. Police officers were able to calm him down, but felt that something was "not right" about him. You arrive to find a calm, but confused man who is sweaty and pale. He has no complaints, but keeps repeating, "I have to get home now." You notice a medical ID bracelet indicating that this patient is an insulin-dependent diabetic.

   How do you best manage this patient?

   _____

   _____

   _____

3. You are dispatched to the residence of a 68-year-old man who is complaining of a "crushing" chest pain radiating down his left arm for the past hour. He is pale, cool, diaphoretic, and is very nauseated. He tells you he had a heart attack several years ago and takes nitroglycerin as needed. He took two tablets prior to your arrival and reports no relief.

   How would you best manage this patient?

   _____

   _____

   _____

CHAPTER

11 Respiratory Emergencies

Workbook Activities

The following activities have been designed to help you. Your instructor may require you to complete some or all of these activities as a regular part of your EMT-B training program. You are encouraged to complete any activity that your instructor does not assign as a way to enhance your learning in the classroom.

Chapter Review

The following exercises provide an opportunity to refresh your knowledge of this chapter.

Matching

Match each of the terms in the left column to the appropriate definition in the right column.

_____	**1.** Asthma	**A.** irritation of the major lung passageways
_____	**2.** Pulmonary edema	**B.** acute spasm of the bronchioles, associated with excessive mucus production and sometimes spasm of the bronchiolar muscles
_____	**3.** Epiglottitis	**C.** accumulation of air in the pleural space
_____	**4.** Emphysema	**D.** fluid build-up within the alveoli and lung tissue
_____	**5.** Pleural effusion	**E.** an infectious disease of the lung that damages lung tissue
_____	**6.** Pneumothorax	**F.** a substance that causes an allergic reaction
_____	**7.** Dyspnea	**G.** difficulty breathing
_____	**8.** Pneumonia	**H.** bacterial infection that can produce severe swelling
_____	**9.** Hypoxia	**I.** a blood clot or other substance in the circulatory system that travels to a blood vessel where it causes blockage
_____	**10.** Bronchitis	**J.** disease of the lungs in which the alveoli stretch, lose elasticity, and are destroyed
_____	**11.** Hyperventilation	**K.** rapid or deep breathing that lowers blood carbon dioxide levels below normal
_____	**12.** Allergen	**L.** fluid outside of the lung
_____	**13.** Embolus	**M.** condition in which the body's cells and tissues do not have enough oxygen

Multiple Choice

Read each item carefully, then select the best response.

_____ **1.** When treating a patient with dyspnea, you must be prepared to treat:

   A. the symptoms.

   B. the underlying problem.

   C. the patient's anxiety.

   D. all of the above

_____ **2.** The oxygen-carbon dioxide exchange takes place in the:

   A. trachea.

   B. bronchial tree.

   C. alveoli.

   D. blood.

_____ **3.** Oxygen-carbon dioxide exchange may be hampered if:

   A. the pleural space is filled with air or excess fluid.

   B. the alveoli are damaged.

   C. the air passages are obstructed.

   D. all of the above

_____ **4.** If carbon dioxide levels drop too low, the person automatically breathes:

   A. normally.

   B. rapidly and deeply.

   C. slower, less deeply.

   D. fast and shallow.

_____ **5.** If the level of carbon dioxide in the arterial blood rises above normal, the patient breathes:

   A. normally.

   B. rapidly and deeply.

   C. slower, less deeply.

   D. fast and shallow.

_____ **6.** The level of carbon dioxide in the arterial blood can rise due to:

   A. emphysema.

   B. chronic bronchitis.

   C. cardiovascular disease.

   D. all of the above

_____ **7.** The second stimulus that develops in patients with normally high levels of carbon dioxide responds to:

   A. increased oxygen levels.

   B. decreased oxygen levels.

   C. increased carbon dioxide levels.

   D. decreased carbon dioxide levels.

_____ **8.** _____ is a sign of hypoxia to the brain.

   A. Altered mental status

   B. Decreased heart rate

   C. Decreased respiratory rate

   D. Delayed capillary refill time

_____ **9.** An obstruction to the exchange of gases between the alveoli and the capillaries may result from:

   A. epiglottitis.

   B. pneumonia.

   C. colds.

   D. all of the above

_____ **10.** Pulmonary edema can develop quickly after a major:

    A. heart attack.

    B. episode of syncope.

    C. brain injury.

    D. all of the above

_____ **11.** In addition to a major heart attack, pulmonary edema may also be produced by:

    A. inhaling large amounts of smoke.

    B. traumatic injuries to the chest.

    C. inhaling toxic chemical fumes.

    D. all of the above

_____ **12.** _____ is a loss of the elastic material around the air spaces as a result of chronic stretching of the alveoli when bronchitic airways obstruct easy expulsion of gases.

    A. Emphysema

    B. Bronchitis

    C. Pneumonia

    D. Diphtheria

_____ **13.** Most patients with COPD will:

    A. chronically produce sputum.

    B. have a chronic cough.

    C. have difficulty expelling air from their lungs.

    D. all of the above

_____ **14.** The patient with COPD usually presents with:

    A. an increased blood pressure.

    B. a green or yellow productive cough.

    C. a decreased heart rate.

    D. all of the above

_____ **15.** A pneumothorax caused by a medical condition without any injury is known as:

    A. a tension pneumothorax.

    B. a subcutaneous pneumothorax.

    C. spontaneous.

    D. none of the above

_____ **16.** Asthma produces a characteristic _____ as patients attempt to exhale through partially obstructed air passages.

    A. rhonchi

    B. stridor

    C. wheezing

    D. rattle

_____ **17.** An allergic response to certain foods or some other allergen may produce an acute:

    A. bronchodilation.

    B. asthma attack.

    C. vasoconstriction.

    D. insulin release.

_____ **18.** Treatment for anaphylaxis and acute asthma attacks include:

    A. epinephrine.

    B. high-flow oxygen.

    C. antihistamines.

    D. all of the above

_____ **19.** A collection of fluid outside the lungs on one or both sides of the chest is called a:

   A. spontaneous pneumothorax.

   B. subcutaneous emphysema.

   C. pleural effusion.

   D. tension pneumothorax.

_____ **20.** Always consider _____ in patients who were eating just before becoming short of breath:

   A. upper airway obstruction

   B. anaphylaxis

   C. lower airway obstruction

   D. bronchoconstriction

_____ **21.** _____ is defined as overbreathing to the point that the level of arterial carbon dioxide falls below normal.

   A. Reactive airway syndrome

   B. Hyperventilation

   C. Tachypnea

   D. Pleural effusion

_____ **22.** Slowing of respirations after administration of oxygen to a COPD patient does not necessarily mean that the patient no longer needs the oxygen; he or she may need:

   A. insulin.

   B. even more oxygen.

   C. mouth-to-mouth resuscitation.

   D. none of the above

Questions 23-27 are derived from the following scenario: You respond to a home of a 78-year-old man having difficulty breathing. He is sitting at the kitchen table in a classic tripod position, wearing a nasal cannula. He is cyanotic, smoking, and has his shirt unbuttoned. His respirations are 30 breaths/min and shallow, his heart rate is 110 beats/min, and his blood pressure is 136/88 mm Hg.

_____ **23.** Your first thought as an EMT-B should be to:

   A. apply a nonrebreathing mask at 15L/min.

   B. call for back-up.

   C. consider BSI precautions.

   D. put the cigarette out.

_____ **24.** His brain stem senses the level of _____ in the arterial blood, causing the rapid respirations.

   A. carbon dioxide

   B. oxygen

   C. insulin

   D. none of the above

_____ **25.** Proper management of this patient should include:

   A. Oxygen via nonrebreathing mask at 15 L/min

   B. Positive-pressure ventilations

   C. Airway positioning

   D. All the above

_____ **26.** Which of the following is <u>NOT</u> a sign or symptom of his inadequate breathing?

   A. His cyanosis

   B. His shirt was unbuttoned

   C. He was in a tripod position

   D. His heart rate was over 100 beats/min (tachycardia)

_____ **27.** What should you do during the ongoing assessment?

    A. Assess vital signs every 5 minutes.

    B. Repeat the initial and focused assessment.

    C. Reassess interventions performed.

    D. All of the above

_____ **28.** Questions to ask during the focused history and physical examination include:

    A. What has the patient already done for the breathing problem?

    B. Does the patient use a prescribed inhaler?

    C. Does the patient have any allergies?

    D. All of the above

_____ **29.** Generic names for popular inhaled medications include:

    A. ventolin.

    B. metaprel.

    C. terbutaline.

    D. all of the above

_____ **30.** Contraindications to helping a patient self-administer any MDI medication include:

    A. not obtaining permission from medical control.

    B. noticing that the inhaler is not prescribed for this patient.

    C. noticing that the patient has already met the maximum prescribed dose.

    D. all of the above

_____ **31.** Possible side effects of over-the-counter cold medications may include:

    A. agitation.

    B. increased heart rate.

    C. increased blood pressure.

    D. all of the above

_____ **32.** A prolonged asthma attack that is unrelieved by epinephrine may progress into a condition known as:

    A. pleural effusion.

    B. status epilepticus.

    C. status asthmaticus.

    D. reactive airway disease.

Labeling

Label the following diagrams with the correct terms.

Obstruction, scarring, and dilation of the alveolar sac

A. _____

B. _____

C. _____

D. _____

E. _____

F. _____

G. _____

H. _____

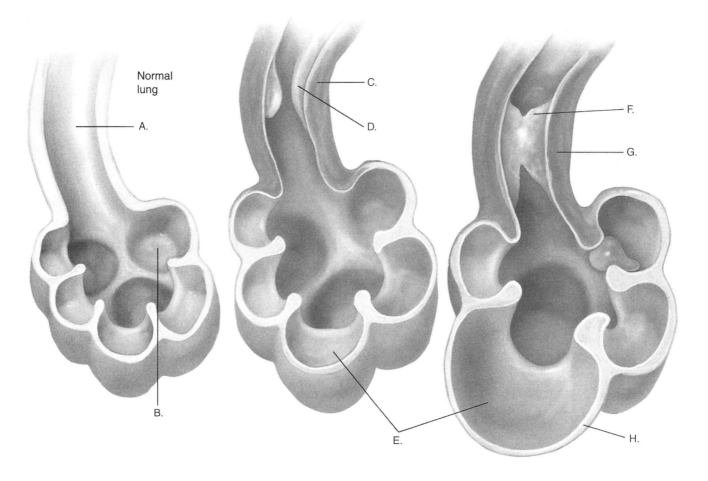

Fill-in

Read each item carefully, then complete the statement by filling in the missing word(s).

1. The level of _____ _____ bathing the brain stem stimulates respiration.

2. The level of _____ in the blood is a secondary stimulus for respiration.

3. _____ _____ entering the alveoli passes into the capillaries, which carry _____

back to the heart.

4. Carbon dioxide and oxygen are exchanged in the _____.

5. Air enters the body through the _____.

6. Abnormal breathing is indicated by a rate slower than _____ breaths/min or faster than

_____ breaths/min.

7. During respiration, oxygen is provided to the blood, and _____ _____ is removed from it.

8. Evaluating the adequacy of the pulse can give you an indication of the patient's _____ _____.

9. The last step in the initial assessment is to make a _____ _____.

10. When asking questions about the present illness during the focused history and physical exam, use

_____ and _____ to guide you in your questioning.

True/False

If you believe the statement to be more true than false, write the letter "T" in the space provided. If you believe the statement to be more false than true, write the letter "F."

_____ **1.** Chronic bronchitis is characterized by spasm and narrowing of the bronchioles due to exposure to allergens.

_____ **2.** With pneumothorax, the lung collapses because the negative vacuum pressure in the pleural space is lost.

_____ **3.** Anaphylactic reactions occur only in patients with a previous history of asthma or allergies.

_____ **4.** Decreased breath sounds in asthma occur because fluid in the pleural space has moved the lung away from the chest wall.

_____ **5.** Pulmonary emboli are difficult to diagnose.

_____ **6.** A patient with aspirin poisoning may hyperventilate in response to acidosis.

_____ **7.** The distinction between hyperventilation and hyperventilation syndrome is straightforward and should guide the EMT-B's treatment choices.

_____ **8.** COPD most often results from cigarette smoking.

_____ **9.** Asthma and COPD are characterized by long inspiratory times.

_____ **10.** SARS is a serious, potentially life-threatening viral infection that usually starts with flu-like symptoms and usually progresses to pneumonia and respiratory failure.

_____ **11.** When assessing a patient, the general impression will help you decide whether the patient's condition is stable or unstable.

_____ **12.** Skin color, capillary refill, level of consciousness, and pain measurement are key in evaluating the respiratory patient.

Short Answer

Complete this section with short written answers using the space provided.

1. List five characteristics of normal breathing.

_____

_____

2. List the five most common mechanisms occurring in lung disorders.

_____

_____

3. Under what conditions should you not assist a patient with a metered-dose inhaler?

_____

_____

4. Describe chronic bronchitis.

_____

_____

5. List five signs of inadequate breathing.

_____

_____

_____

6. Explain carbon dioxide retention.

_____

_____

_____

7. When ventilating a patient, how would you determine if your ventilations are adequate?

_____

_____

Word Fun

The following crossword puzzle is an activity provided to reinforce correct spelling and understanding of medical terminology associated with emergency care and the EMT-B. Use the clues provided to complete the puzzle.

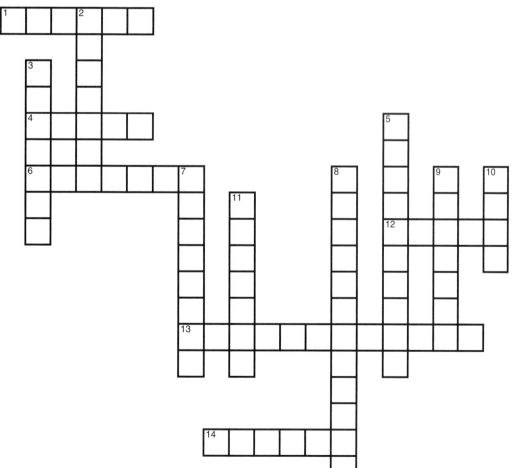

Across

1. High-pitched, whistling sound
4. Crackling, rattling sounds
6. Difficulty breathing
12. Barking cough
13. Inflammation of leaf-shaped airway cover
14. Muscle spasm in small airways

Down

2. Traveling clot
3. Harsh, high-pitched sound
5. Irritation of major airways
7. Substance causing a reaction
8. Air in pleural space
9. Coarse sounds from mucus in airways
10. Slow process of chronic disruption of airways
11. Low oxygen

Ambulance Calls

The following case scenarios will give you an opportunity to explore the concerns associated with patient management. Read each scenario, then answer each question in detail.

1. You are called to the home of a young boy who is reportedly experiencing difficulty swallowing. You arrive to find concerned parents who tell you that their son seems to 'be sick.' He can't swallow, has a high fever and refuses to lie down. As you enter the child's bedroom, you find him standing with arms outstretched onto the footboard of the bed, drooling and with a very frightened look on his face.

   How do you manage this patient?

   _____

   _____

   _____

2. You are dispatched to a 36-year-old woman complaining of shortness of breath. You arrive to find a slightly overweight female patient who tells you she 'can't catch her breath.' She is a smoker whose only medication is birth control pills.

   How would you best manage this patient?

   _____

   _____

   _____

3. You are called to the home of a 73-year-old man complaining of severe dyspnea. The patient has a history of COPD and is on home oxygen at 2 L/min via nasal cannula. His family tells you he has a long history of breathing problems and emphysema. He is cyanotic around his lips and his respirations are 36 breaths/min and shallow.

   How would you best manage this patient?

   _____

   _____

   _____

Skill Drills

Skill Drill 11-1: Assisting a Patient With a Metered-Dose Inhaler

Test your knowledge of this skill drill by filling in the correct words in the photo captions.

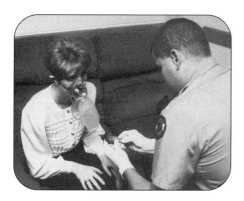 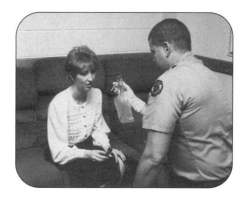

1. Ensure inhaler is at room temperature or _____ .

2. Remove oxygen mask. Hand inhaler to patient. Instruct about breathing and _____ _____ .

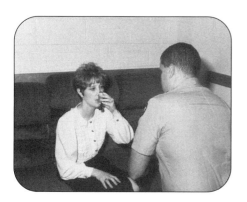 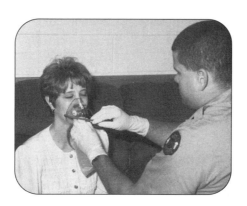

3. Instruct patient to press inhaler and inhale. Instruct about _____ _____ .

3. Reapply _____ . After a few _____ , have patient repeat _____ if order/protocol allows.

Assessment Review

Answer the following questions pertaining to the assessment of the types of emergencies discussed in this chapter.

1. You have been assessing a 17-year-old female in respiratory distress, and you have just obtained her baseline vital signs. Your next step is to:

A. make a transport decision.

B. consider a detailed physical examination.

C. contact medical control.

D. make interventions.

2. You have determined that she is hyperventilating. Your emergency care would include:

A. having her breathe into a small paper sack.

B. providing oxygen.

C. have her run in place until the hyperventilation subsides.

D. none of the above

3. You have been called to a patient who resides in a long-term care facility and who is having difficulty breathing. After assessing and treating life threats to the patient's airway, breathing, and circulation, your next step is to:

A. make a transport decision.

B. obtain a "SAMPLE" history.

C. obtain an "OPQRST" history.

D. obtain baseline vital signs.

4. During the ongoing assessment, vital signs should be taken every _____ minutes for the unstable patient.

A. 3

B. 5

C. 10

D. 15

5. During the ongoing assessment, vital signs should be taken every _____ minutes for the stable patient.

A. 3

B. 5

C. 10

D. 15

Emergency Care Summary

Complete the statements pertaining to emergency care for the types of emergencies discussed in this chapter by filling in the missing word(s).

NOTE: While the steps below are widely accepted, be sure to consult and follow your local protocol.

Respiratory Distress	Asthma	Infection of Upper or Lower Airway
Administer oxygen by placing a _____ mask on the patient and supplying oxygen at a rate of _____ to _____ L/min. For any patient in respiratory distress, use positioning, airway adjuncts (_____ or _____ airway), or positive pressure ventilation as indicated.	Administer oxygen. Allow patient to sit in upright position. Suction large amounts of mucus. Help patient self-administer a _____ inhaler: 1. Obtain order from medical control. 2. Check _____ and whether patient has taken other doses. 3. Ensure inhaler is at room temperature or warmer. 4. Shake inhaler vigorously several times. 5. Remove oxygen mask. Instruct patient to _____ deeply. 6. Instruct patient to press inhaler and inhale. Instruct patient to hold breath as long as is comfortable. 7. Reapply oxygen.	Administer _____ oxygen if available. Do not attempt to suction airway or place an oropharyngeal airway. Transport promptly with patient in position of comfort.

Acute Pulmonary Edema	Chronic Obstructive Pulmonary Disease	Spontaneous Pneumothorax
Administer 100% oxygen and suction any secretions from the airway as necessary. Place in position of comfort and provide _____ _____ as needed. Transport promptly.	Provide _____ oxygen via nonrebreathing mask at _____ /min. If patient is prescribed an inhaler, administer it according to local protocol. Document time and effect on patient with each use. Place in the position of comfort and provide prompt transport.	Provide _____ oxygen and place in position of comfort. Transport promptly. Support airway, breathing, and circulation as necessary.

Pleural Effusions	Obstruction of the Upper Airway	Pulmonary Embolism	Hyperventilation
Provide _____ oxygen at 15 L/min and place in position of comfort. Support airway, breathing, and circulation as necessary. Transport promptly.	For partial or complete foreign body airway obstructions, clear by following _____ guidelines, apply full-flow oxygen at 15 L/min as necessary, and transport promptly.	Clear airway and provide full-flow oxygen at 15 L/min. Place in position of comfort and provide prompt transport. Provide ventilatory support as necessary and be prepared for _____ _____.	Provide full-flow oxygen at 15 L/min and coach _____ slower in a calm manner. Complete an initial assessment and focused history and physical exam. Transport promptly for evaluation.

CHAPTER

12 Cardiovascular Emergencies

Workbook Activities

The following activities have been designed to help you. Your instructor may require you to complete some or all of these activities as a regular part of your EMT-B training program. You are encouraged to complete any activity that your instructor does not assign as a way to enhance your learning in the classroom.

Chapter Review

The following exercises provide an opportunity to refresh your knowledge of this chapter.

Matching

Match each of the terms in the left column to the appropriate definition in the right column.

_____ 1. Atria **A.** absence of all heart electrical activity

_____ 2. Coronary arteries **B.** calcium and cholesterol buildup inside blood vessels

_____ 3. Atrioventricular (AV) node **C.** blood vessels that supply blood to the myocardium

_____ 4. Myocardium **D.** abnormal heart rhythm

_____ 5. Sinus node **E.** unusually slow heart rhythm, less than 60 beats/min

_____ 6. Venae cavae **F.** lack of oxygen

_____ 7. Ventricles **G.** heart muscle

_____ 8. Aorta **H.** lower chambers of the heart

_____ 9. Atherosclerosis **I.** tissue death

_____ 10. Arrhythmia **J.** rapid heart rhythm, more than 100 beats/min

_____ 11. Ischemia **K.** carry oxygen-poor blood back to the heart

_____ 12. Infarction **L.** upper chambers of the heart

_____ 13. Tachycardia **M.** body's main artery

_____ 14. Asystole **N.** electrical impulses begin here

_____ 15. Bradycardia **O.** electrical impulses slow here to allow blood to move from the atria to the ventricles

Multiple Choice

Read each item carefully, then select the best response.

_____ 1. We can help to reduce the number of deaths attributed to cardiovascular disease with:

    A. better public awareness.

    B. early access.

    C. public access defibrillation.

    D. all of the above

_____ 2. The aorta receives its blood supply from the:

    A. right atria.

    B. left atria.

    C. right ventricle.

    D. left ventricle.

_____ 3. Blood enters into the right atrium from the body through the:

    A. vena cava.

    B. aorta.

    C. pulmonary artery.

    D. pulmonary vein.

_____ 4. The only veins in the body to carry oxygenated blood are the:

    A. external jugular veins.

    B. pulmonary veins.

    C. subclavian veins.

    D. inferior vena cava.

_____ 5. Normal electrical impulses originate in the sinus node, just above the:

    A. atria.

    B. ventricles.

    C. AV junction.

    D. Bundle of His.

_____ 6. Dilation of the coronary arteries will _____ blood flow.

    A. shut off

    B. increase

    C. decrease

    D. regulate

_____ 7. The _____ are tiny blood vessels about one cell thick.

    A. arterioles

    B. venules

    C. capillaries

    D. ventricles

_____ 8. _____ carry oxygen to the body's tissues and then remove carbon dioxide.

    A. Red blood cells

    B. White blood cells

    C. Platelets

    D. Veins

_____ 9. _____ is the maximum pressure exerted by the left ventricle as it contracts.

    A. Cardiac output

    B. Diastolic blood pressure

    C. Systolic blood pressure

    D. Stroke volume

_____ **10.** Atherosclerosis can lead to a complete _____ of a coronary artery.

    A. occlusion

    B. disintegration

    C. dilation

    D. contraction

_____ **11.** The lumen of an artery may be partially or completely blocked by the blood-clotting system due to a _____ that exposes the inside of the atherosclerotic wall.

    A. tear

    B. crack

    C. clot

    D. rupture

_____ **12.** Tissues downstream from a blood clot will suffer from lack of oxygen. If blood flow is resumed in a short time, the _____ tissues will recover.

    A. dead

    B. ischemic

    C. necrosed

    D. dry

_____ **13.** Risk factors for myocardial infarction include all of the following except:

    A. male gender.

    B. high blood pressure.

    C. stress.

    D. increased activity level.

_____ **14.** When, for a brief period of time, heart tissues do not get enough oxygen, the pain is called:

    A. AMI.

    B. angina.

    C. ischemia.

    D. CAD.

_____ **15.** Angina pain may be felt in the:

    A. arms.

    B. midback.

    C. epigastrium.

    D. all of the above

_____ **16.** Angina may be associated with:

    A. shortness of breath.

    B. nausea.

    C. sweating.

    D. all of the above

_____ **17.** Because oxygen supply to the heart is diminished with angina, the _____ can be compromised and the person is at risk for significant cardiac rhythm problems.

    A. circulation

    B. cardiac output

    C. electrical system

    D. vasculature

_____ **18.** About _____ minutes after blood flow is cut off, some heart muscle cells begin to die.

    A. 10

    B. 20

    C. 30

    D. 40

_____ **19.** An acute myocardial infarction is more likely to occur in the larger, thick-walled left ventricle, which needs more _____ than in the right ventricle.

    A. oxygen and glucose

    B. force to pump

    C. blood and oxygen

    D. electrical activity

_____ **20.** The pain of AMI differs from the pain of angina because:

    A. it may be caused by exertion.

    B. it is usually relieved by rest.

    C. it does not resolve in a few minutes.

    D. all of the above

_____ **21.** Consequences of AMI may include:

    A. cardiogenic shock.

    B. congestive heart failure.

    C. sudden death.

    D. all of the above

_____ **22.** Sudden death is usually the result of _____, in which the heart fails to generate an effective blood flow.

    A. AMI

    B. atherosclerosis

    C. PVCs

    D. cardiac arrest

_____ **23.** Disorganized, ineffective quivering of the ventricles is known as:

    A. ventricular fibrillation.

    B. asystole.

    C. ventricular stand still.

    D. ventricular tachycardia.

_____ **24.** Causes of congestive heart failure include all of the following except:

    A. chronic hypotension.

    B. heart valve damage.

    C. a myocardial infarction.

    D. longstanding high blood pressure.

_____ **25.** Signs and symptoms of shock include all of the following except:

    A. elevated heart rate.

    B. pale, clammy skin.

    C. air hunger.

    D. elevated blood pressure.

_____ **26.** In patients with CHF, changes in heart function occur, including:

    A. a decrease in heart rate.

    B. enlargement of the left ventricle.

    C. enlargement of the right ventricle.

    D. a decrease in blood pressure.

_____ **27.** Physical findings of AMI include skin that is _____ because of poor cardiac output and the loss of perfusion.

    A. pink

    B. white

    C. gray

    D. red

_____ **28.** All patient assessments begin by determining whether or not the patient:

    A. is breathing.

    B. can talk.

    C. is responsive.

    D. has a pulse.

_____ **29.** To assess chest pain, use the mnemonic:

    A. AVPU.

    B. OPQRST.

    C. SAMPLE.

    D. CHART.

_____ **30.** When using the mnemonic OPQRST, the "P" stands for:

    A. parasthesia.

    B. pain.

    C. provocation.

    D. predisposing factors.

_____ **31.** Nitroglycerin may be in the form of a:

    A. skin patch.

    B. spray.

    C. pill.

    D. all of the above

_____ **32.** When administering nitroglycerin to a patient, you should check the patient's _____ within 5 minutes after each dose.

    A. level of consciousness

    B. breathing

    C. pulse

    D. blood pressure

_____ **33.** In general, a maximum of _____ dose(s) of nitroglycerin are given for any one episode of chest pain.

    A. one

    B. two

    C. three

    D. four

_____ **34.** _____ are inserted when the electrical control system of the heart is so damaged that it cannot function properly.

    A. Stents

    B. Pacemakers

    C. Balloon angioplasties

    D. Defibrillation

_____ **35.** When the battery wears out in a pacemaker, the patient may experience:

    A. syncope.

    B. dizziness.

    C. weakness.

    D. all of the above

_____ **36.** The computer inside the AED is specifically programmed to recognize rhythms that require defibrillation to correct, most commonly:

    A. asystole.

    B. ventricular tachycardia.

    C. ventricular fibrillation.

    D. supraventricular tachycardia.

_____ **37.** You should apply the AED only to unresponsive patients with no:

    A. significant medical problems.

    B. cardiac history.

    C. pulse.

    D. brain activity.

_____ **38.** _____ usually refers to a state of cardiac arrest despite an organized electrical complex.

    A. Asystole

    B. Pulseless electrical activity

    C. Ventricular fibrillation

    D. Ventricular tachycardia

_____ **39.** The links in the chain of survival include all of the following except:

    A. early access and CPR.

    B. early ACLS.

    C. early administration of nitroglycerin.

    D. early defibrillation.

_____ **40.** An AED may fail to function properly due to:

    A. the batteries not working.

    B. improper maintenance.

    C. operator error.

    D. all of the above

Questions 41-45 are derived from the following scenario: At 5:00 in the morning, you respond to the home of a 76-year-old man complaining of chest pain. Upon arrival, the patient states that he has been sleeping in the recliner all night due to indigestion, when the pain woke him up. He also tells you he has taken two nitroglycerin tablets.

_____ **41.** Your first priority is to:

    A. apply an AED.

    B. provide high-flow oxygen.

    C. evaluate the need to administer a third nitroglycerin tablet.

    D. size up the scene.

_____ **42.** His respirations are 16 breaths/min, pulse is 98 beats/min, his blood pressure is 92/76 mm Hg, and he is still complaining of chest pain. What actions should you take to intervene?

    A. Provide high-flow oxygen.

    B. Administer a third nitroglycerin tablet.

    C. Apply an AED.

    D. All of the above

_____ **43.** Without warning, the patient loses consciousness, stops breathing, and has no pulse. After verifying pulselessness and apnea, you should:

    A. begin CPR.

    B. provide two respirations with a BVM device or pocket mask.

    C. call for ALS backup.

    D. apply the AED that is at hand.

_____ **44.** After applying an AED to this patient, the AED states; "No shock advised." What is your next step of action?

    A. Load and transport the patient.

    B. Push to reanalyze.

    C. Perform CPR for 1 minute, then have the AED reanalyze.

    D. None of the above

_____ **45.** Your patient is now conscious and you are en route to the hospital. You are 6 blocks away when the patient stops breathing and no longer has a pulse. You should:

A. continue to the hospital.

B. continue to the hospital and analyze the rhythm.

C. stop the vehicle and analyze the rhythm.

D. none of the above

Labeling
Label the following diagrams with the correct terms.

1. The Right and Left Sides of the Heart
Where arrows appear, indicate the substance and its origin and destination.

Part A:

A. _____

B. _____

C. _____

D. _____

E. _____

F. _____

Part B:

A. _____

B. _____

C. _____

D. _____

E. _____

F. _____

2. Electrical Conduction

A. _____

B. _____

C. _____

D. _____

E. _____

F. _____

G. _____

3. Pulse Points

State the name of the artery that is being assessed at each pulse point below:

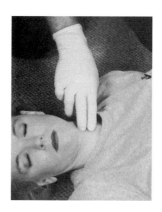

_____

_____

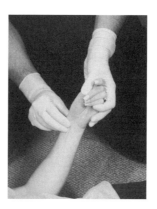

_____

_____

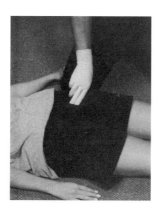

_____

_____

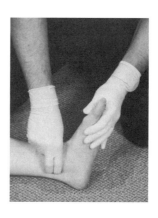

_____

_____

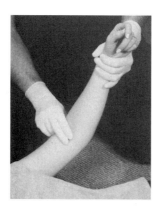

_____

_____

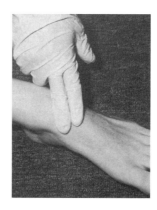

_____

_____

Fill-in

Read each item carefully, then complete the statement by filling in the missing word.

1. The heart is divided down the middle by a wall called the _____.

2. The _____ is the body's main artery.

3. The _____ ventricle pumps blood in through the pulmonary circulation.

4. Electrical impulses spread from the _____ node to the ventricles.

5. Blood supply to the heart is increased by _____ of the coronary arteries.

6. _____ _____ cells remove carbon dioxide from the body's tissues.

7. _____ blood pressure reflects the pressure on the walls of the arteries when the ventricle is at rest.

8. The heart has _____ chambers.

9. The _____ side of the heart is more muscular because it must pump blood into the aorta and all the other arteries of the body.

True/False

If you believe the statement to be more true than false, write the letter "T" in the space provided. If you believe the statement to be more false than true, write the letter "F."

_____ 1. The right side of the heart pumps oxygen-rich blood to the body.

_____ 2. In the normal heart, the need for increased blood flow to the myocardium is easily met by an increase in heart rate.

_____ 3. Atherosclerosis results in narrowing of the lumen of coronary arteries.

_____ 4. Infarction is a temporary interruption of the blood supply to the tissues.

_____ 5. Angina can result from a spasm of the artery.

_____ 6. The pain of angina and the pain of AMI are easily distinguishable.

_____ 7. Nitroglycerin works in most patients within 5 minutes to relieve the pain of AMI.

_____ 8. If an AED malfunctions during use, you must report that problem to the manufacturer and the Department of Human Resources.

_____ 9. Angina occurs when the heart's need for oxygen exceeds its supply.

_____ 10. White blood cells are the most numerous and help the blood to clot.

_____ 11. Cardiac arrest in younger children is less common than in older children and is usually caused by a breathing problem.

_____ 12. An AED with special pediatric pads is indicated for use on pediatric medical patients between the ages of 1 and 7 years who have been assessed to be unresponsive, not breathing, and pulseless.

Short Answer

Complete this section with short written answers in the space provided.

1. Name and describe the two basic types of defibrillators.

_____

_____

2. What are the three most common errors of AED use?

_____

_____

3. If ALS is not responding to the scene, what are the three points at which transport should be initiated for a cardiac arrest patient?

_____

_____

4. List six safety considerations for operating an AED.

_____

_____

5. What is the procedure for assisting a patient with nitroglycerin administration?

_____

_____

6. List three ways in which AMI pain differs from angina pain.

_____

_____

7. List three serious consequences of AMI.

_____

_____

8. Name at least five signs and symptoms associated with AMI.

_____

_____

9. Describe the technique for AED pad placement.

_____

_____

Word Fun

The following crossword puzzle is an activity provided to reinforce correct spelling and understanding of medical terminology associated with emergency care and the EMT-B. Use the clues in the column to complete the puzzle.

Across

1. Less than 60 beats/min

5. Greater than 100 beats/min

6. Lower chamber

7. Lack of oxygen to tissues

8. Widening

9. Absence of electrical activity

Down

2. Irregular heart rhythm

3. To shock the heart

4. Blockage

9. Main artery of body

Ambulance Calls

The following case scenarios provide an opportunity to explore the concerns associated with patient management. Read each scenario, then answer each question in detail.

1. You are dispatched to the residence of a 58-year-old man complaining of chest pain. He states that it feels like "somebody is standing on my chest." He sat down when it started and took a nitroglycerin tablet. He is still a little nauseated and sweaty, but feels better. He is very anxious.

How would you best manage this patient?

_____

_____

_____

2. You are dispatched to the home of a 45-year-old man experiencing chest pain. He told his wife that he was fine, but she decided to call 9-1-1. When you arrive, you find your patient sitting in the living room looking anxious. He is sweaty, pale and admits the pain is worse than just a few moments ago. He tells you that he is a very athletic person, so the pain must just be stress-related and it will go away after he relaxes for a while. He tells you he doesn't want to be taken to the hospital.

How would you best manage this patient?

_____

_____

_____

3. You are dispatched to the home of a 60-year-old woman complaining of sudden weakness. She tells you that she usually has enough energy to perform daily tasks around the house, but today she's suddenly very tired, has some pain in her jaw and has some nausea. She denies any history of recent illness including cough, cold or fever. She is otherwise healthy and does not take any medications.

How would you best manage this patient?

_____

_____

_____

Skill Drills

Skill Drill 12-2: AED and CPR

Test your knowledge of this skill drill by placing the photos below in the correct order. Number the first step with a "1," the second step with a "2," etc.

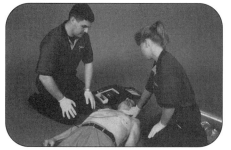

_____

Check pulse.

If pulse is present, check breathing.

Gather additional information on the arrest event.

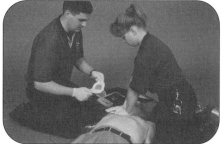

_____

If pulseless, begin CPR.

Prepare the AED pads.

Turn on the AED; begin narrative if needed.

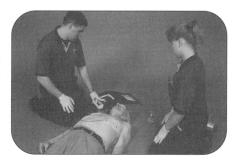

_____

Apply AED pads.

Stop CPR.

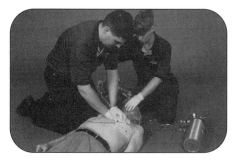

_____

If breathing adequately, give oxygen and transport. If not, open airway, ventilate, and transport.

If no pulse, perform CPR for 1 minute. Clear the patient and analyze again.

If necessary, repeat one cycle of up to three shocks.

Transport and call medical control.

Continue to support breathing or perform CPR, as needed.

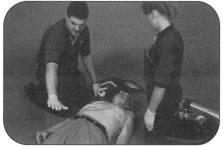

_____

Verbally and visually clear the patient.

Push the Analyze button if there is one.

Wait for the AED to analyze rhythm.

If no shock advised, perform CPR for 1 minute.

If shock advised, recheck that all are clear and push the Shock button.

Push the Analyze button, if needed, to analyze rhythm again.

Press Shock if advised (second shock).

Push the Analyze button, if needed, to analyze rhythm again.

Press Shock if advised (third shock).

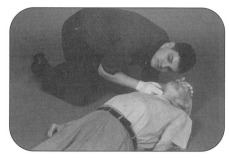

_____

Stop CPR if in progress.

Assess responsiveness.

Check breathing and pulse.

If unresponsive and not breathing adequately, give two slow ventilations.

Assessment Review

Answer the following questions pertaining to the assessment of the types of emergencies discussed in this chapter.

_____ **1.** What type of additional resources may be required for someone with chest pain?

 A. Lift assistance

 B. Advanced life support

 C. Police

 D. All the above

_____ **2.** When taking a SAMPLE history of a conscious person with chest pain, what specific questions should the EMT-B ask of their patient?

 A. Whether he or she has had a heart attack before

 B. How long did he or she stay in the hospital?

 C. Did his or her physician inform him or her of risk factors associated with heart disease?

 D. All of the above

_____ **3.** What steps should be taken to complete a focused history and physical exam on an unconscious patient with a suspected cardiac problem?

 A. Perform a rapid physical exam.

 B. Obtain vital signs.

 C. Obtain history from family or bystanders.

 D. All of the above

_____ **4.** What questions should you ask during the focused history and physical exam of your pulseless, apneic patient?

 A. Have you had a heart attack before?

 B. Have you had heart problems in the past?

 C. Did you take any aspirin today?

 D. None of the above

_____ **5.** What types of BSI should be taken for someone in cardiac arrest?

 A. Gloves

 B. Eye protection

 C. Face mask/shield

 D. All the above

Emergency Care Summary

Complete the statements pertaining to emergency care for the types of emergencies discussed in this chapter by filling in the missing words.

NOTE: While the steps below are widely accepted, be sure to consult and follow your local protocol.

| Chest Pain | Cardiac Arrest |

Chest Pain

Depending on local protocol, prepare to administer baby aspirin and assist with prescribed nitroglycerin. Check condition of medication(s) and expiration date(s).

Aspirin

Administer according to protocols.

Nitroglycerin

1. Obtain permission from medical control.
2. Take patient's blood pressure. Continue only if _____ pressure greater than _____ mm Hg.
3. Check that you have the right medication, right patient, and right delivery route.
4. Question patient about last _____ and effects. Ensure patient understands route of administration. Prepare to have the patient lie down to prevent _____.
5. Ask patient to lift his or her tongue. Place tablet _____ tongue or spray under tongue if medication is in spray form. Have patient keep mouth closed until dissolved/absorbed.
6. Recheck blood pressure within _____ minutes. Record medication and time of administration. If chest pain persists and systolic blood pressure is greater than _____ mm Hg, repeat the dose every 5 minutes as authorized by medical control.

Reevaluate transport decision. Do not delay transport to assist with nitroglycerin.

Cardiac Arrest

Defibrillation

1. Perform initial assessment. If patient is unresponsive and _____, prepare to defibrillate. If patient is responsive, do not apply AED.
2. Stop CPR if it is in progress.
3. Verify pulselessness and _____.
4. Give _____ ventilations using a BVM device or _____ _____.
5. If the AED is not ready, start CPR.
6. Prepare the AED _____.
7. Turn on the machine.
8. Remove clothing from patient's chest area. Apply the pads: one to the right of the _____ just below the _____, one on the left chest.
9. Stop CPR.
10. State aloud, "Clear the patient." Ensure that no one is touching the patient, including yourself.
11. Push the _____ button.
12. Wait for the computer to determine if a shockable _____ is present.
13. If a shock is not needed, go to step 18. If a shock is advised, ensure that no one is touching the patient, including yourself. Push shock button.
14. AED will reanalyze rhythm; if not, push analyze button again.
15. If machine advises a shock, deliver second shock.
16. Reanalyze rhythm.
17. If machine advises a shock, deliver third shock.
18. Check pulse.
19. If pulse is present, check breathing.
20. If breathing adequately, give patient oxygen via _____ mask and transport. If patient is not breathing adequately, open airway and ventilate.
21. If patient has no pulse, perform _____ minute of CPR.
22. Gather additional information on _____ _____.
23. After 1 minute of CPR, ensure no one is touching the patient. Push analyze button.
24. If necessary, repeat one cycle of up to _____ stacked shocks.
25. Transport and check with medical control.
26. Continue to support patient.

CHAPTER

13 Neurologic Emergencies

Workbook Activities

The following activities have been designed to help you. Your instructor may require you to complete some or all of these activities as a regular part of your EMT-B training program. You are encouraged to complete any activity that your instructor does not assign as a way to enhance your learning in the classroom.

Chapter Review

The following exercises provide an opportunity to refresh your knowledge of this chapter.

Matching

Match each of the terms in the left column to the appropriate definition in the right column.

_____ 1. Brain stem	**A.** slurred, hard to understand speech
_____ 2. Foramen magnum	**B.** the back part of this area of the brain processes sight
_____ 3. Spinal nerves	**C.** weakness in an artery wall
_____ 4. Cerebrum	**D.** controls most basic functions of the body
_____ 5. Cranial nerves	**E.** exit at each vertebra and carry messages to and from the body
_____ 6. Cerebellum	**F.** this area of the brain controls muscle and body coordination
_____ 7. Embolism	**G.** hole in the base of the skull
_____ 8. Aneurysm	**H.** low blood glucose
_____ 9. Status epilepticus	**I.** innervate eyes, ears, face
_____ 10. Hypoglycemia	**J.** clot that forms elsewhere and travels to the site of damage
_____ 11. Aphasia	**K.** weakness in a blood vessel that resembles a tiny balloon
_____ 12. Berry aneurysm	**L.** inability to produce or understand speech
_____ 13. Dysarthria	**M.** seizures that recur every few minutes

Multiple Choice

Read each item carefully, then select the best response.

_____ **1.** Seizures may occur as a result of:

    A. metabolic problems.

    B. brain tumor.

    C. a recent or old head injury.

    D. all of the above

_____ **2.** The _____ controls the most basic functions of the body, such as breathing, blood pressure, swallowing, and pupil constriction.

    A. brain stem

    B. cerebellum

    C. cerebrum

    D. spinal cord

_____ **3.** At each vertebra in the neck and back, _____ nerves, called spinal nerves, branch out from the spinal cord and carry signals to and from the body.

    A. two

    B. three

    C. four

    D. five

_____ **4.** Brain disorders include all of the following except:

    A. coma.

    B. infection.

    C. hypoglycemia.

    D. tumor.

_____ **5.** When blood flow to a particular part of the brain is cut off by a blockage inside a blood vessel, the result is:

    A. a hemorrhagic stroke.

    B. atherosclerosis.

    C. an ischemic stroke.

    D. a cerebral embolism.

_____ **6.** Patients who are at the highest risk of hemorrhagic stroke are those who have:

    A. untreated hypertension.

    B. an aneurysm.

    C. a berry aneurysm.

    D. atherosclerosis.

_____ **7.** Patients with a subarachnoid hemorrhage typically complain of a sudden severe:

    A. bout of dizziness.

    B. headache.

    C. altered mental status.

    D. thirst.

_____ **8.** The plaque that builds up in atherosclerosis obstructs blood flow, and interferes with the vessel's ability to:

    A. constrict.

    B. dilate.

    C. diffuse.

    D. exchange gases.

_____ **9.** A TIA, or mini-stroke, is the name given to a stroke when symptoms go away on their own in less than:

   A. half an hour.

   B. 1 hour.

   C. 12 hours.

   D. 24 hours.

_____ **10.** Seizures characterized by unconsciousness and a generalized severe twitching of all the body's muscles that lasts several minutes or longer is called a:

   A. grand mal seizure.

   B. petit mal seizure.

   C. focal motor seizure.

   D. febrile seizure.

_____ **11.** Metabolic seizures may be due to:

   A. epilepsy.

   B. a brain tumor.

   C. high fevers.

   D. hypoglycemia.

_____ **12.** When assessing a patient with a history of seizure activity, it is important to:

   A. determine whether this episode differs from any previous ones.

   B. recognize the postictal state.

   C. look for other problems associated with the seizure.

   D. all of the above

_____ **13.** Signs and symptoms of possible seizure activity include:

   A. altered mental status.

   B. incontinence.

   C. rapid and deep respirations.

   D. all of the above

_____ **14.** Common causes of altered mental status include all of the following, except:

   A. body temperature abnormalities.

   B. hypoxemia.

   C. unequal pupils.

   D. hypoglycemia.

_____ **15.** The principle difference between a patient who has had a stroke and a patient with hypoglycemia almost always has to do with the:

   A. papillary response.

   B. mental status.

   C. blood pressure.

   D. capillary refill time.

_____ **16.** Consider the possibility of _____ in a patient who has had a seizure.

   A. brain injury

   B. hyperglycemia

   C. hypoglycemia

   D. hypertension

_____ **17.** Individuals with chronic alcoholism can have abnormalities in liver function and in their blood-clotting and immune systems, which can predispose them to:

   A. intracranial bleeding.

   B. brain and bloodstream infections.

   C. hypoglycemia.

   D. all of the above

_____ **18.** Low oxygen levels in the bloodstream will affect the entire brain, causing:
   A. anxiety.
   B. restlessness.
   C. confusion.
   D. all of the above

_____ **19.** Patients with _____ may have trouble understanding speech but can speak clearly.
   A. aphasia
   B. receptive aphasia
   C. expressive aphasia
   D. dysarthria

_____ **20.** High blood pressure in stroke patients should not be treated in the field because:
   A. the brain is raising the blood pressure in an attempt to force more oxygen into its injured parts.
   B. quite often, blood pressure will return to normal or may drop significantly on its own.
   C. many times it is a response to bleeding in the brain.
   D. all of the above

_____ **21.** The following conditions may simulate a stroke except:
   A. hyperglycemia.
   B. a postictal state.
   C. hypoglycemia.
   D. subdural bleeding.

_____ **22.** When assessing a patient with a possible CVA, you should check the _____ first.
   A. pulse
   B. airway
   C. pupils
   D. blood pressure

_____ **23.** A patient with a GCS of 12 has:
   A. no dysfunction.
   B. mild dysfunction.
   C. moderate to severe dysfunction.
   D. severe dysfunction.

_____ **24.** Assess the mental status using the mnemonic:
   A. OPQRST.
   B. SAMPLE.
   C. AVPU.
   D. PEARRL.

Questions 25-29 are derived from the following scenario: You are called to a long-term care facility, and find a 92-year-old woman supine in her bed. Though she is able to track your movement with her eyes, she is unresponsive to you and the nurse standing by. The nurse explains this is abnormal behavior for her, as she is normally talkative and very friendly.

_____ **25.** How would you best determine the patient's level of consciousness?
   A. By using AVPU
   B. By using the Cincinnati Stroke Scale
   C. By using the Glasgow Coma Scale
   D. All of the above

_____ **26.** A score of _____ from the Glasgow Coma Scale would indicate severe dysfunction.
   A. 15 or less
   B. 14-15
   C. 11-13
   D. 10 or less

_____ **27.** Your patient may have a hemorrhagic or ischemic stroke. What statement is true regarding the two conditions?

A. Hemorrhagic stroke occurs as a result of bleeding inside the brain.

B. Ischemic stroke occurs when a part of the brain is cut off by a blockage inside a blood vessel.

C. Neither A or B is true.

D. Both A and B are true.

_____ **28.** If the receiving facility told you the cause of her stroke was due to a build up of calcium and cholesterol, forming a plaque inside the walls of her blood vessels, you would know that this patient had:

A. artherosclerosis.

B. a TIA.

C. arteriolosclerosis.

D. a CVA.

_____ **29.** If this patient is having a seizure, what could be the cause?

A. Hypoglycemia

B. Hypoxia

C. Drug overdose

D. All the above

Labeling

Label the following diagrams with the correct terms.

1. Brain

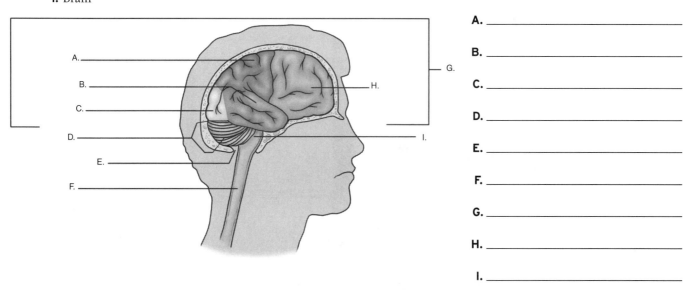

A. _____

B. _____

C. _____

D. _____

E. _____

F. _____

G. _____

H. _____

I. _____

2. Spinal Cord

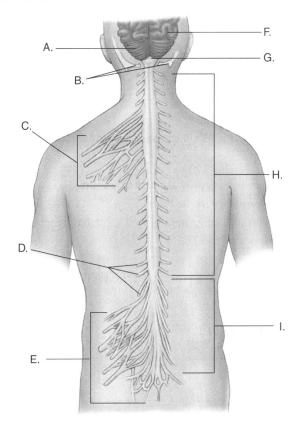

A. _____

B. _____

C. _____

D. _____

E. _____

F. _____

G. _____

H. _____

I. _____

Fill-in

Read each item carefully, then complete the statement by filling in the missing word(s).

1. There are _____ cranial nerves.

2. Playing the piano is coordinated by the _____.

3. The front part of the cerebrum controls _____ and _____.

4. The cranial nerves run to the _____.

5. The brain is divided into _____ major parts.

6. All messages traveling to and from the brain travel along _____.

7. Each hemisphere of the cerebrum controls activities on the _____ side of the body and the _____ side of the face.

8. The _____ is the largest part of the brain.

9. _____ is a loss of bowel and bladder control, and can be due to a generalized seizure.

10. The _____ is the body's computer.

11. Onset of _____ bleeding is usually very rapid after injury.

12. Weakness on one side of the body is known as _____.

13. No matter what the cause, you should consider _____ _____ _____ to be an emergency that requires immediate attention, even when it appears that the cause may simply be alcohol intoxication or a minor car crash or fall.

True/False

If you believe the statement to be more true than false, write the letter "T" in the space provided. If you believe the statement to be more false than true, write the letter "F."

_____ **1.** The postictal state following a seizure commonly lasts only about 3 to 5 minutes.

_____ **2.** Metabolic seizures result from an area of abnormality in the brain.

_____ **3.** Febrile seizures result from sudden high fevers and are generally well tolerated by children.

_____ **4.** Hemiparesis is the inability to speak or understand speech.

_____ **5.** The dura covers the brain.

_____ **6.** Right-sided facial droop is most likely an indication of a problem in the right cerebral hemisphere.

Short Answer

Complete this section with short written answers using the space provided.

1. List and describe the three key tests for assessing stroke.

_____

_____

2. Why is prompt transport of stroke patients critical?

_____

_____

3. Describe the characteristics of a postictal state.

_____

_____

4. What is the difference between infarcted and ischemic cells?

_____

_____

5. List three conditions that may simulate stroke.

_____

_____

Word Fun emtb vocab explorer

The following crossword puzzle is an activity provided to reinforce correct spelling and understanding of medical terminology associated with emergency care and the EMT-B. Use the clues in the column to complete the puzzle.

Across

6. Cholesterol and calcium build-up

7. One-sided weakness

8. Loss of brain function

Down

1. Related to high temperatures, particularly with children

2. Inability to pronounce clearly

3. Low blood glucose level

4. Clotting of vessel

5. Inability to speak

Ambulance Calls

The following case scenarios will give you an opportunity to explore the concerns associated with patient management. Read each scenario, then answer each question in detail.

1. You are dispatched to a private residence for a "confused man." You arrive to find an older man sitting in a recliner. As you begin your assessment, you notice that he has right-sided weakness and doesn't seem to understand your questions. He is alone in the home, and it appears that no one lives with him in the residence. How do you best manage this patient?

_____

_____

_____

2. You are dispatched to a 36-year-old man who had seizure activity at least an hour ago. The patient is incontinent, cold, clammy, and unresponsive. His friends tell you that the "shaking" stopped and he has not woke up. They thought he might just be tired until they discovered they could not wake him. He has no history of seizure activity. He has diabetes for which he takes medication. How would you best manage this patient?

_____

_____

_____

3. You are dispatched to a local business for "woman with severe headache." The 55-year-old patient states that she has had headaches in the past, but this headache is the worst she's ever had in her life. She feels like the room is spinning around; she's seeing "double" and she feels sick to her stomach. She has a history of hypertension. She tells you that she stopped taking her blood pressure medicine about 6-8 months ago because she could no longer afford it.

How do you best manage this patient?

_____

_____

_____

Assessment Review

Answer the following questions pertaining to the assessment of the types of emergencies discussed in this chapter.

You are called to the home of a 52-year-old man who was found unconscious. You have been greeted at the door by an obviously distraught wife who leads you to a bathroom in the master bedroom. As you peer into the room, you see the unresponsive man sitting on the toilet with his pants around his ankles, and your partner finds a small handgun lying on the bedroom floor.

_____ 1. How should you respond?
   A. Determine if he has been shot.
   B. Ask the wife who else is in the home.
   C. Pick-up and secure the gun.
   D. Drop your equipment and leave the home.

_____ 2. After it has been determined this was not a shooting, you begin to assess the patient. He regains consciousness and states he must have fainted while having a bowel movement. What type of exam should you perform?
   A. Rapid physical exam
   B. Focused physical exam
   C. Detailed physical exam
   D. No exam is necessary for this patient.

_____ 3. How should you intervene for this patient?
   A. Provide oxygen.
   B. Determine the patient's glucose level.
   C. Determine the patient's Glasgow Coma Scale score.
   D. All of the above

_____ 4. As you intervene for this patient, his muscles begin to twitch and his eyes roll back into his head. You respond by:
   A. laying him on the floor.
   B. calling for ALS.
   C. obtaining a SAMPLE history.
   D. all the above

_____ 5. He continues to twitch for several minutes. How do you respond?
   A. This is normal, and you need to wait it out.
   B. He is reacting to low blood sugar levels, and needs glucose.
   C. You suspect status epilepticus, and call for ALS.
   D. You suspect a CVA, and provide rapid transport once he is done.

Emergency Care Summary

Complete the statements pertaining to emergency care for the types of emergencies discussed in this chapter by filling in the missing words.

NOTE: While the steps below are widely accepted, be sure to consult and follow your local protocol.

Stroke	Seizure	Altered Mental Status

Stroke

Cincinnati Stroke Scale

1. Ask patient to show _____ or smile to determine facial droop.
2. Ask patient to close eyes and hold both arms out with palms up to measure _____ _____.
3. Ask patient to say, "The sky is blue in _____," to monitor speech.

Seizure

Glasgow Coma Scale

Eye Opening

_____	4
Responsive to speech	3
Responsive to pain	2
None	1

Best Verbal Response

Oriented conversation	5
Confused conversation	4
_____ _____	3
Incomprehensible sounds	2
None	1

Best Motor Response

Obeys commands	6
Localizes pain	5
_____ _____ _____	4
Abnormal flexion	3
Abornormal extension	2
None	1

Add the total points selected from all three categories to determine the patient's

_____ _____ _____

_____.

Altered Mental Status

Use the _____ _____ _____ and/or the _____ _____ _____ to aid in your assessment.

CHAPTER

14 The Acute Abdomen

Workbook Activities

The following activities have been designed to help you. Your instructor may require you to complete some or all of these activities as a regular part of your EMT-B training program. You are encouraged to complete any activity that your instructor does not assign as a way to enhance your learning in the classroom.

Chapter Review

The following exercises provide an opportunity to refresh your knowledge of this chapter.

Matching

Match each of the terms in the left column to the appropriate definition in the right column.

_____ **1.** Aneurysm   **A.** paralysis of the bowel

_____ **2.** Colic   **B.** pain felt in an area of the body other than the actual source

_____ **3.** Retroperitoneal   **C.** protective, involuntary abdominal muscle contractions

_____ **4.** Ulcer   **D.** acute, intermittent cramping abdominal pain

_____ **5.** Hernia   **E.** behind the peritoneum

_____ **6.** Ileus   **F.** vomiting

_____ **7.** Guarding   **G.** common cause of acute abdomen in women

_____ **8.** Anorexia   **H.** a membrane lining the abdomen

_____ **9.** Emesis   **I.** swelling or enlargement of a weakened arterial wall

_____ **10.** Referred pain   **J.** loss of hunger or appetite

_____ **11.** PID   **K.** protrusion of a loop of an organ or tissue through an abnormal body opening

_____ **12.** Cystitis

_____ **13.** Strangulation   **L.** obstruction of blood circulation resulting from compression or entrapment of organ tissue

_____ **14.** Peritonitis

_____ **15.** Peritoneum   **M.** abrasion of the stomach or small intestine

     N. inflammation of the bladder

     O. inflammation of the peritoneum

Multiple Choice
Read each item carefully, then select the best response.

_____ 1. Peritonitis, with associated fluid loss, may lead to _____ shock.
   A. hemorrhagic
   B. septic
   C. hypovolemic
   D. metabolic

_____ 2. Distention of the abdomen is gauged by:
   A. visualization.
   B. auscultation.
   C. palpation.
   D. the patient's complaint of pain around the umbilicus.

_____ 3. A hernia that returns to its proper body cavity is said to be:
   A. reducible.
   B. extractable.
   C. incarcerated.
   D. replaceable.

_____ 4. Sensory nerves from the spinal cord to the skin and muscles are part of the:
   A. somatic nervous system.
   B. peripheral nervous system.
   C. autonomic nervous system.
   D. sympathetic nervous system.

_____ 5. When an organ of the abdomen is enlarged, rough palpation may cause _____ of the organ.
   A. distention
   B. nausea
   C. swelling
   D. rupture

_____ 6. Severe back pain may be associated with which condition?
   A. abdominal aortic aneurysm
   B. PID
   C. appendicitis
   D. mittelschmerz

_____ 7. The _____ are found in the retroperitoneal space.
   A. stomach and gallbladder
   B. kidneys, genitourinary structures, and large vessels
   C. liver and pancreas
   D. adrenal glands and uterus

_____ 8. A(n) _____ may occur as a result of a surgical wound that has failed to heal properly.
   A. ectopic pregnancy
   B. strangulation
   C. hernia
   D. ulcer

_____ 9. The peritoneal membrane that can perceive the sensations of pain, pressure, and cold is the:
   A. meningeal.
   B. parietal.
   C. retroperitoneal.
   D. visceral.

_____ **10.** Common disease(s) that produce(s) signs of an acute abdomen include:

   A. diverticulitis.

   B. cholecystitis.

   C. acute appendicitis.

   D. all of the above

_____ **11.** A patient with peritonitis may present with rapid, shallow breaths due to:

   A. hypovolemia.

   B. ileus.

   C. pain.

   D. inflammation.

Questions 12-16 are derived from the following scenario: You have been dispatched to the home of a 21-year-old woman with severe abdominal pain.

_____ **12.** A possible cause for her pain may be:

   A. peritonitis.

   B. appendicitis.

   C. mittelschmerz.

   D. all of the above

_____ **13.** As you attempt to palpate her abdomen, she pushes your hand away. This is called:

   A. referred pain.

   B. guarding.

   C. protecting.

   D. all of the above

_____ **14.** She informs you that she missed her last menstrual cycle. You may begin to suspect:

   A. mittelschmerz.

   B. cystitis.

   C. ectopic pregnancy.

   D. PID.

_____ **15.** You should transport her:

   A. in the position of comfort.

   B. supine.

   C. left lateral recumbent.

   D. in the recovery position.

_____ **16.** Her respirations are 18 breaths/min, pulse is 78 beats/min, and her blood pressure is 132/80 mm Hg. How often should you reassess her vital signs?

   A. Every 5 minutes

   B. Every 10 minutes

   C. Every 15 minutes

   D. Every 20 minutes

Labeling

Label the following diagrams with the correct terms.

1. Solid Organs

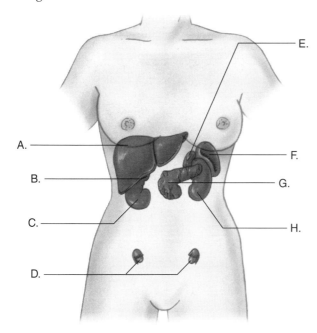

A. _____

B. _____

C. _____

D. _____

E. _____

F. _____

G. _____

H. _____

2. Hollow Organs

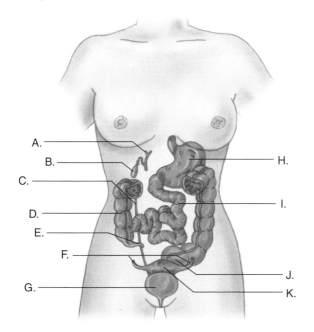

A. _____

B. _____

C. _____

D. _____

E. _____

F. _____

G. _____

H. _____

I. _____

J. _____

K. _____

3. Retroperitoneal Organs

A. _____

B. _____

C. _____

D. _____

E. _____

F. _____

G. _____

H. _____

I. _____

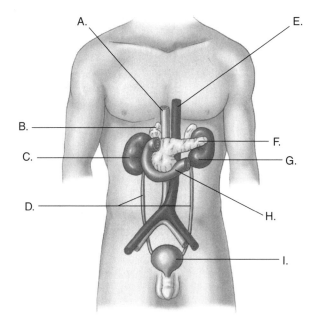

True/False

If you believe the statement to be more true than false, write the letter "T" in the space provided. If you believe the statement to be more false than true, write the letter "F."

_____ **1.** Referred pain is a result of connection between ligaments in the abdominal and chest cavities.

_____ **2.** Abdominal pain in women is usually related to the menstrual cycle and is rarely serious.

_____ **3.** A leading aorta, being retroperitoneal, will not cause peritonitis.

_____ **4.** It is important to accurately diagnose the cause of acute abdominal pain in order to properly treat the patient.

_____ **5.** The parietal peritoneum lines the walls of the abdominal cavity.

_____ **6.** The patient with peritonitis usually reports relief of pain when lying left lateral recumbent with the knees pulled in.

_____ **7.** When palpating the abdomen, always start with the quadrant where the patient complains of the most severe pain.

_____ **8.** Massive hemorrhaging is associated with rupture of an abdominal aortic aneurysm.

_____ **9.** Pneumonia may cause abdominal pain.

Short Answer

Complete this section with short written answers using the space provided.

1. Explain the phenomenon of referred pain.

_____

_____

2. Should an EMT-B attempt to diagnose the cause of abdominal pain? Why or why not?

_____

_____

3. Why does abdominal distention accompany ileus?

_____

_____

4. What two conditions may result in hypovolemic shock in the patient with an acute abdomen?

_____

_____

5. List the general EMT-B emergency care for patients with acute abdomen.

_____

_____

Word Fun emtb vocab explorer

The following crossword puzzle is an activity provided to reinforce correct spelling and understanding of medical terminology associated with emergency care and the EMT-B. Use the clues in the column to complete the puzzle.

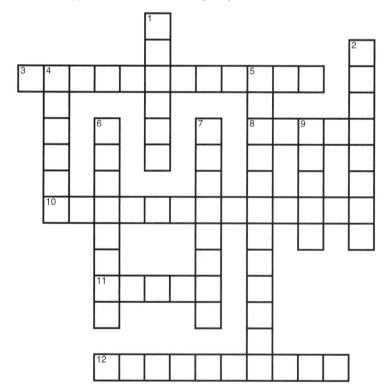

Across

3. Felt elsewhere in the body

8. Abrasion of stomach or small intestine

10. Complete obstruction

11. Paralysis of the bowels

12. Lining of the abdominal cavity

Down

1. Protrusion of a loop of an organ

2. Involuntary muscle contractions for protection

4. Vomiting

5. Sudden onset of pain below diaphragm

6. Lack of appetite

7. Results in the weakening of an arterial wall

9. Acute cramping abdominal pain

Ambulance Calls

The following case scenarios provide an opportunity to explore the concerns associated with patient management. Read each scenario, then answer each question in detail.

1. You are called to the local high school nurse's office for a 16-year-old female complaining of severe, abrupt abdominal pain. She is pale, cool, and clammy with absent radial pulses. The school nurse tells you that the patient found out 4 weeks ago that she is pregnant.

How would you best manage this patient?

_____

_____

_____

2. You are dispatched to a long-term care facility for a geriatric man with abdominal pain. Upon your arrival, one of the staff members tells you that this patient has been bedridden and taking pain medications for the last several weeks, and has recently had problems passing a normal bowel movement. He now has a distended, tender abdomen with nausea, vomiting and tachycardia.

How do you best manage this patient?

_____

_____

_____

3. You are dispatched to the home of another responder for "severe back pain." You arrive to find your coworker writhing in pain on the floor. He tells you that he tried to urinate (unsuccessfully) when he immediately experienced a sharp, cramping sensation in his right side. As you are talking to him he throws up. After vomiting, he tells you the pain is worse and is now spreading to his groin.

How do you best manage this patient?

_____

_____

_____

Assessment Review

Answer the following questions pertaining to the assessment of the types of emergencies discussed in this chapter. Questions 1-5 are derived from the following scenario:

You respond the home of a 6-year-old boy complaining of severe back pain. As you approach the boy, he is in the fetal position crying, and is in obvious pain. As you ask questions of the child, he remains silent and his dad answers your questions.

_____ **1.** What will you determine during the initial assessment?

    A. The priority of care

    B. The child's level of consciousness

    C. Finding and treating any life threats

    D. All of the above

_____ **2.** Your partner takes Dad to a separate room to obtain a SAMPLE history. Which question(s) should she ask?

    A. "Do you know what medications he is currently taking?"

    B. "Where is his mother?"

    C. "Sir, we need to know, did you or your wife hurt him?"

    D. All of the above

_____ **3.** As you take a SAMPLE history of the boy, he admits to you his Dad kicked him in the stomach a few days ago and it has been hurting since. How should you proceed?

    A. Confront the father to see if this is true.

    B. Call for police back-up.

    C. Take the child without the father's knowledge.

    D. All of the above

_____ **4.** Upon examination, you note that his lower right quadrant is distended. The likely cause of the distention is:

    A. strangulation.

    B. cholecystitis.

    C. ileus.

    D. none of the above

_____ **5.** During your ongoing assessment, you should:

    A. repeat the initial assessment.

    B. repeat the focused assessment.

    C. reassure the patient.

    D. all of the above

Emergency Care Summary

Complete the statements pertaining to emergency care for the types of emergencies discussed in this chapter by filling in the missing words.

NOTE: While the steps below are widely accepted, be sure to consult and follow your local protocol.

Acute Abdomen

General Management

1. Explain to the patient what you are about to do.
2. Place the patient in a _____ position with legs drawn up and _____ at the knees unless _____ is suspected.
3. Determine whether the patient is restless or quiet, whether motion causes pain, or whether any characteristic position, _____, or obvious _____ is present.
4. _____ the four _____ of the abdomen.
5. Determine whether the patient can relax the _____ _____ on command.
6. Determine whether the abdomen is tender when _____.

CHAPTER

15 Diabetic Emergencies

Workbook Activities

The following activities have been designed to help you. Your instructor may require you to complete some or all of these activities as a regular part of your EMT-B training program. You are encouraged to complete any activity that your instructor does not assign as a way to enhance your learning in the classroom.

Chapter Review

The following exercises provide an opportunity to refresh your knowledge of this chapter.

Matching

Match each of the terms in the left column to the appropriate definition in the right column.

_____ 1. Hormone

_____ 2. Polydipsia

_____ 3. Type I diabetes

_____ 4. Acidosis

_____ 5. Insulin

_____ 6. Diabetic coma

_____ 7. Polyuria

_____ 8. Type II diabetes

_____ 9. Polyphagia

_____ 10. Insulin shock

_____ 11. Glucose

_____ 12. Kussmaul respirations

_____ 13. Hyperglycemia

_____ 14. Diabetes

A. altered level of consciousness caused by insufficient glucose in the blood

B. diabetes that usually starts in childhood; requires insulin

C. excessive eating

D. deep, rapid breathing

E. excessive urination

F. excessive thirst persisting for a long period of time

G. diabetes with onset later in life; may be controlled by diet and oral medication

H. chemical produced by a gland that regulates body organs

I. literal meaning: "A passer through; a siphon"

J. extremely high blood glucose level

K. pathologic condition resulting from the accumulation of acids in the body

L. hormone that enables glucose to enter the cells

M. primary fuel, along with oxygen, for cellular metabolism

N. state of unconsciousness resulting from several problems, including ketoacidosis, dehydration, and hyperglycemia

Multiple Choice

Read each item carefully, then select the best response.

_____ **1.** Patients with which type of diabetes are more likely to have metabolic problems and organ damage?

    A. Type I

    B. Type II

    C. Sugar diabetes

    D. HHNC

_____ **2.** Normal blood glucose levels range from _____ mg/dL.

    A. 80 to 120

    B. 90 to 140

    C. 70 to 110

    D. 60 to 100

_____ **3.** Patients with diabetes mellitus and a lack of insulin excrete excess glucose through their:

    A. lymphatic system.

    B. sweat.

    C. respiratory efforts.

    D. urine.

_____ **4.** Diabetes is a metabolic disorder in which the hormone _____ is missing or ineffective.

    A. estrogen

    B. adrenaline

    C. insulin

    D. epinephrine

_____ **5.** Complications of diabetes include:

    A. paralysis.

    B. cardiovascular disease.

    C. brittle bones.

    D. hepatitis.

_____ **6.** The accumulation of ketones and fatty acids in blood tissue can lead to a dangerous condition in diabetic patients known as:

    A. diabetic ketoacidosis.

    B. insulin shock.

    C. HHNC.

    D. hypoglycemia.

_____ **7.** The term for excessive eating as a result of cellular "hunger" is:

    A. polyuria.

    B. polydipsia.

    C. polyphagia.

    D. polyphony.

_____ **8.** Insulin is produced by the:

    A. adrenal glands.

    B. hypothalamus.

    C. spleen.

    D. pancreas.

_____ **9.** Factors that may contribute to diabetic coma include:

  A. infection.

  B. alcohol consumption.

  C. insufficient insulin.

  D. all of the above

_____ **10.** The only organ that does not require insulin to allow glucose to enter its cells is the:

  A. liver.

  B. brain.

  C. pancreas.

  D. heart.

_____ **11.** The sweet or fruity odor on the breath of a diabetic patient is caused by _____ in the blood.

  A. acetone

  B. ketones

  C. alcohol

  D. insulin

_____ **12.** The term for excessive thirst is:

  A. polyuria.

  B. polydipsia.

  C. polyphagia.

  D. polyphony.

_____ **13.** Oral diabetic medications include:

  A. Micronase.

  B. Glucotrol.

  C. Diabinase.

  D. all of the above

_____ **14.** _____ is one of the basic sugars in the body.

  A. Dextrose

  B. Sucrose

  C. Fructose

  D. Syrup

_____ **15.** _____ is the hormone that is normally produced by the pancreas that enables glucose to enter the cells

  A. Insulin

  B. adrenaline

  C. Estrogen

  D. Epinephrine

_____ **16.** The term for excessive urination is:

  A. polyuria.

  B. polydipsia.

  C. polyphagia.

  D. polyphony.

_____ **17.** When fat is used as an immediate energy source, _____ and fatty acids are formed as waste products.

  A. dextrose

  B. sucrose

  C. ketones

  D. bicarbonate

_____ **18.** When using a glucometer, the patient tests his or her glucose level in a drop of:

  A. urine.

  B. blood.

  C. saliva.

  D. cerebrospinal fluid.

_____ **19.** The onset of hypoglycemia can occur within:

    A. seconds.

    B. minutes.

    C. hours.

    D. days.

_____ **20.** Without _____, or with very low levels, brain cells rapidly suffer permanent damage.

    A. epinephrine

    B. ketones

    C. bicarbonate

    D. glucose

_____ **21.** _____ is/are a potentially life-threatening complication of insulin shock.

    A. Kussmaul respirations

    B. Hypotension

    C. Seizures

    D. Polydipsia

_____ **22.** Blood glucose levels are measured in:

    A. micrograms per deciliter.

    B. milligrams per deciliter.

    C. milliliters per decigram.

    D. microliters per decigram.

_____ **23.** Diabetic coma may develop as a result of:

    A. too little insulin.

    B. too much insulin.

    C. overhydration.

    D. metabolic alkalosis.

_____ **24.** Always suspect hypoglycemia in any patient with:

    A. Kussmaul respirations.

    B. an altered mental status.

    C. nausea and vomiting.

    D. all of the above

_____ **25.** The most important step in caring for the unresponsive diabetic patient is to:

    A. give oral glucose immediately.

    B. perform a focused assessment.

    C. open the airway.

    D. obtain a SAMPLE history.

_____ **26.** Determination of diabetic coma or insulin shock should:

    A. be made before transport of the patient.

    B. be made before administration of oral glucose.

    C. be determined by a urine glucose test.

    D. be based upon your knowledge of the signs and symptoms of each condition.

_____ **27.** An unresponsive patient involved in a motor vehicle crash with a diabetic identification bracelet should be suspected to be _____ until proven otherwise.

    A. hypoglycemic

    B. hyperglycemic

    C. intoxicated

    D. in shock

_____ **28.** Contraindications for the use of oral glucose include:

    A. unconsciousness.

    B. known alcoholic.

    C. insulin shock.

    D. all of the above

_____ **29.** When reassessing the diabetic patient after administration of oral glucose, watch for:

    A. airway problems.

    B. seizures.

    C. sudden loss of consciousness.

    D. all of the above

_____ **30.** Signs and symptoms associated with hypoglycemia include:

    A. warm, dry skin.

    B. rapid, weak pulse.

    C. Kussmaul respirations.

    D. anxious or combative behavior.

_____ **31.** The patient in insulin shock is experiencing:

    A. hyperglycemia.

    B. hypoglycemia.

    C. diabetic ketoacidosis.

    D. a low production of insulin.

_____ **32.** Signs of dehydration include:

    A. good skin turgor.

    B. elevated blood pressure.

    C. sunken eyes.

    D. all of the above

_____ **33.** Diabetic patients who complain of "not feeling so well" should:

    A. have their glucose level checked.

    B. have a rapid trauma assessment completed.

    C. be rapidly transported to the closest medical facility.

    D. immediately be given oral glucose.

_____ **34.** Causes of insulin shock include:

    A. taking too much insulin.

    B. vigorous exercise without sufficient glucose intake.

    C. nausea, vomiting, anorexia.

    D. all of the above

_____ **35.** Insulin shock can develop more often and more severely in children than in adults due to their:

    A. high activity level and failure to maintain a strict schedule of eating.

    B. genetic makeup.

    C. smaller body size.

    D. all of the above

_____ **36.** Because diabetic coma is a complex metabolic condition that usually develops over time and involves all the tissues of the body, correcting this condition may:

    A. be accomplished quickly through the use of oral glucose.

    B. require rapid infusion of IV fluid to prevent permanent brain damage.

    C. take many hours in a hospital setting.

    D. include a reduction in the amount of insulin normally taken by the patient.

_____ **37.** A patient in insulin shock or a diabetic coma may appear to be:

    A. having a heart attack.

    B. perfectly normal.

    C. intoxicated.

    D. having a stroke.

Questions 38-42 are derived from the following scenario: A 54-year-old golfer collapsed on the 17th green at the golf course. His friend said he wasn't feeling well after the 8th hole, but insisted on walking and finishing out the game. He is pale, cool and diaphoretic, and answers incoherently to your questions.

_____ **38.** During your rapid physical exam, you discover a medical alert necklace around his neck that reads "Type 2 Diabetic". This tells you that:

    A. he developed diabetes later in life.

    B. his body produces inadequate amounts of insulin.

    C. he is likely to be taking non-insulin type of oral medications.

    D. all of the above

_____ **39.** His blood glucose level is 65 mg/dL. You:

    A. do not suspect hypoglycemia and begin to think cardiac in nature.

    B. suspect hyperglycemia and proceed to give oral glucose.

    C. suspect hypoglycemia and proceed to give oral glucose.

    D. suspect hypoglycemia but oral glucose is contraindicated for him.

_____ **40.** The patient loses consciousness and a second blood glucose level reads 48 mg/dL. You should:

    A. call for, or transport to, ALS.

    B. ensure a patent airway.

    C. provide high-flow oxygen.

    D. all of the above

_____ **41.** Because of his blood glucose level and rapid respirations, you suspect:

    A. insulin shock.

    B. diabetic coma.

    C. renal failure.

    D. mittelschmerz.

_____ **42.** Since the patient is unconscious and his blood glucose level is 48 mg/dL, how should the glucose be delivered?

    A. Between the cheek and gum

    B. Placed on the back of the tongue

    C. Placed on the tip of the tongue

    D. None of the above

Fill-in

Read each item carefully, then complete the statement by filling in the missing word(s).

1. The full name of diabetes is _____ _____.

2. Diabetes is considered to be a(n) _____ problem, in which the body becomes allergic to its own tissues and literally destroys them.

3. Diabetes is defined as a lack of or _____ action of insulin.

4. Too much blood glucose by itself does not always cause _____ _____, but on some occasions, it can lead to it.

5. A patient in insulin shock needs _____ immediately and a patient in a diabetic coma needs _____ and IV fluid therapy.

True/False

If you believe the statement to be more true than false, write the letter "T" in the space provided. If you believe the statement to be more false than true, write the letter "F."

_____ **1.** When patients use fat for energy, the fat waste products increase the amount of acid in the blood and tissue.

_____ **2.** The level of consciousness can be affected if a patient has not exercised enough.

_____ **3.** If blood glucose levels remain low, a patient may lose consciousness or have permanent brain damage.

_____ **4.** Signs and symptoms can develop quickly in children because their level of activity can exhaust their glucose levels.

_____ **5.** Diabetic emergencies can occur when a patient's blood glucose level gets too high or when it drops too low.

_____ **6.** Diabetic patients may require insulin to control their blood glucose.

_____ **7.** Glucose is a hormone that enables insulin to enter the cells of the body.

_____ **8.** Insulin is one of the basic sugars essential for cell metabolism in humans.

_____ **9.** Diabetes can cause kidney failure, blindness, and damage to blood vessels.

_____ **10.** Most children with diabetes are insulin dependent.

_____ **11.** Many adults with diabetes can control their blood glucose levels with diet alone.

Short Answer

Complete this section with short written answers using the space provided.

1. What is insulin and what is its role in metabolism?

_____

_____

2. What are two trade names for oral glucose?

_____

_____

3. When should you not give oral glucose to a patient experiencing a suspected diabetic emergency?

_____

_____

4. List the trade names of three oral medications used by diabetics.

_____

_____

5. What are the three problems associated with the development of diabetic coma?

_____

_____

6. List the physical signs of diabetic coma.

_____

_____

7. If a diabetic patient was "fine" 2 hours ago and now is unconscious and unresponsive, which diabetes-related condition would you suspect and why?

_____

_____

8. Why should oral glucose be given to any diabetic patient with an altered level of consciousness?

_____

_____

Word Fun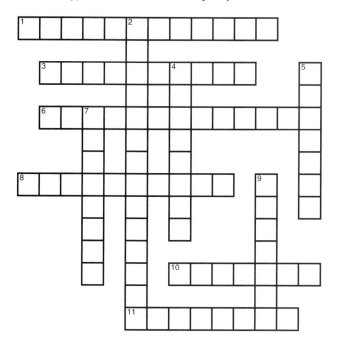

The following crossword puzzle is an activity provided to reinforce correct spelling and understanding of medical terminology associated with emergency care and the EMT-B. Use the clues in the column to complete the puzzle.

Across

1. Unconscious state with high glucose levels
3. Excessive eating
6. Disease that usually starts early in life, generally requires daily injections
8. Excessive thirst
10. Chemical substance produced by a gland
11. May result from hypoglycemia

Down

2. Disease that starts later in life, usually controlled by diet and oral medications
4. Opposite of alkalosis
5. Hormone produced in pancreas
7. Excessive urination
9. One of the basic sugars

Ambulance Calls

The following case scenarios provide an opportunity to explore the concerns associated with patient management. Read each scenario, then answer each question in detail.

1. You are called to a local residence where you find a 22-year-old woman supine in bed, unresponsive to your attempts to rouse her. She is cold and clammy with gurgling respirations. Her mother tells you that her only history is diabetes, which she has had since she was a small child. What steps would you take in managing this patient?

_____

_____

_____

2. You are requested by local law enforcement to assist with "a man acting strangely." You arrive to find a man in the back of the patrol car, singing and rocking back and forth. The officer tells you he thinks this man is "off his rocker." Apparently, the man was walking down Main Street when he decided to remove all of his clothing. He continued to walk around downtown, naked, until restrained by law enforcement officers.

How do you best manage this patient?

_____

_____

_____

3. You are dispatched to assist with a diabetic patient well known in your department for being noncompliant with his medications and diet. You have responded numerous times to his residence, all for instances of low blood sugar. Family members greet you at the door and say, "It's Jon again. Just give him some sugar like you usually do." You walk into the patient's bedroom to discover him unconscious with snoring respirations.

How do you best manage this patient?

_____

_____

_____

Skill Drills
Skill Drill 15-1: Administering Glucose
Test your knowledge of this skill drill by filling in the correct words in the photo captions.

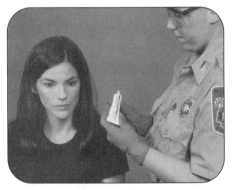
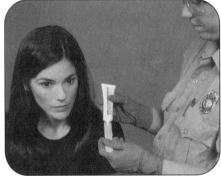
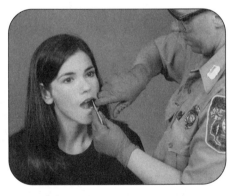

1. Make sure that the tube of glucose is intact and has not _____.

2. Squeeze a generous amount of oral glucose onto the _____ _____ of a _____ _____ or tongue depressor.

3. Open the patient's _____. Place the tongue depressor on the _____ _____ between the cheek and the gum with the _____ _____ next to the cheek. Repeat until the entire tube has been used.

Comparison Table

Complete the following table on the characteristics of diabetic emergencies.

	Hyperglycemia	Hypoglycemia
History Food intake Insulin dosage Onset Skin Infection		
Gastrointestinal Tract Thirst Hunger Vomiting		
Respiratory System Breathing Odor of breath		
Cardiovascular System Blood pressure Pulse		
Nervous System Consciousness		
Urine Sugar Acetone		
Treatment Response		

Assessment Review

Answer the following questions pertaining to the assessment of the types of emergencies discussed in this chapter. Questions 1-5 are derived from the following scenario:

While driving back to the station, you and your partner find an unconscious person lying on the grass in front of a home.

_____ **1.** After completing scene size-up, your fist step is to:

　　A. take appropriate BSI precautions.

　　B. form a general impression of the patient.

　　C. apply oxygen.

　　D. none of the above

_____ **2.** The patient appears to be a woman in her mid 30s, and she is unresponsive to verbal or painful stimulus. Because there is no one around, you are unable to complete a focused history. Which physical exam should you perform first?

　　A. Focused physical exam

　　B. Rapid physical exam

　　C. Detailed physical exam

　　D. Blood glucose level

_____ **3.** Her respirations are 28 breaths/min, her pulse is 110 beats/min, and her blood pressure is 94/52 mm Hg. How should you intervene for her?

　　A. Give her oral glucose.

　　B. Give her insulin.

　　C. Provide high-flow oxygen.

　　D. All of the above

_____ **4.** Your protocols do not allow you to measure blood glucose levels, and you are unsure as to the nature of her illness. You should:

　　A. provide oral glucose anyway.

　　B. provide insulin found in her purse.

　　C. provide nitroglycerin found in her purse.

　　D. none of the above

_____ **5.** When relaying information to medical control, you should inform them of:

　　A. the patient's condition.

　　B. any changes of consciousness.

　　C. any difficulty the patient may experience in breathing.

　　D. all of the above

Emergency Care Summary

Complete the statements pertaining to emergency care for the types of emergencies discussed in this chapter by filling in the missing words.

NOTE: While the steps below are widely accepted, be sure to consult and follow your local protocol.

Diabetic Emergencies

Administering Glucose

1. Examine the tube to ensure that it is not open or broken. Check the _____ _____.

2. Squeeze a _____ amount onto the bottom _____ of a bite stick or tongue depressor.

3. Open the patient's mouth. Place the tongue depressor on the _____ _____ between the cheek and gum, with the gel side next to the _____.

CHAPTER

16 Allergic Reactions and Envenomations

Workbook Activities

The following activities have been designed to help you. Your instructor may require you to complete some or all of these activities as a regular part of your EMT-B training program. You are encouraged to complete any activity that your instructor does not assign as a way to enhance your learning in the classroom.

Chapter Review

The following exercises provide an opportunity to refresh your knowledge of this chapter.

Matching

Match each of the terms in the left column to the appropriate definition in the right column.

_____ **1.** Allergic reaction

_____ **2.** Leukotrienes

_____ **3.** Wheezing

_____ **4.** Urticaria

_____ **5.** Stridor

_____ **6.** Allergen

_____ **7.** Wheal

_____ **8.** Toxin

A. substance made by body; released in anaphylaxis

B. harsh, high-pitched inspiratory sound, usually resulting from upper airway obstruction

C. raised, swollen area on skin resulting from an insect bite or allergic reaction

D. an exaggerated immune response to any substance

E. multiple raised areas on the skin that itch or burn

F. a poison or harmful substance

G. substance that causes an allergic reaction

H. high-pitched, whistling breath sound usually resulting from blockage of the airway and typically heard on expiration

Multiple Choice
Read each item carefully, then select the best response.

_____ 1. Steps for assisting a patient with administration of an EpiPen include:
   A. taking body substance isolation precautions.
   B. placing the tip of the auto-injector against the medial part of the patient's thigh.
   C. recapping the injector before placing it in the trash.
   D. all of the above

_____ 2. Allergens may include:
   A. food.
   B. animal bites.
   C. semen.
   D. all of the above

_____ 3. Anaphylaxis is not always life threatening, but it typically involves:
   A. multiple organ systems.
   B. wheezing.
   C. urticaria.
   D. wheals.

_____ 4. Signs and symptoms of insect stings or bites include:
   A. swelling.
   B. wheals.
   C. localized heat.
   D. all of the above

_____ 5. Prolonged respiratory difficulty can cause _____, shock, and even death.
   A. tachypnea
   B. pulmonary edema
   C. tachycardia
   D. airway obstruction

_____ 6. Speed is essential because more than two-thirds of patients who die of anaphylaxis do so within the first:
   A. 10 minutes.
   B. 30 minutes.
   C. hour.
   D. 3 hours.

_____ 7. Questions to ask when obtaining a history from a patient appearing to have an allergic reaction include:
   A. whether the patient has a history of allergies.
   B. what the patient was exposed to.
   C. how the patient was exposed.
   D. all of the above

_____ 8. The dosage of epinephrine in an adult EpiPen is:
   A. 0.10 mg.
   B. 0.15 mg.
   C. 0.30 mg.
   D. 0.50 mg.

_____ 9. Epinephrine, whether made by the body or by a drug manufacturer, works rapidly to:
   A. raise the pulse rate and blood pressure.
   B. inhibit an allergic reaction.
   C. dilate the bronchioles.
   D. all of the above

_____ **10.** Because the stinger of the honeybee is barbed and remains in the wound, it can continue to inject venom for up to:

    A. 1 minute.

    B. 15 minutes.

    C. 20 minutes.

    D. several hours.

_____ **11.** You should not use tweezers or forceps to remove an embedded stinger because:

    A. squeezing may cause the stinger to inject more venom into the wound.

    B. the stinger may break off in the wound.

    C. the tweezers are not sterile and may cause infection.

    D. removing the stinger may cause bleeding.

_____ **12.** Your assessment of the patient experiencing an allergic reaction should include evaluations of the:

    A. respiratory system.

    B. circulatory system.

    C. skin.

    D. all of the above

_____ **13.** Eating certain foods, such as shellfish or nuts, may result in a relatively _____ reaction that still can be quite severe.

    A. mild

    B. fast

    C. slow

    D. rapid

_____ **14.** In dealing with allergy-related emergencies, you must be aware of the possibility of acute _____ and cardiovascular collapse.

    A. hypotension

    B. tachypnea

    C. airway obstruction

    D. shock

_____ **15.** Wheezing occurs because excessive _____ and mucus are secreted into the bronchial passages.

    A. fluid

    B. carbon dioxide

    C. blood

    D. all of the above

Questions 16-20 are derived from the following scenario: You have been called to a park where a local church is holding a pot-luck dinner. As you exit your ambulance, a woman is holding her 7-year-old son who is wheezing and having difficulty breathing. She informs you that he had inadvertently eaten a brownie with nuts, and he is allergic to nuts.

_____ **16.** You lift his shirt and find small, raised areas that he is trying to itch. They are likely to be:

    A. leukotrienes.

    B. histamines.

    C. urticaria.

    D. none of the above

_____ **17.** Why is he wheezing?

    A. He has had an envenomation.

    B. His bronchioles are constricting.

    C. His bronchioles are dilating.

    D. His uvula has swollen.

_____ **18.** His mother has two different EpiPens. Which dosage of insulin should be given to the child?

    A. 0.1 to 0.3 mL

    B. 0.3 to 0.5 mL

    C. 0.5 to 0.7 mL

    D. none of the above

_____ **19.** When assisting with an auto-injector, how long should you hold the pen against the thigh?

    A. 3 minutes

    B. 5 minutes

    C. 10 minutes

    D. none of the above

_____ **20.** After removing the auto-injector from his thigh, you should:

    A. record the time.

    B. record the dose.

    C. reassess his vital signs.

    D. all of the above

Fill-in

Read each item carefully, then complete the statement by filling in the missing word(s).

1. Wheezing occurs because excessive fluid and mucus are secreted into the _____ _____.

2. Small areas of generalized itching or burning that appear as multiple, small, raised areas on the skin are called _____.

3. The stinger of the honeybee is _____, so the bee cannot withdraw it.

4. A reaction involving the entire body is called _____.

5. The presence of _____ or respiratory distress indicates that the patient is having a severe enough allergic reaction to lead to death.

6. Epinephrine inhibits the allergic reaction and dilates the _____.

7. Your ability to recognize and manage the many signs and symptoms of allergic reactions may be the only thing standing between a patient and _____ _____.

True/False

If you believe the statement to be more true than false, write the letter "T" in the space provided. If you believe the statement to be more false than true, write the letter "F."

_____ **1.** Allergic reactions can occur in response to almost any substance.

_____ **2.** An allergic reaction occurs when the body has an immune response to a substance.

_____ **3.** Wheezing is a high-pitched breath sound usually resulting from blockage of the airway and heard on expiration.

_____ **4.** For a patient appearing to have an allergic reaction, give 100% oxygen via nasal cannula.

Short Answer

Complete this section with short written answers using the space provided.

1. Common side effects of epinephrine include:

_____

_____

2. What are five stimuli that most often cause allergic reactions?

_____

_____

3. What are the steps for administering or assisting with administration of an epinephrine auto-injector?

_____

_____

4. What are the common respiratory and circulatory signs or symptoms of an allergic reaction?

_____

_____

Word Fun

The following crossword puzzle is an activity provided to reinforce correct spelling and understanding of medical terminology associated with emergency care and the EMT-B. Use the clues in the column to complete the puzzle.

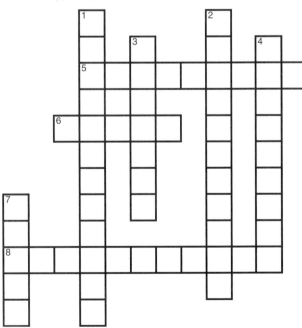

Across

5. Small spots; itching, raised areas

6. Poison or harmful substance

8. Adrenaline

Down

1. Chemical substance made by the body, leads to anaphylaxis

2. Severe allergic reaction

3. Harsh, high-pitched airway sounds

4. Responsible for allergy symptoms

7. Raised, swollen area from a sting

Ambulance Calls

The following case scenarios provide an opportunity to explore the concerns associated with patient management. Read each scenario, then answer each question in detail.

1. You are dispatched to care for a wanted suspect who was fleeing from police and was eventually subdued by a canine officer. The man has several puncture wounds on his left arm and no gross bleeding is present. How do you best manage this patient?

_____

_____

_____

2. You are dispatched to assist a 12-year-old child who was climbing a tree and apparently disturbed a wasp nest. When you arrive, the child is lying under the tree and the nest is on the ground next to her. How do you best manage this patient?

_____

_____

_____

3. You are dispatched to a local seafood restaurant for a person who is having difficulty breathing. Upon arrival, you find a 22-year-old woman with facial edema, cyanosis around the lips, audible wheezing, and urticaria on her face and upper body. Her boyfriend tells you she ate shrimp and she is allergic to them. He also tells you she has some medicine in her purse and hands you an EpiPen prescribed to her. How would you best manage this patient?

_____

_____

_____

Skill Drills

Skill Drill 16-1: Using an Auto-injector

Test your knowledge of this skill drill by filling in the correct words in the photo captions.

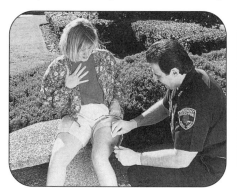 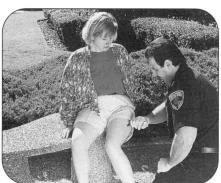 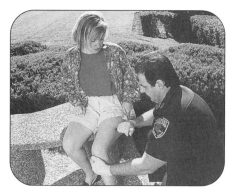

1. Remove the auto-injector's _____ _____, and quickly wipe the thigh with _____.

2. Place the tip of the auto-injector against the _____ part of the thigh.

3. Push the _____ firmly against the _____, and hold it in place until all the medication is injected.

Skill Drill 16-2: Using an AnaKit

Test your knowledge of this skill drill by placing the following photos in the correct order. Number the first step with a "1," the second step with a "2," etc.

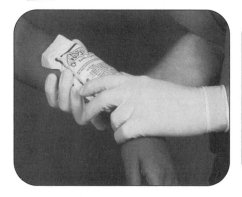

_____

If available, apply a cold pack to the sting site.

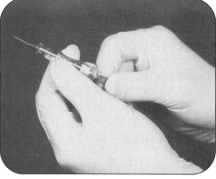

_____

Turn the plunger one-quarter turn.

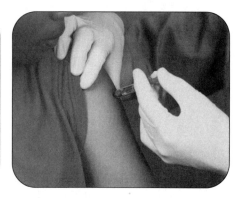

_____

Hold the syringe steady, and push the plunger until it stops.

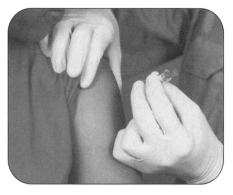

_____

Quickly insert the needle into the muscle.

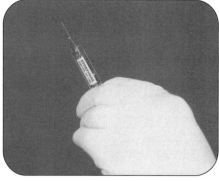

_____

Hold the syringe upright, and carefully use the plunger to remove air.

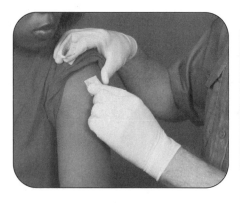

_____

Prepare the injection site with antiseptic, and remove the needle cover.

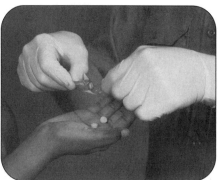

_____

Have the patient chew and swallow the Chlo-Amine antihistamine tablets provided in the kit.

Assessment Review

Answer the following questions pertaining to the assessment of the types of emergencies discussed in this chapter.

_____ **1.** As you begin to assess a patient suspected of anaphylactic shock, what should be done first?

A. Assist with an EpiPen.

B. Take a set of vital signs.

C. Provide high-flow oxygen.

D. Obtain a pulse oximetry reading.

_____ **2.** After assisting with an EpiPen:

A. apply high-flow oxygen if it has not been done already.

B. take a set of vital signs.

C. place the used EpiPen in a biohazard container.

D. all of the above

_____ **3.** When using the auto-injector:

A. remove the safety cap.

B. wipe the thigh with antiseptic.

C. push the autoinjector firmly against the thigh for about 10 seconds.

D. all of the above

_____ **4.** What does the letter "M" stand for in SAMPLE history?

A. Money—how will they pay for this?

B. Maintenance—have they been compliant with their medications?

C. Medications—what medications are they currently taking?

D. None of the above

_____ **5.** What does the letter "P" stand for in SAMPLE history?

A. Pain—rate your pain from 1-10

B. Probable cause—what caused this to happen?

C. Priority—is this a high or low priority patient?

D. Past pertinent history

Emergency Care Summary

Complete the statements pertaining to emergency care for the types of emergencies discussed in this chapter by filling in the missing words.

> *NOTE:* While the steps below are widely accepted, be sure to consult and follow your local protocol.

Allergic Reactions

Using an Auto-injector

1. Remove the auto-injector's safety cap, and quickly wipe the thigh with antiseptic.

2. Place the tip of the auto-injector against the _____ part of the thigh.

3. Push the auto-injector firmly against the thigh, and hold it in place until all the medication is injected (about _____ seconds).

Using an Anakit

1. Prepare the injection site with antiseptic, and remove the needle cover.

2. Hold the syringe _____, and carefully use the plunger to remove the air.

3. Turn the plunger _____ turn.

4. Quickly insert the needle into the _____.

5. Hold the syringe steady, and push the plunger until it stops.

6. Have the patient chew and swallow the Chlo-Amine _____ tablets provided in the kit.

7. If available, apply a _____ _____ to the sting site.

CHAPTER

17 Substance Abuse and Poisoning

Workbook Activities

The following activities have been designed to help you. Your instructor may require you to complete some or all of these activities as a regular part of your EMT-B training program. You are encouraged to complete any activity that your instructor does not assign as a way to enhance your learning in the classroom.

Chapter Review

The following exercises provide an opportunity to refresh your knowledge of this chapter.

Matching

Match each of the terms in the left column to the appropriate definition in the right column.

_____ **1.** Poison

_____ **2.** Substance abuse

_____ **3.** Antidote

_____ **4.** Tolerance

_____ **5.** Cholinergic

_____ **6.** Ingestion

_____ **7.** Hematemesis

_____ **8.** Stimulant

_____ **9.** Opioid

_____ **10.** Sedative-hypnotic

_____ **11.** Anticholinergic

A. Xanax, Librium, Valium

B. drug or agent with actions similar to morphine

C. Atropine, Benadryl, some cyclic antidepressants

D. need for increasing amounts of a drug to obtain the same effect

E. agent that produces an excited state

F. any substance whose chemical action can damage body structures or impair body functions

G. a substance that will counteract the effects of a particular poison

H. the misuse of any substance to produce a desired effect

I. taking a substance by mouth

J. overstimulates body functions controlled by parasympathetic nerves

K. vomiting blood

Multiple Choice

Read each item carefully, then select the best response.

_____ **1.** Activated charcoal is in the form of a(n):

    A. elixir.

    B. suspension.

    C. syrup.

    D. emulsion.

_____ **2.** The presence of burning or blistering of the mucous membranes suggests:

    A. ingestion of depressants.

    B. ingestion of poison.

    C. overdose of heroin.

    D. the patient may be a heavy smoker.

_____ **3.** Treatment for ingestion of poisonous plants includes:

    A. assessing the ABCs.

    B. taking the plant to the emergency department.

    C. prompt transport.

    D. all of the above

_____ **4.** The most important consideration in caring for a patient who has been exposed to an organophosphate insecticide or some other cholinergic agent is to:

    A. maintain the airway.

    B. apply high-flow oxygen.

    C. avoid exposure yourself.

    D. initiate CPR.

_____ **5.** Objects that may provide clues to the nature of the poison include:

    A. a needle or syringe.

    B. scattered pills.

    C. chemicals.

    D. all of the above

_____ **6.** The most worrisome avenue of poisoning is:

    A. ingestion.

    B. inhalation.

    C. injection.

    D. absorption.

_____ **7.** The major side effect of ingesting activated charcoal is:

    A. depressed respirations.

    B. overproduction of stomach acid.

    C. black stools.

    D. increased blood pressure.

_____ **8.** Alcohol is a powerful CNS depressant. It:

    A. sharpens the sense of awareness.

    B. slows reflexes.

    C. increases reaction time.

    D. all of the above

_____ **9.** Frequently abused synthetic opioids include:

    A. heroin.

    B. morphine.

    C. Demerol.

    D. all of the above

_____ **10.** Treatment of patients who have overdosed with sedative-hypnotics and have respiratory depression is to:

    A. provide airway clearance.

    B. provide ventilatory assistance.

    C. provide prompt transport.

    D. all of the above

_____ **11.** Anticholinergic medications have properties that block the _____ nerves.

    A. parasympathetic

    B. sympathetic

    C. adrenergic

    D. parasympatholytic

_____ **12.** _____ crack produces the most rapid means of absorption and therefore the most potent effect.

    A. Injected

    B. Absorbed

    C. Smoked

    D. Ingested

_____ **13.** "Nerve gases" overstimulate normal body functions that are controlled by parasympathetic nerves causing:

    A. increased salivation.

    B. increased heart rate.

    C. increased urination.

    D. all of the above

_____ **14.** Signs and symptoms of staphylococcal food poisoning include:

    A. difficulty in speaking.

    B. nausea, vomiting, diarrhea.

    C. blurred vision.

    D. all of the above

_____ **15.** Inhalant effects range from mild drowsiness to coma, but unlike most other sedative-hypnotics, these agents may often cause:

    A. seizures.

    B. vomiting.

    C. swelling of the tongue.

    D. all of the above

_____ **16.** Cocaine may be taken via:

    A. inhalation.

    B. injection.

    C. absorption.

    D. all of the above

_____ **17.** Abusable substances include:

    A. vitamins.

    B. nasal decongestants.

    C. food.

    D. all of the above

_____ **18.** A person who has been using marijuana rarely needs transport to the hospital. Exceptions may include someone who is:

   A. hallucinating.

   B. very anxious.

   C. paranoid.

   D. all of the above

_____ **19.** Sympathomimetics are CNS stimulants that frequently cause:

   A. hypotension.

   B. tachycardia.

   C. pinpoint pupils.

   D. all of the above

_____ **20.** Carbon monoxide:

   A. is odorless.

   B. produces severe hypoxia.

   C. does not damage or irritate the lungs.

   D. all of the above

_____ **21.** Chlorine:

   A. is odorless.

   B. does not damage or irritate the lungs.

   C. causes pulmonary edema.

   D. all of the above

_____ **22.** Localized signs and symptoms of absorbed poisoning include:

   A. a history of exposure.

   B. burns, irritation of the skin.

   C. dyspnea.

   D. all of the above

_____ **23.** Poisoning by injection is almost always the result of:

   A. repetitive bee stings.

   B. pit viper envenomation.

   C. deliberate drug overdose.

   D. homicide.

_____ **24.** When dealing with substances such as phosphorous and elemental sodium, you should:

   A. brush the chemical off the patient.

   B. remove contaminated clothing.

   C. apply a dry dressing to the burn area.

   D. all of the above

_____ **25.** Injected poisons are impossible to dilute or remove, as they are usually _____ or cause intense local tissue destruction.

   A. absorbed quickly into the body

   B. bound to hemoglobin

   C. large compounds

   D. combined with the cerebrospinal fluid

_____ **26.** Medical problems that may cause the patient to present as intoxicated include:

   A. head trauma.

   B. toxic reactions.

   C. uncontrolled diabetes.

   D. all of the above

_____ 27. Signs and symptoms of alcohol withdrawal include:
  A. agitation and restlessness.
  B. fever, sweating.
  C. seizures.
  D. all of the above

_____ 28. Treatments for inhaled poisons include:
  A. moving the patient into fresh air.
  B. apply an SCBA to the patient.
  C. covering the patient to prevent spread of the poison.
  D. all of the above

_____ 29. Signs and symptoms of chlorine exposure include:
  A. cough.
  B. chest pain.
  C. wheezing.
  D. all of the above

_____ 30. Ingested poisons include:
  A. contaminated food.
  B. household cleaners.
  C. plants.
  D. all of the above

_____ 31. Ingestion of an opiate, sedative, or barbituate can cause depression of the CNS and:
  A. paralysis of the extremities.
  B. dilation of the pupils.
  C. carpopedal spasms.
  D. slow breathing.

_____ 32. Inhaled poisons include:
  A. chlorine.
  B. venom.
  C. dieffenbachia.
  D. all of the above

_____ 33. The most important treatment for poisoning is _____ and/or physically removing the poisonous agent.
  A. administering a specific antidote
  B. high-flow oxygen
  C. diluting
  D. syrup of ipecac

Questions 34-38 are derived from the following scenario: You have responded to home of a 26-year-old woman who had reportedly taken a large amount of pills in an attempt to commit suicide. As you enter the living room, you see her sleeping in her chair, with several empty alcohol containers. She is breathing heavily.

_____ 34. You are able to arouse her consciousness for a short period of time. Which course of action takes priority?
  A. Apply 15 L/min oxygen via nasal cannula.
  B. Apply 12 L/min oxygen via nonrebreathing mask.
  C. Have her take activated charcoal while she is conscious.
  D. Call for ALS.

_____ 35. You have determined to give her activated charcoal. How much should you give her?
  A. A half glass
  B. 12.5 to 25 mL
  C. 25 to 50 mL
  D. None of the above

_____ **36.** What would be the desired goal of giving her activated charcoal?

    A. To vomit the drugs and alcohol

    B. To bind the toxin and prevent absorption

    C. To teach her a lesson

    D. None of the above

_____ **37.** If she does not want to take the activated charcoal, you should:

    A. Restrain her, pinch her nose, and make her drink it.

    B. Have her sign a patient refusal form.

    C. Persuade her.

    D. All of the above

_____ **38.** Side effects of ingesting activated charcoal include:

    A. vomiting.

    B. black stools.

    C. nausea.

    D. all of the above

Fill-in

Read each item carefully, then complete the statement by filling in the missing word(s).

1. When dealing with exposure to chemicals, treatment focuses on support: assessing and maintaining the patient's

_____.

2. The most commonly abused drug in the United States is _____.

3. Activated charcoal works by _____, or sticking to, many commonly ingested poisons, preventing the toxin

from being absorbed into the body.

4. If the patient has a chemical agent in the eyes, you should irrigate them quickly and thoroughly, at least

_____ for acid substances and _____ for alkalis.

5. Opioid analgesics are CNS depressants and can cause severe _____ _____.

6. Severe acute alcohol ingestion may cause _____.

7. Your primary responsibility to the patient who has been poisoned is to _____ that a poisoning occurred.

8. The usual dosage for activated charcoal for an adult or child is _____ of activated charcoal per

_____ of body weight.

9. As you irrigate the eyes, make sure that the fluid runs from the bridge of the nose _____.

10. Approximately 80% of all poisoning is by _____, including plants, contaminated food, and most drugs.

11. Patients experiencing alcohol withdrawal may develop _____ _____ if they no longer have their daily

source of alcohol.

12. Phosphorus and elemental sodium _____ when they come in contact with water.

13. Increasing tolerance of a substance can lead to _____.

14. _____ may develop from sweating, fluid loss, insufficient fluid intake, or vomiting associated with DTs.

True/False

If you believe the statement to be more true than false, write the letter "T" in the space provided. If you believe the statement to be more false than true, write the letter "F."

_____ **1.** The usual adult dose of activated charcoal is 25 to 50 g.

_____ **2.** The general treatment of a poisoned patient is to induce vomiting.

_____ **3.** Activated charcoal is a standard of care in all ingestions.

_____ **4.** Inhaled chlorine produces profound hypoxia without lung irritation.

_____ **5.** Shaking activated charcoal decreases its effectiveness.

_____ **6.** Opioid overdose typically presents with pinpoint pupils.

_____ **7.** Cholinergics are chemicals such as nerve gases, organophosphate insecticides, or certain wild mushrooms.

_____ **8.** Alcohol is a stimulant.

_____ **9.** Demerol, Dilaudid, and Vicodin are all examples of opioids.

_____ **10.** Cocaine is one of the most addicting substances known.

Short Answer

Complete this section with short written answers using the space provided.

1. How does activated charcoal work to counteract ingested poison?

_____

_____

2. What are four routes of contact for poisoning?

_____

_____

3. List the typical signs and symptoms of an overdose of sympathomimetics.

_____

_____

4. What are the two main types of food poisoning?

_____

_____

5. What differentiates the presentation of acetaminophen poisoning from that of other substances? What does this mean to the prehospital caregiver?

_____

_____

6. What condition do the mnemonics DUMBELS and SLUDGE pertain to, and what do they mean?

_____

_____

7. In addition to alcohol and marijuana, what are the seven categories of drugs seen in overdoses/poisoning?

_____

_____

8. What five questions should you ask a possible poisoning victim?

_____

_____

9. Why should phosphorous or elemental sodium poisoning victims not be irrigated?

_____

_____

Word Fun

The following crossword puzzle is an activity provided to reinforce correct spelling and understanding of medical terminology associated with emergency care and the EMT-B. Use the clues in the column to complete the puzzle.

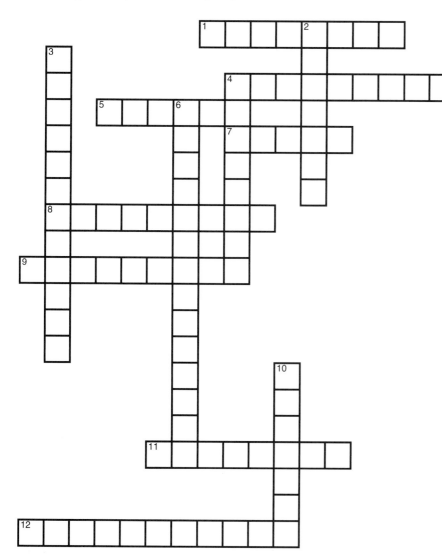

Across

1. Induces sleep

4. Overwhelming obsession or physical need

5. Substance whose chemical action causes damage

7. Poison or harmful substance; produced by animals, plants

8. Swallowing

9. Need for increasing amounts of a drug

11. Decreases activity and excitement

12. Vomiting blood

Down

2. Similar to morphine

3. Produces false perceptions

4. Used to neutralize or counteract a poison

6. Misuse of any substance to produce a desired effect

10. Material in emesis

Ambulance Calls

The following case scenarios provide an opportunity to explore the concerns associated with patient management. Read each scenario, then answer each question in detail.

1. You are dispatched to a private residence for "accidental ingestion." You arrive to find a 3-year-old, who parents tell you "got into some rat poison." The child is alert, crying and responding appropriately to parents and environmental stimulus.

How do you best manage this patient?

_____

_____

_____

2. You are dispatched to the sidewalk in front of a small business for "an intoxicated male." You arrive to find a 60-year-old man sitting on the curb, holding a bottle inside a paper bag. He is not fully alert, and can only tell you that his name is Andy. He allows you to take his blood pressure, and as you roll up his sleeve you notice needle marks along his veins.

How do you best manage this patient?

_____

_____

_____

3. You are called to a possible suicide attempt. You arrive on the scene to find police and a neighbor in the home of a 25-year-old woman who is unresponsive, supine on her bed. The neighbor tells you that the patient recently broke up with her boyfriend and has been very distraught. There is an empty pill bottle on the nightstand. When you look at the label you see that the prescription was filled yesterday and there were 30 tablets dispensed. There is also an empty liquor bottle on the floor.

How would you best manage this patient?

_____

_____

_____

Assessment Review

Answer the following questions pertaining to the assessment of the types of emergencies discussed in this chapter.

_____ **1.** When would it be more important to provide activated charcoal before applying oxygen?

    A. It wouldn't. Oxygen is always the top priority.

    B. When there's a life threat

    C. When oxygen is contraindicated

    D. None of the above

_____ **2.** What life threat can occur from applying a nonrebreathing mask after a patient has consumed activated charcoal?

 A. Vomiting into the nonrebreathing mask

 B. Aspirating the vomitus

 C. Choking on the vomitus

 D. All of the above

_____ **3.** The "O" in OPQRST stands for:

 A. OPQRST is for trauma only.

 B. On a scale of 1 to 10, rate your pain.

 C. Onset

 D. None of the above

_____ **4.** Why is "T" important in OPQRST?

 A. You will learn what Triggered the event.

 B. You will learn what Time the event started.

 C. You will obtain the patient's Temperature.

 D. You will find out what the patient has Taken.

_____ **5.** When would you not give activated charcoal?

 A. If the patient drank gasoline

 B. If the patient overdosed on aspirin

 C. If the patient overdosed on antidepressants

 D. None of the above

Emergency Care Summary

Complete the statements pertaining to emergency care for the types of emergencies discussed in this chapter by filling in the missing words.

 NOTE: While the steps below are widely accepted, be sure to consult and follow your local protocol.

Substance Abuse and Poisoning

General Management

1. Have trained rescuers remove patient from any poisonous environment.

2. Establish and maintain airway, _____ as needed. Provide _____ _____.

3. Obtain _____ history and _____ _____. Ascertain which drug(s) have been taken.

4. Request _____ when available.

5. Take all containers, bottles, and labels of poisons to the receiving hospital.

For patients who have taken _____, provide calm, prompt transport.

For _____ agents, it is critical to take sufficient body substance isolation precautions.

For patients who have _____ poisoning, notify regional poison control center for assistance in identifying the plant.

For patients who have _____ poisoning, if there are more than two patients with the same illness, transport the food suspected to be responsible for the poisoning.

Administer _____ _____ for poisonous ingestions according to local protocol. Follow these steps:

1. Do not give if the patient exhibits _____ _____ _____, has ingested acids or alkalis, or is unable to _____.

2. Obtain order from medical direction or follow protocol.

3. Shake container.

4. Place in cup with straw and have patient drink _____ to 25 g (for infants and children) or 25 to _____ g (for adults).

CHAPTER

18 Environmental Emergencies

Workbook Activities

The following activities have been designed to help you. Your instructor may require you to complete some or all of these activities as a regular part of your EMT-B training program. You are encouraged to complete any activity that your instructor does not assign as a way to enhance your learning in the classroom.

Chapter Review

The following exercises provide an opportunity to refresh your knowledge of this chapter.

Matching

Match each of the terms in the left column to the appropriate definition in the right column.

_____ **1.** Conduction	**A.** slowing of heart rate caused by sudden immersion in cold water
_____ **2.** Air embolism	**B.** salts and other chemicals dissolved in body fluids
_____ **3.** Evaporation	**C.** severe constriction of the larynx and vocal cords
_____ **4.** Hyperthermia	**D.** death from suffocation after submersion in water
_____ **5.** Diving reflex	**E.** heat loss resulting from standing in a cold room
_____ **6.** Core temperature	**F.** core temperature greater than 101°F
_____ **7.** Convection	**G.** condition when the entire body temperature falls
_____ **8.** Laryngospasm	**H.** condition caused by air bubbles in the blood vessels
_____ **9.** Electrolytes	**I.** heat loss that occurs from helicopter rotor blade downwash
_____ **10.** Radiation	**J.** heat loss resulting from sitting on snow
_____ **11.** Hypothermia	**K.** heat loss resulting from sweating
_____ **12.** Ambient temperature	**L.** painful muscle spasms that occur after vigorous exercise
_____ **13.** Heat cramps	**M.** temperature of the surrounding environment
_____ **14.** Drowning	**N.** temperature of the central part of the body

Multiple Choice

Read each item carefully, then select the best response.

_____ 1. _____ causes body heat to be lost, as warm air in the lungs is exhaled into the atmosphere and cooler air is inhaled.

    A. Convection

    B. Conduction

    C. Radiation

    D. Respiration

_____ 2. Evaporation, the conversion of any liquid to a gas, is a process that requires:

    A. energy.

    B. circulating air.

    C. a warmer ambient temperature.

    D. all of the above

_____ 3. The rate and amount of heat loss by the body can be modified by:

    A. increasing heat production.

    B. moving to an area where heat loss is decreased.

    C. wearing insulated clothing.

    D. all of the above

_____ 4. The characteristic appearance of blue lips and/or fingertips seen in hypothermia is the result of:

    A. lack of oxygen in venous blood.

    B. frostbite.

    C. blood vessels constricting.

    D. bruising.

_____ 5. Signs and symptoms of severe systemic hypothermia include all of the following, except:

    A. weak pulse.

    B. coma.

    C. confusion.

    D. very slow respirations.

_____ 6. Hypothermia is more common among:

    A. older individuals.

    B. infants and children.

    C. those who are already ill.

    D. all of the above

_____ 7. To assess a patient's general temperature, pull back your glove and place the back of your hand on the patient's:

    A. abdomen, underneath the clothing.

    B. forehead.

    C. forearm, on the inside of the wrist.

    D. neck, at the area where you check the carotid pulse.

_____ 8. Never assume that a(n) _____, pulseless patient is dead.

    A. apneic

    B. cyanotic

    C. cold

    D. hyperthermic

_____ **9.** Management of hypothermia in the field consists of all of the following except:

    A. stabilizing vital functions.

    B. removing wet clothing.

    C. preventing further heat loss.

    D. massaging the cold extremities.

_____ **10.** When exposed parts of the body become very cold but not frozen, the condition is called:

    A. frostnip.

    B. chilblains.

    C. immersion foot.

    D. all of the above

_____ **11.** When the body is exposed to more heat energy than it loses, _____ results.

    A. hyperthermia

    B. heat cramps

    C. heat exhaustion

    D. heatstroke

_____ **12.** Contributing factors to the development of heat illnesses include:

    A. high air temperature.

    B. vigorous exercise.

    C. high humidity.

    D. all of the above

_____ **13.** Keeping yourself hydrated while on duty is very important. Drink at least _____ of water per day, and more when exertion or heat is involved.

    A. 8 glasses

    B. 1 liter

    C. 2 liters

    D. 3 liters

_____ **14.** The following statements concerning heat cramps are true except:

    A. they only occur when it is hot outdoors.

    B. they may be seen in well-conditioned athletes.

    C. the exact cause of heat cramps is not well understood.

    D. dehydration may play a role in the development of heat cramps.

_____ **15.** Signs and symptoms of heat exhaustion and associated hypovolemia include:

    A. cold, clammy skin with ashen pallor.

    B. dizziness, weakness, or faintness.

    C. normal vital signs.

    D. all of the above

_____ **16.** Be prepared to transport the patient to the hospital for aggressive treatment of hyperthermia if:

    A. the symptoms do not clear up promptly.

    B. the level of consciousness improves.

    C. the temperature drops.

    D. all of the above

_____ **17.** Often, the first sign of heatstroke is:

    A. a change in behavior.

    B. an increase in pulse rate.

    C. an increase in respirations.

    D. hot, dry, flushed skin.

_____ **18.** The least common but most serious illness caused by heat exposure, occurring when the body is subjected to more heat than it can handle and normal mechanisms for getting rid of the excess heat are overwhelmed, is:

A. hyperthermia.

B. heat cramps.

C. heat exhaustion.

D. heatstroke.

_____ **19.** _____ is the body's attempt at self-preservation by preventing water from entering the lungs.

A. Bronchoconstriction

B. Laryngospasm

C. Esophageal spasms

D. Swelling in the oropharynx

_____ **20.** Treatment of drowning/near drowning begins with:

A. opening the airway.

B. ventilation with 100% oxygen via BVM device.

C. suctioning the lungs to remove the water.

D. rescue and removal from the water.

_____ **21.** After removing a near drowning patient from the water, it may be difficult to find a pulse because of:

A. dilation of peripheral blood vessels.

B. body temperature at the core.

C. low cardiac output.

D. all of the above

_____ **22.** If the near drowning victim has evidence of upper airway obstruction by foreign matter, attempt to clear it by:

A. removing the obstruction manually.

B. suction.

C. using abdominal thrusts.

D. all of the above

_____ **23.** You should never give up on resuscitating a cold-water drowning victim because:

A. when the patient is submerged in water colder than body temperature, heat is maintained in the body.

B. the resulting hypothermia can protect vital organs from the lack of oxygen.

C. the resulting hypothermia raises the metabolic rate.

D. all of the above

_____ **24.** The three phases of a dive, in the order they occur, are:

A. ascent, descent, bottom.

B. descent, bottom, ascent.

C. orientation, bottom, ascent.

D. descent, orientation, ascent.

_____ **25.** Areas usually affected by descent problems include:

A. the lungs.

B. the skin.

C. the joints.

D. vision.

_____ **26.** Potential problems associated with rupture of the lungs include:

A. air emboli.

B. pneumomediastinum.

C. pneumothorax.

D. all of the above

_____ **27.** The organs most severely affected by air embolism are the:

    A. brain and spinal cord.

    B. brain and heart.

    C. heart and lungs.

    D. brain and lungs.

_____ **28.** Black widow spiders may be found in:

    A. New Hampshire.

    B. woodpiles.

    C. Georgia.

    D. all of the above

_____ **29.** Coral snakes may be found in:

    A. Florida.

    B. Kansas.

    C. New Jersey.

    D. all of the above

_____ **30.** Rocky Mountain spotted fever and Lyme disease are both spread through the tick's:

    A. saliva.

    B. blood.

    C. hormones.

    D. all of the above

_____ **31.** Signs of envenomation by a pit viper include:

    A. swelling.

    B. severe burning pain at the site of the injury.

    C. ecchymosis.

    D. all of the above

_____ **32.** Removal of a tick should be accomplished by:

    A. suffocating it with gasoline.

    B. burning it with a lighted match to cause it to release its grip.

    C. using fine tweezers to pull it straight out of the skin.

    D. suffocating it with Vaseline.

_____ **33.** Treatment for a black widow spider bite consists of maintaining:

    A. the airway.

    B. breathing.

    C. circulation.

    D. all of the above

_____ **34.** Treatment of a snake bite from a pit viper includes:

    A. calming the patient.

    B. providing BLS as needed if the patient shows no sign of envenomation.

    C. marking the skin with a pen over the swollen area to note whether swelling is spreading.

    D. all of the above

Questions 35-39 are derived from the following scenario: At 2:00 in the afternoon in July, the weather is 105°F and very humid. You have been called for a "man down" at the park. As you arrive, you recognize him as an alcoholic who has been a "frequent-flyer" with your service. It looks like he had been sitting under a tree when he fell over, unconscious.

_____ **35.** As you assess the patient, he has cold, clammy skin and a dry tongue. You suspect that:

    A. he is dehydrated.

    B. he has suffered heat exhaustion.

    C. he is hypothermic.

    D. all of the above

_____ **36.** As you look closer, you note that he is shivering and his respirations are 20 breaths/min. You begin to have a stronger suspicion that he is:

    A. hyperthermic.

    B. hypothermic.

    C. drunk.

    D. none of the above

_____ **37.** The direct transfer of heat from his body to the cold ground is called:

    A. conduction.

    B. convection.

    C. radiation.

    D. evaporation.

_____ **38.** You pull back on your glove and place the back of your hand on his skin at the abdomen, and the skin feels cool. Again, you suspect:

    A. hyperthermia.

    B. hypothermia.

    C. that he is drunk.

    D. none of the above

_____ **39.** How will you treat this patient?

    A. Prevent conduction heat loss.

    B. Prevent convection heat loss.

    C. Remove the patient from the environment.

    D. All of the above

Fill-in

Read each item carefully, then complete the statement by filling in the missing word.

1. Do not attempt to rewarm patients who have _____ _____ _____ hypothermia, because they are prone to developing arrhythmias unless handled very carefully.

2. Most significant diving injuries occur during _____.

3. When treating a patient with frostbite, never attempt _____ if there is any chance that the part may freeze again before the patient reaches the hospital.

4. As with so many hazards, you cannot help others if you do not practice _____.

5. _____, a common effect of hypothermia, is the body's attempt to maintain heat.

6. Whenever a person dives or jumps into very cold water, the _____ _____ may cause immediate bradycardia.

True/False

If you believe the statement to be more true than false, write the letter "T" in the space provided. If you believe the statement to be more false than true, write the letter "F."

_____ **1.** Normal body temperature is 98.6°F (37.0°C).

_____ **2.** To assess the skin temperature in a patient experiencing a generalized cold emergency, you should feel the patient's skin.

_____ **3.** Mild hypothermia occurs when the core temperature drops to 85°F.

_____ **4.** The body's most efficient heat-regulating mechanisms are sweating and dilation of skin blood vessels.

_____ **5.** People who are at greatest risk for heat illnesses are the elderly and children.

_____ **6.** The strongest stimulus for breathing is an elevation of oxygen in the blood.

_____ **7.** Immediate bradycardia after jumping in cold water is called the diving reflex.

_____ **8.** Ice should be promptly applied to any insect sting or snake bite with swelling.

_____ **9.** The most common type of pit viper is the copperhead.

_____ **10.** Cottonmouths are known for aggressive behavior.

_____ **11.** Ticks should be removed by firmly grasping them with tweezers while rotating them counterclockwise.

_____ **12.** The pain of coelenterate stings may respond to flushing with cold water.

Short Answer

Complete this section with short written answers using the space provided.

1. What are three ways to modify heat loss? Give an example of each.

_____

_____

2. What are the steps in treating heatstroke?

_____

_____

3. What is an air embolism and how does it occur?

_____

_____

4. For what diving emergencies are hyperbaric chambers used?

_____

_____

5. How should a frostbitten foot be treated?

_____

_____

6. What are four "Do Nots" in relation to local cold injuries?

_____

_____

7. What treatments for a snake bite assist with slowing and monitoring the spread of venom?

_____

_____

8. What are the two most common poisonous spiders in the United States and how do their bites differ?

_____

_____

Word Fun

The following crossword puzzle is an activity provided to reinforce correct spelling and understanding of medical terminology associated with emergency care and the EMT-B. Use the clues in the column to complete the puzzle.

Across

1. Slowing heart from sudden submersion in cold water
3. Loss of heat by direct contact
5. Less than 60 beats/min
7. Salts and chemicals in body fluids
8. Used for breathing underwater
9. Loss of heat by air movement
10. Temperature greater than 101°F

Down

2. Loss of heat to colder environment
4. Excessive heat problem, may be fatal
6. Air bubbles in blood vessels

Ambulance Calls

The following case scenarios provide an opportunity to explore the concerns associated with patient management. Read each scenario, then answer each question in detail.

1. You are called to the local airport for a 52-year-old man who is the pilot of his own aircraft. He tells you he is having severe abdominal pain and joint pain. History reveals that the patient is returning from a dive trip off the coast. He says he has had "the bends" before and this feels similar.

   How would you best manage this patient?

   _____

   _____

   _____

2. You are dispatched to a long-term care facility for an Alzheimer patient with an "unknown problem." You arrive to find several staff members who greet you at the front door. They explain that the patient wandered out the back exit door of the Alzheimer unit when the nurse was on her other rounds. They aren't sure how this happened as each patient wears a necklace that triggers an alarm if patients leave this specialized wing of the facility. They found him outside in the snow, and he has possibly been outdoors for 45 minutes.

   How do you best manage this patient?

   _____

   _____

   _____

3. You are dispatched to an unconscious female at a local beauty spa locally known for its "body wraps." You arrive to find a conscious, yet confused, 17-year-old female. A friend tells you that the patient has been using over-the-counter 'water pills' and laxative agents, along with strenuous exercise, in order to lose weight for the prom. She tells you that her friend is otherwise healthy, but she complained of feeling dizzy prior to undergoing the spa treatment.

How would you best manage this patient?

_____

_____

_____

Skill Drills
Skill Drill 18-1: Treating for Heat Exhaustion
Test your knowledge of this skill drill by filling in the correct words in the photo captions.

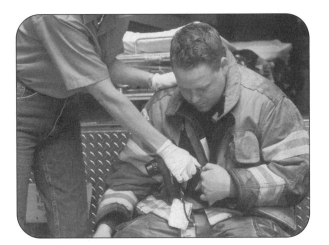

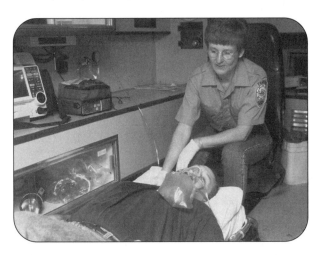

1. Remove _____ _____.

2. Move the patient to a _____ _____.
Give _____.
Place the patient in a _____ position,
elevate the legs, and _____ the patient.

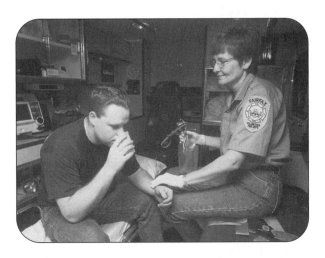

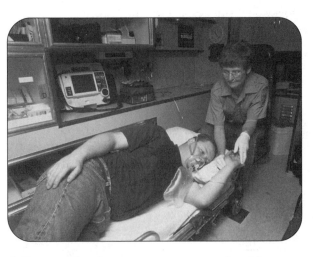

3. If the patient is _____ _____, give water by mouth.

4. If nausea develops, _____ on the side.

Skill Drill 18-2: Stabilizing a Suspected Spinal Injury in the Water
Test your knowledge of this skill drill by placing the photos below in the correct order. Number the first step with a "1," the second step with a "2," etc.

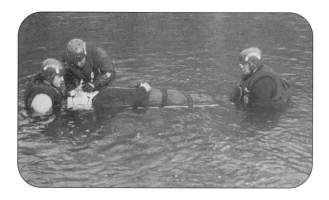

Secure the patient to the backboard.

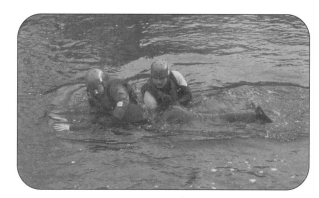

Turn the patient to a supine position by rotating the entire upper half of the body as a single unit.

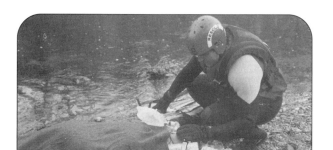

Cover the patient with a blanket and apply oxygen if breathing. Begin CPR if breathing and pulse are absent.

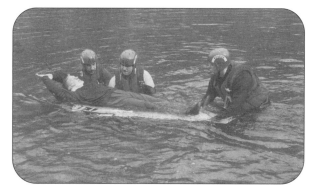

Float a buoyant backboard under the patient.

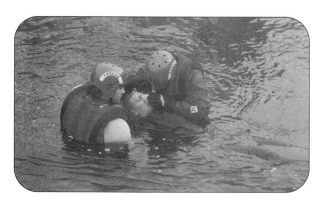

As soon as the patient is turned, begin artificial ventilation using the mouth-to-mouth method or a pocket mask.

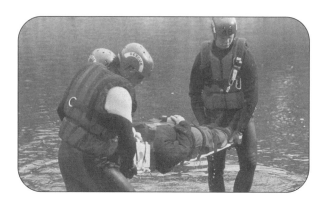

Remove the patient from the water.

Assessment Review

Answer the following questions pertaining to the assessment of the types of emergencies discussed in this chapter.

_____ 1. When assessing the circulation of a patient with cold injuries, how long should you evaluate the pulse?

A. 15 seconds

B. 30 seconds

C. 60 seconds

D. 90 seconds

_____ 2. If a patient has a cold skin temperature, he or she likely is:

A. hypothermic.

B. hyperthermic.

C. alcoholic.

D. none of the above

_____ 3. If a patient has a hot skin temperature, he or she likely is:

A. hypothermic.

B. hyperthermic.

C. alcoholic.

D. none of the above

_____ 4. When treating multiple victims of lightning strikes, who should you concentrate your efforts on first?

A. Conscious patients

B. Unconscious patients in respiratory or cardiac arrest

C. All unconscious patients

D. None of the above

_____ 5. What is the best method of inactivating a jellyfish sting?

A. Urinating

B. Flushing the site with cold water

C. Applying vinegar

D. Applying an ice pack

Emergency Care Summary

Complete the statements pertaining to emergency care for the types of emergencies discussed in this chapter by filling in the missing words.

NOTE: While the steps below are widely accepted, be sure to consult and follow your local protocol.

Cold Injuries	Heat Injuries	Drowning and Diving Injuries
1. Remove wet clothing and keep the patient dry. 2. Prevent heat loss. Move the patient away from any wet or cold surface. 3. _____ all exposed body parts by wrapping them in a blanket or dry, bulky material. 4. Prevent _____ heat loss by erecting a wind barrier around the patient. 5. Remove the patient from the _____ _____ as promptly as possible.	1. Remove any excess layers of clothing. 2. Move the patient promptly from the hot environment and out of the sun. 3. Provide _____, if not already done during the initial assessment. 4. Encourage the patient to lie _____ with legs _____. Loosen any tight clothing and _____ the patient. 5. If the patient is alert, encourage him or her to sit up and slowly drink a _____ of water if _____ does not develop. 6. Transport patient in the _____ _____ recumbent position.	1. Turn the patient to a _____ position by rotating the entire upper half of the body as a single unit. 2. Begin artificial ventilation using the mouth-to-mouth method or a _____ _____. 3. Float a buoyant _____ under the patient. 4. Secure the patient to the backboard. 5. Remove the patient from the water. 6. Cover the patient with a blanket and apply _____ if breathing. Begin CPR if breathing and pulse are absent.

Lightning Injuries	Spider Bites	Snake Bites	Injuries From Marine Animals
1. Move patient to a sheltered area. 2. Those who are _____ following a lightning strike are much less likely to develop delayed respiratory or _____ _____; most of these victims will survive. Therefore, you should focus your efforts on those who are in respiratory or _____ _____.	**Black Widow Spider** 1. Provide _____ for patient in respiratory distress. 2. Transport the patient to the emergency department as soon as possible for treatment of pain and muscle _____. 3. If possible, bring the _____. **Brown Recluse Spider** If bite causes systemic symptoms: 1. Provide BLS. 2. Transport to emergency department. 3. If possible, bring the spider.	**Using an AnaKit** 1. Prepare the injection site with antiseptic, and remove the needle cover. 2. Hold the syringe upright, and carefully use the _____ to remove air. 3. Turn the plunger _____ _____ turn. 4. Quickly insert the needle into the _____. 5. Holding the syringe steady, push the plunger until it stops. 6. Have the patient chew and swallow the Chlo-Amine _____ tablets provided in the kit. 7. If available, apply a _____ _____ to the sting site.	1. Limit further _____ of nematocysts by avoiding fresh water, wet sand, showers, or careless manipulation of the tentacles. Keep the patient calm and _____ motion of the affected extremity. 2. Inactivate the nematocysts by applying _____. 3. Remove the remaining tentacles by scraping them off with the edges of a sharp, stiff object such as a _____ _____. 4. Provide prompt transport.

CHAPTER

19 Behavioral Emergencies

Workbook Activities

The following activities have been designed to help you. Your instructor may require you to complete some or all of these activities as a regular part of your EMT-B training program. You are encouraged to complete any activity that your instructor does not assign as a way to enhance your learning in the classroom.

Chapter Review

The following exercises provide an opportunity to refresh your knowledge of this chapter.

Matching

Match each of the terms in the left column to the appropriate definition in the right column.

_____ **1.** Behavioral crisis

_____ **2.** Psychogenic

_____ **3.** Organic brain syndrome

_____ **4.** Depression

_____ **5.** Functional disorder

_____ **6.** Behavior

A. what you can see of a person's response to the environment; his or her actions

B. temporary or permanent dysfunction of the brain caused by a disturbance in brain tissue function

C. any reaction to events that interferes with activities of daily living or is unacceptable to the patient or others

D. a persistent mood of sadness, despair, or discouragement

E. abnormal operation of an organ that cannot be traced to an obvious change in structure or physiology of the organ

F. a symptom or illness caused by mental factors as opposed to physical ones

Multiple Choice

Read each item carefully, then select the best response.

_____   **1.** A psychological or behavioral crisis may be due to:

    A. mind-altering substances.

    B. the emergency situation.

    C. stress.

    D. all of the above

_____   **2.** A normal reaction to a crisis situation would be:

    A. Monday morning blues that last until Friday.

    B. feeling "blue" after the break up of a long-term relationship.

    C. feeling depressed week after week with no discernible cause.

    D. all of the above

_____   **3.** The cause of a behavioral crisis experienced by an unmanageable patient may be:

    A. drug use.

    B. a history of mental illness.

    C. alcohol abuse.

    D. all of the above

_____   **4.** Learning to adapt to a variety of situations in daily life, including stresses and strains, is called:

    A. disruption.

    B. adjustment.

    C. behavior.

    D. functional.

_____   **5.** If the interruption of daily routine tends to recur on a regular basis, the behavior is also considered a _____ problem.

    A. mental health

    B. functional disorder

    C. behavioral

    D. psychogenic

_____   **6.** If an abnormal or disturbing pattern of behavior lasts for at least _____, it is regarded as a matter of concern from a mental health standpoint.

    A. 6 weeks

    B. a month

    C. 6 months

    D. a year

_____   **7.** A person who is no longer able to respond appropriately to the environment may be having what is called a psychological or _____ emergency.

    A. psychiatric

    B. behavioral

    C. functional

    D. adjustment

_____   **8.** Mental disorders may be caused by a:

    A. social disturbance.

    B. chemical disturbance.

    C. biological disturbance.

    D. all of the above

_____ **9.** An altered mental status may arise from:

    A. an oxygen saturation of 98%.

    B. moderate temperatures.

    C. an inadequate blood flow to the brain.

    D. adequate glucose levels in the blood.

_____ **10.** Organic brain syndrome may be caused by:

    A. hypoglycemia.

    B. excessive heat or cold.

    C. lack of oxygen.

    D. all of the above

_____ **11.** An example of a functional disorder would be:

    A. schizophrenia.

    B. organic brain syndrome.

    C. Alzheimer's.

    D. all of the above

_____ **12.** When documenting abnormal behavior, it is important to:

    A. record detailed, subjective findings.

    B. avoid judgmental statements.

    C. avoid quoting the patient's own words.

    D. all of the above

_____ **13.** Safety guidelines for behavioral emergencies include:

    A. assessing the scene.

    B. being prepared to spend extra time.

    C. encouraging purposeful movement.

    D. all of the above

_____ **14.** In evaluating a situation that is considered a behavioral emergency, the first things to consider are:

    A. airway and breathing.

    B. scene safety and patient response.

    C. history of medications.

    D. respiratory and circulatory status.

_____ **15.** Psychogenic circumstances may include:

    A. severe depression.

    B. death of a loved one.

    C. a history of mental illness.

    D. all of the above

_____ **16.** Risk factors for suicide may include:

    A. denial of alcohol use.

    B. recent marriage.

    C. holidays.

    D. all of the above

_____ **17.** Suicidal patients may also be:

    A. homicidal.

    B. hypoxic.

    C. joking.

    D. seeking attention.

_____ **18.** Causes of altered behavior in geriatric patients may include:

 A. constipation.

 B. diabetes.

 C. stroke.

 D. all of the above

_____ **19.** Restraint of a person must be ordered by:

 A. a physician.

 B. a court order.

 C. a law enforcement officer.

 D. all of the above

_____ **20.** When restraining a patient without an appropriate order, legal actions may involve charges of:

 A. abandonment.

 B. negligence.

 C. battery.

 D. breach of duty.

_____ **21.** When restraining a patient face down on a stretcher, it is necessary to constantly reassess the patient's:

 A. level of consciousness.

 B. airway.

 C. emotional status.

 D. pulse rate.

Questions 22-26 are derived from the following scenario: Dean, a man in his 50s, is acting irrationally. His wife states he thinks he is a dictator of a small country, and is wearing nothing but a baseball cap and a belt with a small handgun attached to it.

_____ **22.** What is your best course of action?

 A. Call ALS.

 B. Assess Dean from a distance.

 C. Have his wife take the gun from him.

 D. Call for police back-up.

_____ **23.** The scene is safe. Dean now tells you he is "God," and can do anything he wants to. Is this a psychiatric emergency?

 A. Yes.

 B. No.

 C. This is normal behavior.

 D. None of the above

_____ **24.** How should you approach Dean?

 A. Identify yourself.

 B. Be direct.

 C. Express interest in Dean's story.

 D. All of the above

_____ **25.** Dean becomes agitated and states, "You'll never take me alive." Ordinarily, who can order restraint?

 A. Physician

 B. Court

 C. Law enforcement officer

 D. All of the above

_____ **26.** How many people should be present to restrain Dean?

 A. 2

 B. 4

 C. 6

 D. None of the above

Fill-in

Read each item carefully, then complete the statement by filling in the missing word.

1. _____ is what you can see of a person's response to the environment; his or her actions.

2. A _____ _____ or emergency is any reaction to events that interferes with the activities of daily living or has become unacceptable to the patient, family, or community.

3. Chronic _____, or a persistent feeling of sadness or despair, may be a symptom of a mental or physical disorder.

4. _____ _____ _____ is a temporary or permanent dysfunction of the brain caused by a disturbance in the physical or physiologic functioning of the brain.

5. Any time you encounter an emotionally depressed patient, you must consider the possibility of _____.

True/False

If you believe the statement to be more true than false, write the letter "T" in the space provided. If you believe the statement to be more false than true, write the letter "F."

_____ 1. Depression lasting 2 to 3 weeks after being fired from a job is a normal mental health response.

_____ 2. Low blood glucose or lack of oxygen to the brain may cause behavioral changes, but not to the degree that a psychiatric emergency could exist.

_____ 3. From a mental health standpoint, a pattern of abnormal behavior must last at least 3 months to be a matter of concern.

_____ 4. A disturbed patient should always be transported with restraints.

_____ 5. It is sometimes helpful to allow a patient with a behavioral emergency some time alone to calm down and collect their thoughts.

_____ 6. It is important to avoid looking directly at the patient when dealing with a behavioral crisis.

_____ 7. A patient should never be asked if he or she is considering suicide.

_____ 8. Urinary tract infections can cause behavioral changes in elderly patients.

_____ 9. All individuals with mental health disorders are dangerous, violent, or otherwise unmanageable.

_____ 10. When completing the documentation, it is important to record detailed, subjective findings that support the conclusion of abnormal behavior.

_____ 11. When restraining a patient, at least four people should be present to carry out the restraint.

Short Answer

Complete this section with short written answers using the space provided.

1. What is the distinction between a behavioral crisis and a mental health problem?

_____

_____

2. What three major areas should be considered in evaluating the possible source of a behavioral crisis?

_____

_____

3. What are three factors to consider in determining the level of force required to restrain a patient?

_____

_____

4. List ten safety guidelines for dealing with behavioral emergencies.

_____

_____

5. List ten risk factors for suicide.

_____

_____

Word Fun

The following crossword puzzle is a good way to review correct spelling and meaning of medical terminology associated with emergency care and the EMT-B. Use the clues in the column to complete the puzzle.

Across

3. Reactions interfere with normal activities

5. Illness with psychological symptoms

6. Caused by mental factors; not physical

7. Persistent sadness; despair

Down

1. A change in behavior

2. No known physiologic reason for abnormality

4. Basic doings of a normal person

Ambulance Calls

The following case scenarios provide an opportunity to explore the concerns associated with patient management. Read each scenario, then answer each question in detail.

1. You are dispatched to a non-emergency transport of a female from a local hospital emergency department to a care facility that provides treatment for emotionally disturbed teenagers. She became violent in the ED and was placed in 4-point restraints. As you begin transporting the patient, she begins to cry and asks you to remove the restraints.

How do you best manage this patient?

_____

_____

_____

2. You are dispatched to a "suicide attempt" at a private residence. When you arrive on scene, you are greeted by a calm, middle-aged man who appears to have been crying. He tells you that he was on the phone with his sister who lives out of state, and that she must have called for the ambulance. Dispatch informed you via cellular phone that this man recently lost his wife of 15 years to breast cancer.

How do you best manage this patient?

_____

_____

_____

3. You are dispatched to the residence of a 40-year-old woman who is upset over the loss of her mother 5 weeks ago. She tells you that she has no family and has cared for her elderly mother for the past 7 years. She has not eaten for several days and is severely depressed.

How would you best manage this patient?

_____

_____

_____

Assessment Review

Answer the following questions pertaining to the assessment of the types of emergencies discussed in this chapter. Questions 1-5 are based on risk factors in assessing the level of danger in a behavior call.

_____ **1.** When assessing the history, what past behavior(s) do you want to know the patient has exhibited?

  A. Hostile behavior

  B. Overly aggressive behavior

  C. Violent behavior

  D. All of the above

_____ **2.** Physical tension is often a warning signal of impeding hostility. What sign might warn you of physical tension?

  A. Posture

  B. Eye movement

  C. Facial expression

  D. Laughter

_____ **3.** What warning signs can be detected from the scene?

  A. Is the patient holding a potentially lethal object?

  B. Is he or she near a potentially lethal object?

  C. Does he or she keep looking at a potentially lethal object?

  D. All of the above

_____ **4.** What kind of speech may be an indicator of emotional distress?

  A. Loud speech

  B. Obscene speech

  C. Erratic and bizarre speech

  D. All of the above

_____ **5.** What type of physical activity may be an indicator of risk to the EMT-B?

  A. Tense muscles

  B. Clenched fists

  C. Pacing or glaring eyes

  D. All of the above

Emergency Care Summary

Complete the statements pertaining to emergency care for the types of emergencies discussed in this chapter by filling in the missing words.

> _NOTE:_ While the steps below are widely accepted, be sure to consult and follow your local protocol.

Behavioral Emergencies

The main task is to diffuse and _____ the situation and _____ _____ the patient. Risk factors to assess the level of danger include:

1. **History**—Has the patient previously exhibited hostile, overly aggressive, or violent behavior?

2. **Posture**—Physical _____ is often a warning signal of impending hostility.

3. **The scene**—Is the patient holding or near potentially lethal objects?

4. **Vocal activity**—What kind of speech is the patient using? Loud, obscene, erratic, and bizarre speech patterns usually indicate _____ _____.

5. **Physical activity**—The patient who has tense muscles, clenched fists, or glaring eyes; is pacing; cannot sit still; or is fiercely protecting personal space requires careful watching. Agitation may predict a quick escalation to _____.

CHAPTER

20 Obstetric and Gynecologic Emergencies

Workbook Activities

The following activities have been designed to help you. Your instructor may require you to complete some or all of these activities as a regular part of your EMT-B training program. You are encouraged to complete any activity that your instructor does not assign as a way to enhance your learning in the classroom.

Chapter Review

The following exercises provide an opportunity to refresh your knowledge of this chapter.

Matching

Match each of the terms in the left column to the appropriate definition in the right column.

_____ **1.** Cervix

_____ **2.** Perineum

_____ **3.** Placenta

_____ **4.** Amniotic sac

_____ **5.** Fetus

_____ **6.** Birth canal

_____ **7.** Uterus

_____ **8.** Umbilical cord

_____ **9.** Vagina

_____ **10.** Breech presentation

_____ **11.** Limb presentation

_____ **12.** Multipara

_____ **13.** Nuchal cord

_____ **14.** Presentation

_____ **15.** Miscarriage

A. an umbilical cord that is wrapped around the infant's neck

B. a fluid-filled, bag-like membrane inside the uterus that grows around the developing fetus

C. the area of skin between the vagina and the anus

D. the neck of the uterus

E. Connects mother and infant

F. the outermost part of a woman's reproductive system

G. the part of the infant that appears first

H. the vagina and lower part of the uterus

I. a woman who has had more than one live birth

J. spontaneous abortion

K. delivery in which the presenting part is a single arm, leg, or foot

L. tissue that develops on the wall of the uterus and is connected to the fetus

M. the hollow organ inside the female pelvis where the fetus grows

N. the developing baby in the uterus

O. delivery in which the buttocks come out first

Multiple Choice

Read each item carefully, then select the best response.

_____ **1.** In the event of a nuchal cord, proper procedure is to:

   A. gently slip the cord over the infant's head or shoulder.

   B. clamp the cord and cut it before delivering the infant.

   C. clamp the cord and cut it, then gently unwind it from around the neck if wrapped around more than once.

   D. all of the above

_____ **2.** If the amniotic fluid is greenish instead of clear or has a foul odor, this is called:

   A. nuchal rigidity.

   B. meconium staining.

   C. placenta previa.

   D. bloody show.

_____ **3.** Once the entire infant is delivered, you should immediately:

   A. wrap it in a towel and place it on one side with head lowered.

   B. be sure the head is covered and keep the neck in a neutral position.

   C. use a sterile gauze pad to wipe the infant's mouth, then suction again.

   D. all of the above

_____ **4.** You may help control bleeding by massaging the _____ after delivery of the placenta.

   A. perineum

   B. fundus

   C. lower back

   D. inner thighs

_____ **5.** The APGAR score should be calculated at _____ minutes after birth.

   A. 1 and 5

   B. 3 and 7

   C. 2 and 10

   D. 4 and 8

_____ **6.** Once the infant is delivered, feel for a brachial pulse or the pulsations in the umbilical cord. The pulse rate should be at least _____ beats/min and if not, begin artificial ventilations.

   A. 60

   B. 80

   C. 100

   D. 120

_____ **7.** When assisting ventilations in a newborn with a BVM device, the rate is _____ breaths/min.

   A. 20 to 30

   B. 30 to 50

   C. 35 to 45

   D. 40 to 60

_____ **8.** When performing CPR on a newborn, you should perform a combined total of _____ ventilations and compressions per minute.

   A. 90

   B. 100

   C. 110

   D. 120

_____ **9.** You cannot successfully deliver a _____ presentation in the field.

    A. limb

    B. breech

    C. vertex

    D. all of the above

_____ **10.** Care for a mother with a prolapsed cord includes:

    A. positioning the mother to keep the weight of the infant off the cord.

    B. high-flow oxygen and rapid transport.

    C. use your hand to physically hold the infant's head off the cord.

    D. all of the above

_____ **11.** When handling a delivery of a drug- or alcohol-addicted mother, your first concern should be for:

    A. the airway of the mother.

    B. your personal safety.

    C. the airway of the infant.

    D. the need for CPR for the infant.

_____ **12.** The stages of labor include:

    A. dilation of the cervix.

    B. expulsion of the baby.

    C. delivery of the placenta.

    D. all of the above

_____ **13.** The first stage of labor begins with the onset of contractions and ends when:

    A. the infant is born.

    B. the cervix is fully dilated.

    C. the water breaks.

    D. the placenta is delivered.

_____ **14.** Signs of the beginning of labor include:

    A. bloody show.

    B. contractions of the uterus.

    C. rupture of the amniotic sac.

    D. all of the above

_____ **15.** The second stage of labor begins when the cervix is fully dilated and ends when:

    A. the infant is born.

    B. the water breaks.

    C. the placenta delivers.

    D. the uterus stops contracting.

_____ **16.** The third stage of labor begins with the birth of the infant and ends with the:

    A. release of milk from the breasts.

    B. cessation of uterine contractions.

    C. delivery of the placenta.

    D. cutting of the umbilical cord.

_____ **17.** The difference between pre-eclampsia and eclampsia is the onset of:

    A. seeing spots.

    B. seizures.

    C. swelling in the hands and feet.

    D. headaches.

_____ **18.** You should consider the possibility of a(n) _____ in women who have missed a menstrual cycle and complain of a sudden stabbing and usually unilateral pain in the lower abdomen.

   A. PID

   B. ectopic pregnancy

   C. miscarriage

   D. placenta abruptio

_____ **19.** Consider delivery of the fetus at the scene when:

   A. delivery can be expected within a few minutes.

   B. when a natural disaster, or other problem, makes it impossible to reach the hospital.

   C. no transportation is available.

   D. all of the above

_____ **20.** When in doubt about the possibility of an imminent delivery:

   A. go for help if you are alone.

   B. insert two fingers into the vagina to feel for the head.

   C. contact medical control for further guidance.

   D. all of the above

_____ **21.** Low blood pressure resulting from compression of the inferior vena cava by the weight of the fetus when the mother is supine is called:

   A. pregnancy-induced hypertension.

   B. placenta previa.

   C. placenta abruptio.

   D. supine hypotensive syndrome.

_____ **22.** _____ is a situation in which the umbilical cord comes out of the vagina before the infant.

   A. Eclampsia

   B. Placenta previa

   C. Placenta abruptio

   D. Prolapsed cord

_____ **23.** Premature separation of the placenta from the wall of the uterus is known as:

   A. eclampsia.

   B. placenta previa.

   C. placenta abruptio.

   D. prolapsed cord.

_____ **24.** _____ is a condition in which the placenta develops over and covers the cervix.

   A. Eclampsia

   B. Placenta previa

   C. Placenta abruptio

   D. Prolapsed cord

_____ **25.** _____ is heralded by the onset of convulsions, or seizures, resulting from severe hypertension in the pregnant woman.

   A. Eclampsia

   B. Placenta previa

   C. Placenta abruptio

   D. Supine hypotensive syndrome

_____ **26.** _____ is a condition of infants who are born to alcoholic mothers; it is characterized by physical and mental retardation and a variety of congenital abnormalities.

   A. Pregnancy-induced hypertension

   B. Ectopic pregnancy

   C. Fetal alcohol syndrome

   D. Supine hypotensive syndrome

Questions 27-31 are derived from the following scenario: You have been dispatched to the side of a highway where a woman is reported to be delivering a baby. As you approach the vehicle, you see her lying down in the back seat.

_____ **27.** Which of the following signs/symptoms tell you that the birth is imminent?
   A. Her water has broken.
   B. Her contractions are 30 to 60 minutes apart.
   C. Multigravida 4, Multipara 3
   D. All of the above

_____ **28.** As you prepare her for delivery, what position should she be placed in?
   A. Supine, on the back seat
   B. Supine, on the ground
   C. Supine, one foot on the ground and one foot on the seat
   D. Seated

_____ **29.** As you perform a visual exam, you note crowning. This means that:
   A. the baby is making a crowing-type of sound.
   B. the baby cannot be visualized.
   C. you can visualize the baby's head.
   D. the father is excited and needs care.

_____ **30.** Once the head has been delivered:
   A. suction the nose, and then the mouth.
   B. apply oxygen over the vagina.
   C. suction the mouth, then the nose.
   D. apply a nasal cannula at 3 L/min to the child.

_____ **31.** Concerning the delivery of the placenta, which of the following are emergency situations?
   A. More than 30 minutes have elapsed and the placenta has not delivered.
   B. There is more than 500 mL of bleeding before delivery of the placenta.
   C. There is significant bleeding after delivery of the placenta.
   D. All of the above

Tables

Complete the following table for the APGAR scoring system by listing the characteristics for each score.

Area of Activity	Score		
	2	1	0
Appearance			
Pulse			
Grimace or Irritability			
Activity or Muscle Tone			
Respiration			

Labeling

Label the following diagram with the correct terms.

1. Anatomic structures of the pregnant woman

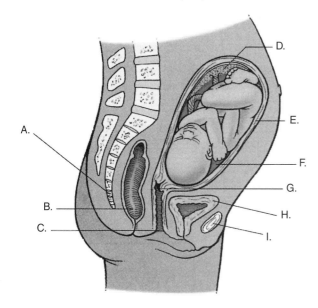

A. _____

B. _____

C. _____

D. _____

E. _____

F. _____

G. _____

H. _____

I. _____

Fill-in

Read each item carefully, then complete the statement by filling in the missing word(s).

1. After delivery, the _____, or afterbirth, separates from the uterus and is delivered.

2. The umbilical cord contains two _____ and one _____.

3. The amniotic sac contains about _____ _____ _____ of amniotic fluid, which helps to insulate and protect the floating fetus as it develops.

4. A full-term pregnancy is from _____ to _____ weeks, counting from the first day of the last menstrual cycle.

5. The pregnancy is divided into three _____ of about 3 months each.

6. There is a high potential of exposure due to _____ _____ released during childbirth.

7. The leading cause of maternal death in the first trimester is internal hemorrhage into the abdomen following rupture of an _____ _____.

8. In serious trauma, the only chance to save the infant is to adequately _____ the mother.

9. During the delivery, be careful that you do not poke your fingers into the infant's eyes or into the two soft spots, called _____, on the head.

True/False

If you believe the statement to be more true than false, write the letter "T" in the space provided. If you believe the statement to be more false than true, write the letter "F."

_____ **1.** The small mucous plug from the cervix that is discharged from the vagina, often at the beginning of labor, is called a bloody show.

_____ **2.** Crowning occurs when the baby's head obstructs the birth canal, preventing normal delivery.

_____ **3.** Labor begins with the rupture of the amniotic sac and ends with the delivery of the baby's head.

_____ **4.** A woman who is having her first baby is called a multigravida.

_____ **5.** Once labor has begun, it can be slowed by holding the patient's legs together.

_____ **6.** Delivery of the buttocks before the baby's head is called a breech delivery.

_____ **7.** After delivery, the baby should be kept at the same level as the mother's vagina until after the cord is cut.

_____ **8.** The placenta and cord should be properly disposed of in a biohazard container after delivery.

_____ **9.** The umbilical cord may be gently pulled to aid in delivery of the placenta.

_____ **10.** A limb presentation occurs when the baby's arm, leg, or foot is emerging from the vagina first.

_____ **11.** Multiple births may have more than one placenta.

Short Answer

Complete this section with short written answers using the space provided.

1. What are some possible causes of vaginal hemorrhage in early and late pregnancy?

_____

_____

2. In what position should pregnant patients who are not delivering be transported and why?

_____

_____

3. List three signs that indicate the beginning of labor.

_____

_____

4. Under what three circumstances should you consider delivering the patient at the scene?

_____

_____

5. Once the baby's head emerges, what actions should be taken to prevent too rapid a delivery?

_____

_____

6. Why is it important to avoid pushing on the fontanels?

_____

_____

7. How can you help decrease perineal tearing?

_____

_____

8. What are the two situations in which an EMT-B may insert his or her fingers into a patient's vagina?

_____

_____

9. What are three fetal effects of maternal drug or alcohol addiction?

_____

_____

Word Fun

The following crossword puzzle is an activity provided to reinforce correct spelling and understanding of medical terminology associated with emergency care and the EMT-B. Use the clues in the column to complete the puzzle.

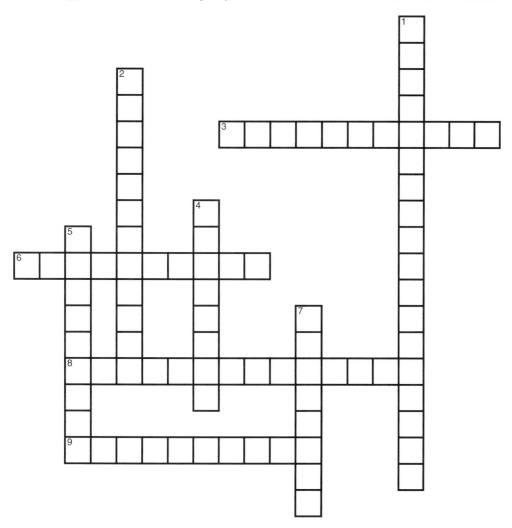

Across

3. Fluid-filled bag for developing fetus

6. Umbilicus wrapped around baby's neck

8. Develops over and covers the cervix

9. Rating of newborn on 5 factors

Down

1. Buttocks first

2. Previously given birth

4. Head showing during labor

5. Convulsions from hypertension in pregnant woman

7. Area of skin between anus and vagina, subject to tearing during birth process

Ambulance Calls

The following case scenarios provide an opportunity to explore the concerns associated with patient management. Read each scenario, then answer each question in detail.

1. You are dispatched to a grocery store for an "unknown medical problem." You arrive to find a 20-year-old woman who is in her 22nd week of pregnancy. She tells you that this is her first pregnancy and she had made an appointment to see her obstetrician later that day because she was not feeling well. She's been experiencing a headache, swelling in her hands and feet, and transient problems with her vision. She states that she suddenly felt lightheaded and had to sit down. She appears unhurt.

How do you best manage this patient?

_____

_____

_____

2. You are enjoying a quiet lunch at the fire station when you hear the back doorbell ring. As you look out the window, you see a young woman running away from the building. You open the door to call to her and when you look down, you see something bundled in a wet sheet. It's a newborn; she's wet with amniotic fluid and she's not breathing very well.

How do you best manage this patient?

_____

_____

_____

3. You are on the scene with a 32-year-old woman who is 38 weeks pregnant and delivery is imminent. As the infant starts to crown, you notice that the amniotic sac is still intact.

How would you best manage this patient?

_____

_____

_____

Skill Drills

Skill Drill 20-1: Delivering the Baby

Test your knowledge of this skill drill by placing the photos below in the correct order. Number the first step with a "1," the second step with a "2," etc. Also, fill in the correct words in the photo captions.

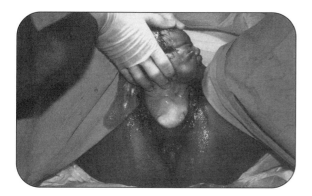

Support the head and upper body as the _____ _____ delivers, guiding the head _____ if needed.

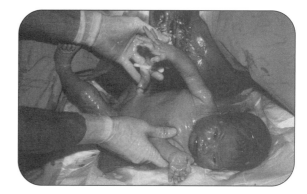

Place the umbilical cord clamps _____ inch(es) to _____ inch(es) apart, and _____ between them.

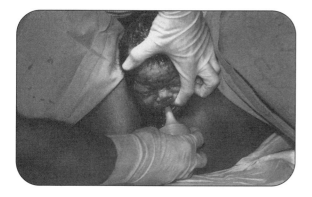

Support the _____ parts of the head with your hands as it emerges. Suction fluid from the _____, then _____.

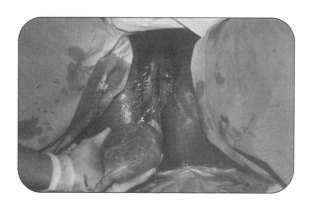

Allow the _____ to deliver itself. Do not pull on the _____ to speed delivery.

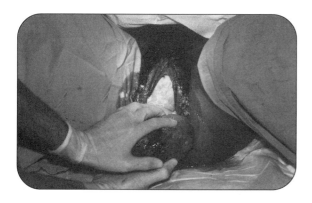

As the _____ _____ appears, guide the head _____ slightly, if needed, to deliver the _____.

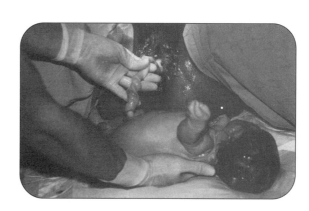

Handle the slippery, delivered infant firmly but gently, keeping the neck in _____ position to _____ the airway.

Skill Drill 20-2: Giving Chest Compressions to an Infant
Test your knowledge of this skill drill by filling in the correct words in the photo captions.

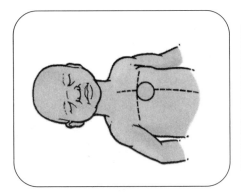
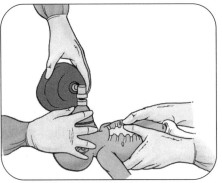
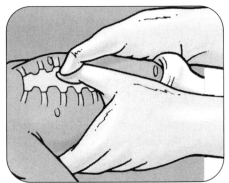

1. Find the proper position: just below the _____ _____, middle or _____ _____ of the sternum.

2. Wrap your hands around the body, with your _____ resting at that position.

3. Press your thumbs gently against the sternum, compressing _____ inch(es) to _____ inch(es) deep.

Assessment Review

Answer the following questions pertaining to the assessment of the types of emergencies discussed in this chapter.

_____ 1. After the head has been delivered and the shoulder appears:
   A. guide the head down slightly, to deliver the shoulder.
   B. apply a nasal cannula to the child.
   C. guide the head up slightly, to deliver the shoulder.
   D. pull gently.

_____ 2. When giving chest compressions to an infant:
   A. press the palm of your hand over the sternum, compressing ½ to ¾ inches deep.
   B. press the palm of your hand over the sternum, compressing 1 to 1½ inches deep.
   C. compress at a rate of 60 to 80 times a minute.
   D. compress the sternum ½ to ¾ inches deep.

_____ 3. Which exam will you perform before delivery?
   A. Focused physical
   B. Rapid physical
   C. Detailed physical
   D. All of the above

_____ 4. What should the focused physical exam include?
   A. The abdomen
   B. The length and frequency of contractions
   C. The vagal opening
   D. All of the above

_____ 5. When cutting the umbilical cord:
   A. place the clamps 7 to 10 inches apart.
   B. place the clamps 2 to 4 inches apart.
   C. tie the cord with shoelaces if you don't have any clamps.
   D. tie the cord with string if you don't have any clamps.

Emergency Care Summary

Complete the statements pertaining to emergency care for the types of emergencies discussed in this chapter by filling in the missing words.

NOTE: While the steps below are widely accepted, be sure to consult and follow your local protocol.

Delivering the Baby

1. Support the _____ parts of the head with your hands as it emerges. Suction fluid from the baby's _____, then _____.

2. As the upper shoulder appears, guide the head _____ slightly, if needed, to deliver the shoulder.

3. Support the head and upper body as the lower shoulder delivers, guiding the head _____ if needed.

4. Handle the slippery, delivered infant firmly but gently, keeping the neck in _____ position to maintain the airway.

5. Place the umbilical cord clamps ___" to ___" apart, and cut between them.

6. Allow the placenta to deliver itself. Do not pull on the cord to speed delivery.

Giving Chest Compressions to an Infant

1. Find the proper position——just below the nipple line, _____ or _____ third of the sternum.

2. Wrap your hands around the body, with your thumbs resting at that position.

3. Press the two thumbs against the sternum, compressing ___" to ___" deep.

Premature Infant

1. Keep the infant warm. Keep the infant in a place where the temperature is between ___°F and ___°F (between ___°C and ___°C).

2. Keep the mouth and nose clear of mucus with a

   _____ _____.

3. Inspect the cut end of the cord attached to the infant for

   _____.

4. Give _____ into a small tent over the infant's head.

5. Do not infect the infant. Wear a mask to help prevent you from breathing on the infant.

6. Notify the hospital of a neonatal transport.

CHAPTER

21 Kinematics of Trauma

Workbook Activities

The following activities have been designed to help you. Your instructor may require you to complete some or all of these activities as a regular part of your EMT-B training program. You are encouraged to complete any activity that your instructor does not assign as a way to enhance your learning in the classroom.

Chapter Review

The following exercises provide an opportunity to refresh your knowledge of this chapter.

Matching

Match each of the terms in the left column to the appropriate definition in the right column.

_____ 1. Cavitation

_____ 2. Deceleration

_____ 3. Kinetic energy

_____ 4. Mechanism of injury

_____ 5. Potential energy

_____ 6. Blunt trauma

_____ 7. Penetrating trauma

_____ 8. Work

A. impact on the body by objects that cause injury without penetrating soft tissue or internal organs and cavities

B. force acting over a distance

C. product of mass, gravity, and height

D. injury caused by objects that pierce the surface of the body

E. how trauma occurs

F. energy of moving object

G. slowing

H. emanation of pressure waves that can damage nearby structures

Multiple Choice

Read each item carefully, then select the best response.

_____ 1. The following are concepts of energy typically associated with injury, except:

    A. potential energy.

    B. thermal energy.

    C. kinetic energy.

    D. work.

_____ 2. The energy of a moving object is called:

    A. potential energy.

    B. thermal energy.

    C. kinetic energy.

    D. work.

_____ 3. Energy may be:

    A. created.

    B. destroyed.

    C. converted.

    D. all of the above

_____ 4. The amount of kinetic energy that is converted to do work on the body dictates the _____ of the injury.

    A. location

    B. severity

    C. cause

    D. speed

_____ 5. Potential energy is mostly associated with the energy of:

    A. falling objects.

    B. motor vehicle crashes.

    C. pedestrian vs. bicycle crashes.

    D. gun shot wounds.

_____ 6. Motor vehicle crashes are classified traditionally as:

    A. frontal.

    B. rollover.

    C. lateral.

    D. all of the above

_____ 7. The three collisions in a frontal impact include all of the following, except:

    A. car vs. object.

    B. passenger vs. vehicle.

    C. flying objects vs. passengers.

    D. internal organs vs. solid structures of the body.

_____ 8. The mechanism of injury provides information about the severity of the collision and therefore has a(n) _____ effect on patient care.

    A. direct

    B. positive

    C. indirect

    D. negative

_____ **9.** Your index of suspicion for the presence of life-threatening injuries should automatically increase if you see:

    A. seats torn from their mountings.

    B. collapsed steering wheels.

    C. intrusion into the passenger compartment.

    D. all of the above

_____ **10.** In a motor vehicle crash, as the passenger's head hits the windshield, the brain continues to move forward until it strikes the inside of the skull resulting in a _____ injury.

    A. compression

    B. laceration

    C. lateral

    D. motion

_____ **11.** Your quick initial assessment of the patient and the evaluation of the _____ can help to direct lifesaving care and provide critical information to the hospital staff.

    A. scene

    B. index of suspicion

    C. mechanism of injury

    D. abdominal area

_____ **12.** A contusion to a patient's forehead along with a spiderwebbed windshield suggests possible injury to the:

    A. nose.

    B. brain.

    C. face.

    D. heart.

_____ **13.** Significant mechanisms of injury include:

    A. moderate intrusions from a lateral impact.

    B. severe damage from the rear.

    C. collisions in which rotation is involved.

    D. all of the above

_____ **14.** Significant clues to the possibility of severe injuries include:

    A. death of a passenger.

    B. a blown out tire.

    C. broken glass.

    D. a deployed airbag.

_____ **15.** When properly applied, seat belts are successful in:

    A. restraining the passengers in a vehicle.

    B. preventing a second collision inside the motor vehicle.

    C. decreasing the severity of the third collision.

    D. all of the above

_____ **16.** Air bags decrease injury to all of the following, except:

    A. chest.

    B. heart.

    C. face.

    D. head.

_____ **17.** Signs of most injuries sustained in a motor vehicle crash can be found by simply inspecting the _____ during extrication of the patient.

    A. head and neck

    B. chest

    C. interior of the vehicle

    D. torso

_____ **18.** _____ impacts are probably the number one cause of death associated with motor vehicle crashes.

    A. Frontal

    B. Lateral

    C. Rear-end

    D. Rollover

_____ **19.** The most common life-threatening event in a rollover is _____ or partial ejection of the passenger from the vehicle.

    A. "sandwiching"

    B. centrifugal force

    C. ejection

    D. spinal cord injury

_____ **20.** A fall from more than _____ times the patient's height is considered to be significant.

    A. two

    B. three

    C. four

    D. five

Questions 21-25 are derived from the following scenario: A young boy was riding his bicycle down the street when he hit a parked car.

_____ **21.** How many collisions took place?

    A. 1

    B. 2

    C. 3

    D. 4

_____ **22.** What was the first collision?

    A. The bike hitting the car

    B. The bide rider hitting his bike/car

    C. The bike rider's internal organs against the solid structures of the body.

    D. None of the above

_____ **23.** What was the second collision?

    A. The bike hitting the car

    B. The bide rider hitting his bike/car

    C. The bike rider's internal organs against the solid structures of the body.

    D. None of the above

_____ **24.** "For every action, there is an equal and opposite reaction" is:

    A. Newton's first law

    B. Newton's second law

    C. Newton's third law

    D. A statement that is not true.

_____ **25.** What will rate your index of suspicion for this collision?

    A. The MOI

    B. The NOI

    C. How loudly he's crying

    D. A quick visual assessment

Fill-in

Read each item carefully, then complete the statement by filling in the missing word(s).

1. _____ are the leading cause of death and disability in the United States among children and young adults.

2. Certain injury _____ occur with certain types of injury _____.

3. _____ _____ occurs to the body when the body's tissues are exposed to energy levels beyond their tolerance.

4. The formula for calculating kinetic energy is _____.

5. _____ of the crash scene may provide valuable information to the staff and treating physicians of the trauma center.

6. Air bags provide the final capture point of the passengers and decrease the severity of _____ injuries.

7. Seat belts that buckle automatically at the shoulder but require the passengers to buckle the lap portion can result in the body _____ forward underneath the shoulder restraint when the lap portion is not attached.

True/False

If you believe the statement to be more true than false, write the letter "T" in the space provided. If you believe the statement to be more false than true, write the letter "F."

_____ 1. Work is defined as force acting over distance.
_____ 2. Energy can be both created and destroyed.
_____ 3. The energy of a moving object is called potential energy.
_____ 4. Rear-end collisions often cause whiplash injuries.
_____ 5. The cervical spine has little tolerance for lateral bending.
_____ 6. The injury potential of a fall is related to the height from which the patient fell.
_____ 7. Injuries are the leading cause of death and injuries among 1- to 34-year-olds in the United States.

Short Answer

Complete this section with short written answers using the space provided.

1. Describe potential energy.

_____

_____

2. List the three series of collisions typical with motor vehicles.

_____

_____

3. List the three factors to consider when evaluating a fall.

_____

_____

4. Describe the phenomenon of cavitation as it relates to an injury from a bullet.

_____

_____

5. Why is it important to try to determine the type of gun and ammunition used when you are caring for a gunshot victim?

_____

_____

Word Fun

The following crossword puzzle is an activity provided to reinforce correct spelling and understanding of medical terminology associated with emergency care and the EMT-B. Use the clues in the column to complete the puzzle.

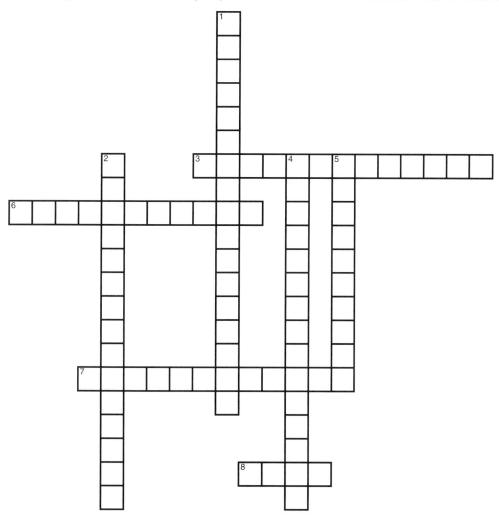

Across

3. Energy from a moving object

6. Impact on the body without penetrating soft tissues

7. Slowing down

8. Force acting over a distance

Down

1. Cause or reason for injury

2. Product of mass 3 gravity 3 height

4. The result of body tissues being exposed to energy levels beyond their tolerance

5. Pressure waves from speed

Ambulance Calls

The following case scenarios provide an opportunity to explore the concerns associated with patient management. Read each scenario, then answer each question in detail.

1. You are dispatched to a one-car MVC. As you arrive, you notice that the car hit a large deer that is lying in the road, dead. Highway speed limits on this road are 65 mph. The driver was restrained with a lap belt only, and his vehicle was not equipped with airbags. He is complaining of head and neck pain, and tells you that he doesn't remember what happened.

   How do you best manage this patient?

   _____

   _____

   _____

2. As December 25th approaches, many people in your community enjoy hanging lights and decorating their front yards. You are dispatched to assist a man who fell from a ladder as he was hanging lights from the roof of his two-story home. You arrive to find an unconscious middle-aged man lying in the snow. He is breathing and has a pulse. The call to 9-1-1 was placed after the man was found by a neighbor.

   _____

   _____

   _____

3. You are called to the residence of a 19-year-old male who was stabbed in the abdomen with an ice pick. The scene is safe and the patient is lying on the floor with the ice pick impaled in his left lower quadrant. Bystanders tell you he did not fall. He is alert and complaining of severe pain.

   How would you best manage this patient?

   _____

   _____

   _____

CHAPTER

22 Bleeding

Workbook Activities

The following activities have been designed to help you. Your instructor may require you to complete some or all of these activities as a regular part of your EMT-B training program. You are encouraged to complete any activity that your instructor does not assign as a way to enhance your learning in the classroom.

Chapter Review

The following exercises provide an opportunity to refresh your knowledge of this chapter.

Matching

Match each of the terms in the left column to the appropriate definition in the right column.

_____ 1. Pulmonary artery

_____ 2. Heart

_____ 3. Ventricle

_____ 4. Aorta

_____ 5. Atrium

_____ 6. Pulmonary vein

_____ 7. Coagulation

_____ 8. Ecchymosis

_____ 9. Epistaxis

_____ 10. Hematoma

_____ 11. Hemophilia

_____ 12. Hemorrhage

_____ 13. Hypovolemic shock

A. mass of blood in the soft tissues beneath the skin

B. formation of clot to plug opening in injured blood vessel and stop blood flow

C. upper chamber

D. a congenital condition in which a patient lacks one or more of the blood's normal clotting factors

E. hollow muscular organ

F. largest artery in body

G. a condition in which low blood volume results in inadequate perfusion

H. oxygenated blood travels through this

I. bruising

J. deoxygenated blood travels through this

K. lower chamber

L. bleeding

M. nosebleed

Multiple Choice

Read each item carefully, then select the best response.

_____ **1.** The function of the blood is to _____ all of the body's cells and tissues.

    A. deliver oxygen to

    B. deliver nutrients to

    C. carry waste products away from

    D. all of the above

_____ **2.** The cardiovascular system consists of:

    A. a pump.

    B. a container.

    C. fluid.

    D. all of the above

_____ **3.** Blood leaves each chamber of a normal heart through a:

    A. vein.

    B. artery.

    C. one-way valve.

    D. capillary.

_____ **4.** Blood enters into the right atrium from the:

    A. coronary arteries.

    B. lungs.

    C. vena cava.

    D. coronary veins.

_____ **5.** Blood enters into the left atrium from the:

    A. coronary arteries.

    B. lungs.

    C. vena cava.

    D. coronary veins.

_____ **6.** The only arteries in the body to carry deoxygenated blood are the:

    A. pulmonary arteries.

    B. coronary arteries.

    C. femoral arteries.

    D. subclavian arteries.

_____ **7.** The _____ is the thickest chamber of the heart.

    A. right atrium

    B. right ventricle

    C. left atrium

    D. left ventricle

_____ **8.** The _____ link(s) the arterioles and the venules.

    A. aorta

    B. capillaries

    C. vena cava

    D. valves

_____ 9. At the arterial end of the capillaries, the muscles dilate and constrict in response to conditions such as:

    A. fright.

    B. a specific need for oxygen.

    C. a need to dispose of metabolic wastes.

    D. all of the above

_____ 10. Blood contains all of the following, except:

    A. white cells.

    B. plasma.

    C. cerebrospinal fluid.

    D. platelets.

_____ 11. _____ is the circulation of blood within an organ or tissue in adequate amounts to meet the cells' current needs for oxygen, nutrients, and waste removal.

    A. Anatomy

    B. Perfusion

    C. Physiology

    D. Conduction

_____ 12. The _____ only require a minimal blood supply when at rest.

    A. lungs

    B. kidneys

    C. muscles

    D. heart

_____ 13. The term _____ means constantly adapting to changing conditions.

    A. perfusion

    B. conduction

    C. dynamic

    D. autonomic

_____ 14. _____ is inadequate tissue perfusion.

    A. Shock

    B. Hyperperfusion

    C. Hypertension

    D. Contraction

_____ 15. The brain and spinal cord cannot go for more than _____ minutes without perfusion, or the nerve cells will be permanently damaged.

    A. 30 to 45

    B. 12 to 20

    C. 8 to 10

    D. 4 to 6

_____ 16. An organ or tissue that is considerably _____ is much better able to resist damage from hypoperfusion.

    A. warmer

    B. colder

    C. younger

    D. older

_____ 17. The body will not tolerate an acute blood loss of greater than _____ of blood volume.

    A. 10%

    B. 20%

    C. 30%

    D. 40%

_____ **18.** If the typical adult loses more than 1 L of blood, significant changes in vital signs such as _____ will occur.

    A. increased heart rate

    B. increased respiratory rate

    C. decreased blood pressure

    D. all of the above

_____ **19.** _____ is a condition in which low blood volume results in inadequate perfusion and even death.

    A. Hypovolemic shock

    B. Metabolic shock

    C. Septic shock

    D. Psychogenic shock

_____ **20.** You should consider bleeding to be serious if all of the following conditions are present, except:

    A. blood loss is rapid.

    B. there is no mechanism of injury.

    C. the patient has a poor general appearance.

    D. assessment reveals signs and symptoms of shock.

_____ **21.** Significant blood loss demands your immediate attention as soon as the _____ has been managed.

    A. fractures

    B. extrication

    C. airway

    D. none of the above

_____ **22.** The process of blood clotting and plugging the hole is called:

    A. conglomeration.

    B. configuration.

    C. coagulation.

    D. coalition.

_____ **23.** Even though the body is very efficient at controlling bleeding on its own, it may fail in situations such as:

    A. when medications interfere with normal clotting.

    B. when damage to the vessel may be so large that a clot cannot completely block the hole.

    C. when sometimes only part of the vessel wall is cut, preventing it from constricting.

    D. all of the above

_____ **24.** A lack of one or more of the blood's clotting factors is called:

    A. a deficiency.

    B. hemophilia.

    C. platelet anomaly.

    D. anemia.

_____ **25.** You respond to a 25-year-old man who has cut his arm with a circular saw. The bleeding appears to be bright red and spurting. The patient is alert and oriented and converses with you freely. He appears to be stable at this point. What is your first step in controlling his bleeding?

    A. Direct pressure

    B. Maintaining the airway

    C. BSI precautions

    D. Elevation

_____ **26.** When applying a bandage to hold a dressing in place, stretch the bandage tight enough to control bleeding, but not so tight as to decrease _____ to the extremity.

    A. blood flow

    B. pulses

    C. oxygen

    D. CRTs

_____ **27.** If bleeding continues after applying a pressure dressing, you should do all of the following, except:

    A. remove the dressing and apply another sterile dressing.

    B. apply manual pressure through the dressing.

    C. add more gauze pads over the first dressing.

    D. secure both dressings tighter with a roller bandage.

_____ **28.** When using an air splint to control bleeding in a fractured extremity, you should reassess the _____ frequently.

    A. airway

    B. breathing

    C. circulation in the injured extremity

    D. fracture site

_____ **29.** Contraindications to the use of the PASG include:

    A. pulmonary edema.

    B. pregnancy.

    C. penetrating chest injuries.

    D. all of the above

_____ **30.** You and your partner respond to a patient who has had his hand nearly severed by a drill press. As you approach the patient he is pale and there appears to be a lot of blood on the floor. The wound continues to bleed massively. You consider applying a tourniquet but know they are rarely needed and often:

    A. resolve the problem.

    B. decrease the problem.

    C. create more problems.

    D. all of the above

_____ **31.** In the above call, all methods of trying to control the bleeding are unsuccessful and it is decided to apply the tourniquet. You know that the patient will probably lose the injured extremity but you feel it necessary to save his life. You know you must be sure to:

    A. use the narrowest bandage possible to minimize the area restricted.

    B. cover the tourniquet with a bandage.

    C. never pad underneath the tourniquet.

    D. not loosen the tourniquet after you have applied it.

_____ **32.** You are called to the local playground for an 8-year-old girl who has an uncontrolled nose bleed. The child is crying uncontrollably and will not converse with you. The baby sitter is not able to tell you if there was any trauma involved but there is a bump on the temporal portion of her head. The baby sitter does state that she has had a cold for several days, but can give you no further information on the medical history. All the children playing with her deny any trauma. What could be the possible cause(s) of the bleeding?

    A. A skull fracture

    B. Sinusitis

    C. Coagulation disorders

    D. All of the above

_____ **33.** You respond to a 33-year-old man who was hit in the ear by a line drive during a softball game. He is complaining of a severe headache, ringing in his ears, and being dizzy. He has blood draining from his ear. Why would you not apply pressure to control bleeding?

    A. It should be collected to be reinfused at the hospital.

    B. It could collect within the head and increase the pressure in the brain.

    C. It is contaminated.

    D. You could fracture the skull with the pressure needed to staunch the flow of blood.

_____ **34.** When treating a patient with signs and symptoms of hypovolemic shock and no outward signs of bleeding, always consider the possibility of bleeding into the:

A. thoracic cavity.

B. abdomen.

C. skull.

D. chest.

_____ **35.** Nontraumatic internal bleeding may be caused by:

A. an ulcer.

B. a ruptured ectopic pregnancy.

C. an aneurysm.

D. all of the above

_____ **36.** The most common symptom of internal abdominal bleeding is:

A. bruising around the abdomen.

B. distention of the abdomen.

C. rigidity of the abdomen.

D. acute abdominal pain.

_____ **37.** Signs and symptoms of internal bleeding in both trauma and medical patients include:

A. hematochezia.

B. melena.

C. hemoptysis.

D. all of the above

_____ **38.** The first sign of hypovolemic shock is a change in:

A. respirations.

B. heart rate.

C. mental status.

D. blood pressure.

Labeling

Label the following diagrams with the correct terms. Where arrows appear, indicate the substance and its origin and destination.

1. The Left and Right Sides of the Heart

A. _____

B. _____

C. _____

D. _____

E. _____

F. _____

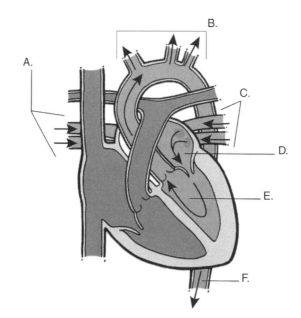

A. _____

B. _____

C. _____

D. _____

E. _____

F. _____

2. Perfusion

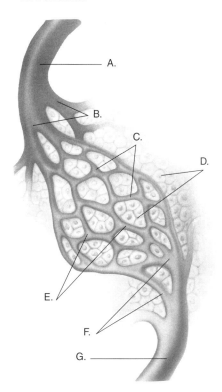

A. _____

B. _____

C. _____

D. _____

E. _____

F. _____

G. _____

3. Arterial Pressure Points

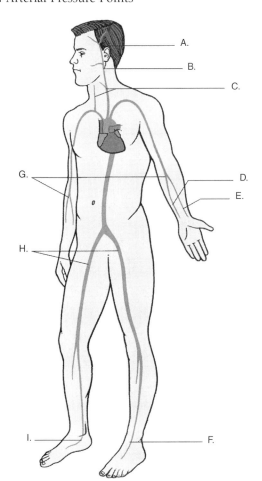

A. _____

B. _____

C. _____

D. _____

E. _____

F. _____

G. _____

H. _____

I. _____

Fill-in

Read each item carefully, then complete the statement by filling in the missing word(s).

1. The circulation of blood in adequate amounts to meet cellular needs is called _____.

2. The heart is a(n) _____ muscle, which is controlled by the autonomic nervous system.

3. Exchange of oxygen and carbon dioxide occurs in the _____.

4. Shock is a condition related to _____.

5. Blood returning to the heart from the lower body is first collected in the _____ vena cava.

6. Blood contains four major components, which are _____ _____ _____ _____.

7. The left ventricle receives _____ blood while the right ventricle receives deoxygenated blood.

8. During a state of shock, the autonomic nervous system directs blood away from some organs and distributes it to the _____ _____ _____ _____.

9. The brain and spinal cord generally cannot go longer than _____ minutes without adequate perfusion, or permanent nerve cell damage may occur.

10. If the patient has a significant mechanism of injury that may affect multiple systems, he or she should receive a _____ _____ assessment.

True/False

If you believe the statement to be more true than false, write the letter "T" in the space provided. If you believe the statement to be more false than true, write the letter "F."

_____ 1. Venous blood tends to spurt and is difficult to control.
_____ 2. The human body is tolerant of blood losses greater than 20% of blood volume.
_____ 3. The first step in controlling external bleeding is application of the PASG.
_____ 4. The first step in preparing to treat a bleeding patient is BSI.
_____ 5. A properly applied tourniquet should be loosened by the EMT-B every ten minutes.
_____ 6. A patient who has swallowed a lot of blood may become nauseated and vomit.
_____ 7. You should check with medical control every time a PASG may be indicated.
_____ 8. If a wound continues to bleed after it is bandaged, you should remove the bandage and start over again.
_____ 9. A tourniquet is always required for massive spurting blood loss.
_____ 10. Do not use PASG if the transport time is less than 30 minutes.

Short Answer

Complete this section with short written answers in the space provided.

1. Describe how the autonomic nervous system responds to severe bleeding.

_____

_____

2. Describe the characteristics of bleeding from each type of vessel (artery, vein, capillary).

_____

3. List, in the proper sequence, the methods in which an EMT-B should attempt to control external bleeding.

_____

4. List ten signs and symptoms of hypovolemic shock.

_____

5. List, in the proper sequence, the general EMT-B emergency care for patients with internal bleeding.

_____

Word Fun

The following crossword puzzle is an activity provided to reinforce correct spelling and understanding of medical terminology associated with emergency care and the EMT-B. Use the clues in the column to complete the puzzle.

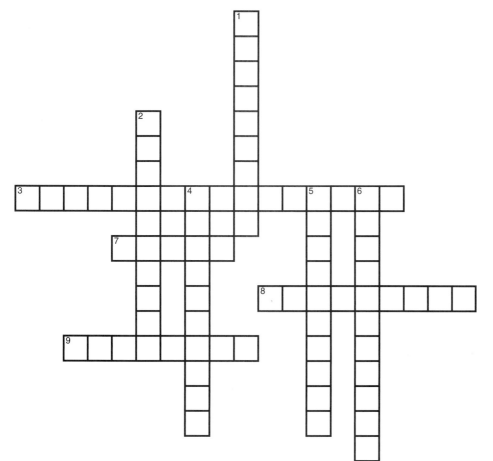

Across

3. Low blood volume, inadequate perfusion

7. Circulatory system failure

8. Circulation of blood within the body

9. Mass of blood in soft tissues

Down

1. Nosebleed

2. Lacks normal clotting factors

4. Discoloration of skin from closed wound

5. Bleeding

6. Formation of clots to stop bleeding

Ambulance Calls

The following case scenarios provide an opportunity to explore the concerns associated with patient management. Read each scenario, then answer each question in detail.

1. You are dispatched to a school playground for an 8-year-old boy complaining of a minor laceration to his left wrist with uncontrollable hemorrhaging. The teacher tells you that he has a history of hemophilia. The blood is steady, but not spurting, and dark in color.

How would you best manage this patient?

_____

_____

_____

2. You are dispatched to a local lumberyard for an "unknown accident." Upon your arrival you see that a man sitting on the ground, his coworkers surrounding him. His shirt got caught in a machine, and his arm was severed from the elbow down. He is holding a blood-soaked towel to the end of his right arm.

How do you best manage this patient?

_____

_____

_____

3. You are dispatched to the local jail for a male prisoner who has jabbed his arm with a ballpoint pen. He is bleeding continuously from the wound that is in the area of his antecubital vein on his left arm.

How do you best manage this patient?

_____

_____

_____

Skill Drills

Skill Drill 22-1: Controlling External Bleeding

Test your knowledge of this skill drill by filling in the correct words in the photo captions.

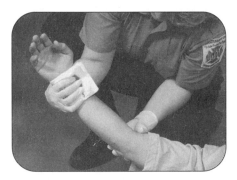
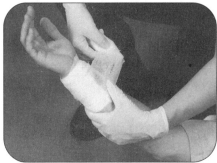
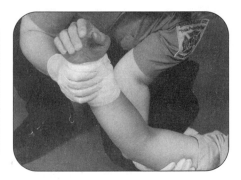

1. Apply _____ _____
   over the wound.
   Elevate the injury above the
   _____ of the _____ if
   no _____ is suspected.

2. Apply a _____
   _____ .

3. Apply pressure at the appropriate
   _____ _____ while
   continuing to hold _____
   _____ .

Skill Drill 22-2: Applying a Pneumatic Antishock Garment (PASG)

Test your knowledge of this skill drill by placing the photos below in the correct order. Number the first step with a "1", the second step with a "2", etc.

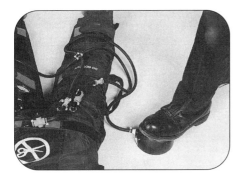

_____

Inflate with the foot pump, and close the stopcocks when the patient's systolic blood pressure reaches 100 mm Hg or the Velcro crackles.

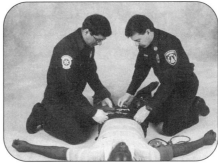

_____

Enclose both legs and the abdomen.

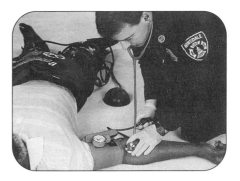

_____

Check the patient's blood pressure again. Monitor the vital signs.

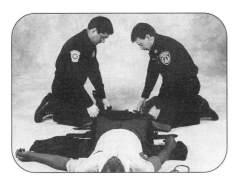

_____

Apply the garment so that the top is below the lowest rib.

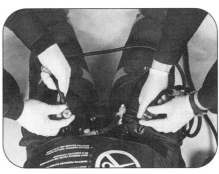

_____

Open the stopcocks.

Assessment Review

Answer the following questions pertaining to the assessment of the types of emergencies discussed in this chapter.

_____ 1. When you are performing a scene size-up on a patient with external bleeding, the minimum BSI that should be taken is:

   A. gloves and gown.

   B. gown and eye protection.

   C. gloves and eye protection.

   D. gown and face mask.

_____ 2. For a patient with suspected internal bleeding, you should assess circulation by checking the pulse for:

   A. rate and quality.

   B. rate and rhythm.

   C. quality and rhythm.

   D. presence.

_____ 3. If you have completed your initial assessment and transport decision on an unresponsive patient with a significant mechanism of injury, how should the focused history and physical exam be performed?

   A. Just check the injury

   B. Rapid trauma assessment

   C. Just like any other patient

   D. Move to the ongoing assessment

_____ 4. Your external bleeding patient needs a detailed physical exam. When should it be performed?

   A. Immediately after the initial assessment

   B. During the focused physical exam

   C. When you arrive at the patient's side

   D. En route to the hospital

_____ 5. What should be included in the communications to the hospital when dealing with a patient with suspected internal bleeding?

   A. Amount of blood loss

   B. Location of the bleeding

   C. Interventions performed

   D. Patient's blood type

Emergency Care Summary

Fill in the following chart pertaining to the management of the types of emergencies discussed in this chapter.

NOTE: While the steps below are widely accepted, be sure to consult and follow your local protocol.

External Bleeding	Internal Bleeding

External Bleeding

Follow BSI precautions—minimum of gloves and eye protection.

Ensure that patient has open airway.

Maintain the _____ stabilization if MOI suggests possible spinal injury.

Provide high-flow oxygen.

Control bleeding using one of the following methods:
- Direct pressure and elevation
- Pressure dressings
- Pressure points
- Splints
- Air splints
- PASG
- Tourniquets

Controlling External Bleeding

1. Apply direct local pressure to bleeding site.
2. Elevate the bleeding extremity.
3. Create a _____ dressing.
4. Apply pressure at the appropriate pressure point while continuing to hold direct pressure.
5. If the wound continues to bleed, elevate extremity and place additional pressure over proximal pressure point.

Using PASG for Control of Massive Soft-tissue

Bleeding in the Extremities

1. Apply the garment.
2. Close and fasten both leg compartments and the abdominal compartment.
3. Open the stopcocks.
4. Inflate the compartments similar to an _____ _____.
5. Check the patient's circulation, motor function, and sensation in distal lower extremities.

Applying a Tourniquet

1. Fold a triangular bandage.
2. Wrap the bandage around the extremity _____.
3. Tie one know in the bandage. Place a stick or rod on top of the knot. Tie the ends of the bandage on the stick in a _____ knot.
4. Use the stick as a handle and twist it to tighten the tourniquet until bleeding has stopped.
5. Secure the stick in place with another triangular bandage.
6. Write "TK" and the exact time the tourniquet was applied on a piece of adhesive tape. Fasten the tape to the patient's forehead.
7. As an alternative, use a blood pressure cuff. Inflate enough to stop bleeding.

Treating Epistaxis

1. Follow BSI precautions.
2. Help the patient to sit, leaning forward.
3. Apply direct pressure for at least _____ minutes by pinching nostrils together.
4. Keep the patient calm and quiet.
5. Apply ice over the nose.
6. Maintain the pressure until bleeding is completely controlled.
7. Provide prompt transport.
8. If bleeding cannot be controlled, transport patient immediately. Treat for _____ and administer oxygen via mask if necessary.

Internal Bleeding

Steps to Caring for Patient With Internal Bleeding

1. Follow BSI precautions.
2. Maintain the airway with cervical immobilization if MOI suggests possible spinal injury.
3. Administer high-flow oxygen.
4. Control all obvious external bleeding.
5. Apply a _____ to an extremity where internal bleeding is suspected.
6. Monitor and record vital signs at least every 5 minutes.
7. Give the patient _____ by mouth.
8. Elevate the legs 6″ to 12″ in significant trauma patients.
9. Keep the patient warm.
10. Provide immediate transport for patients with signs and symptoms of shock. Report changes in condition to hospital personnel.

Using PASG for Treatment of Shock

1. Apply the garment.
2. Close and fasten both leg compartments and the _____ compartment.
3. Open the stopcocks.
4. Contact medical control for specific verbal orders to inflate or use standing order specific to inflation of PASG.
5. Inflate the compartments based on the patient's blood pressure.
6. Recheck the patient's blood pressure and inflate more based on patient _____ and blood pressure.

CHAPTER

23 Shock

Workbook Activities

The following activities have been designed to help you. Your instructor may require you to complete some or all of these activities as a regular part of your EMT-B training program. You are encouraged to complete any activity that your instructor does not assign as a way to enhance your learning in the classroom.

Chapter Review

The following exercises provide an opportunity to refresh your knowledge of this chapter.

Matching

Match each of the terms in the left column to the appropriate definition in the right column.

_____ **1.** Shock   **A.** severe allergy

_____ **2.** Perfusion   **B.** hypoperfusion

_____ **3.** Sphincters   **C.** regulates involuntary body functions

_____ **4.** Autonomic nervous system   **D.** early stage of shock

_____ **5.** Blood pressure   **E.** provides a rough measure of perfusion

_____ **6.** Anaphylaxis   **F.** severe bacterial infection

_____ **7.** Septic shock   **G.** sufficient circulation to meet cell needs

_____ **8.** Syncope   **H.** regulate blood flow in capillaries

_____ **9.** Compensated shock   **I.** fainting

Multiple Choice

Read each item carefully, then select the best response.

_____ **1.** Shock:

   A. refers to a state of collapse and failure of the cardiovascular system.

   B. results in the inadequate flow of blood to the body's cells.

   C. results in failure to rid cells of metabolic wastes.

   D. all of the above

_____ **2.** Blood flow through the capillary beds is regulated by:

   A. systolic pressure.

   B. the capillary sphincters.

   C. perfusion.

   D. diastolic pressure.

_____ **3.** The autonomic nervous system regulates involuntary functions such as:

   A. sweating.

   B. digestion.

   C. constriction and dilation of capillary sphincters.

   D. all of the above

_____ **4.** Regulation of blood flow is determined by:

   A. oxygen intake.

   B. systolic pressure.

   C. cellular need.

   D. diastolic pressure.

_____ **5.** Perfusion requires having a working cardiovascular system as well as:

   A. adequate oxygen exchange in the lungs.

   B. adequate nutrients in the form of glucose in the blood.

   C. adequate waste removal.

   D. all of the above

_____ **6.** The action of the hormones stimulates _____ to maintain pressure in the system and, as a result, perfusion of all vital organs.

   A. an increase in heart rate

   B. an increase in the strength of cardiac contractions

   C. vasoconstriction in nonessential areas

   D. all of the above

_____ **7.** Basic causes of shock include:

   A. poor pump function.

   B. blood or fluid loss.

   C. blood vessel dilation.

   D. all of the above

_____ **8.** Noncardiovascular causes of shock include respiratory insufficiency and:

   A. sepsis.

   B. metabolic.

   C. anaphylaxis.

   D. hypovolemia.

_____ **9.** You are called to the residence of a 67-year-old man who is complaining of chest pain. He is alert and oriented. During your assessment process the patient tells you he has had two previous heart attacks. He is taking medication for fluid retention. As you listen to his lungs, you notice that he has fluid in his lungs. This is known as pulmonary:

    A. edema.

    B. overload.

    C. cessation.

    D. failure.

_____ **10.** _____ develops when the heart muscle can no longer generate enough pressure to circulate the blood to all organs.

    A. Pump failure

    B. Cardiogenic shock

    C. A myocardial infarction

    D. Congestive heart failure

_____ **11.** You are called to a construction site where a 27-year-old worker has fallen from the second floor. He landed on his back and is drifting in and out of consciousness. A quick assessment reveals no bleeding or blood loss. His blood pressure is 90/60 mm Hg with a pulse rate of 110 beats/min. His airway is open and breathing is within normal limits. You realize the patient is in shock. The patient's shock is due to an injury to the:

    A. cervical vertebrae.

    B. skull.

    C. spinal cord.

    D. peripheral nerves.

_____ **12.** Neurogenic shock usually results from damage to the spinal cord at the:

    A. cervical level.

    B. thoracic level.

    C. lumbar level.

    D. sacral level.

_____ **13.** You respond to the local nursing home of an 85-year-old woman who has altered mental status. During your assessment you notice that the patient has an elevated body temperature. She is hypotensive and the pulse is tachycardic. The nursing staff tells you that she has been sick for several days and that they called because of her mental status that continued to decline. You suspect the patient is in septic shock. The shock is due to:

    A. pump failure.

    B. massive vasoconstriction.

    C. widespread dilation.

    D. increased volume.

_____ **14.** In septic shock:

    A. there is an insufficient volume of fluid in the container.

    B. the fluid that has leaked out often collects in the respiratory system.

    C. there is a larger-than-normal vascular bed to contain the smaller-than-normal volume of intravascular fluid.

    D. all of the above

_____ **15.** Neurogenic shock is caused by:

    A. a radical change in the size of the vascular system.

    B. massive vasoconstriction.

    C. low volume.

    D. fluid collecting around the spinal cord causing compression of the cord.

_____ **16.** Hypovolemic shock is a result of:
  A. widespread vasodilation.
  B. low volume.
  C. massive vasoconstriction.
  D. pump failure.

_____ **17.** An insufficient concentration of _____ in the blood can produce shock as rapidly as vascular causes.
  A. oxygen
  B. hormones
  C. epinephrine
  D. histamine

_____ **18.** In anaphylactic shock, the combination of poor oxygenation and poor perfusion is a result of:
  A. widespread vasodilation.
  B. low volume.
  C. massive vasoconstriction.
  D. pump failure.

_____ **19.** Causes of syncope include:
  A. generalized vascular dilation.
  B. the sight of blood.
  C. cardiac arrhythmias.
  D. all of the above

_____ **20.** You are called to a motor vehicle collision. Your patient is a 19-year-old female who was not wearing her seat belt. She is conscious but confused. Her airway is open and respirations are within normal limits. She pulse is slightly tachycardic but regular. The blood pressure is within normal limits. She is complaining of being thirsty and appears very anxious. You know that the last measurable factor to change to indicate shock is:
  A. mental status.
  B. blood pressure.
  C. pulse rate.
  D. respirations.

_____ **21.** You should suspect shock in all of the following except:
  A. an allergic reaction.
  B. multiple severe fractures.
  C. a severe infection.
  D. abdominal or chest injury.

_____ **22.** When treating a suspected shock patient, vital signs should be recorded approximately every _____ minutes.
  A. 2
  B. 5
  C. 10
  D. 15

_____ **23.** The Golden Hour refers to the first 60 minutes after:
  A. medical help arrives on scene.
  B. transport begins.
  C. the injury occurs.
  D. 9-1-1 is called.

_____ **24.** Signs of cardiogenic shock include all of the following except:

    A. cyanosis.

    B. strong, bounding pulse.

    C. nausea.

    D. anxiety.

_____ **25.** You respond to a 17-year-old football player who was hit by numerous opponents and while walking off the field became unconscious. He is currently unconscious. You take c-spine control and start your assessment. You know that in the treatment of shock you must:

    A. secure and maintain an airway.

    B. provide respiratory support.

    C. assisted ventilations.

    D. all of the above

_____ **26.** When assessing the patient who has psychogenic shock, be sure to consider possible _____ if the patient fell.

    A. extremity fractures

    B. cervical spine injury

    C. paralysis

    D. pelvic fractures

Fill-in

Read each item carefully, then complete the statement by filling in the missing word(s).

1. _____ refers to the failure of the cardiovascular system.

2. Pressure in the arteries during cardiac _____ is known as systolic pressure.

3. In shock conditions, the body redirects blood from _____ organs to _____ organs.

4. Blood pressure is a rough measurement of _____.

5. The cardiovascular system consists of the _____, _____, and _____.

6. Inadequate circulation that does not meet the body's needs is known as _____.

7. _____ are circular muscle walls in capillaries, causing the walls to _____ and _____.

8. _____ pressure occurs during cardiac relaxation, while _____ pressure occurs during cardiac contractions.

9. _____ pressure is the pressure in the blood vessels at all times.

10. The autonomic nervous system controls the _____ actions of the body.

True/False

If you believe the statement to be more true than false, write the letter "T" in the space provided. If you believe the statement to be more false than true, write the letter "F".

_____ **1.** Life-threatening allergic reactions can occur in response to almost any substance that a patient may encounter.

_____ **2.** Bleeding is the most common cause of shock following an injury.

_____ **3.** Shock occurs when oxygen and nutrients cannot get to the body's cells.

_____ **4.** A person in shock, left untreated, will most likely survive.

_____ **5.** Compensated shock is related to the last stages of shock.

_____ **6.** An injection of epinephrine is the only really effective treatment for anaphylactic shock.

_____ **7.** Septic shock is a combination of vessel and content failure.

_____ **8.** Metabolism is the cardiovascular system's circulation of blood and oxygen to all cells in different tissues and organs of the body.

_____ **9.** Shock only occurs with massive blood loss from the body.

_____ **10.** Decompensated shock occurs when the systolic blood pressure falls below 120 mm Hg.

Short Answer

Complete this section with short written answers using the space provided.

1. List the causes, signs and symptoms, and treatment of anaphylactic shock.

_____

_____

2. List the causes, signs and symptoms, and treatment of cardiogenic shock.

_____

_____

3. List the causes, signs and symptoms, and treatment of hypovolemic shock.

_____

_____

4. List the causes, signs and symptoms, and treatment of metabolic shock.

_____

_____

5. List the causes, signs and symptoms, and treatment of neurogenic shock.

_____

_____

6. List the causes, signs and symptoms, and treatment of psychogenic shock.

_____

_____

7. List the causes, signs and symptoms, and treatment of septic shock.

_____

_____

8. List the three basic physiologic causes of shock.

_____

_____

9. List the signs and symptoms of decompensated shock.

_____

_____

10. List the steps for using an autoinjector.

_____

_____

Word Fun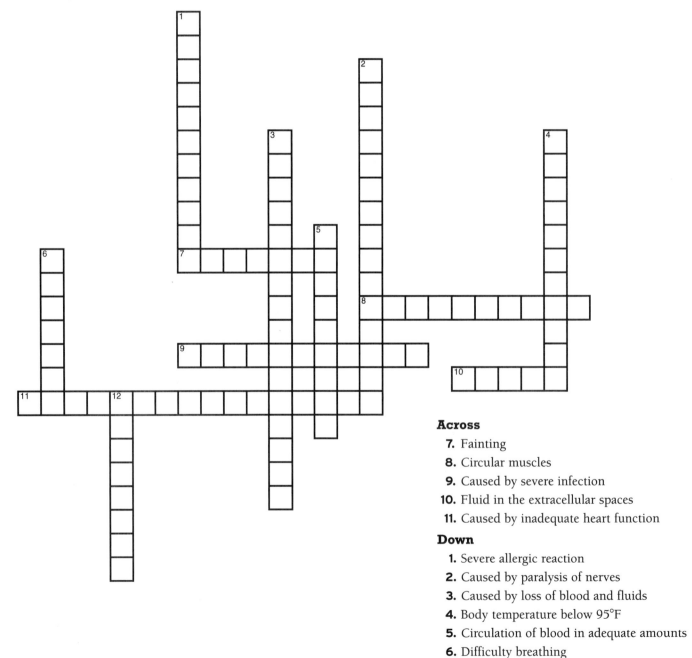

The following crossword puzzle is an activity provided to reinforce correct spelling and understanding of medical terminology associated with emergency care and the EMT-B. Use the clues in the column to complete the puzzle.

Across

7. Fainting
8. Circular muscles
9. Caused by severe infection
10. Fluid in the extracellular spaces
11. Caused by inadequate heart function

Down

1. Severe allergic reaction
2. Caused by paralysis of nerves
3. Caused by loss of blood and fluids
4. Body temperature below 95°F
5. Circulation of blood in adequate amounts
6. Difficulty breathing
12. Lack of oxygen

Ambulance Calls

The following case scenarios provide an opportunity to explore the concerns associated with patient management. Read each scenario, then answer each question in detail.

1. You are dispatched to the victim of a fall at the local community college theater. One of the students involved in rigging the theater backgrounds fell from the platform above the stage. He landed directly on his back, and is now complaining of numbness and tingling in his lower body.

How do you best manage this patient?

_____

_____

_____

2. You are dispatched to a local long-term care facility for an older man with a history of fever. You arrive to find an 80-year-old man who is responsive to painful stimuli and has the following vital signs: blood pressure 80/40 mm Hg, weak radial pulse of 140 beats/min and irregular, respirations of 60 breaths/min and shallow, and pulse oximetry of 80% on 4 L/min nasal cannula.

How do you best manage this patient?

_____

_____

_____

3. You are dispatched to a residence where a 16-year-old female was stung by a bee. Her mother tells you she is severely allergic to bees. She is voice responsive, covered in hives, and is wheezing audibly. She has a very weak radial pulse and is blue around the lips.

How would you best manage this patient?

_____

_____

_____

Skill Drills

Skill Drill 23-1: Treating Shock

Test your knowledge of this skill drill by placing the photos below in the correct order. Number the first step with a "1", the second step with a "2", etc.

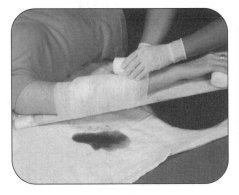

_____

Splint any broken bones or joint injuries.

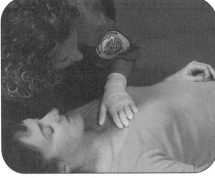

_____

Keep the patient supine, open the airway, and check breathing and pulse.

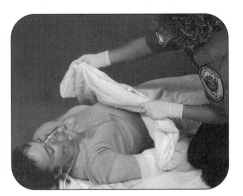

_____

Give high-flow oxygen if you have not already done so, and place blankets under and over the patient.

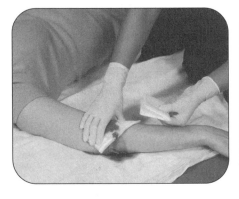

_____

Control obvious external bleeding.

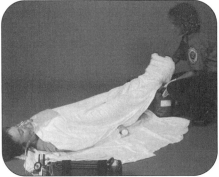

_____

If no fractures are suspected, elevate the legs 6″ to 12″.

Assessment Review

Answer the following questions pertaining to the assessment of the types of emergencies discussed in this chapter.

_____ **1.** In the scene size-up for a patient/patients who you think may be susceptible to shock, you should:

    A. ensure scene safety.

    B. determine the number of patients.

    C. consider c-spine stabilization.

    D. All of the above

_____ **2.** During the initial assessment of a patient in shock you should:

    A. treat any immediate life threats.

    B. obtain a SAMPLE history.

    C. get a complete set of vital signs.

    D. inform medical control of the situation.

_____ **3.** You have completed your initial assessment of a patient who stepped off a curb and heard her ankle pop. Your focused history should include:

A. a rapid trauma assessment.

B. an assessment of the affected area.

C. a detailed physical exam.

D. an ongoing assessment.

_____ **4.** Interventions for the treatment of shock should include:

A. giving the patient something to drink.

B. maintaining normal body temperature.

C. positioning the patient in the Fowler's position for transport.

D. delayed transport to splint fractures.

_____ **5.** You are transporting an unstable patient who you feel in going into shock. How often do you recheck his vital signs?

A. Every 3 minutes

B. Every 10 minutes

C. Every 5 minutes

D. Every 15 minutes

Emergency Care Summary

Fill in the following chart pertaining to the management of the types of emergencies discussed in this chapter.

NOTE: While the steps below are widely accepted, be sure to consult and follow your local protocol.

General Shock	Anaphylactic Shock
Minimum treatment for shock, with the exception of anaphylactic shock, is as follows:	Follow the steps for using an auto-injector (discussed in Chapter 16):
1. Provide _____ stabilization if needed.	1. Remove the auto-injector's safety cap, and quickly wipe the thigh with antiseptic.
2. Keep the patient _____, open the airway, and check breathing and pulse.	2. Place the tip of the auto-injector against the _____ part of the thigh.
3. Control obvious external bleeding.	3. Push the auto-injector firmly against the thigh, and hold it in place until all the medication is _____.
4. Splint any broken bones or joint injuries.	
5. Give high-flow oxygen if you have not already done so, and place blankets under and over the patient.	
6. If no extremity fractures are suspected, elevate the legs 6" to 12".	
7. Provide rapid transport in a position that best supports _____ and breathing.	
Treatment for cardiogenic shock also requires the following:	
For cardiogenic shock, place the patient in a position of comfort. Assist with ventilation and suction as needed. Monitor the _____ closely and provide rapid, calm transport.	

CHAPTER

24 Soft-Tissue Injuries

Workbook Activities

The following activities have been designed to help you. Your instructor may require you to complete some or all of these activities as a regular part of your EMT-B training program. You are encouraged to complete any activity that your instructor does not assign as a way to enhance your learning in the classroom.

Chapter Review

The following exercises provide an opportunity to refresh your knowledge of this chapter.

Matching

Match each of the terms in the left column to the appropriate definition in the right column.

_____ 1. Dermis

_____ 2. Sweat glands

_____ 3. Epidermis

_____ 4. Mucous membranes

_____ 5. Sebaceous glands

_____ 6. Abrasion

_____ 7. Laceration

_____ 8. Penetrating wound

_____ 9. Avulsion

_____ 10. Evisceration

A. gunshot wound

B. cool the body by discharging a substance through the pores

C. tissue hanging as a flap from wound

D. tough external layer forming a watertight covering for the body

E. razor cut

F. secrete a watery substance that lubricates the openings of the mouth and nose

G. inner layer of skin that contains the structures that give skin its characteristic appearance

H. produce oil, which waterproofs the skin and keeps it supple

I. exposed intestines

J. skinned knee

Multiple Choice

Read each item carefully, then select the best response.

_____ 1. The _____ is (are) our first line of defense against external fractures.
- **A.** extremities
- **B.** hair
- **C.** skin
- **D.** lips

_____ 2. The skin covering the _____ is quite thick.
- **A.** lips
- **B.** scalp
- **C.** ears
- **D.** eyelids

_____ 3. As the cells on the surface of the skin are worn away, new cells form in the _____ layer.
- **A.** dermal
- **B.** germinal
- **C.** epidermal
- **D.** subcutaneous

_____ 4. The hair follicles, sweat glands, and sebaceous glands are found in the:
- **A.** dermis.
- **B.** germinal layer.
- **C.** epidermis.
- **D.** subcutaneous layer.

_____ 5. The skin regulates temperature in a cold environment by:
- **A.** secreting sweat through sweat glands.
- **B.** constricting the blood vessels.
- **C.** dilating the blood vessels.
- **D.** increasing the amount of heat that is radiated from the body's surface.

_____ 6. Closed soft-tissue injuries are characterized by all of the following except:
- **A.** pain at the site of injury.
- **B.** swelling beneath the skin.
- **C.** damage of the protective layer of skin.
- **D.** a history of blunt trauma.

_____ 7. A(n) _____ occurs whenever a large blood vessel is damaged and bleeds.
- **A.** contusion
- **B.** hematoma
- **C.** crushing injury
- **D.** avulsion

_____ 8. A(n) _____ is usually associated with extensive tissue damage.
- **A.** contusion
- **B.** hematoma
- **C.** crushing injury
- **D.** avulsion

_____ 9. A hematoma can result from:
- **A.** a soft-tissue injury.
- **B.** a fracture.
- **C.** any injury to a large blood vessel.
- **D.** all of the above

_____ **10.** A(n) _____ occurs when a great amount of force is applied to the body for a long period of time.

A. contusion

B. hematoma

C. crushing injury

D. avulsion

_____ **11.** More extensive closed injuries may involve significant swelling and bleeding beneath the skin, which could lead to:

A. compartment syndrome.

B. contamination.

C. hypovolemic shock.

D. hemothorax.

_____ **12.** You respond to a 14-year-old female who was playing softball and slid into second base. She states she felt and heard a loud pop. There is no obvious bleeding but there is swelling present. Her pulse is 86 beats/min and her blood pressure is 114/74 mm Hg. You decide you can manage this situation and decide to use the RICES method of treatment. The S stands for:

A. swelling.

B. soft-tissue.

C. splinting.

D. shock.

_____ **13.** Open soft-tissue wounds include all of the following, except:

A. abrasions.

B. contusions.

C. lacerations.

D. avulsions.

_____ **14.** In doing a more detailed exam on your patient in question 12, you notice that she has an abrasion on her left knee that she sustained when she slid. The abrasion is covered with dirt and is oozing blood. You know that this injury is classified as _____:

A. superficial.

B. deep.

C. full-thickness.

D. none of the above

_____ **15.** A laceration may be:

A. superficial.

B. deep.

C. jagged.

D. all of the above

_____ **16.** You decide to manage the injury for the patient in question 14. You flush the site with sterile water and it continues to bleed. What would be the best way to control the bleeding from the site?

A. Elevation

B. Pressure dressings

C. Tourniquets

D. Pressure points

_____ **17.** You respond to a 24-year-old man who has been shot. Law enforcement is on scene and the scene is safe. As you approach the victim, you notice that he is bleeding from the lower right abdominal area. He is alert and oriented but seems confused. His airway is open and he is breathing at a normal rate. His pulse is 120 beats/min, weak and regular. His blood pressure is 98/60 mm Hg. You ask the police officer about the weapon. You need the information due to the fact that the amount of damage is related to the:

A. size of the entrance wound.

B. size of the bullet.

C. size of the exit wound.

D. speed of the bullet.

_____ **18.** Because shootings usually end up in court, it is important to factually and completely document:

A. the circumstances surrounding any gunshot injury.

B. the patient's condition.

C. the treatment given.

D. all of the above

_____ **19.** All open wounds are assumed to be _____ and present a risk of infection.

A. contaminated

B. life-threatening

C. minimal

D. extensive

_____ **20.** Before you begin caring for a patient with an open wound, you should:

A. survey the scene.

B. follow BSI precautions.

C. be sure the patient has an open airway.

D. all of the above

_____ **21.** Splinting an extremity even when there is no fracture can help by:

A. reducing pain.

B. minimizing damage to an already-injured extremity.

C. making it easier to move the patient.

D. all of the above

_____ **22.** Treatment for an abdominal evisceration includes:

A. pushing the exposed organs back into the abdominal cavity.

B. covering the organs with dry dressings.

C. flexing the knees and legs to relieve pressure on the abdomen.

D. applying moist, adherent dressings.

_____ **23.** An open neck injury may result in _____ if enough air is sucked into a blood vessel.

A. hypovolemic shock

B. tracheal deviation

C. air embolism

D. subcutaneous emphysema

_____ **24.** Burns may result from:

A. heat.

B. toxic chemicals.

C. electricity.

D. all of the above

_____ **25.** Factors in helping to determine the severity of a burn include:

A. the depth of the burn.

B. the extent of the burn.

C. whether or not there are critical areas involved.

D. all of the above

_____ **26.** _____ burns involve only the epidermis.

    A. Full-thickness

    B. Second-degree

    C. Superficial

    D. Third-degree

_____ **27.** _____ burns cause intense pain.

    A. First-degree

    B. Second-degree

    C. Superficial

    D. Third-degree

_____ **28.** _____ burns may involve subcutaneous layers, muscle, bone, or internal organs.

    A. Superficial

    B. Partial-thickness

    C. Full-thickness

    D. Second-degree

_____ **29.** You respond to a house fire with the local fire department. They bring a 48-year-old woman out of the house. She is unconscious but her airway is open. Her breathing is shallow and at 30 beats/min. Her pulse is 110 beats/min strong and regular. Her blood pressure is 108/72 mm Hg. She has been burned over 40% of her body. The burned area appears to be dry and leathery. It looks charred and has pieces of fabric embedded in the flesh. You know that this type of burn is called:

    A. first-degree.

    B. second-degree.

    C. partial-thickness.

    D. third-degree.

_____ **30.** Significant airway burns may be associated with:

    A. singeing of the hair within the nostrils.

    B. hoarseness.

    C. hypoxia.

    D. all of the above

_____ **31.** The most important consideration when dealing with electrical burns is:

    A. BSI precautions.

    B. scene safety.

    C. level of responsiveness.

    D. airway.

_____ **32.** Treatment of electrical burns includes:

    A. maintaining the airway.

    B. monitoring the patient closely for respiratory or cardiac arrest.

    C. splinting any suspected injuries.

    D. all of the above

_____ **33.** All of the following, except _____, may be used as an occlusive dressing:

    A. gauze pads

    B. Vaseline gauze

    C. aluminum foil

    D. plastic

_____ **34.** Using elastic bandages to secure dressings may result in _____ if the injury swells or if improperly applied.

    A. additional tissue damage

    B. loss of a limb

    C. impaired circulation

    D. all of the above

Labeling

Label the following diagrams with the correct terms.

1. The Skin

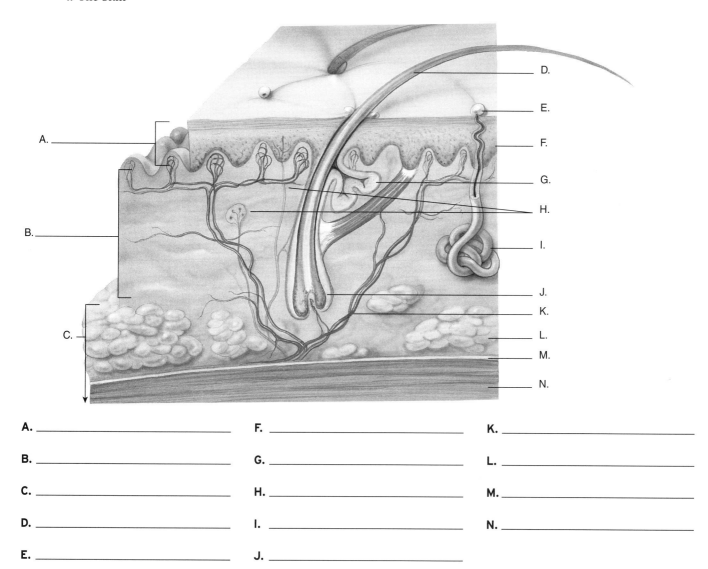

A. _____	F. _____	K. _____
B. _____	G. _____	L. _____
C. _____	H. _____	M. _____
D. _____	I. _____	N. _____
E. _____	J. _____	

2. The Rule of Nines

A. _____

B. _____

C. _____

D. _____

E. _____

F. _____

G. _____

H. _____

A. _____

B. _____

C. _____

D. _____

E. _____

F. _____

G. _____

H. _____

Fill-in

Read each item carefully, then complete the statement by filling in the missing word(s).

1. Mucous membranes are _____.

2. A person will sweat in an effort to _____ the body.

3. Nerve endings are located in the _____.

4. Below the dermis lies the _____ tissue.

5. In cold weather, skin blood vessels will _____.

6. The skin protects the body by keeping _____ out and _____ in.

7. Because nerve endings are present, injury to the _____ may be painful.

8. A major function of the skin is regulating body _____.

9. The external layer of skin is the _____ and the inner layer is the _____.

10. When the vessels of the skin dilate, heat is _____ from the body.

True/False

If you believe the statement to be more true than false, write the letter "T" in the space provided. If you believe the statement to be more false than true, write the letter "F".

_____ **1.** Partial-thickness burns involve the epidermis and some portion of the dermis.

_____ **2.** Blisters are commonly seen with superficial burns.

_____ **3.** Severe burns are usually a combination of superficial, partial-thickness, and full-thickness burns.

_____ **4.** The Rule of Nines allows you to estimate the percentage of body surface area that has been burned.

_____ **5.** Two factors, depth and extent, are critical in assessing the severity of a burn.

_____ **6.** Your first responsibility with a burn patient is to stop the burning process.

_____ **7.** Burned areas should be immersed in cool water for up to 30 minutes.

_____ **8.** Electrical burns are always more severe than the external signs indicate.

_____ **9.** The universal dressing is ideal for covering large open wounds.

_____ **10.** Occlusive dressings are usually made of Vaseline gauze, aluminum foil, or plastic.

_____ **11.** Gauze pads prevent air and liquids from entering or exiting the wound.

_____ **12.** Elastic bandages can be used to secure dressings.

_____ **13.** Soft roller bandages are slightly elastic and the layers adhere somewhat to one another.

_____ **14.** Ecchymosis is associated with open wounds.

_____ **15.** A laceration is considered a closed wound.

Short Answer

Complete this section with short written answers using the space provided.

1. List the three major classifications of depth of burns.

_____

_____

2. List the three general classifications of soft-tissue injuries.

_____

_____

3. Define the acronym RICES.

R: _____

I: _____

C: _____

E: _____

S: _____

4. Describe the classifications of a critical burn for an infant or child.

_____

_____

5. What treatment should be used with a patient burned by a dry chemical?

_____

_____

6. Why are electrical burns particularly dangerous to a patient?

_____

_____

7. Describe a sucking chest wound.

_____

_____

8. List the three primary functions of dressings and bandages.

_____

_____

9. List the four types of open soft-tissue injuries.

_____

_____

10. List the five factors used to determine the severity of a burn.

_____

_____

Word Fun

The following crossword puzzle is an activity provided to reinforce correct spelling and understanding of medical terminology associated with emergency care and the EMT-B. Use the clues in the column to complete the puzzle.

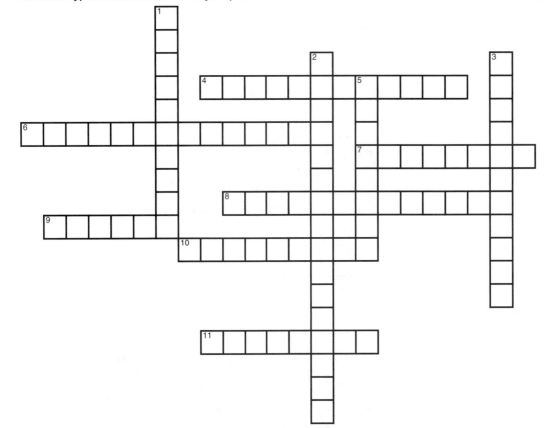

Across

4. Displacement of organs outside body
6. Lining of body cavities and passages with contact to outside
7. Torn completely loose or hanging as a flap
8. Presence of infective organisms
9. Inner layer of skin
10. Bruise
11. Blood collected in soft tissues

Down

1. Discoloration associated with closed injury
2. Injury from sharp, pointed object
3. Assigns percentages to burns
5. Scraping wound

Ambulance Calls

The following case scenarios provide an opportunity to explore the concerns associated with patient management. Read each scenario, then answer each question in detail.

1. You are dispatched to a residence where a 10-year-old girl fell onto a jagged piece of metal and has a gaping laceration to the right upper arm that is spurting bright red blood. The mother tried to control bleeding with a towel, but it kept soaking through.

   How would you best manage this patient?

   _____

   _____

   _____

2. You are dispatched to the home of a 3-year-old for an unknown problem. You arrive to find a young mother screaming for your help. Apparently, she was cooking a meal for her other children when the phone rang. While she was talking, the 3-year-old child grabbed the pot handle, pulling boiling hot water onto his body.

   How do you best manage this patient?

   _____

   _____

   _____

3. You are watching TV at the station when a fire fighter comes into the room holding his left hand. His wedding ring got caught in a piece of small machinery at the stationhouse, resulting in a 'degloving' of his ring finger.

   How do you best manage this patient?

   _____

   _____

   _____

Skill Drills

Skill Drill 24-1: Controlling Bleeding from a Soft-Tissue Injury

Test your knowledge of this skill drill by filling in the correct words in the photo captions.

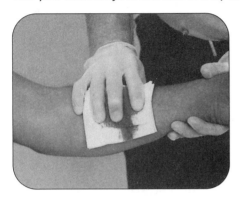

1. Apply _____ _____ with a _____ bandage.

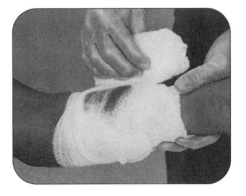

2. Maintain pressure with a _____ bandage.

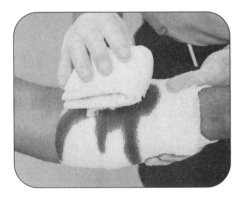

3. If bleeding continues, apply a second _____ and _____ bandage over the first.

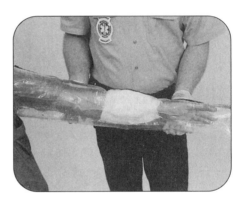

4. _____ the extremity.

Skill Drill 24- 2: Stabilizing an Impaled Object

Test your knowledge of this skill drill by filling in the correct words in the photo captions.

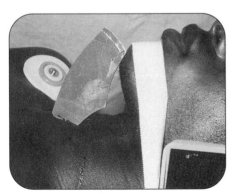

1. Do not attempt to _____ or _____ the object. Stabilize the impaled body part.

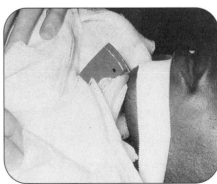

2. Control _____ and _____ the object in place using _____ _____, _____, and/or _____.

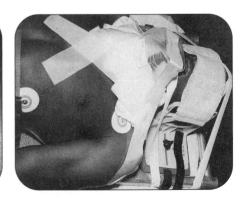

3. Tape a _____ item over the stabilized object to protect it from _____ during transport.

Skill Drill 24- 3: Caring for Burns

Test your knowledge of this skill drill by placing the photos below in the correct order. Number the first step with a "1", the second step with a "2", etc.

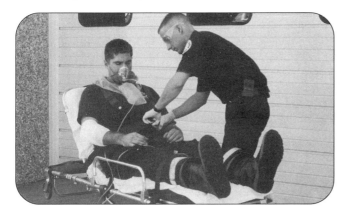

Prepare for transport.

Treat for shock.

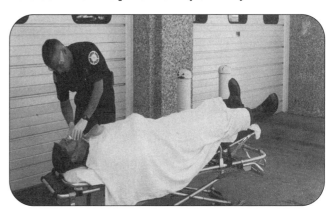

Estimate the severity of the burn, then cover the area with a dry, sterile dressing or clean sheet.

Assess and treat the patient for any other injuries.

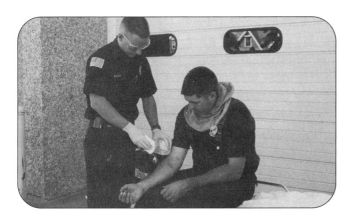

Follow BSI precautions to help prevent infection.

If it is safe to do so, remove the patient from the burning area; extinguish or remove hot clothing and jewelry as needed.

If the wound(s) is still burning or hot, immerse the hot area in cool, sterile water, or cover with a wet, cool dressing.

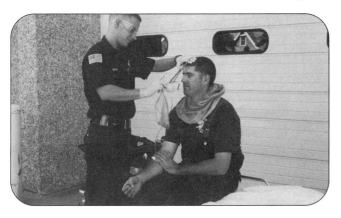

Provide high-flow oxygen and continue to assess the airway.

Cover the patient with blankets to prevent loss of body heat. Transport promptly.

Assessment Review

Answer the following questions pertaining to the assessment of the types of emergencies discussed in this chapter.

_____ **1.** During the initial assessment of burns, it is important to remember to:

    A. determine scene safety.

    B. obtain vital signs.

    C. prevent heat loss.

    D. estimate the amount of body surface injuries.

_____ **2.** You have been dispatched to a residence for a 24-year old woman who splashed cooking grease on her arm while cooking. As you approach her she is crying and yelling that it hurts. Her pulse is 130 beats/min and regular. Her blood pressure is 126/86 mm Hg. You decide that she is not an immediate transport. The focused history and physical exam should be:

    A. rapid trauma assessment.

    B. an examination of the burned arm.

    C. a detailed physical exam.

    D. done during transport to the hospital.

_____ **3.** During the rapid trauma assessment of a burn patient with a significant mechanism of injury you should:

    A. splint all fractures.

    B. determine the transport decision.

    C. open all blisters.

    D. estimate the amount of body surface injured.

_____ **4.** During the intervention step of patient assessment for a burn patient, the first intervention should be:

    A. stop the burning process.

    B. provide complete spinal stabilization.

    C. treat for shock.

    D. cover burns with moist sterile dressings.

_____ **5.** You respond to a patient who has been stabbed in the neck. You arrive to find the patient in police custody and bleeding moderately from the neck wound. The patient is alert, oriented, and swearing loudly. His pulse is 120 beats/min and blood pressure is 124/76 mm Hg. You start to bandage the wound. What type of bandage should you use?

    A. Triangular bandage

    B. Adhesive bandage

    C. Roller bandage

    D. Occlusive bandage

Emergency Care Summary

Fill in the following chart pertaining to the management of the types of emergencies discussed in this chapter.

NOTE: While the steps below are widely accepted, be sure to consult and follow your local protocol.

Closed Injuries	Open Injuries	Burns
1. Keep the patient as quiet comfortable as possible.	1. Apply direct pressure with a sterile bandage.	1. Follow BSI precautions.
2. Apply ice (or cold packs).	2. Maintain pressure with a _____ bandage.	2. Move the patient away from the burning area.
3. Apply direct pressure.	3. If bleeding continues, apply a second dressing and _____ bandage over the first.	3. Innerse the burned skin in cool, _____ water.
4. Elevate the injured part just above the level of the patient's _____.	4. Splint the extremity.	4. Provide high-flow oxygen.
5. Splint the injured area.		5. Cover the patient with a clean blanket.
		6. Rapidly estimate the burn's severity.
		7. Check for _____ injuries.
		8. Treat the patient for shock.
		9. Provide prompt transport.

Abdominal Injuries	Impaled Objects	Neck Wounds
1. Do not touch or move exposed organs.	1. Do not attempt to move or remove the object.	1. Cover wound with _____ dressing.
2. Keep organs moist. Use moist sterile dressing, cover and secure in place.	2. Control bleeding and stabilize the object in place using soft dressings _____, and/or tape.	2. Apply manual pressure, but do not compress both _____ vessels at the same time.
3. If the patient's legs and knees are uninjured, flex them to relieve pressure on the _____.	3. Tape a rigid item over the stabilized object to protect it from movement during transport.	3. Secure dressing over the wound.

Chemical Burns	Electrical Burns	Small Animal and Human Bites
1. Stop the burning process; safely remove any chemical from the patient, always brushing off a dry chemical.	1. Ensure that the scene is safe.	1. Promptly stabilize the area with a splint or bandage.
2. Remove all of patient's clothing.	2. If indicated, begin CPR and apply the _____.	2. Apply a dry, sterile dressing.
3. Flush the burn area with large amounts of water for _____ to _____ minutes after the patient says the burning has stopped.	3. Treat soft-tissue areas by placing dry, sterile dressings on all burn wounds and splinting fractures.	3. Provide transport to the emergency department for surgical cleansing of the wound and _____ therapy.

CHAPTER
25 Eye Injuries

Workbook Activities

The following activities have been designed to help you. Your instructor may require you to complete some or all of these activities as a regular part of your EMT-B training program. You are encouraged to complete any activity that your instructor does not assign as a way to enhance your learning in the classroom.

Chapter Review

The following exercises provide an opportunity to refresh your knowledge of this chapter.

Matching

Match each of the terms in the left column to the appropriate definition in the right column.

_____ 1. Cornea	**A.** membrane that covers the exposed surface of the eye
_____ 2. Iris	**B.** focuses light
_____ 3. Lens	**C.** muscle behind cornea
_____ 4. Pupil	**D.** transparent tissue in front of pupil and iris
_____ 5. Sclera	**E.** circular opening in iris
_____ 6. Orbit	**F.** the eyeball
_____ 7. Conjunctiva	**G.** eye socket
_____ 8. Globe	**H.** the light-sensitive area of the eye where images are projected
_____ 9. Lacrimal glands	**I.** tear glands
_____ 10. Retina	**J.** white portion of eye

Multiple Choice

Read each item carefully, then select the best response.

_____ **1.** The conjunctiva covers the:

    A. outer surface of the eyelids.

    B. exposed surface of the eye.

    C. lens.

    D. iris.

_____ **2.** The purpose of the _____, an extremely tough, fibrous tissue, is to help maintain the eye's globular shape.

    A. cornea

    B. lens

    C. retina

    D. sclera

_____ **3.** The _____ allows light to enter the eye.

    A. cornea

    B. lens

    C. retina

    D. sclera

_____ **4.** The circular muscle that adjusts the size of the opening behind the cornea to regulate the amount of light that enters the eye is called the:

    A. iris.

    B. lens.

    C. retina.

    D. sclera.

_____ **5.** You respond to a 78-year-old man who is unresponsive. His pulse is 126 beats/min and blood pressure is 184/96 mm Hg. His respirations are 22 breaths/min and regular. His wife tells you he was complaining of a severe headache. She tells you that he told her it was the worst headache he ever had and then he collapsed. During your focused exam you notice that one pupil is constricted and the other dilated. You know that a normal, uninjured eye would have pupils that:

    A. are round.

    B. are equal in size.

    C. react equally when exposed to light.

    D. all of the above

_____ **6.** Important signs and symptoms to record include all of the following, except:

    A. how the injury occurred.

    B. any changes in vision.

    C. any history of color blindness.

    D. the use of any eye medications.

_____ **7.** The delicate tissues of the eye can be burned by _____, often causing permanent damage.

    A. chemicals

    B. heat

    C. light rays

    D. all of the above

_____ **8.** You respond with the local fire department to a house fire. The fire fighters bring you a 25-year-old woman who was trying to light a propane stove when it exploded in her face. She is alert and oriented and able to converse with you. Her pulse rate is 110 beats/min and her blood pressure is 126/76 mm Hg. She is complaining that her eyes burn and it feels like she has gravel in her eyes. You decide that you need to bandage the injury. You need to remember to:

    A. cover both eyes with a sterile dressing moistened with sterile saline.

    B. apply eye shields over the dressing.

    C. transport promptly.

    D. all of the above

_____ **9.** You are called to the residence of a 48-year-old man who was watching a solar eclipse. He was looking directly at the eclipse without using protective eyewear. He states that it feels like there is something in his eye but has not been able to find anything. His vital signs are all within normal limits. Your assessment reveals no apparent injury. The patient states that he does not want to go to the hospital. You try and convince him to go because you know that retinal damage caused by exposure to extremes of light are not _____ but may result in permanent damage to vision.

    A. deep

    B. painful

    C. lacerated

    D. none of the above

_____ **10.** Superficial burns of the eyes can result from:

    A. light from prolonged exposure to a sunlamp.

    B. reflected light from a bright snow-covered area.

    C. ultraviolet rays from an arc welding unit.

    D. all of the above

_____ **11.** You respond to a 38-year-old man who is employed in a local metal shop. A piece of metal hit him in the face, lacerating the eyelid. He is alert and oriented but extremely anxious. His pulse is 140 beats/min and his blood pressure is 138/86 mm Hg. His respirations are 24 breaths/min and regular. He has heavy bleeding coming from the eye. You know that most bleeding from the eyelid can be controlled by:

    A. firm pressure.

    B. gentle pressure.

    C. pressure dressings.

    D. flushing the eyes.

_____ **12.** You respond to the same patient in question 11 but this time the patient has lacerated the globe of the eye. How much pressure would you apply to control the bleeding?

    A. Firm pressure

    B. Gentle pressure

    C. No pressure

    D. Pressure dressings

_____ **13.** Important guidelines in treating penetrating injuries of the eye include all of the following, except:

    A. Never exert pressure on or manipulate the globe in any way.

    B. If part of the eyeball is exposed, gently apply a moist, sterile dressing to prevent drying.

    C. Cover the injured eye with a protective metal eye shield or sterile dressing.

    D. Gently replace the eyeball if it is displaced out of its socket.

_____ **14.** A black eye is a result of:

    A. bleeding into tissue around the orbit.

    B. a fracture of the orbit.

    C. a torn retina.

    D. none of the above

_____ **15.** Bleeding into the anterior chamber of the eye that obscures part or all of the iris is called:

    A. hematemesis.

    B. hyphema.

    C. hyphoma.

    D. hemoptysis.

_____ **16.** Fracture of the orbit, particularly of the bones that form its floor and support of the globe is known as a:

    A. blowout fracture.

    B. retinal detachment.

    C. hyphema.

    D. black eye.

_____ **17.** Eye findings that should alert you to the possibility of a head injury include:

    A. one pupil larger than the other.

    B. bleeding under the conjunctiva.

    C. protrusion or bulging of one eye.

    D. all of the above

_____ **18.** The only time that contact lenses should be removed immediately in the field is in the case of a _____ the eye.

    A. blowout fracture of

    B. retinal detachment of

    C. chemical burn in

    D. broken contact lens in

Fill-in

Read each item carefully, then complete the statement by filling in the missing word(s).

1. The glands that produce fluids to keep the eye moist are called _____ _____.

2. A cranial nerve that transmits visual information to the brain is called an _____ _____.

3. The eye works like a _____, with the iris and pupil making adjustments to light and the retina acting like film.

4. Never remove contact lenses from an injured eye unless the injury is a _____ _____.

5. The _____ is composed of the adjacent bones of the face and skull.

6. When performing an examination, you are looking for specific _____ or conditions that may suggest the nature of the problem.

7. Large objects are prevented from penetrating the eye by the protective _____ that surrounds it.

8. _____ is inflammation and redness of the conjunctiva.

9. The delicate membrane that covers the inside of the eyelid and the surface of the eye is the _____.

10. The tough, fibrous tissue that helps maintain the eye's globular shape is called the _____.

True/False

If you believe the statement to be more true than false, write the letter "T" in the space provided. If you believe the statement to be more false than true, write the letter "F."

_____ **1.** Objects impaled in the eye should be removed before applying dressing.

_____ **2.** Vitreous humor can be replaced.

_____ **3.** Aqueous humor can be replaced.

_____ **4.** Lacrimal glands help keep the eye dry.

_____ **5.** Contact lenses should always be removed in the field.

_____ **6.** Foreign objects stuck to the cornea should be removed prior to transport.

_____ **7.** Bleeding soon after irritation or injury can result in a bright yellow conjunctiva.

_____ **8.** In a normal, uninjured eye the entire circle of the iris is visible.

_____ **9.** If a small foreign object is lying on the surface of the patient's eye, you should use a dextrose solution to gently irrigate the eye.

_____ **10.** The iris gives the eye its characteristic color.

Short Answer

Complete this section with short written answers using the space provided.

1. Describe a retinal detachment, including common signs and symptoms.

_____

_____

2. List the three guidelines for treating penetrating eye injuries.

_____

_____

3. List assessment findings in the eye that may indicate head injury.

_____

_____

Word Fun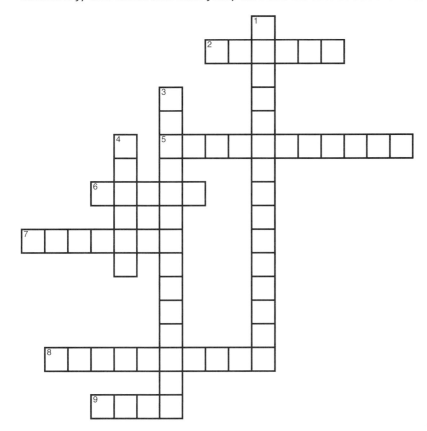

The following crossword puzzle is an activity provided to reinforce correct spelling and understanding of medical terminology associated with emergency care and the EMT-B. Use the clues in the column to complete the puzzle.

Across

2. White portion of eye
5. Membrane that lines eyelids and surface of eye
6. Eye socket
7. Bleeding into anterior chamber of eye
8. Transmits visual sensations to the brain
9. Muscle regulating light into eye

Down

1. Break in the bones of the orbit
3. Tear producer
4. Transparent tissue in front of pupil

Ambulance Calls

The following case scenarios provide an opportunity to explore the concerns associated with patient management. Read each scenario, then answer each question in detail.

1. You are dispatched to a local school playground for an eye injury. Two of the children were "play sword fighting" with two sticks. One child lunged forward with the stick, accidentally poking the other in the eye. You arrive to find the child holding his eye and crying vigorously.

   How do you best manage this patient?

   _____

   _____

   _____

2. You are called to an industrial site where a 32-year-old man had acid splashed in his eyes. Coworkers have tried pouring water into his eyes, but he is still unable to see and is in severe pain.

   How would you best manage this patient?

   _____

   _____

   _____

3. You are dispatched to a construction site for an "injury to the face." You arrive to find a young man who was accidentally hit in the face with a ladder. He tells you that the end of the ladder hit him in the face when a coworker swung around to see someone who called his name. Your patient is complaining of pain with eye movement and double vision.

How do you best manage this patient?

_____

_____

_____

Skill Drills

Skill Drill 25-1: Removing a Foreign Object From Under the Upper Eyelid
Test your knowledge of skill drills by filling in the correct words in the photo captions.

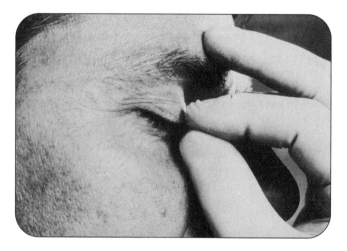

1. Have the patient look _____, grasp the _____ _____, and gently pull the lid away from the eye.

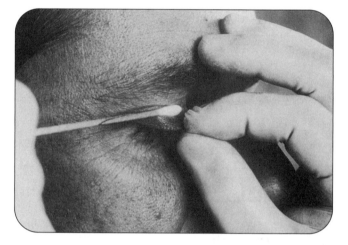

2. Place a _____ _____ on the outer surface of the upper lid.

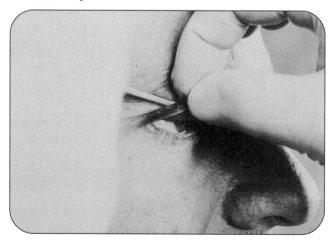

3. Pull the lid _____ and _____, folding it back over the applicator.

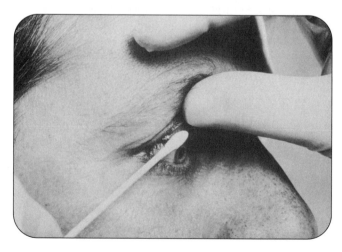

4. Gently remove the foreign object from the eyelid with a _____, _____ applicator.

Skill Drill 25-2: Stabilizing a Foreign Object Impaled in the Eye

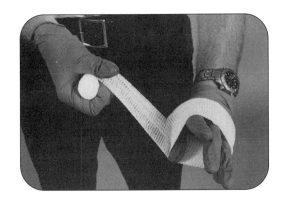

1. To prepare a doughnut ring, wrap a _____ roll around your fingers and thumb _____ or _____ times. Adjust the diameter by _____ your fingers.

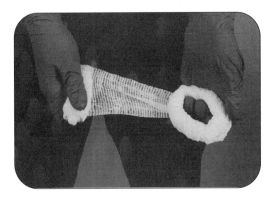

2. Wrap the remainder of the roll . . .

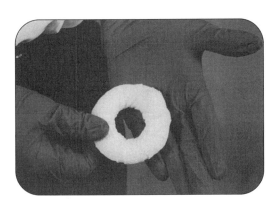

3. . . . working around the ring.

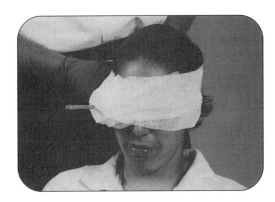

4. Place the dressing over the _____ to hold the impaled object in place, then _____ it with a _____ dressing.

Assessment Review

Answer the following questions pertaining to the assessment of the types of emergencies discussed in this chapter.

_____ 1. You have been dispatched to an 18-year-old male patient who has a blowout fracture of the left orbit. He is alert and oriented. His respirations, pulse, and blood pressure are within normal limits. During the rapid trauma assessment, what intervention should be performed?

  A. Spinal immobilization to a backboard

  B. Airway management

  C. Hemorrhage control

  D. AVPU

_____ 2. You respond to a 23-year-old woman who was an unrestrained passenger in an automobile collision. The windshield is spider webbed and she has significant facial damage. You are in the focused history and physical exam, how do you get a SAMPLE history?

  A. Family members

  B. Friends

  C. Bystanders

  D. All of the above

_____ 3. Your patient is a factory worker who has metal shavings in his right eye. You have assessed the airway, breathing, and circulation and all are within the normal limits for a patient his age. You decide that bandaging is necessary; how would you accomplish this?

  A. Bandage the right eye only.

  B. Bandage the left eye only.

  C. Bandage both eyes.

  D. Apply a pressure bandage.

_____ 4. You respond to the local high school where a 16-year-old female working in the chemistry lab has gotten an unknown substance in her eyes. She is alert and oriented. She is able to converse with you and tells you her eyes are burning. Her pulse is 124 beats/min, respirations 18 breaths/min, and blood pressure is 118/76 mm Hg. She was cleaning the shelf in the storage room when it collapsed and several chemicals fell on top of her. How long should you irrigate the eyes?

  A. 2 to 3 minutes

  B. 5 to 20 minutes

  C. 20 to 30 minutes

  D. 30 to 45 minutes

_____ 5. Your patient is a 15-year-old who was playing baseball and was hit in the right eye. The impact resulted in a blowout fracture with the eyeball partially exposed. How should you bandage the injury?

  A. Dry sterile dressing

  B. Moist sterile dressing

  C. Occlusive dressing

  D. Multitrauma dressing

Emergency Care Summary

Fill in the following chart pertaining to the management of the types of emergencies discussed in this chapter.

NOTE: While the steps below are widely accepted, be sure to consult and follow your local protocol.

Foreign Objects	Burns	Lacerations	Blunt Trauma
1. Tell the patient to look down while you grasp the _____ of the upper eyelid with your thumb and index finger. Gently pull the eyelid away from the eyeball. 2. Gently place a cotton-tipped applicator horizontally along the center of the outer surface of the upper eyelid. 3. If you see a foreign object, gently remove it with a moistened, sterile, cotton-tipped applicator. **Stabilizing a Foreign Object Impaled in the Eye** 1. To prepare a doughnut rung, wrap a _____ around your fingers and thumb seven or eight times. 2. Wrap the remainder of the roll, working around the ring. 3. Place the dressing over the eye to hold the impaled object in place and then secure it with a gauze dressing.	**Chemical Burns** 1. Holding the eyelid open, irrigate the eye for _____ to _____ minutes. 2. Apply a clean, dry sterile dressing to cover the eye. **Thermal Burns** 1. Cover both eyes with a sterile dressing moistened with sterile _____. **Light Burns** 1. Cover each eye with a sterile, moist pad and eye shield. 2. Transport supine and prevent further exposure to bright light.	1. Never exert pressure on or manipulate the injured eye in any way. 2. If part of the eyeball is exposed, gently apply a _____ sterile dressing to prevent drying. 3. Cover the injured eye with a protective metal eye shield or sterile dressing.	1. Protect the eye from further injury with a _____ _____. 2. Cover the other eye to minimize movement on the injured side.

CHAPTER

26 Face and Throat Injuries

Workbook Activities

The following activities have been designed to help you. Your instructor may require you to complete some or all of these activities as a regular part of your EMT-B training program. You are encouraged to complete any activity that your instructor does not assign as a way to enhance your learning in the classroom.

Chapter Review

The following exercises provide an opportunity to refresh your knowledge of this chapter.

Matching

Match each of the terms in the left column to the appropriate definition in the right column.

_____ **1.** Cranium   **A.** upper jaw

_____ **2.** Occiput   **B.** posterior cranium

_____ **3.** Pinna   **C.** contains the brain

_____ **4.** Zygomas   **D.** pull/tear away

_____ **5.** Mandible   **E.** visible part of ear

_____ **6.** Avulse   **F.** cheekbones

_____ **7.** Maxilla   **G.** lower jawbone

Multiple Choice

Read each item carefully, then select the best response.

_____ **1.** As an EMT-B, your objective is to:

   A. prevent further injury.

   B. manage any acute airway problems.

   C. control bleeding.

   D. all of the above

_____ **2.** The head is divided into two parts: the cranium and the:

   A. brain.

   B. face.

   C. skull.

   D. medulla oblongata.

_____ **3.** The brain connects to the spinal cord through a large opening at the base of the skull known as the:

   A. eustachian tube.

   B. spinous process.

   C. foramen magnum.

   D. vertebral foramina.

_____ **4.** Approximately _____ of the nose is composed of bone. The remainder is composed of cartilage.

   A. 9/10

   B. 2/3

   C. 3/4

   D. 1/3

_____ **5.** Motion of the mandible occurs at the:

   A. temporomandibular joint.

   B. mastoid process.

   C. chin.

   D. mandibular angle.

_____ **6.** You respond to a 71-year-old woman who is unresponsive. You try to get her to respond but have no success. Her airway is open and she is breathing at a rate of 14 breaths/min. You know you can check a pulse in either side of the neck. You know that the jugular veins and several nerves run through the neck next to the trachea. What structure are you trying to locate to take a pulse?

   A. Hypothalamus

   B. Subclavian arteries

   C. Cricoid cartilage

   D. Carotid arteries

_____ **7.** The _____ connects the cricoid cartilage and thyroid cartilage.

   A. larynx

   B. cricoid membrane

   C. cricothyroid membrane

   D. thyroid membrane

_____ **8.** You respond to a 68-year-old man who was involved in a motor vehicle collision. He is unresponsive and as you approach you notice he is not breathing. He was unrestrained and has massive facial injuries. When you check his airway, it is obstructed. You know that upper airway obstructions can be caused by:

   A. heavy bleeding.

   B. loosened teeth or dentures.

   C. soft-tissue swelling.

   D. all of the above

_____ **9.** You are dispatched to a residential neighborhood for a 6-year-old who was bitten by the family pet. The mother meets you at the door with the child who is crying uncontrollably and has blood covering the right side of her head. You look at the child and notice that the lower right ear has been completely avulsed. You control the bleeding with direct pressure and bandage the injury. You follow the blood trail back to where the incident occurred and find the avulsed part. How do you manage the avulsed tissue?

    A. Wrap the skin in a moist, sterile dressing/place in a plastic bag in ice water/transport with patient.

    B. Place the skin in plastic "biohazard" bag and dispose of properly.

    C. Place the skin in a plastic bag filled with ice and transport to the ER.

    D. Leave it at the scene to be disposed of later.

_____ **10.** The nasal cavity is divided into two chambers by the:

    A. frontal sinus.

    B. middle turbinate.

    C. zygoma.

    D. nasal septum.

_____ **11.** You are called to the home of a 48-year-old woman who has a history of high blood pressure and now has a major nose bleed. She is alert and oriented and converses freely with you. Her respirations and pulse are within normal limits. Her blood pressure is 194/108 mm Hg. You have been able to rule out trauma. How would you manage the nose bleed?

    A. Apply a sterile dressing.

    B. Pinch the nostrils together.

    C. Put the patient in a supine position.

    D. Have the patient hold ice in her mouth.

_____ **12.** The middle ear is connected to the nasal cavity by the:

    A. frontal sinus.

    B. zygomatic process.

    C. eustachian tube.

    D. superior trachea.

_____ **13.** You are called to a motor vehicle collision that was the result of a lateral impact. The patient is conscious but extremely confused. The airway is open and the patient is breathing at 16 breaths/min and unlabored. The pulse is 110 beats/min strong and regular. The blood pressure is 136/90 mm Hg. The patient has bleeding from the left temple area. You start to examine the head and you know that basilar skull fracture may present with:

    A. leakage of CSF from the ears and nose.

    B. distended neck veins.

    C. Battle's signs.

    D. periorbital ecchymosis.

_____ **14.** Signs of a possible facial fracture include:

    A. bleeding in the mouth.

    B. absent or loose teeth.

    C. loose and/or moveable bone fragments.

    D. all of the above

_____ **15.** The presence of air in the soft tissues of the neck that produces a crackling sensation is called:

    A. the "Rice Krispy" effect.

    B. a pneumothorax.

    C. rales.

    D. subcutaneous emphysema.

_____ **16.** Most bleeding from the neck can be controlled by:

    A. direct pressure.

    B. a pressure point.

    C. elevation.

    D. a tourniquet.

Labeling

Label the following diagrams with the correct terms.

1. Face/Skull

A. _____   F. _____   J. _____

B. _____   G. _____   K. _____

C. _____   H. _____   L. _____

D. _____   I. _____   M. _____

E. _____

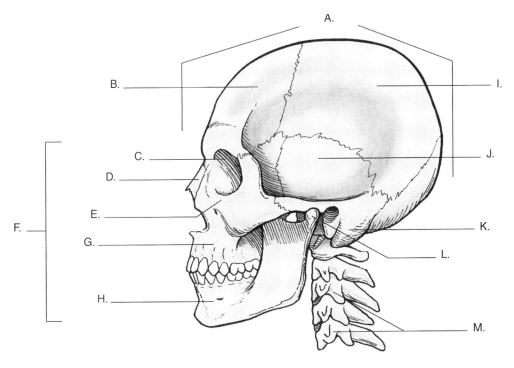

Fill-in

Read each item carefully, then complete the statement by filling in the missing word(s).

1. Pulsations in the neck are felt in the _____ vessels.

2. The _____ vertebrae are in the neck.

3. The _____ lobes of the cranium are located on the lateral portion of the head.

4. The _____ is located in the anterior portion of the neck.

5. The rings of the trachea are made of _____.

6. The Adam's Apple is more prominent in _____ than in _____.

7. The _____ _____ is a large opening at the base of the skull.

8. The _____ is the upper part of the jaw.

9. The _____ lobes lie laterally between the temporal and occipital lobes.

10. The _____ connects the larynx with the main air passage.

True/False

If you believe the statement to be more true than false, write the letter "T" in the space provided. If you believe the statement to be more false than true, write the letter "F."

_____ 1. Injuries to the face often lead to airway problems.

_____ 2. Care for facial injuries begins with BSI precautions and the ABCs.

_____ 3. Exposed eye or brain injuries are covered with a dry dressing.

_____ 4. Clear fluid in the outer ear is normal.

_____ 5. Any crushing injury of the upper part of the neck likely involves the larynx or the trachea.

_____ 6. Soft-tissue injuries to the face are common.

_____ 7. The opening that the spinal core leaves the head through is called the occiput.

_____ 8. The muscle that allows movement of the head is the temporomandibular.

_____ 9. BSI for assessing face and throat injuries should include eye and oral protection.

_____ 10. The airway of choice with facial injuries is the nasopharyngeal.

Short Answer

Complete this section with short written answers using the space provided.

1. Describe bleeding control methods for facial injuries.

_____

_____

2. Describe bleeding control methods for lacerations to veins or arteries in the neck.

_____

_____

Word Fun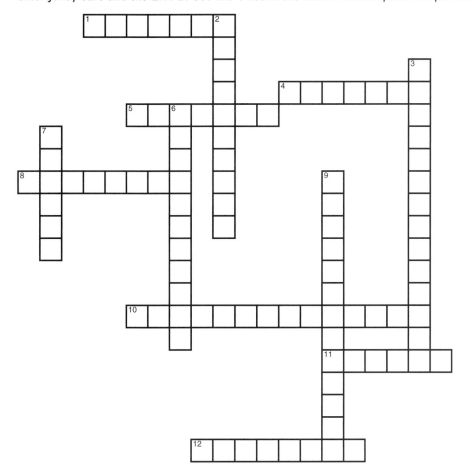

The following crossword puzzle is a good way to review correct spelling and meaning of medical terminology associated with emergency care and the EMT-B. Use the clues in the column to complete the puzzle.

Across

1. Posterior portion of skull
4. Upper jawbone
5. Skull
8. Lower jawbone
10. Connects middle ear to nasal cavity
11. To pull or tear away
12. Blood accumulated in soft tissue

Down

2. Layers of bones in nasal cavity
3. Bony mass about 1″ posterior to ear
6. Air in the veins
7. Fleshy bulge anterior to ear canal
9. Large opening in base of skull

Ambulance Calls

The following case scenarios provide an opportunity to explore the concerns associated with patient management. Read each scenario, then answer each question in detail.

1. You are dispatched to assist a small child who was attacked by his family's dog. The dog bit his face and neck repeatedly, then grabbed him by the neck and shook him violently. The mother found the boy "making funny breathing sounds" and called for help. She has removed the dog from the area.

   How do you best manage this patient?

   _____

   _____

   _____

2. You are dispatched to a 37-year-old man with a large laceration to the right side of his neck. Bleeding is dark and heavy. He is alert, but weak.

   How would you best manage this patient?

   _____

   _____

   _____

3. You are dispatched to a Little League baseball game to assist an assault victim. Apparently, emotions were running high when two parents began to argue. You arrive to find a 40-year-old man with a bloody nose.

How do you best manage this patient?

_____

_____

_____

Skill Drills
Skill Drill 26-1: Controlling Bleeding From a Neck Injury
Test your knowledge of skill drills by filling in the correct words in the photo captions.

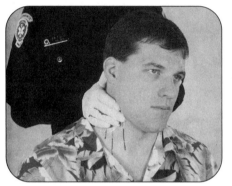

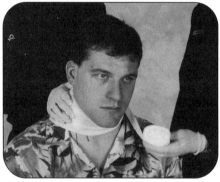

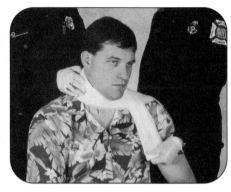

1. Apply _____ _____ to control bleeding.

2. Use _____ _____ to secure a dressing in place.

3. Wrap the bandage around and under the patient's _____.

Assessment Review

Answer the following questions pertaining to the assessment of the types of emergencies discussed in this chapter.

_____ **1.** You have responded to an automobile collision and found a 21-year-old man who has massive facial trauma. There is heavy bleeding and he is unconscious. The first thing that you do in your treatment of this patient is:

    A. take c-spine precautions.

    B. open the airway.

    C. assess his breathing.

    D. take BSI precautions.

_____ **2.** For the patient described above, how often would you reassess the vitals during your ongoing assessment?

    A. Every 3 minutes

    B. Every 5 minutes

    C. Every 10 minutes

    D. Every 15 minutes

_____ **3.** You have a patient who has severe epistaxis. You have been able to rule out trauma. How would you position this patient to help control the bleeding?

    A. Supine

    B. Prone

    C. Sitting leaning back

    D. Sitting leaning forward

_____ **4.** You have a patient who has had a tooth knocked out. You find the tooth; how would you transport it to the hospital?

    A. In the patient's saliva

    B. In dextrose

    C. In ice

    D. In a dry sterile dressing

_____ **5.** You respond to a child who has placed a pebble in his ear. He is complaining that it is hurting. You should:

    A. remove it with a Q-tip.

    B. have the child try and shake it out.

    C. leave it and transport.

    D. no load because this is not an emergency.

Emergency Care Summary

Fill in the following chart pertaining to the management of the types of emergencies discussed in this chapter.

NOTE: While the steps below are widely accepted, be sure to consult and follow your local protocol.

Nose Injuries	Ear Injuries	Facial Fractures	Neck Injuries
Controlling Epistaxis (See Skill Drill 22-4) 1. Position the patient sitting, leaning _____. 2. Apply direct pressure, pinching the fleshy part of the nostrils for 15 minutes. 3. Keep the patient calm and quiet. 4. Apply ice over the nose.	1. Place a soft, padded dressing between the ear and the scalp. 2. If the ear is avulsed, wrap it in a _____, sterile dressing and place in a plastic bag. 3. Leave any foreign object within the ear for the physician to remove. 4. Note any clear fluid coming from the ear.	1. Remove and save loose teeth and _____ fragment from the mouth and transport them with you. 2. Remove dentures and dental bridges to protect them against airway obstruction. 3. Maintain an open airway. 4. When transporting dislodged teeth, place them in a container of the patient's _____ or milk, if possible.	1. Apply direct pressure to control bleeding. 2. Use _____ _____ to secure a dressing in place. 3. Wrap the bandage around and under the patient's shoulder.

CHAPTER

27 Chest Injuries

Workbook Activities

The following activities have been designed to help you. Your instructor may require you to complete some or all of these activities as a regular part of your EMT-B training program. You are encouraged to complete any activity that your instructor does not assign as a way to enhance your learning in the classroom.

Chapter Review

The following exercises provide an opportunity to refresh your knowledge of this chapter.

Matching

Match each of the terms in the left column to the appropriate definition in the right column.

_____ 1. Thoracic cage   **A.** chest rises

_____ 2. Diaphragm   **B.** chest

_____ 3. Exhalation   **C.** chest falls

_____ 4. Inhalation   **D.** separates chest from abdomen

_____ 5. Aorta   **E.** major artery in the chest

_____ 6. Closed chest injury   **F.** penetrating wound

_____ 7. Hemoptysis   **G.** rapid respirations

_____ 8. Pericardium   **H.** unusually blunt trauma

_____ 9. Open chest injury   **I.** coughing up blood

_____ 10. Tachypnea   **J.** sac around the heart

Multiple Choice

Read each item carefully, then select the best response.

_____ **1.** Air is supplied to the lungs via the:

    A. esophagus.

    B. trachea.

    C. nares.

    D. oropharynx.

_____ **2.** The _____ separates the thoracic cavity from the abdominal cavity.

    A. diaphragm

    B. mediastinum

    C. xyphoid process

    D. inferior border of the ribs

_____ **3.** On inhalation, all of the following occur, except:

    A. the intercostal muscles contract, elevating the rib cage.

    B. the diaphragm contracts.

    C. the pressure inside the chest increases.

    D. air enters through the nose and mouth.

_____ **4.** You respond to the local rodeo arena for a bull rider. The scene is safe and the patient is lying in the middle of the arena unconscious. His airway is open and he is breathing at 20 breaths/min. His pulse is 128 beats/min and blood pressure is 110/64 mm Hg. There is no obvious bleeding. Bystanders tell you he was thrown into the air and landed on the bull's head. He was not wearing a vest. You know that blunt trauma to the chest may:

    A. bruise the lungs and heart.

    B. fracture whole areas of the chest wall.

    C. damage the aorta.

    D. all of the above

_____ **5.** You respond to a motor vehicle collision and have a 29-year-old woman who is complaining of chest pain. Her chest struck the steering wheel. Her airway is open, she is breathing at 24 breaths/min, and coughing up blood. Her pulse is 130 beats/min rapid and weak, and blood pressure is 90/58 mm Hg. You notice cyanosis around the lips and her fingers are also blue. When you expose the chest, she tells you it hurts and points to a bruised spot. Which of these is a symptom?

    A. Cyanosis around the lips or fingertips

    B. Rapid, weak pulse

    C. Hemoptysis

    D. Pain at the site of injury

_____ **6.** Common causes of dyspnea include:

    A. airway obstruction.

    B. lung compression.

    C. damage to the chest wall.

    D. all of the above

_____ **7.** You respond to an 18-year-old male who has been assaulted with a baseball bat. He was hit in the chest. He is conscious but is having difficulty breathing. His airway is open and his respirations are 30 breaths/min. His pulse is 126 beats/min and blood pressure is 114/72 mm Hg. You quickly expose the chest and there is heavy bruising. The chest wall does not expand on each side when the patient inhales. This is known as:

    A. flail segment.

    B. paradoxical motion.

    C. pneumothorax.

    D. hemoptysis.

_____ **8.** The principle reason for concern about a patient who has a chest injury is:

   A. hemoptysis.

   B. cyanosis.

   C. that the body has no means of storing oxygen.

   D. a rapid, weak pulse and low blood pressure.

_____ **9.** A _____ results when an injury allows air to enter through a hole in the chest wall or the surface of the lung as the patient attempts to breathe, causing the lung on that side to collapse.

   A. tension pneumothorax

   B. hemothorax

   C. hemopneumothorax

   D. pneumothorax

_____ **10.** A sucking chest wound should be treated:

   A. after assessing ABCs.

   B. after confirming mental status.

   C. immediately by covering with a gloved hand, then an occlusive dressing.

   D. by using a stack of gauze dressings.

_____ **11.** You respond to a 20-year-old man who was playing basketball and suddenly developed chest pain and respiratory difficulty. He is alert and oriented and complaining of chest pain and breathing at 24 breaths/min. His pulse is 140 beats/min and blood pressure is 160/90 mm Hg. Upon listening to the chest, you notice diminished breath sounds on the left. There is no obvious injury anywhere to the chest. You are thinking that the patient has a spontaneous pneumothorax. A spontaneous pneumothorax:

   A. presents with a sudden sharp chest pain.

   B. presents with increasing difficulty breathing.

   C. should be treated the same as a traumatic pneumothorax.

   D. all of the above

_____ **12.** You know that if you do not treat the patient properly and transport them rapidly to the hospital they could develop a tension pneumothorax. What effect does the development of a tension pneumothorax have on the body?

   A. Air gradually increases the pressure in the chest.

   B. It causes the complete collapse of the affected lung.

   C. It prevents blood from returning through the venae cavae to the heart.

   D. All of the above

_____ **13.** Common signs and symptoms of tension pneumothorax include:

   A. increasing respiratory distress.

   B. distended neck veins.

   C. tracheal deviation away from the injured site.

   D. all of the above

_____ **14.** A hemothorax results from blood collecting in the pleural space from:

   A. a bleeding rib cage.

   B. a bleeding lung.

   C. a bleeding great vessel.

   D. all of the above

_____ **15.** A fractured rib that penetrates into the pleural space may lacerate the surface of the lung, causing a:

   A. tension pneumothorax.

   B. hemothorax.

   C. hemopneumothorax.

   D. all of the above

_____ **16.** In what is called paradoxical movement, the detached portion of the chest wall:

    A. moves opposite of normal.

    B. moves out instead of in during inhalation.

    C. moves in instead of out during expiration.

    D. all of the above

_____ **17.** Traumatic asphyxia:

    A. is bruising of the lung.

    B. occurs when three or more adjacent ribs are fractured in two or more places.

    C. is a sudden, severe compression of the chest.

    D. all of the above

_____ **18.** Traumatic asphyxia results in a very characteristic appearance, including:

    A. distended neck veins.

    B. cyanosis.

    C. hemorrhage into the sclera of the eye.

    D. all of the above

_____ **19.** Signs and symptoms of a pericardial tamponade include:

    A. low blood pressure.

    B. a weak pulse.

    C. muffled heart tones.

    D. all of the above

_____ **20.** Large blood vessels in the chest that can result in massive hemorrhaging include all of the following, except:

    A. the pulmonary arteries.

    B. the femoral arteries.

    C. the aorta.

    D. four main pulmonary veins.

Labeling

Label the following diagrams with the correct terms.

    1. Anterior Aspect of the Chest

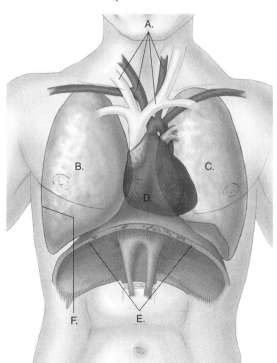

A. _____

B. _____

C. _____

D. _____

E. _____

F. _____

2. The Ribs

A. _____

B. _____

C. _____

D. _____

E. _____

F. _____

G. _____

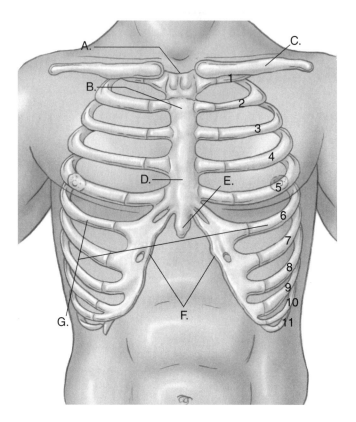

Fill-in

Read each item carefully, then complete the statement by filling in the missing word.

1. The esophagus is located in the _____ of the chest.

2. During inhalation, the pressure in the chest _____.

3. In the anterior chest, ribs connect to the _____.

4. The trachea divides into the right and left main stem _____.

5. The _____ nerves supply the diaphragm.

6. Contents of the chest are protected by the _____.

7. The chest extends from the lower end of the neck to the _____.

8. _____ line the area between the lungs and chest wall.

9. The great vessel located in the chest is the _____.

10. During inhalation, the diaphragm _____.

True/False

If you believe the statement to be more true than false, write the letter "T" in the space provided. If you believe the statement to be more false than true, write the letter "F."

_____ **1.** Dyspnea is difficulty with breathing.

_____ **2.** Tachypnea is slow respirations.

_____ **3.** Distended neck veins may be a sign of a tension pneumothorax.

_____ **4.** Rib fractures are common in children.

_____ **5.** Narrowing pulse pressure is related to spontaneous pneumothorax.

_____ **6.** Laceration of the large blood vessels in the chest can cause minimal hemorrhage.

_____ **7.** The thoracic cage extends from the lower end of the neck to the umbilicus.

_____ **8.** Patients with spinal cord injuries at C3 or above can lose their ability to breathe entirely.

_____ **9.** Almost one third of people who are killed immediately in car crashes die as a result of traumatic rupture of the myocardium.

_____ **10.** Open chest injury is caused by penetrating trauma.

Short Answer

Complete this section with short written answers using the space provided.

1. List the signs and symptoms associated with a chest injury.

_____

_____

2. Describe the two methods for sealing a sucking chest wound.

_____

_____

3. Describe the method(s) for immobilizing a flail chest wall segment.

_____

_____

4. Define traumatic asphyxia and describe its signs.

_____

_____

Word Fun

The following crossword puzzle is an activity provided to reinforce correct spelling and understanding of medical terminology associated with emergency care and the EMT-B. Use the clues in the column to complete the puzzle.

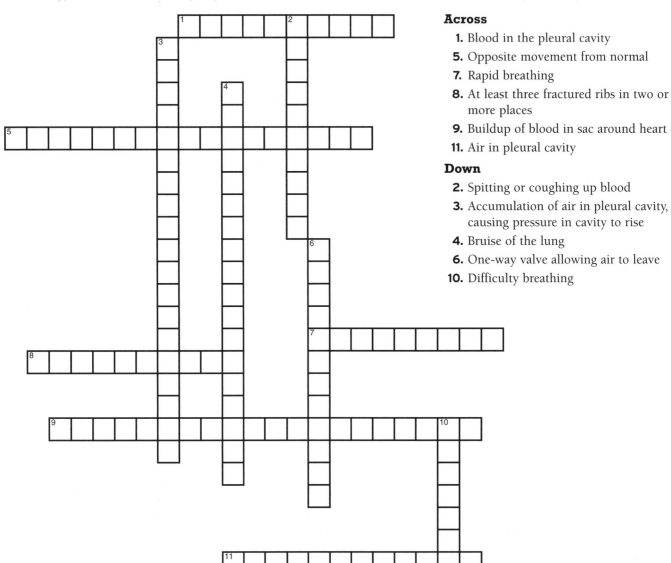

Across

1. Blood in the pleural cavity
5. Opposite movement from normal
7. Rapid breathing
8. At least three fractured ribs in two or more places
9. Buildup of blood in sac around heart
11. Air in pleural cavity

Down

2. Spitting or coughing up blood
3. Accumulation of air in pleural cavity, causing pressure in cavity to rise
4. Bruise of the lung
6. One-way valve allowing air to leave
10. Difficulty breathing

Ambulance Calls

The following case scenarios provide an opportunity to explore the concerns associated with patient management. Read each scenario, then answer each question in detail.

1. You are dispatched to an area horse ranch for an injury to a rider. You arrive to find that a horse has kicked one of the riders in the chest. He is having significant difficulty breathing and appears to be in extreme pain.

How do you best manage this patient?

_____

_____

_____

2. You are dispatched for a man trapped under a car. As you travel to the location, the dispatcher informs you that your patient is now free, but is experiencing significant chest and mid-back pain.

How do you best manage this patient?

_____

_____

_____

3. You are dispatched to a lumberyard where a 27-year-old man was crushed by a piece of heavy equipment. Coworkers pulled the equipment off the patient. He presents with distended neck veins, cyanosis, and bloodshot eyes.

How would you best manage this patient?

_____

_____

_____

Assessment Review

Answer the following questions pertaining to the assessment of the types of emergencies discussed in this chapter.

1. You respond to an accidental shooting of a 37-year-old man. During the initial assessment you find his airway to be open and breathing is labored at 24 breaths/min. His pulse is rapid and weak. Upon exposing the chest you find a sucking chest wound. You should:
   A. take a blood pressure.
   B. cover the wound.
   C. continue your assessment.
   D. transport immediately.

2. You respond to a 17-year-old female who was hit in the chest with a lawn dart. Upon arrival she is conscious and able to converse with you. Her airway is open and her breathing is becoming progressivly more difficult. Her pulse is rapid and weak. You can palpate a radial pulse. Upon examining the chest, she has a penetrating injury to the chest and there is a sucking sound as she breathes. How do you manage this wound?
   A. Apply oxygen by nasal cannula.
   B. Stabilize the c-spine.
   C. Use a gauze 4 × 4.
   D. Occlusive dressing.

3. When bandaging an open chest wound, what is the minimum number of sides that have to be taped down?
   A. 1
   B. 2
   C. 3
   D. 4

4. Dispatch sends you to a farm on the edge of town. The 57-year-old man was kicked in the chest by a horse. He walked into his house and collapsed. He is alert and oriented. His breathing is labored at 20 breaths/min, pulse is rapid and regular, and you are able to palpate a radial pulse. Upon examination of his chest you notice paradoxical movement on the right chest wall. You should:
   A. take spinal precautions.
   B. put the patient in a position of comfort.
   C. provide oxygen by nasal cannula.
   D. stabilize the flail segment.

5. A 16-year-old male patient walks into a pipe gate that hits him in the ribs on the left side. Upon your arrival he is alert and oriented. His breathing is shallow at 22 breaths/min. His pulse is regular and strong. You palpate a radial pulse. You are able to rule out spinal trauma. What position do you transport him in?
   A. Position of comfort
   B. Supine
   C. Prone
   D. Lateral recumbent

Emergency Care Summary

Fill in the following chart pertaining to the management of the types of emergencies discussed in this chapter.

NOTE: While the steps below are widely accepted, be sure to consult and follow your local protocol.

Pneumothorax	Hemothorax	Rib Fractures	Flail Chest
1. Clear and maintain an open airway. 2. Provide high-flow oxygen. 3. Seal the wound with an _____ dressing, using a large enough dressing so that it is not pulled or sucked into the chest cavity. 4. Depending on your local protocol, you may tape the dressing down on all four sides, or create a _____ _____ by taping only three sides of the dressing.	1. Clear and maintain an open airway. 2. Provide high-flow oxygen. Cover the patient with a blanket. 3. Treat the patient for _____.	1. Clear and maintain an open airway. 2. Provide high-flow oxygen. Cover the patient with a blanket. 3. Place in a position of comfort to support breathing unless a _____ _____ is suspected.	1. Clear and maintain an open airway. 2. Provide respiratory support if necessary. 3. Provide _____ oxygen. 4. Stabilize flail segment by securing (or having the patient hold) a pillow firmly against the chest wall.

CHAPTER

28 Abdomen and Genitalia Injuries

Workbook Activities

The following activities have been designed to help you. Your instructor may require you to complete some or all of these activities as a regular part of your EMT-B training program. You are encouraged to complete any activity that your instructor does not assign as a way to enhance your learning in the classroom.

Chapter Review

The following exercises provide an opportunity to refresh your knowledge of this chapter.

Matching

Match each of the terms in the left column to the appropriate definition in the right column.

_____ **1.** Hollow organs   **A.** blood in urine
_____ **2.** Solid organs   **B.** organs outside of the body
_____ **3.** Peritonitis   **C.** abdominal lining inflammation
_____ **4.** Genitourinary system **D.** kidneys, liver, spleen
_____ **5.** Filtering system   **E.** kidneys
_____ **6.** Evisceration   **F.** abdomen
_____ **7.** Hematuria   **G.** stomach, bladder, ureters
_____ **8.** Peritoneal cavity   **H.** controls reproductive functions and the waste discharge system

Multiple Choice
Read each item carefully, then select the best response.

_____ 1. The abdomen contains several organs that make up the:
   A. digestive system.
   B. urinary system.
   C. genitourinary system.
   D. all of the above

_____ 2. Hollow organs of the abdomen include the:
   A. stomach.
   B. ureters.
   C. bladder.
   D. all of the above

_____ 3. Solid organs of the abdomen include all of the following, except the:
   A. liver.
   B. spleen.
   C. gallbladder.
   D. pancreas.

_____ 4. The first signs of peritonitis include:
   A. severe abdominal pain.
   B. tenderness.
   C. muscular spasm.
   D. all of the above

_____ 5. Late signs of peritonitis may include:
   A. a soft abdomen.
   B. nausea.
   C. normal bowel sounds.
   D. all of the above

_____ 6. _____ takes place in the solid organs.
   A. Digestion
   B. Excretion
   C. Energy production
   D. all of the above

_____ 7. Because solid organs have a rich supply of blood, any injury can result in major:
   A. hemorrhaging.
   B. damage.
   C. pain.
   D. guarding.

_____ 8. You are dispatched to an auto collision. You see a 25-year-old woman who was restrained but is complaining of abdominal pain. She is alert and oriented. Airway is open and patient is breathing normally. Her pulse is regular but weak and rapid. She has a radial pulse. You inspect the abdomen for possible bleeding. You would expect to see all of the following except:
   A. pain or tenderness.
   B. rigidity.
   C. urticaria.
   D. distention.

_____ **9.** The major soft-tissue landmark is (are) the _____, which overlie(s) the fourth lumbar vertebra.

    A. iliac crests

    B. umbilicus

    C. pubic symphysis

    D. anterior iliac spines

_____ **10.** The abdomen is divided into four:

    A. quadrants.

    B. planes.

    C. sections.

    D. angles.

_____ **11.** Injuries to the abdomen may involve:

    A. hollow organs.

    B. open injuries.

    C. solid organs.

    D. all of the above

_____ **12.** Open abdominal injuries are also known as:

    A. blunt injuries.

    B. eviscerations.

    C. penetrating injuries.

    D. peritoneal injuries.

_____ **13.** Closed abdominal injuries may result from:

    A. a stab wound.

    B. seat belts.

    C. a gunshot wound.

    D. all of the above

_____ **14.** The major complaint of patients with abdominal injury is:

    A. pain.

    B. tachycardia.

    C. rigidity.

    D. swelling.

_____ **15.** The most common sign of significant abdominal injury is:

    A. pain.

    B. tachycardia.

    C. rigidity.

    D. distention.

_____ **16.** Late signs of abdominal injury include all of the following, except:

    A. distention.

    B. increased blood pressure.

    C. rigidity.

    D. shallow respirations.

_____ **17.** Your primary concern when dealing with an unresponsive patient with an open abdominal injury is:

    A. covering the wound with a moist dressing.

    B. maintaining the airway.

    C. controlling the bleeding.

    D. monitoring vital signs.

_____ **18.** You respond to an 18-year-old high school football player who was hit in the abdominal area with a helmet. He is complaining of pain in the area. He is alert and oriented. His airway is open and his respirations are within normal limits. His pulse is rapid and regular. He has a radial pulse. You know that blunt abdominal trauma may result in:

    A. severe bruises on the abdominal wall.

    B. laceration of the liver or spleen.

    C. rupture of the intestine.

    D. all of the above

_____ **19.** For the patient in the question above, how would you provide treatment for him?

    A. Log roll onto a backboard.

    B. Transport rapidly.

    C. Give oxygen.

    D. All of the above

_____ **20.** When used alone, diagonal shoulder safety belts can cause:

    A. a bruised chest.

    B. a lacerated liver.

    C. decapitation.

    D. all of the above

_____ **21.** You are dispatched to a motor vehicle collision. Your patient is a 42-year-old restrained woman. The airbag did deploy and she has abrasions on her face. She is complaining of pain to both her chest and abdomen. Her airway is open and respirations are within normal limits. Her pulse is a little rapid but strong and regular. She has distal pulses. It is important to look at/for:

    A. debris inside the vehicle.

    B. the condition of the tires.

    C. damage to the steering column underneath the airbag.

    D. all of the above

_____ **22.** Patients with penetrating abdominal injuries often complain of:

    A. pain.

    B. nausea.

    C. vomiting.

    D. all of the above

_____ **23.** You are called to the local bar where a fight has taken place. The police department tells you that you have a 36-year-old man who has been stabbed twice in the abdomen. Upon arrival the patient is alert and oriented. His airway is open and his respirations are at 24 breaths/min, pulse is rapid, regular, and weak. He has distal pulses. With the penetrating trauma, you should assume that the object:

    A. has penetrated the peritoneum.

    B. entered the abdominal cavity.

    C. possibly injured one or more organs.

    D. all of the above

_____ **24.** When treating a patient with an evisceration, you should:

    A. attempt to replace the abdominal contents.

    B. cover the protruding organs with a dry, sterile dressing.

    C. cover the protruding organs with moist, adherent dressings.

    D. cover the protruding contents with moist, sterile gauze compresses.

_____ **25.** The solid organs of the urinary system include the:

    A. kidneys.

    B. ureters.

    C. bladder.

    D. urethra.

_____ **26.** All of the male genitalia lie outside the pelvic cavity with the exception of the:

    A. urethra.

    B. penis.

    C. seminal vesicles.

    D. testes.

_____ **27.** Suspect kidney damage if the patient has a history or physical evidence of:

    A. an abrasion, laceration, or contusion in the flank.

    B. a penetrating wound in the region of the lower rib cage or the upper abdomen.

    C. fractures on either side of the lower rib cage.

    D. all of the above

_____ **28.** Signs of injury to the kidney may include:

    A. bruises or lacerations on the overlying skin.

    B. shock.

    C. hematuria.

    D. all of the above

_____ **29.** Suspect a possible injury of the urinary bladder in all of the following findings, except:

    A. bruising to the left upper quadrant.

    B. blood at the urethral opening.

    C. blood at the tip of the penis or a stain on the patient's underwear.

    D. physical signs of trauma on the lower abdomen, pelvis, or perineum.

_____ **30.** When treating a patient with an amputation of the penile shaft, your top priority is:

    A. locating the amputated part.

    B. controlling bleeding.

    C. keeping the remaining tissue dry.

    D. delaying transport until bleeding is controlled.

_____ **31.** Treatment of injuries involving the external male genitalia includes:

    A. making the patient as comfortable as possible.

    B. using sterile, moist compresses to cover areas that have been stripped of skin.

    C. applying direct pressure with dry, sterile gauze dressings to control bleeding.

    D. all of the above

_____ **32.** In cases of sexual assault, you must treat the medical injuries but also provide:

    A. privacy.

    B. support.

    C. reassurance.

    D. all of the above

Labeling

Label the following diagrams with the correct terms.

1. Hollow Organs

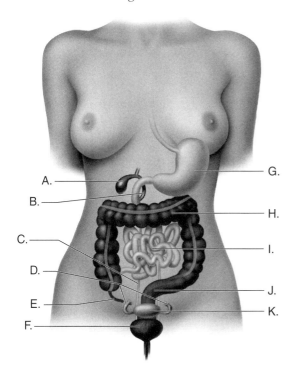

A. _____

B. _____

C. _____

D. _____

E. _____

F. _____

G. _____

H. _____

I. _____

J. _____

K. _____

2. Solid Organs

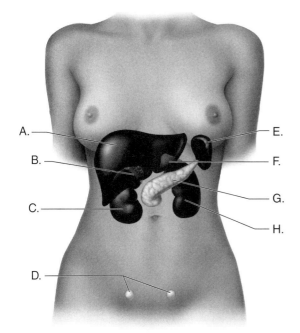

A. _____

B. _____

C. _____

D. _____

E. _____

F. _____

G. _____

H. _____

Fill-in

Read each item carefully, then complete the statement by filling in the missing word.

1. Severe bleeding may occur with injury to _____ organs.

2. The _____ system is responsible for filtering waste.

3. Kidneys are located in the _____ space.

4. Injuries to the kidneys or bladder will not have obvious _____ _____, but there are usually more

subtle clues such as lower rib pain or a possible pelvic fracture.

5. When ruptured, the organs of the abdominal cavity can spill their contents into the peritoneal cavity, causing an

intense inflammatory reaction called _____.

6. Blood within the peritoneal cavity does not provoke a(n) _____ _____, and may not cause pain or

tenderness.

7. Closed abdominal injuries are also known as _____ _____.

8. Open abdominal injuries are also known as _____ _____.

9. Another name for the right and left upper quadrants is _____.

10. An open wound that allows internal organs or fat to protrude though the wound is called _____.

True/False

If you believe the statement to be more true than false, write the letter "T" in the space provided. If you believe the statement to be more false than true, write the letter "F."

_____ **1.** Hollow organs will bleed profusely if injured.
_____ **2.** The most common sign of an abdominal injury is an elevated heart rate.
_____ **3.** Patients with abdominal injuries should be kept supine with head elevated.
_____ **4.** Peritoneal irritation is in response to hollow organ injury.
_____ **5.** Eviscerated organs should be covered with a dry dressing.
_____ **6.** Injuries to the kidneys usually occur in isolation.
_____ **7.** Peritonitis is an inflammation of the peritoneum.
_____ **8.** The abdomen is divided into two quadrants.
_____ **9.** Small children can be injured by air bags.
_____ **10.** Patients with peritonitis will want to lie still with their legs drawn up.

Short Answer

Complete this section with short written answers using the space provided.

1. List the hollow organs of the abdomen and urinary system.

_____

_____

2. List the solid organs of the abdomen and urinary system.

_____

_____

3. List the signs and symptoms of an abdominal injury.

_____

_____

4. List the steps to care for a penetrating abdominal injury.

_____

_____

5. List the steps to care for an open abdominal wound with exposed organs.

_____

_____

6. List the major history or physical findings associated with possible kidney damage.

_____

_____

Word Fun

The following crossword puzzle is an activity provided to reinforce correct spelling and understanding of medical terminology associated with emergency care and the EMT-B. Use the clues in the column to complete the puzzle.

Across

4. Contracting of muscle to protect
5. Stomach, small intestines, bladder
7. Displacement of organs outside of abdomen
8. Inflammation of abdominal lining

Down

1. Liver, spleen, pancreas
2. Abdominal cavity
3. Penetrating wound of belly
6. Blood in urine

Ambulance Calls

The following case scenarios provide an opportunity to explore the concerns associated with patient management. Read each scenario, then answer each question in detail.

1. You are dispatched to a local bar where your patient, a 26-year-old man, was involved in an altercation. He has several superficial lacerations to his arms, and a knife is impaled in his right upper quadrant. He is lying supine on the floor. He is alert and bar patrons tell you that he did not fall; they helped him to the floor.

How would you best manage this patient?

_____

_____

_____

2. You are dispatched to assist police with a mentally ill patient who as threatened harm to himself and others. Police officers found the man running around his home with a knife and blood all over his lower body. The man tells you "the voices" told him to cut his penis off.

How do best manage this patient?

_____

_____

_____

3. You are dispatched to a construction site, where a man has fallen onto a piece of rebar. You arrive to find a man sitting on the ground with his legs drawn toward his chest. He tells you that he fell from a ladder onto a piece of rebar. He tells you, "Something's sticking out of me." As you visualize his abdomen, you can clearly see a portion of his bowel on the outside of his body.

How do you best manage this patient?

_____

_____

_____

Assessment Review

Answer the following questions pertaining to the assessment of the types of emergencies discussed in this chapter.

_____ **1.** If you are treating a patient with an abdominal evisceration you should use a(n):

    A. moist, sterile dressing.

    B. dry, sterile dressing.

    C. adhesive dressing.

    D. occlusive dressing.

_____ **2.** You have a male patient who has no immediate life threat, but does have a genitalia bleeding. You should bandage with a(n):

    A. dry dressing.

    B. moist dressing.

    C. occlusive dressing.

    D. adhesive dressing.

_____ **3.** You have a patient with suspected kidney injury but no spinal injury. How should he be positioned?

    A. supine

    B. prone

    C. lateral recumbent

    D. position of comfort

_____ **4.** Your patient has his penis caught in his zipper. What do you need to do to relieve pressure?

    A. Pull the pants off the patient.

    B. Force the zipper open.

    C. Remove the foreskin.

    D. Cut the zipper out of the pants.

_____ **5.** Whenever possible you should always provide the sexual assault patient with:

    A. police escort.

    B. rape crisis intervention.

    C. same gender attendant.

    D. name of the assailant.

Emergency Care Summary

Fill in the following chart pertaining to the management of the types of emergencies discussed in this chapter.

NOTE: While the steps below are widely accepted, be sure to consult and follow your local protocol.

Kidney and Urinary Bladder Injuries

1. Treat for shock early and aggressively.
2. Place patient in position of comfort unless spinal injury is suspected.
3. Provide prompt transport.
4. Monitor _____ _____ en route.

External Male Genitalia Injuries

Avulsion

1. Wrap the penis in a soft, sterile dressing moistened with sterile _____ solution.
2. Use direct pressure to control any bleeding.
3. Try to save and preserve the avulsed skin, but do not delay transport for more than a few _____ to do so.

Amputation

1. Manage blood loss using local pressure with a sterile dressing on the remaining stump.
2. Wrap the amputated part in a moist, sterile dressing; place it in a plastic bag; transport in a cooled container without allowing it to come in direct contact with _____.

Fractured or Severely Angled

1. Provide prompt transport.

Lacerated Head or the Penis

1. Stop the hemorrhage with a _____ _____ and local pressure.

Penis Caught in a Zipper

1. Attempt to unzip pants.
2. If unable to unzip pants, explain to the patient that you are going to cut the zipper out of the pants to relieve pressure.

Urethral Injuries

1. Save any voided _____ for examination.

Avulsion of Scrotum Skin

1. Preserve avulsed skin in moist, sterile dressing.
2. Wrap scrotal contents or the perineal area with a sterile, moist dressing to control bleeding.

Rupture of a Testicle or Significant Accumulation of Blood Around the Testes

1. Apply ice pack to the scrotal area.

External Female Genitalia Injuries	Internal Female Genitalia Injuries, Pregnancy	Rectal Bleeding
1. Treat with moist, sterile _____. 2. Apply local pressure to control the bleeding and a diaper-type bandage to hold dressings in place.	1. Carefully place patient on her _____ side. 2. If the patient is on the backboard, tilt the board to the _____.	1. Pack the crease between the buttocks with _____ and consult with medical control to determine the need for transport.

Sexual Assault

1. Document the patient's history, assessment, treatment, and response to treatment in detail.
2. Make _____ _____ a major priority.
3. Complete the SAMPLE history in an objective, nonjudgmental way.
4. If the patient will tolerate being wrapped in a sterile burn sheet, this may help investigators to find any hair, fluid, or fiber from the alleged offender.
5. Do not examine the genitalia unless there is _____ _____. If an object has been inserted into the vagina or rectum, do not attempt to remove it.
6. Make sure the EMT-B is the same gender as the patient whenever possible.
7. Discourage the patient from bathing, voiding, or cleaning any wounds until hospital staff has completed an assessment. Handle the patient's clothes as little as possible, placing articles and any other evidence in _____ bags. Do not use _____ bags. If the female patient insists on urinating, have her do so in a sterile urine container (if available). Also, have her deposit the toilet paper in a paper bag. Seal and mark the bag for the police. This can be critical evidence.

C H A P T E R

29 Musculoskeletal Care

Workbook Activities

The following activities have been designed to help you. Your instructor may require you to complete some or all of these activities as a regular part of your EMT-B training program. You are encouraged to complete any activity that your instructor does not assign as a way to enhance your learning in the classroom.

Chapter Review

The following exercises provide an opportunity to refresh your knowledge of this chapter.

Matching

Match each of the terms in the left column to the appropriate definition in the right column.

_____ **1.** Striated	**A.** any injury that makes the limb appear in an unnatural position
_____ **2.** Tendons	**B.** any fracture in which the skin has not been broken
_____ **3.** Smooth	**C.** a thin layer of cartilage, covering the articular surface of bones in synovial joints
_____ **4.** Joint	
_____ **5.** Ligaments	**D.** involuntary muscle
_____ **6.** Closed fracture	**E.** any break in the bone in which the overlying skin has been damaged as well
_____ **7.** Point tenderness	
_____ **8.** Displaced fracture	**F.** hold joints together
_____ **9.** Articular cartilage	**G.** skeletal muscle
_____ **10.** Open fracture	**H.** the act of exerting a pulling force on a structure
_____ **11.** Traction	**I.** where two bones contact
	J. attach muscle to bone
	K. tenderness sharply located at the site of an injury

Multiple Choice

Read each item carefully, then select the best response.

_____ 1. Blood in the urine is known as a:

    A. hematuria.

    B. hemotysis.

    C. hematocrit.

    D. hemoglobin.

_____ 2. Smooth muscle is found in the:

    A. back.

    B. blood vessels.

    C. heart.

    D. all of the above

_____ 3. The bones in the skeleton produce _____ in the bone marrow.

    A. red blood cells

    B. minerals

    C. electrolytes

    D. white blood cells

_____ 4. _____ are held together in a tough fibrous structure known as a capsule.

    A. Tendons

    B. Joints

    C. Ligaments

    D. Bones

_____ 5. Joints are bathed and lubricated by _____ fluid.

    A. cartilaginous

    B. articular

    C. synovial

    D. cerebrospinal

_____ 6. A _____ is a disruption of a joint in which the bone ends are no longer in contact.

    A. torn ligament

    B. dislocation

    C. fracture dislocation

    D. sprain

_____ 7. A _____ is a joint injury in which there is both some partial or temporary dislocation of the bone ends and partial stretching or tearing of the supporting ligaments.

    A. dislocation

    B. strain

    C. sprain

    D. torn ligament

_____ 8. A _____ is a stretching or tearing of the muscle.

    A. strain

    B. sprain

    C. torn ligament

    D. split

_____ **9.** The zone of injury includes the:

   A. adjacent nerves.

   B. adjacent blood vessels.

   C. surrounding soft tissue.

   D. all of the above

_____ **10.** A(n) _____ fractures the bone at the point of impact.

   A. direct blow

   B. indirect force

   C. twisting force

   D. high-energy injury

_____ **11.** A(n) _____ may cause a fracture or dislocation at a distant point.

   A. direct blow

   B. indirect force

   C. twisting force

   D. high-energy injury

_____ **12.** When caring for patients who have fallen, you must identify the _____ and the mechanism of injury so that you will not overlook associated injuries.

   A. site of injury

   B. height of fall

   C. point of contact

   D. twisting forces

_____ **13.** _____ produce severe damage to the skeleton, surrounding soft tissues, and vital internal organs.

   A. Direct blows

   B. Indirect forces

   C. Twisting forces

   D. High-energy injuries

_____ **14.** Regardless of the extent and severity of the damage to the skin, you should treat any injury that breaks the skin as a possible:

   A. closed fracture.

   B. open fracture.

   C. nondisplaced fracture.

   D. displaced fracture.

_____ **15.** A _____ is also known as a hairline fracture.

   A. closed fracture

   B. open fracture

   C. nondisplaced fracture

   D. displaced fracture

_____ **16.** A _____ produces actual deformity, or distortion, of the limb by shortening, rotating, or angulating it.

   A. closed fracture

   B. open fracture

   C. nondisplaced fracture

   D. displaced fracture

_____ **17.** You respond to a 19-year-old female who was kicked in the leg by a horse. She is alert and oriented. Respirations are 20 breaths/min regular and unlabored. Pulse is 110 beats/min and regular. Distal pulses are present. She has point tenderness at the site of the injury. You should compare the limb to:

   A. the opposite uninjured limb.

   B. one of your limbs or one of your partner's limbs.

   C. an injury chart.

   D. none of the above

_____ **18.** _____ is the most reliable indicator of an underlying fracture.

   A. Crepitus

   B. Deformity

   C. Point tenderness

   D. Absence of distal pulse

_____ **19.** A(n) _____ is a fracture that occurs in a growth section of a child's bone, which may prematurely stop growth if not properly treated.

   A. greenstick fracture

   B. comminuted fracture

   C. pathological fracture

   D. epiphyseal fracture

_____ **20.** A(n) _____ is an incomplete fracture that passes only partway through the shaft of a bone but may still cause severe angulation.

   A. greenstick fracture

   B. comminuted fracture

   C. pathological fracture

   D. epiphyseal fracture

_____ **21.** You are called to the local assisted living facility where a 94-year-old man has fallen. He is alert and oriented and denies passing out. His respirations are 18 breaths/min and regular. Pulse is 106 beats/min, regular, and strong. Distal pulses are present. He states he was walking and heard a pop and fell to the floor. You suspect a(n):

   A. greenstick fracture.

   B. comminuted fracture.

   C. pathological fracture.

   D. epiphyseal fracture.

_____ **22.** A(n) _____ is a fracture in which the bone is broken into two or more fragments.

   A. greenstick fracture

   B. comminuted fracture

   C. pathological fracture

   D. epiphyseal fracture

_____ **23.** Your 24-year-old patient fell off a balance beam and landed on his arm. His is complaining of pain in the upper arm and there is obvious swelling. You know that swelling is a sign of:

   A. bleeding.

   B. laceration.

   C. locked joint.

   D. compartment syndrome.

_____ **24.** Fractures are almost always associated with _____ of the surrounding soft tissue.

   A. laceration

   B. crepitus

   C. ecchymosis

   D. swelling

_____ **25.** Signs and symptoms of a dislocated joint include:

    A. marked deformity.

    B. tenderness or palpation.

    C. locked joint.

    D. all of the above

_____ **26.** Signs and symptoms of sprains include all of the following, except:

    A. point tenderness.

    B. pain prevents the patient from moving or using the limb normally.

    C. marked deformity.

    D. instability of the joint is indicated by increased motion.

_____ **27.** Assessment of patients with musculoskeletal injuries must include:

    A. initial assessment followed by a focused physical exam.

    B. evaluation of neurovascular function.

    C. applying oxygen as needed.

    D. all of the above

_____ **28.** Compartment syndrome:

    A. occurs within 6 to 12 hours after injury.

    B. usually is a result of excessive bleeding, a severely crushed extremity, or the rapid return of blood to an ischemic limb.

    C. is characterized by pain that is out of proportion to the injury.

    D. all of the above

_____ **29.** Always check neurovascular function:

    A. after any manipulation of the limb.

    B. before applying a splint.

    C. after applying a splint.

    D. all of the above

_____ **30.** You respond to a 19-year-old female who was involved in a motor vehicle collision. She is alert and oriented. Her airway is open and respirations are 18 breaths/min and unlabored. Pulse is 94 beats/min, strong, and regular. Distal pulses are present. Her upper are has obvious deformity. You splint the upper arm. You know that splinting will help:

    A. excessive bleeding of the tissues at the injury site caused by broken bone ends.

    B. laceration of the skin by broken bone ends.

    C. increased pain from movement of bone ends.

    D. all of the above

_____ **31.** In-line _____ is the act of exerting a pulling force on a body structure in the direction of its normal alignment.

    A. stabilization

    B. immobilization

    C. traction

    D. direction

_____ **32.** Basic types of splints include:

    A. rigid.

    B. formable.

    C. traction.

    D. all of the above

_____ **33.** Do not use traction splints for any of the following conditions, except:

    A. injuries of the pelvis.

    B. an isolated femur fracture.

    C. partial amputation or avulsions with bone separation.

    D. lower leg or ankle injury.

_____ **34.** While transporting the patient in question 30, you continue to recheck the splint you applied. You know that improperly applying a splint can cause:

    A. compression of nerves, tissues, and blood vessels.

    B. delay in transport of a patient with a life-threatening injury.

    C. reduction of distal circulation if the splint is too tight.

    D. all of the above

_____ **35.** The _____ is one of the most commonly fractured bones in the body.

    A. scapula

    B. clavicle

    C. humerus

    D. radius

_____ **36.** Indications that blood vessels have likely been injured include:

    A. a cold, pale hand.

    B. weak or absent pulse.

    C. poor capillary refill.

    D. all of the above

_____ **37.** Signs and symptoms associated with hip dislocation include:

    A. severe pain in the hip.

    B. lateral and posterior aspects of the hip region will be tender on palpation.

    C. being able to palpate the femoral head deep within the muscles of the buttock.

    D. all of the above

_____ **38.** There is always a significant amount of blood loss, as much as _____ mL, after a fracture of the shaft of the femur.

    A. 100 to 250

    B. 250 to 500

    C. 500 to 1,000

    D. 100 to 1,500

_____ **39.** The knee is especially susceptible to _____ injuries, which occur when abnormal bending or twisting forces are applied to the joint.

    A. tendon

    B. ligament

    C. dislocation

    D. fracture-dislocation

_____ **40.** Signs and symptoms of knee ligament injury include:

    A. swelling.

    B. point tenderness.

    C. joint effusion.

    D. all of the above

_____ **41.** Although substantial ligament damage always occurs with a knee dislocation, the more urgent injury is to the _____ artery, which is often lacerated or compressed by the displaced tibia.

    A. tibial

    B. femoral

    C. popliteal

    D. dorsalis pedis

_____ **42.** Because of local tenderness and swelling, it is easy to confuse a nondisplaced or minimally displaced fracture about the knee with a:

A. tendon injury.

B. ligament injury.

C. dislocation.

D. fracture-dislocation.

_____ **43.** Fracture of the tibia and fibula are often associated with _____ as a result of the distorted positions of the limb following injury.

A. vascular injury

B. muscular injury

C. tendon injury

D. ligament injury

_____ **44.** The _____ is the most commonly injured joint.

A. knee

B. elbow

C. ankle

D. hip

Labeling

Label the following diagram with the correct terms.

A. _____

B. _____

C. _____

D. _____

E. _____

F. _____

G. _____

H. _____

I. _____

J. _____

K. _____

L. _____

M. _____

N. _____

O. _____

P. _____

1. The Human Skeleton

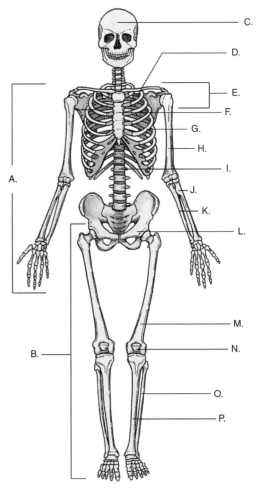

Fill-in

Read each item carefully, then complete the statement by filling in the missing word.

1. Atrophy is the _____ of muscle tissue.

2. Bone marrow produces _____ blood cells.

3. The knee and elbow are _____ and socket joints.

4. The _____ is one of the most commonly fractured bones in the body.

5. Always carefully assess the _____ _____ _____ to try to determine the amount of kinetic

energy that an injured limb has absorbed.

6. Penetrating injury should alert you to the possibility of a(n) _____ _____ .

7. The _____ _____ is the most important nerve in the lower extremity; it controls the activity of

muscles in the thigh and below the knee.

8. The _____ is the longest and largest bone in the body.

9. A grating or grinding sensation known as _____ can be felt and sometimes even heard when fractured

bone ends rub together.

10. A dislocated joint sometimes will spontaneously _____ , or return to its normal position.

11. If you suspect that a patient has compartment syndrome, splint the affected limb, keeping it at the level of the

heart, and provide immediate transport, checking _____ _____ frequently during transport.

True/False

If you believe the statement to be more true than false, write the letter "T" in the space provided. If you believe the statement to be more false than true, write the letter "F."

_____ **1.** All extremity injuries should be splinted before moving a patient unless the patient's life is in
immediate danger.

_____ **2.** Splinting reduces pain and prevents the motion of bone fragments.

_____ **3.** You should use traction to reduce a fracture and force all bone fragments back into alignment.

_____ **4.** When applying traction, the direction of pull is always along the axis of the limb.

_____ **5.** Cover wounds with a dry, sterile dressing before applying a splint.

_____ **6.** When splinting a fracture, you should be careful to immobilize only the joint above the injury site.

_____ **7.** One of the steps of the neurological examination is to palpate the pulse distal to the point of injury.

_____ **8.** Assessment of neurovascular function should be repeated every 5 to 10 minutes until the patient arrives
at the hospital.

_____ **9.** A patient's ability to sense light touch in the fingers and toes distal to the injury site is a good indication
that the nerve supply is intact.

_____ **10.** If the hand or foot is involved in the injury, you should check motor function.

Short Answer

Complete this section with short written answers using the space provided.

1. List the four types of forces that may cause injury to a limb.

_____

_____

2. List five of the signs associated with a possible fracture.

_____

_____

3. List the four items to check when assessing neurovascular function.

_____

_____

4. List the general principles of splinting.

_____

_____

5. What are the three goals of in-line traction?

_____

_____

Word Fun

The following crossword puzzle is an activity provided to reinforce correct spelling and understanding of medical terminology associated with emergency care and the EMT-B. Use the clues in the column to complete the puzzle.

Across

3. Exerting a pulling force

5. Major lower extremity nerve

6. Hand position for splinting

7. Elevation of pressure within fibrous tissues

8. Blood in urine

11. Collarbone

12. Joint between the two pubic bones

13. Forearm bone on small finger side

14. Striated, attached to bones

Down

1. Part of the scapula that joins with the humerus

2. Broken bone with overlying skin injured

4. Bone fragments are separated

9. Discoloration from bleeding under skin

10. Grating sound of bone ends

Ambulance Calls

The following case scenarios provide an opportunity to explore the concerns associated with patient management. Read each scenario, then answer each question in detail.

1. You are dispatched to care for a 17-year-old male who jumped from the top of a three-story home into a pool. He landed directly on his feet just short of the pool. He is now complaining of low back pain and numbness and tingling of his legs.

How do you best manage this patient?

_____

_____

_____

2. You are called to a local park where an 11-year-old girl fell off the parallel bars onto her right elbow. She is cradling the arm to her chest. She has obvious swelling and deformity in the area. She has good pulse, motor, and sensation at the wrist. ABCs are normal.

How would you best manage this patient?

_____

_____

_____

3. You are dispatched to an attempted suicide at the local prison. The inmate attempted to kill himself by strangling himself with an electrical cord. When you arrive he is cyanotic and not breathing.

How do you best manage this patient?

_____

_____

_____

Skill Drills

Skill Drill 29-1: Assessing Neurovascular Status
Test your knowledge of this skill drill by filling in the correct words in the photo captions.

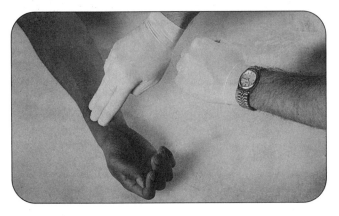

1. Palpate the _____ pulse in the upper extremity.

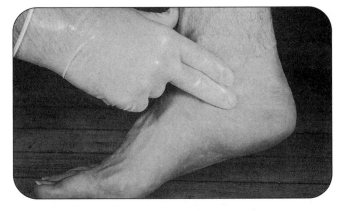

2. Palpate the _____ _____ pulse in the lower extremity.

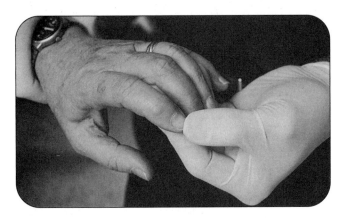

3. Assess capillary refill by blanching a fingernail or _____.

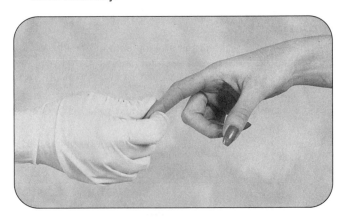

4. Assess sensation on the flesh near the _____ of the _____ finger.

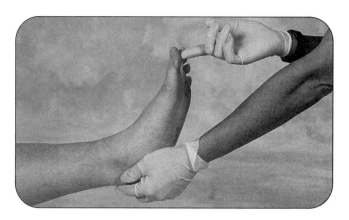

5. On the foot, first check sensation on the flesh near the _____ of the _____ _____.

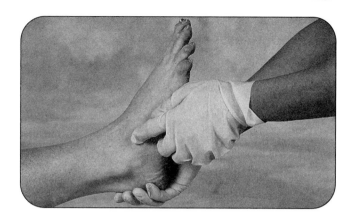

6. Also check foot sensation on the _____ _____.

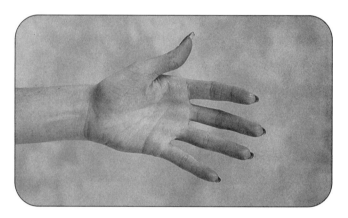

7. Evaluate motor function by asking the patient to _____ the hand. (Perform motor tests only if the hand or foot is not _____. _____ a test if it causes pain.)

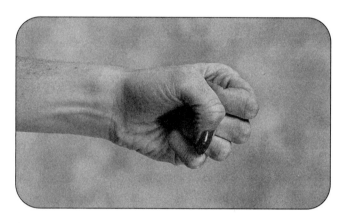

8. Also ask the patient to _____ _____ _____.

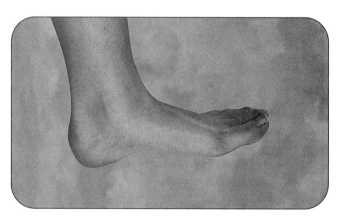

9. To evaluate motor function in the foot, ask the patient to _____ the foot.

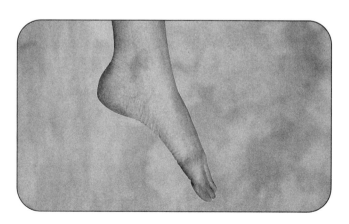

10. Also have the patient _____ the foot and _____ the toes.

Skill Drill 29-2: Caring for Musculoskeletal Injuries
Test your knowledge of this skill drill by filling in the correct words in the photo captions.

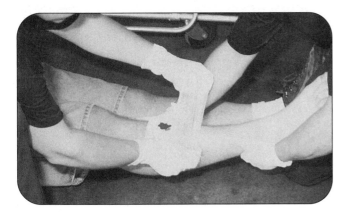

1. Cover open wounds with a _____,
   _____ dressing, and _____
   _____ to control bleeding.

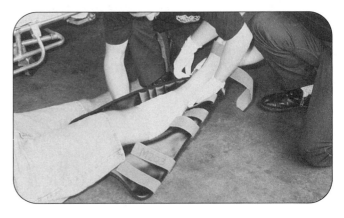

2. Apply a splint and elevate the extremity about
   _____" (slightly above the level of the
   _____).

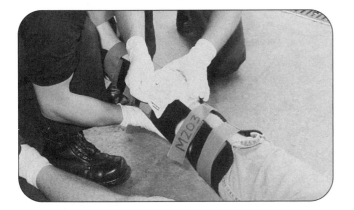

3. Apply _____ _____ if there is swelling,
   but do not place them _____ on the skin.

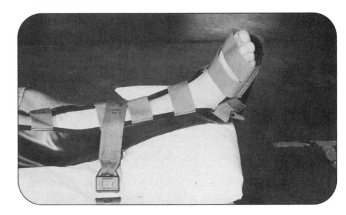

4. _____ the patient for transport and
   _____ the injured area.

Skill Drill 29-3: Applying a Rigid Splint
Test your knowledge of this skill drill by filling in the correct words in the photo captions.

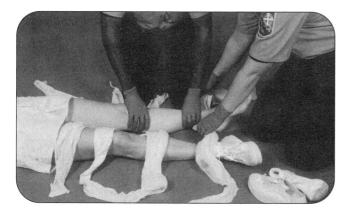

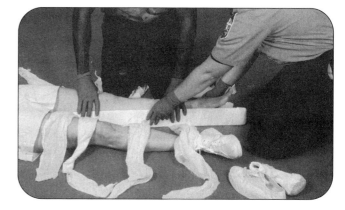

1. Provide gentle _____ and _____ _____ for the limb.

2. Second EMT-B places the splint _____ or _____ the limb. _____ between the limb and the splint as needed to ensure even pressure and contact.

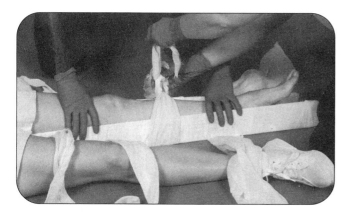

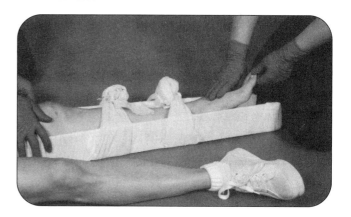

3. Secure the splint to the limb with _____.

4. Assess and record _____ _____ function.

Skill Drill 29-4: Applying a Zippered Air Splint
Test your knowledge of this skill drill by filling in the correct words in the photo captions.

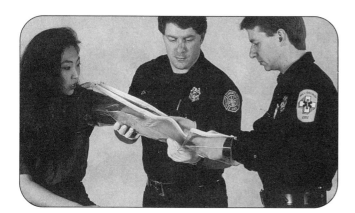

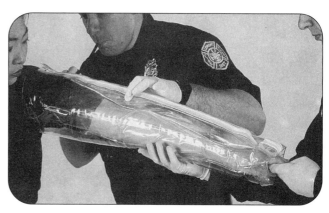

1. Support the injured limb and apply gentle _____ as your partner applies the open, deflated splint.

2. Zip up the splint, inflate it by _____ or by _____, and test the _____. Check and record _____ _____ function.

Skill Drill 29-5: Applying an Unzipped Air Splint

Test your knowledge of this skill drill by filling in the correct words In the photo captions.

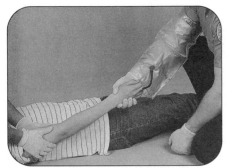

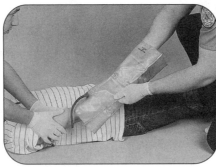

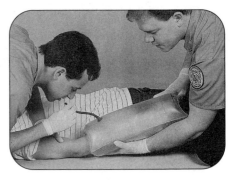

1. _____ the injured limb. Have your partner place his or her arm through the splint to grasp the patient's _____ or _____.

2. Apply gentle _____ while sliding the splint onto the injured limb.

3. _____ the splint.

Skill Drill 29-6: Applying a Vacuum Splint

Test your knowledge of this skill drill by filling in the correct words in the photo captions.

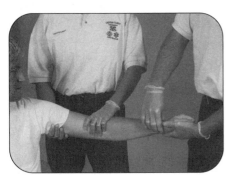

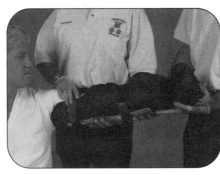

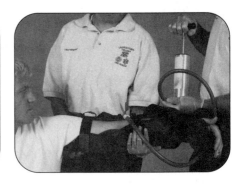

1. _____ and _____ the injury.

2. Place the splint and _____ it around the limb.

3. _____ the air _____ _____ the splint through the suction valve, and then _____ the valve.

Skill Drill 29-7: Applying a Hare Traction Splint

Test your knowledge of this skill drill by placing the photos below in the correct order. Number the first step with a "1," the second step with a "2," etc.

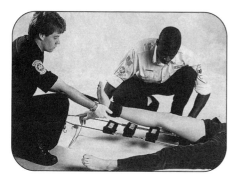

_____

Slide the splint into position under the injured limb.

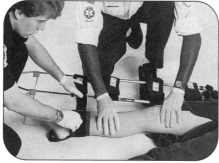

_____

Support the injured limb as your partner fastens the ankle hitch about the foot and ankle.

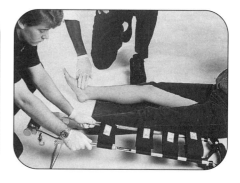

_____

Expose the injured limb and check pulse, motor, and sensory function. Place the splint beside the uninjured limb, adjust the splint to proper length, and prepare the straps.

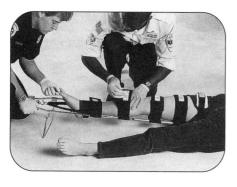

_____

Secure and check support straps. Assess pulse, motor, and sensory functions.

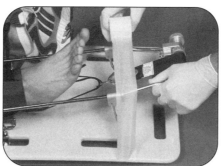

_____

Secure the patient and splint to the backboard in a way that will prevent movement of the splint during patient movement and transport.

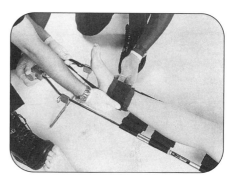

_____

Connect the loops of the ankle hitch to the end of the splint as your partner continues to maintain traction. Carefully tighten the ratchet to the point that the splint holds adequate traction.

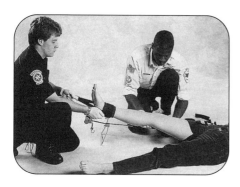

_____

Continue to support the limb as your partner applies gentle in-line traction to the ankle hitch and foot.

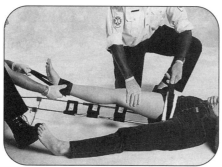

_____

Pad the groin and fasten the ischial strap.

Skill Drill 29-8: Applying a Sager Traction Splint
Test your knowledge of this skill drill by placing the photos below in the correct order. Number the first step with a "1," the second step with a "2," etc.

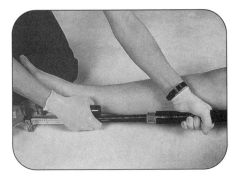

_____

Estimate the proper length of the splint by placing it next to the injured limb. Fit the ankle pads to the ankle.

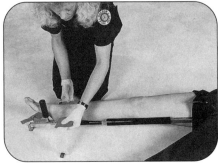

_____

Tighten the ankle harness just above the malleoli.
Snug the cable ring against the bottom of the foot.

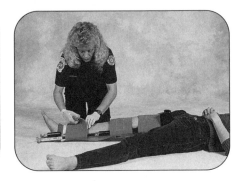

_____

Secure the splint with elasticized cravats.

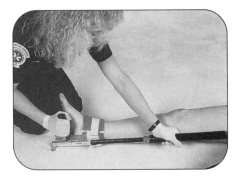

_____

Extend the splint's inner shaft to apply traction of about 10% of body weight.

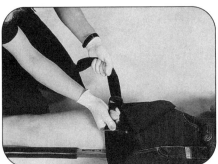

_____

Place the splint at the inner thigh, apply the thigh strap at the upper thigh, and secure snugly.

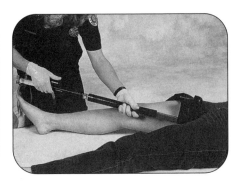

_____

After exposing the injured area, check the patient's pulse and motor and sensory function.
Adjust the thigh strap so that it lies anteriorly when secured.

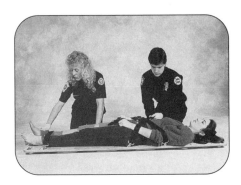

_____

Secure the patient to a long backboard. Check pulse, motor, and sensory functions.

Skill Drill 29-9: Splinting the Hand and Wrist
Test your knowledge of this skill drill by filling in the correct words in the photo captions.

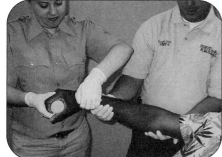 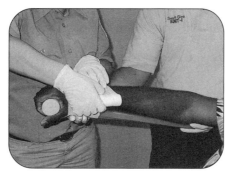 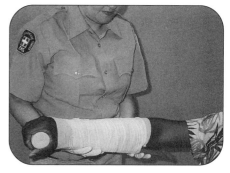

1. Move the hand into the

   _____ _____

   _____ . Place a soft

   _____ _____ in the

   palm.

2. Apply a _____

   _____ splint on the

   _____ side with fingers

   _____ .

3. Secure the splint with a

   _____ _____ .

Assessment Review

Answer the following questions pertaining to the assessment of the types of emergencies discussed in this chapter.

_____ **1.** You respond to a motorcycle accident for a 41-year-old man who is unconscious. He has obvious deformity to both lower legs and is bleeding moderately from an open fracture. His airway is open and he is making gurgling noises. Pulse is rapid and weak. Distal pulses are very weak. Your first priority with this patient is to:

A. control bleeding.

B. apply splints.

C. maintain an airway.

D. apply PASG.

_____ **2.** You have loaded the patient in the question above and are on the way to the hospital. You have secured the airway and immobilized the fractures. How often would you reassess his vital signs?

A. Every 3 minutes

B. Every 5 minutes

C. Every 10 minutes

D. Every 15 minutes

_____ **3.** You are called to a 16-year-old female patient who was injured in a basketball game. She is alert and oriented. Her airway is open and respirations are within normal limits. Her pulse is strong and regular. Distal pulses are present. She states that she felt her ankle pop and she immediately became nauseated. You decide to assess neurovascular status. When would you not perform the motor test?

A. When you get a pain response

B. When the patient walks away

C. When you feel a distal pulse

D. When the patient feels your touch

_____ **4.** You are called to the local junior high school where a 12-year-old boy fell and hurt his wrist. There is obvious deformity. He is alert and oriented. Respirations and pulse are within normal limits. Distal pulse is present. It is important to remember to:

A. use a zippered air splint.

B. splint in position of function.

C. splint the wrist only.

D. completely cover the wrist and hand.

_____ **5.** When you have applied a traction splint, the last thing that you do is:

A. check pulse, motor, and sensation.

B. release traction if the pulse disappears.

C. apply elasticized straps.

D. secure to a backboard.

Emergency Care Summary

Complete the statements pertaining to emergency care for the types of emergencies discussed in this chapter by filling in the missing words.

Please note that only two sections of the Emergency Care Summary are included here.

NOTE: While the steps below are widely accepted, be sure to consult and follow your local protocol.

Musculoskeletal Injuries

Applying a Hare Traction Splint

1. Expose the injured limb and check pulse, motor, and _____ function. Place the splint beside the uninjured limb, adjust the splint to proper length, and prepare the straps.
2. Support the injured limb as your partner fastens the ankle hitch about the foot and ankle.
3. Continue to support the limb as your partner applies gentle _____ _____ to the ankle hitch and foot.
4. Slide the splint into position under the injured limb.
5. Pad the groin and fasten the _____ strap.
6. Connect the loops of the ankle hitch to the end of the splint as your partner continues to maintain traction. Carefully tighten the ratchet to the point that the splint holds adequate traction.
7. Secure and check _____ _____. Assess pulse, motor, and sensory functions.
8. Secure the patient and splint to the backboard in a way that will prevent movement of the splint during patient movement and transport.

Applying a Sager Traction Splint

1. After exposing the injured area, check the patient's pulse and motor and sensory function. Adjust the thigh strap so that it lies _____ when secured.
2. Estimate the proper length of the splint by placing it next to the injured limb. Fit the ankle pads to the ankle.
3. Place the splint at the _____ thigh, apply the thigh strap at the _____ thigh, and secure snugly.
4. Tighten the ankle harness just above the _____. Snug the cable ring against the bottom of the foot.
5. Extend the splint's inner shaft to apply traction of about _____ of body weight.
6. Secure the splint with elasticized cravats.
7. Secure the patient to a long backboard. Check pulse, motor, and sensory functions.

CHAPTER

30 Head and Spine Injuries

Workbook Activities

The following activities have been designed to help you. Your instructor may require you to complete some or all of these activities as a regular part of your EMT-B training program. You are encouraged to complete any activity that your instructor does not assign as a way to enhance your learning in the classroom.

Chapter Review

The following exercises provide an opportunity to refresh your knowledge of this chapter.

Matching

Match each of the terms in the left column to the appropriate definition in the right column.

_____ 1. Cerebellum

_____ 2. Brain stem

_____ 3. Somatic nervous system

_____ 4. Autonomic nervous system

_____ 5. Spinal column

_____ 6. Central nervous system

_____ 7. Cerebral edema

_____ 8. Connecting nerves

_____ 9. Intervertebral disk

_____ 10. Meninges

A. consists of 33 bones

B. swelling of the brain

C. the brain and spinal cord

D. controls movement

E. the part of the central nervous system that controls virtually all the functions that are absolutely necessary for life

F. three distinct layers of tissue that surround and protect the brain and spinal cord within the skull and spinal cord

G. the part of the nervous system that regulates involuntary functions

H. the part of the nervous system that regulates voluntary activities

I. located in the brain and spinal cord, these connect the motor and sensory nerves

J. cushion that lies between the vertebrae

Multiple Choice

Read each item carefully, then select the best response.

_____ 1. The nervous system includes:

    A. the brain.

    B. the spinal cord.

    C. billions of nerve fibers.

    D. all of the above

_____ 2. The nervous system is divided into two parts: the central nervous system and the:

    A. autonomic nervous system.

    B. peripheral nervous system.

    C. sympathetic nervous system.

    D. somatic nervous system.

_____ 3. The brain is divided into three major areas: the cerebrum, the cerebellum, and the:

    A. foramen magnum.

    B. meninges.

    C. brain stem.

    D. spinal column.

_____ 4. Injury to the head and neck may indicate injury to the:

    A. thoracic spine.

    B. lumbar spine.

    C. cervical spine.

    D. sacral spine.

_____ 5. The _____ is composed of three layers of tissue that surround the brain and spinal cord within the skull and spinal canal.

    A. meninges

    B. dura mater

    C. pia mater

    D. arachnoid space

_____ 6. The skull is divided into two large structures: the cranium and the:

    A. occipital.

    B. face.

    C. parietal.

    D. foramen magnum.

_____ 7. Peripheral nerves include:

    A. connecting nerves.

    B. sensory nerves.

    C. motor nerves.

    D. all of the above

_____ 8. The brain and spinal cord float in cerebrospinal fluid (CSF), which:

    A. acts as a shock absorber.

    B. bathes the brain and spinal cord.

    C. buffers them from injury.

    D. all of the above

_____ **9.** The autonomic nervous system is composed of two parts: the sympathetic nervous system and the:

A. peripheral nervous system.

B. central nervous system.

C. parasympathetic nervous system.

D. somatic nervous system.

_____ **10.** The most prominent and the most easily palpable spinous process is at the _____ cervical vertebra at the base of the neck.

A. 7th

B. 6th

C. 5th

D. 4th

_____ **11.** You respond to a 14-year-old male who fell out of a tree at a local park. He is unresponsive. His airway is open and respirations are 16 breaths/min and regular. His pulse is strong and regular. Distal pulses are present. You manage the c-spine. Who should you ask for help in determining how the injury happened?

A. First responders

B. Family members

C. Bystanders

D. All of the above

_____ **12.** Emergency medical care of a patient with a possible spinal injury begins with:

A. opening the airway.

B. level of consciousness.

C. scene of safety.

D. BSI precautions.

_____ **13.** The _____ is a tunnel running the length of the spine, which encloses and protects the spinal cord.

A. foramen magnum

B. spinal canal

C. foramen foramina

D. meninges

_____ **14.** Once the head and neck are manually stabilized, you should assess:

A. pulse.

B. motor function.

C. sensation.

D. all of the above

_____ **15.** You are called to a motor vehicle collision where you have a 27-year-old woman who has a bump on her head. You immediately take manual stabilization of the head. Her airway is open and respirations are within normal limits. Her pulse is a little fast but strong and regular. Distal pulses are present. You can release manual stabilization when:

A. the patient's head and torso are in line.

B. the patient is secured to a backboard with the head immobilized.

C. the rigid cervical collar is in place.

D. the patient arrives at the hospital.

_____ **16.** The ideal procedure for moving a patient from the ground to the backboard is the:

A. four-person log roll.

B. lateral slide.

C. four-person lift.

D. push and pull maneuver.

_____ 17. You respond to a motor vehicle collision with a 29-year-old woman who struck the rearview mirror and has serious bleeding from the scalp. Her airway is open and respirations are normal. The pulse is a little rapid but strong and regular. Distal pulses are present and there is no deformity to the skull. Most bleeding from the scalp can be controlled by:

  A. direct pressure.

  B. elevation.

  C. pressure point.

  D. tourniquet.

_____ 18. Exceptions to using a short spinal extrication device include all of the following, except:

  A. you or the patient is in danger.

  B. the patient is conscious and complaining of lumbar pain.

  C. you need to gain immediate access to other patients.

  D. the patient's injuries justify immediate removal.

_____ 19. Your patient in question 17 has the same presentation except that she has an open skull fracture. You know that excessive pressure to the wound site could:

  A. increase intracranial pressure.

  B. push bone fragments into the brain.

  C. increase the size of the soft-tissue injury.

  D. all of the above

_____ 20. A _____ is a temporary loss or alteration of a part or all of the brain's abilities to function without actual physical damage to the brain:

  A. contusion

  B. concussion

  C. hematoma

  D. subdural hematoma

_____ 21. Symptoms of a concussion include:

  A. dizziness.

  B. weakness.

  C. visual changes.

  D. all of the above

_____ 22. Intracranial bleeding outside of the dura and under the skull is known as a(n):

  A. concussion.

  B. intracerebral hemorrhage.

  C. subdural hematoma.

  D. epidural hematoma.

_____ 23. The difference in signs and symptoms of traumatic vs. nontraumatic brain injuries is the:

  A. lack of altered mental status.

  B. lack of mechanism of injury.

  C. lack of swelling.

  D. increase in blood pressure.

_____ 24. _____ is the most reliable sign of a closed head injury.

  A. Vomiting

  B. Decreased LOC

  C. Seizures

  D. Numbness and tingling in extremities

_____ 25. _____ is one of the most common, and one of the most serious, complications of a head injury.

  A. Cyanosis

  B. Hypoxia

  C. Vomiting

  D. Cerebral edema

_____ **26.** Common causes of head injuries include all of the following, except:

    A. direct blows.

    B. motor vehicle crashes.

    C. seizure activity.

    D. sports injuries.

_____ **27.** Assessment of mental status is accomplished through the use of the mnemonic:

    A. SAMPLE.

    B. OPQRST.

    C. AVPU.

    D. AEIOU-TIPS.

_____ **28.** You respond to an 18-year-old male who fell while rock climbing. He is unconscious with an open airway. The respiration rate and pulse rates are within normal limits. His distal pulses are intact. You check his pupils and they are unequal. You know this could be a sign of:

    A. increased intracranial pressure.

    B. a congenital problem.

    C. damage to the nerves that control dilation and constriction.

    D. all of the above

_____ **29.** Patients with head injuries often have injuries to the _____ as well.

    A. face

    B. torso

    C. cervical spine

    D. extremities

_____ **30.** Proper order of treatment for traumatic head injuries includes:

    A. scene safety, airway, LOC with c-spine control, breathing, circulation.

    B. LOC with c-spine control, airway, breathing, circulation.

    C. LOC, airway, breathing, circulation, c-spine.

    D. BSI, ABCs, LOC, c-spine control.

_____ **31.** A cervical collar should be applied to a patient with a possible spinal injury based on:

    A. the mechanism of injury.

    B. the history.

    C. signs and symptoms.

    D. all of the above

_____ **32.** Helmets must be removed in all of the following cases, except:

    A. cardiac arrest.

    B. when the helmet allows for excessive movement.

    C. when there are no impending airway or breathing problems.

    D. when a shield cannot be removed.

_____ **33.** Your best choice of action for a child involved in a motor vehicle crash and found in their car seat is to:

    A. immobilize the child in the car seat.

    B. rule out spinal injury and place the child with a parent.

    C. pad sides of car seat but leave space to allow for lateral movement.

    D. move the child to a pediatric immobilization device.

Labeling

Label the following diagrams with the correct terms.

1. The Brain

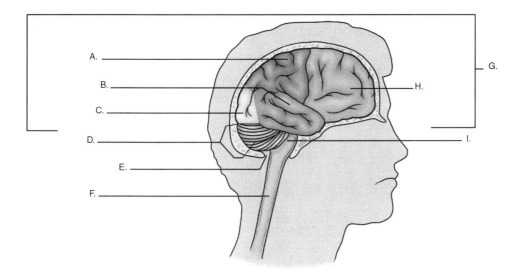

A. _____

B. _____

C. _____

D. _____

E. _____

F. _____

G. _____

H. _____

I. _____

2. The Connecting Nerves in the Spinal Cord

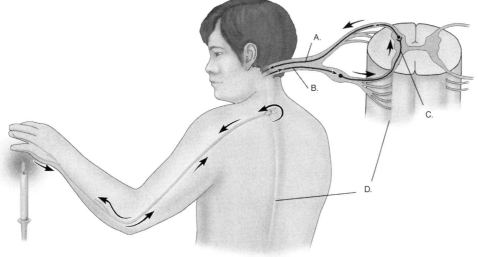

A. _____

B. _____

C. _____

D. _____

E. _____

F. _____

G. _____

H. _____

I. _____

J. _____

3. The Spinal Column

A. _____

B. _____

C. _____

D. _____

E. _____

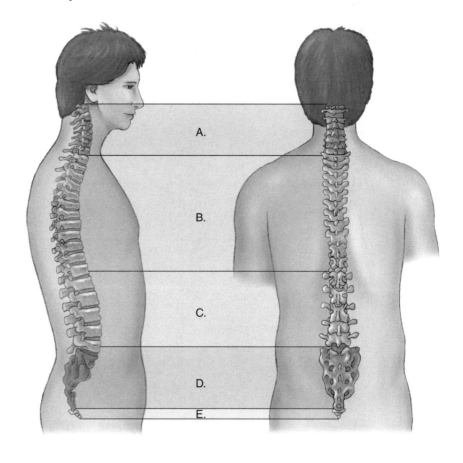

Fill-in

Read each item carefully, then complete the statement by filling in the missing word(s).

1. The _____ nerves carry information to the muscles.

2. The dura mater, arachnoid, and pia mater are layers of _____ within the skull and spinal canal.

3. The brain and spinal cord are part of the _____ nervous system.

4. Within the peripheral nervous system, there are _____ pairs of spinal nerves.

5. The _____ nerves pass through holes in the skull and transmit sensations directly to the brain.

6. Vertebrae are separated by cushions called _____ _____.

7. The skull has two large structures of bone, the _____ and the _____.

8. The _____ and _____ produce cerebrospinal fluid (CSF).

9. The _____ nervous system reacts to stress.

10. The _____ nervous system causes the body to relax.

True/False

If you believe the statement to be more true than false, write the letter "T" in the space provided. If you believe the statement to be more false than true, write the letter "F."

_____ **1.** A distracted spine has been moved laterally.

_____ **2.** If a sensory nerve in the reflex arc detects an irritating stimulus, it will bypass the motor nerve and send a message directly to the brain.

_____ **3.** Voluntary activities are those actions we perform unconsciously.

_____ **4.** The autonomic nervous system is composed of the sympathetic nervous system and the parasympathetic nervous system.

_____ **5.** The parasympathetic nervous system reacts to stress with the fight-or-flight response whenever it is confronted with a threatening situation.

_____ **6.** All patients with suspected head and/or spine injuries should have their head realigned to an in-line neutral position.

_____ **7.** When assessing a patient for possible spinal injury, you should begin with a focused history and physical exam.

_____ **8.** Your ideal procedure for moving a patient from the ground to a backboard is the four-person log roll.

_____ **9.** You should not try to put a patient on a short board if they are in danger.

_____ **10.** To properly measure a cervical collar, use the manufacturer's specifications.

Short Answer

Complete this section with short written answers using the space provided.

1. List the five basic questions to ask a conscious patient when conducting an assessment of a head or head and spine injury.

_____

_____

2. List the reasons for not placing the head/spine injury patient's head into a neutral in-line position.

_____

_____

3. List the three major types of brain injuries.

_____

_____

4. List at least five signs and symptoms of a head injury.

_____

_____

5. List the three general principles for treating a head injury.

_____

_____

6. List the six questions to ask yourself when deciding whether or not to remove a helmet.

_____

_____

Word Fun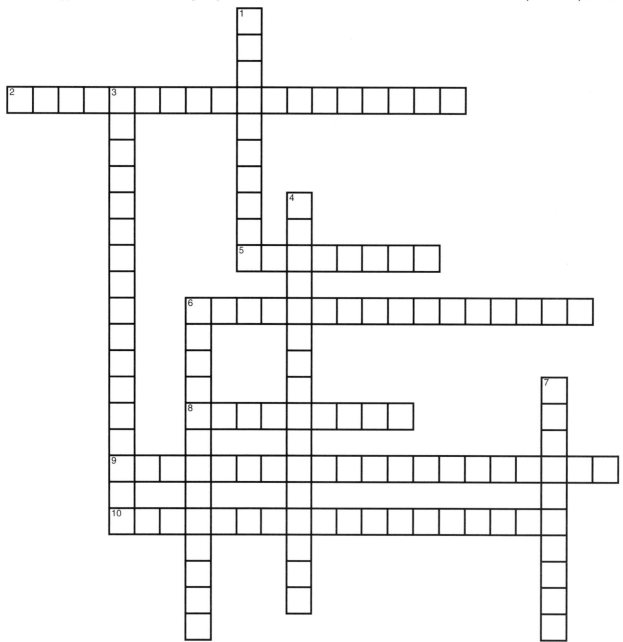

The following crossword puzzle is an activity provided to reinforce correct spelling and understanding of medical terminology associated with emergency care and the EMT-B. Use the clues in the column to complete the puzzle.

Across

2. Cushion between vertebrae
5. Layers of tissues surrounding the brain
6. Cerebral trauma without broken skin
8. Controls primary life functions
9. Voluntary part of CNS
10. Inability to remember after the event

Down

1. Coordinates body movement
3. Inability to remember the event
4. Join motor and sensory nerves
6. Swelling of the brain
7. Pulling the spine along its length

Ambulance Calls

The following case scenarios provide an opportunity to explore the concerns associated with patient management. Read each scenario, then answer each question in detail.

1. You are dispatched to a bicycle versus car. The driver of the car is uninjured, but the bicyclist is reported as "severely injured." You arrive to find the patient lying in the street, unconscious and with an apparent head injury. The patient was not wearing a helmet when she was struck by the car. Witnesses say she was launched into the windshield, and then landed in the road.

How do you best manage this patient?

_____

_____

_____

2. You are dispatched to assist a "young child fallen." You arrive to find a frantic parent who tells you her child was playing on the family's trampoline in the back yard. She was bouncing very high and accidentally launched herself off the trampoline, landing face down onto a concrete pad in the neighbor's yard. She responds to painful stimuli and has snoring respirations.

How do you best manage this patient?

_____

_____

_____

3. You are dispatched to a motor vehicle crash with major damage to the patient compartment. Your patient, an 18-month-old boy, is still in his car seat in the center of the back seat. He responds appropriately and there is no damage to his seat. He has no visible injuries, but a front seat passenger was killed.

How would you best manage this patient?

_____

_____

_____

Skill Drills

Skill Drill 30-1: Performing Manual In-Line Stabilization

Test your knowledge of this skill drill by filling in the correct words in the photo captions.

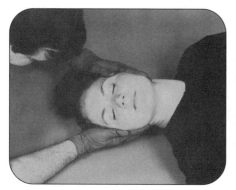

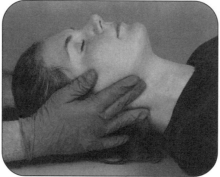

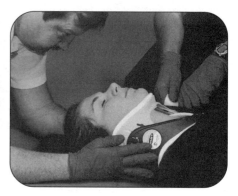

1. Kneel behind the patient and place your hands firmly around the _____ of the _____ on either _____ .

2. Support the lower jaw with your _____ and _____ fingers, and the head with your _____. Gently _____ the head into a _____, _____ position, aligned with the torso. Do not _____ the head or neck excessively, forcefully, or rapidly.

3. Continue to _____ the head manually while your partner places a rigid _____ _____ around the neck. Maintain _____ _____ until you have completely secured the patient to a backboard.

Skill Drill 30-2: Immobilizing a Patient to a Long Backboard

Test your knowledge of this skill drill by placing the photos below in the correct order. Number the first step with a "1," the second step with a "2," etc. Also, fill in the correct words in the photo captions.

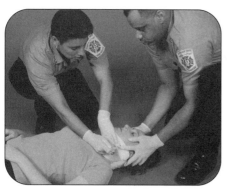

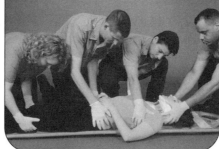

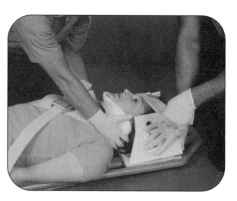

_____

Apply a _____ _____ .

_____ the patient on the board.

Place _____ across the patient's forehead.

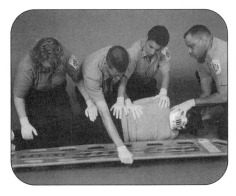

On command, rescuers _____ the patient toward themselves, quickly examine the _____, slide the backboard under the patient, and roll the patient onto the board.

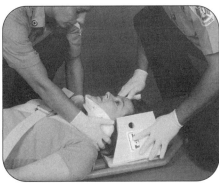

Begin to secure the patient's head using a commercial immobilization device or _____ _____ .

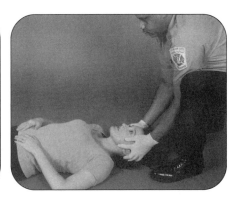

Apply and maintain _____ _____ .
Assess _____ _____ in all extremities.

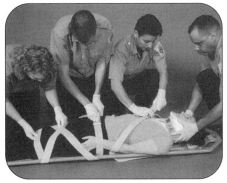

Secure the _____ , _____ , and _____ _____ .

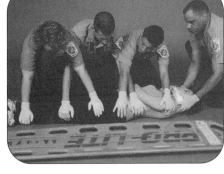

Rescuers _____ on one side of the patient and place _____ on the far side of the patient.

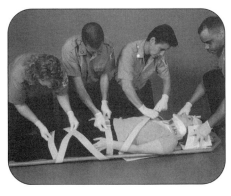

Check all _____ and readjust as needed.
Reassess _____ _____ in all extremities.

Secure the _____ _____ first.

Skill Drill 30-3: Immobilizing a Patient Found in a Sitting Position
Test your knowledge of this skill drill by placing the photos below in the correct order. Number the first step with a "1," the second step with a "2," etc.

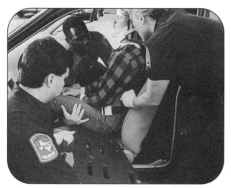

Wedge a long backboard next to the patient's buttocks.

_____

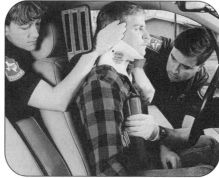

Open the side flaps, and position them around the patient's torso, snug around the armpits.

_____

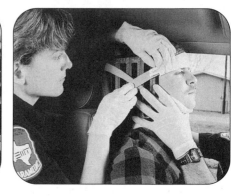

Pad between the head and the device as needed.
Secure the forehead strap and fasten the lower head strap around the collar.

_____

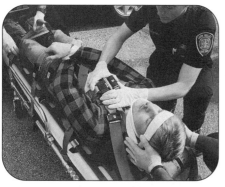

Secure the immobilization devices to each other.
Reassess pulse, motor, and sensory functions in each extremity.

_____

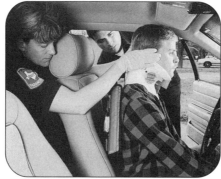

Insert a short spine immobilization device between the patient's upper back and the seat.

_____

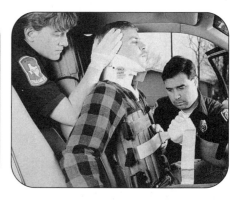

Secure the upper torso flaps, then the midtorso flaps.

_____

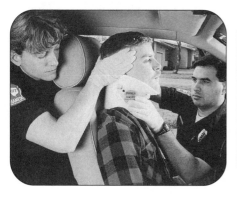

Stabilize the head and neck in a neutral, in-line position.
Assess pulse, motor, and sensory function in each extremity.
Apply a cervical collar.

_____

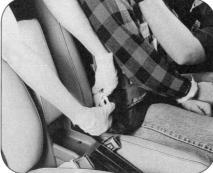

Secure the groin (leg) straps. Check and adjust torso straps.

_____

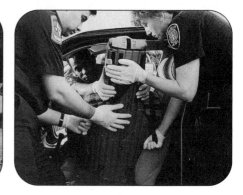

Turn and lower the patient onto the long board.
Lift the patient, and slip the long board under the spine device.

Skill Drill 30-4: Immobilizing a Patient Found in a Standing Position
Test your knowledge of this skill drill by filling in the correct words in the photo captions.

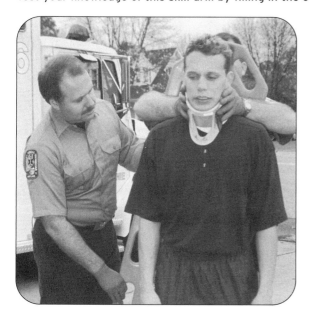

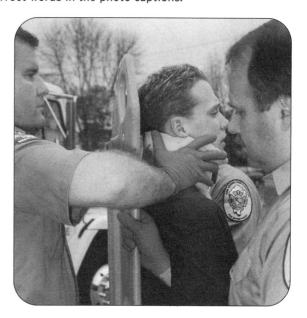

1. While _____ stabilizing the head and neck, apply a ___ ___. Position the board _____ the patient.

2. Position EMT-Bs at _____ and _____ the patient.
   Side EMT-Bs reach under patient's _____ and grasp _____ at or slightly above _____ level.

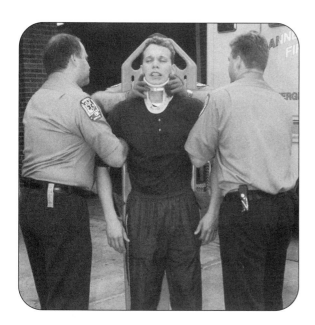

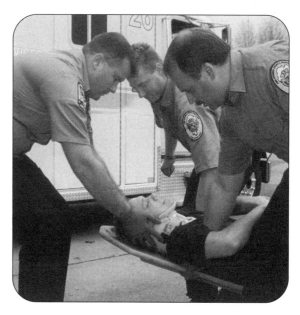

3. Prepare to lower the patient. EMT-Bs on the sides should be _____ the EMT-B at the head and _____ for his or her _____ .

4. On command, _____ the backboard to the ground.

Skill Drill 30-5: Application of a Cervical Collar

Test your knowledge of this skill drill by filling in the correct words in the photo captions.

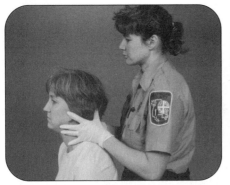

1. Apply _____ stabilization.

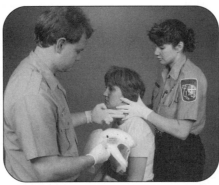

2. Measure the proper _____ _____.

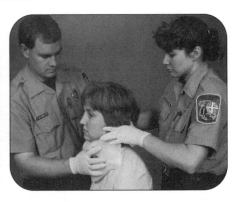

3. Place the _____ _____ first.

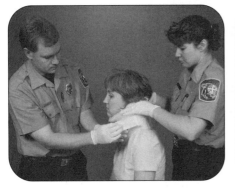

4. _____ the collar around the neck and _____ the collar.

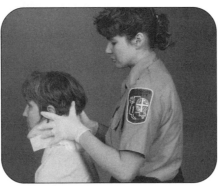

5. Ensure proper _____ and maintain _____, _____ stabilization.

Skill Drill 30-6: Removing a Helmet

Test your knowledge of this skill drill by placing the photos below in the correct order. Number the first step with a "1," the second step with a "2," etc. Also, fill in the correct words in the photo captions.

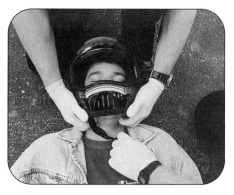

_____

Prevent head movement by placing your _____ on either side of the helmet and fingers on the _____ _____. Have your partner _____ the strap.

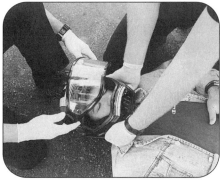

_____

Kneel down at the patient's head with your _____ at one side. Open the face shield to assess _____ and _____. Remove _____ if present.

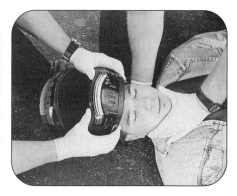

_____

Have your partner slide the hand from the _____ to the _____ of the head to prevent it from snapping back.

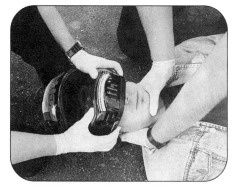

_____

Gently slip the helmet about _____ off, then stop.

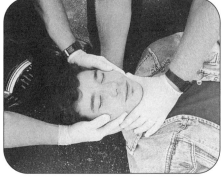

_____

Remove the helmet and _____ the cervical spine.
Apply a _____ _____ and secure the patient to a _____ _____ .
_____ as needed to prevent neck flexion or extension.

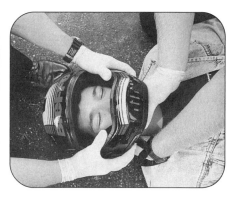

_____

Have your partner place one hand at the _____ of the _____ and the other at the _____ .

Assessment Review

Answer the following questions pertaining to the assessment of the types of emergencies discussed in this chapter.

_____ 1. You respond to a patient who was assaulted and is unconscious. Upon reaching his side you check his airway and it is open. The breathing is at 18 breaths/min and regular. Pulse is strong and regular with distal pulses present. You want to administer oxygen. How would you give it?

   A. 2 L/min

   B. 6 L/min

   C. 10 L/min

   D. 15 L/min

_____ 2. You and your partner have determined that you need to put the patient above in full immobilization. When can your partner release manual stabilization of the head?

   A. When the C-collar is applied

   B. When the torso is secured to the board

   C. When the patient is completely secured to the board

   D. When you arrive at the hospital

_____ 3. You decide to put the patient on a long backboard and will use the logroll technique to accomplish the task. When do you check the back of the patient?

   A. After being secured to the board

   B. As the patient is rolled onto their side

   C. Before any movement is attempted

   D. When you move them to the hospital bed

_____ 4. If you respond to a patient who is in a sitting position and stable, how would you immobilize them?

   A. Lay them down and log roll them.

   B. Use a scoop stretcher.

   C. Use a short board.

   D. Have them lay down on your backboard.

_____ 5. You respond to a motorcycle accident. You decide that you need to remove the rider's helmet. What is the minimum number of people required to remove the helmet?

   A. 2

   B. 3

   C. 4

   D. 5

Emergency Care Summary

Complete the statements pertaining to emergency care for the types of emergencies discussed in this chapter by filling in the missing words.
Please note that only two sections of the Emergency Care Summary are included here.

NOTE: While the steps below are widely accepted, be sure to consult and follow your local protocol.

Head and Spine Injuries

Immobilizing a Patient Found in a Sitting Position

1. Stabilize the head and neck in a _____, _____ position. Assess pulse, motor, and sensory function in each extremity. Apply a _____ _____.

2. Insert a _____ _____ immobilization device between the patient's upper back and the seat.

3. Open the side flaps, and position them around the patient's torso, snug around the armpits.

4. Secure the upper torso flaps, then the midtorso flaps.

5. Secure the groin (leg) straps. Check and adjust torso straps.

6. Pad between the head and the device as needed. Secure the forehead strap and fasten the _____ _____ _____ around the collar.

7. Wedge a _____ _____ next to the patient's buttocks.

8. Turn and lower the patient onto the long board. Lift the patient, and slip the long board under the spine device.

9. Secure the immobilization devices to each other. Reassess pulse, motor, and sensory functions in each _____.

CHAPTER

31 Pediatric Emergencies

Workbook Activities

The following activities have been designed to help you. Your instructor may require you to complete some or all of these activities as a regular part of your EMT-B training program. You are encouraged to complete any activity that your instructor does not assign as a way to enhance your learning in the classroom.

Chapter Review

The following exercises provide an opportunity to refresh your knowledge of this chapter.

Matching

Match each of the terms in the left column to the appropriate definition in the right column.

_____ **1.** Gastrostomy tube   **A.** ages 12 to 18 years

_____ **2.** Shunt   **B.** ages 3 to 6 years

_____ **3.** Tracheostomy tube   **C.** soft openings within the skull of an infant

_____ **4.** Toddler   **D.** specialized medical practice devoted to the care of children

_____ **5.** Preschool-age children   **E.** used for breathing

_____ **6.** Adolescents   **F.** diverts excess cerebrospinal fluid

_____ **7.** Infancy   **G.** first month after birth

_____ **8.** Neonate   **H.** the first year of life

_____ **9.** Fontanels   **I.** used for feeding

_____ **10.** Pediatrics   **J.** after infancy, until about 3 years of age

Multiple Choice

Read each item carefully, then select the best response.

_____ 1. In addition to the tongue, the _____ help(s) to produce a smaller opening to move air easily.

    A. tonsils

    B. adenoids

    C. soft pallet

    D. all of the above

_____ 2. A respiratory rate of _____ breaths/min is normal for the newborn.

    A. 12 to 20

    B. 20 to 40

    C. 30 to 50

    D. 40 to 60

_____ 3. Breathing requires the use of the _____ and diaphragm.

    A. chest muscles

    B. neck muscles

    C. subclavian muscles

    D. abdominal muscles

_____ 4. You respond to an automobile accident involving a 3-year-old boy. You remove the patient from the vehicle and prepare to secure him to a long backboard. You should be careful not to cause respiratory compromise by putting a strap across the:

    A. thorax.

    B. air.

    C. diaphragm.

    D. lungs.

_____ 5. The primary method for the body to compensate for decreased oxygenation is to:

    A. increase the respiratory rate.

    B. increase the heart rate.

    C. increase the blood pressure.

    D. increase diaphragm contractions.

_____ 6. Signs of vasoconstriction can include:

    A. weak peripheral pulses.

    B. delayed capillary refill.

    C. cool hands or feet.

    D. all of the above

_____ 7. Infants respond mainly to _____ stimuli.

    A. social

    B. mental

    C. physical

    D. all of the above

_____ 8. You respond to a call for a sick 10-month-old. As you enter the residence, you would begin your initial assessment from across the room. What would you be checking?

    A. Work of breathing

    B. Skin color and alertness

    C. Level of activity

    D. All of the above

_____ **9.** Injuries in the _____ age group are more frequent.

    A. infant

    B. toddler

    C. preschool

    D. school

_____ **10.** At the _____ age, children are easily distracted with counting games and small toys.

    A. infant

    B. toddler

    C. preschool

    D. adolescent

_____ **11.** You are called to a local residence for a child on a home ventilator. The parents state he has been having trouble with his breathing. You should first determine:

    A. baseline vital signs.

    B. normal baseline status.

    C. previous injuries.

    D. over-the-counter medications.

_____ **12.** For the patient above, your first priority in treating a special-needs child includes:

    A. obtaining an extensive history.

    B. determining mode of transportation.

    C. assessing the airway.

    D. obtaining the patient's medications to take to the hospital.

_____ **13.** You are called to the home of a 13-year-old girl with altered mental status. Upon arrival, you notice the child has a tracheostomy tube. You perform your initial assessment. You know that potential problems associated with the tracheostomy tube include:

    A. obstruction of the tube by mucous plugs.

    B. bleeding.

    C. air leakage around the tube.

    D. all of the above

_____ **14.** Tubes that extend from the brain to the abdomen to drain excess cerebrospinal fluid that may accumulate near the brain are called:

    A. shunts.

    B. central lines.

    C. G-tubes.

    D. tracheostomy tubes.

Fill-in

Read each item carefully, then complete the statement by filling in the missing word.

1. The specialized medical practice devoted to the care of the young is called _____.

2. The _____ is longer and more rounded compared to the size of the mandible, or lower jaw, in younger children.

3. In a child, the _____ is softer and narrower.

4. An infant's heart rate can become as high as _____ beats or more per minute if the body needs to compensate for injury or illness.

5. _____ _____ is an early sign that the child may be compensating for decreased perfusion.

6. Infants have two soft openings within the skull called _____.

7. Most _____ are able to think abstractly and can participate in decision making.

True/False

If you believe the statement to be more true than false, write the letter "T" in the space provided. If you believe the statement to be more false than true, write the letter "F."

_____ **1.** Toddlers often resist separation and demonstrate stranger anxiety.

_____ **2.** The skeletal system contains growth plates at the ends of long bones, which enable these bones to grow during childhood.

_____ **3.** Adulthood begins at age 18.

_____ **4.** Infants are usually afraid of strangers, because they are the center of attention in most families.

_____ **5.** Preschool-age children have a rich fantasy life, which can make them particularly fearful of pain and change involving their bodies.

_____ **6.** The parent or caregiver of a special-needs child will be an important part of your assessment.

_____ **7.** Children with diabetes who receive insulin and tube feedings may become hyperglycemic quickly if tube feedings are discontinued.

_____ **8.** If a shunt becomes clogged due to infection, changes in mental status and respiratory arrest may occur.

Short Answer

Complete this section with short written answers using the space provided.

1. Discuss developmental considerations for infancy and approach for caregivers.

_____

_____

2. Give four examples of special-needs children.

_____

_____

3. Discuss developmental considerations for toddlers and approach for caregivers.

_____

_____

4. Discuss developmental considerations for the school-age child and approach for caregivers.

_____

_____

5. Discuss developmental considerations for the adolescent and approach for caregivers.

_____

_____

Word Fun

The following crossword puzzle is an activity provided to reinforce correct spelling and understanding of medical terminology associated with emergency care and the EMT-B. Use the clues in the column to complete the puzzle.

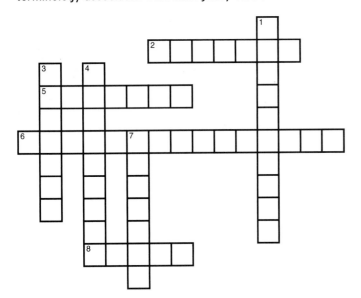

Across

2. Terrible twos stage

5. First month after birth

6. Feeding tube placed through abdominal wall

8. Tube diverting cerebrospinal fluid to abdomen

Down

1. Specialized medical practice devoted to care of children

3. First year of life

4. Two soft openings within the skull

7. Back of the head

Ambulance Calls

The following case scenarios provide an opportunity to explore the concerns associated with patient management. Read each scenario, then answer each question in detail.

1. You are dispatched to the residence of a toddler with a history of fever who is now unresponsive. You arrive to find a 13-year-old babysitter who tells you she is not sure what is wrong with the 2-year-old boy. She tells you he started "shaking all over" and she didn't know what to do. He is currently responsive to painful stimuli and warm to the touch.

How do you best manage this patient?

_____

_____

_____

2. You are dispatched to the residence of a 3-year-old child with a history of lung problems. The child, a very small boy, is cyanotic and lethargic. He is pain responsive. He has copious mucous secretions in his airway. The grandmother, who was sitting with the child, is hysterical.

How would you best manage this patient?

_____

_____

_____

3. You are dispatched to assist a young girl with shortness of breath. You arrive to find a 16-year-old female patient who is obviously having difficulty breathing. She is holding a metered-dose inhaler and is so air-starved, she cannot answer your questions.

How do you best manage this patient?

_____

_____

_____

CHAPTER

32 Pediatric Assessment and Management

Workbook Activities

The following activities have been designed to help you. Your instructor may require you to complete some or all of these activities as a regular part of your EMT-B training program. You are encouraged to complete any activity that your instructor does not assign as a way to enhance your learning in the classroom.

Chapter Review

The following exercises provide an opportunity to refresh your knowledge of this chapter.

Matching

Match each of the terms in the left column to the appropriate definition in the right column.

_____ 1. Croup

_____ 2. Wheezing

_____ 3. Epiglottis

_____ 4. Rales

_____ 5. Stridor

_____ 6. Septum

_____ 7. Shock

_____ 8. Apnea

_____ 9. Blanching

_____ 10. Xiphoid process

_____ 11. Febrile seizure

_____ 12. Tripod position

_____ 13. Jaw-thrust maneuver

A. leaning forward on two arms stretched forward

B. seizure relating to a fever

C. absence of breathing

D. infection of the airway below the level of the vocal cords

E. turning white

F. whistling sound made from air moving through narrowed bronchioles

G. the lower tip of the sternum

H. infection of soft tissue in the area above the vocal cords

I. the central divider in the nose

J. crackling sound caused by flow of air through liquid

K. insufficient blood to body organs

L. high-pitched sound usually caused by swelling around vocal cords

M. used to open the airway with suspected spinal injuries

Multiple Choice

Read each item carefully, then select the best response.

_____   **1.** Positioning the airway in a neutral sniffing position:
   A. keeps the trachea from kinking when the neck is hyperextended.
   B. keeps the trachea from kinking when the neck is flexed.
   C. maintains the proper alignment if you have to immobilize the spine.
   D. all of the above

_____   **2.** Benefits of using a nasopharyngeal airway include all of the following, except:
   A. it is usually well tolerated.
   B. it may be used in the presence of head trauma.
   C. it is not as likely as the oropharyngeal airway to cause vomiting.
   D. it is used for conscious patients or those with altered levels of consciousness.

_____   **3.** Indications for assisting ventilations in a child include:
   A. respiratory rate of less than 12 breaths/min.
   B. respiratory rate of greater than 60 breaths/min.
   C. inadequate tidal volume.
   D. all of the above

_____   **4.** Errors in technique, when providing ventilations with a BVM device, that may result in gastric distention include:
   A. providing too much volume.
   B. squeezing the bag too forcefully.
   C. ventilating too fast.
   D. all of the above

_____   **5.** _____ is an infection of the airway below the level of the vocal cords, usually caused by a virus.
   A. Croup
   B. Tonsillitis
   C. Epiglottitis
   D. Pharyngitis

_____   **6.** Signs of complete airway obstruction include:
   A. inability to speak or cry.
   B. increasing respiratory difficulty with stridor.
   C. cyanosis.
   D. all of the above

_____   **7.** You are called to a 3-year-old in respiratory distress. As you approach the child, you would expect the early signs of respiratory distress to include all of the following, except:
   A. combativeness.
   B. anxiety.
   C. cyanosis.
   D. restlessness.

_____   **8.** If the child's condition in the question above were to get worse, you would expect the signs of increased work of breathing to include:
   A. nasal flaring.
   B. wheezing, stridor, or other abnormal airway sounds.
   C. accessory muscle use.
   D. all of the above

_____ **9.** You are called to the home of a 14-year-old girl with seizures. Upon your arrival, she is actively seizing. The parents tell you she seems to have had two seizures without regaining consciousness; one stopped and then the other started. This is her third. She has been seizing for approximately 2 minutes. You know this condition as:

    A. status epilepticus.

    B. grand mal seizure.

    C. absence seizure.

    D. focal motor seizure.

_____ **10.** During the postictal period, the patient may appear:

    A. sleepy.

    B. confused.

    C. unresponsive.

    D. all of the above

_____ **11.** Most pediatric seizures are due to _____, which is why they are called febrile seizures.

    A. infection

    B. fever

    C. ingestion

    D. trauma

_____ **12.** Signs that a patient is not breathing adequately include:

    A. very slow respirations.

    B. very shallow breaths.

    C. cyanosis or pale lips.

    D. all of the above

_____ **13.** Care of the actively seizing child includes all of the following, except:

    A. assessing and managing the ABCs.

    B. noting the type of movement and position of the eyes.

    C. cooling the patient with alcohol if there is fever.

    D. making sure the patient is protected from hitting anything.

_____ **14.** Nonverbal infants may demonstrate consciousness by:

    A. tracking.

    B. babbling and cooing.

    C. crying.

    D. all of the above

_____ **15.** You respond to an 11-year-old boy who is unconscious. Nobody has any information on what happened. His respirations are rapid, pulse weak and rapid, and distal pulses are weak but present. His skin is cool and clammy. You know that common causes of shock in children include all of the following except:

    A. heart attack.

    B. head trauma.

    C. dehydration.

    D. pneumothorax.

_____ **16.** At birth, most infants only need stimulation to:

    A. cry.

    B. wake up.

    C. breathe.

    D. move.

_____ **17.** You respond to a 24-year-old woman who gave birth at home. Your partner takes responsibility for the mother. He assigns you the newborn. The baby is crying and you want to check a pulse. You know you can check the brachial; where else can you check the pulse in a neonate?

    A. Carotid artery

    B. Radial artery

    C. Femoral artery

    D. The base of the umbilical cord

_____ **18.** Respiratory problems leading to cardiopulmonary arrest in children may be caused by:

    A. a foreign body in the airway.

    B. near drowning.

    C. sudden infant death syndrome.

    D. all of the above

_____ **19.** _____ will decrease the risk of gastric distention and aspiration of vomitus by pushing the larynx back to compress and close off the esophagus.

    A. Using a BVM device

    B. The Sellick maneuver

    C. Abdominal compression

    D. none of the above

_____ **20.** While checking a pulse, you may observe other signs of circulation including:

    A. breathing.

    B. coughing.

    C. movement.

    D. all of the above

_____ **21.** When approaching a child, you should look for all of the following, except:

    A. work of breathing.

    B. pulse.

    C. level of activity.

    D. skin color.

_____ **22.** When caring for children with sports-related injuries, you should remember to:

    A. elevate the extremities.

    B. assist ventilations.

    C. immobilize the cervical spine.

    D. remove all helmets.

_____ **23.** Your single most important step in caring for a child with a head injury is to:

    A. immobilize the cervical spine.

    B. bandage all wounds.

    C. ensure an open airway.

    D. obtain a SAMPLE history.

_____ **24.** Signs of shock in children include all of the following, except:

    A. tachycardia.

    B. hypotension.

    C. poor capillary refill.

    D. mental status changes.

_____ **25.** For children who have had traumatic injuries, use a child-sized BVM device at a rate of one breath every _____ seconds.

    A. 2

    B. 3

    C. 4

    D. 5

_____ **26.** If _____—an abnormal airway sound made by turbulent airflow—is present, use the jaw-thrust maneuver to keep the airway open.

    A. rales

    B. rhonchi

    C. stridor

    D. wheezing

Fill-in

Read each item carefully, then complete the statement by filling in the missing word.

1. The term _____ _____ is used to describe a continuous seizure, or multiple seizures without a return to consciousness, for 30 minutes or more.

2. Because a young child might not be able to speak, your assessment of his or her condition must be based in large part on what you can _____ and _____.

3. _____ occurs when fluid losses are greater than fluid intake.

4. _____ _____ are devices that help to maintain the airway or assist in providing artificial ventilation.

5. An oropharyngeal airway should be used in neither conscious patients nor those who have a decreased level of consciousness, because both will have a _____ _____.

6. _____ _____ indicates the amount of oxygen getting to the organs of the body.

7. The _____ _____ is the amount of air that is delivered to the lungs and airways in one inhalation.

8. _____ should be considered as a possible cause of airway obstruction if a child has congestion, fever, drooling, and cold symptoms.

9. A _____ is the result of disorganized electrical activity in the brain.

10. Because a child's _____ is proportionately larger than an adult's, it exerts greater stress on the neck structures during a deceleration injury.

11. Children can lose a greater proportion of their blood volume than adults can before signs and symptoms of _____ develop.

True/False

If you believe the statement to be more true than false, write the letter "T" in the space provided. If you believe the statement to be more false than true, write the letter "F."

_____ 1. You must always assist ventilations in all pediatric patients who have respiratory rates greater than 60 breaths/min.

_____ 2. Febrile seizures are self-limiting and do not need transport unless they recur.

_____ 3. Febrile seizures may not be accompanied by a postictal phase.

_____ 4. Alcohol applied to skin is a recommended method of cooling a patient.

_____ 5. Infants with severe dehydration may present with sunken fontanels.

_____ 6. Young children with severe dehydration will have delayed capillary refill.

_____ 7. Children with moderate dehydration should be rehydrated at home.

_____ 8. Children younger than 1 year should not have an AED applied.

_____ 9. Children can lose a greater proportion of blood than adults before showing signs or symptoms of shock.

Short Answer

Complete this section with short written answers using the space provided.

1. How is urine output assessed in infants?

_____

_____

2. List four signs of increased work of breathing in children.

_____

_____

Word Fun emtb. vocab explorer

The following crossword puzzle is an activity provided to reinforce correct spelling and understanding of medical terminology associated with emergency care and the EMT-B. Use the clues in the column to complete the puzzle.

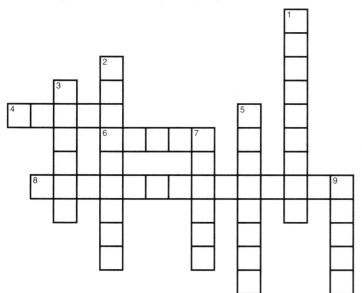

Across

4. Absence of breathing

6. External openings of nasal passages

8. The lower tip of the sternum

Down

1. Increased respiratory rate

2. Turning white

3. Deficiency of red blood cells or hemoglobin

5. Dark green material in amniotic fluid

7. Central divider of the nose

9. Inadequate tissue perfusion

Ambulance Calls

The following case scenarios provide an opportunity to explore the concerns associated with patient management. Read each scenario, then answer each question in detail.

1. You are dispatched to assist an unconscious 11-year-old boy. You arrive to find a home filled with several teenagers who appear to have been having an unsupervised party. You see several beer cans and bottles of whiskey on the floor. They tell you that they "think" the 11-year-old was drinking beer, but they're "not sure." They noticed he was sleeping and tried to wake him up without success. You see that he has vomited and is currently lying on his back with snoring respirations. How do you best manage this patient?

_____

_____

2. You are called to a residence for a 2-year-old child with difficulty breathing. The little girl has stridor and expiratory wheezes, as well as intercostal retractions. She is very upset by your arrival and clings to her mother. Her breathing worsens with agitation. Her mother tells you she is currently taking medication for an upper respiratory infection and has spent much of her life in and out of hospitals with respiratory problems.

How would you best manage this patient?

_____

_____

_____

3. It's 5:30 A.M. and you are dispatched to the home of a 6-month-old girl who is not breathing. You arrive to find a crying, young mother holding a lifeless baby. The infant is not breathing, is cold to the touch, and appears to have dependent lividity.

How do you best manage this patient?

_____

_____

_____

Skill Drills
Skill Drill 32-1: Positioning the Airway in a Child
Test your knowledge of this skill drill by filling in the correct words in the photo captions.

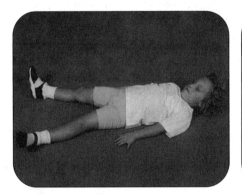

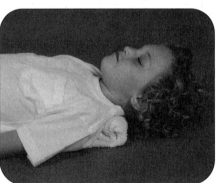

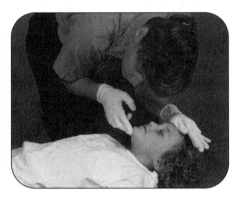

1. Position the child on a _____ surface.

2. Place a _____ towel about _____ inch(es) thick under the _____ and _____.

3. _____ the forehead to limit _____ and use the head tilt-chin lift to open the airway

Skill Drill 32-2: Inserting an Oropharyngeal Airway in a Child
Test your knowledge of this skill drill by filling in the correct words in the photo captions.

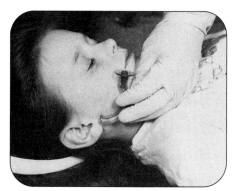

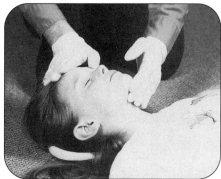

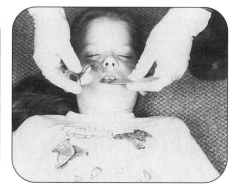

1. Determine the _____ _____ airway. Confirm the correct size _____, by placing it next to the patient's _____.

2. Position the patient's _____ with the appropriate method.

3. Open the mouth. Insert the airway until the _____ rests against the _____. _____ the airway.

Skill Drill 32-3: Inserting a Nasopharyngeal Airway in a Child
Test your knowledge of this skill drill by filling in the correct words in the photo captions.

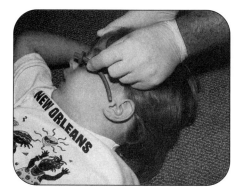

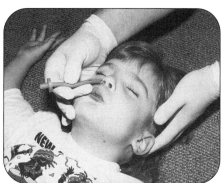

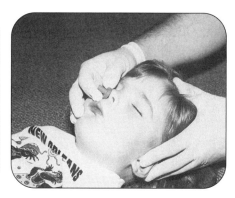

1. Determine the correct airway size by comparing its _____ to the opening of the _____ (naris). Place the airway next to the patient's _____ to confirm correct _____. _____ the airway.

2. _____ the airway. Insert the _____ into the right naris with the bevel pointing toward the _____.

3. Carefully move the tip forward until the _____ rests against the _____ of the nostril. Reassess the _____.

Skill Drill 32-4: One-rescuer BVM Ventilation on a Child
Test your knowledge of this skill drill by placing the photos below in the correct order. Number the first step with a "1," the second step with a "2," etc.

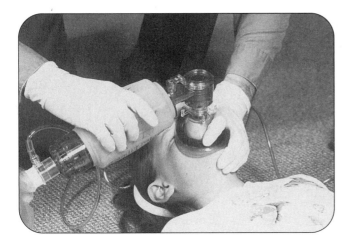

Hold the mask on the patient's face with a one-handed head tilt-chin lift technique (E-C grip).
Ensure a good mask-face seal while maintaining the airway.

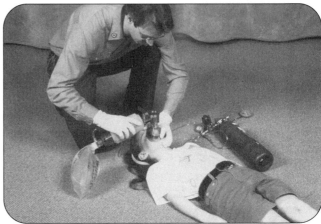

Assess effectiveness of ventilation by watching bilateral rise and fall of the chest.

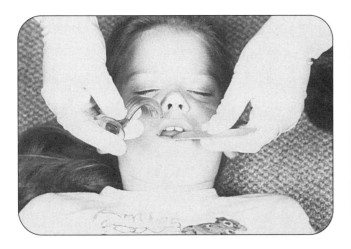

Open the airway and insert the appropriate airway adjunct.

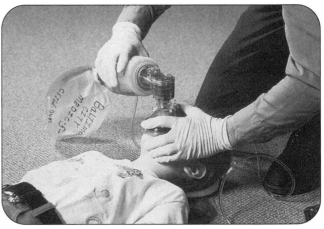

Squeeze the bag 20 times/min for a child or 30 times/min for an infant. Allow adequate time for exhalation.

Skill Drill 32-5: Removing a Foreign Body Airway Obstruction in an Unconscious Child

Test your knowledge of this skill drill by placing the photos below in the correct order. Number the first step with a "1," the second step with a "2," etc.

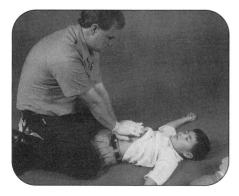

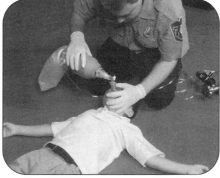

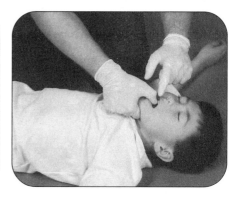

_____

If ventilation is unsuccessful, position your hands on the abdomen above the navel and well below the chest cage. Give five abdominal thrusts.

_____

Attempt rescue breathing. If unsuccessful, reposition the head and try again.

_____

Open the airway again to try to see the object. Only try to remove the obstruction if you can see it.
Attempt rescue breathing. If unsuccessful, reposition the head and try again.
Repeat abdominal thrusts if obstruction persists.

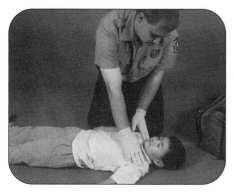

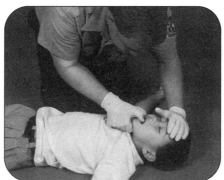

_____

Position the child on a firm, flat surface.

_____

Inspect the airway. Remove any visible foreign object that you can see.

Skill Drill 32-6: Performing Infant Chest Compressions

Test your knowledge of this skill drill by filling in the correct words in the photo captions.

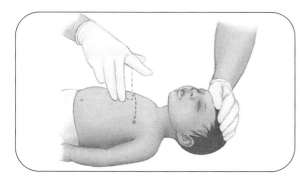

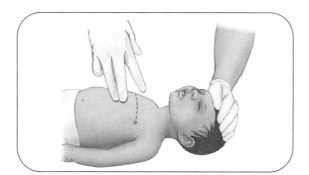

1. Position the infant on a _____ surface while

_____ the airway.

Place two _____ in the _____ of

the sternum just below a line between the

_____ .

2. Use two fingers to _____ the chest about

_____ inch(es) to _____ inch(es) at

a rate of _____ times/min.

Allow the sternum to return _____ to its

_____ position between compressions.

Skill Drill 32-7: Performing CPR on a Child
Test your knowledge of this skill drill by filling in the correct words in the photo captions.

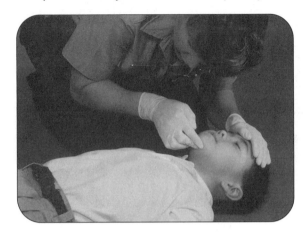

1. Place the child on a _____ surface and maintain the airway with one _____.

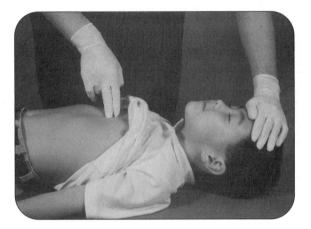

2. Using two fingers of the other hand, locate the bottom of the _____ by tracing the lower margin of the rib cage to the notch where the ribs and sternum meet. Place the _____ of your other hand over the lower half of the _____, avoiding the _____.

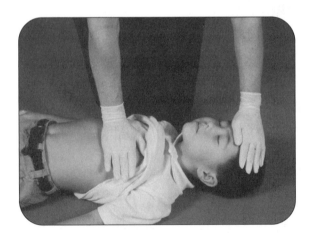

3. Compress the chest about _____ inch(es) to _____ inch(es) at a rate of _____ /min (about _____ /min with pauses for ventilations). Coordinate compressions with ventilations in a _____ ratio, pausing for _____.

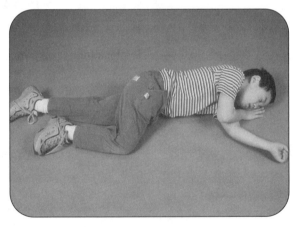

4. Reassess for _____ and _____ after about _____ minute(s), and then every _____ minute(s). If the child resumes _____ breathing, place him or her in the _____ position.

Skill Drill 32-8: Immobilizing a Child

Test your knowledge of this skill drill by filling in the correct words in the photo captions.

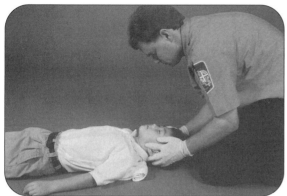

1. Use a towel under the back, from the

_____ to the _____, to maintain

the head in a _____ position.

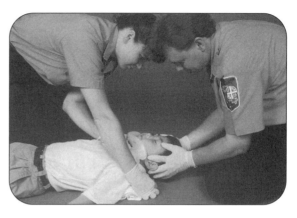

2. Apply an appropriately sized _____

_____.

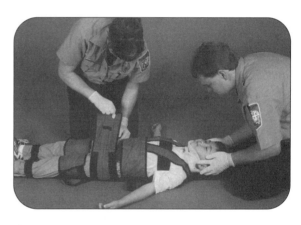

3. _____ _____ the child onto the

_____ device.

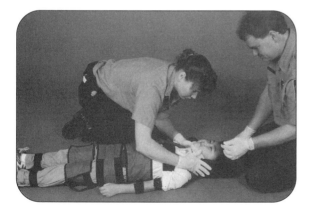

4. Secure the _____ first.

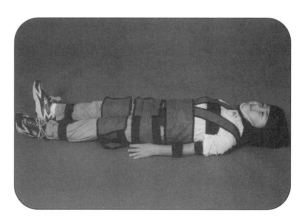

5. Secure the _____.

6. Ensure that the child is _____ in properly.

Skill Drill 32-10: Immobilizing an Infant Out of a Car Seat
Test your knowledge of this skill drill by placing the photos below in the correct order. Number the first step with a "1," the second step with a "2," etc.

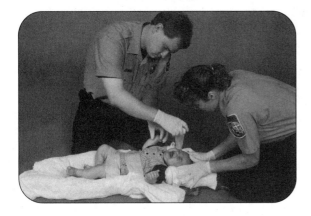

Secure the head.

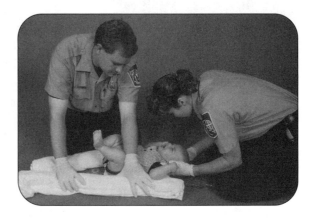

Slide the infant onto the board.

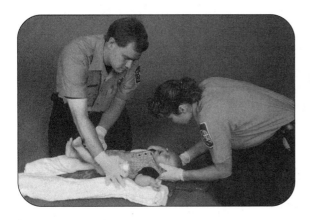

Place a towel under the back, from the shoulders to the hips, to ensure neutral head position.

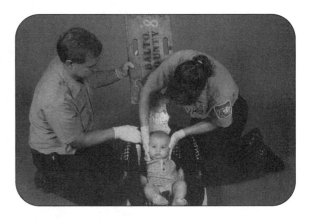

Stabilize the head in neutral position.

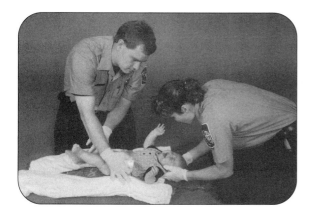

Secure the torso first; pad any voids.

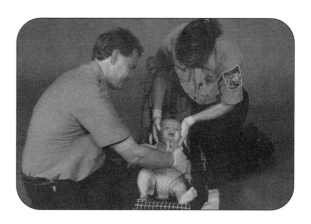

Place an immobilization device between the patient and the surface he or she is resting on.

CHAPTER

33 Geriatric Emergencies

Workbook Activities

The following activities have been designed to help you. Your instructor may require you to complete some or all of these activities as a regular part of your EMT-B training program. You are encouraged to complete any activity that your instructor does not assign as a way to enhance your learning in the classroom.

Chapter Review

The following exercises provide an opportunity to refresh your knowledge of this chapter.

Matching

Match each of the terms in the left column to the appropriate definition in the right column.

_____ **1.** Aneurysm

_____ **2.** Cataract

_____ **3.** Delirium

_____ **4.** Dementia

_____ **5.** Syncope

_____ **6.** Dyspnea

_____ **7.** Compensated shock

_____ **8.** Decompensated shock

_____ **9.** Collagen

_____ **10.** Vasoconstriction

A. a protein that is the chief component of connective tissue and bones

B. narrowing of a blood vessel

C. clouding of the lens of the eye

D. early shock

E. abnormal blood-filled dilation of a blood vessel

F. difficulty breathing

G. inability to focus, think logically, or maintain attention

H. late shock

I. slow onset of progressive disorientation

J. fainting

Multiple Choice
Read each item carefully, then select the best response.

_____ 1. Leading causes of death in the older population include all of the following, except:

A. heart disease.

B. AIDS.

C. cancer.

D. diabetes.

_____ 2. You are called the residence of an 86-year-old man who lives alone and seems to be confused. His airway is open and respirations are regular and unlabored. His pulse is strong and regular with good distal pulses. He is oriented and does not want to go to the hospital. You are worried about his well-being. You know that lifesaving interventions for geriatric patients may include:

A. reviewing the home environment.

B. providing information on preventing falls.

C. making referrals to appropriate social services agencies.

D. all of the above

_____ 3. Simple preventive measures can help older people to avoid:

A. further injury.

B. costly medical treatment.

C. death.

D. all of the above

_____ 4. Acute illness and trauma are more likely to involve _____ beyond those initially involved.

A. organ systems

B. bones

C. fractures

D. vessels

_____ 5. Risk factors that affect mortality in geriatric patients include all of the following, except:

A. living alone.

B. unsound mind.

C. regular exercise.

D. recent hospitalization.

_____ 6. Loss of collagen makes the skin:

A. wrinkled.

B. thinner.

C. more susceptible to injury.

D. all of the above

_____ 7. Driving and walking become more hazardous because the pupils of the eyes begin to lose the ability to:

A. dilate.

B. handle changes in light.

C. constrict.

D. detect color.

_____ 8. Problems with balance are usually related to changes in the:

A. blood pressure.

B. vision.

C. inner eyes.

D. cardiovascular system.

_____ **9.** Although the alveoli became enlarged, their elasticity decreases, resulting in a decreased ability to:

   A. cough and thereby increasing the chance of infection.

   B. exchange oxygen and carbon dioxide.

   C. monitor the changes in oxygen and carbon dioxide.

   D. force carbon dioxide out of the lungs.

_____ **10.** Compensation for an increased demand on the cardiovascular system is accomplished by:

   A. increasing heart rate.

   B. increasing contraction of the heart.

   C. constricting the blood vessels to nonvital organs.

   D. all of the above

_____ **11.** Aging decreases a person's ability to _____ because of stiffer vessels.

   A. vasoconstrict

   B. vasodilate

   C. circulate blood

   D. exchange oxygen

_____ **12.** An accumulation of fatty materials in the arteries is known as:

   A. myocardial infarction.

   B. stroke.

   C. atherosclerosis.

   D. aneurysm.

_____ **13.** You respond to a 68-year-old woman who is just not feeling well. She is alert and oriented. Her airway is open and there is no indication of any respiration problem. Pulse is regular and strong. Her blood pressure is 140/86 mm Hg. When asked about medications, she gives you a box that contains multiple medications from multiple doctors. She tells you she has been taking medications for years with no ill effects. She also mentions that on her last visit the doctor seemed a little concerned about her kidney function. You know that with a decrease in renal function, levels of _____ may rise, creating the impression of an overdose.

   A. medications

   B. toxins

   C. acid

   D. alkali

_____ **14.** By age 85, a 10% reduction in brain weight can result in:

   A. increased risk of head trauma.

   B. short-term memory impairment.

   C. slower reflex times.

   D. all of the above

_____ **15.** As a person ages, fractures are more likely to occur because of a decrease in bone:

   A. cartilage.

   B. density.

   C. length.

   D. tissue.

_____ **16.** The best rule of thumb when assessing mental status is to always compare the patient's current level of consciousness or ability to function with the level or ability:

   A. of another adult in the household.

   B. before the problem began.

   C. of a person of the same age.

   D. none of the above

_____ **17.** The _____ is usually the key in helping to assess the older patient's problem.

   A. history

   B. medication

   C. environment

   D. all of the above

_____ **18.** An older patient's diminished _____ may hamper communication.

   A. sight

   B. hearing

   C. speaking ability

   D. all of the above

_____ **19.** The term applied to prescribing multiple medications is:

   A. hypermedicating.

   B. hyperpharmacy.

   C. polypharmacy.

   D. overmedicating.

_____ **20.** You are called to the residence of a 71-year-old woman. She is complaining of not feeling well. She is alert and oriented. Her airway is open and she is breathing at 22 breaths/min but seems a little pale. Her pulse is 112 beats/min, irregular and weak. Her distal pulse is diminished. You know that the sensation of pain may be _____ in a geriatric patient, leading to "silent" heart attacks.

   A. enhanced

   B. diminished

   C. overstated

   D. false

_____ **21.** You must consider the body's decreasing ability to _____ simple trauma when you are assessing and caring for an older patient.

   A. isolate

   B. separate

   C. heal

   D. recognize

_____ **22.** An isolated hip fracture in an 85-year-old patient can produce a systemic impact that results in:

   A. deterioration.

   B. shock.

   C. life-threatening conditions.

   D. all of the above

_____ **23.** When assessing an older patient who has fallen, it is important to determine why the fall occurred because it may have been the result of a medical problem such as:

   A. fainting.

   B. a cardiac rhythm disturbance.

   C. a medication interaction.

   D. all of the above

_____ **24.** Your assessment of the patient's condition and stability must include past medical conditions, even if they are not currently acute or:

   A. symptomatic.

   B. asymptomatic.

   C. complaining.

   D. on medication.

_____ **25.** A common complaint from the patient experiencing an abdominal aortic aneurysm (AAA) is pain in the:

   A. abdomen.

   B. back.

   C. leg with decreased blood flow.

   D. all of the above

_____ **26.** All of the following are true of delirium, except:

   A. it may have metabolic causes.

   B. the patient may be hypoglycemic.

   C. it develops slowly over a period of years.

   D. the memory remains mostly intact.

_____ **27.** You respond to a residence for a difficulty breathing call. Upon arrival the 86-year-old patient is pulseless and apneic. The family tells you he has a DNR. For a DNR order to be valid, it must:

   A. be signed by the patient or legal guardian.

   B. be signed by one or more physicians.

   C. be dated within the preceding 12 months.

   D. all of the above

_____ **28.** When in doubt about whether an advance directive is valid, or if one is in place, your best course of action is to:

   A. call medical control to see if an order is needed.

   B. take resuscitation action that is appropriate to the situation.

   C. wait for the family or caregivers to produce the appropriate document.

   D. none of the above

_____ **29.** Signs and symptoms of possible abuse include all of the following, except:

   A. chronic pain.

   B. no history of repeated visits to the emergency department or clinic.

   C. depression or lack of energy.

   D. self-destructive behavior.

_____ **30.** Signs of neglect include:

   A. lack of hygiene.

   B. poor dental hygiene.

   C. lack of reasonable amenities in the home.

   D. all of the above

Fill-in

Read each item carefully, then complete the statement by filling in the missing word.

1. Geriatric patients are individuals who are older than _____ years.

2. The aging body of the geriatric person may _____ serious medical conditions.

3. Common _____ about older people include the presence of mental confusion, illness, a sedentary lifestyle, and immobility.

4. Older skin feels dry due to fewer _____ _____.

5. _____ _____ is a measure of the workload of the heart.

6. An _____ is an abnormal blood-filled dilation of the wall of a blood vessel.

7. Flexion at the neck and a forward curling of the shoulders produce a condition called _____.

True/False

If you believe the statement to be more true than false, write the letter "T" in the space provided. If you believe the statement to be more false than true, write the letter "F."

_____ **1.** Vasodilation is a narrowing of a blood vessel.

_____ **2.** Cardiovascular disease is one of the leading causes of death in the older population.

_____ **3.** Mental confusion and immobility are common stereotypes about the older population.

_____ **4.** Assessment of an older patient usually takes less time than a middle-aged person.

_____ **5.** The sensation of pain in an older patient may be diminished.

_____ **6.** Older people are more prone to hypothermia than younger people.

_____ **7.** Elder abuse is on the decline in the United States.

Short Answer

Complete this section with short written answers using the space provided.

1. List the three major categories of elder abuse.

_____

_____

2. Briefly describe the three possible causes of syncope in an older patient.

_____

_____

3. List at least five informational items that may be important in assessing possible elder abuse.

_____

_____

4. Name three common signs and symptoms of a heart attack in an older patient.

_____

_____

Word Fun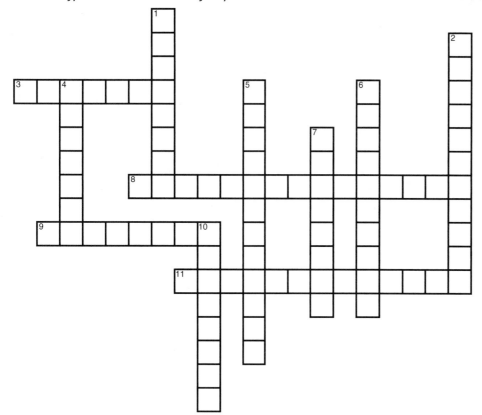

The following crossword puzzle is an activity provided to reinforce correct spelling and understanding of medical terminology associated with emergency care and the EMT-B. Use the clues in the column to complete the puzzle.

Across

3. Difficulty breathing

8. Fatty materials deposited

9. Slow onset of progressive disorientation

11. Late shock

Down

1. Clouding of the lens

2. Early shock

4. Fainting

5. Generalized bone disease

6. Taking advantage (physical, emotional, etc.) of an elder

7. Chief component of connective tissue

10. Abnormal blood-filled dilation of blood vessel

Ambulance Calls

The following case scenarios provide an opportunity to explore the concerns associated with patient management. Read each scenario, then answer each question in detail.

1. You are called to the residence of an 87-year-old woman who is "not acting right." Family members tell you they think she may have taken her medication twice this morning. She is lethargic, confused, and hypotensive.

How would you best manage this patient?

_____

_____

_____

2. It's 3:00 A.M., and you are dispatched to a long-term care facility for a geriatric woman with an "unknown emergency." You arrive to find no staff around, but you hear someone crying for help. You follow the voice and find an older woman lying on the floor holding her right hip. Her bed is made and the side rails are up. When a staff member finally appears, you ask how long she's been lying there. They respond, "We don't know. How are we supposed to know that? We don't have enough help around here."

How do you best manage this patient?

_____

_____

_____

3. You are dispatched to the home of a 65-year-old woman who is complaining of severe back pain. She tells you that she tried to pick up the lawnmower when she "heard a pop and felt a crack in her back." She is experiencing intense pain in her lower back and feels some numbness in her legs.

How do you best manage this patient?

_____

_____

_____

CHAPTER

34 Geriatric Assessment and Management

Workbook Activities

The following activities have been designed to help you. Your instructor may require you to complete some or all of these activities as a regular part of your EMT-B training program. You are encouraged to complete any activity that your instructor does not assign as a way to enhance your learning in the classroom.

Chapter Review

The following exercises provide an opportunity to refresh your knowledge of this chapter.

Matching

Match each of the terms in the left column to the appropriate definition in the right column.

_____ **1.** Acetabulum

_____ **2.** Bacteremia

_____ **3.** Central cord syndrome

_____ **4.** Compression fractures

_____ **5.** Polypharmacy

_____ **6.** Septicemia

_____ **7.** Stable spinal injury

_____ **8.** Vasodilation

A. The disease state that results from the presence of microorganisms in the bloodstream

B. Stable spinal cord injuries in which often only the anterior third of the vertebra is collapsed

C. Simultaneous use of many medications

D. Spinal injury that has a low risk of leading to permanent neurologic deficit or structural deformity

E. The depression on the lateral pelvis where its three component bones join

F. Incomplete spinal cord injury in which some of the signals from the brain to the body are not received

G. The presence of bacteria in the blood

H. widening of a blood vessel

Multiple Choice

Read each item carefully, then select the best response.

_____ **1.** Scene clues that can provide important information include:
   A. the general condition of the home.
   B. the number and type of pill bottles around.
   C. any hazards that could cause a fall.
   D. all of the above

_____ **2.** You are called to the local nursing home for a 91-year-old man with altered mental status. He is very confused. His airway is open and respirations are unlabored. His pulse is strong, regular, and distal pulses are good. In order to understand a patient's baseline condition and how today's behavior differs from it, you should ask the nursing home staff questions concerning the patient's:
   A. mobility.
   B. activities of daily living.
   C. ability to speak.
   D. all of the above

_____ **3.** The S in the GEMS diamond stands for:
   A. seriousness.
   B. severity.
   C. social situation.
   D. resuscitative.

_____ **4.** You respond to a 96-year-old man who is alert and oriented. His airway is open with no respiratory distress. Pulses are present and strong and regular. You are having difficulty with communication. All of the following will help with communication except:
   A. standing directly over the patient.
   B. standing in a well lit area.
   C. turning off all radios and televisions.
   D. talking in a normal tone of voice.

_____ **5.** The average patient age 65 or older will be taking how many medications?
   A. Four
   B. Three
   C. Two
   D. One

_____ **6.** Common complaints of the geriatric patient include:
   A. diarrhea.
   B. chest pain.
   C. shortness of breath.
   D. all of the above

_____ **7.** You respond to an auto accident in which your patient is a 71-year-old woman. She is complaining of severe back pain. She is alert and oriented and respirations are normal and unlabored. Her pulses are present and strong. After applying a C-collar, you start your assessment of the injured area. Upon palpation, you notice a bulged area and the patient reacts by screaming when you touch the area. You know that you have to be extremely careful with the patient because:
   A. she has an unstable spinal injury.
   B. she has a stable spinal injury.
   C. she has no pain tolerance.
   D. you don't want to get sued.

_____ **8.** Because of the presence of arthritis, relatively small hyperextension injuries can cause the spinal cord to be squeezed, leading to a dysfunction known as:

    A. compression fractures.

    B. burst fractures.

    C. unstable spine.

    D. central cord syndrome.

_____ **9.** You are called to the residence of an 84-year-old man who fell and hit his head. He is alert and oriented with no sign of obvious injury. His respirations and pulses are within normal limits. He takes blood thinners daily. You should:

    A. assume everything is alright and release the patient.

    B. treat for a head injury and transport.

    C. check pupil response and if normal, release the patient.

    D. release him to a family member.

_____ **10.** Nearly _____ of all older patients will die within 12 months of hip fracture.

    A. 10%

    B. 15%

    C. 20%

    D. 25%

_____ **11.** You respond to a 90-year-old woman who is complaining of difficulty breathing. She is alert and oriented and respirations are at 26 breaths/min and regular. Pulse is 110 beats/min and irregular. She is not complaining of any pain; just not feeling well. You should be alert for:

    A. septicemia.

    B. aortic abdominal aneurysm.

    C. cardiovascular emergency.

    D. infectious disease.

_____ **12.** When responding to a nursing facility for a patient, what information do you need to get from the staff before you transport?

    A. patient's mobility

    B. patient's daily activities

    C. patient's ability to speak

    D. all of the above

Fill-in

Read each item carefully, then complete the statement by filling in the missing word.

1. _____ occurs when a patient takes multiple medications that can interact.

2. A spinal injury that has a low risk for leading to permanent neurologic deficit or structural deformity is called _____.

3. A spinal injury that has a high risk of permanent neurologic deficit or structural deformity is called _____.

4. The site of pelvic injuries that result from high-energy trauma in older people is the _____.

5. Because of the presence of arthritis, relatively small hyperextension injuries can cause the spinal cord to be squeezed, leading to a dysfunction known as _____ _____ _____.

6. A stable injury in which often only the anterior third of the vertebra is collapsed is the _____ _____.

7. _____ fractures typically result from a higher energy mechanism such as a motor vehicle crash or fall from substantial height.

8. The fracture that involves flexion and distraction component that cause a fracture through the entire vertebral body and bony arch is called _____ _____ _____.

9. The disease state that results from the presence of microorganisms or their toxic products in the bloodstream is _____.

10. The presence of bacteria in the blood is called _____.

True/False

If you believe the statement to be more true than false, write the letter "T" in the space provided. If you believe the statement to be more false than true, write the letter "F."

_____ 1. Approximately 20% to 30% of older people have "silent" heart attacks.

_____ 2. Most nursing facilities will send transfer records along with a patient being transported. These records contain the patient's history, medication lists, and dosages.

_____ 3. The "E" in the GEMS diamond stands for energy level.

_____ 4. You should never assume that an altered mental status is normal for a geriatric patient.

_____ 5. One of the best tools for assessing the geriatric patient is their history.

_____ 6. Geriatric patients often stop taking medications without talking to their doctor.

_____ 7. A rapid physical exam is typically performed before obtaining the vital signs.

_____ 8. Compression fractures are unstable injuries.

_____ 9. Prehospital treatment of older head-injured patients should be aimed at maintaining the heart rate.

Short Answer

Complete this section with short written answers using the space provided.

1. List the steps in immobilizing a kyphotic patient.

_____

_____

2. List the steps for immobilizing a patient with a hip fracture.

_____

_____

3. What critical information do you need to get from nursing staff at a nursing facility?

_____

_____

Word Fun

The following crossword puzzle is an activity provided to reinforce correct spelling and understanding of medical terminology associated with emergency care and the EMT-B. Use the clues in the column to complete the puzzle.

Across

3. Compression fractures of the vertebrae
5. Simultaneous use of many medications
6. Depression on the lateral pelvis where its three component bones join

Down

1. Results from the presence of microorganisms in the bloodstream
2. Presence of bacteria in the blood
4. Sudden unconsciousness

Ambulance Calls

The following case scenarios provide an opportunity to explore the concerns associated with patient management. Read each scenario, and then answer each question in detail.

1. You are dispatched to an unknown medical emergency at 222 Orchid Lane. You arrive to find an older woman who greets you at the front door. She tells you her husband is laying on the bathroom floor, and he's too heavy for her to lift. As you enter the small bathroom, you notice a large laceration and hematoma on the man's forehead. He tells you that he was on the toilet and must have fallen, but doesn't remember exactly what happened. How would you best manage this patient?

_____

_____

_____

2. You are dispatched to a private residence for a woman who has fallen. She tells you that she tripped over her granddaughter's toys and fell onto the hardwood floor. She tried to get up several times but couldn't. She denies any head, neck, back pain, or loss of consciousness. Her only complaint is pain in her right hip. How would you best manage this patient?

_____

_____

3. It is early evening, and you are dispatched to the parking lot of a popular shopping mall. Over the past several hours, local weather conditions have consisted of a combination of freezing rain and snow, making for very icy road conditions. Your patient is an older woman who has fallen and now complains of back pain and shortness of breath. She has severe kyphosis and will not tolerate traditional methods of spinal immobilization.

How would you best manage this patient?

_____

_____

_____

C H A P T E R

35 Ambulance Operations

Workbook Activities

The following activities have been designed to help you. Your instructor may require you to complete some or all of these activities as a regular part of your EMT-B training program. You are encouraged to complete any activity that your instructor does not assign as a way to enhance your learning in the classroom.

Chapter Review

The following exercises provide an opportunity to refresh your knowledge of this chapter.

Matching

Match each of the terms in the left column to the appropriate definition in the right column.

_____ 1. Medivac	**A.** the use of lights and sirens
_____ 2. Emergency mode	**B.** the killing of pathogenic agents by direct application of chemicals
_____ 3. Spotter	**C.** the process of removing dirt, dust, blood, or other visible contaminants
_____ 4. Sterilization	**D.** medical evacuation of a patient by helicopter
_____ 5. Ambulance	**E.** a person who assists a driver in backing up an ambulance
_____ 6. Cleaning	**F.** specialized vehicle for treating and transporting sick and injured patients
_____ 7. Disinfection	**G.** removes microbial contamination

Multiple Choice

Read each item carefully, then select the best response.

_____ 1. Ambulances today are designed according to strict government regulations based on _____ standards.

    A. local

    B. state

    C. national

    D. individual

_____ 2. Features of the modern ambulance include all of the following, except:

    A. self-contained breathing apparatus.

    B. a patient compartment.

    C. two-way radio communication.

    D. a driver's compartment.

_____ 3. You report to work and the first thing you do each day that you arrive is to make sure all equipment and supplies are functioning and in their assigned place. This is the _____ phase of ambulance operations.

    A. preparation

    B. dispatch

    C. arrival at scene

    D. transport

_____ 4. The Type _____ ambulance is a standard van with a forward-control integral cab body.

    A. I

    B. II

    C. III

    D. IV

_____ 5. Items needed to care for life-threatening conditions include:

    A. equipment for airway management.

    B. equipment for artificial ventilation.

    C. oxygen delivery devices.

    D. all of the above

_____ 6. Oropharyngeal airways can be used for:

    A. adults.

    B. children.

    C. infants.

    D. all of the above

_____ 7. A BVM device, when attached to oxygen supply with the oxygen reservoir in place, is able to supply almost _____ oxygen.

    A. 100%

    B. 95%

    C. 90%

    D. 85%

_____ 8. BVM devices should be transparent so that you can:

    A. monitor the patient's respirations.

    B. notice any color changes in the patient.

    C. detect vomiting.

    D. all of the above

_____ **9.** Oxygen masks, with and without nonbreathing bags, should be transparent and disposable and in sizes for:

  A. adults.

  B. children.

  C. infants.

  D. all of the above

_____ **10.** Basic wound care supplies include all of the following, except:

  A. sterile sheets.

  B. an OB kit.

  C. an assortment of band-aids.

  D. large safety pins.

_____ **11.** Your supervisor approaches you and tells you he wants you to make up jump kits for each ambulance. He has told you that he will leave it up to you as to what goes in the kit. You would want to put everything it in that you might need within the first _____ minutes of arrival at the patient's side.

  A. 2

  B. 3

  C. 4

  D. 5

_____ **12.** Deceleration straps over the shoulders prevent the patient from continuing to move _____ in case the ambulance suddenly slows or stops.

  A. forward

  B. backwards

  C. laterally

  D. down

_____ **13.** The ambulance inspection should include checks of:

  A. fuel levels.

  B. brake fluid.

  C. wheels and tires.

  D. all of the above

_____ **14.** You are hired at the local EMS service. During your orientation, you are given a tour of the station and the ambulances you will be riding on. Your duties include station cleanup and checking the unit for mechanical problems. You should also check all medical equipment and supplies:

  A. after every call.

  B. after every emergency transport.

  C. every 12 hours.

  D. every day.

_____ **15.** For every emergency request, the dispatcher should gather and record all of the following, except:

  A. the nature of the call.

  B. the location of the patient(s).

  C. medications that the patient is currently taking.

  D. the number of patients and possible severity of their condition.

_____ **16.** During the _____ phase, the team should review dispatch information and assign specific initial duties and scene management tasks to each team member.

  A. preparation

  B. dispatch

  C. en route

  D. transport

_____ **17.** Basic requirements for the driver to safely operate an ambulance include:
   A. physical fitness.
   B. emotional fitness.
   C. proper attitude.
   D. all of the above

_____ **18.** The _____ phase may be the most dangerous part of the call.
   A. preparation
   B. en route
   C. transport
   D. on scene

_____ **19.** In order to operate an emergency vehicle safely, you must know how it responds to _____ under various conditions.
   A. steering
   B. braking
   C. acceleration
   D. all of the above

_____ **20.** You must always drive:
   A. offensively.
   B. defensively.
   C. under the speed limit.
   D. all of the above

_____ **21.** When driving with lights and siren, you are _____ drivers to yield the right-of-way.
   A. requesting
   B. demanding
   C. offering
   D. none of the above

_____ **22.** Vehicle size and _____ will greatly influence braking and stopping distances.
   A. length
   B. height
   C. weight
   D. width

_____ **23.** When on an emergency call, before proceeding past a stopped school bus with its lights flashing, you should stop before reaching the bus and wait for the driver to:
   A. make sure the children are safe.
   B. close the bus door.
   C. turn off the warning lights.
   D. all of the above

_____ **24.** The _____ is probably the most overused piece of equipment on an ambulance.
   A. stethoscope
   B. siren
   C. cardiac monitor
   D. stretcher

_____ **25.** The _____ is the most visible, effective warning device for clearing traffic in front of the vehicle.
   A. front light bar
   B. rear light bar
   C. high-beam flasher unit
   D. standard headlight

_____ **26.** If you are involved in a motor vehicle crash while operating an emergency vehicle and are found to be at fault, you may be charged:

A. civilly.

B. criminally.

C. both civilly and criminally.

D. neither civilly nor criminally.

_____ **27.** _____ crashes are the most common and usually the most serious type of collision in which ambulances are involved.

A. T-bone

B. Intersection

C. Lateral

D. Rollover

_____ **28.** You respond to a multiple vehicle collision. You and your partner are reviewing dispatch information en route to the scene. You will be in a major intersection of two state highways. As you approach the scene, you review the guidelines for sizing up the scene. The guidelines include:

A. looking for safety hazards.

B. evaluating the need for additional units or other assistance.

C. evaluating the need to stabilize the spine.

D. all of the above

_____ **29.** The main objectives in directing traffic include:

A. warning other drivers.

B. preventing additional crashes.

C. keeping vehicles moving in an orderly fashion.

D. all of the above

_____ **30.** Transferring the patient to receiving staff member occurs during the _____ phase.

A. arrival

B. transport

C. delivery

D. postrun

_____ **31.** Cleaning the vehicle inside and out, refueling the vehicle, disposing of contaminated waste, and replacing equipment and supplies all are accomplished during the _____ phase.

A. preparation

B. transport

C. delivery

D. postrun

_____ **32.** You have called for an air ambulance. While your partner is monitoring the patient, he tells you to go set up a landing zone for the helicopter. When clearing a landing site for an approaching helicopter, look for:

A. loose debris.

B. electric or telephone wires.

C. poles.

D. all of the above

Fill-in

Read each item carefully, then complete the statement by filling in the missing word.

1. A _____ _____ is a portable kit containing items that are used in the initial care of the patient.

2. The six-pointed star that identifies vehicles that meet federal specifications as licensed or certified ambulances is known as the _____ _____ _____.

3. For many decades after 1906, a _____ was the vehicle that was most often used as an ambulance.

4. _____ _____ _____ respond initially to the scene with personnel and equipment to treat the sick and injured until an ambulance can arrive.

5. An ambulance call has _____ phases.

6. Devices should be either disposable or easy to clean and _____, which means to remove radiation, chemical, or other hazardous materials.

7. Suction tubing must reach the patient's _____, regardless of the patient's position.

8. A _____ _____ provides a firm surface under the patient's torso so that you can give effective chest compressions.

True/False

If you believe the statement to be more true than false, write the letter "T" in the space provided. If you believe the answer to be more false than true, write the letter "F."

_____ **1.** Equipment and supplies should be placed in the unit according to their relative importance and frequent use.
_____ **2.** A CPR board is a pocket-sized reminder that the EMT-B carries to help recall CPR procedures.
_____ **3.** Having the ability to exchange equipment between units or between your unit and the emergency department decreases the time that you and your unit must stay at the hospital.
_____ **4.** The en route or response phase of the emergency call is the least dangerous for the EMT-B.
_____ **5.** When the siren is on, you can speed up and assume that you have the right-of-way.
_____ **6.** Use the "4-second rule" to help you maintain a safe following distance.
_____ **7.** Always approach a helicopter from the front.
_____ **8.** Fixed-wing air ambulances are generally used for short-haul patient transfers.
_____ **9.** A clear landing zone of 50' by 50' is recommended for EMS helicopters.

Short Answer

Complete this section with short written answers using the space provided.

1. Describe the three basic ambulance designs.

_____

_____

2. List the phases of an ambulance call.

_____

_____

3. List the five factors that contribute to the use of excessive speed.

_____

_____

4. Describe the three basic principles that govern the use of warning lights and sirens.

_____

_____

5. List four guidelines for safe ambulance driving.

_____

_____

6. Describe the correct technique for approaching a helicopter that is "hot" (rotors turning).

_____

_____

7. List the general considerations used for selecting a helicopter landing site.

_____

_____

_____

_____

Word Fun emtb vocab explorer

The following crossword puzzle is an activity provided to reinforce correct spelling and understanding of medical terminology associated with emergency care and the EMT-B. Use the clues in the column to complete the puzzle.

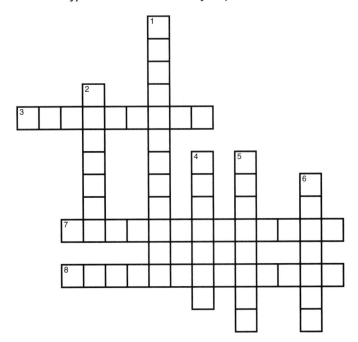

Across

3. Specialized vehicle for transporting sick and injured patients

7. Process that removes microbial contamination

8. Remove or neutralize radiation

Down

1. Killing of pathogenic agents with chemicals

2. Portable kit used in initial care of patient

4. Medical evacuation of a patient by helicopter

5. Process of removing visible contaminants from a surface

6. Person who assists a driver in backing up an ambulance

Ambulance Calls

The following case scenarios provide an opportunity to explore the concerns associated with patient management. Read each scenario, then answer each question in detail.

1. You are cross-trained as a fire fighter and your station has been dispatched to a working structure fire. As you near the scene, another call is dispatched for "an unknown medical emergency." You are the closest unit to the medical emergency.

   How would you best manage this situation?

   _____

   _____

   _____

2. Your department's coverage area is quite large, including ALS coverage for the entire county as well as surrounding areas out of state. You are dispatched to an unfamiliar address for "CPR in progress" and are working with a newly hired partner who is not familiar with your coverage area.

   How would you best manage this situation?

   _____

   _____

   _____

3. You are called to the scene of a motor vehicle crash. The car is situated in a curve and traffic is heavy. Police are not on the scene. Your patient is alert and looking around, but stuck in the vehicle due to traffic. You see blood smeared across her face, but it appears to be minimal.

   How would you best manage this situation?

   _____

   _____

   _____

CHAPTER

36 Gaining Access

Workbook Activities

The following activities have been designed to help you. Your instructor may require you to complete some or all of these activities as a regular part of your EMT-B training program. You are encouraged to complete any activity that your instructor does not assign as a way to enhance your learning in the classroom.

Chapter Review

The following exercises provide an opportunity to refresh your knowledge of this chapter.

Matching

Match each of the terms in the left column to the appropriate definition in the right column.

_____ 1. Extrication

_____ 2. Simple access

_____ 3. Complex access

_____ 4. Access

_____ 5. Incident commander

_____ 6. Structure fire

_____ 7. Hazardous material

A. access requiring no special tools and training

B. individual who has overall command of the scene in the field

C. a substance that causes injury or death with exposure

D. access requiring special tools and training

E. removal from entrapment or a dangerous situation or position

F. gaining entry to an enclosed area to reach a patient

G. fire in a house, apartment building, or other building

Multiple Choice

Read each item carefully, then select the best response.

_____ 1. You are dispatched to an automobile accident with reports of trapped patients. There are also reports of fluid spills. From this information you know that you will need what other rescuers at the crash scene?
   A. Firefighters
   B. Law enforcement
   C. A rescue group
   D. All of the above

_____ 2. In the scenario above, which of the four teams is responsible for investigating the crash?
   A. Firefighter
   B. Law enforcement
   C. Rescue group
   D. EMS personnel

_____ 3. In the scenario of question 1, which of the four teams at a crash scene is responsible for properly securing and stabilizing the vehicle?
   A. Firefighter
   B. Law enforcement
   C. Rescue group
   D. EMS personnel

_____ 4. In the scenario of question 1, which of the four teams at a crash scene is responsible for washing down any spilled fuel?
   A. Firefighter
   B. Law enforcement
   C. Rescue group
   D. EMS personnel

_____ 5. Before proceeding with an extrication, you should:
   A. position your unit in a safe location.
   B. make sure the scene is properly marked.
   C. determine if any additional resources will be needed.
   D. all of the above

_____ 6. While you are gaining access to the patient and during extrication, you must make sure that the patient:
   A. remains safe.
   B. stays conscious.
   C. holds his/her head completely still.
   D. all of the above

_____ 7. When dealing with multiple patients, you should locate and rapidly _____ each patient.
   A. treat
   B. triage
   C. transport
   D. extricate

_____ 8. When preparing for patient removal, you should determine:
   A. how urgently the patient must be extricated.
   B. where you should be positioned during extrication.
   C. how you will best move the patient from the vehicle.
   D. all of the above

_____ **9.** Once the patient has been extricated, additional assessment should be completed:

    A. once the patient has been placed on the stretcher.

    B. inside the ambulance inclement weather.

    C. en route if the patient's condition requires rapid transport.

    D. all of the above

_____ **10.** Even when a technical rescue group includes a paramedic or physician, generally nothing but essential _____ is provided until the rescuers can bring the patient to the nearest point where a safe, stable setting exists.

    A. bandaging

    B. triage

    C. simple care

    D. splinting

_____ **11.** When called to a person lost outdoors, your role involves:

    A. standing by at the search base until the lost person is found.

    B. preparing necessary equipment.

    C. obtaining any medical history from relatives on scene.

    D. all of the above

_____ **12.** Tactical situations involve all of the following, except:

    A. an armed hostage situation.

    B. a structure fire.

    C. the presence of a sniper.

    D. an exchange of shots.

Fill-in

Read each item carefully, then complete the statement by filling in the missing word(s).

1. _____ is the final phase of extrication, and this usually results in the patient being placed on the ambulance stretcher.

2. During all phases of rescue, your primary concern is _____.

3. Good _____ among team members and clear leadership are essential to safe, efficient provision of proper emergency care.

4. You should not attempt to gain access to the patient or enter the vehicle until you are sure that the vehicle is _____.

5. When gaining access, it is up to you to identify the _____, most efficient way to gain access.

6. Moving the patient in one fast, continuous step increases the risk of _____ and confusion.

7. Search and rescue is performed by teams of firefighters wearing full turnout gear and _____ _____ _____ _____ (SCBA), and carrying tools and fully charged hose lines.

True/False

If you believe the statement to be more true than false, write the letter "T" in the space provided. If you believe the statement to be more false than true, write the letter "F."

_____ **1.** There should be no talking throughout the extrication process.

_____ **2.** You should maintain at least a 10" clearance around driver airbags that have not deployed.

_____ **3.** If you will be involved with extrication, you should wear leather gloves over your disposable gloves.

_____ **4.** Simple access is trying to get to the patient as quickly as possible using tools or other forcible entry methods.

_____ **5.** You should not try to access the patient until you are sure that the vehicle is stable and that hazards have been identified and properly controlled.

Short Answer

Complete this section with short written answers using the space provided.

1. Explain the four different basic functions that must be addressed at any crash scene.

_____

_____

2. To determine the exact location and position of the patient, you and your team should consider what questions?

_____

_____

3. List the steps for assessing and caring for a patient who is entrapped once access has been gained.

_____

_____

4. When examining the exposed area of the limb or other part of the patient that is trapped, explain what you are assessing for.

_____

_____

5. Explain the proper technique for patient removal once they are disentangled.

_____

_____

Word Fun emtb.com

The following crossword puzzle is an activity provided to reinforce correct spelling and understanding of medical terminology associated with emergency care and the EMT-B. Use the clues in the column to complete the puzzle.

Across

3. Danger zone

6. To be caught with no way out

8. Requires tools and special training

9. Cave rescue, dive rescue, etc.

Down

1. Substance that causes injury or death with exposure

2. Person responsible for overall incident management

4. Removal from trapped area

5. Fire in a house, office, or other building

7. Gaining entry to an enclosed area

Ambulance Calls

The following case scenarios provide an opportunity to explore the concerns associated with patient management. Read each scenario, then answer each question in detail.

1. You are dispatched to "chest pain" by a third party caller. No one answers the front door when you knock, and the door is locked. You hear a dog barking inside. The dispatcher informs you that the call was placed by the man's wife who is not on the premises. She told the dispatcher that her husband called her cellular phone complaining of chest pain, and he has recently been released from the hospital.

   How would you best manage this situation?

   _____

   _____

   _____

2. It is spring, and the water run off from melting snow has caused the local viaduct to swell with cold, fast moving waters. You are off duty when you hear a tone out for "small boy swept away by flood waters." You arrive to the scene before your department's on-duty responders. You see a boy of approximately 13 years old who is clinging to life in the middle of the channel, holding onto a trapped log. His mother is hysterical and screaming for you to "jump in and get him." You have no safety equipment available.

   How would you best manage this patient?

   _____

   _____

   _____

3. You are dispatched to a chemical spill where a train car derailed. The patient is the engineer who went back to look at the damage. He is lying beside the tracks and appears to be breathing from your vantage point at the staging area. HazMat team members are suiting up to go in and retrieve the patient. They will decontaminate him before bringing him to the staging area.

   How will you best manage this situation and patient?

   _____

   _____

   _____

CHAPTER

37 Special Operations

Workbook Activities

The following activities have been designed to help you. Your instructor may require you to complete some or all of these activities as a regular part of your EMT-B training program. You are encouraged to complete any activity that your instructor does not assign as a way to enhance your learning in the classroom.

Chapter Review

The following exercises provide an opportunity to refresh your knowledge of this chapter.

Matching

Match each of the terms in the left column to the appropriate definition in the right column.

_____ 1. Mass-casualty incident

_____ 2. Incident command

_____ 3. Toxicity level

_____ 4. Triage

_____ 5. Chemical Transportation

_____ 6. Protection level

_____ 7. Casualty collection area

_____ 8. Disaster

_____ 9. Hazardous materials

_____ 10. Rehabilitation area

_____ 11. Transportation area

_____ 12. Treatment officer

A. incident in which a hazardous material is no longer properly contained and isolated

B. area where patients can receive further system triage and medical care

C. individual who is in charge of and directs EMS personnel at the treatment area

D. the process of sorting patients based on the severity of injury and medical need, to establish treatment and transportation priorities

E. a measure of the amount and type of Emergency Center protective equipment that an individual (CHEMTREC) needs to avoid injury during contact with a hazardous material

F. provides protection and treatment to firefighters and other personnel working at an emergency

G. area where ambulances and crews are organized

H. an agency that assists emergency personnel in identifying and handling hazardous materials transport incidents

I. widespread event that disrupts community incident resources and functions

J. an emergency situation involving more than one patient, and which can place such demand on equipment or personnel that the system is stretched to its limit or beyond

K. an organizational system to help control, direct, and coordinate emergency responders and resources; known more generally as an incident management system (IMS)

L. a measure of the risk that a hazardous material poses to the health of an individual who comes in contact with it

Multiple Choice

Read each item carefully, then select the best response.

_____ 1. Functions normally centered at the command post include:

    A. information.

    B. safety.

    C. liaison with other agencies and groups who are responding.

    D. all of the above

_____ 2. In extended operations, the typical incident command structure may have multiple sectors including:

    A. operations.

    B. planning.

    C. logistics.

    D. all of the above

_____ 3. You are dispatched to a major airline crash. Initial reports state that the plane exploded into a fireball. Multiple agencies have been alerted and are in route. With a major airplane crash, the leading agency is typically the:

    A. EMS department.

    B. law enforcement.

    C. fire department.

    D. HazMat team.

_____ 4. As you approach the crash site there is a lot of activity with multiple agencies arriving at the same time. You report to incident commander and he tells you to report to the holding area for arriving ambulances and crews until they can be assigned a particular task. This area is know as a:

    A. staging area.

    B. treatment area.

    C. transportation area.

    D. rehabilitation area.

_____ 5. The _____ provides protection and treatment to firefighters and other personnel working at the emergency scene.

    A. staging area

    B. treatment area

    C. transportation area

    D. rehabilitation area

_____ **6.** For the scenario in question 3, you have been asked to move forward and pickup patients for removal to a hospital. The area you report to is the:

A. staging area.

B. treatment area.

C. transportation area.

D. rehabilitation area.

_____ **7.** For the scenario in question 3, you and your partner pick up your patients and prepare to transport them to the hospital. As you load the patients into the ambulance, what should the transport officer log?

A. Each patient's mass-casualty tag number

B. Each patient's overall condition

C. The hospital to which they will be taken

D. All of the above

_____ **8.** The _____ is where a more thorough assessment is made and on-scene treatment is begun while transport is being arranged.

A. staging area

B. treatment area

C. transportation area

D. rehabilitation area

_____ **9.** Examples of mass-casualty incidents include:

A. airplane crashes.

B. earthquakes.

C. railroad crashes.

D. all of the above

_____ **10.** To make decontaminating the ambulance easier after a HazMat incident:

A. tape the cabinet doors shut.

B. place any equipment that will not be used en route in the front of the truck.

C. turn on the power vent ceiling fan and patient compartment air conditioning unit fan.

D. all of the above

_____ **11.** You respond to a HazMat call. Upon arrival, the incident commander tells you they have a critical patient whom they don't have time to decontaminate. You should do all of the following except:

A. wear two pairs of gloves.

B. remove goggles.

C. wear a protective coat.

D. wear respiratory protection.

_____ **12.** EMT-Bs providing care in the treatment area should assess and treat the patient:

A. as contaminated.

B. with respect.

C. from the point where the previous caregiver left off.

D. in the same way as a patient who has not previously been assessed or treated.

_____ **13.** To avoid entrapment and communication of contaminants, only _____ are applied, until the "clean" patient has been moved to the treatment area.

A. pressure dressings that are needed to control bleeding

B. bandages

C. splints

D. cervical collars

_____ 14. When toxic gas, fumes, or airborne droplets or particles are involved, the safe area is upwind and at least _____ from the site of any visible cloud or other discharge.

   A. 50'

   B. 100'

   C. 150'

   D. 200'

_____ 15. If you can see and read the placard or other warning sign, note _____, and, if included, the four-digit number that appears on it or on any orange panel near it.

   A. its color

   B. its wording

   C. any symbols that it contains

   D. all of the above

_____ 16. Once you have reached a safe place, try to rapidly assess the situation and provide as much information as possible when calling for the HazMat team, including:

   A. your specific location.

   B. the size and shape of the containers of the hazardous material.

   C. what you have observed and been told has occurred.

   D. all of the above

_____ 17. In the event of a leak or spill, a hazardous materials incident is often indicated by presence of:

   A. a visible cloud or strange-looking smoke resulting from the escaping substance.

   B. a leak or spill from a tank, etc., with or without HazMat placards or labels.

   C. an unusual, strong, noxious, acrid odor in the area.

   D. all of the above

_____ 18. Safety of _____ must be your most important concern.

   A. you and your team

   B. the other responders

   C. the public

   D. all of the above

_____ 19. In some incidents, a large number of people are _____ and may be injured or killed before the presence of a hazardous materials incident is identified.

   A. transported

   B. exposed

   C. injected

   D. decontaminated

_____ 20. Often, the presence of hazardous materials is easily recognized from warning signs, placards, or labels found:

   A. on buildings or areas where hazardous materials are produced, used, or stored.

   B. on trucks and railroad cars that carry any amount of hazardous material.

   C. on barrels or boxes that contain hazardous material.

   D. all of the above

For the remainder of the multiple-choice section, the following answers are to be applied:

A. First priority (red)
B. Second priority (yellow)
C. Third priority (green)
D. Fourth priority (black)

Classify the following emergencies according to triage priority:

21. Shock _____

22. Major or multiple bone or joint injuries _____

23. Cardiac arrest _____

24. Minor fractures _____

25. Decreased level of consciousness _____

26. Obvious death _____

27. Airway and breathing difficulties _____

28. Burns without airway problems _____

29. Major open brain trauma _____

30. Minor soft-tissue injuries _____

Fill-in

Read each item carefully, then complete the statement by filling in the missing word(s).

1. The _____ _____ _____ is more effective when used to organize large numbers of personnel at complex incidents such as hazardous materials spills and mass-casualty incidents.

2. The incident commander usually remains at a _____ _____, the designated field command center.

3. The _____ _____ is responsible for protecting all personnel and any victims of the incident.

4. When you arrive at the scene of a possible _____ _____ _____, you must first step back and assess the situation.

5. If patients are entrapped, _____ is required.

6. A _____ is a widespread event that disrupts functions and resources of a community and threatens lives and property.

7. _____ is the sorting of patients based on the severity of their conditions to establish priorities for care based on available resources.

8. Transporting a _____ patient merely increases the size of the event.

9. Most serious injuries and deaths from hazardous materials result from _____ and _____ problems.

10. _____ is the process of removing or neutralizing and properly disposing of hazardous materials from equipment, patients, and rescue personnel.

11. When dealing with a HazMat situation, be sure to check the wind direction periodically, and _____ if a change in wind direction dictates.

12. Some substances are not hazardous; however, when mixed with another substance, they may become _____ or volatile.

13. In most cases, the package or tank must contain a certain amount of a hazardous material before a _____ is required.

True/False

If you believe the statement to be more true than false, write the letter "T" in the space provided. If you believe the statement to be more false than true, write the letter "F."

_____ 1. When you are responding to a hazardous materials incident, you must first take time to accurately assess the scene.

_____ 2. Moving patients from the contaminated area is your main responsibility in a hazardous materials situation.

_____ 3. Toxicity level 1 is more dangerous than level 4.

_____ 4. Protective clothing level A is the least level of protection.

_____ 5. Patients with major or multiple bone or joint injuries should be assigned to the second priority triage category.

_____ 6. Patients with severe burns should be assigned to the black triage category.

_____ 7. A large number of hazardous gases and fluids are essentially odorless.

_____ 8. Only the original patients who leave the hazard zone must pass through the decontamination area.

_____ 9. Most hazardous materials have specific antidotes or treatments for exposure.

_____ 10. The success of any incident command system depends on all personnel performing their assigned tasks and working within the system.

Short Answer

Complete this section with short written answers using the space provided.

1. Define the five levels of toxicity as classified by the NFPA.

_____

_____

2. Describe the four levels of protection and the type of protective gear required for each level.

_____

_____

3. List the eight major EMS-related positions within an incident command system.

_____

_____

4. List and define the four triage priorities.

_____

_____

5. For each of the following hazardous materials classifications, list the general category of hazard.

Class	Type
Class 1	
Class 2	
Class 3	
Class 4	
Class 5	
Class 6	
Class 7	
Class 8	
Class 9	

6. Define and describe the process of decontamination and the decontamination area.

Word Fun emtb.com vocab explorer

The following crossword puzzle is an activity provided to reinforce correct spelling and understanding of medical terminology associated with emergency care and the EMT-B. Use the clues in the column to complete the puzzle.

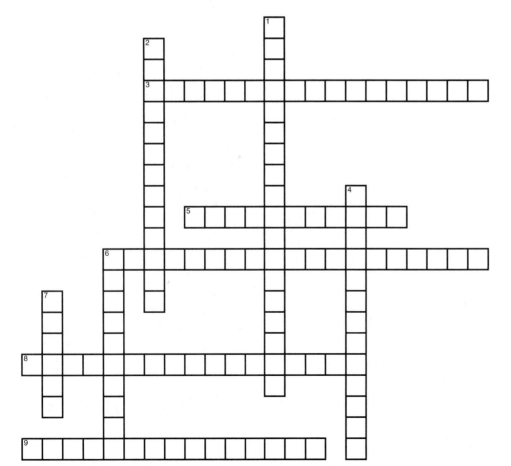

Across

3. Person responsible for overall incident management

5. Designated field command center

6. Zone where contaminants are removed

8. Any harmful substance

9. Determines amount of gear to be worn around a given hazard

Down

1. Zone for loading of patients into ambulances

2. Responsible for sorting of patients

4. Measures of health risk of a substance

6. Area of least safety, exposure to harm possible

7. Sorting by priority

Ambulance Calls

The following case scenarios will give you an opportunity to explore the concerns associated with patient management. Read each scenario, then answer each question in detail.

1. You are dispatched to a multi-vehicle crash where you encounter three patients: a 4-year-old boy with bilateral femur fractures and absent radial pulse, a 27-year-old woman with a laceration to the head and a humerus fracture, and a 42-year-old man who is apneic and pulseless with an open skull fracture.

   How should you triage these patients?

   _____

   _____

   _____

2. Your response area contains a large portion of farming and other agricultural lands, including many orchards and vineyards. Right at shift change, there is a tone out for a "crop duster accident" in a remote area of your jurisdiction. It appears that 15-30 agricultural workers were accidentally sprayed with pesticides and other chemicals from a crop dusting plane. They are now experiencing a variety of signs and symptoms including: nausea, vomiting, eye and upper airway irritation.

   How would you best manage this situation?

   _____

   _____

   _____

3. You and your partner are enjoying an unusually uneventful evening at work when you receive a dispatch for "overturned semi truck." As you approach the scene, you see a semi tractor trailer that has left the roadway and rolled down a steep embankment. You see the driver attempting to climb up to the roadway where many passersby have stopped to see what happened. He is vigorously coughing, and you can see a liquid dripping from the truck's tank.

   How would you best manage this situation?

   _____

   _____

   _____

CHAPTER

38 Response to Terrorism and Weapons of Mass Destruction

Workbook Activities

The following activities have been designed to help you. Your instructor may require you to complete some or all of these activities as a regular part of your EMT-B training program. You are encouraged to complete any activity that your instructor does not assign as a way to enhance your learning in the classroom.

Chapter Review

The following exercises provide an opportunity to refresh your knowledge of this chapter.

Matching

Match each of the terms in the left column to the appropriate definition in the right column.

_____ 1. Mutagen

_____ 2. Vesicants

_____ 3. Disease vector

_____ 4. Phosgene

_____ 5. Neurotoxins

_____ 6. Bacteria

_____ 7. Volatility

_____ 8. Cyanide

_____ 9. Vapor hazard

_____ 10. Lymph nodes

A. pulmonary agent that is a product of combustion

B. describes how long a chemical agent will stay on a surface before it evaporates

C. microorganisms that reproduce by binary fission

D. agent that enters the body through the respiratory tract

E. animal that, once infected, spreads the disease to another animal

F. agent that affects the body's ability to use oxygen

G. blister agents

H. area of the lymphatic system where infection-fighting cells are housed

I. substance that mutates and damages the structures of DNA in the body's cells

J. biological agents that are the most deadly substances known to humans

Multiple Choice
Read each item carefully, then select the best response.

_____ **1.** Examples of terrorist groups include:

A. violent religious groups.

B. extremist political groups.

C. technology groups.

D. all of the above

_____ **2.** An example of a single issue group is:

A. antiabortion groups.

B. separatist groups.

C. Aum Shinrikyo.

D. KKK.

_____ **3.** When were chemical agents first introduced?

A. Spanish-American War

B. World War I

C. World War II

D. Korean War

_____ **4.** When the U. S. Department of Homeland Security Advisory System is at yellow, what does that mean?

A. Severe risk of terrorist attack

B. Significant risk of terrorist attack

C. High risk of terrorist attack

D. General risk of terrorist attack

_____ **5.** You are called to the scene of an unexplained explosion at the local shopping mall. The reports are that there are multiple injuries. You are the first unit to arrive on the scene. Your first responsibility is:

A. scene safety.

B. set up the incident command system.

C. start triage.

D. request additional resources.

_____ **6.** In the previous scenario, you have been informed that there are numerous agencies responding with many different types of apparatus. They are approaching the scene from all directions and will be arriving shortly. You need to:

A. set up a staging area.

B. separate the different types of apparatus.

C. let them continue as they are.

D. have them come in from downwind.

_____ **7.** You have been called to an explosion that has released a gas cloud into the air. What are some of the possible hazards at the location?

A. Suspicious package

B. Change in wind direction

C. Contaminated patients

D. All of the above

_____ **8.** A brownish, yellowish oily substance that is generally considered very persistent is:

A. lewisite.

B. phosgene oxime.

C. sulfur mustard.

D. vesicant.

_____ **9.** An example of a pulmonary agent is:

    A. chlorine.

    B. phosgene oxime.

    C. G agents.

    D. lewisite.

_____ **10.** The most lethal of all the nerve agents is:

    A. V agent.

    B. sarin.

    C. soman.

    D. tabun.

_____ **11.** What two medications do MARK 1 antidote kits contain?

    A. atropine and 2-PAM chloride

    B. atropine and epinephrine

    C. epinephrine and 2-PAM chloride

    D. lidocaine and atropine

_____ **12.** You are dispatched to a local farm where a 41-year-old man has been discovered unconscious. The airway is open but the patient has been vomiting. Respirations are within normal limits and distal pulses are present. The patient has muscle twitches and has urinated on himself. There is a funny odor that seems to be coming from the clothing of the patient. You would suspect:

    A. alcohol poisoning.

    B. organophosphate poisoning.

    C. nerve agent.

    D. respiratory agent.

_____ **13.** You are dispatched to a patient who is having respiratory problems. He is awake but is working so hard to breathe that he can't answer questions. His distal pulses are present and strong. There is an odor of almonds in the air. You would suspect:

    A. cyanide.

    B. sarin.

    C. soman.

    D. tabun.

_____ **14.** The period of time between the person becoming exposed to an agent and when symptoms begin is called:

    A. contagious.

    B. incubation.

    C. communicability.

    D. remission.

_____ **15.** Examples of viral hemorrhagic fevers include:

    A. Ebola.

    B. Rift Valley.

    C. Yellow Fever.

    D. all of the above.

_____ **16.** The infectious disease that has killed the most humans is:

    A. anthrax.

    B. bacteria.

    C. virus.

    D. plague.

_____ **17.** Bubonic plague infects the:

    A. respiratory system.

    B. circulatory system.

    C. lymphatic system.

    D. digestive system.

_____ **18.** The deadliest substances know to humans are:

   A. neurotoxins.

   B. hemotoxins.

   C. plagues.

   D. bacteria.

_____ **19.** The least toxic route for ricin is:

   A. oral.

   B. inhalation.

   C. injection.

   D. absorption.

_____ **20.** The EMS role in helping to determine a biological event is to:

   A. administer medications.

   B. be aware of an unusual number of calls for unexplainable flu.

   C. quarantine infected individuals.

   D. set up field hospitals.

_____ **21.** The most powerful of all radiation is:

   A. alpha.

   B. neutron.

   C. beta.

   D. gamma.

_____ **22.** To protect yourself from radiation exposure, you should:

   A. limit the time of exposure.

   B. increase distance between yourself and the source.

   C. use shielding.

   D. all of the above

Fill-in

Read each item carefully, then complete the statement by filling in the missing word.

   1. The bombing of the Alfred P. Murrah Federal Building in Oklahoma City is an example of _____

   _____.

   2. Any agent designed to bring about mass death, casualties, and/or massive damage to property and infrastructure is

   a _____ _____ _____ _____.

   3. _____ _____ is when a nation has close ties with terrorist groups.

   4. If there is a high risk of a terrorist attack, the Homeland Security Advisory system will be at threat level

   _____.

   5. _____ occurs when you come into contact with a contaminated person who has not been decontaminated.

   6. _____ _____ _____ is a term used to describe how the agent most effectively enters the

   body.

   7. An agent that gives off very little or no vapor and enters the body through the skin is called _____

   _____.

8. _____ _____ are among the most deadly chemicals developed.

9. _____ means that vapors are continuously released over a period of time.

10. _____ is the means by which a terrorist will spread the agent.

11. _____ is a germ that requires a living host to multiply and survive.

12. The group of viruses that cause the blood in the body to seep out from the tissues and blood vessels are called

    _____ _____ _____.

13. _____ is a deadly bacterium that lays dormant in a spore.

14. Buboes are formed when the _____ _____ become infected and grow.

15. The most potent neurotoxin is _____.

16. _____ _____ _____ are strategically placed facilities that have been preestablished for the

    mass distribution of medications and supplies.

17. Any device that is designed to disperse a radioactive device is called a _____ _____ _____.

True/False

If you believe the statement to be more true than false, write the letter "T" in the space provided. If you believe the statement to be more false than true, write the letter "F."

_____ 1. Atlanta's Centennial Park bombing during the 1996 Summer Olympics is an example of international terrorism.

_____ 2. WMDs are easy to obtain or create.

_____ 3. Most acts of terrorism occur after a warning is given to the general public.

_____ 4. Understanding and being aware of the current threat is only the beginning of responding safely.

_____ 5. Failure to park your ambulance in a safe location can place you and your partner in danger.

_____ 6. You should have all units responding to an explosion converge on the main entrance to the building.

_____ 7. Vapor hazards enter the body through the pores in the skin.

_____ 8. The primary route of exposure of vesicants is through inhalation.

_____ 9. Phosgene and phosgene oxime are two different classes of agents.

_____ 10. Tabun looks like baby oil.

_____ 11. Seizures are the most common symptom of nerve agent exposure.

_____ 12. Organophosphate is the basic ingredient in nerve agents.

_____ 13. Cyanide binds with the body's cells, preventing oxygen from being used.

_____ 14. When dealing with smallpox, gloves are all the BSI you need.

_____ 15. Outbreaks of the viral hemorrhagic fevers are extremely rare worldwide.

_____ 16. Pulmonary anthrax infections are associated with a 90% death rate if untreated.

_____ 17. Pneumonic plague is deadlier than bubonic plague.

_____ 18. Ricin is deadlier than botulinum.

_____ 19. Ingestion of ricin causes necrosis of the lungs.

_____ 20. Large containers called "life packs" are delivered during a biological event.

_____ 21. The dirty bomb is an ineffective WMD.

_____ 22. Being exposed to a radiation source does not make a patient contaminated or radioactive.

Short Answer

Complete this section with short written answers using the space provided.

1. What are the key questions you should ask yourself about dealing with WMDs?

   _____

   _____

2. List the four classes of chemical agents.

   _____

   _____

3. What things should you observe on every call to determine the potential for a terrorist attack?

   _____

   _____

4. List the signs of vesicant exposure to the skin.

   _____

   _____

5. What are some of the later signs and symptoms of chlorine inhalation?

   _____

   _____

6. What does the mnemonic SLUDGEM stand for?

   _____

   _____

7. What are the signs and symptoms of high doses of cyanide?

   _____

   _____

8. List the signs and symptoms of ricin ingestion.

   _____

   _____

9. List three places that radioactive waste may be found.

   _____

   _____

10. The best way to protect yourself from the effects of radiation is to use:

   _____

   _____

Word Fun

The following crossword puzzle is an activity provided to reinforce correct spelling and understanding of medical terminology associated with emergency care and the EMT-B. Use the clues in the column to complete the puzzle.

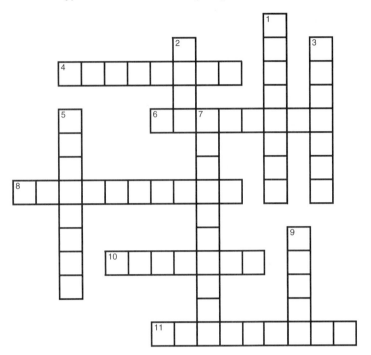

Across

4. Pulmonary agent that is a product of combustion
6. Microorganisms that reproduce by binary fission
8. Describes how long a chemical agent will stay on a surface before it evaporates
10. Agent that affects the body's ability to use oxygen
11. Blister agents

Down

1. First chemical agent ever used in warfare
2. Energy that is emitted from a strong radiological source
3. Substance that damages and changes the DNA structures in the body's cells
5. Highly contagious disease
7. Person infected with a disease that is highly communicable
9. Neurotoxin derived from mash that is left from the castor bean

Ambulance Calls

The following case scenarios provide an opportunity to explore the concerns associated with patient management. Read each scenario, then answer each question in detail.

1. You are dispatched to an explosion at a nearby shopping mall. No other information is available regarding the nature of the explosion, only that there are possibly upwards of five fatally wounded and fifty severely injured. How would you best manage this situation?

2. Your emergency system is suddenly inundated with numerous calls for people experiencing fever, chills, headache, muscle aches, nausea/vomiting, diarrhea, severe abdominal cramping, and GI bleeding. All of the patients attended a local indoor sporting event some six hours earlier. How would you best manage this situation?

3. You are dispatched to treat numerous patients with known exposure to cyanide. This occurred in a neighboring jurisdiction, and they have requested your assistance. The local fire department has set up a decontamination area, and you are asked to transport patients to the nearest appropriate medical facility.

What are important considerations to note about cyanide exposure?

_____

_____

_____

CHAPTER

39 Advanced Airway Management

Workbook Activities

The following activities have been designed to help you. Your instructor may require you to complete some or all of these activities as a regular part of your EMT-B training program. You are encouraged to complete any activity that your instructor does not assign as a way to enhance your learning in the classroom.

Chapter Review

The following exercises provide an opportunity to refresh your knowledge of this chapter.

Matching

Match each of the terms in the left column to the appropriate definition in the right column.

_____ **1.** Pharynx	**A.** a plastic-coated wire that adds rigidity and shape to the endotracheal tube
_____ **2.** Larynx	
_____ **3.** Epiglottis	**B.** passive phase of breathing
_____ **4.** Inhalation	**C.** gas exchanged in body
_____ **5.** Alveolar/capillary	**D.** an instrument that provides a direct view of the vocal cords
_____ **6.** Capillary/cellular	**E.** active phase of breathing
_____ **7.** Exhalation	**F.** the space between the base of the tongue and the epiglottis
_____ **8.** End tidal carbon dioxide detector	**G.** vocal cords
	H. rigid, ring-shaped cartilage
_____ **9.** Cricoid	**I.** the placement of a tube into the trachea to maintain the airway
_____ **10.** Stylet	**J.** gas exchanged in the lungs
_____ **11.** Intubation	**K.** throat
_____ **12.** Laryngoscope	**L.** leaf-shaped structure that prevents food/liquids from entering the lower airway
_____ **13.** Vallecula	
	M. a plastic disposable indicator that signals, by color change, that an ETT is in the proper place

Multiple Choice

Read each item carefully, then select the best response.

_____ 1. To maintain a patent airway, patients whose consciousness is altered may require:
  A. an oropharyngeal airway.
  B. a nasopharyngeal airway.
  C. suctioning.
  D. all of the above

_____ 2. The purpose of advanced airway management is to protect and improve _____ in patients by using a tube to create a direct channel to the trachea.
  A. respiration
  B. ventilation
  C. oxygenation
  D. patency

_____ 3. The upper airway includes all of the following, except:
  A. nose.
  B. mouth.
  C. larynx.
  D. pharynx.

_____ 4. The _____ is located at the glottic opening and prevents food and liquid from entering the lower airway during swallowing.
  A. larynx
  B. vocal cords
  C. epiglottis
  D. carina

_____ 5. Gas exchange occurs in the:
  A. alveoli.
  B. nares.
  C. bronchioles.
  D. trachea.

_____ 6. The mechanical process of breathing occurs through the nose of the diaphragm and:
  A. ribs.
  B. intercostal muscles.
  C. lung parenchyma.
  D. trachea.

_____ 7. The diaphragm and intercostal muscles _____ during inhalation, increasing the size of the chest cavity.
  A. expand
  B. contract
  C. dilate
  D. spasm

_____ 8. During inspiration:
  A. the diaphragm contracts and the ribs move up and out.
  B. the diaphragm relaxes and the ribs move up and out.
  C. the diaphragm contracts and the ribs move down and in.
  D. the diaphragm relaxes and the ribs move down and in.

_____ **9.** During expiration:

    A. the diaphragm contracts and the ribs move up and out.

    B. the diaphragm relaxes and the ribs move up and out.

    C. the diaphragm contracts and the ribs move down and in.

    D. the diaphragm relaxes and the ribs move down and in.

_____ **10.** After _____ minutes without oxygen, cells in the brain and nervous system may die.

    A. 2 to 3

    B. 3 to 5

    C. 4 to 6

    D. 5 to 8

_____ **11.** The first step in airway management is:

    A. suctioning.

    B. c-spine control.

    C. applying oxygen.

    D. opening the airway.

_____ **12.** Patients with gastric distention are prone to:

    A. gas.

    B. vomiting.

    C. sepsis.

    D. hypoxia.

_____ **13.** A nasogastric tube can cause:

    A. nasal trauma.

    B. a basilar skull fracture.

    C. gastric distention.

    D. facial trauma.

_____ **14.** To perform the Sellick maneuver, apply pressure to the:

    A. thyroid cartilage.

    B. cricoid cartilage.

    C. cricothyroid membrane.

    D. trachea.

_____ **15.** You should not immediately intubate a patient who is unresponsive or in cardiac arrest, but you must try:

    A. to open the airway with the appropriate BLS maneuver.

    B. to clear the airway.

    C. to ventilate the patient with a BVM or oxygen-powered breathing device.

    D. all of the above

_____ **16.** _____ is the most effective way to control a patient's airway and has many advantages over other airway management techniques.

    A. An oropharyngeal adjunct

    B. Orotracheal intubation

    C. A nasopharyngeal adjunct

    D. A jaw thrust

_____ **17.** Remember that _____ is the priority for patients in cardiac arrest from ventricular fibrillation.

    A. airway

    B. breathing

    C. circulation

    D. defibrillation

_____ **18.** The purpose of a _____ is to sweep the tongue out of the way and align the airway so that you can see the vocal cords and pass the ET tube through them.

   A. laryngoscope

   B. lighted stylet

   C. Magill forceps

   D. 10-mL syringe

_____ **19.** The curved laryngoscope blade is inserted just in front of the epiglottis, into the _____, allowing you to see the glottic opening and vocal cords.

   A. uvula

   B. vallecula

   C. larynx

   D. pharynx

_____ **20.** The proper sized tube for adult male patients ranges from _____ mm.

   A. 6.5 to 8.0

   B. 7.0 to 8.0

   C. 7.5 to 8.5

   D. 8.0 to 9.0

_____ **21.** The proper sized tube for adult female patients ranges from _____ mm.

   A. 6.5 to 8.0

   B. 7.0 to 8.0

   C. 7.5 to 8.5

   D. 8.0 to 9.0

_____ **22.** A good rule of thumb is to always have a _____ mm ETT on hand; this size tube will fit most male or female adult patients.

   A. 6.5

   B. 7.0

   C. 7.5

   D. 8.0

_____ **23.** In children younger than 8 years, the circular narrowing of the trachea at the level of the _____ functions as a cuff.

   A. larynx

   B. cricoid cartilage

   C. pharynx

   D. thyroid cartilage

_____ **24.** A plastic-coated wire called a _____ may be inserted into the ETT to add rigidity and shape to the tube.

   A. Murphy eye

   B. stylet

   C. pipe cleaner

   D. vallecula

_____ **25.** You will use the _____ to test for air holes in the ETT before intubation.

   A. 10-mL syringe

   B. lighted stylet

   C. Murphy eye

   D. pilot balloon

_____ **26.** Equipment used for airway and ventilation assistance include:

   A. oxygen.

   B. a suctioning unit.

   C. a ventilation device.

   D. all of the above

_____ **27.** Do not let go of the ETT until:

    A. the distal cuff is inflated.

    B. placement is confirmed.

    C. it is secured.

    D. the stylet is removed.

_____ **28.** Confirm placement of the ETT by listening with a stethoscope over both lungs and over the _____ as you ventilate the patient through the tube.

    A. stomach

    B. heart

    C. diaphragm

    D. ribs

_____ **29.** The best way to confirm placement of an ETT is by:

    A. X-ray.

    B. auscultating over both lung fields and over the epigastrium.

    C. visualizing the cuff passing through the vocal cords.

    D. seeing the chest rise and fall.

_____ **30.** The first step in nasotracheal intubation is to:

    A. check for a gag reflex.

    B. turn the stylet on.

    C. hyperventilate the patient.

    D. use BSI precautions.

_____ **31.** Complications of endotracheal intubation include:

    A. mechanical failure.

    B. intubating the esophagus.

    C. causing soft-tissue trauma.

    D. all of the above

_____ **32.** Benefits of endotracheal intubation include all of the following, except:

    A. it provides complete protection of the airway.

    B. patient intolerance.

    C. it prevents gastric distention and aspiration.

    D. it delivers better oxygen concentration than a BVM device.

_____ **33.** Always check for a gag reflex before intubation by using:

    A. a tongue blade.

    B. the laryngoscope blade.

    C. an oral airway.

    D. all of the above

_____ **34.** Benefits of using a multi-lumen airway include all of the following, except:

    A. no mask seal necessary.

    B. requires deeply comatose patient.

    C. may be inserted blindly.

    D. ease of proper placement.

_____ **35.** Contraindications of the ETC include:

    A. patients with a gag reflex.

    B. children younger than 16 years.

    C. patients who have ingested a caustic substance.

    D. all of the above

_____ **36.** To remove the ETC, you should _____ prior to removal.

    A. turn the patient on his or her side

    B. deflate both balloon cuffs

    C. have suction available

    D. all of the above

_____ **37.** Contraindications of the PtL include all of the following, except:

    A. patients with a gag reflex.

    B. children younger than 14 years.

    C. children older than 16 years.

    D. patients who have a known esophageal disease.

_____ **38.** Potential contraindications when using an LMA include:

    A. when positive pressure ventilation with high airway pressures occur, the mask may leak.

    B. active vomiting may dislodge the device.

    C. esophageal disease.

    D. all of the above

Labeling

Label the following diagram with the correct terms.

    1. The Upper and Lower Airways

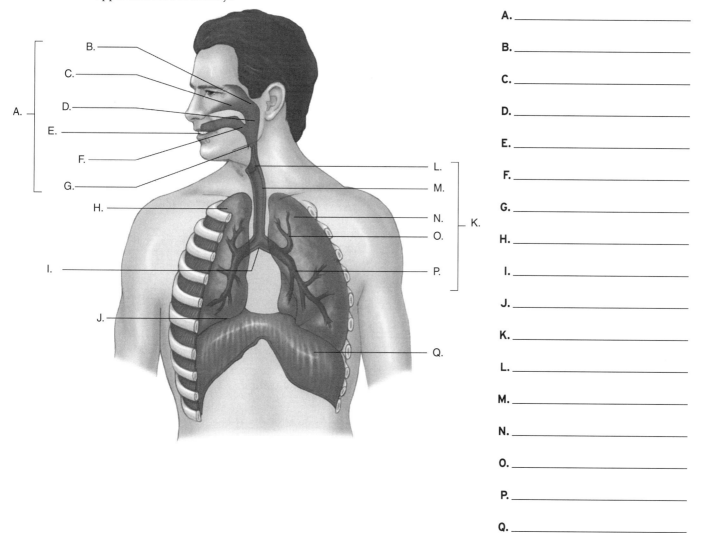

A. _____

B. _____

C. _____

D. _____

E. _____

F. _____

G. _____

H. _____

I. _____

J. _____

K. _____

L. _____

M. _____

N. _____

O. _____

P. _____

Q. _____

Fill-in

Read each item carefully, then complete the statement by filling in the missing word.

1. During _____, the diaphragm contracts.

2. The _____ branch off from the trachea.

3. During the _____ phase of breathing, the intercostal muscles relax.

4. _____ in the alveoli crosses over into the blood.

5. _____ _____ in the blood crosses over into the alveoli.

6. Cells in the brain and nervous system may die after _____ minutes without oxygen.

7. The _____ are the smallest air passages leading to the alveoli.

8. Alveoli are surrounded by _____, which bring deoxygenated blood to the lungs.

True/False

If you believe the statement to be more true than false, write the letter "T" in the space provided. If you believe the statement to be more false than true, write the letter "F."

_____ 1. The light in the laryngoscope will not work unless the blade is attached correctly.
_____ 2. Endotracheal intubation is usually most appropriate for unconscious patients.
_____ 3. There are three different sizes of ETTs.
_____ 4. The balloon cuff around the end of an ETT holds 25 mL of air.
_____ 5. Uncuffed tubes are used in children younger than 8 years.
_____ 6. When a wire stylet is used, it should stick out 1/2" beyond the tip of the ETT.

Short Answer

Complete this section with short written answers using the space provided.

1. Describe how to perform the Sellick maneuver.

_____

_____

2. List three advantages of orotracheal intubation.

_____

_____

3. List nine possible complications associated with endotracheal intubation.

_____

_____

4. List five contraindications for an Esophageal Tracheal Combitube.

_____

_____

5. List three benefits and three complications of multi-lumen airways.

_____

_____

Word Fun

The following crossword puzzle is an activity provided to reinforce correct spelling and understanding of medical terminology associated with emergency care and the EMT-B. Use the clues in the column to complete the puzzle.

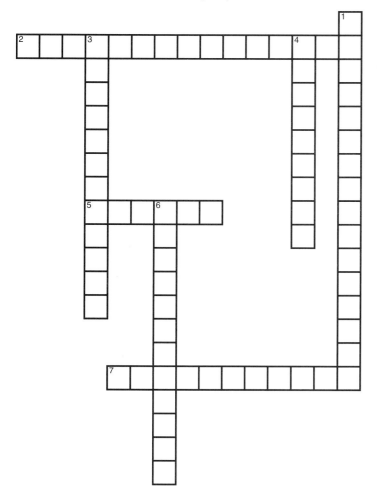

Across

   2. Pressure on cricoid cartilage

   5. Small metal rod inserted into an ET tube

   7. Removes substances from stomach

Down

   1. Rigid, ring-shaped structure at larynx

   3. Vocal cord spasm

   4. Between base of tongue and epiglottis

   6. Used to gain direct view of patient's throat

Ambulance Calls

The following case scenarios provide an opportunity to explore the concerns associated with patient management. Read each scenario, then answer each question in detail.

   1. You are dispatched to a pulseless, apneic 45-year-old man. After assessing the patient, your partner decides to perform endotracheal intubation (a newly allowed skill by your medical program director). This is the first field intubation either you or your partner has attempted without supervision of a paramedic or physician on-scene. Your partner tells you that he "thinks" he passed through the cords. As you auscultate the chest, you do not hear breath sounds, but you do hear gurgling over the epigastrium.

   How would you best manage this situation?

_____

_____

_____

2. You are dispatched to "CPR in progress" at a local restaurant. You arrive to find laypersons feverishly attempting CPR. You also notice that the patient's stomach is rather distended. Witnesses tell you that the man complained of chest pain just prior to collapse when he was assisted to the floor without suffering any trauma. Your local protocols allow for placement of gastric tubes.

How would you best manage this situation?

_____

_____

_____

3. You are dispatched to the scene of a motor vehicle crash where your patient, the unrestrained 18-year-old driver, is breathing at a rate of 4 breaths/min and has weak radial pulses. He is also trapped in the vehicle and the fire department has not yet arrived.

How would you best manage this patient?

_____

_____

_____

Skill Drills
Skill Drill 39-1: Performing the Sellick Maneuver
Test your knowledge of this skill drill by filling in the correct words in the photo captions.

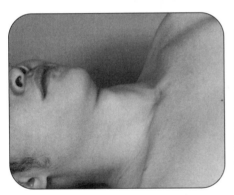

1. Visualize the _____ cartilage.

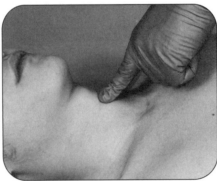

2. _____ to confirm its location.

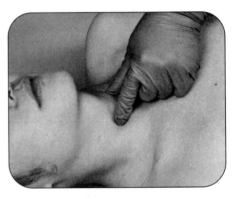

3. Apply _____ pressure on the cricoid _____ with your thumb and index finger on either side of the _____. Maintain pressure until the patient is

_____ .

Skill Drill 39-2: Performing Orotracheal Intubation

Test your knowledge of this skill drill by placing the photos below in the correct order. Number the first step with a "1," the second step with a "2," etc.

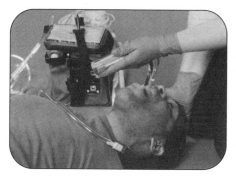

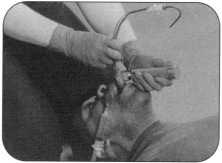

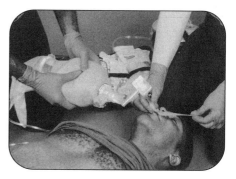

Confirm adequate preoxygenation, and remove the oral airway.

If available, have another rescuer perform the Sellick maneuver to improve visualization of the cords.

Use the head tilt-chin lift maneuver to position the nontrauma patient for insertion of the laryngoscope.

Insert the laryngoscope from the right side of mouth, and move the tongue to the left. Lift the laryngoscope away from the posterior pharynx to visualize the vocal cords. *Do not pry or use the teeth as a fulcrum.*

Insert the ET tube from the right side until the ET tube cuff passes between the vocal cords. Remove the laryngoscope and stylet. Hold the tube carefully until it is secured.

Secure the tube, and continue to ventilate.

Note and record depth of insertion (centimeter marking at the teeth), and reconfirm position after each time you move the patient.

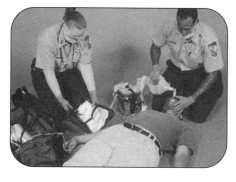

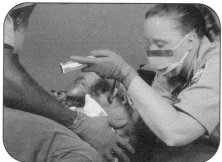

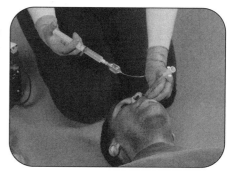

Open and clear the airway.

Place an oropharyngeal airway, and preoxygenate with a BVM device.

In a trauma patient, maintain the cervical spine in-line and neutral as your partner lies down or straddles the patient's head to visualize the vocal cords.

Inflate the balloon cuff, and remove the syringe as your partner prepares to ventilate.

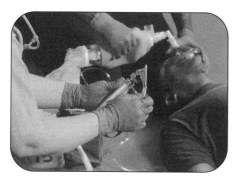

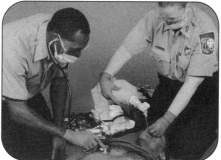

Assemble and test intubation equipment as your partner continues to ventilate.

Begin ventilating, and confirm placement of the ET tube by listening over the stomach and both lungs. Also confirm placement with an end-tidal carbon dioxide detector or EDD, if available.

CHAPTER

40 Assisting With Intravenous Therapy

Workbook Activities

The following activities have been designed to help you. Your instructor may require you to complete some or all of these activities as a regular part of your EMT-B training program. You are encouraged to complete any activity that your instructor does not assign as a way to enhance your learning in the classroom.

Chapter Review

The following exercises provide an opportunity to refresh your knowledge of this chapter.

Matching

Match each of the terms in the left column to the appropriate definition in the right column.

_____ **1.** Saline lock

_____ **2.** Proximal tibia

_____ **3.** Local reaction

_____ **4.** Access port

_____ **5.** Infiltration

_____ **6.** Vasovagal reaction

_____ **7.** Gauge

_____ **8.** Systemic complication

A. mild to moderate reaction to an irritant without systemic consequence

B. sudden hypotension and fainting associated with traumatic or medical events

C. special type of IV apparatus

D. escape of fluid into the surrounding tissue

E. moderate to severe complication affecting the systems of the body

F. measure of the interior diameter of the catheter

G. anatomic location for intraosseous catheter insertion

H. sealed hub on an administration set designed for sterile access to the IV fluid

Multiple Choice
Read each item carefully, then select the best response.

_____ **1.** IV administration requires the use of a(n):

  A. solution.

  B. administration set.

  C. catheter.

  D. all of the above

_____ **2.** When an IV solution is taken out of its protective sterile plastic bag, it must be used within:

  A. 12 hours.

  B. 24 hours.

  C. 36 hours.

  D. 48 hours.

_____ **3.** A microdrip administration set requires _____ drops to flow 1 mL.

  A. 15

  B. 30

  C. 45

  D. 60

_____ **4.** The gauge of a catheter refers to the:

  A. diameter of the needle.

  B. length of the needle.

  C. strength of the needle.

  D. use of the needle.

_____ **5.** Intraosseous IVs are started in the:

  A. external jugular.

  B. proximal tibia.

  C. hand.

  D. antecubital vein.

_____ **6.** Risk associated with starting an IV includes:

  A. infiltration.

  B. phlebitis.

  C. occlusion.

  D. all of the above

_____ **7.** An accumulation of blood in the tissues surrounding an IV site is called a:

  A. contusion.

  B. hematoma.

  C. bruise.

  D. rupture.

_____ **8.** Circulatory overload occurs most commonly in patients with:

  A. an altered mental status.

  B. diabetes.

  C. kidney dysfunction.

  D. dialysis.

_____ **9.** The best administration set to use when giving fluids to a pediatric patient is the:

   A. macrodrip.

   B. Volutrol.

   C. microdrip.

   D. whatever you have closest.

_____ **10.** If fluid replacement is not an issue, what size catheter would be best to use in a geriatric patient?

   A. 14 gauge

   B. 16 gauge

   C. 20 gauge

   D. Butterfly

Fill-in

Read each item carefully, then complete the statement by filling in the missing word.

1. A(n) _____ _____ moves fluid from the IV bag into the patient's vascular system.

2. _____ _____ are best used for rapid fluid replacement.

3. _____ _____ are a way to maintain an active IV site without having to run fluids through the vein.

4. Intraosseous IVs are started with a special needle called a _____ _____.

5. An inflammation of the vein is called _____.

6. _____ _____ occurs when part of the catheter is pinched against the needle and the needle slices

through the catheter, creating a free-floating segment.

True/False

If you believe the statement to be more true than false, write the letter "T" in the space provided. If you believe the statement to be more false than true, write the letter "F."

_____ **1.** The most important thing to remember about IV techniques and fluid administration is to keep the IV equipment sterile.

_____ **2.** The more common prehospital volumes are 250 ml and 100 ml.

_____ **3.** The most common types of catheters found in the prehospital setting are central-line catheters.

_____ **4.** A 14-gauge catheter has a greater diameter than a 22-gauge catheter.

_____ **5.** Starting an external jugular IV requires a different technique than starting other IVs.

_____ **6.** An occlusion is the physical blockage of a vein.

_____ **7.** If a hematoma develops when an IV catheter insertion is attempted, the procedure should stop.

_____ **8.** Healthy adults can handle as much as 4 to 5 extra liters of fluid without compromise.

_____ **9.** For pediatric patients, the best catheters for insertions are 20, 22, 24, or 26 gauge.

_____ **10.** Fluid overload is not a problem with geriatric patients.

Short Answer

Complete this section with short written answers using the space provided.

1. List the steps for assembling IV equipment.

_____

_____

2. What are some examples of common local reactions when starting an IV?

_____

_____

3. List the common systemic complications associated with IV insertion.

_____

_____

4. What treatment should a patient suffering a vasovagal reaction be given?

_____

_____

5. What items do you check if your IV is not flowing properly?

_____

_____

Word Fun emtb vocab explorer

The following crossword puzzle is an activity provided to reinforce correct spelling and understanding of medical terminology associated with emergency care and the EMT-B. Use the clues in the column to complete the puzzle.

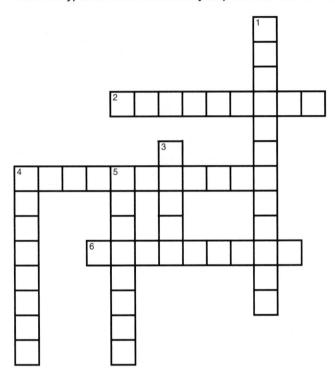

Across

2. Blockage; usually of a tubular structure such as a blood vessel

4. Area of administration set where fluid accumulates

6. Inflammation of a vein

Down

1. Escape of fluid into the surrounding tissue

3. Measure of the interior diameter of the catheter

4. Another name for administration sets

5. Flexible, hollow structure that drains or delivers fluids

Ambulance Calls

1. You are in the patient compartment with your EMT-B partner who is taking care of a patient with congestive heart failure. Your partner has initiated IV therapy and is now giving a radio report to the receiving hospital. You notice the IV tubing is still running wide open and that nearly the entire liter of fluid has been administered over a few minutes. The patient states his shortness of breath is worsening.

   How would you best manage this situation?

   _____

   _____

   _____

2. Your fire department provides "ride alongs" for paramedic students attending school at the local community college. You watch the paramedic student as she starts the IV; she appears to follow all of the appropriate steps, but the IV fails to flow properly.

   What could be the problem with this IV?

   _____

   _____

   _____

3. You are caring for a patient who begins to complain of pain at the IV insertion site. The paramedic asks you to inspect her IV for problems. You see swelling around the catheter.

   What is this condition and what does it signify?

   _____

   _____

   _____

CHAPTER

41 Assisting With Cardiac Monitoring

Workbook Activities

The following activities have been designed to help you. Your instructor may require you to complete some or all of these activities as a regular part of your EMT-B training program. You are encouraged to complete any activity that your instructor does not assign as a way to enhance your learning in the classroom.

Chapter Review

The following exercises provide an opportunity to refresh your knowledge of this chapter.

Matching

Match each of the terms in the left column to the appropriate definition in the right column.

_____ **1.** Sinus tachycardia

_____ **2.** Ventricular tachycardia

_____ **3.** Electrical conduction system

_____ **4.** Arrhythmia

_____ **5.** Sinus bradycardia

_____ **6.** Ventricular fibrillation

_____ **7.** Sinus rhythm

A. network of special cells in the heart through which an electrical current flows

B. consistent P waves, consistent P-R intervals, and a regular heart rate that is less than 60 beats/min

C. consistent P waves, consistent P-R intervals, and a regular heart rate that is more than 100 beats/min

D. rapid, disorganized ventricular rhythm with chaotic characteristics

E. abnormal heart rhythm

F. presence of three or more abnormal ventricular complexes in a row with a rate of more than 100 beats/min

G. rhythm in which the SA node acts as the pacemaker

Multiple Choice

Read each item carefully, then select the best response.

_____ 1. Studies have indicated a 95% or better accuracy rate in the diagnosis of myocardial infarction with the use of a:
   A. 3-lead ECG.
   B. 4-lead ECG.
   C. 6-lead ECG.
   D. 12-lead ECG.

_____ 2. The part of the electrical pathway that leads to the right side of the interventricular septum is the:
   A. left bundle.
   B. Purkinje system.
   C. AV node.
   D. right bundle.

_____ 3. In the normally functioning heart, the electrical impulse originates at the:
   A. AV node.
   B. SA node.
   C. internodal pathway.
   D. Bundle of His.

_____ 4. On the ECG paper, how many boxes equal one second?
   A. 5 big boxes
   B. 5 little boxes
   C. 2 big boxes
   D. 2 little boxes

_____ 5. Tachycardia refers to a heart rate:
   A. below 60 beats/min.
   B. above 100 beats/min.
   C. above 60 beats/min.
   D. below 100 beats/min.

_____ 6. Maximum heart rate is figured as:
   A. 220 beats/min – age (in years).
   B. 210 beats/min – age (in years).
   C. 200 beats/min – age (in years).
   D. 220 beats/min + age (in years).

_____ 7. It is not uncommon for ventricular tachycardia to deteriorate into:
   A. sinus tachycardia.
   B. ventricular fibrillation.
   C. asystole.
   D. ventricular bradycardia.

_____ 8. The reason for using a 12-lead ECG is for early identification of:
   A. vessel blockage.
   B. prolapsed valves.
   C. myocardial ischemia.
   D. embolism.

_____ 9. Which leads have to be placed exactly?
   A. Positive leads
   B. Negative leads
   C. Chest leads
   D. Limb leads

Fill-in

Read each item carefully, then complete the statement by filling in the missing word(s).

1. The heart contains a network of specialized tissue that is capable of conduction of electrical current through the heart, it is known as _____ _____ _____.

2. _____ _____ is a rhythm is which the SA node acts as the pacemaker.

3. _____ is an abnormal rhythm of the heart and is sometimes called a dysrhythmia.

4. _____ _____ is a rapid, completely disorganized ventricular rhythm with chaotic characteristics.

5. _____ refers to the complete absence of any electrical cardiac activity.

6. The leads that are placed on the arms and legs are referred to as _____ _____.

7. _____ _____ are only used in 12-lead ECGs.

True/False

If you believe the statement to be more true than false, write the letter "T" in the space provided. If you believe the statement to be more false than true, write the letter "F."

_____ 1. When the heart is deprived of oxygen, blood pressure increases.

_____ 2. The fastest pacer of the heart is the AV node.

_____ 3. The normal heart rate is between 60 and 100 beats/min.

_____ 4. Bradycardia is a heart rate above 60 beats/min.

_____ 5. Ventricular tachycardia and ventricular fibrillation account for more than 300,000 sudden cardiac deaths in the United States each year.

_____ 6. Immediate defibrillation is the most effective treatment for ventricular fibrillation.

_____ 7. One of the immediate advantages of 12-lead ECG monitoring is early identification of acute ischemia.

_____ 8. You should use alcohol preps to keep leads attached.

Short Answer

Complete this section with short written answers using the space provided.

1. Trace the electrical pathway of the heart.

_____

_____

2. List the ECG tracing through the cardiac cycle.

_____

_____

Word Fun

The following crossword puzzle is an activity provided to reinforce correct spelling and understanding of medical terminology associated with emergency care and the EMT-B. Use the clues in the column to complete the puzzle.

Across

2. Electrocardiogram
4. Complete absence of any electrical cardiac activity
5. An abnormal rhythm of the heart; sometimes called a dysrhythmia
6. Four leads used with a 4-lead ECG

Down

1. Refers to a fast heart rate
3. Leads that are used only with a 12-lead ECG

Ambulance Calls

The following case scenarios provide an opportunity to explore the concerns associated with patient management. Read each scenario, then answer each question in detail.

1. You are dispatched to assist with a patient who is experiencing chest pain and dizziness. You notice another EMT on the scene assist with the application of the ECG. As the paramedic's attention is focused on starting an IV, you see that the EMT has forgotten to attach one of the leads. The paramedic now begins assessing the patient's cardiac rhythm, but he appears confused by what he sees.

   How would you best manage this situation?

2. You and your paramedic partner are dispatched to a "syncopal episode." You arrive to find an older woman who is now awake, but is complaining of lightheadedness and nausea. You notice that her pulse rate is 40 beats/min. As the paramedic applies the ECG machine, you see that her rhythm is regular, with consistent, upright 'P' waves and consistent P-R intervals.

   Is this considered normal, and if not, what is this arrhythmia?

3. You and your paramedic partner are assessing a patient experiencing chest pain and shortness of breath. Your partner asks you to apply a 12-Lead ECG. As you bare the man's chest, you notice that he is very sweaty and has chest hair.

   How will his skin condition and chest hair impact the effectiveness of the ECG, and how can you correct these problems?

A   BLS Review

Workbook Activities

The following activities have been designed to help you. Your instructor may require you to complete some or all of these activities as a regular part of your EMT-B training program. You are encouraged to complete any activity that your instructor does not assign as a way to enhance your learning in the classroom.

Chapter Review

The following exercises provide an opportunity to refresh your knowledge of this chapter.

Matching

Match each of the terms in the left column to the appropriate definition in the right column.

_____ **1.** Artificial ventilation

_____ **2.** Abdominal-thrust

_____ **3.** Basic life support (BLS)

_____ **4.** Advanced life support

_____ **5.** Cardiopulmonary resuscitation

A. steps used to establish artificial ventilation and circulation in a patient who is not breathing and has no pulse

B. noninvasive emergency lifesaving care used maneuver for patients in respiratory or cardiac arrest

C. procedures, such as cardiac monitoring, starting IV fluids, and using advanced airway adjuncts

D. a method of dislodging food or other (ALS) material from the throat of a choking victim

E. opening the airway and restoring breathing resuscitation (CPR) by mouth-to-mask ventilation and by the use of mechanical devices

Multiple Choice

Read each item carefully, then select the best response.

_____ 1. Basic life support is noninvasive emergency lifesaving care that is used to treat:

   A. airway obstruction.

   B. respiratory arrest.

   C. cardiac arrest.

   D. all of the above

_____ 2. Exhaled gas from you to the patient contains _____ oxygen.

   A. 8%

   B. 12%

   C. 16%

   D. 21%

_____ 3. BLS differs from advanced life support by involving advanced lifesaving procedures including all of the following, except:

   A. cardiac monitoring.

   B. mouth-to-mouth.

   C. administration of IV fluids and medications.

   D. use of advanced airway adjuncts.

_____ 4. In some instances such as _____, early BLS measures may be all that a patient needs to be resuscitated.

   A. choking

   B. near drowning

   C. lightning injuries

   D. all of the above

_____ 5. In addition to checking level of consciousness, it is also important to protect the _____ from further injury while assessing the patient and performing CPR.

   A. spinal cord

   B. ribs

   C. internal organs

   D. facial structures

_____ 6. In most cases, cardiac arrest in children younger than 9 years results from:

   A. choking.

   B. aspiration.

   C. congenital heart disease.

   D. respiratory arrest.

_____ 7. Causes of respiratory arrest in infants and children include:

   A. aspiration of foreign bodies.

   B. airway infections.

   C. sudden infant death syndrome (SIDS).

   D. all of the above

_____ 8. Signs of irreversible or biological death include clinical death along with:

   A. rigor mortis.

   B. dependent lividity.

   C. decapitation.

   D. all of the above

_____ **9.** Once you begin CPR in the field, you must continue until:

    A. the fire department arrives.

    B. the funeral home arrives.

    C. a physician arrives who assumes responsibility.

    D. law enforcement arrives and assumes responsibility.

_____ **10.** Once the patient is properly positioned, you can easily assess:

    A. airway.

    B. breathing.

    C. disability.

    D. all of the above

_____ **11.** The chin lift has the added advantage of holding _____ in place, making obstruction by the lips less likely.

    A. loose dentures

    B. the tongue

    C. the mandible

    D. the maxilla

_____ **12.** To perform a _____, place your fingers behind the angles of the patient's lower jaw and then move the jaw forward.

    A. head tilt-chin lift maneuver

    B. jaw-thrust maneuver

    C. tongue-jaw lift maneuver

    D. all of the above

_____ **13.** Providing slow, deliberate inhalations over 2 seconds prevents:

    A. overexpansion of the lungs.

    B. rupture of the bronchial tree.

    C. gastric distention.

    D. rupture of the alveoli.

_____ **14.** A _____ is an opening that connects the trachea directly to the skin.

    A. tracheostomy

    B. stoma

    C. laryngectomy

    D. none of the above

_____ **15.** The _____ position helps to maintain a clear airway in a patient with a decreased level of consciousness who has not had traumatic injuries and is breathing on his or her own.

    A. recovery

    B. lithotomy

    C. Trendelenburg's

    D. Fowler's

_____ **16.** Excessive pressure applied to the carotid artery can:

    A. obstruct the carotid circulation.

    B. dislodge blood clots.

    C. produce marked reflex slowing of heart rate.

    D. all of the above

_____ **17.** The lower tip of the breastbone is the:

    A. xiphoid process.

    B. sternum.

    C. manubrium.

    D. intercostal space.

_____ **18.** Complications from chest compressions can include:

    A. fractured ribs.

    B. a lacerated liver.

    C. a fractured sternum.

    D. all of the above

_____ **19.** When checking for a pulse in an infant, you should palpate the _____ artery.

    A. radial

    B. brachial

    C. carotid

    D. femoral

_____ **20.** The technique for chest compressions in infants and children differs because of a number of anatomic differences, including:

    A. the position of the heart.

    B. the size of the chest.

    C. the fragile organs.

    D. all of the above

_____ **21.** The rate of compressions for an infant is at least _____ compressions per minute.

    A. 70

    B. 80

    C. 90

    D. 100

_____ **22.** The rate of compression to ventilation for infants and children is _____ for both one-rescuer and two-rescuer CPR.

    A. 1:5

    B. 5:1

    C. 15:2

    D. 2:15

_____ **23.** Sudden airway obstruction is usually easy to recognize in someone who is eating or has just finished eating because they suddenly:

    A. are unable to speak or cough.

    B. turn cyanotic.

    C. make exaggerated efforts to breathe.

    D. all of the above

_____ **24.** You should suspect an airway obstruction in the unresponsive patient if:

    A. the standard maneuvers to open the airway and ventilate the lungs are not effective.

    B. you feel resistance to blowing into the patient's lungs.

    C. pressure builds up in your mouth.

    D. all of the above

_____ **25.** You should use _____ for women in advanced stages of pregnancy, patients who are very obese, and children younger than 1 year.

    A. the Heimlich maneuver

    B. chest thrusts

    C. the abdominal-thrust maneuver

    D. any of the above

_____ **26.** For a patient with a partial airway obstruction, you should:

    A. perform the Heimlich maneuver.

    B. attempt a finger sweep to remove the foreign body.

    C. not interfere with the patient's attempt to expel the foreign body.

    D. all of the above

Fill-in

Read each item carefully, then complete the statement by filling in the missing word.

1. Permanent brain damage may occur if the brain is without oxygen for _____ to _____ minutes.

2. CPR does not require any equipment; however, you should use a _____ device to perform rescue breathing.

3. Because of the urgent need to start CPR in a pulseless, nonbreathing patient, you must complete an initial assessment as soon as possible, evaluating the patient's _____.

4. The most important element for successful CPR is immediate _____ of the airway.

5. _____ _____, such as living wills, may express the patient's wishes, but these documents are not binding for all health care providers.

6. For CPR to be effective, the patient must be lying supine on a _____ surface.

7. Without an open _____, rescue breathing will not be effective.

True/False

If you believe the statement to be more true than false, write the letter "T" in the space provided. If you believe the statement to be more false than true, write the letter "F."

_____ 1. During the initial assessment, you need to quickly evaluate the patient's airway, breathing, circulation, and level of consciousness.

_____ 2. All unconscious patients need all elements of BLS.

_____ 3. A patient who is not fully conscious often needs some degree of BLS.

_____ 4. The recovery position should be used to maintain an open airway in a patient with a head or spinal injury.

_____ 5. You should always remove a patient's dentures before initiating artificial ventilation.

_____ 6. You should not start CPR if the patient has obvious signs of irreversible death.

_____ 7. After you apply pressure to depress the sternum, you must follow with an equal period of relaxation so that the chest returns to normal position.

_____ 8. The ratio of compressions to ventilations for one-person CPR on an adult is 2:1.

_____ 9. When performed correctly, external chest compressions provide 50% of the blood normally pumped by the heart.

_____ 10. For infants, the preferred technique of artificial ventilation is mouth-to-nose-and-mouth ventilation with a mask or other barrier device.

_____ 11. You need to use less ventilatory pressure to inflate a child's lungs because the airway is smaller than that of an adult.

Short Answer

Complete this section with short written answers using the space provided.

1. List the four obvious signs of death, in addition to absence of pulse and breathing, that are used as a general rule to not start CPR.

_____

_____

2. Complete the following table regarding pediatric BLS by listing the procedure parameters or guidelines for each age group as they relate to the action noted on the left.

Procedure	Infants (younger than age 1 year)	Children (1 to 8 years)
Airway		
Breathing Initial breaths Subsequent breaths		
Circulation Pulse check Compression area Compression width Compression depth Compression rate Ratio of Compressions to Ventilations Foreign Body Obstruction		

3. List the four acceptable reasons for stopping CPR.

_____

_____

4. Describe how to perform a head tilt-chin lift maneuver.

_____

_____

5. Describe how to perform a jaw-thrust maneuver.

_____

_____

6. Describe the process of chest compressions during one-rescuer adult CPR.

_____

_____

7. List and describe the method for "switching positions" during two-rescuer adult CPR.

_____

_____

8. Describe the process of abdominal thrusts for a standing patient and a supine patient.

_____

_____

9. Describe the process for chest thrusts on a standing and a supine patient.

_____

_____

10. Describe the process for removing a foreign body airway obstruction in an infant.

_____

_____

Word Fun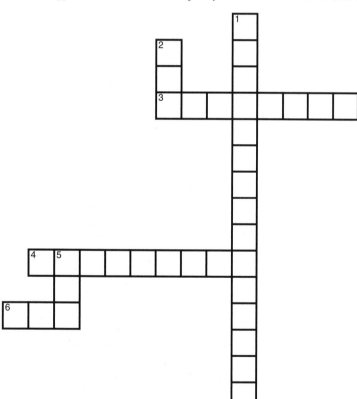

The following crossword puzzle is an activity provided to reinforce correct spelling and understanding of medical terminology associated with emergency care and the EMT-B. Use the clues in the column to complete the puzzle.

Across

3. Position after patient regains consciousness

4. Opening airway by moving lower bone forcibly forward

6. First level of care

Down

1. Preferred method to remove airway obstruction

2. Chest compression and artificial ventilation

5. High level of care, beyond basic

Ambulance Calls

The following case scenarios provide an opportunity to explore the concerns associated with patient management. Read each scenario, then answer each question in detail.

1. You are dispatched to a "person down". The dispatcher informs you that the caller said the patient is not breathing. Upon arrival, you find a 78-year-old woman in bed, apneic and pulseless. In the process of moving the patient to place a CPR board underneath her, you note the discoloration of her back and hips known as dependent lividity.

How would you best manage this patient?

_____

_____

_____

2. You are off-duty when you hear a dispatch for "chest pain" at a private residence near you. You arrive to find the patient's family members attempting to apply an AED they bought over the Internet.

How would you best manage this situation?

_____

_____

_____

3. You are dispatched to "unconscious male" at a private residence. You arrive to find the man lying in the grass in the backyard. Due to the ladder and equipment on the rooftop, it appears he was working on the roof of his two-story home. No one witnessed the event.

How would you best manage this patient?

_____

_____

_____

Skill Drills

Skill Drill A-1: Positioning the Patient

Test your knowledge of this skill drill by placing the photos below in the correct order. Number the first step with a "1," the second step with a "2," etc.

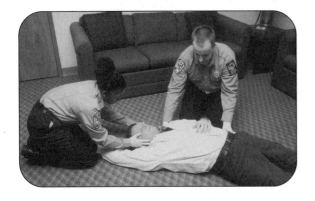

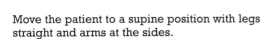

Move the patient to a supine position with legs straight and arms at the sides.

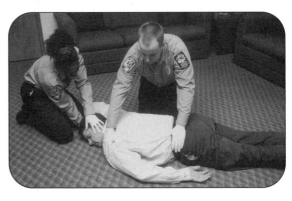

Grasp the patient, stabilizing the cervical spine if needed.

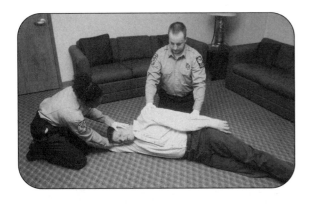

Move the head and neck as a unit with the torso as your partner pulls on the distant shoulder and hip.

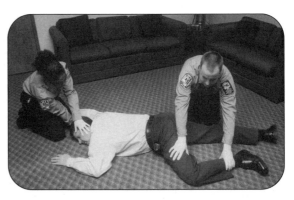

Kneel beside the patient, leaving room to roll the patient toward you.

Skill Drill A-2: Performing Chest Compressions

Test your knowledge of this skill drill by filling in the correct words in the photo captions.

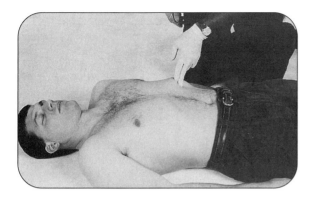

1. Slide your _____ and _____ fingers along the rib cage to the _____ in the _____ of the chest.

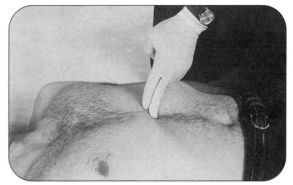

2. Push the middle finger high into the notch, and lay the index finger on the _____ _____ of the sternum.

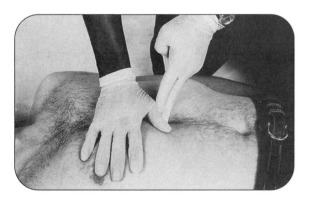

3. Place the _____ of the second hand on the lower half of the sternum, touching the _____ _____ of your first hand.

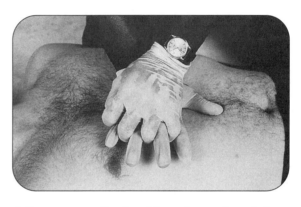

4. Remove your first hand from the notch, and place it over the _____ on the sternum.

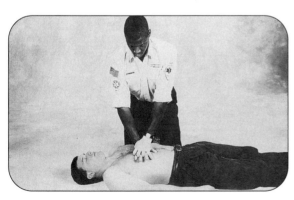

5. With your arms straight, _____ your elbows, and position your shoulders directly _____ your hands. Depress the sternum _____ inch(es) to _____ inch(es) using a rhythmic motion.

Skill Drill A-3: Performing One-rescuer Adult CPR

Test your knowledge of this skill drill by placing the photos below in the correct order. Number the first step with a "1," the second step with a "2," etc.

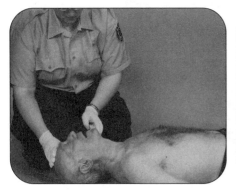

Open the airway.

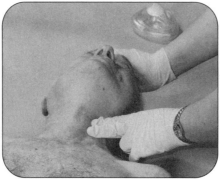

Check for a carotid pulse.

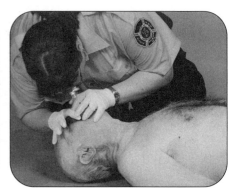

If not breathing, give two breaths of 2 seconds each.

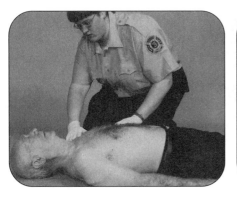

Establish unresponsiveness, and call for help.

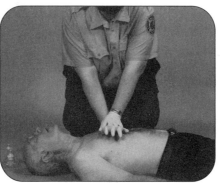

If no pulse is found, apply your AED. If there is no AED, place your hands in the proper position for chest compressions. Give 15 compressions at a rate of about 100/min.

Open the airway, and give two ventilations of 2 seconds each.

Perform four cycles of compressions. Stop CPR, and check for return of the carotid pulse.

Depending on patient condition, continue CPR, continue rescue breathing only, or place the patient in the recovery position and monitor breathing and pulse.

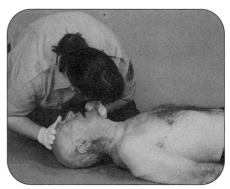

Look, listen, and feel for breathing. If breathing is adequate, place the patient in the recovery position and monitor.

Skill Drill A-4: Performing Two-rescuer Adult CPR

Test your knowledge of this skill drill by filling in the correct words in the photo captions.

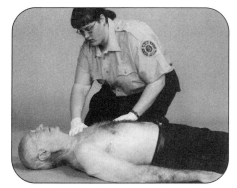

1. Establish _____, and take positions.

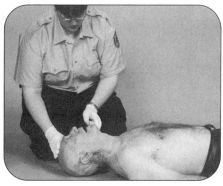

2. _____ the airway.

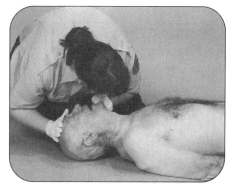

3. Look, listen, and feel for breathing. If breathing is adequate, place the patient in the _____ position and _____.

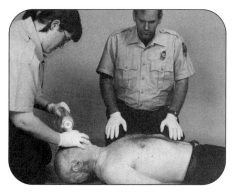

4. If not breathing, give _____ breaths of _____ seconds each.

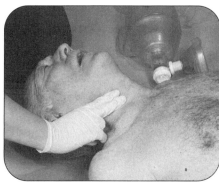

5. Check for a _____ pulse.

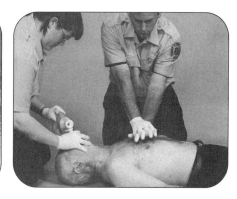

6. If there is no pulse but an AED is available, apply it now. If no AED is available, begin _____ _____ at about _____/min (_____ compressions to _____ ventilations). After _____ minute(s), check for a _____ pulse. Check every few _____ thereafter. Depending on patient _____, continue CPR, continue rescue breathing only, or place in the recovery position and monitor.

Chapter 1: Introduction to Emergency Medical Care

Matching

1. H (page 8)
2. F (page 5)
3. M (page 4)
4. G (page 4)
5. A (page 4)
6. K (page 12)
7. B (page 13)
8. C (page 4)
9. L (page 13)
10. E (page 13)
11. I (page 12)
12. D (page 12)
13. J (page 6)

Multiple Choice

1. B (page 6)
2. A (page 12)
3. D (page 13)
4. C (page 13)
5. A (page 17)
6. C (page 12)
7. D (page 12)
8. D (page 10)
9. A (page 8)
10. B (page 9)

Fill-in

1. the U.S. DOT 1994 EMT-B National Standard Curriculum (page 5)
2. life-threatening, non-life threatening (page 5)
3. medications (page 10)
4. 9-1-1 (page 10)
5. medical control (page 12)

True/False

1. F (page 4)
2. T (page 10)
3. F (page 13)
4. T (page 16)
5. T (page 17)
6. T (page 18)

Short Answer

1. The EMT-B is one of the five levels of prehospital care. The EMT-B provides basic life support skills and may also provide some ALS skills, such as advanced airways and defibrillation. (page 10)
2. The Department of Transportation (DOT) has developed a series of guidelines, curriculum, funding sources, and assessment tools, all designed to develop and improve EMS in the United States. (page 9)
3. –Ensuring your own safety and the safety of your fellow EMT-Bs, the patient, and others at the scene
   –Locating and safely driving to the scene
   –Sizing up the scene and situation
   –Rapidly assessing the patient's gross neurologic, respiratory, and circulatory status
   –Providing any essential immediate intervention

–Performing a thorough, accurate patient assessment

–Obtaining an expanded SAMPLE history

–Reaching a clinical impression and providing prompt, efficient, prioritized patient care based on your assessment

–Communicating effectively with and advising the patient of any procedures you will perform

–Properly interacting and communicating with fire, rescue, and law enforcement responders at the scene

–Identifying patients who require rapid packaging and initiating transport without delay

–Identifying patients who do not need emergency care and will benefit from further detailed assessment and care before they are moved and transported

–Properly packaging the patients

–Safely lifting and moving the patient to the ambulance and loading the patient into it

–Providing safe appropriate transport to the hospital emergency department or other ordered facility

–Giving the necessary radio report to the medical control center or receiving hospital emergency department

–Providing any additional assessment or treatment while en route

–Monitoring the patient and checking vital signs while en route

–Documenting all findings and care on the run report

–Unloading the patient safely and, after giving a proper verbal report, transferring the patient's care to the emergency department staff

–Safeguarding the patient's rights (page 6)

4. On-line medical direction is provided through radio or telephone connections between the EMT-B and the medical control facility. Off-line medical direction is provided through written protocols, procedures, and standing orders. (page 12)

Word Fun

Ambulance Calls

1. You cannot release a minor to their own care unless they are considered an "emancipated minor." You should examine this patient thoroughly, treat him using rules of implied consent and make every attempt to contact his parents or legal guardians. If you cannot immediately contact his parents, you must release him to local law enforcement.

2. Call the dispatcher to send police if the environment appears hostile. Wait for them to arrive and then proceed to care for the patient. It would also be appropriate for the boy to come to you. Ask someone close by to bring the boy to the ambulance so that you can examine his injury. If in any doubt, wait for law enforcement.

3. Leaving any patient for any reason (without releasing him to the care of equally trained providers or the hospital) is legally viewed as abandonment. This scenario presents a dilemma. Obviously you are close to the scene, so you must make a quick decision based on the following questions. Is another ambulance en route, and if so, how long will their response time be? Can you split your crew? Can you place your patient in the back of the ambulance, respond to the other call, and continue caring for the patient while your partner assesses the unconscious assault victim? You will run into real world scenarios that require quick thinking, may not be "cut and dried," and may require you to think outside the box. You must however, always obey local protocols.

Chapter 2: The Well-Being of the EMT-B

Matching

1. D (page 64)
2. A (page 36)
3. C (page 43)
4. F (page 33)
5. B (page 44)
6. E (page 42)
7. M (page 42)
8. G (page 53)
9. L (page 52)
10. I (page 51)
11. J (page 44)
12. N (page 55)
13. H (page 52)
14. K (page 51)

Multiple Choice

1. C (page 25)
2. C (page 26)
3. A (page 26)
4. D (page 26)
5. B (page 26)
6. A (page 27)
7. D (page 27)
8. C (page 27)
9. B (page 27)
10. D (page 28)
11. D (page 28)
12. D (page 29)
13. D (page 30)
14. A (page 31)
15. B (page 32)
16. D (page 32)
17. D (page 33)
18. B (page 33)
19. D (page 33)
20. D (page 31)
21. D (page 34)
22. B (page 33)
23. D (page 36)
24. A (page 41)
25. A (page 34)
26. D (page 35)
27. D (page 36)
28. B (page 37)
29. C (page 35)
30. D (page 35)
31. D (page 33)
32. D (page 39)
33. B (page 40)
34. C (page 41)
35. B (page 44)

36. D (page 44)

37. A (page 47)

38. C (page 45)

39. D (page 49)

40. D (page 54)

41. B (page 56)

42. C (page 57)

43. D (page 65)

Fill-in

1. well-being (page 24)

2. emotional stress (page 24)

3. heart disease (page 25)

4. physician (page 25)

5. warm (page 21)

6. Fear (page 26)

7. depression (page 26)

8. minor (page 32)

9. high-stress (page 32)

True/False

1. T (page 24)

2. T (page 51)

3. T (page 26)

4. F (pages 42-43)

5. F (page 32)

6. T (page 34)

Short Answer

1. An infection control practice that assumes all body fluids are potentially infectious. (page 44)

2. **1.** Denial

2. Anger/hostility

3. Bargaining

4. Depression

5. Acceptance

(page 26)

3. –Irritability toward coworkers, family and friends

–Inability to concentrate

–Difficulty sleeping, increased sleeping, or nightmares

–Anxiety; indecisiveness; guilt

–Loss of appetite (gastrointestinal disturbances)

–Loss of interest in sexual activities

–Isolation

–Loss of interest in work

–Increased use of alcohol

–Recreational drug use (page 36)

4. –Change or eliminate stressors

–Change partners to avoid a negative or hostile personality

–Change work hours

–Cut back on overtime

–Change your attitude about the stressor

–Stop wasting your energy complaining or worrying about things you cannot change

–Try to adopt a more relaxed, philosophical outlook

–Expand your social support system apart from your coworkers

–Sustain friends and interests outside emergency services

–Minimize the physical response to stress by employing various techniques (page 35)

5. **1.** Use soap and water.

2. Rub hands together for at least 10 to 15 seconds to work up a lather.

3. Rinse hands and dry with a paper towel.

4. Use paper towel to turn off faucet. (page 44)

6. (page 57)

Level	Hazard	Protection Needed
0	Little to no hazard	None
1	Slightly hazardous	SCBA only (level C suit)
2	Slightly hazardous	SCBA only (level C suit)
3	Extremely hazardous	Full protection, with no exposed skin (level A or B suit)
4	Minimal exposure causes death	Special HazMat gear (level A suit)

7. **1.** Thin inner layer

2. Thermal middle layer

3. Outer layer

(page 60)

8. **1.** Past history

2. Posture

3. Vocal activity

4. Physical activity

(pages 64-65)

Word Fun

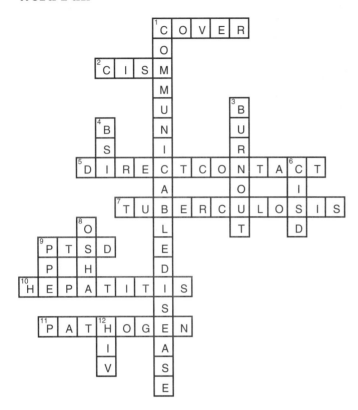

Ambulance Calls

1. Although family members understand that their loved one is terminally ill, it is common for a sudden feeling of panic to occur when the patient begins to deteriorate and you may be called to respond. This will be an emotionally charged event that will only heighten with the arrival of EMS personnel. Do not resuscitate orders apply to persons in cardiorespiratory arrest, and this patient is breathing and has a pulse. You will need to review the advance directives (living will documents), and this paperwork should be available along with the DNR orders. If the hospice nurse is available, you should speak directly with that person. If that person is not available, explain your concern for the patient and family members and explain your legal duties/requirements and notify medical control of the situation.

2. You must triage your patients. You may find this situation difficult, especially given that the crowd of onlookers will not understand any delay in patient care. You must treat the critical patients who will benefit from your care the most. This will likely prevent you from engaging in any sort of care for the patient who has the open head injury. You must regularly practice triaging patients, so that it will become an automatic response in the field. Patients like the one in this scenario can and do 'suck in' even the most seasoned providers. If you had plenty of resources, you could assist this patient not because it would change the patient's outcome but for other reasons (harvesting organs/PR issues). Always follow local protocols.

3. –Continue to treat your patient appropriately, including c-spine stabilization and transport.
   –Allow your cut to bleed as long as it is minimal and it will help to wash/clean it out.
   –Clean your wound with an alcohol gel if available.
   –Once patient care has been transferred at the receiving facility, immediately wash thoroughly with soap and water and report to your supervisor.
   –Follow up with prompt medical attention.

Skill Drills

Skill Drill 2-1: Proper Glove Removal Technique (page 46)

1. Partially remove the first glove by pinching at the wrist. Be careful to touch only the outside of the glove.
2. Remove the second glove by pinching the exterior with the partially gloved hand.
3. Pull the second glove inside-out toward the fingertips.
4. Grasp both gloves with your free hand touching only the clean, interior surfaces.

Chapter 3: Medical, Legal, and Ethical Issues

Matching

1. H (page 75)
2. I (page 75)
3. G (page 79)
4. E (page 75)
5. L (page 74)
6. A (page 75)
7. D (page 75)
8. F (page 74)
9. B (page 75)
10. C (page 76)
11. M (page 75)
12. N (page 76)
13. J (page 74)
14. K (page 73)

Multiple Choice

1. C (page 72)
2. A (page 72)
3. D (page 74)
4. D (page 74)
5. C (page 75)
6. B (page 78)
7. D (page 80)
8. D (page 81)
9. B (page 75)
10. A (page 75)
11. A (page 75)
12. C (page 76)
13. B (page 74)
14. D (page 83)
15. A (page 83)
16. D (page 84)
17. B (page 81)

Fill-in

1. scope of practice (page 72)
2. standard of care (page 73)
3. duty to act (page 74)
4. negligence (page 74)
5. termination (page 75)
6. expressed, implied (page 75)
7. assault, battery (page 75)
8. advance directive, DNR order (page 79)
9. refuse treatment (page 77)
10. special reporting (page 81)

True/False

1. T (page 74)
2. F (page 75)
3. T (page 75)
4. T (page 76)
5. T (page 75)

Short Answer

1. If the minor is emancipated, married, or pregnant (page 76)
2. You must continue to care for the patient until the patient is transferred to another medical professional of equal or higher skill level, or another medical facility. (page 75)

3. 1. Obtain refusing party's signature on an official medical release form that acknowledges refusal.

2. Obtain a signature from a witness of the refusal.

3. Keep the refusal form with the incident report.

4. Note the refusal on the incident report.

5. Keep a department copy of the records for future reference. (page 78)

4. 1. If it wasn't documented, it did not happen.

2. Incomplete or disorderly records equate to incomplete or inexpert medical care. (page 81)

5. 1. Inform medical control.

2. Treat the patient as you would any patient.

3. Take any steps necessary to preserve life.

4. If saving the patient is not possible, take steps to make sure the organ remains viable. (page 84)

Word Fun

Ambulance Calls

1. This patient needs to be evaluated at the hospital. Her parents will likely feel a right to be informed of their child's medical conditions and medical care. Laws regarding reproductive rights of minors vary from state to state. Some states allow minors to make decisions regarding birth control, prenatal care, or pregnancy termination without consenting parents, while others do not. You must know your local laws. You will have to provide information regarding the pregnancy to other health care providers directly involved in her care, and you should explain that fact and the necessity of such. Be tactful. Don't unnecessarily break your patient's trust by immediately sharing this knowledge with her parents. Document carefully and consult medical control.

2. You have a duty to act regardless of your current off-duty status (some states/provider levels/paid status varies) and you did the right thing by stopping to help the child. Once you have initiated care, you must ensure the child's parent(s) or legal guardian is notified. Although the grandfather is home, you now have another dilemma. The condition of the house/capability of the grandfather to care for the child while the mother is away is such that the question of neglect arises. You should speak with the grandfather and attempt to contact the mother of the child. If you believe that neglect or abuse of a child is occurring, you are legally required to intervene. You should document the condition of the house and notify medical control and/or child protective serves in accordance with your local protocols.

3. Assess the patient's mental status. If he is intoxicated, or has an altered mental status, he is treated under implied consent. If he is alert and oriented, you may attempt to talk him into being treated by explaining what you feel is necessary and what may happen if he does not receive care. If he has an altered mental status, orders from medical control may be obtained to restrain the patient with the help of law enforcement and transport him to the hospital.

Chapter 4: The Human Body

Matching

1.	F (page 92)	**20.**	B (page 106)
2.	K (page 123)	**21.**	A (page 107)
3.	D (page 92)	**22.**	A (page 107)
4.	G (page 93)	**23.**	A (page 110)
5.	E (page 92)	**24.**	B (page 111)
6.	L (page 123)	**25.**	B (page 111)
7.	A (page 93)	**26.**	A (page 110)
8.	C (page 93)	**27.**	A (page 110)
9.	M (page 123)	**28.**	C (page 111)
10.	J (page 93)	**29.**	B (page 111)
11.	O (page 123)	**30.**	C (page 111)
12.	B (page 93)	**31.**	A (page 109)
13.	H (page 93)	**32.**	C (page 111)
14.	N (page 93)	**33.**	A (page 99)
15.	I (page 92)	**34.**	C (page 126)
16.	B (page 100)	**35.**	E (page 128)
17.	B (page 100)	**36.**	B (page 128)
18.	A (page 100)	**37.**	F (page 126)
19.	B (page 106)	**38.**	D (page 128)

Multiple Choice

1. B (page 92)
2. C (page 93)
3. B (page 113)
4. B (page 131)
5. D (page 119)
6. C (page 96)
7. A (page 99)
8. A (page 103)
9. D (page 95)
10. A (page 95)

Labeling

1. Directional Terms (page 93)

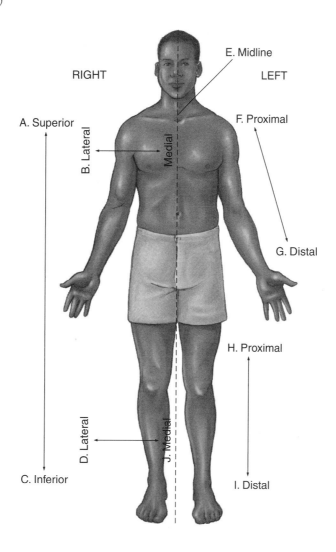

2. Anatomic Positions (page 95)

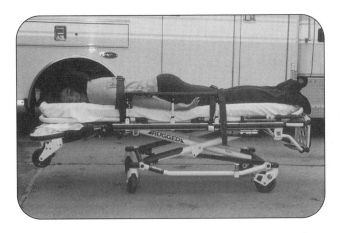

Prone

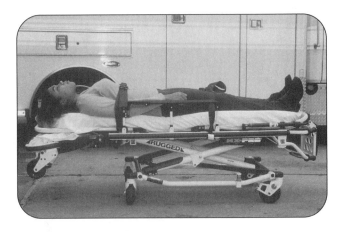

Supine

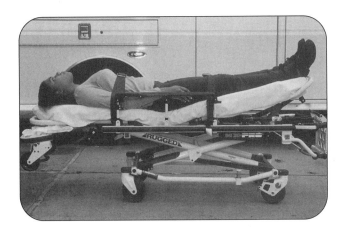

Shock position (modified Trendelenburg's position)

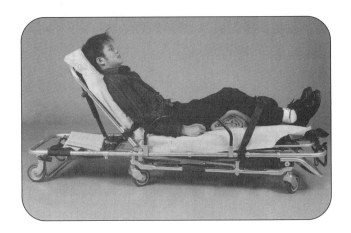

Fowler's position

3. Skeletal System (page 96)

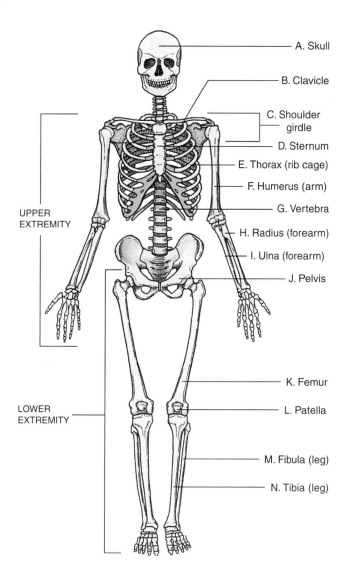

A. Skull
B. Clavicle
C. Shoulder girdle
D. Sternum
E. Thorax (rib cage)
F. Humerus (arm)
G. Vertebra
H. Radius (forearm)
I. Ulna (forearm)
J. Pelvis
K. Femur
L. Patella
M. Fibula (leg)
N. Tibia (leg)

UPPER EXTREMITY

LOWER EXTREMITY

4. The Skull (page 97)

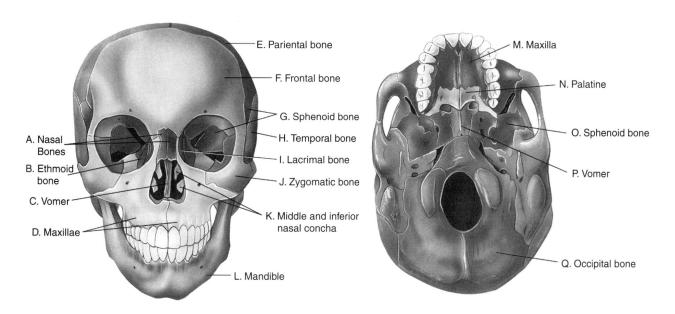

E. Pariental bone
F. Frontal bone
G. Sphenoid bone
H. Temporal bone
I. Lacrimal bone
J. Zygomatic bone
K. Middle and inferior nasal concha
A. Nasal Bones
B. Ethmoid bone
C. Vomer
D. Maxillae
L. Mandible

M. Maxilla
N. Palatine
O. Sphenoid bone
P. Vomer
Q. Occipital bone

5. The Spinal Column (page 99)

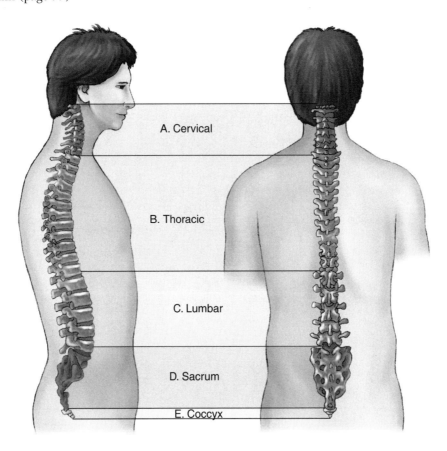

A. Cervical

B. Thoracic

C. Lumbar

D. Sacrum

E. Coccyx

6. The Thorax (page 101)

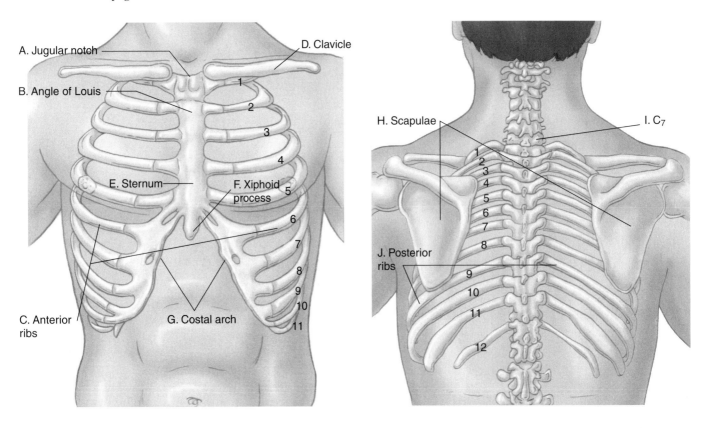

A. Jugular notch

B. Angle of Louis

D. Clavicle

E. Sternum

F. Xiphoid process

C. Anterior ribs

G. Costal arch

H. Scapulae

I. C_7

J. Posterior ribs

7. The Pelvis (page 104)

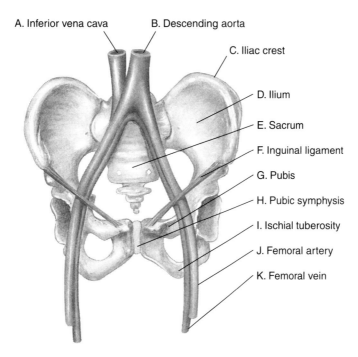

A. Inferior vena cava   B. Descending aorta

C. Iliac crest

D. Ilium

E. Sacrum

F. Inguinal ligament

G. Pubis

H. Pubic symphysis

I. Ischial tuberosity

J. Femoral artery

K. Femoral vein

8. The Lower Extremity (page 106)

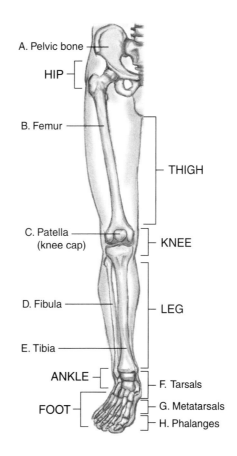

A. Pelvic bone

HIP

B. Femur

THIGH

C. Patella
(knee cap)

KNEE

D. Fibula

LEG

E. Tibia

ANKLE

FOOT

F. Tarsals

G. Metatarsals

H. Phalanges

9. The Shoulder Girdle (page 107)

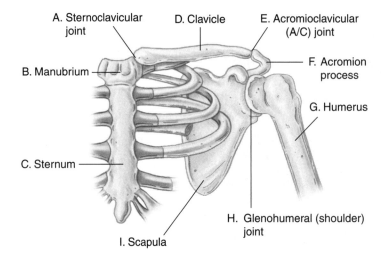

A. Sternoclavicular joint
D. Clavicle
E. Acromioclavicular (A/C) joint
B. Manubrium
F. Acromion process
G. Humerus
C. Sternum
H. Glenohumeral (shoulder) joint
I. Scapula

10. The Upper Extremity (page 107)

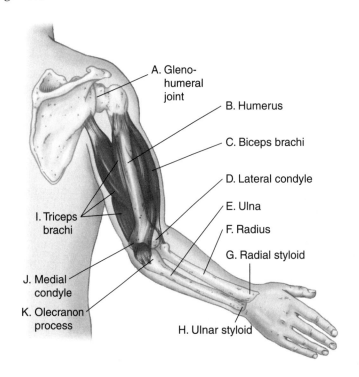

A. Gleno-humeral joint
B. Humerus
C. Biceps brachi
D. Lateral condyle
E. Ulna
F. Radius
G. Radial styloid
I. Triceps brachi
J. Medial condyle
K. Olecranon process
H. Ulnar styloid

11. Wrist and Hand (page 108)

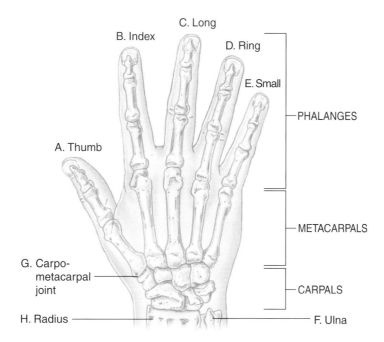

B. Index
C. Long
D. Ring
E. Small
A. Thumb
PHALANGES
G. Carpo-
metacarpal
joint
METACARPALS
CARPALS
H. Radius
F. Ulna

12. The Respiratory System (page 112)

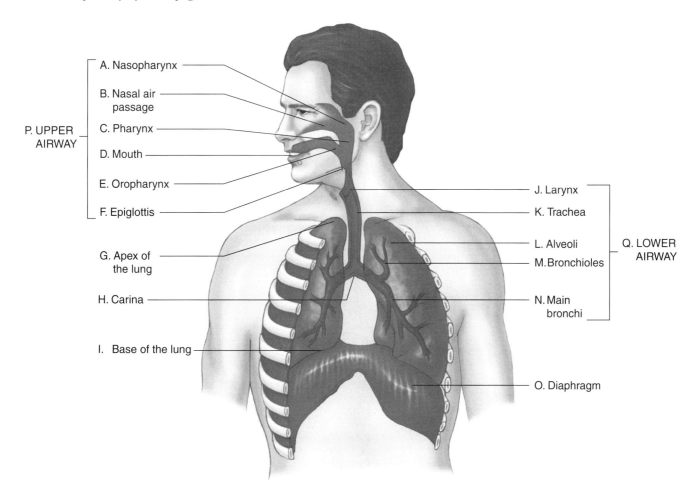

A. Nasopharynx
B. Nasal air passage
P. UPPER AIRWAY
C. Pharynx
D. Mouth
E. Oropharynx
F. Epiglottis
G. Apex of the lung
H. Carina
I. Base of the lung
J. Larynx
K. Trachea
L. Alveoli
M. Bronchioles
Q. LOWER AIRWAY
N. Main bronchi
O. Diaphragm

13. The Circulatory System (page 119)

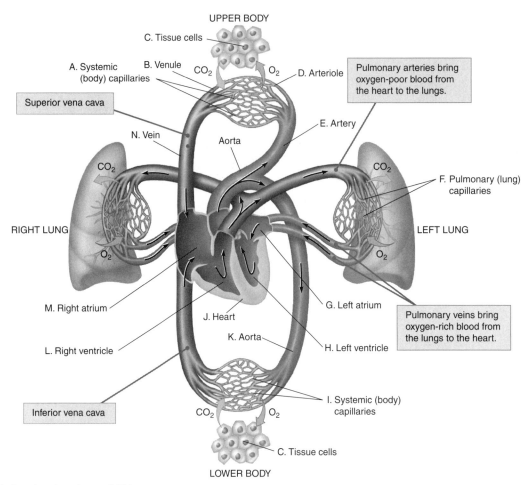

UPPER BODY

C. Tissue cells

A. Systemic (body) capillaries

B. Venule

CO_2 O_2

D. Arteriole

Pulmonary arteries bring oxygen-poor blood from the heart to the lungs.

Superior vena cava

E. Artery

N. Vein

Aorta

CO_2

CO_2

RIGHT LUNG

LEFT LUNG

F. Pulmonary (lung) capillaries

O_2

O_2

M. Right atrium

G. Left atrium

J. Heart

Pulmonary veins bring oxygen-rich blood from the lungs to the heart.

L. Right ventricle

K. Aorta

H. Left ventricle

Inferior vena cava

CO_2 O_2

I. Systemic (body) capillaries

C. Tissue cells

LOWER BODY

14. Electrical Conduction (page 121)

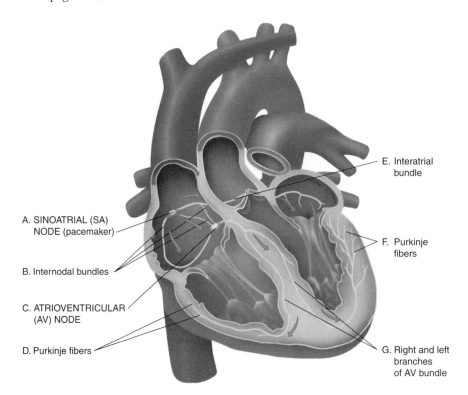

E. Interatrial bundle

A. SINOATRIAL (SA) NODE (pacemaker)

F. Purkinje fibers

B. Internodal bundles

C. ATRIOVENTRICULAR (AV) NODE

D. Purkinje fibers

G. Right and left branches of AV bundle

15. Central and Peripheral Pulses (page 124)

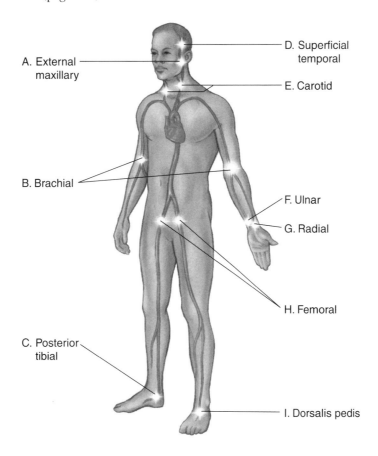

A. External maxillary

D. Superficial temporal

E. Carotid

B. Brachial

F. Ulnar

G. Radial

H. Femoral

C. Posterior tibial

I. Dorsalis pedis

16. Brain (page 126)

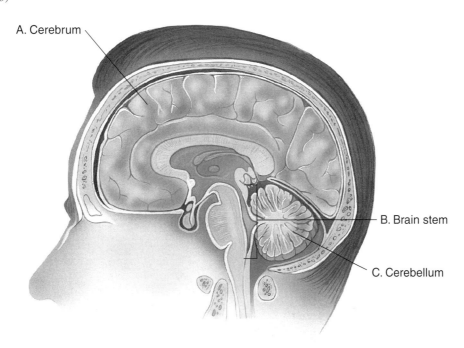

A. Cerebrum

B. Brain stem

C. Cerebellum

17. Anatomy of the Skin (page 130)

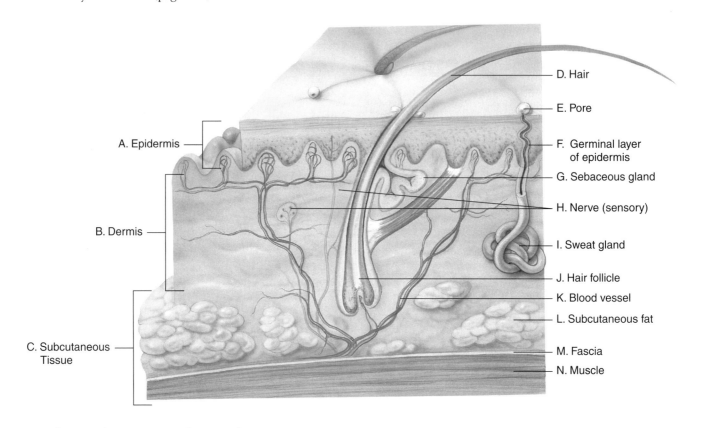

A. Epidermis

B. Dermis

C. Subcutaneous Tissue

D. Hair

E. Pore

F. Germinal layer of epidermis

G. Sebaceous gland

H. Nerve (sensory)

I. Sweat gland

J. Hair follicle

K. Blood vessel

L. Subcutaneous fat

M. Fascia

N. Muscle

18. Male Reproductive System (page 136)

FRONT VIEW

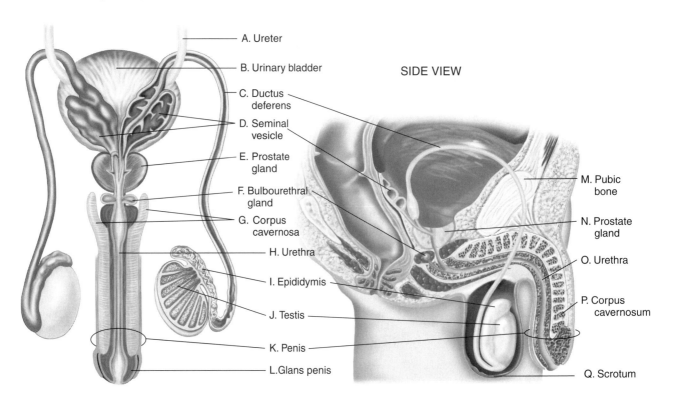

A. Ureter

B. Urinary bladder

C. Ductus deferens

D. Seminal vesicle

E. Prostate gland

F. Bulbourethral gland

G. Corpus cavernosa

H. Urethra

I. Epididymis

J. Testis

K. Penis

L. Glans penis

SIDE VIEW

M. Pubic bone

N. Prostate gland

O. Urethra

P. Corpus cavernosum

Q. Scrotum

19. Female Reproductive System (page 136)

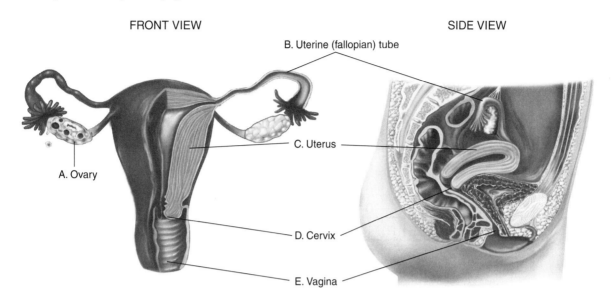

FRONT VIEW   SIDE VIEW

B. Uterine (fallopian) tube

A. Ovary

C. Uterus

D. Cervix

E. Vagina

Fill-in

1. 7 (page 99)
2. mandible (page 97)
3. 5 (page 113)
4. 12 (page 100)
5. 33 (page 100)
6. talus (page 106)
7. floating ribs (page 100)

True/False

1. F (page 122)
2. T (page 108)
3. T (pages 106-108)
4. F (page 120)
5. F (page 100)

Short Answer

1. Plasma – is a sticky, yellow fluid that carries the blood cells and nutrients
Red blood cells – give blood its red color and carry oxygen
White blood cells – play a role in the body's immune defense mechanism against infection
Platelets – essential in the formation of blood clots (pages 123 to 124)

2. Cervical spine – 7
Thoracic spine – 12
Lumbar spine – 5
Sacrum – 5
Coccyx – 4 (page 100)

3. RUQ – liver, gallbladder, portion of the colon
LUQ – stomach, spleen, portion of the colon
RLQ – large intestine, small intestine, appendix, ascending colon
LLQ – large intestine, small intestine, descending and the sigmoid portions of the colon (page 103)

4. **1.** superior and inferior vena cava

2. right atrium

3. right ventricle

4. pulmonary artery

5. lungs

6. pulmonary vein

7. left atrium

8. left ventricle

9. aorta (page 120)

Word Fun

Ambulance Calls

1. Lacerated liver, gall bladder, small intestine, large intestine, pancreas, diaphragm, right lung if the pathway is up, right kidney depending on length of knife. You could also have involvement of the other four quadrants based on the direction of travel of the blade.

   The description would be a puncture wound or stab wound.

2. There is significant mechanism of injury in this scenario. Not only did the patient's vehicle impact a solid, stationary object but also with enough force to deform the steering wheel. This patient was not restrained and the abrupt deceleration caused driver's chest to impact the steering wheel with significant force. He could have numerous internal injuries including: pneumo and/or hemothorax, cardiac or pulmonary contusions, fractured ribs/sternum (not to mention spinal and head injuries). Immediate transport with full spinal precautions and high-flow oxygen is required.

3. Depending upon the condition of the track, the rider's use of protective gear, and the speed and height of the fall, he may or may not have sustained significant injuries. Given his self-splinting, it can be assumed that he has (at minimum) fractures to the left humerus, radius and/or ulna and clavicle. Treat and transport according to local protocols.

Chapter 5: Baseline Vital Signs and SAMPLE History

Matching

1. N (page 152)
2. E (page 157)
3. D (page 158)
4. L (page 154)
5. A (page 156)
6. H (page 148)
7. K (page 157)
8. F (page 155)
9. M (page 154)
10. O (page 154)
11. B (page 155)
12. G (page 158)
13. I (page 158)
14. C (page 155)
15. J (page 154)

Multiple Choice

1. C (page 147)
2. A (page 147)
3. B (page 149)
4. D (page 149)
5. A (page 149)
6. D (page 149)
7. D (page 150)
8. B (page 151)
9. C (page 151)
10. B (page 151)
11. C (pages 152-153)
12. C (page 153)
13. A (page 153)
14. D (page 154)
15. D (page 154)
16. D (page 154)
17. D (page 154)
18. B (page 155)
19. D (page 155)
20. D (page 155)
21. B (page 156)
22. D (page 156)
23. B (page 156)
24. A (page 157)
25. C (page 158)
26. A (page 160)
27. B (page 160)
28. D (page 160)
29. D (page 162)
30. C (page 149)
31. A (page 147)
32. B (page 158)
33. C (page 161)
34. C (page 162)
35. B (page 154)

Fill-in

1. Tidal volume (page 152)
2. conjunctiva (page 155)
3. deductive (page 146)
4. symptom (page 147)
5. spontaneous respirations (page 149)
6. Vital signs (page 149)
7. quality (page 150)
8. labored breathing (page 151)
9. fluid (page 151)
10. perfusion (page 154)

True/False

1. T (page 153)
2. T (page 158)
3. F (page 158)
4. T (page 151)
5. T (page 150)
6. F (page 153)
7. F (page 154)
8. T (page 154)
9. T (page 154)
10. T (page 155)
11. F (page 155)
12. F (page 161)
13. F (page 154)

Short Answer

1. 1. Pulse
   2. Respirations
   3. Pupils
   4. Blood pressure
   5. Skin
   6. Level of consciousness
   7. Capillary refill (page 149)
2. 1. Flushed (red)
   2. Pale (white, ashen, or graying)
   3. Jaundice (yellow)
   4. Cyanotic (blue-gray) (pages 154-155)
3. 1. Rate
   2. Rhythm
   3. Quality
   4. Depth (tidal volume) (pages 150-152)
4. Pressure exerted against the walls of the artery when the left ventricle contracts (page 157)
5. Pressure remaining against the walls of the artery when the left ventricle is at rest (page 157)
6. 1. Rate
   2. Strength
   3. Regularity (pages 153-154)
7. 1. Color
   2. Temperature
   3. Moisture (pages 154-155)
8. Gently compress the fingertip until it blanches. Release the fingertip, and count until it returns to its normal pink color. (page 155)
9. Pupils Equal And Round, Regular in size, react to Light (page 162)
10. A sign is a condition that can be seen, heard, felt, smelled, or measured. A symptom is something that the patient reports to you as a problem or feeling. (page 147)

Word Fun

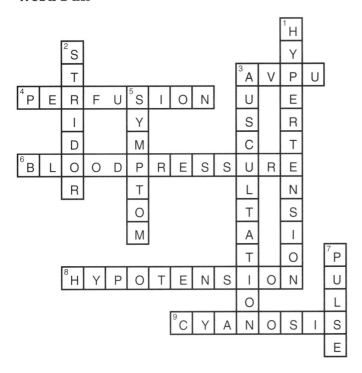

Ambulance Calls

1. You must closely monitor this patient's airway as its patency could change at any time. You should not take any actions to clear her airway unless it becomes blocked again (or partially blocked to the point of ineffective airway exchange). Obviously, no attempt should be made to pull the foreign body out of her airway. You must gently transport this patient in a position she finds most comfortable and be prepared to administer abdominal thrusts at any point should it become necessary.

2. Shoveling snow is very physical work (especially wet, heavy snow). The first snowfall often brings 9-1-1 calls for chest pain. People often don't fully understand how strenuous this activity is, and normally sedentary individuals will attempt to shovel snow without thought. This man isn't simply having angina, he is having a heart attack. He likely has heart disease, and although he reports his pain is "better," his chest heaviness continues despite rest. He should be transported immediately according to local protocols.

3. –Open and assess the airway.
   –Apply high-flow oxygen via nonrebreathing mask or BVM.
   –Assess carotid pulse.
   –If no pulse, initiate chest compressions.
   –If patient has a pulse, treat for shock and rapid transport.
   –Place patient in Trendelenburg position and cover to keep warm.
   –Continue assessment and obtain SAMPLE history en route.
   –Monitor vital signs and take a complete set every 5 minutes.

Skill Drills

Skill Drill 5-1: Obtaining a Blood Pressure by Auscultation or Palpation (page 159)

1. Apply the cuff snugly.
2. Palpate the brachial artery.
3. Place the stethoscope over the brachial artery, and grasp the ball-pump and turn-valve.
4. Close the valve and pump to 20 mm Hg above the point at which you stop hearing pulse sounds. Note the systolic and diastolic pressures as you let air escape slowly.
5. Open the valve, and quickly release remaining air.
6. When using the palpitation method, you should place your fingertips on the radial artery so that you feel the radial pulse.

Chapter 6: Lifting and Moving Patients

Matching

1. C (page 191)
2. G (page 200)
3. H (page 197)
4. E (page 202)
5. A (page 202)

6. I (page 197)
7. F (page 190)
8. B (page 200)
9. D (page 197)

Multiple Choice

1. D (page 204)
2. D (page 184)
3. D (page 171)
4. D (page 171)
5. D (page 173)
6. A (page 173)
7. B (page 176)
8. B (page 176)
9. D (page 179)
10. A (page 179)
11. D (page 182)
12. D (page 181)
13. D (page 182)
14. C (page 182)
15. D (page 183)
16. B (page 184)
17. A (page 185)
18. D (page 184)
19. C (page 185)
20. D (page 186)
21. D (page 185)
22. C (page 193)
23. A (page 202)
24. D (page 202)
25. D (page 197)
26. B (page 184)
27. A (page 174)
28. D (page 193)
29. B (page 193)
30. B (page 196)

Fill-in

1. body mechanics (page 170)
2. upright (page 171)
3. power lift (page 172)
4. palm (page 173)
5. locked-in (page 176)
6. 250 (page 180)
7. sideways (page 182)
8. locked (page 197)
9. overhead (page 198)
10. less strain (page 184)
11. spine movement (page 186)
12. direct ground lift (page 190)
13. extremity lift (page 191)
14. fluid resistant (page 198)
15. scoop stretcher (page 202)

True/False

1. T (page 200)
2. T (page 172)
3. F (page 180)
4. F (page 193)
5. T (page 184)
6. F (page 202)
7. F (page 197)
8. F (page 186)
9. F (page 190)
10. T (page 196)

Short Answer

1. –Front cradle
   –Firefighter's drag
   –One-person walking assist
   –Firefighter's carry
   –Pack strap (page 187)

2. –The vehicle or scene is unsafe.
   –The patient cannot be properly assessed before being removed from the car.
   –The patient needs immediate intervention that requires a supine position.
   –The patient's condition requires immediate transport to the hospital.
   –The patient blocks the EMT-B's access to another seriously injured patient. (page 186)

3. –Make sure there is sufficient lifting power.
   –Follow the manufacturer's directions for safe and proper use of the cot.
   –Make sure that all cots and patients are fully secured before you move the ambulance. (page 199)

4. –Be sure that you know or can find out the weight to be lifted and the limitations of the team's abilities.
   –Coordinate your movements with those of the other team members while constantly communicating with them.
   –Do not twist your body as you are carrying the patient.
   –Keep the weight that you are carrying as close to your body as possible while keeping your back in a locked-in position.
   –Be sure to flex at the hips, not at the waist, and bend at the knees, while making sure that you do not hyperextend your back by leaning back from your waist. (page 175)

5. Always keep your back in a straight, upright position and lift without twisting. (page 171)

Word Fun

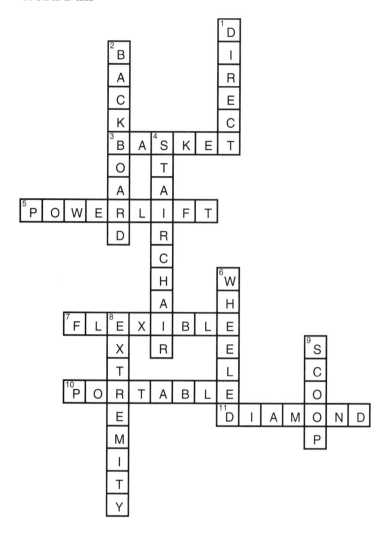

Ambulance Calls

1. –Immobilize the patient on a long spine board and apply high-flow oxygen.
   –Use four persons to carry the board back up the ledge.
   –Plan the route and brief your helpers before moving the patient.
   –Clarify whether you will move on "three" or count to three then move.
   –Coordinate the move until the patient is loaded into the ambulance.

2. It is highly unlikely that you will be able to move this patient, especially without significantly hurting yourself or your partner. You should immediately request additional personnel. You can attempt to move the patient, but if you cannot successfully do so, you will have to open his airway, etc. in his current position. Do the best you can until the patient can be moved.

3. Patients whose conditions will be exacerbated by physical activity should not walk to the gurney or ambulance. If a patient's condition is not such that it is medically necessary that you carry them, it is safer for them to walk on their own power to the ambulance. This patient should not/cannot walk. This produces a safety issue for you and your partner especially given the fact there is no elevator. Fortunately, this patient can sit upright and the use of a stair chair would be appropriate in this situation. Regardless, you should ask for more personnel given the patient's large size. Back injuries are very common in EMS. In order for providers to avoid these injuries, correct lifting techniques should be used and assistance should be requested whenever the patient is large or in a position not conducive to correct lifting procedures.

Skill Drills

Skill Drill 6-1: Performing the Power Lift (page 174)

1. Lock your back into an **upright**, inward curve. **Spread** and bend your legs. Grasp the backboard, palms up and just in front of you. **Balance** and center the weight between your arms.
2. Position your feet, **straddle** the object, and **distribute** weight.
3. **Straighten** your legs and lift, keeping your back locked in.

Skill Drill 6-2: Performing the Diamond Carry (page 176)

1. Position yourselves facing the patient.
2. After the patient has been lifted, the EMT-B at the foot turns to face forward.
3. EMT-Bs at the side each turn the head-end hand palm down and release the other hand.
4. EMT-Bs at the side turn toward the foot end.

Skill Drill 6-3: Performing the One-Handed Carrying Technique (page 177)

1. **Face** each other and use both **hands**.
2. Lift the backboard to **carrying height**.
3. **Turn** in the direction you will walk and **switch** to using one hand.

Skill Drill 6-4: Carrying a Patient on Stairs (page 178)

1. **Strap** the patient securely. Make sure one strap is tight across the **upper torso**, under the arms, and secured to the handles to prevent the patient from **sliding**.
2. Carry a patient down stairs with the **foot** end first, **head** elevated.
3. Carry the **head** end first going up stairs, always keeping the head elevated.

Skill Drill 6-5: Using a Stair Chair (page 181)

1. Position and secure the patient on the chair with **straps**.
2. Take your places at the **head** and **foot** of the chair.
3. A third **rescuer** "backs up" the rescuer carrying the **foot**.
4. **Lower** the chair to roll on landings, or for transfer to the cot.

Skill Drill 6-6: Performing the Rapid Extrication Technique (page 188)

1. First EMT-B provides in-line manual support of the head and cervical spine.
2. Second EMT-B gives commands, applies a cervical collar, and performs the initial assessment.
3. Second EMT-B supports the torso.
   Third EMT-B frees the patient's legs from the pedals and moves the legs together, without moving the pelvis or spine.
4. Second and Third EMT-Bs rotate the patient as a unit in several short, coordinated moves.
   First EMT-B (relieved by Fourth EMT-B or bystander as needed) supports the head and neck during rotation (and later steps).
5. First (or Fourth) EMT-B places the backboard on the seat against patient's buttocks.
6. Third EMT-B moves to an effective position for sliding the patient.
   Second and Third EMT-Bs slide the patient along the backboard in coordinated, 8" to 12" moves until the hips rest on the backboard.
7. Third EMT-B exits the vehicle, moves to the backboard opposite Second EMT-B, and they continue to slide the patient until patient is fully on the board.
8. First (or Fourth) EMT-B continues to stabilize the head and neck while Second and Third EMT-Bs carry the patient away from the vehicle.

Skill Drill 6-7: Extremity Lift (page 192)

1. Patient's hands are **crossed** over the chest.
   First EMT-B grasps patient's wrists or **forearms** and pulls patient to a **sitting** position.

2. When the patient is sitting, First EMT-B passes his or her arms through patient's **armpits** and grasps the patient's opposite (or his or her own) **forearms** or **wrists**.
   Second EMT-B kneels between the **legs**, facing in the same direction as the patient, and places his or her hands under the **knees**.

3. Both EMT-Bs rise to **crouching**.
   On **command**, both lift and begin to move.

Skill Drill 6-8: Using a Scoop Stretcher (page 194)

1. Adjust stretcher **length**.

2. **Lift** patient slightly and **slide** stretcher into place, one side at a time.

3. **Lock** the stretcher ends together, avoiding **pinching**.

4. **Secure** the patient to the scoop stretcher and **transfer** it to the cot.

Skill Drill 6-9: Loading a Cot into an Ambulance (page 199)

1. Tilt the head of the cot **upward**, and place it into the patient compartment with the wheels on the floor.

2. Second rescuer on the side of the cot releases the **undercarriage** lock and lifts the undercarriage.

3. **Roll** the cot into the back of the ambulance.

4. Secure the cot to the **brackets** mounted in the ambulance.

Chapter 7: Airway

Matching

1. C (page 216)
2. I (page 216)
3. H (page 216)
4. G (page 216)
5. K (page 220)
6. E (page 216)
7. A (page 216)
8. F (page 216)
9. L (page 214)
10. D (page 214)
11. J (page 219)
12. B (page 193)

Multiple Choice

1. D (page 218)
2. B (pages 223-225)
3. B (page 221)
4. D (page 220)
5. A (page 220)
6. A (page 222)
7. C (page 227)
8. D (page 245)
9. C (page 246)
10. C (page 232)
11. B (page 225)
12. D (page 231)
13. C (page 226)
14. D (page 246)
15. A (page 242)
16. A (page 242)
17. C (page 218)
18. D (page 221)
19. A (page 222)
20. C (page 234)

Labeling

1. Upper and Lower Airways (page 215)

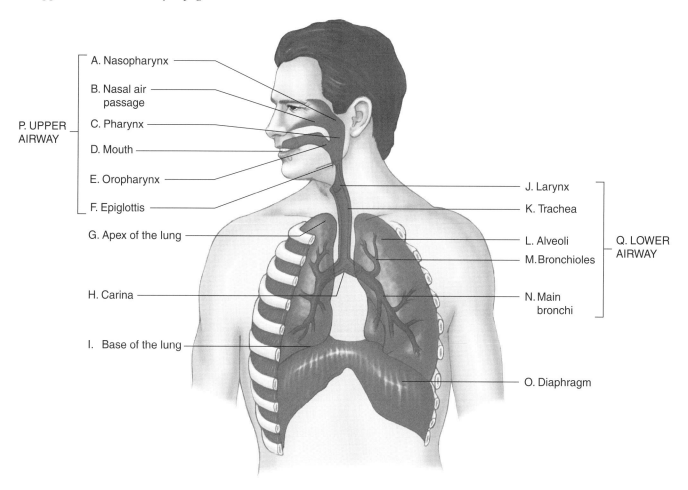

P. UPPER AIRWAY

A. Nasopharynx
B. Nasal air passage
C. Pharynx
D. Mouth
E. Oropharynx
F. Epiglottis

G. Apex of the lung
H. Carina
I. Base of the lung

J. Larynx
K. Trachea
L. Alveoli
M. Bronchioles
N. Main bronchi
O. Diaphragm

Q. LOWER AIRWAY

2. Thoracic Cage (page 215)

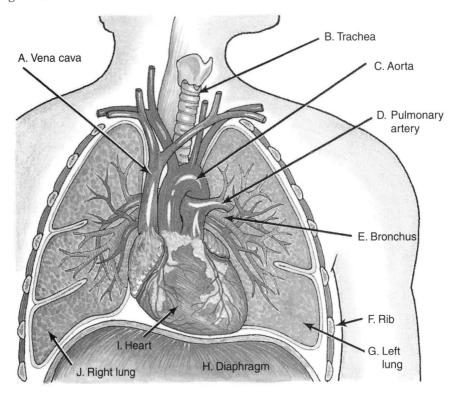

Fill-in

1. trachea (page 216)

2. higher (page 216)

3. 21, 78 (page 218)

4. carbon dioxide (page 219)

5. diaphragm, intercostal muscles (page 216)

6. low oxygen, high carbon dioxide (pages 218-219)

7. hypoxia (page 219)

True/False

1. F (page 226)

2. T (page 241)

3. F (page 227)

4. F (page 237)

5. F (page 236)

Short Answer

1. Nervousness, tachycardia, irritability, fear, apprehension. (Other signs: Mental status changes, use of accessory muscles for breathing, breathing difficulty, possible chest pain.) (page 222)

2. Adults: 12 to 20 breaths/min
Children: 15 to 30 breaths/min
Infants: 25 to 50 breaths/min (page 221)

3. Give slow, gentle breaths. (page 248)

4. **1.** Kneel above the patient's head.

    2. Extend the patient's neck unless you suspect a cervical spine injury.

    3. Open the mouth and suction as needed. Insert an airway adjunct as needed.

    4. Select a proper-sized mask.

    5. Position the mask on the patient's face.

    6. Use the C-clamp technique to hold the mask, then squeeze the bag every 5 seconds for adults, every 3 seconds for children and infants. (page 245)

5. 1. Respiratory rate of less than 8 breaths/min or greater than 24 breaths/min
    2. Accessory muscle use
    3. Skin pulling in around the ribs during inspiration
    4. Pale, cyanotic, or cool (clammy) skin
    5. Irregular pattern of inhalation and exhalation
    6. Lung sounds that are decreased, unequal, or "wet"
    7. Labored breathing
    8. Shallow and/or uneven chest movement
    9. Two- or three-word sentences spoken (page 222)
6. They are the secondary muscles of respiration. They are not used in normal breathing. They include:
    1. Sternocleidomastoid (neck)
    2. Pectoralis major (chest)
    3. Abdominal muscles (page 222)
7. When the patient has severe trauma to the head or face. (page 227)
8. 1. Select the proper-size airway and apply a water-soluble lubricant.
    2. Place the airway in the larger nostril with the curvature following the curve of the floor of the nose.
    3. Advance the airway gently.
    4. Continue until the flange rests against the skin. (page 227)
9. Tonsil tips are best because they have a large diameter and do not collapse. In addition, they are curved, which allows easy, rapid placement. (page 231)
10. 15 seconds. (page 232)

Word Fun

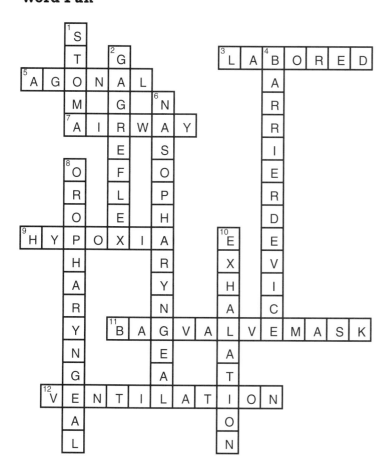

Ambulance Calls

1. Maintain cervical spine stabilization.
   Immediately open the airway with a modified jaw thrust.
   Suction to remove obstruction.
   Assess the airway for breathing (rate, rhythm, quality) and provide oxygen via nonrebreathing mask or BVM.
   Continue initial assessment, rapid extrication, and rapid transport.

2. You should reposition the head and attempt to re-ventilate the patient. If you are unsuccessful in your second attempt, you must take action to clear her airway. If you fail to clear her airway, she will like go into cardiac arrest as well. Choking victims have been known to walk away from others without indicating that they are choking and when this occurs in a restaurant setting, many of these people will go into a bathroom. If you find a patient in a restroom who cannot be ventilated, they likely have a foreign body airway obstruction (FBAO) most often as a result of ingested food.

3. The most common cause of airway obstruction in an unconscious patient is the tongue. The patient's husband told you that he helped her to the ground without injury, so it is safe to place her in the recovery position. If you were unsure of the presence of trauma, this position would not be used, instead using the jaw-thrust maneuver to manage her airway. In either case, you must continually monitor her condition and be prepared for vomitus.

Skill Drills

Skill Drill 7-1: Positioning the Unconscious Patient (page 224)

1. Support the head while your partner straightens the patient's legs.
2. Have your partner place his or her hand on the patient's far shoulder and hip.
3. Roll the patient as a unit with the person at the head calling the count to begin the move.
4. Open and assess the patient's airway and breathing status.

Chapter 8: Patient Assessment

Matching

1. P (page 268)
2. D (page 278)
3. M (page 289)
4. N (page 289)
5. B (page 278)
6. H (page 289)
7. L (page 276)
8. A (page 276)
9. O (page 272)
10. J (page 279)
11. G (page 278)
12. E (page 274)
13. F (page 283)
14. I (page 277)
15. K (page 274)
16. C (page 289)

Multiple Choice

1. C (pages 265-269)
2. D (page 226)
3. B (page 267)
4. C (page 267)
5. D (page 267)
6. A (page 267)
7. D (page 268)
8. B (page 269)
9. B (page 270)
10. C (page 274)
11. D (page 275)
12. A (page 276)
13. D (page 278)
14. B (page 277)
15. A (page 278)
16. C (page 278)
17. D (page 278)
18. D (page 278)
19. D (page 278)
20. C (page 279)
21. D (page 283)
22. B (page 268)
23. B (page 283)
24. C (page 289)
25. A (page 290)
26. D (page 263)
27. D (page 302)
28. B (page 307)
29. D (page 308)
30. A (page 264)
31. D (page 264)
32. D (page 270)
33. B (page 282)
34. B (page 294)

Fill-in

1. decisions (page 263)
2. body substance isolation (page 265)
3. victim (page 266)
4. safety (page 266)
5. Triage (page 268)
6. general impression (page 271)
7. life-threatening (page 271)
8. patency (page 275)
9. reevaluate (page 276)
10. wrist (page 278)
11. initial assessment (page 279)

True/False

1. F (page 284)
2. F (page 272)
3. T (page 272)
4. T (page 277)
5. T (page 279)

Short Answer

1. To identify and initiate treatment of immediate or potential life threats. (page 271)
2. Immediate assessment of the environment, the patient's presenting signs and symptoms, and the patient's chief complaint. (page 271)
3. A-Airway

   B-Breathing

   C-Circulation (page 271)
4. Orientation to person, place, time, and event. Person (name) evaluates long-term memory. Place and time evaluate intermediate-term memory. Event evaluates short-term memory. (page 274)
5. 1. Identify the patient's chief complaint.

   2. Understand the circumstances surrounding the chief complaint.

   3. Direct further physical examination. (page 274)
6. Deformities, Contusions, Abrasions, Punctures/penetrations, Burns, Tenderness, Lacerations, Swelling (page 284)
7. 1. Ejection from a vehicle

   2. Death in the passenger compartment

   3. Fall greater than 15 to 20 feet

   4. Vehicle rollover

   5. High-speed vehicle collision

   6. Vehicle-pedestrian collision

   7. Motorcycle crash

   8. Unresponsiveness or altered mental status following trauma

   9. Penetrating head, chest, or abdominal trauma (page 267)

Word Fun

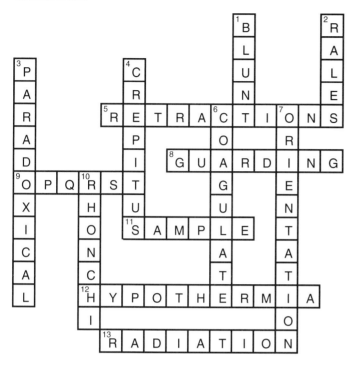

Ambulance Calls

1. –Maintain cervical spine control
   –Immediately manage the airway by suction and oxygen
   –Rapid survey and transport

   This patient is a load-and-go based on:
   • Mechanism of injury
   • Level of consciousness
   • Airway compromise

   Damage to vehicle indicates possible occult injuries.

2. This patient is having a very serious asthma attack. Accessory muscle use (nasal flaring, tracheal tugging, suprasternal and intercostal muscle retractions), work of breathing, wheezing, and one- to two-word responses all point to the seriousness of his attack. You should transport immediately, apply high-flow oxygen, and assist with MDI administration according to your local protocols.

3. Mechanism of injury is significant for this patient. Not only did he fall down a flight of wooden stairs, but he landed on a cement floor. His head injury is likely more significant than the bruising and laceration you can see. He could also have skull fractures, contusions, or intracranial bleeding. With any significant trauma to the head comes the likelihood for cervical spine fractures. You should also question the mechanism of his fall as medical conditions can sometimes precipitate injuries. Full c-spine precautions must be taken along with application of high-flow oxygen and prompt transport.

Skill Drills

Skill Drill 8-1: Performing a Rapid Physical Exam (pages 285 to 286)

1. Assess the head. Have your partner maintain in-line stabilization.
2. Assess the neck.
3. Apply a cervical spinal immobilization device on trauma patients.
4. Assess the chest. Listen to breath sounds on both sides of the chest.
5. Assess the abdomen.
6. Assess the pelvis. If there is no pain, gently compress the pelvis downward and inward to look for tenderness or instability.

7. Assess all four extremities. Assess pulse, motor, and sensory function.
8. Assess the back. In trauma patients, roll the patient in one motion.

Skill Drill 8-3: Performing the Detailed Physical Exam (pages 301 to 303)

1. Observe the face.
2. Inspect the area around the eyes and eyelids.
3. Examine the eyes for redness, contact lenses. Check pupil function.
4. Look behind the ear for Battle's sign.
5. Check the ears for drainage or blood.
6. Observe and palpate the head.
7. Palpate the zygomas.
8. Palpate the maxillae.
9. Palpate the mandible.
10. Assess the mouth and nose.
11. Check for unusual breath odors.
12. Inspect the neck.
13. Palpate the front and back of the neck.
14. Observe for jugular vein distention.
15. Inspect the chest and observe breathing motion.
16. Gently palpate over the ribs.
17. Listen to anterior breath sounds (midaxillary, midclavicular).
18. Listen to posterior breath sounds (bases, apices).
19. Observe the abdomen and pelvis.
20. Gently palpate the abdomen.
21. Gently compress the pelvis from the sides.
22. Gently press the iliac crests.
23. Inspect the extremities; assess distal circulation and motor sensory function.
24. Log roll the patient and inspect the back.

Chapter 9: Communications and Documentation

Matching

1. M (page 316)
2. G (page 317)
3. J (page 317)
4. K (page 317)
5. H (page 318)
6. L (page 317)
7. I (page 317)
8. C (page 318)
9. A (page 317)
10. F (page 319)
11. E (page 318)
12. D (page 317)
13. B (page 327)

Multiple Choice

1. D (pages 316-317)
2. A (page 317)
3. D (pages 316-317)
4. B (page 317)
5. B (page 318)
6. D (page 318)
7. C (page 319)
8. D (pages 319-320)
9. B (page 321)
10. D (page 322)
11. A (page 322)
12. B (page 323)
13. D (page 324)
14. D (page 324)
15. D (page 322)
16. A (page 323)
17. A (page 323)
18. A (page 325)
19. C (page 325)
20. D (page 324)
21. B (page 326)
22. D (page 326)
23. D (pages 326-327)
24. D (page 327)
25. C (pages 330-331)
26. D (page 330)
27. C (page 331)
28. A (pages 331-332)
29. B (page 332)
30. D (page 333)
31. D (page 333)
32. A (page 333)
33. D (page 336)
34. C (page 336)
35. D (page 334)
36. A (page 335)
37. D (page 335)
38. C (page 336)

Fill-in

1. patient care report (page 316)
2. transmitter, receiver (pages 316-317)
3. dedicated line (page 317)
4. telemetry (page 318)
5. cell phones (page 318)
6. Pagers (page 321)
7. importance (pages 320-321)
8. medical control (page 322)
9. slander (page 323)
10. medical control (page 323)
11. repeat (page 324)
12. standing orders (page 326)
13. eye contact (page 327)
14. honest (page 330)
15. interpreter (page 332)
16. minimum data set (page 332)
17. Competent (page 336)

True/False

1. T (pages 316-317)
2. T (pages 316-317)
3. T (page 318)
4. F (page 317)
5. T (page 317)
6. T (pages 332-333)
7. F (page 318)
8. F (page 319)
9. F (page 332)
10. T (page 329)

Short Answer

1. –Allocating specific radio frequencies for use by EMS providers
   –Licensing base stations and assigning appropriate radio call signs for those stations
   –Establishing licensing standards and operating specifications for radio equipment used by EMS providers
   –Establishing limitations for transmitter power output
   –Monitoring radio operations (pages 319-320)

2. –Monitor the channel before transmitting.
   –Plan your message.
   –Press the push-to-talk (PTT) button.
   –Hold the microphone 2 to 3 inches from your mouth and speak clearly.
   –Identify the person or unit you are calling, then identify your unit as the sender.
   –Acknowledge a transmission as soon as you can.
   –Use plain English.
   –Keep your message brief.
   –Avoid voicing negative emotions.
   –When transmitting a number with two or more digits, say the entire number first, then each digit separately.
   –Do not use profanity on the radio.
   –Use EMS frequencies only for EMS communications.
   –Reduce background noise.
   –Be sure other radios on the same frequency are turned down. (page 325)

3. –Continuity of care
   –Legal documentation
   –Education
   –Administrative
   –Research
   –Evaluation and continuous quality improvement (page 333)

4. –Traditional, written form with check boxes and a narrative section
   –Computerized, using electronic clipboard or similar device (page 335)

Word Fun

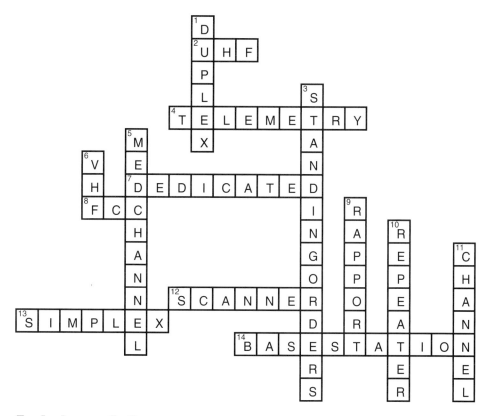

Ambulance Calls

1. –Go ahead and dispatch the closest ambulance for an emergency response.
   –Call for assistance from the fire department and local law enforcement.
   –Try to calm the caller down to obtain additional information.
   –If the caller is still of no help, ask her to get someone else to the phone.
   –Relay any additional information to the responding units.

2. You should determine if anyone on scene can translate for you (children will often speak both English and Spanish). If no one on scene can translate, you should contact a department translator. Every department should have a group of translators for different languages common to your community. (Ideally, you should speak languages commonly heard in your area.) If neither of these options is available, you should attempt as much nonverbal communication as possible, obtain baseline vital signs, and perform a physical exam to determine the nature of the problem. If the patient appears to refuse your help, you are in a tough situation. You cannot leave without knowing what the medical emergency is (if any), and you cannot obtain an informed refusal if clear communication does not occur.

3. Attempt to locate any identification that he may have on his person. If this is not possible or you cannot locate any forms of identification, you should notify law enforcement officers. The child should undergo a medical examination to ensure no injuries or other medical emergencies are present. Take care to communicate in a non-intimidating manner (taking care in level/tone of voice and posture) and attempt to establish trust with the patient.

Chapter 10: General Pharmacology

Matching

1. I (page 345)
2. J (page 344)
3. F (page 344)
4. G (page 350)
5. D (page 344)
6. H (page 344)
7. B (page 344)
8. C (page 344)
9. E (page 346)
10. A (page 348)

Multiple Choice

1. C (page 344)
2. A (page 355)
3. A (page 345)
4. A (page 345)
5. D (page 346)
6. D (page 347)
7. B (page 349)
8. D (page 351)
9. B (page 351)
10. A (pages 354-355)
11. D (pages 354-355)
12. C (page 349)
13. C (page 351)
14. A (page 344)
15. B (page 344)
16. D (page 350)

Fill-in

1. Glucose (page 350)
2. Epinephrine (page 351)
3. sublingually (page 355)
4. intravenous injection (page 345)
5. solutions (page 347)
6. medication (page 344)

True/False

1. F (page 349)
2. F (page 350)
3. F (page 351)
4. T (page 354)
5. F (page 345)
6. T (page 356)
7. F (page 353)
8. F (page 354)

Short Answer

1. Intravenous   Intramuscular   Transcutaneous
   Oral   Intraosseous   Inhalation
   Sublingual   Subcutaneous   Per rectum (pages 345-346)

2. 1. Obtain an order from medical control.

   2. Verify the proper medication and prescription.

   3. Verify the form, dose, and route.

   4. Check the expiration date and condition of medication.

   5. Reassess vital signs, especially heart rate and blood pressure, at least every 5 minutes or as the patient's condition changes.

   6. Document. (pages 355-356)

3. Many drugs adsorb (stick to) activated charcoal, preventing the drugs from being absorbed by the body. It needs to be shaken because it is a suspension and should be given in a covered container with a straw. (page 350)

4. 1. Dilates lung passages

   2. Constricts blood vessels

   3. Increases heart rate and blood pressure (page 351)

5. By pressing it into the skin (page 351)

6. **1.** Relaxes coronary arteries and veins

   2. Less blood is returned to the heart

   3. Decreases blood pressure

   4. Relaxes veins throughout the body

   5. May cause headaches (page 355)

7. To aim the spray properly (page 354)

Word Fun

Across:
3. TRANSCUTANEOUS
5. ABSORPTION
6. INTRAVENOUS
7. EPINEPHRINE
8. INTRAOSSEOUS
9. NITROGLYCERIN

Down:
1. INDICATION
2. SUBLINGUAL
4. ADSORPTION
5. ATOMIZER
7. EPINEPHRINE (ETION)

Ambulance Calls

1. This patient is in serious trouble. The history of the events combined with his level of consciousness, stridor, and hypotension are obvious signs of an anaphylactic reaction. You must immediately administer epinephrine in order to counteract the effects of the insect stings, i.e. histamine release. If available, ALS providers should be requested. If not available, transport to the nearest appropriate facility should occur without delay. With the presence of multiple stings, this patient will likely need repeat doses of epinephrine as well as the administration of antihistamines, breathing treatments, and possibly advanced airway maneuvers. Your partner should apply high-flow oxygen and remove any remaining stingers in the neck or face by scraping them from the skin. Your prompt action is essential to patient survival.

2. This patient is suffering from hypoglycemia. Although this patient is confused, he is able to talk and swallow. Some states allow EMT-B's to perform blood glucose tests, and this would provide information regarding this patient's blood glucose level. If your local protocols do not allow for this skill, you can gather much information about this patient through his physical signs and medical history (all indicative of low blood sugar). You should administer (at least) one tube of oral glucose and reassess his mentation and vital signs. Provide treatment and transport according to local protocols.

3. –Place patient in position of comfort.

  –Give 100% oxygen via nonrebreathing mask.

  –Check blood pressure!

  –Check expiration date on nitroglycerin.

  –Contact medical control for permission to assist patient with 1 nitroglycerin tablet SL.

  –Monitor vital signs.

  –Rapid transport.

Chapter 11: Respiratory Emergencies

Matching

1. B (page 373)
2. D (page 369)
3. H (page 370)
4. J (page 372)
5. L (page 374)
6. C (page 373)
7. G (page 368)
8. E (page 370)
9. M (page 389)
10. A (page 370)
11. K (page 376)
12. F (page 373)
13. I (page 375)

Multiple Choice

1. D (page 384)
2. C (page 366)
3. D (page 368)
4. C (page 366)
5. B (page 367)
6. D (page 368)
7. B (page 368)
8. A (page 389)
9. B (page 370)
10. A (page 369)
11. D (page 371)
12. A (page 372)
13. D (pages 372-373)
14. B (pages 372-373)
15. C (page 374)
16. C (page 373)
17. B (page 373)
18. D (pages 389-390)
19. C (page 374)
20. A (page 375)
21. B (page 376)
22. B (page 368)
23. D (page 377)
24. A (page 366)
25. D (page 384)
26. B (page 379)
27. D (page 392)
28. D (page 380)
29. C (page 385)
30. D (page 385)
31. D (page 385)
32. C (page 390)

Labeling

Obstruction, scarring, and dilation of the alveolar sac (page 372)

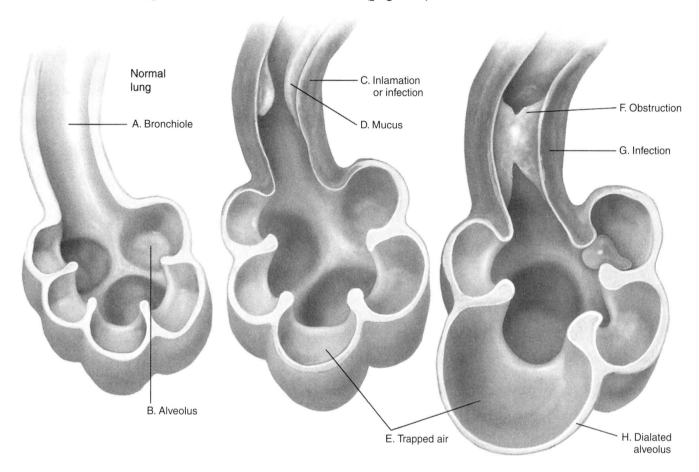

Normal lung

A. Bronchiole

C. Inlamation or infection

D. Mucus

F. Obstruction

G. Infection

B. Alveolus

E. Trapped air

H. Dialated alveolus

Fill-in

1. carbon dioxide (page 366)
2. oxygen (page 367)
3. Carbon dioxide, oxygen (page 368)
4. alveoli (page 366)
5. trachea (page 366)
6. 12, 20 (page 367)
7. carbon dioxide (page 366)
8. breathing status (page 379)
9. transport decision (page 379)
10. SAMPLE, OPQRST (page 380)

True/False

1. F (page 370)
2. T (page 373)
3. F (page 373)
4. F (page 373)
5. T (page 375)
6. T (page 376)

7. F (page 376)
8. T (page 389)
9. F (pages 373 & 379)
10. T (page 370)
11. T (page 378)
12. T (page 382)

Short Answer

1. 1. Normal rate and depth
   2. Regular pattern of inhalation and exhalation
   3. Good audible breath sounds on both sides of the chest
   4. Regular rise and fall on both sides of the chest
   5. Pink, warm, dry skin (page 367)

2. 1. Pulmonary vessels are obstructed from absorbing oxygen and releasing carbon dioxide by fluid, infection, or collapsed air spaces.
   2. Damaged alveoli
   3. Air passages obstructed by muscle spasm, mucus, weakened airway walls
   4. Blood flow to the lungs obstructed
   5. Pleural space is filled with air or excess fluid (page 368)

3. 1. Patient is unable to coordinate administration and inhalation.
   2. Inhaler is not prescribed for patient.
   3. You did not obtain permission from medical control or local protocol.
   4. Patient has already met maximum prescribed dose before your arrival. (page 385)

4. An ongoing irritation of the respiratory tract; excess mucus production obstructs small airways and alveoli. Protective mechanisms are impaired. Repeated episodes of irritation and pneumonia can cause scarring and alveolar damage, leading to COPD. (page 370)

5. 1. Respiratory rate of slower than 12 breaths/min or faster than 20 breaths/min
   2. Muscle retractions above the clavicles between ribs, below rib cage, especially in children
   3. Pale or cyanotic skin
   4. Cool, damp (clammy) skin
   5. Shallow or irregular respirations
   6. Pursed lips
   7. Nasal flaring (pages 379)

6. A condition characterized by a chronically high blood level of carbon dioxide in which the respiratory center no longer responds to high blood levels of carbon dioxide. In these patients, low blood oxygen causes the respiratory center to respond and stimulate respiration. If the arterial level of oxygen is then raised, as happens when the patient is given additional oxygen, there is no longer any stimulus to breathe; both the high carbon dioxide and low oxygen drives are lost. (page 368)

7. 1. Is the air going in?
   2. Does the chest expand with each breath?
   3. Does the chest fall with each breath?
   4. Is the rate adequate for the age of your patient? (page 378)

Word Fun

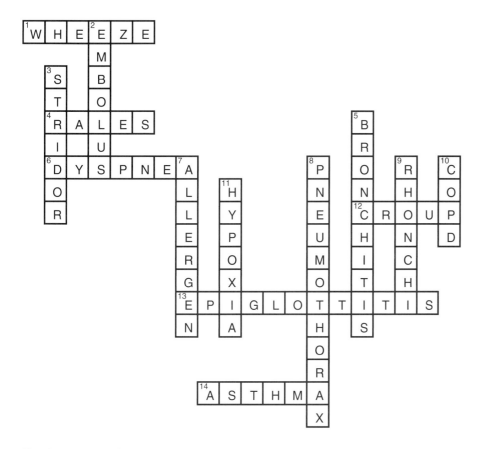

Ambulance Calls

1. This child has all the classics signs of epiglottitis. You should do nothing to excite or frighten the child as doing so will likely cause his airway to spasm and close. Remember to use non-threatening body language (place yourself below his or her eye level), give the child distance (until you establish trust) and perform any exam using the toe-to-head method. This is a true emergency that requires immediate transport to the hospital, but you must do so tactfully. Use parents to assist with patient care efforts such as applying humidified oxygen (blow-by or mask).

2. This patient's chief complaint, age, weight, smoking and birth control use all place her at risk of pulmonary embolism. PE patients most often experience a sudden onset of shortness of breath that they describe as sharp and worsening with inspiration. You should provide high flow oxygen, obtain vital signs, perform a secondary exam en route to the hospital (including auscultation of lung sounds) and prompt transport to the nearest appropriate facility.

3. –Place patient in position of comfort.
   –Provide high-flow oxygen via nonrebreathing mask.
   –Monitor vital signs.
   –Provide rapid transport.

Skill Drills

Skill Drill 11-1: Assisting a Patient With a Metered-Dose Inhaler (page 388)

1. Ensure inhaler is at room temperature or **warmer**.
2. Remove oxygen mask. Hand inhaler to patient. Instruct about breathing and **lip seal**.
3. Instruct patient to press inhaler and inhale. Instruct about **breath holding**.
4. Reapply **oxygen**. After a few **breaths**, have patient repeat **dose** if order/protocol allows.

Assessment Review

1. D (page 392)
2. B (page 393)
3. A (page 392)
4. B (page 393)
5. D (page 393)

Emergency Care Summary

Respiratory Distress

nonrebreathing
10 to 15
oropharyngeal
nasopharyngeal

Asthma

metered-dose
expiration date
exhale

Infection of Upper or Lower Airway

humidified

Acute Pulmonary Edema

ventilatory support

Chronic Obstructive Pulmonary Disease

full-flow
15 L

Spontaneous Pneumothorax

supplemental

Pleural Effusions

high-flow

Obstruction of the Upper Airway

BLS

Pulmonary Embolism

cardiac arrest

Hyperventilation

respirations
(page 393)

Chapter 12: Cardiovascular Emergencies

Matching

1. L (page 402)
2. C (page 403)
3. O (page 403)
4. G (page 403)
5. N (page 403)
6. K (page 404)
7. H (page 402)
8. M (page 402)
9. B (page 405)
10. D (page 409)
11. F (page 404)
12. I (page 407)
13. J (page 410)
14. A (page 410)
15. E (page 410)

Multiple Choice

1. D (page 402)
2. D (page 402)
3. A (page 402)
4. B (page 402)
5. A (page 403)
6. B (page 404)
7. C (page 404)
8. A (page 404)
9. C (page 404)
10. A (page 405)
11. B (page 407)
12. B (page 407)
13. D (page 408)
14. B (page 408)
15. D (page 408)
16. D (page 408)
17. C (page 408)
18. C (page 408)
19. C (page 408)
20. C (page 409)
21. D (page 409)
22. D (page 409)
23. A (page 409)
24. A (page 412)
25. D (page 411)
26. B (page 412)
27. C (page 409)
28. C (page 413)
29. B (page 414)
30. C (page 415)
31. D (page 415)
32. D (page 415)
33. C (page 415)
34. B (page 419)
35. D (page 419)
36. C (page 421)
37. C (page 421)
38. B (page 421)
39. C (page 422)
40. D (page 421)
41. D (page 423)
42. A (page 432)
43. B (page 426)
44. C (page 427)
45. C (page 429)

Labeling

1. The Right and Left Sides of Heart (page 403)

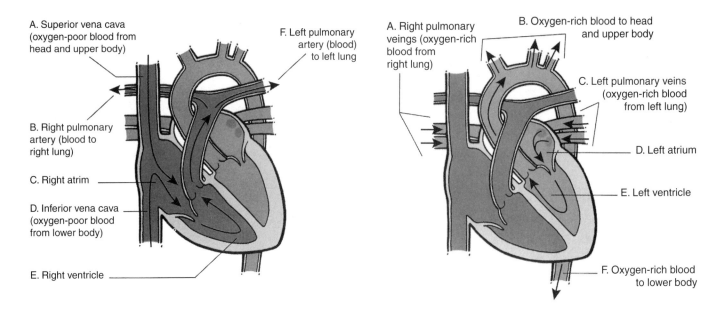

A. Superior vena cava (oxygen-poor blood from head and upper body)

F. Left pulmonary artery (blood) to left lung

B. Right pulmonary artery (blood to right lung)

C. Right atrim

D. Inferior vena cava (oxygen-poor blood from lower body)

E. Right ventricle

A. Right pulmonary veings (oxygen-rich blood from right lung)

B. Oxygen-rich blood to head and upper body

C. Left pulmonary veins (oxygen-rich blood from left lung)

D. Left atrium

E. Left ventricle

F. Oxygen-rich blood to lower body

2. Electrical Conduction (page 403)

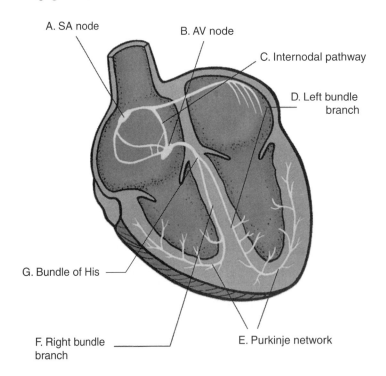

A. SA node

B. AV node

C. Internodal pathway

D. Left bundle branch

G. Bundle of His

F. Right bundle branch

E. Purkinje network

3. Pulse Points (page 406)

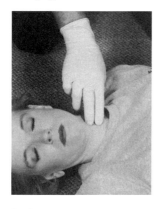

A. Carotid

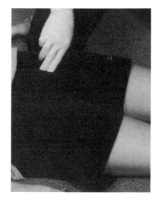

B. Femoral

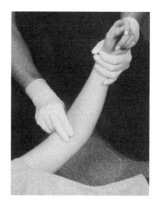

C. Brachial

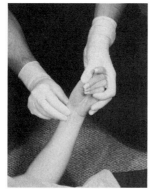

D. Radial

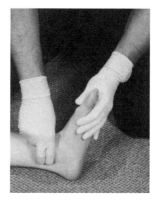

E. Posterior tibial

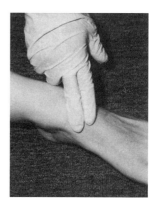

F. Dorsalis pedis

Fill-in

1. septum (page 402)
2. aorta (page 402)
3. right (page 402)
4. AV (page 403)
5. dilation (page 403)
6. Red blood (page 404)
7. Diastolic (page 404)
8. four (page 402)
9. left (page 402)

True/False

1. F (page 402)
2. F (page 403)
3. T (page 405)
4. F (page 407)
5. T (page 408)
6. F (page 408)
7. F (page 415)
8. F (page 424)
9. T (page 408)
10. F (page 404)
11. T (page 420)
12. T (page 420)

Short Answer

1. Automated: Operator needs only to apply pads and turn on the machine. It performs all functions for analyzing and shocking. This type of defibrillator often has a computer voice synthesizer to advise the EMT which steps to take.

   Semi-automated: Operator applies pads, turns on the machine, and pushes button to shock. (pages 420–421)

2. 1. Not having a charged battery
   2. Applying the AED to a patient who is moving
   3. Applying the AED to a responsive patient with a rapid heart rate (page 421)

3. **1.** If the patient regains a pulse

   2. After six to nine shocks have been delivered

   3. If the machine gives three consecutive "no shock" messages (page 427)

4. **1.** Place pads correctly.

   2. Make sure no one is touching the patient.

   3. Do not defibrillate a patient who is in pooled water.

   4. Dry the chest before defibrillating a wet patient.

   5. Do not defibrillate a patient who is touching metal that others are touching.

   6. Remove nitroglycerin patches and wipe the area with a dry towel before defibrillation. (pages 426-427)

5. **1.** Obtain an order from medical direction.

   2. Take the patient's blood pressure; continue with administration only if the systolic blood pressure is greater than 100 mm Hg.

   3. Check that you have the right medication, right patient, and right delivery route.

   4. Check the expiration date of the nitroglycerin.

   5. Question the patient about the last dose he or she took and its effects.

   6. Be prepared to have the patient lie down.

   7. Give the medication sublingually.

   8. Advise the patient to keep his or her mouth closed to allow the medication to dissolve.

   9. Recheck blood pressure within 5 minutes.

  10. Record each medication and the time of administration.

  11. Perform continued assessment. (page 417)

6. **1.** It may or may not be caused by exertion, but can occur at any time.

   2. It does not resolve in a few minutes.

   3. It may or may not be relieved by rest or nitroglycerin. (page 408)

7. **1.** Sudden death

   2. Cardiogenic shock

   3. Congestive heart failure (page 409)

8. **1.** Sudden onset of weakness, nausea, or sweating without an obvious cause

   2. Chest pain/discomfort that does not change with each breath

   3. Pain in lower jaw, arms, or neck

   4. Sudden arrhythmia with syncope

   5. Pulmonary edema

   6. Sudden death

   7. Increased and/or irregular pulse

   8. Normal, increased, or decreased blood pressure

   9. Normal or labored respirations

  10. Pale or gray skin

  11. Feelings of apprehension (pages 408-409)

9. Remove clothing from the patient's chest area. Apply the pads to the chest: one just to the right of the sternum, just below the clavicle, the other on the left chest with the top of the pad 2 to 3 inches below the armpit. Ensure that the pads are attached to the patient cables (and that they are attached to the AED in some models). (page 426)

Word Fun

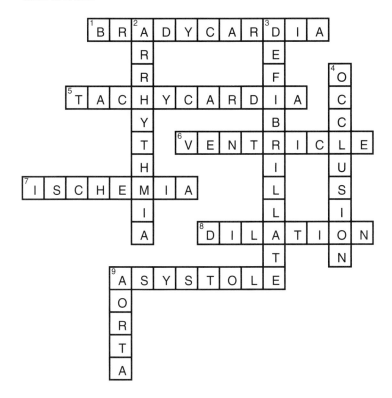

Ambulance Calls

1. –Place patient in the position of comfort.
   –Provide high-flow oxygen via nonrebreathing mask.
   –Monitor vital signs.
   –Provide normal transport.

2. Denial is one of the biggest indicators of heart attack. Although this patient is considered "younger" and otherwise healthy, he is having signs and symptoms of a myocardial infarction. It may take some convincing of the need for treatment and transport, but you must be clear on the potential consequences of his refusal of care (informed refusal). If he initially refuses, explain what physical signs you see that lead you to believe he is likely having a heart attack, express genuine concern for his well-being and speak directly with medical control. More often than not, when patients hear the same or similar information from a physician, it makes a different impact. If he allows you to examine, treat and transport him, apply high-flow oxygen, transport promptly and follow local protocols.

3. This patient could be having a heart attack. A common symptom that women (especially post-menopausal women) experience when having a heart attack is the sudden onset of generalized weakness. Although chest pain is a common indicator of heart attack, if a patient is not experiencing pain or pressure it does not necessarily mean they are not experiencing a cardiac event. It is important to note that heart disease is the number one killer of women in the United States, taking more lives than cancer and killing more women than men every year. If your patient exhibits any combination of the "associated symptoms" of heart attack such as nausea, vomiting, shortness of breath, pain or numbness in the neck, jaw, back, arm(s) or cool, pale, sweaty skin, you should suspect the possibility of a heart attack. You should apply high-flow oxygen, obtain vital signs, allow the patient to maintain a position of comfort, and provide immediate transport to the nearest appropriate facility.

Skill Drills

Skill Drill 12-2: AED and CPR (pages 428–429)

1. Stop CPR if in progress.
   Assess responsiveness.
   Check breathing and pulse.
   If unresponsive and not breathing adequately, give two slow ventilations.

2. If pulseless, begin CPR.
   Prepare the AED pads.
   Turn on the AED; begin narrative if needed.

3. Apply AED pads.
   Stop CPR.

4. Verbally and visually clear the patient.
   Push the Analyze button if there is one.
   Wait for the AED to analyze rhythm.
   If no shock advised, perform CPR for 1 minute.
   If shock advised, recheck that all are clear and push the Shock button.
   Push the Analyze button, if needed, to analyze rhythm again.
   Press Shock if advised (second shock).
   Push the Analyze button, if needed, to analyze rhythm again.
   Press Shock if advised (third shock).

5. Check pulse.
   If pulse is present, check breathing.
   Gather additional information on the arrest event.

6. If breathing adequately, give oxygen and transport.
   If not, open airway, ventilate, and transport.
   If no pulse, perform CPR for 1 minute.
   Clear the patient and analyze again.
   If necessary, repeat one cycle of up to three shocks.
   Transport and call medical control.
   Continue to support breathing or perform CPR, as needed.

Assessment Review

1. D (page 432)   **4.** D (page 432)
2. A (page 432)   **5.** D (page 432)
3. D (page 432)

Emergency Care Summary

Chest Pain	Cardiac Arrest
Nitroglycerin	Defibrillation
systolic	pulseless
100	apnea
dose	two
fainting	pocket mask
underneath	pads
5	breastbone
100	collarbone
	analyze
	rhythm
	nonrebreathing
	1
	arrest event
	three
	(page 433)

Chapter 13: Neurologic Emergencies

Matching

1. D (page 440)   **8.** C (page 442)
2. G (page 441)   **9.** M (page 451)
3. E (page 441)   **10.** H (page 451)
4. B (page 440)   **11.** L (page 444)
5. I (page 441)   **12.** K (page 442)
6. F (page 441)   **13.** A (page 444)
7. J (page 442)

Multiple Choice

1. D (page 440)   **16.** C (page 457)
2. A (page 440)   **17.** D (page 457)
3. A (page 441)   **18.** D (pages 457-458)
4. C (page 442)   **19.** B (page 444)
5. C (page 442)   **20.** D (page 444)
6. A (page 442)   **21.** A (pages 444-445)
7. B (page 442)   **22.** B (page 445)
8. B (page 443)   **23.** C (page 428)
9. D (page 444)   **24.** C (page 445)
10. A (page 451)   **25.** A (page 445)
11. D (page 451)   **26.** D (page 448)
12. D (page 453)   **27.** D (pages 442-443)
13. D (page 451)   **28.** A (page 443)
14. C (page 440)   **29.** D (page 451)
15. B (page 457)

Labeling

1. Brain (page 441)

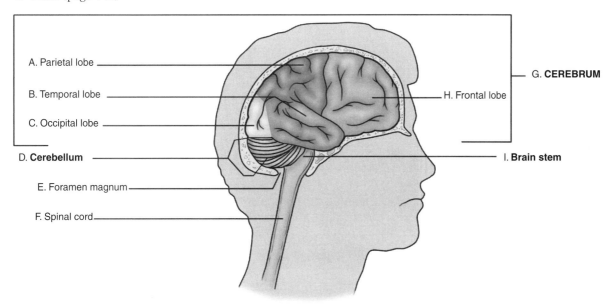

2. Spinal Cord (page 441)

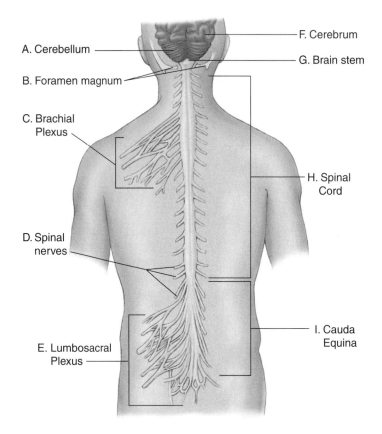

A. Cerebellum
B. Foramen magnum
C. Brachial Plexus
D. Spinal nerves
E. Lumbosacral Plexus
F. Cerebrum
G. Brain stem
H. Spinal Cord
I. Cauda Equina

Fill-in

1. twelve (page 441)
2. cerebellum (page 440)
3. emotion and thought (page 440)
4. head (page 441)
5. three (page 440)
6. nerves (page 441)
7. opposite, same (page 440)
8. cerebrum (page 440)
9. Incontinence (page 452)
10. brain (page 440)
11. epidural (page 445)
12. hemiparesis (page 452)
13. altered mental status (page 458)

True/False

1. F (page 444)
2. F (page 451)
3. T (page 451)
4. F (page 451)
5. T (page 452)
6. F (page 444)

Short Answer

1. **1.** Facial droop—Ask patient to show teeth or smile.
2. Arm drift—Ask patient to close eyes and hold arms out with palms up.
3. Speech—Ask patient to say, "The sky is blue in Cincinnati." (page 448)

2. Newer clot-busting therapies may be helpful in reversing damage in certain kinds of strokes, but treatment must be started within 3 hours after onset of the event. (page 450)

3. A period of time after a seizure, generally lasting from 5 to 30 minutes, that is characterized by some degree of altered mental status and labored respirations (page 452)

4. Infarcted cells are dead. Ischemic cells are still alive, although they are not functioning properly because of hypoxia. (page 442)

5. **1.** Hypoglycemia
2. Postictal state
3. Subdural or epidural bleeding (pages 444-445)

Word Fun

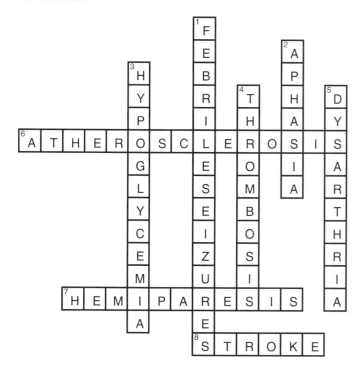

Ambulance Calls

1. Given these signs, your patient is likely experiencing a left hemispheric stroke. Any problems related to his ability to understand or use language will be frustrating for both you and the patient. After performing your initial assessment, the Cincinnati Stoke Scale can provide valuable information regarding the presence of a stroke. This assessment measures abnormalities in speech and the presence of facial droop and arm drift. Stroke is a true emergency that requires prompt transport. You should apply high-flow oxygen and take care during transport to prevent injury of affected body parts as the patient will not be able to protect them on their own. It is helpful to place the patient on the affected side and elevate their heads approximately 6" to facilitate swallowing. Be sure to relate your positive findings of stroke to the hospital to avoid any unnecessary delays in patient care upon arrival to the emergency department.

2. Maintain the airway—high-flow oxygen.
Suction if necessary or position lateral recumbent to clear secretions.
Check glucose level.
Provide rapid transport.

3. This patient's signs and symptoms cause you to suspect the presence of a hemorrhagic stroke. You should apply high-flow oxygen and provide immediate transport. This patient will be more likely to experience seizure activity than patients suffering from ischemic stroke. There is no way for you to determine the type or extent of her stroke, as this can be accomplished only in the hospital. Your job is to recognize the seriousness of the situation, provide supportive measures within your scope of practice, and provide prompt transport and notification to the receiving facility.

Assessment Review

1. D (page 459)
2. B (page 459)
3. D (page 459)
4. D (page 459)
5. C (page 459)

Emergency Care Summary
Stroke
teeth
arm drift
Cincinnati

Seizure
Spontaneous
Inappropriate words
Withdraws to pain
Glasgow Coma Scale score

Altered Mental Status
Cincinnati Stroke Scale
Glasgow Coma Scale
(page 460)

Chapter 14: The Acute Abdomen

Matching

1. I (page 469)		**9.** F (page 470)	
2. D (page 466)		**10.** B (page 466)	
3. E (page 466)		**11.** G (page 469)	
4. M (page 467)		**12.** N (page 468)	
5. K (page 469)		**13.** L (page 470)	
6. A (page 470)		**14.** O (page 466)	
7. C (page 471)		**15.** H (page 466)	
8. J (page 470)			

Multiple Choice

1. C (page 470)	**9.** B (page 466)
2. A (page 470)	**10.** D (page 466)
3. A (page 469)	**11.** C (page 471)
4. A (page 466)	**12.** D (pages 468-469)
5. D (page 473)	**13.** B (page 471)
6. A (page 469)	**14.** C (page 469)
7. B (page 466)	**15.** A (page 474)
8. C (page 469)	**16.** C (page 476)

Labeling

1. Solid Organs (page 467)

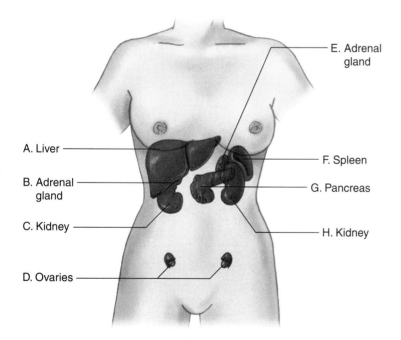

A. Liver
B. Adrenal gland
C. Kidney
D. Ovaries
E. Adrenal gland
F. Spleen
G. Pancreas
H. Kidney

2. Hollow Organs (page 467)

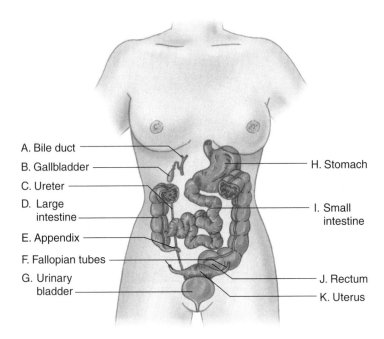

A. Bile duct
B. Gallbladder
C. Ureter
D. Large intestine
E. Appendix
F. Fallopian tubes
G. Urinary bladder

H. Stomach
I. Small intestine
J. Rectum
K. Uterus

3. Retroperitoneal Organs (page 467)

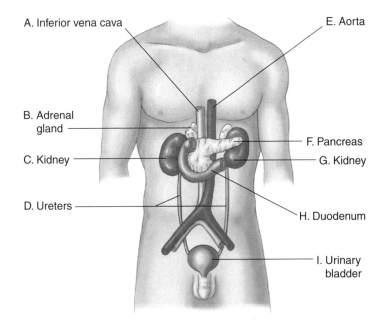

A. Inferior vena cava
B. Adrenal gland
C. Kidney
D. Ureters

E. Aorta
F. Pancreas
G. Kidney
H. Duodenum
I. Urinary bladder

True/False

1. F (page 466)
2. F (pages 468-469)
3. F (page 468)
4. F (page 466)
5. T (page 466)

6. F (page 471)
7. F (page 472)
8. T (page 469)
9. T (page 469)

Short Answer

1. Occurs because of connections between the body's two nervous systems. The abdominal organs are supplied by autonomic nerves, which, when irritated, stimulate close-lying sensory (somatic) nerves. (page 466)

2. No. It is too complex and treatment is the same. (page 466)

3. Paralysis of muscular contractions in the bowel results in retained gas and feces. Nothing can pass through. (page 470)

4. Bleeding and fluid shifts. (page 470)

5. 1. Explain to the patient what you are about to do.
   2. Place the patient in a supine position with the legs drawn up and flexed at the knees unless trauma is suspected.
   3. Determine whether the patient is restless or quiet, whether motion causes pain, or whether any characteristic position, distention, or obvious abnormality is present.
   4. Palpate the four quadrants of the abdomen.
   5. Determine whether the patient can relax the abdominal wall on command.
   6. Determine whether the abdomen is tender when palpated. (page 476)

Word Fun

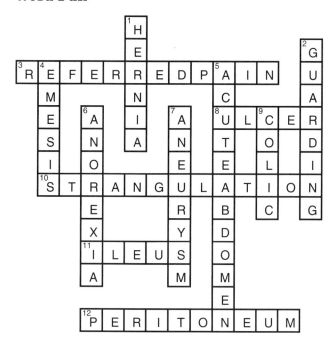

Ambulance Calls

1. Possible appendicitis.
   Place patient in the position of comfort.
   Apply high-flow oxygen.
   Keep patient warm.
   Rapid transport.
   Obtain a SAMPLE history.
   Document OPQRST.
   Monitor patient closely.

2. This patient has a bowel obstruction (fecal impaction) that is causing his pain and tenderness. If left untreated, his condition will deteriorate. When assessing his abdomen, explain what you will do, place him with knees slightly toward his abdomen and gently palpate all four quadrants to determine the presence of rigidity or masses. If a patient points to a specific location of pain, palpate that area last. You must take great care in moving and transporting him, as it will be particularly painful if he is bumped or jostled. Apply high-flow oxygen, allow him to find his position of comfort, and move him gently. Do not delay transport to attempt to determine the cause of abdominal pain.

3. Individuals who have experienced a kidney stone(s) will tell you that it is an extremely painful experience. Provide prompt, gentle transport. Monitor his airway, breathing and circulation, be prepared for continued vomiting, apply oxygen (which can ease nausea), obtain vital signs, do not give anything by mouth, and keep the patient as comfortable as possible. Be sure to thoroughly document all information regarding their signs and symptoms as well as any treatment you provide. Always follow local protocols.

Assessment Review

1. D (page 476)
2. A (page 476)
3. B (page 476)
4. C (page 470)
5. D (page 476)

Emergency Care Summary

supine
flexed
trauma
distention
abnormality
Palpate
quadrants
abdominal wall
palpated
(page 476)

Chapter 15: Diabetic Emergencies

Matching

1.	H (page 482)	**8.**	G (page 483)
2.	F (page 483)	**9.**	C (page 483)
3.	B (page 482)	**10.**	A (page 485)
4.	K (page 484)	**11.**	M (page 482)
5.	L (page 482)	**12.**	D (page 485)
6.	N (page 485)	**13.**	J (page 484)
7.	E (page 483)	**14.**	I (page 482)

Multiple Choice

1.	A (page 483)	**22.**	B (page 484)
2.	A (page 484)	**23.**	A (page 485)
3.	D (page 482)	**24.**	B (pages 484-485)
4.	C (page 482)	**25.**	C (page 487)
5.	B (page 482)	**26.**	D (page 485)
6.	A (page 484)	**27.**	A (page 493)
7.	C (page 483)	**28.**	A (page 490)
8.	D (page 482)	**29.**	D (page 490)
9.	D (page 485)	**30.**	D (page 408)
10.	B (page 483)	**31.**	B (page 485)
11.	B (page 486)	**32.**	C (page 485)
12.	B (page 483)	**33.**	A (page 487)
13.	D (page 483)	**34.**	D (page 485)
14.	A (page 482)	**35.**	A (page 485)
15.	A (page 482)	**36.**	C (page 492)
16.	A (page 483)	**37.**	C (page 485)
17.	C (page 483)	**38.**	D (page 483)
18.	B (page 484)	**39.**	C (page 488)
19.	B (page 484)	**40.**	D (page 494)
20.	D (page 483)	**41.**	A (page 488)
21.	C (page 485)	**42.**	D (page 488)

Fill-in

1.	diabetes mellitus (page 482)	**4.**	diabetic coma (page 485)
2.	autoimmune (page 483)	**5.**	sugar, insulin (pages 488-489)
3.	ineffective (page 483)		

True/False

1.	T (page 483)	**7.**	F (page 482)
2.	F (page 483)	**8.**	F (page 482)
3.	T (page 484)	**9.**	F (page 492)
4.	T (page 485)	**10.**	T (page 482)
5.	T (page 485)	**11.**	T (page 483)
6.	T (page 483)		

Short Answer

1. Insulin is a hormone that enables glucose to enter body cells. (page 482)
2. **1.** Glucose
   2. Insta-Glucose (page 488)
3. A patient who is unconscious or not able to swallow should not be given oral glucose. (page 490)
4. **1.** Diabinase
   2. Orinase
   3. Micronase
   4. Glucotrol (page 483)
5. **1.** Ketoacidosis
   2. Dehydration
   3. Hyperglycemia (page 485)
6. Kussmaul respirations; dehydration; fruity odor on breath; rapid, weak pulse; normal or slightly low blood pressure; varying degrees of unresponsiveness. (page 485)
7. Insulin shock; it develops rapidly as opposed to diabetic coma, which takes longer to develop. (page 484)
8. It will immediately benefit the patient in insulin shock and is unlikely to worsen the condition of the patient in a diabetic coma. (page 490)

Word Fun

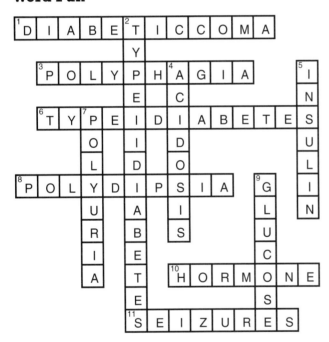

Ambulance Calls

1. Turn the patient on her side immediately or use suction to clear the airway.
   Insert an oral or nasal airway and apply high-flow oxygen.
   Attempt to obtain a blood glucose level.
   Transport patient rapidly, since you should never give anything by mouth to an unresponsive patient.
   Monitor the patient closely.
2. When experiencing hypoglycemia, diabetics can exhibit very strange behavior. Some family members can be quite surprised to see or hear their loved ones doing and saying things quite out of their normal behavior. When patients are experiencing low blood sugar, they may act as if they are intoxicated or mentally unstable. Perform a physical exam and look for clues regarding potential medical conditions. Some EMT-Bs can perform blood glucose testing, and this should be done for any patients with decreased levels of consciousness. If this patient is alert enough to swallow, administer oral glucose and provide prompt transport. Continue to monitor their ABCs for any changes.

3. You cannot give this patient anything by mouth as he is unconscious and therefore unable to protect his own airway. If available, you should request ALS providers, as they can administer intravenous dextrose (glucose). If you have no emergency providers available with this scope of practice within your system, you must transport this patient immediately. You may encounter family members who do not understand why you cannot "just give him some sugar." Hopefully, there will be no delays in explaining his need for transport or the seriousness of his condition. Perform a thorough assessment (including blood glucose testing if permitted), provide high-flow oxygen, monitor his ABCs (using airway adjuncts, positive pressure ventilations and suctioning as needed), and provide prompt transport.

Skill Drills
Skill Drill 15-1: Administering Glucose (page 491)
1. Make sure that the tube of glucose is intact and has not **expired**.
2. Squeeze a generous amount of oral glucose onto the **bottom third** of a **bite stick** or tongue depressor.
3. Open the patient's **mouth**. Place the tongue depressor on the **mucous membranes** between the cheek and the gum with the **gel side** next to the cheek. Repeat until the entire tube has been used.

Comparison Table

	Hyperglycemia	Hypoglycemia
History		
Food intake	Excessive	Insufficient
Insulin dosage	Insufficient	Excessive
Onset	Gradual (hours to days)	Rapid, within minutes
Skin	Warm and dry	Pale and moist
Infection	Common	Uncommon
Gastrointestinal Tract		
Thirst	Intense	Absent
Hunger	Absent	Intense
Vomiting	Common	Uncommon
Respiratory System		
Breathing	Rapid, deep (Kussmaul respirations)	Normal or rapid
Odor of breath	Sweet, fruity	Normal
Cardiovascular System		
Blood pressure	Normal to low	Low
Pulse	Normal or rapid and full	Rapid, weak
Nervous System		
Consciousness	Restless merging to coma	Irritability, confusion, seizure, or coma
Urine		
Sugar	Present	Absent
Acetone	Present	Absent
Treatment		
Response	Gradual, within 6 to 12 hours following medical treatment	Immediately after administration of glucose

Assessment Review

1. B (page 494)
2. B (page 494)
3. C (page 494)
4. D (page 494)
5. D (page 494)

Emergency Care Summary

expiration date

generous

third

mucous membranes

cheek

(page 494)

Chapter 16: Allergic Reactions and Envenomations

Matching

1. D (page 500)
2. A (page 500)
3. H (page 500)
4. E (page 500)
5. B (page 505)
6. G (page 500)
7. C (page 502)
8. F (page 502)

Multiple Choice

1. A (page 508)
2. D (page 500)
3. A (page 500)
4. D (page 502)
5. C (pages 505-506)
6. B (page 503)
7. D (page 505)
8. C (page 508)
9. D (page 507)
10. C (page 502)
11. A (page 503)
12. D (page 513)
13. C (page 501)
14. C (page 500)
15. A (page 500)
16. C (page 500)
17. B (page 500)
18. D (page 512)
19. D (page 508)
20. D (page 508)

Fill-in

1. bronchial passages (page 500)
2. urticaria (page 500)
3. barbed (page 501)
4. anaphylactic (page 500)
5. hypoperfusion (page 505)
6. bronchioles (page 507)
7. imminent death (page 500)

True/False

1. T (page 500)
2. T (page 500)
3. T (page 500)
4. F (page 504)

Short Answer

1. Increased blood pressure, tachycardia, pallor, dizziness, chest pain, headache, nausea, vomiting (page 512)

2. 1. Insect bites/stings
   2. Medications
   3. Plants
   4. Food
   5. Chemicals (pages 500-501)

3. 1. Obtain order from medical control.
   2. Follow BSI techniques.
   3. Make sure medication was prescribed for that patient.
   4. Check for discoloration or expiration of medications.
   5. Remove cap.
   6. Wipe thigh with alcohol if possible.
   7. Place tip against lateral midthigh.
   8. Push firmly until activation.
   9. Hold in place until medication is injected.
   10. Remove and dispose.
   11. Record the time and dose.
   12. Reassess and record patient's vital signs. (page 508)

4. Respiratory: Sneezing or itchy, runny nose; chest or throat tightness; dry cough; hoarseness; rapid, noisy, or labored respirations; wheezing and/or stridor

   Circulatory: Decreased blood pressure; increased pulse (initially); pale skin and dizziness; loss of consciousness and coma (page 506)

Word Fun

Ambulance Calls

1. Scene safety is not an issue in this case as it was a police dog that caused the patient's injuries. Rabies is a non-issue as well, because this dog has been inoculated. Because there is still the chance for infection and the need for wound care/sutures, the patient should be evaluated by a physician. You should cover the wound with sterile dressings and provide transport to the emergency department.

2. Based on the information you have, there is no way to determine if the child fell out of the tree or climbed down. You should assume that the child fell, which will require the use of full spinal precautions. You also have the issue of scene safety, as the damaged hive is now lying on the ground next to the patient. You must take care not to receive multiple stings yourself, so proceed with caution. If the child is having a severe allergic reaction, hopefully you will have access to an EpiPen Junior. Provide high flow oxygen and prompt transport according to local protocols.

3. –Check the EpiPen for clarity, expiration date, etc.
   –Obtain a physician's order to administer the EpiPen to the patient.
   –Administer the EpiPen and promptly dispose of auto-injector.
   –Apply high-flow oxygen.
   –Rapid transport.
   –Monitor the patient and assess vital signs frequently.

Skill Drills

Skill Drill 16-1: Using an Auto-injector (page 509)

1. Remove the auto-injector's **safety cap**, and quickly wipe the thigh with **antiseptic**.
2. Place the tip of the auto-injector against the **lateral** part of the thigh.
3. Push the **injector** firmly against the **thigh**, and hold it in place until all the medication is injected.

Skill Drill 16-2: Using an AnaKit (pages 510-511)

1. Prepare the injection site with antiseptic, and remove the needle cover.
2. Hold the syringe upright, and carefully use the plunger to remove air.
3. Turn the plunger one-quarter turn.
4. Quickly insert the needle into the muscle.
5. Hold the syringe steady, and push the plunger until it stops.
6. Have the patient chew and swallow the Chlo-Amine antihistamine tablets provided in the kit.
7. If available, apply a cold pack to the sting site.

Assessment Review

1. A (page 513)
2. D (page 513)
3. D (page 513)
4. C (page 513)
5. D (page 513)

Emergency Care Summary

Using an Auto-injector

lateral

10

Using an AnaKit

upright

one-quarter

muscle

antihistamine

cold pack

(page 513)

Chapter 17: Substance Abuse and Poisoning

Matching

1. F (page 518)
2. H (page 518)
3. G (page 519)
4. D (page 528)
5. J (page 533)
6. I (page 518)
7. K (page 529)
8. E (page 531)
9. B (page 518)
10. A (page 528)
11. C (page 532)

Multiple Choice

1. B (page 523)
2. B (page 518)
3. D (page 536)
4. C (page 533)
5. D (pages 518-519)
6. C (page 520)
7. C (page 527)
8. B (pages 528-529)
9. C (page 529)
10. D (page 530)
11. A (page 532)
12. C (page 531)
13. D (page 533)
14. B (page 535)
15. A (page 521)
16. D (page 531)
17. D (page 533)
18. D (page 532)
19. B (page 531)
20. D (page 521)
21. C (page 521)
22. B (page 521)
23. C (page 523)
24. D (page 522)
25. A (page 524)
26. D (page 528)
27. D (page 529)
28. A (page 521)
29. D (page 521)
30. D (page 522)
31. D (page 523)
32. A (page 520)
33. C (page 520)
34. C (page 538)
35. D (page 527)
36. B (page 527)
37. C (page 527)
38. D (page 527)

Fill-in

1. ABCs (pages 521-522)
2. alcohol (page 528)
3. adsorbing (page 527)
4. 5 to 10 minutes, 15 to 20 minutes (page 522)
5. respiratory depression (page 529)
6. hypoglycemia (page 528)
7. recognize (page 520)
8. 1 gram, kilogram (page 527)
9. outward (page 522)
10. ingestion (page 522)
11. delirium tremens (DTs) (page 529)
12. ignite (page 522)
13. addiction (page 522)
14. Hypovolemia (page 529)

True/False

1. T (page 527)

2. F (pages 520-523)

3. F (page 527)

4. F (page 521)

5. F (page 523)

6. T (page 529)

7. T (page 533)

8. F (page 528)

9. T (page 529)

10 T (page 532)

Short Answer

1. Activated charcoal adsorbs (binds to) the toxin and keeps it from being absorbed in the gastrointestinal tract. (page 523)

2. **1.** Ingestion

　　2. Inhalation

　　3. Injection

　　4. Absorption (page 521)

3. Hypertension, tachycardia, dilated pupils, and agitation/seizures (page 531)

4. **1.** The organism itself causes the disease.

　　2. The organism produces toxins that cause disease. (page 534)

5. Symptoms of acetaminophen overdose do not appear until the damage is irreversible, up to a week later. Finding evidence at the scene can save a patient's life. (page 533)

6. They describe patient presentation in cholinergic poisoning (organophosphate insecticides, wild mushrooms).
DUMBELS: Defecation, urination, miosis, bronchorrhea, emesis, lacrimation, salivation
SLUDGE: Salivation, lacrimation, urination, defecation, gastrointestinal irritation, eye constriction/emesis (page 533)

7. **1.** Opioid analgesics

　　2. Sedative-hypnotics

　　3. Inhalants

　　4. Sympathomimetics

　　5. Hallucinogens

　　6. Anticholinergic agents

　　7. Cholinergic agents (pages 528-533)

8. **1.** What substance did you take?

　　2. When did you take it or become exposed to it?

　　3. How much did you ingest?

　　4. What actions have been taken?

　　5. How much do you weigh? (page 518)

9. Because they ignite when they come into contact with water (page 522)

Word Fun

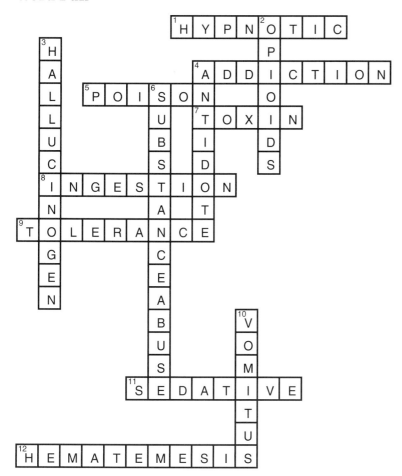

Ambulance Calls

1. You should attempt to identify the substance. Some rat poisons are actually "blood thinning agents" or anticoagulants, such as Coumadin. You should collect the substance and call the poison control center (1-800-222-1222) and/or the hospital emergency department for patient care instructions. Some substances require the administration of activated charcoal, while others do not. Perform your initial assessment, and provide high flow oxygen (blow by) and prompt transport. Know your local protocols.

2. This patient obviously abuses alcohol and illegal substances. However, you cannot automatically assume that his decrease in mentation is directly related to alcohol intoxication or influence of other substances. He may have other medical conditions, which may mimic intoxication or even be obscured by it. You should perform a thorough assessment including vital signs, monitor his ABCs (as these could change at any time), and transport to the nearest appropriate medical facility for evaluation. It is also important to be aware of the possibility of used needles when performing assessments and/or removal of clothing when visualizing any potential injuries. Protect yourself.

3. Maintain the airway with an adjunct and high-flow oxygen via BVM device or nonrebreathing mask with 100% oxygen. Monitor vital signs and provide supportive measures.
   Provide rapid transport.
   Take the pill bottle along to the emergency department.
   Be alert for possible vomiting.
   Monitor patient closely and be prepared for the possible need for CPR.

Assessment Review

1. B (page 538)
2. D (page 538)
3. C (page 538)
4. B (page 538)
5. A (page 538)

Emergency Care Summary

suctioning

high-flow oxygen

SAMPLE

vital signs

ALS

hallucinogens

cholinergic

plant

food

activated charcoal

altered mental status

swallow

12.5

50

Chapter 18: Environmental Emergencies

Matching

1. J (page 545)
2. H (page 564)
3. K (page 545)
4. F (page 554)
5. A (page 562)
6. N (page 546)
7. I (page 545)
8. C (page 560)
9. B (page 554)
10. E (page 545)
11. G (page 545)
12. M (page 553)
13. L (page 554)
14. D (page 560)

Multiple Choice

1. D (page 545)
2. A (page 545)
3. D (page 545)
4. C (page 546)
5. C (page 547)
6. D (page 546)
7. A (page 546)
8. C (page 547)
9. D (page 551)
10. D (pages 551-552)
11. A (page 554)
12. D (page 554)
13. D (page 554)
14. A (page 554)
15. D (page 555)
16. A (page 557)
17. A (page 557)
18. D (page 557)
19. B (page 560)
20. D (page 566)
21. C (page 562)
22. D (page 566)
23. B (page 562)
24. B (page 564)
25. A (page 564)
26. D (page 564)
27. A (page 564)
28. D (page 569)
29. A (page 573)
30. A (page 574)
31. D (page 572)
32. C (page 574)
33. D (page 569)
34. D (page 572)
35. D (page 555)
36. B (page 546)
37. A (page 545)
38. B (page 546)
39. D (page 551)

Fill-in

1. moderate to severe (pages 549-550)
2. ascent (page 564)
3. rewarming (page 552)
4. self-protection (page 553)
5. Shivering (page 564)
6. diving reflex (page 567)

True/False

1. T (page 553)
2. T (page 547)
3. F (page 546)
4. T (page 553)
5. T (page 554)
6. F (page 555)
7. T (page 567)
8. F (page 572)
9. F (page 572)
10. T (page 572)
11. F (page 574)
12. F (page 574)

Short Answer

1. **1.** Increase heat production: shiver, jump, walk around, etc.
   2. Move to another area where heat loss decreases: out of wind, into sun, etc.
   3. Wear insulated clothing: layer with wool, down, synthetics, etc. (pages 545-546)
2. **1.** Move the patient out of the hot environment and into the ambulance.
   2. Set air conditioning to maximum cooling.
   3. Remove patient's clothing.
   4. Administer high-flow oxygen.
   5. Apply cool packs to patient's neck, groin, and armpits.
   6. Cover patient with wet towels, or spray with cool water and fan.
   7. Keep fanning.
   8. Transport immediately.
   9. Notify the hospital. (pages 555-556)
3. An air embolism is a bubble of air in the blood vessels caused by breath-holding during rapid ascent. The resulting high pressure in the lungs causes alveolar rupture. (page 564)
4. Treatment of air embolism and decompression sickness (page 565)
5. **1.** Remove the patient from the cold.
   2. Handle injured part gently and protect from further injury.
   3. Administer oxygen.
   4. Remove wet or restricting clothing. (page 552)
6. **1.** Do not break blisters.
   2. Do not rub or massage area.
   3. Do not apply heat or rewarm unless instructed by medical control.
   4. Do not allow patient to stand or walk on a frostbitten foot. (page 552)
7. **1.** Have the patient lie flat and stay quiet.
   2. Wash the bite area with soapy water.
   3. Splint the extremity.
   4. Mark the skin with a pen to monitor advancing swelling. (page 572)
8. Black widow: Bite has a systemic effect (venom is neurotoxic).
   Brown recluse: Bite destroys tissue locally (venom is cytotoxic). (pages 569-570)

Word Fun

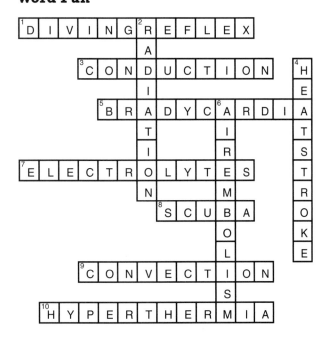

Ambulance Calls

1. Provide BLS.
   Administer oxygen.
   Transport the patient in the left lateral recumbent position with the head down.
   Transport to a facility with hyperbaric chamber access.

2. Your main concern for this patient is hypothermia. Although this patient could also likely have localized cold injuries such as frostbite or frostnip, hypothermia can be fatal. You must handle this patient carefully, remove them from the cold environment, remove any wet clothing, and prevent further heat loss. Assessing the extent of the hypothermia through mentation will be difficult in this case, as your patient is likely confused. Take note of the presence of shivering (this protective mechanism stops at core temperatures <90° F), and if possible take their temperature (rectally). Assess airway, breathing and circulation; provide warm, humidified oxygen (if possible) and passive rewarming measures, such as increasing the heat in the patient compartment and prompt transport.

3. This patient has severe dehydration. Her use of diuretics and laxatives combined with strenuous exercise and a "body wrap," have depleted her body's volume. There is also the possibility that she is suffering from hyperthermia, as her lack of fluids will affect her body's thermoregulatory mechanisms. She needs fluid replacement therapy and assessment of her core temperature. You should remove excess layers of clothing (in this case, the body wrap), give high flow oxygen, encourage oral fluid replacement if fully alert, and provide non-aggressive cooling measures.

Skill Drills

Skill Drill 18-1: Treating for Heat Exhaustion (page 556)

1. Remove **extra clothing**.

2. Move the patient to a **cooler environment**.
   Give **oxygen**.
   Place the patient in a **supine** position, elevate the legs, and **fan** the patient.

3. If the patient is **fully alert**, give water by mouth.

4. If nausea develops, **transport** on the side.

Skill Drill 18-2: Stabilizing a Suspected Spinal Injury in the Water (page 563)

1. Turn the patient to a supine position by rotating the entire upper half of the body as a single unit.

2. As soon as the patient is turned, begin artificial ventilation using the mouth-to-mouth method or a pocket mask.

3. Float a buoyant backboard under the patient.

4. Secure the patient to the backboard.

5. Remove the patient from the water.

6. Cover the patient with a blanket and apply oxygen if breathing. Begin CPR if breathing and pulse are absent.

Assessment Review

1. B (page 576)
2. A (page 576)
3. B (page 576)
4. B (page 576)
5. C (page 578)

Emergency Care Summary

Cold Injuries

Insulate

convection

cold environment

Heat Injuries

oxygen

supine

elevated

fan

liter

nausea

left-lateral

Drowning and Diving Injuries

supine

pocket-mask

backboard

oxygen

Lightning Injuries

conscious

cardiac arrest

cardiac arrest

Spider Bites

BLS

rigidity

spider

Snake Bites

plunger

one-quarter

muscle

antihistamine

cold pack

Injuries From Marine Animals

discharge

reduce

vinegar

credit card

(page 578)

Chapter 19: Behavioral Emergencies

Matching

1. C (page 584)
2. F (page 588)
3. B (page 586)
4. D (page 585)
5. E (page 586)
6. A (page 584)

Multiple Choice

1. D (page 584)
2. B (page 584)
3. D (page 584)
4. B (page 585)
5. A (page 585)
6. B (page 585)
7. A (page 584)
8. D (page 585)
9. C (page 586)
10. D (page 586)
11. A (page 586)
12. B (page 590)
13. D (page 586)
14. B (page 587)
15. D (page 588)
16. C (page 590)
17. A (page 590)
18. D (page 592)
19. D (page 592)
20. C (page 593)
21. B (page 593)
22. D (page 586)
23. B (page 585)
24. D (page 586)
25. D (page 592)
26. B (page 593)

Fill-in

1. Behavior (page 584)
2. behavioral crisis (page 584)
3. depression (page 585)
4. Organic brain syndrome (page 586)
5. suicide (page 590)

True/False

1. T (page 585)
2. F (page 586)
3. F (page 585)
4. F (page 593)
5. F (page 586)
6. F (page 589)
7. F (page 590)
8. T (page 592)
9. F (page 584)
10. F (page 590)
11. T (page 593)

Short Answer

1. A behavioral crisis is a temporary change in behavior that interferes with ADL or that is unacceptable to the patient or others. A mental health problem is this kind of behavioral change recurring on a regular basis. (page 584-585)

2.
   1. Improper functioning of the central nervous system.
   2. Drugs or alcohol
   3. Psychogenic circumstances (page 586)

3.
   1. The degree of force necessary to keep the patient from injuring self or others
   2. Patient's gender, size, strength, and mental status
   3. The type of abnormal behavior the patient is exhibiting (page 593)

4.
   1. Be prepared to spend extra time.
   2. Have a definite plan of action.
   3. Identify yourself calmly.
   4. Be direct.
   5. Assess the scene.
   6. Stay with the patient.
   7. Encourage purposeful movement.
   8. Express interest in the patient's story.
   9. Do not get too close to the patient.
   10. Avoid fighting with the patient.
   11. Be honest and reassuring.
   12. Do not judge. (page 586)

5.
   1. Depression at any age
   2. Previous suicide attempt
   3. Current expression of wanting to commit suicide or sense of hopelessness
   4. Family history of suicide
   5. Age older than 40 years, particularly for single, widowed, divorced, alcoholic, or depressed individuals
   6. Recent loss of spouse, significant other, family member, or support system
   7. Chronic debilitating illness or recent diagnosis of serious illness
   8. Holidays
   9. Financial setback, loss of job, police arrest, imprisonment, or some sort of social embarrassment
   10. Substance abuse, particularly with increasing usage
   11. Children of an alcoholic parent
   12. Severe mental illness
   13. Anniversary of death of loved one, job loss, marriage, etc.
   14. Unusual gathering or new acquisition of things that can cause death, such as purchase of a gun, a large volume of pills, or increased use of alcohol (page 590)

Word Fun

```
1              2
 A              F
 L              U
 T              N
 E              C
 R              T
3                            4
 B  E  H  A  V  I  O  R  A  L  C  R  I  S  I  S
 D              O        D
 M     5        
       M  E  N  T  A  L  D  I  S  O  R  D  E  R
 E              A
 N              L
 T              D
 A              I
 L              S
6                
 P  S  Y  C  H  O  G  E  N  I  C
 T              R
 A              7
                D  E  P  R  E  S  S  I  O  N
 T              E
 U              R
 S
```

Ambulance Calls

1. Removing restraints (especially when the patient has a known history of recent violence) is ill advised and potentially against local protocols. Restraints, although uncomfortable, afford you and your patient a safe environment. You should continually monitor the restraints to ensure they are not too tight and that no manner of restraints (whether applied initially by you in the field or by hospital personnel for an interfacility transport) affects the patient's ability to breathe. Know your local laws regarding the use of restraints and your local protocols for appropriate use and discontinuation.

2. Although he tells you that he is fine, you cannot simply walk away. Those individuals who contemplate suicide often tell people they are "fine." With information passed along by his sister, you must take action. Because there is no evidence that the patient has tried to harm himself and he did not express directly to you that he intends to, you must use persuasive techniques to gain consent to treatment and transport.

3. –Be understanding and listen.
   –Explain to the patient that she needs medical care.
   –Monitor vital signs and reassure patient en route.

Assessment Review

1. D (page 595)
2. A (page 595)
3. D (page 595)
4. D (page 595)
5. D (page 595)

Emergency Care Summary

control
safely transport
tension
emotional distress
violence
(page 595)

Chapter 20: Obstetric and Gynecologic Emergencies

Matching

1. D (page 600)		**9.** F (page 600)	
2. C (page 600)		**10.** O (page 616)	
3. L (page 600)		**11.** K (page 618)	
4. B (page 601)		**12.** I (page 602)	
5. N (page 600)		**13.** A (page 611)	
6. H (page 600)		**14.** G (page 616)	
7. M (page 600)		**15.** J (page 603)	
8. E (page 601)			

Multiple Choice

1. D (page 611)	**17.** B (page 603)
2. B (page 605)	**18.** B (page 603)
3. D (page 612)	**19.** D (page 602)
4. B (page 613)	**20.** C (page 602)
5. A (page 614)	**21.** D (page 603)
6. C (page 615)	**22.** D (page 618)
7. D (page 615)	**23.** C (page 603)
8. D (page 616)	**24.** B (page 603)
9. A (page 618)	**25.** A (page 603)
10. D (page 618)	**26.** C (page 620)
11. B (page 620)	**27.** D (page 602)
12. D (page 602)	**28.** C (page 608)
13. B (page 602)	**29.** C (page 602)
14. D (page 602)	**30.** C (page 611)
15. A (page 602)	**31.** D (page 613)
16. C (page 602)	

Tables

Apgar Scoring System

Area of Activity	Score		
	2	1	0
Appearance	Entire infant is pink.	Body is pink, but hands and feet remain blue.	Entire infant is blue and pale.
Pulse	More than 100 beats/min	Fewer than 100 beats/min	Absent pulse.
Grimace or Irritability	Infant cries and tries to move foot away from finger snapped against its sole.	Infant gives a weak cry in response to stimulus.	Infant does not cry or react to stimulus.
Activity or Muscle Tone	Infant resists attempts to straighten out hips and knees.	Infant makes weak attempts to resist straightening.	Infant is completely limp, with no muscle tone.
Respiration	Rapid respirations	Slow respirations	Absent respirations

Labeling

1. Anatomic Structures of the Pregnant Woman (page 600)

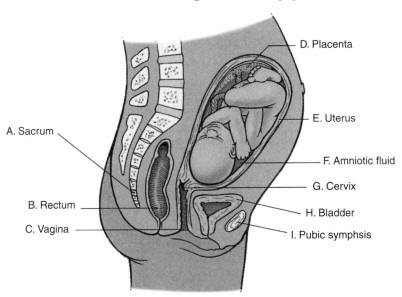

D. Placenta

E. Uterus

F. Amniotic fluid

G. Cervix

H. Bladder

I. Pubic symphsis

A. Sacrum

B. Rectum

C. Vagina

Fill-in

1. placenta (page 613)
2. arteries, vein (page 601)
3. 500 to 1000 mL (page 601)
4. 36, 40 (page 602)
5. trimesters (page 602)
6. body fluids (page 603)
7. ectopic pregnancy (page 603)
8. resuscitate (page 604)
9. fontanels (page 611)

True/False

1. T (page 600)
2. F (page 602)
3. F (page 602)
4. F (page 602)
5. F (page 607)
6. T (page 616)
7. T (page 612)
8. F (page 613)
9. F (page 613)
10. T (page 618)
11. T (page 620)

Short Answer

1. Early: spontaneous abortion (miscarriage) or ectopic pregnancy
   Later: Placenta previa or placenta abruptio (page 603)
2. On the left side, to prevent supine hypotensive syndrome (low blood pressure occurring from the weight of the fetus compressing the inferior vena cava) (page 603)

3. **1.** Uterine contractions

    2. Bloody show

    3. Rupture of amniotic sac (page 602)

4. **1.** When delivery can be expected in a few minutes.

    2. When some natural disaster or catastrophe makes it impossible to reach the hospital.

    3. When no transportation is available. (page 607)

5. Exert gentle pressure on the head as it emerges to prevent rapid expulsion with a strong contraction. (page 607)

6. The brain is covered by only skin and membrane at the fontanels. (page 611)

7. Exerting gentle pressure horizontally across the perineum with a sterile gauze pad may reduce the risk of perineal tearing. (page 611)

8. **1.** During a breech delivery to protect the infant's airway

    2. When the umbilical cord is prolapsed (pages 617-618)

9. **1.** Prematurity

    2. Low birth weight

    3. Severe respiratory depression (page 620)

Word Fun

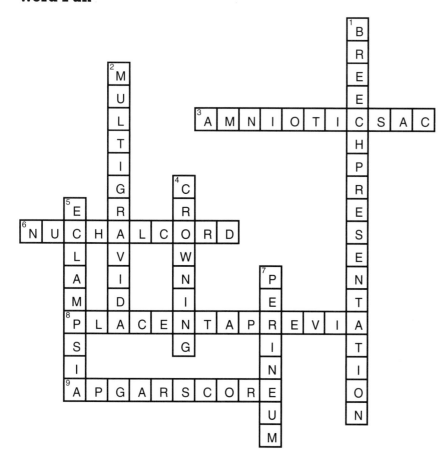

Ambulance Calls

1. This patient has classic signs of pre-eclampsia. If she does not receive medical care soon to control her hypertension, she will likely experience seizure activity. Provide high flow oxygen, obtain a set of vital signs (especially blood pressure), and provide prompt transport with the patient on her left side.

2. Recent laws have been enacted to provide protection for new mothers who do not wish to keep their babies. They can release their newborns and infants to fire stations and hospitals without fear of criminal charges (as the young woman in this scenario chose to do). You should notify other providers in your station as you begin measures to dry, warm, stimulate, and suction the baby's airway. These measures are very effective in improving a newborn's oxygenation and perfusion status. Blow-by oxygen will help immensely, but if those measures fail to quickly improve the newborn's status, bag valve mask ventilations should be initiated. Provide chest compressions if the newborn's heart rate is <100 beats/min, and take note of the condition of the umbilical cord to ensure no blood loss occurs. Provide prompt transport and notify the hospital of the incoming patient.

3. –Position the mother for delivery and apply high-flow oxygen.
   –As crowning occurs, use a clamp to puncture the sac, away from the baby's face.
   –Push the ruptured sac away from the infant's face as the head is delivered.
   –Clear the baby's mouth and nose immediately.
   –Continue with the delivery as normal.

Skill Drills

Skill Drill 20-1: Delivering the Baby (page 610)

1. Support the **bony** parts of the head with your hands as it emerges. Suction fluid from the **mouth**, then **nostrils**.
2. As the **upper shoulder** appears, guide the head **down** slightly, if needed, to deliver the **shoulder**.
3. Support the head and upper body as the **lower shoulder** delivers, guiding the head **up** if needed.
4. Handle the slippery, delivered infant firmly but gently, keeping the neck in **neutral** position to **maintain** the airway.
5. Place the umbilical cord clamps **2"** to **4"** apart and **cut** between them.
6. Allow the **placenta** to deliver itself. Do not pull on the **cord** to speed delivery.

Skill Drill 20-2: Giving Chest Compressions to an Infant (page 617)

1. Find the proper position: just below the **nipple line**, middle or **lower third** of the sternum.
2. Wrap your hands around the body, with your **thumbs** resting at that position.
3. Press your thumbs gently against the sternum, compressing **1/2"** to **3/4"** deep.

Assessment Review

1. A (page 624)
2. D (page 624)
3. A (page 623)
4. D (page 623)
5. B (page 623)

Emergency Care Summary

Delivering the Baby

bony

mouth

nostrils

down

up

neutral

2, 4

Giving Chest Compressions to an Infant

middle

lower

1/2, 3/4

Premature Infant

90, 95

32.2, 35

bulb syringe

bleeding

oxygen

(page 624)

Chapter 21: Kinematics of Trauma

Matching

1. H (page 643)   **5.** C (page 633)
2. G (page 638)   **6.** A (page 633)
3. F (page 632)   **7.** D (page 633)
4. E (page 632)   **8.** B (page 632)

Multiple Choice

1. B (page 632)   **14.** A (page 638)
2. C (page 632)   **15.** D (page 638)
3. C (page 632)   **16.** B (page 638)
4. B (page 633)   **17.** C (page 638)
5. A (page 633)   **18.** B (page 640)
6. D (pages 637-640) **19.** C (page 640)
7. C (pages 637-640) **20.** B (page 641)
8. C (page 633)   **21.** C (page 634)
9. D (page 636)   **22.** A (page 634)
10. A (page 636)   **23.** B (page 636)
11. C (page 636)   **24.** C (page 635)
12. B (page 636)   **25.** A (page 632)
13. D (page 638)

Fill-in

1. Injuries (page 632)
2. patterns, events (page 632)
3. Traumatic injury (page 632)
4. KE = 1/2 MV^2 (page 634)
5. Polaroids (page 637)
6. deceleration (page 638)
7. submarining (page 638)

True/False

1. T (page 632)
2. F (page 632)
3. F (page 633)
4. T (page 639)
5. T (page 639)
6. T (page 633)
7. T (page 632)

Short Answer

1. Potential energy is the product of mass (weight), force of gravity, and height, and is mostly associated with the energy of falling objects. (page 633)

2. **1.** Collision of the car against another car or other object

   2. Collision of the passenger against the interior of the car

   3. Collision of the passenger's internal organs against the solid structures of the body (pages 637-639)

3. **1.** The height of the fall

   2. The surface struck

   3. The part of the body that hits first, followed by the path of energy displacement (page 642)

4. A bullet, because of its speed, creates pressure waves that emanate from its path, causing distant damage. (page 643)

5. The size (mass) and speed (velocity) of the projectile affect the potential damage. If the mass is doubled, the potential energy is doubled. If the velocity is doubled, the potential energy is quadrupled. (page 633)

Word Fun

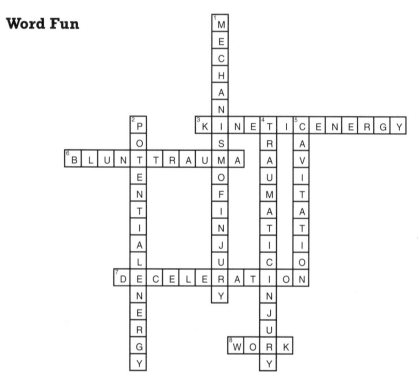

Ambulance Calls

1. Given the highway speeds and lack of a shoulder belt and airbag along with his complaints of head and neck pain, your index of suspicion for head and spinal injuries is very high. It is a positive sign that he is awake and able to communicate, however, this should not encourage you to spend any more time on scene than is necessary to extricate this patient and place him in full spinal precautions. His condition could change at any time, and his inability to remember the details of the event likely indicate the presence of a closed head injury. Provide high-flow oxygen and prompt transport.

2. Each story is 10 feet, so this patient fell approximately 20 feet from the ladder to the hard ground (assuming you live in an area with cold winter weather). He is now unconscious and lying in the snow. He not only has significant injuries, but now the high possibility of hypothermia, the severity of which will depend upon the length of time he has been exposed to the elements as well as local weather conditions. Assume he has significant head and spinal injuries; determine if he is responsive, and manage his airway, as he will be unable to protect it. Provide high-flow oxygen and prompt transport to the nearest appropriate facilities, taking care not to waste time in determining other injuries.

3. –Apply high-flow oxygen.

   –Stabilize object in place with bulky dressings.

   –Monitor vital signs.

   –Transport in a supine position.

   –Rapid transport due to abdominal penetration.

Chapter 22: Bleeding

Matching

1. J (page 650)

2. E (page 650)

3. K (page 650)

4. F (page 651)

5. C (page 650)

6. H (page 650)

7. B (page 655)

8. I (page 668)

9. M (page 666)

10. A (page 668)

11. D (page 656)

12. L (page 654)

13. G (page 655)

Multiple Choice

1. D (page 652)

2. D (page 650)

3. C (page 650)

4. C (page 650)

5. B (page 650)

6. A (page 650)

7. D (page 650)

8. B (page 651)

9. D (page 652)

10. C (page 652)

11. B (page 653)

12. C (page 653)

13. C (page 653)

14. A (page 653)

15. D (page 654)

16. B (page 654)

17. B (page 655)

18. D (page 655)

19. A (page 655)

20. B (page 655)

21. C (page 655)

22. C (page 655)

23. D (page 656)

24. B (page 656)

25. C (page 659)

26. A (page 660)

27. A (page 660)

28. C (page 661)

29. D (page 662)

30. C (page 663)

31. D (page 656)

32. D (page 666)

33. B (page 666)

34. B (page 667)

35. D (page 668)

36. D (page 668)

37. D (page 668)

38. C (page 669)

Labeling

1. The left and right sides of the heart (page 651)

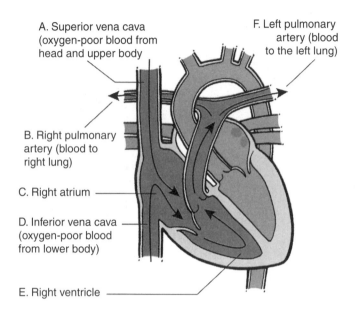

A. Superior vena cava (oxygen-poor blood from head and upper body

F. Left pulmonary artery (blood to the left lung)

B. Right pulmonary artery (blood to right lung)

C. Right atrium

D. Inferior vena cava (oxygen-poor blood from lower body)

E. Right ventricle

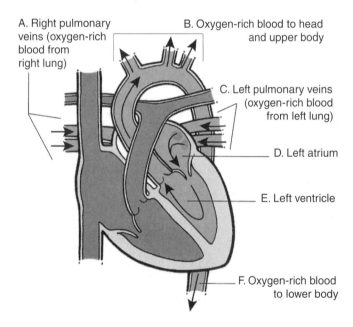

A. Right pulmonary veins (oxygen-rich blood from right lung)

B. Oxygen-rich blood to head and upper body

C. Left pulmonary veins (oxygen-rich blood from left lung)

D. Left atrium

E. Left ventricle

F. Oxygen-rich blood to lower body

2. Perfusion (page 653)

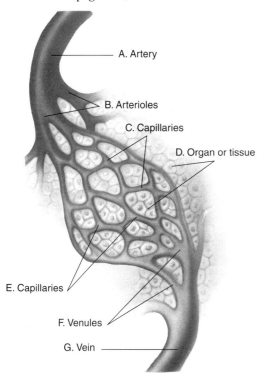

A. Artery

B. Arterioles

C. Capillaries

D. Organ or tissue

E. Capillaries

F. Venules

G. Vein

3. Arterial pressure points (page 662)

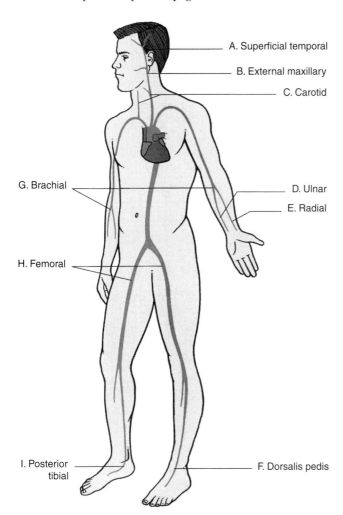

A. Superficial temporal

B. External maxillary

C. Carotid

G. Brachial

D. Ulnar

E. Radial

H. Femoral

I. Posterior tibial

F. Dorsalis pedis

Fill-in

1. perfusion (page 653)
2. involuntary (page 650)
3. lungs (page 653)
4. hypoperfusion (page 653)
5. inferior (page 651)
6. white cells, red cells, platelets, and plasma (page 652)
7. oxygenated (page 650)
8. heart, brain, lungs, and kidneys (page 653)
9. 4 to 6 (page 654)
10. rapid trauma assessment (page 658)

True/False

1. F (page 655)
2. F (page 655)
3. F (page 659)
4. T (page 659)
5. F (page 666)
6. T (page 666)
7. T (page 661)
8. F (page 660)
9. F (page 663)
10. T (page 662)

Short Answer

1. It redirects blood away from nonessential organs to the heart, brain, lungs, and kidneys. (page 653)
2. Artery: Bright red, spurting

   Vein: Dark color with steady flow

   Capillary: Darker color, oozes (page 655)
3.   1. Direct pressure and elevation
     2. Pressure dressings
     3. Pressure points (for upper and lower extremities)
     4. Splints
     5. Air splints
     6. PASG
     7. Tourniquets (page 659)
4.   1. Change in mental status (restlessness, anxiety, combativeness)
     2. Weakness, fainting, or dizziness on standing (early sign) or at rest (later sign)
     3. Tachycardia
     4. Thirst
     5. Nausea and vomiting
     6. Cold, moist (clammy) skin
     7. Shallow, rapid breathing
     8. Dull eyes
     9. Slightly dilated pupils, slow to respond to light
     10. Capillary refill in infants and children of more than 2 seconds
     11. Weak, rapid (thready) pulse
     12. Decreasing blood pressure
     13. Altered level of consciousness (page 669)
5.   1. BSI
     2. Maintain the airway.
     3. Administer high-flow oxygen.
     4. Control all obvious external bleeding.

5. Apply splints to extremity, if a limb is involved.
6. Monitor and record the patient's vital signs.
7. Give the patient nothing by mouth.
8. Elevate the legs 6 to 12 inches in nontrauma patients.
9. Keep the patient warm.
10. Provide immediate transport. (page 670)

Word Fun

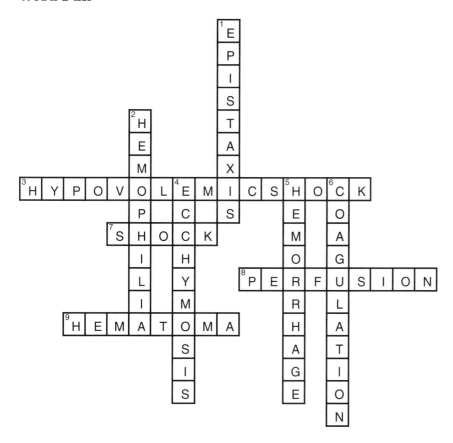

Ambulance Calls

1. Control bleeding with direct pressure, elevation, pressure point, and a tourniquet as a LAST resort.
Apply high-flow oxygen.
Place patient in the position of comfort.
Monitor vital signs.
Provide rapid transport.

2. You must control bleeding through direct pressure, elevation, pressure dressings and pressure points as needed. You must also transport the amputated portion of the limb with the patient to the hospital. Quickly attempt to determine how much blood has been lost and assess his skin and vital signs as these will provide accurate indicators of the significance of blood loss. Place the patient in the Trendelenburg position as needed; apply high-flow oxygen and provide prompt transport.

3. This is an isolated injury that, depending upon the severity of the laceration to the antecubital vein, can result in significant blood loss. Attempt to control bleeding through direct pressure, elevation, pressure dressings and pressure points as needed. Something as benign as a pen can cause significant damage in the hands of a determined person.

Skill Drills

Skill Drill 22-1: Controlling External Bleeding (page 661)

1. Apply **direct pressure** over the wound.
   Elevate the injury above the **level** of the **heart** if no **fracture** is suspected.
2. Apply a **pressure dressing**.
3. Apply pressure at the appropriate **pressure point** while continuing to hold **direct pressure**.

Skill Drill 22-2: Applying a Pneumatic Antishock Garment (PASG) (page 664)

1. Apply the garment so that the top is below the lowest rib.
2. Enclose both legs and the abdomen.
3. Open the stopcocks.
4. Inflate with the foot pump, and close the stopcocks when the patient's systolic blood pressure reaches 100 mm Hg or the Velcro crackles.
5. Check the patient's blood pressure again. Monitor the vital signs.

Assessment Review

1. C (page 672)
2. A (page 672)
3. B (page 672)
4. D (page 672)
5. C (page 672)

Emergency Care Summary

External Bleeding

cervical

Controlling External Bleeding

pressure

Using PASG for Control of Massive Soft-Tissue Bleeding in the Extremities

air splint

Applying a Tourniquet

twice
square

Treating Epistaxis

15
shock

Internal Bleeding
Steps to Caring for Patient with Internal Bleeding

splint
nothing

Using PASG for Treatment of Shock

abdominal
response
(page 673)

Chapter 23: Shock

Matching

1. B (page 678)
2. G (page 678)
3. H (page 678)
4. C (page 678)
5. E (page 681)
6. A (page 681)
7. F (page 682)
8. I (page 683)
9. D (page 684)

Multiple Choice

1. D (page 678)
2. B (page 678)
3. D (page 680)
4. C (page 680)
5. D (page 680)
6. D (page 680)
7. D (page 680)
8. C (page 683)
9. A (page 681)
10. B (page 681)
11. C (page 690)
12. A (page 682)
13. C (page 682)
14. D (page 682)
15. A (page 682)
16. B (page 682)
17. A (page 683)
18. A (page 683)
19. D (page 683)
20. B (page 684)
21. A (page 683)
22. B (page 688)
23. C (page 688)
24. B (page 689)
25. D (page 694)
26. B (page 691)

Fill-in

1. Hypoperfusion (page 678)
2. contraction (page 678)
3. nonessential, essential (page 678)
4. perfusion (page 678)
5. heart, vessels, blood (page 678)
6. shock (hypoperfusion) (page 678)
7. Sphincters, contract, dilate (page 678)
8. Diastolic, systolic (page 678)
9. Blood (page 678)
10. involuntary (page 680)

True/False

1. T (page 683)
2. T (page 682)
3. T (page 678)
4. F (page 678)
5. F (page 684)

6. T (page 691)
7. T (page 682)
8. F (page 678)
9. F (page 680)
10. F (page 684)

Short Answer

1. Causes: allergic reaction (most severe form)
   Signs/Symptoms: Can develop within seconds; mild itching/rash; burning skin; vascular dilation; generalized edema; profound coma; rapid death
   Treatment: Manage airway. Assist ventilations. Administer high-flow oxygen. Determine cause. Assist with administration of epinephrine. Transport promptly.
   (page 689)

2. Causes: Inadequate heart function; disease of muscle tissue; impaired electrical system; disease or injury
   Signs/Symptoms: Chest pains; irregular pulse; weak pulse; low blood pressure; cyanosis (lips, under nails); anxiety
   Treatment: Position comfortably. Administer oxygen. Assist ventilations. Transport promptly.
   (page 689)

3. Causes: Loss of blood or fluid
   Signs/Symptoms: Rapid, weak pulse; low blood pressure; change in mental status; cyanosis (lips, under nails); cool, clammy skin; increased respiratory rate
   Treatment: Secure airway. Assist ventilations. Administer high-flow oxygen. Control external bleeding. Elevate legs. Keep warm. Transport promptly.
   (page 689)

4. Causes: Excessive loss of fluid and electrolytes due to vomiting, urination, or diarrhea
   Signs/Symptoms: Rapid, weak pulse; low blood pressure; change in mental status; cyanosis (lips, under nails); cool, clammy skin; increased respiratory rate
   Treatment: Secure airway. Assist ventilations. Administer high-flow oxygen. Determine illness. Transport promptly.
   (page 689)

5. Causes: Damaged cervical spine, which causes widespread blood vessel dilation
   Signs/Symptoms: Bradycardia (slow pulse); low blood pressure; signs of neck injury
   Treatment: Secure airway. Spinal immobilization. Assist ventilations. Administer high-flow oxygen. Transport promptly.
   (page 689)

6. Causes: Temporary, generalized vascular dilation; anxiety; bad news; sight of injury/blood; prospect of medical treatment; severe pain; illness; tiredness
   Signs/Symptoms: Rapid pulse; normal or low blood pressure
   Treatment: Determine duration of unconsciousness. Record initial vital signs and mental status. Suspect head injury if patient is confused or slow to regain consciousness. Transport promptly.
   (page 689)

7. Causes: Severe bacterial infection
   Signs/Symptoms: Warm skin; tachycardia; low blood pressure
   Treatment: Transport promptly. Administer oxygen en route. Provide full ventilatory support. Elevate legs. Keep patient warm. (page 689)

8. **1.** Poor pump function
   2. Blood or fluid loss from blood vessels
   3. Poor vessel function (blood vessels dilate) (page 681)

9. Falling blood pressure, labored or irregular breathing, ashen, mottled, or cyanotic skin, thready or absent peripheral pulses, dull eyes or dilated pupils, and poor urinary output. (page 684)

10. **1.** Remove the autoinjector's safety cap, and quickly wipe the thigh with antiseptic.
    2. Place the tip of the autoinjector against the lateral part of the thigh.
    3. Push the autoinjector firmly against the thigh, and hold it in place until all the medication is injected. (page 693)

Word Fun

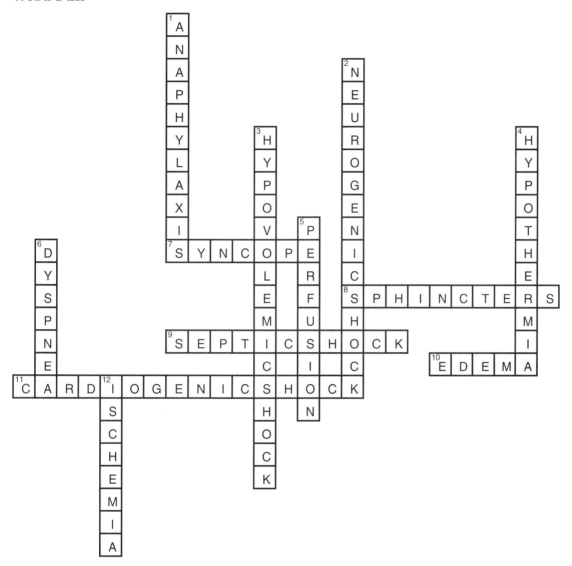

Ambulance Calls

1. When assessing the victim of a fall, you must take into consideration not only the patient's complaints and obvious injuries, but also the mechanism of injury including the height of the fall, the surface on which he or she landed, the position in which he or she landed, and any medical and/or previous traumatic injuries that could exacerbate the injuries. This patient landed on a hard surface, most likely a wooden floor, and now presents with numbness and tingling of his lower body. These are all indicators of spinal cord injury. Assume spinal fractures are present; ensure that you assess pulse, motor, and sensation of all extremities prior to placing him in full spinal precautions and reassess again after immobilized. Document your findings and continue this assessment en route to the hospital.

2. This patient is in shock and it seems to be related to an infectious organism (septic shock). In this case, although he has not lost blood volume through hemorrhage, his vessels or 'container' has become too large, making his available blood volume inadequate. Immediate transport is required. The patient should be given high-flow oxygen and placed in the Trendelenburg position to facilitate available perfusion to essential organs (heart, lungs, brain, and kidneys).

3. –Treat for anaphylactic shock.
   –Apply high-flow oxygen while inquiring if the patient has an EpiPen.
   –Obtain orders and administer EpiPen.
   –Monitor vital signs.
   –Rapid transport.

Skill Drills

Skill Drill 23-1: Treating Shock (page 687)

1. Keep the patient supine, open the airway, and check breathing and pulse.
2. Control obvious external bleeding.
3. Splint any broken bones or joint injuries.
4. Give high-flow oxygen if you have not already done so, and place blankets under and over the patient.
5. If no fractures are suspected, elevate the legs 6 to 12 inches.

Assessment Review

1. D (page 692)
2. A (page 692)
3. B (page 692)
4. B (page 692)
5. C (page 692)

Emergency Care Summary

General Shock

spinal

supine

circulation

pulse

Anaphylactic Shock

lateral

injected

(page 693)

Chapter 24: Soft-Tissue Injuries

Matching

1. G (page 698)
2. B (page 698)
3. D (page 698)
4. F (page 699)
5. H (page 698)
6. J (page 705)
7. E (page 705)
8. A (page 706)
9. C (page 705)
10. I (page 711)

Multiple Choice

1. C (page 698)
2. B (page 698)
3. B (page 698)
4. A (page 698)
5. B (page 699)
6. C (page 699)
7. B (page 700)
8. B (page 700)
9. D (page 700)
10. C (page 700)
11. C (page 702)
12. C (page 703)
13. B (page 700)
14. A (page 705)
15. D (page 705)
16. B (page 710)
17. D (page 707)
18. D (page 707)
19. A (page 704)
20. D (page 707)
21. D (page 711)
22. C (page 712)
23. C (page 714)
24. D (page 715)
25. D (page 715)
26. C (page 716)
27. B (page 716)
28. C (page 716)
29. D (page 716)
30. D (page 718)
31. B (page 723)
32. D (page 724)
33. A (page 726)
34. D (page 727)

Labeling

1. The Skin (page 699)

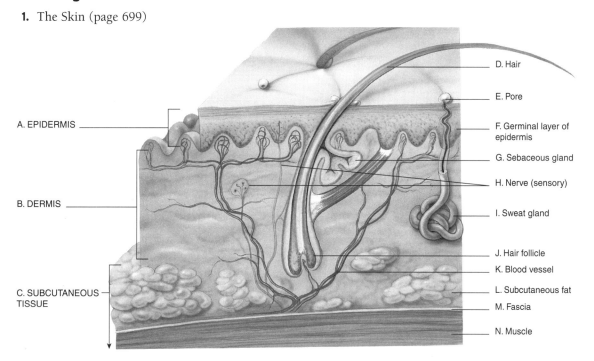

A. EPIDERMIS

B. DERMIS

C. SUBCUTANEOUS TISSUE

D. Hair

E. Pore

F. Germinal layer of epidermis

G. Sebaceous gland

H. Nerve (sensory)

I. Sweat gland

J. Hair follicle

K. Blood vessel

L. Subcutaneous fat

M. Fascia

N. Muscle

2. The Rule of Nines (page 718)

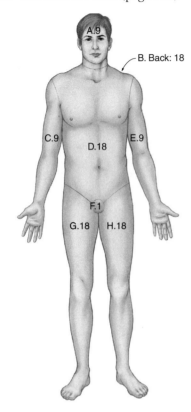
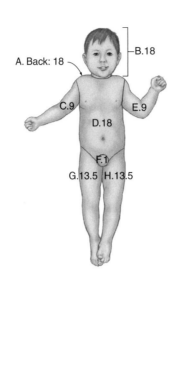

Fill-in

1. moist (page 699)

2. cool (page 698)

3. dermis (page 698)

4. subcutaneous (page 699)

5. constrict (page 699)

6. bacteria, water (page 699)

7. dermis (page 698)

8. temperature (page 699)

9. epidermis, dermis (page 698)

10. radiated (page 699)

True/False

1. T (page 716)

2. F (page 716)

3. T (page 716)

4. T (page 718)

5. T (page 715)

6. T (page 719)

7. F (page 720)

8. T (page 724)

9. T (page 726)

10. T (page 726)

11. F (page 726)

12. F (page 727)

13. T (page 727)

14. F (page 700)

15. F (page 705)

Short Answer

1. **1.** superficial

    2. partial-thickness

    3. full-thickness (page 716)

2. **1.** closed

    2. open

    3. burns (page 699)

3. R=rest

I=ice

C=compression

E=elevation

S=splinting (page 703)

4. –Full- or partial-thickness burns covering more than 20% of total body surface area

–Burns involving the hands, feet, face, airway, or genitalia (page 717)

5. Brush off dry chemicals and/or remove clothing, then flush the burned area with large amounts of water. (page 722)

6. First, there may be deep tissue injury not visible on the outside. Second, there is a danger of cardiac arrest from the electrical shock. (page 724)

7. A wound caused by a penetrating object into the chest that causes air to enter the chest. The air enters the chest area through the wound, but remains in the pleural space and the lung does not expand. With exhalation, air passes back through the wound, making a "sucking" sound. (page 708)

8. **1.** Control bleeding

2. Protect from further damage

3. Prevent further contamination and infection (page 726)

9. **1.** Abrasions

2. Lacerations

3. Avulsions

4. Penetrating (page 704)

10. **1.** Depth (superficial/partial/full)

2. Extent (% of body burned)

3. Involvement of critical areas (face, upper airway, hands, feet, genitalia)

4. Pre-existing medical conditions or other injuries

5. Age of younger than 5 years or older than 55 years (page 715)

Word Fun

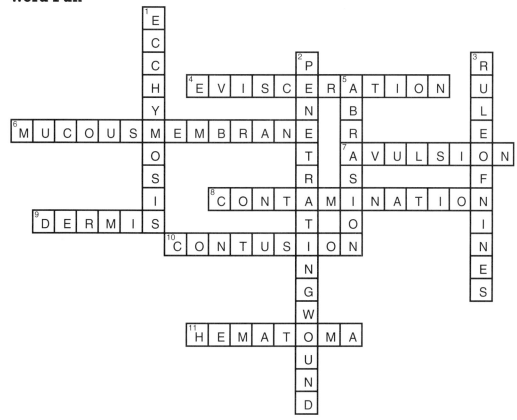

Ambulance Calls

1. –BSI precautions
   –Apply direct pressure.
   –Elevate the extremity and apply a pressure dressing.
   –Try a pressure point if bleeding is not controlled (tourniquet as a last resort).
   –Once bleeding is controlled, splint the arm to decrease movement.
   –Apply high-flow oxygen.
   –Transport in position of comfort, normal response.
   –Monitor vital signs.

2. Unfortunately, this scenario has occurred in households throughout the country. This is why it is so important to 'turn pot handles in' when cooking in the home of a small, inquisitive child. You must evaluate the child quickly to determine the extent and severity of the burns. Assess airway, breathing, and circulation, and quickly apply sterile dressings and high-flow oxygen. Promptly transport the patient according to local protocols.

3. Apply direct pressure to control any bleeding using sterile dressings. Have the patient lie down; as this injury will be quite painful and even the toughest of people can suddenly feel faint, especially if they look at the injury. Find the piece of avulsed tissue, wrap it in sterile dressings, and transport it with you to the hospital. Oxygen via nasal cannula can assist with nausea that the patient may experience.

Skill Drills

Skill Drill 24-1: Controlling Bleeding from a Soft-Tissue Injury (page 711)

1. Apply **direct pressure** with a **sterile** bandage.
2. Maintain pressure with a **roller** bandage.
3. If bleeding continues, apply a second **dressing** and **roller** bandage over the first.
4. **Splint** the extremity.

Skill Drill 24-2: Stabilizing an Impaled Object (page 713)

1. Do not attempt to **move** or **remove** the object. Stabilize the impaled body part.
2. Control **bleeding** and **stabilize** the object in place using **soft dressings**, **gauze**, and/or **tape**.
3. Tape a **rigid** item over the stabilized object to protect it from **movement** during transport.

Skill Drill 24-3: Caring for Burns (page 721)

1. Follow BSI precautions to help prevent infection.
   If it is safe to do so, remove the patient from the burning area; extinguish or remove hot clothing and jewelry as needed.
   If the wound(s) is still burning or hot, immerse the hot area in cool, sterile water, or cover with a wet, cool dressing.
2. Provide high-flow oxygen and continue to assess the airway.
3. Estimate the severity of the burn, then cover the area with a dry, sterile dressing or clean sheet.
   Assess and treat the patient for any other injuries.
4. Prepare for transport.
   Treat for shock.
5. Cover the patient with blankets to prevent loss of body heat.
   Transport promptly.

Assessment Review

1. C (page 728)
2. B (page 728)
3. D (page 728)
4. A (page 728)
5. D (page 730)

Emergency Care Summary
Closed Injuries
heart

Open Injuries
roller

roller

Burns
sterile

traumatic

Abdominal Injuries
abdomen

Impaled objects
gauze

Neck Wounds
occlusive

carotid

Chemical Burns
15

20

Electrical Burns
AED

Small Animal and Human Bites
antibiotic

(page 730)

Chapter 25: Eye Injuries

Matching

1. D (page 736)
2. C (page 737)
3. B (page 737)
4. E (page 737)
5. J (page 736)
6. G (page 736)
7. A (page 736)
8. F (page 736)
9. I (page 736)
10. H (page 737)

Multiple Choice

1. B (page 736)
2. D (page 736)
3. A (page 736)
4. A (page 737)
5. D (page 739)
6. C (page 738)
7. D (page 744)
8. D (page 745)
9. B (page 745)
10. D (page 745)
11. B (page 746)
12. C (page 746)
13. D (page 747)
14. A (page 747)
15. B (page 747)
16. A (page 748)
17. D (page 749)
18. C (page 750)

Fill-in

1. lacrimal glands (page 736)
2. optic nerve (page 737)
3. camera (page 737)
4. chemical burn (page 750)
5. orbit (page 736)
6. abnormalities (page 740)
7. orbit (page 741)
8. Conjunctivitis (page 741)
9. conjunctiva (page 736)
10. sclera (page 736)

True/False

1. F (page 742)
2. F (page 736)
3. T (page 736)
4. F (page 736)
5. F (page 750)
6. F (page 742)
7. F (page 741)
8. T (page 737)
9. F (page 741)
10. T (page 736)

Short Answer

1. A condition in which the retina is separated from its attachments at the back of the eye. Common findings include flashing lights, floaters, or a cloud or shade over the patient's vision. However, pain is not a common complaint. (page 749)

2. **1.** Never exert pressure on the eye.

   2. If part of the eyeball is exposed, gently apply a moist, sterile dressing to prevent drying.

   3. Cover the eye with a protective shield or sterile dressing. (page 747)

3. **1.** One pupil larger than the other

   2. Eyes not moving together or pointing in different directions

   3. Failure of the eyes to follow movement when instructed

   4. Bleeding under the conjunctiva

   5. Protrusion or bulging of the eye (page 749)

Word Fun

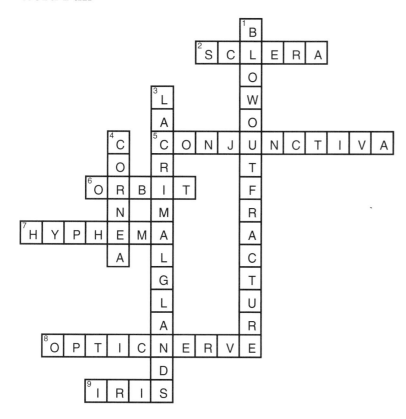

Ambulance Calls

1. You may find examination of the eye to be difficult as the child is very upset and frightened. To prevent any further injury to the eye, the other eye must be covered. This will also likely frighten the child. Anxiety will be lessened if the child is accompanied to the hospital with an adult who knows him. Request that the teacher ride with the child to the emergency department. Notify the receiving facility of the seriousness of the injury.

2. Position patient supine on stretcher.
   Set up IV bags to use as irrigation hoses.
   Connect IV line to a nasal cannula and place the prongs over the nose so that the fluid runs into the eyes.
   Monitor patient and flush eyes continuously en route to the hospital.
   Provide rapid transport.

3. This patient could have sustained facial fractures surrounding his eye (orbital fractures) as well as trauma to the eye itself. Note if the eye has held its shape or if you see any drainage from the eye, or swelling or deformity of the facial bones. Take spinal precautions as appropriate; cover both eyes to prevent further damage; apply oxygen and transport to the nearest appropriate facility.

Skill Drills

Skill Drill 25-1: Removing a Foreign Object From Under the Upper Eyelid (page 743)

1. Have the patient look **down**, grasp the **upper lashes**, and gently pull the lid away from the eye.
2. Place a **cotton-tipped applicator** on the outer surface of the upper lid.
3. Pull the lid **forward** and **up**, folding it back over the applicator.
4. Gently remove the foreign object from the eyelid with a **moistened, sterile** applicator.

Skill Drill 25-2: Stabilizing a Foreign Object Impaled in the Eye (page 745)

1. To prepare a doughnut ring, wrap a 2" roll around your fingers and thumb **seven** or **eight** times. Adjust the diameter by **spreading** your fingers.
2. Wrap the remainder of the roll, . . .
3. . . . working around the ring.
4. Place the dressing over the **eye** to hold the impaled object in place, then **secure** it with a **gauze** dressing.

Assessment Review

1. A (page 751)
2. D (page 751)
3. C (page 751)
4. B (page 752)
5. B (page 752)

Emergency Care Summary

Foreign Objects

lashes
2" roll

Burns

5, 20
saline

Lacerations

moist

Blunt Trauma

metal shield
(page 752)

Chapter 26: Face and Throat Injuries

Matching

1. C (page 758)
2. B (page 758)
3. E (page 758)
4. F (page 758)
5. G (page 758)
6. D (page 760)
7. A (page 758)

Multiple Choice

1. D (page 758)
2. B (page 758)
3. C (page 758)
4. D (page 758)
5. A (page 758)
6. D (page 759)
7. C (page 759)
8. D (page 760)
9. A (page 765)
10. D (page 765)
11. B (page 766)
12. C (page 766)
13. B (page 767)
14. D (page 767)
15. D (page 768)
16. A (page 769)

Labeling

Face/Skull (page 759)

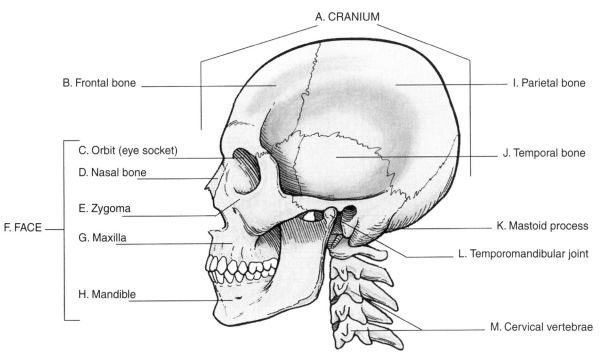

A. CRANIUM
B. Frontal bone
C. Orbit (eye socket)
D. Nasal bone
E. Zygoma
F. FACE
G. Maxilla
H. Mandible
I. Parietal bone
J. Temporal bone
K. Mastoid process
L. Temporomandibular joint
M. Cervical vertebrae

Fill-in

1. carotid (page 760)
2. cervical (page 758)
3. temporal (page 758)
4. trachea (page 759)
5. cartilage (page 759)
6. men, women (page 759)
7. foramen magnum (page 758)
8. maxilla (page 758)
9. parietal (page 758)
10. trachea (pages 759)

True/False

1. T (page 760)
2. T (page 761)
3. F (page 764)
4. F (page 767)
5. T (page 768)
6. T (page 758)
7. F (page 758)
8. F (page 760)
9. T (page 761)
10. F (page 765)

Short Answer

1. Direct manual pressure with a dry dressing. Use roller gauze around the circumference of the head to hold pressure dressing in place. (page 764)
2. Apply direct pressure above and below the injury. (page 769)

Word Fun

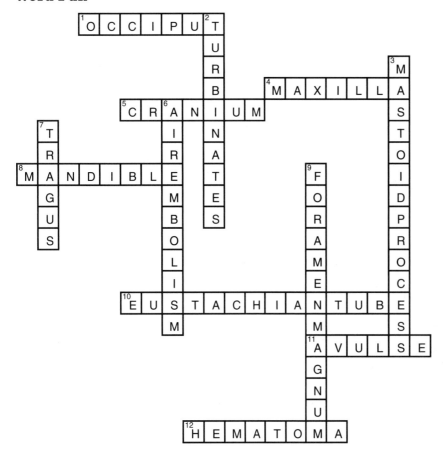

Ambulance Calls

1. –Have patient lean forward while pinching the nostrils together.
   –Assess the airway to assure patency.

2. Depending upon where the dog's teeth have punctured the skin, you may have a variety of soft-tissue injuries and swelling. If you notice the presence of subcutaneous emphysema, the dog punctured or perforated the child's trachea. You must also assume the presence of cervical spine injuries and must take appropriate precautions. Assess his level of consciousness, airway, breathing, and circulation. Control any bleeding and apply other dressings as needed after airway management is accomplished and while en route to the hospital. Always follow local protocols.

3. You should determine what objects were used to cause injury to this man's face. Baseball bats would be readily available and would increase your index of suspicion. You should determine the presence of head and neck pain. If the area of injury is limited to his nose, and the need for spinal precautions are not indicated, you can instruct the patient in controlling his bleeding by ensuring he is pushing on the cartilage of his nose and does not lean his head backwards. Swallowing blood will cause nausea. Do not allow the patient to blow his nose and use ice as needed to reduce swelling and pain. Transport according to local protocols.

Skill Drills

Skill Drill 26-1: Controlling Bleeding From a Neck Injury (page 770)

1. Apply **direct pressure** to control bleeding.
2. Use **roller gauze** to secure a dressing in place.
3. Wrap the bandage around and under the patient's **shoulder**.

Assessment Review

1. D (page 771)
2. B (page 771)
3. D (page 772)
4. A (page 772)
5. C (page 772)

Emergency Care Summary

Nose Injuries

forward

Ear Injuries

moist

Facial Fractures

bone

saliva

Neck Injuries

roller gauze

(page 772)

Chapter 27: Chest Injuries

Matching

1. B (page 778)
2. D (page 779)
3. C (page 779)
4. A (page 779)
5. E (page 779)

6. H (page 780)
7. I (page 780)
8. J (page 789)
9. F (page 780)
10. G (page 780)

Multiple Choice

1. B (page 779)
2. A (page 779)
3. C (page 779)
4. D (page 780)
5. D (page 780)
6. D (page 781)
7. B (page 787)
8. C (page 787)
9. D (page 784)
10. C (page 785)

11. D (page 786)
12. D (page 786)
13. D (page 786)
14. D (page 786)
15. D (page 787)
16. A (page 787)
17. C (page 788)
18. D (page 788)
19. D (page 789)
20. B (page 789)

Labeling

Anterior Aspect of the Chest (page 778)

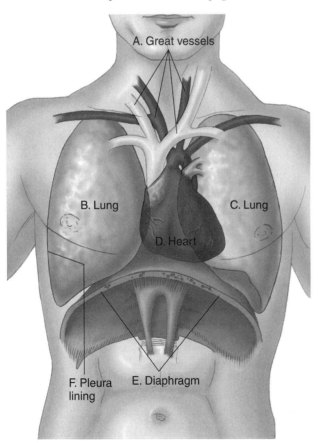

A. Great vessels
B. Lung
C. Lung
D. Heart
E. Diaphragm
F. Pleura lining

The Ribs (page 779)

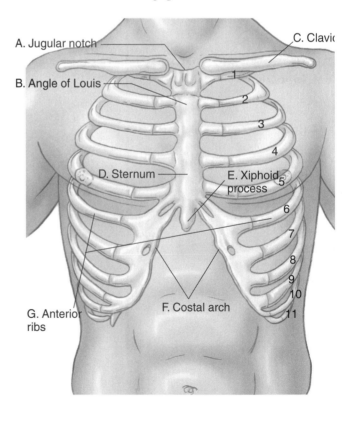

A. Jugular notch
B. Angle of Louis
C. Clavic
D. Sternum
E. Xiphoid process
F. Costal arch
G. Anterior ribs

Fill-in

1. back (page 779)

2. decreases (page 779)

3. sternum (page 779)

4. bronchi (page 779)

5. phrenic (page 779)

6. ribs (page 779)

7. diaphragm (page 778)

8. Pleura (page 779)

9. aorta (page 779)

10. contracts (page 779)

True/False

1. T (page 780)

2. F (page 780)

3. T (page 786)

4. F (page 787)

5. F (page 786)

6. F (page 789)

7. F (page 778)

8. T (page 779)

9. F (page 780)

10. T (page 780)

Short Answer

1. –Pain at the site of injury

–Pain localized at the site of injury that is aggravated by or increased with breathing

–Dyspnea (difficulty breathing, shortness of breath)

–Hemoptysis (coughing up blood)

–Failure of one or both sides of the chest to expand normally with inspiration

–Rapid, weak pulse and low blood pressure

–Cyanosis around the lips or fingernails. (page 780)

2. **1.** Seal the wound with a large airtight dressing that seals all four sides.

2. Seal the wound with a dressing that seals three sides with the fourth side as a flutter valve.

Your local protocol will dictate the way you are to care for this injury. (page 785)

3. Tape a bulky pad against the segment of the chest. (page 788)

4. Sudden severe compression of the chest, causing a rapid increase of pressure within the chest. Characteristic signs include distended neck veins, facial and neck cyanosis, and hemorrhage in the sclera of the eye. (page 788)

Word Fun

Crossword answers:

1. HEMOTHORAX
2. HEMOPTYSIS
3. TENSPNEUMOTHORAT (TENSION PNEUMOTHORAX)
4. PUMONARYCONTUSION (PULMONARY CONTUSION)
5. PARADOXICAL MOTION
6. FLUTTERVALVE
7. TACHYPNEA
8. FLAIL CHEST
9. PERICARDIAL TAMPONADE
10. DYSPNEA
11. PNEUMOTHORAX

Ambulance Calls

1. You should be concerned with the presence of rib and sternal fractures as well as pulmonary contusions and pneumothoracies. This patient may require assistance in breathing as it will be extremely painful for him to breathe in. If he requires assistance with a BVM device, you must be careful not to become too aggressive in your ventilations. Time your ventilations with the patient's respirations and be gentle. Provide high-flow oxygen and take spinal precautions according to your local protocols.

2. This patient's chest has been crushed with a significant amount of weight. This mechanism of injury indicates the high potential for rib, sternal, thoracic fractures and other soft-tissue injuries as well. Patients who experience sternal fractures will find it difficult to be placed supine, as this will likely increase their pain. There will be little you can do to ease this pain as they should be immobilized on a long backboard. Provide prompt transport, high-flow oxygen, and monitor the pulse, motor, and sensations particularly distal to the suspected spinal injury.

3. –Apply high-flow oxygen via nonrebreathing mask or BVM device.
   –Fully c-spine immobilized patient.
   –Rapid transport
   –Monitor vital signs en route.

Assessment Review

1. B (page 791)
2. D (page 792)
3. C (page 792)
4. D (page 792)
5. A (page 792)

Emergency Care Summary

Pneumothorax

occlusive

flutter valve

Hemothorax

shock

Rib Fracture

spinal injury

Flail Chest

high-flow

(page 792)

Chapter 28: Abdomen and Genitalia Injuries

Matching

1. G (page 798)   **5.** E (page 807)
2. D (page 798)   **6.** B (page 802)
3. C (page 798)   **7.** A (page 809)
4. H (page 807)   **8.** F (page 798)

Multiple Choice

1. D (page 798)
2. D (page 798)
3. C (page 798)
4. D (page 798)
5. B (page 798)
6. D (page 798)
7. A (page 798)
8. C (page 799)
9. B (page 799)
10. A (page 799)
11. D (page 799)
12. C (page 799)
13. B (page 799)
14. A (page 800)
15. B (page 800)
16. B (page 800)
17. B (page 804)
18. D (page 800)
19. D (page 800)
20. D (page 801)
21. C (page 801)
22. D (page 802)
23. D (page 802)
24. D (page 802)
25. A (page 807)
26. C (page 808)
27. D (page 809)
28. D (page 809)
29. A (page 809)
30. B (page 809)
31. D (page 810)
32. D (page 812)

Labeling

1. Hollow organs (page 798)

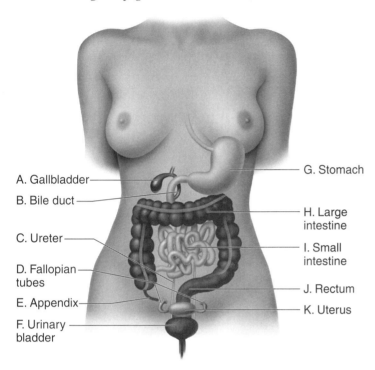

A. Gallbladder
B. Bile duct
C. Ureter
D. Fallopian tubes
E. Appendix
F. Urinary bladder
G. Stomach
H. Large intestine
I. Small intestine
J. Rectum
K. Uterus

2. Solid organs (page 799)

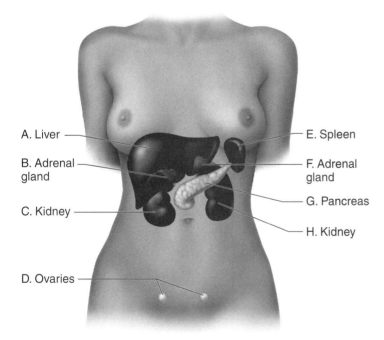

A. Liver
B. Adrenal gland
C. Kidney
D. Ovaries
E. Spleen
F. Adrenal gland
G. Pancreas
H. Kidney

Fill-in

1. solid (page 798)
2. urinary (page 807)
3. retroperitoneal (page 807)
4. external signs (page 809)
5. peritonitis (page 798)

6. inflammatory response (page 798)
7. blunt injuries (page 799)
8. penetrating injuries (page 799)
9. flank (page 800)
10. evisceration (page 802)

True/False

1. F (page 798)
2. T (page 800)
3. F (page 801)
4. T (page 809)
5. F (page 798)
6. F (page 799)
7. T (page 798)
8. F (page 799)
9. T (page 801)
10. T (page 802)

Short Answer

1. Stomach, intestines, ureters, bladder, gallbladder, and rectum (page 798)
2. Liver, spleen, pancreas, and kidneys (page 798)
3. Pain, shock signs, bruises, lacerations, bleeding, tenderness, guarding, and difficulty with movement because of pain (page 800)
4. –Inspect the patient's back and sides for exit wounds.
   –Apply a dry, sterile dressing to all open wounds.
   –If the penetrating object is still in place, apply a stabilizing bandage around it to control external bleeding and to minimize movement of the object. (page 802)
5. –Cover with moistened sterile dressing.
   –Secure dressing with bandage.
   –Secure bandage with tape. (page 802)
6. –An abrasion, laceration, or contusion in the flank
   –A penetrating wound in the region of the lower rib cage (the flank) or the upper abdomen
   –Fractures on either side of the lower rib cage or of the lower thoracic or upper lumbar vertebrae (page 809)

Word Fun

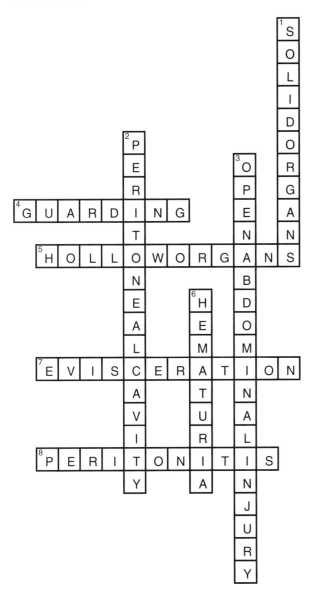

Ambulance Calls

1. Assess the ABCs.
   Apply high-flow oxygen.
   Control any bleeding.
   Stabilize the knife in place with bulky dressings—DO NOT REMOVE.
   Keep movement of patient to the bare minimum, so as not to create further injury. (Sliding the patient very carefully onto a backboard may help to minimize movement.)
   Monitor vital signs.
   Provide rapid transport.
   Bandage minor lacerations en route.

2. Quickly visualize the area to determine how badly he has cut himself, and if he has in fact amputated any portion of his penis. You will need to control bleeding, as blood loss in this area can be significant. Use pressure dressings/pressure points as needed to control bleeding; provide high-flow oxygen and prompt transport. Also, request the presence of a police officer during transport as this patient will likely need to be restrained and could be unpredictable during transport.

3. Cover the abdomen and the portion of the protruding bowel with a moistened, sterile dressing and/or an occlusive dressing. Secure these dressings with tape; allow the patient to draw his knees up as needed for comfort; apply high-flow oxygen; cover the patient to preserve warmth and promptly transport to the hospital.

Assessment Review

1. A (page 813)
2. B (page 813)
3. D (page 814)
4. D (page 814)
5. C (page 814)

Emergency Care Summary

Kidney and Urinary Bladder Injuries

vital signs

External Male Genitalia Injuries

Avulsion

saline

minutes

Amputation

ice

Lacerated Head of the Penis

sterile dressing

Urethral Injuries

urine

External Female Genitalia Injuries

compress

Internal Female Genitalia Injuries, Pregnancy

left

left

Rectal Bleeding

compresses

Sexual Assault

airway maintenance

major bleeding

paper

plastic

(page 814)

Chapter 29: Musculoskeletal Care

Matching

1. G (page 820)
2. J (page 820)
3. D (page 821)
4. I (page 822)
5. F (page 822)
6. B (page 824)
7. K (page 825)
8. A (page 825)
9. C (page 822)
10. E (page 824)
11. H (page 838)

Multiple Choice

1. A (page 856)
2. B (page 821)
3. A (page 821)
4. B (page 822)
5. C (page 822)
6. B (page 822)
7. C (page 823)
8. A (page 823)
9. D (page 824)
10. A (page 824)
11. B (page 824)
12. C (page 824)
13. D (page 824)
14. B (page 824)
15. C (page 825)
16. D (page 825)
17. A (page 825)
18. C (page 825)
19. D (page 825)
20. A (page 825)
21. C (page 825)
22. B (page 825)
23. A (page 826)
24. C (page 826)
25. D (page 828)
26. C (page 828)
27. D (page 830)
28. D (page 829)
29. D (page 832)
30. D (page 836)
31. C (page 838)
32. D (page 838)
33. B (page 841)
34. D (page 846)
35. B (page 848)
36. D (page 853)
37. D (page 857)

38. C (page 859)
39. B (page 859)
40. D (page 860)
41. C (page 860)
42. B (page 860)
43. A (page 861)
44. C (page 862)

Labeling

The Human Skeleton (page 822)

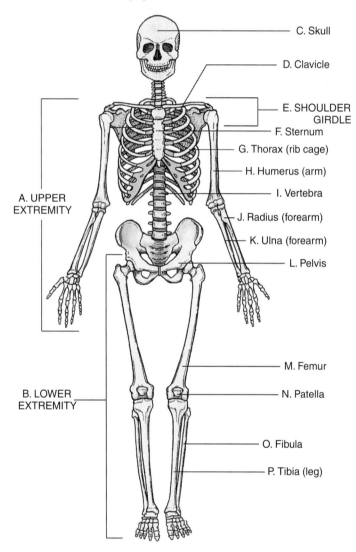

A. UPPER EXTREMITY

B. LOWER EXTREMITY

C. Skull
D. Clavicle
E. SHOULDER GIRDLE
F. Sternum
G. Thorax (rib cage)
H. Humerus (arm)
I. Vertebra
J. Radius (forearm)
K. Ulna (forearm)
L. Pelvis
M. Femur
N. Patella
O. Fibula
P. Tibia (leg)

Fill-in

1. wasting (page 821)
2. red (page 821)
3. hinge (page 822)
4. clavicle (page 848)
5. mechanism of injury (page 834)
6. open fracture (page 824)
7. sciatic nerve (page 857)
8. femur (page 856)
9. crepitus (page 827)
10. reduce (page 828)
11. neurovascular status (page 829)

True/False

1. T (page 836)   **6.** F (page 837)

2. T (page 836)   **7.** T (page 837)

3. F (page 838)   **8.** T (page 837)

4. T (page 838)   **9.** T (page 832)

5. T (page 837)   **10.** F (page 832)

Short Answer

1. **1.** Direct

    2. Indirect

    3. Twisting

    4. High-energy (page 824)

2. Deformity
Tenderness (point)
Guarding
Swelling
Bruising
Crepitus
False motion
Exposed fragments
Pain
Locked joint (page 825)

3. **1.** Pulse

    2. Capillary refill

    3. Sensation

    4. Motor function (page 832)

4. **1.** Remove clothing from the area.

    2. Note and record the patient's neurovascular status distal to the site of the injury.

    3. Cover all wounds with a dry, sterile dressing before splinting.

    4. Do not move the patient before splinting.

    5. For a suspected fracture, immobilize the joints above and below the fracture.

    6. For a joint injury, immobilize the bones above and below the injured joint.

    7. Pad all rigid splints.

    8. Maintain manual immobilization to minimize movement of the limb and to support the injury site.

    9. Use a constant, gentle manual traction to align the limb.

    10. If you encounter resistance to limb alignment, splint the limb in its deformed position.

    11. Immobilize all suspected spinal injuries in a neutral in-line position on a backboard.

    12. If the patient has signs of shock, align the limb in the normal anatomic position and provide transport.

    13. When in doubt, splint. (page 836)

5. **1.** Stabilize the fracture.

    2. Align the limb.

    3. Avoid potential neurovascular compromise. (page 838)

Word Fun

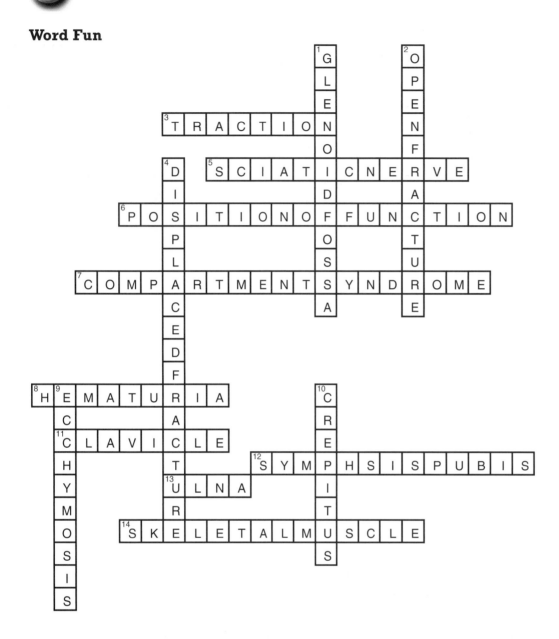

Ambulance Calls

1. This patient likely has a compression injury to his lumbar spine. The force exerted on his body from the landing will be transferred up from his feet through his legs to his pelvis and spine. You must take all spinal precautions, apply high-flow oxygen, and provide prompt transport to the nearest appropriate facility. Continue to monitor any changes in the pulse, motor, and sensation, specifically in his lower body.

2. –Splint the arm in position found, since circulation is intact.
   –Use a board splint for support with a sling and swathe.
   –Immobilize hand in the position of function.
   –Apply oxygen as needed.
   –Transport in the position of comfort.
   –Normal transport.
   –Monitor vital signs.

3. This man not only has probable injuries and swelling to his airway but significant likelihood for distraction injuries to his cervical spine. You must take c-spine precautions as you open his airway and determine the presence of breathing. The information provided does not include whether he has a pulse. Assess airway, breathing, and circulation; apply full spinal precautions, high-flow oxygen, positive pressure ventilations, and CPR as needed.

Skill Drills

Skill Drill 29-1: Assessing Neurovascular Status (pages 833-834)

1. Palpate the **radial** pulse in the upper extremity.
2. Palpate the **posterior tibial** pulse in the lower extremity.
3. Assess capillary refill by blanching a fingernail or **toenail.**
4. Assess sensation on the flesh near the **tip** of the **index** finger.
5. On the foot, first check sensation on the flesh near the **tip** of the **great toe.**
6. Also check foot sensation on the **lateral side.**
7. Evaluate motor function by asking the patient to **open** the hand. (Perform motor tests only if the hand or foot is not **injured. Stop** a test if it causes pain.)
8. Also ask the patient to **make a fist.**
9. To evaluate motor function in the foot, ask the patient to **extend** the foot.
10. Also have the patient **flex** the foot and **wiggle** the toes.

Skill Drill 29-2: Caring for Musculoskeletal Injuries (page 837)

1. Cover open wounds with a **dry, sterile** dressing, and **apply pressure** to control bleeding.
2. Apply a splint and elevate the extremity about 6" (slightly above the level of the **heart**).
3. Apply **cold packs** if there is swelling, but do not place them **directly** on the skin.
4. **Position** the patient for transport and **secure** the injured area.

Skill Drill 29-3: Applying a Rigid Splint (page 839)

1. Provide gentle **support** and **in-line traction** of the limb.
2. Second EMT-B places the splint **alongside** or **under** the limb.
   Pad between the limb and the splint as needed to ensure even pressure and contact.
3. Secure the splint to the limb with **bindings.**
4. Assess and record **distal neurovascular** functions.

Skill Drill 29-4: Applying a Zippered Air Splint (page 841)

1. Support the injured limb and apply gentle **traction** as your partner applies the open, deflated splint.
2. Zip up the splint, inflate it by **pump** or by **mouth**, and test the **pressure.** Check and record **distal neurovascular** function.

Skill Drill 29-5: Applying an Unzipped Air Splint (page 842)

1. **Support** the injured limb. Have your partner place his or her arm through the splint to grasp the patient's **hand** or **foot.**
2. Apply gentle **traction** while sliding the splint onto the injured limb.
3. **Inflate** the splint.

Skill Drill 29-6: Applying a Vacuum Splint (page 843)

1. **Stabilize** and **support** the injury.
2. Place the splint and **wrap** it around the limb.
3. **Draw** the air **out of** the splint through the suction valve, and then **seal** the valve.

Skill Drill 29-7: Applying a Hare Traction Splint (page 844)

1. Expose the injured limb and check pulse, motor, and sensory function.
   Place the splint beside the uninjured limb, adjust the splint to proper length, and prepare the straps.
2. Support the injured limb as your partner fastens the ankle hitch about the foot and ankle.
3. Continue to support the limb as your partner applies gentle in-line traction to the ankle hitch and foot.
4. Slide the splint into position under the injured limb.
5. Pad the groin and fasten the ischial strap.

6. Connect the loops of the ankle hitch to the end of the splint as your partner continues to maintain traction. Carefully tighten the ratchet to the point that the splint holds adequate traction.

7. Secure and check support straps.
Assess pulse, motor, and sensory functions.

8. Secure the patient and splint to the backboard in a way that will prevent movement of the splint during patient movement and transport.

Skill Drill 29-8: Applying a Sager Traction Splint (page 846)

1. After exposing the injured area, check the patient's pulse and motor and sensory function.
Adjust the thigh strap so that it lies anteriorly when secured.

2. Estimate the proper length of the splint by placing it next to the injured limb.
Fit the ankle pads to the ankle.

3. Place the splint at the inner thigh, apply the thigh strap at the upper thigh, and secure snugly.

4. Tighten the ankle harness just above the malleoli.
Snug the cable ring against the bottom of the foot.

5. Extend the splint's inner shaft to apply traction of about 10% of body weight.

6. Secure the splint with elasticized cravats.

7. Secure the patient to a long backboard.
Check pulse, motor, and sensory functions.

Skill Drill 29-9: Splinting the Hand and Wrist (page 855)

1. Move the hand into the **position of function**. Place a soft **roller bandage** in the palm.

2. Apply a **padded board** splint on the **palmar** side with fingers **exposed**.

3. Secure the splint with a **roller bandage**.

Assessment Review

1. C (page 864)
2. B (page 864)
3. A (page 865)
4. B (page 865)
5. D (page 865)

Emergency Care Summary
Applying a Hare Traction Splint

sensory

in-line traction

ischial

support straps

Applying a Sager Traction Splint

anteriorly

inner

upper

malleoli

10%

(page 865)

Chapter 30: Head and Spine Injuries

Matching

1. D (page 872)

2. E (page 872)

3. H (page 875)

4. G (page 875)

5. A (page 876)

6. C (page 872)

7. B (page 880)

8. I (page 874)

9. J (page 877)

10. F (page 872)

Multiple Choice

1. D (page 872)

2. B (page 874)

3. C (page 872)

4. C (page 890)

5. A (page 872)

6. B (page 876)

7. D (page 874)

8. D (page 872)

9. C (page 875)

10. A (page 877)

11. D (page 882)

12. D (page 881)

13. B (page 877)

14. D (page 890)

15. B (page 889)

16. A (page 891)

17. A (page 886)

18. B (page 893)

19. D (page 886)

20. B (page 879)

21. D (page 879)

22. D (page 879)

23. B (page 880)

24. B (page 880)

25. D (page 880)

26. C (page 880)

27. C (page 882)

28. D (page 884)

29. C (page 890)

30. B (page 890)

31. D (page 898)

32. C (page 900)

33. A (page 905)

Labeling

1. The Brain (page 873)

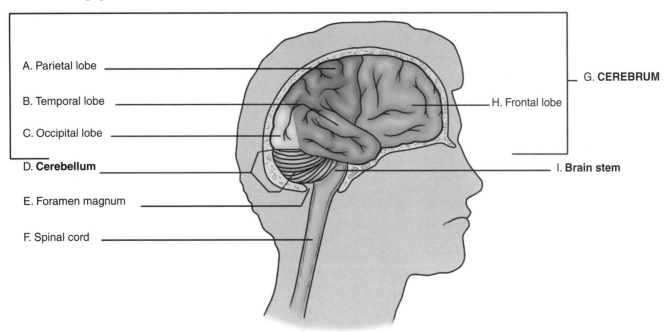

A. Parietal lobe

B. Temporal lobe

C. Occipital lobe

D. **Cerebellum**

E. Foramen magnum

F. Spinal cord

G. **CEREBRUM**

H. Frontal lobe

I. **Brain stem**

2. The Connecting Nerves in the Spinal Cord (page 875)

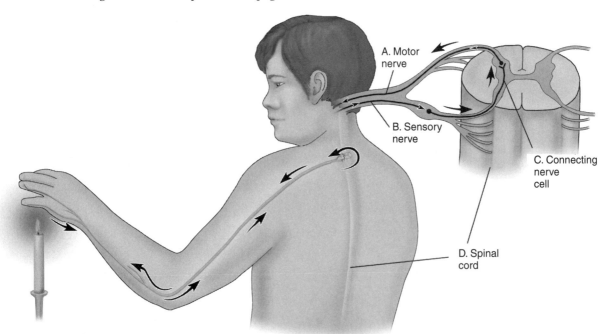

A. Motor nerve

B. Sensory nerve

C. Connecting nerve cell

D. Spinal cord

3. The Spinal Column (page 877)

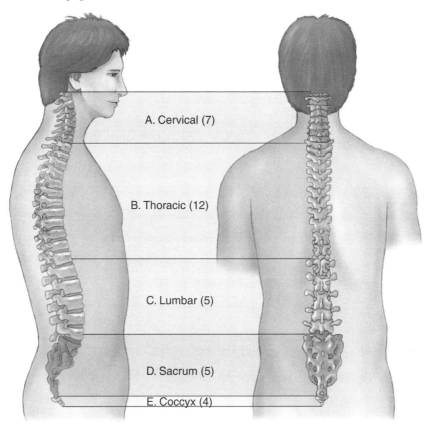

A. Cervical (7)

B. Thoracic (12)

C. Lumbar (5)

D. Sacrum (5)

E. Coccyx (4)

Fill-in

1. motor (page 874)
2. meninges (page 872)
3. central (page 872)
4. 31 (page 874)
5. cranial (page 874)
6. intervertebral discs (page 877)
7. cranium, face. (page 876)
8. arachnoid, pia mater (page 872)
9. sympathetic (page 875)
10. parasympathetic (page 876)

True/False

1. T (page 880)
2. F (page 875)
3. F (page 875)
4. T (page 875)
5. F (page 876)
6. F (page 890)
7. F (page 881)
8. T (page 891)
9. T (page 893)
10. T (page 898)

Short Answer

1. **1.** Does your neck or back hurt?

    2. What happened?

    3. Where does it hurt?

    4. Can you move your hands and feet?

    5. Can you feel me touching your fingers? Your toes? (page 881)

2. –Muscle spasms in the neck
    –Increased pain
    –Numbness, tingling, or weakness
    –Compromised airway or ventilations (page 890)

3. **1.** Concussion

    2. Contusion

    3. Intracranial bleeding (page 879)

4. –Lacerations, contusions, or hematomas to the scalp
    –Soft area or depression upon palpation
    –Visible fractures or deformities of the skull
    –Ecchymosis about the eyes or behind the ear over the mastoid process
    –Clear or pink cerebrospinal fluid leakage from a scalp wound, the nose, or the ear
    –Failure of the pupils to respond to light
    –Unequal pupil size
    –Loss of sensation and/or motor function
    –A period of unconsciousness
    –Amnesia
    –Seizures
    –Numbness or tingling in the extremities
    –Irregular respirations
    –Dizziness
    –Visual complaints
    –Combative or other abnormal behavior
    –Nausea or vomiting (page 880)

5. **1.** Establish an adequate airway.

    2. Control bleeding.

    3. Assess the patient's baseline level of consciousness. (page 890)

6. **1.** Is the patient's airway clear?

    2. Is the patient breathing adequately?

    3. Can you maintain the airway and assist ventilations if the helmet remains in place?

    4. How well does the helmet fit?

    5. Can the patient move within the helmet?

    6. Can the spine be immobilized in a neutral position with the helmet on? (page 900)

Word Fun

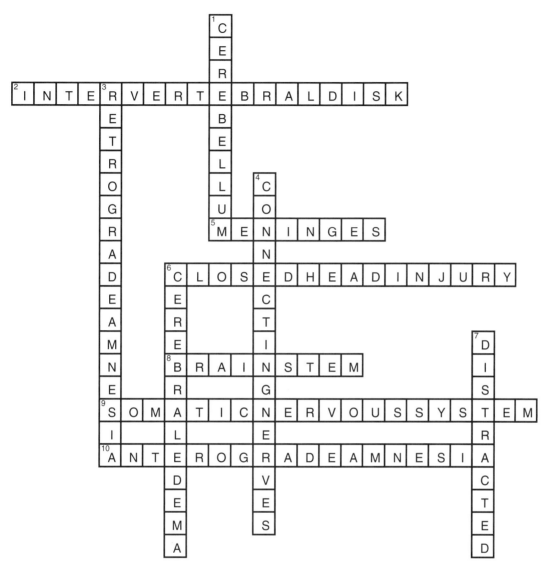

Ambulance Calls

1. There is significant mechanism of injury involved in this incident. The impact with the car, the lack of a helmet, the obvious head trauma, and the patient's decreased level of consciousness all indicate significant life-threatening injuries. You must quickly apply full spinal precautions and manage her airway. Provide prompt transport, high-flow oxygen and perform ongoing assessments while en route to the nearest appropriate medical facility.

2. This child landed face down on a concrete surface with significant force. She is now unconscious with a partially obstructed airway. You must move her to a supine position to manage her airway. Take note of any apparent injuries to her back as you reposition her. Ideally, you will have the appropriate equipment and adequate staffing to quickly and safely move her to a long backboard immediately. However, do not delay appropriately moving her to a supine position as you must do this to assess and manage her airway. This may be difficult as she likely has facial fractures and possibly broken teeth, blood, and secretions in her airway. Be prepared to suction her airway and apply positive pressure ventilations (this may be especially challenging in the presence of significant facial fractures). Use high-flow oxygen and promptly transport her to the nearest appropriate facility according to your local protocols.

3. –Leave the patient in his car seat.

   –Pad appropriately to immobilize the patient.

   –Use blow-by oxygen if the patient will tolerate it.

   –Monitor vital signs.

   –Continue assessment.

   –Rapid transport due to mechanism of injury and death in vehicle

Skill Drills

Skill Drill 30-1: Performing Manual In-Line Stabilization (page 889)

1. Kneel behind the patient and place your hands firmly around the **base** of the **skull** on either **side**.
2. Support the lower jaw with your **index** and **long** fingers, and the head with your **palms**. Gently **lift** the head into a **neutral, eyes-forward** position, aligned with the torso. Do not **move** the head or neck excessively, forcefully, or rapidly.
3. Continue to **support** the head manually while your partner places a rigid **cervical collar** around the neck. Maintain **manual support** until you have completely secured the patient to a backboard.

Skill Drill 30-2: Immobilizing a Patient to a Long Backboard (page 892)

1. Apply and maintain **cervical stabilization**.

   Assess **distal functions** in all extremities.
2. Apply a **cervical collar**.
3. Rescuers **kneel** on one side of the patient and place **hands** on the far side of the patient.
4. On command, rescuers **roll** the patient toward themselves, quickly examine the **back**, slide the backboard under the patient, and roll the patient onto the board.
5. **Center** the patient on the board.
6. Secure the **upper torso** first.
7. Secure the **chest, pelvis**, and **upper legs**.
8. Begin to secure the patient's head using a commercial immobilization device or **rolled towels**.
9. Place **tape** across the patient's forehead.
10. Check all **straps** and readjust as needed.

    Reassess **distal functions** in all extremities.

Skill Drill 30-3: Immobilizing a Patient Found in a Sitting Position (page 895)

1. Stabilize the head and neck in a neutral, in-line position.

   Assess pulse, motor, and sensory function in each extremity.

   Apply a cervical collar.
2. Insert a short spine immobilization device between the patient's upper back and the seat.
3. Open the side flaps, and position them around the patient's torso, snug around the armpits.
4. Secure the upper torso flaps, then the midtorso flaps.
5. Secure the groin (leg) straps. Check and adjust torso straps.
6. Pad between the head and the device as needed.

   Secure the forehead strap and fasten the lower head strap around the collar.
7. Wedge a long backboard next to the patient's buttocks.
8. Turn and lower the patient onto the long board.

   Lift the patient, and slip the long board under the spine device.
9. Secure the immobilization devices to each other.

   Reassess pulse, motor, and sensory functions in each extremity.

Skill Drill 30-4: Immobilizing a Patient found in a Standing Position (page 897)

1. While **manually** stabilizing the head and neck, apply a **cervical collar**. Position the board **behind** the patient.
2. Position EMT-Bs at **sides** and **behind** the patient.
   Side EMT-Bs reach under patient's **arms** and grasp **handholds** at or slightly above **shoulder** level.
3. Prepare to lower the patient. EMT-Bs on the sides should be **facing** the EMT-B at the head and **wait** for his or her **direction**.
4. On command, **lower** the backboard to the ground.

Skill Drill 30-5: Application of a Cervical Collar (page 899)

1. Apply **in-line** stabilization.
2. Measure the proper **collar size**.
3. Place the **chin support** first.
4. **Wrap** the collar around the neck and **secure** the collar.
5. Assure proper **fit** and maintain **neutral, in-line** stabilization.

Skill Drill 30-6: Removing a Helmet (page 903)

1. Kneel down at the patient's head with your **partner** at one side.
   Open the face shield to assess **airway** and **breathing**. Remove **eyeglasses** if present.
2. Prevent head movement by placing your **hands** on either side of the helmet and fingers on the **lower jaw**. Have your partner **loosen** the strap.
3. Have your partner place one hand at the **angle** of the **lower jaw** and the other at the **occiput**.
4. Gently slip the helmet about **halfway** off, then stop.
5. Have your partner slide the hand from the **occiput** to the **back** of the head to prevent it from snapping back.
6. Remove the helmet and **stabilize** the cervical spine.
   Apply a **cervical collar** and secure the patient to a **long backboard**.
   Pad as needed to prevent neck flexion or extension.

Assessment Review

1. D (page 906)
2. C (page 907)
3. B (page 907)
4. C (page 907)
5. A (page 907)

Emergency Care Summary
Immobilizing a Patient Found in a Sitting Position

neutral, in-line
cervical collar
short spine
lower head strap
long backboard
extremity
(page 907)

Chapter 31: Pediatric Emergencies

Matching

1. I (page 934)
2. F (page 935)
3. E (page 934)
4. J (page 918)
5. B (page 919)
6. A (page 920)
7. H (page 918)
8. G (page 918)
9. C (page 918)
10. D (page 916)

Multiple Choice

1. D (page 917)
2. D (page 917)
3. A (page 917)
4. C (page 917)
5. B (page 917)
6. D (page 917)
7. C (page 918)
8. D (page 918)
9. B (page 918)
10. C (page 919)
11. B (page 933)
12. C (page 933)
13. D (page 934)
14. A (page 935)

Fill-in

1. pediatrics (page 916)
2. tongue (page 917)
3. trachea (page 917)
4. 200 (page 917)
5. pale skin (page 917)
6. fontanels (page 917)
7. adolescents (page 920)

True/False

1. T (page 918)
2. T (page 918)
3. F (page 920)
4. F (page 918)
5. T (page 919)
6. T (page 933)
7. F (page 935)
8. T (page 935)

Short Answer

1. At first, infants respond mainly to physical stimuli. Crying is the main avenue of expression. Later, infants learn to coo, smile, roll over, and recognize caregivers. Usually, they demonstrate no stranger anxiety. Observe infants from a distance first and allow the caregiver to hold the baby as you perform the examination. (page 918)

2. –Children who were born prematurely and have associated lung disease problems
   –Small children or infants with congenital heart disease
   –Children with neurologic disease, such as cerebral palsy
   –Children with chronic disease or with functions that have been altered since birth (page 933)

3. Toddlers begin to walk and explore the environment. Because they are able to open doors, boxes, and so forth, injuries in this age group are more frequent. Stranger anxiety develops early in this period. They are also developing their own ideas about almost everything. Make as many observations as you can before touching the child. When appropriate, examine the child on the caregiver's lap and use a distraction. Allowing the child to examine your equipment may be enough distraction to allow you to complete an assessment. (page 918)

4. These children are beginning to act more like adults and can think in concrete terms, respond sensibly to direct questions, and help take care of themselves. Talk to the child, not just the parent, when obtaining a history. Give the child choices and explain any procedures. Give them simple explanations and carry on a conversation to distract them. Reward the child after a procedure. (page 920)

5. Adolescents are able to think abstractly, can participate in decision making, and are more susceptible to peer pressure. They are very concerned about body image and how they appear to peers and others. Respect their privacy at all times. They can understand complex concepts and treatment options and should be included on decision making concerning their care. Advise them in advance of painful procedures and talk with them about their interests to distract them. (page 920)

Word Fun

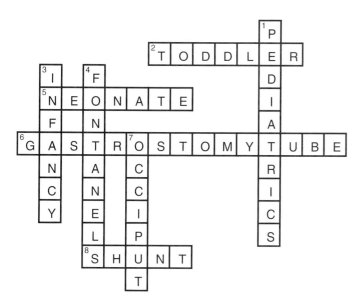

Ambulance Calls

1. Young children typically experience febrile seizures when their temperature rises rapidly, not simply the temperature of the fever itself. As with any call, you should assess airway, breathing, and circulation of this 2-year-old. Ensure that his airway is patent, assist him with breathing using a BVM device and airway adjunct as necessary, apply high-flow oxygen, and remove excessive clothing. The child's level of consciousness should improve, but if it doesn't or the child experiences additional seizure activity, this is a very serious sign that should be relayed to the receiving emergency department.

2. –Immediately open and suction the airway.

    –Assess breathing and apply high-flow oxygen by nonrebreathing mask or BVM device.

    –Assess patient further en route.

    –Rapid transport

    –Obtain history from grandmother en route.

    –Reassess patient's airway and vital signs en route.

3. When a patient cannot answer questions at all or can only respond in one- or two-word responses, this is a true emergency. She obviously has a history of respiratory disease or condition that requires her use of a metered-dose inhaler. You can ask her "yes" or "no" responses to aid in clarification of her medical history. Provide rapid transport and high-flow oxygen and assist her with her MDI in accordance with your local protocols.

Chapter 32: Pediatric Assessment and Management

Matching

1. D (page 958)
2. F (page 959)
3. H (page 958)
4. J (page 959)
5. L (page 959)
6. I (page 952)
7. K (page 976)
8. C (page 976)
9. E (page 981)
10. G (page 968)
11. B (page 978)
12. A (page 975)
13. M (page 944)

Multiple Choice

1. D (page 950)
2. B (page 952)
3. D (page 954)
4. D (page 957)
5. A (page 958)
6. D (page 959)
7. C (page 944)
8. D (page 975)
9. A (page 977)
10. D (page 977)
11. B (page 978)
12. D (page 978)
13. C (page 978)
14. D (page 943)
15. A (page 976)
16. C (page 963)
17. D (page 964)
18. D (page 970)
19. B (page 967)
20. D (page 968)
21. B (page 943)
22. C (page 971)
23. C (page 944)
24. B (page 977)
25. B (page 957)
26. C (page 945)

Fill-in

1. status epilepticus (page 977)
2. see, hear (page 942)
3. Dehydration (page 978)
4. Airway adjuncts (page 950)
5. gag reflex (page 951)
6. Skin condition (page 944)
7. tidal volume (page 955)

8. Infection (page 958)
9. seizure (page 977)
10. head (page 971)
11. shock (page 976)

True/False

1. F (page 956)
2. F (page 978)
3. T (page 978)
4. F (page 978)
5. T (page 978)
6. T (page 978)
7. F (page 978)
8. T (page 969)
9. T (page 976)

Short Answer

1. By the number of wet diapers: 6 to 10 per day is normal. (page 753)
2. –Nasal flaring
   –Grunting
   –Wheezing, stridor, or other abnormal airway sounds
   –Use of accessory muscles
   –Retractions
   –Tripod position (page 746)

Word Fun

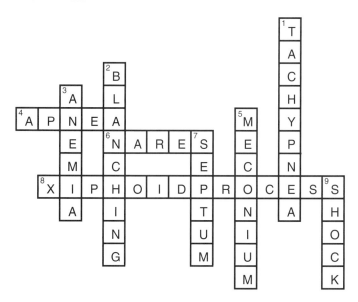

Ambulance Calls

1. This child has very likely aspirated vomitus into his lungs. You must immediately assess and manage his airway. This will require suctioning, use of airway adjuncts, and assisting his ventilations with high-flow oxygen and a BVM device. It appears that this boy has consumed alcohol and/or drugs, and the condition and situation of the scene require your notification of law enforcement. Ensure that no trauma has occurred or recently occurred to this patient; when in doubt, apply full c-spine precautions. You may find that obtaining information regarding medical conditions or history of recent trauma or illness is challenging in situations dealing with minors who fear punishment from their parents or guardians or consequences with law enforcement.

2. –Allow the child to remain in the mother's arms to decrease her anxiety.
   –Offer oxygen via a nonrebreathing mask with the mother holding it.
   –If she will not tolerate the nonrebreathing mask, use blow-by oxygen.
   –Allow the mother to ride in the patient compartment to comfort the child.
   –Provide rapid transport in position of comfort with as much oxygen as she will tolerate.
   –Continually assess patient for signs of altered mental status and decreasing tidal volume; be prepared to assist ventilations.
   –Obtain further history en route.

3. This infant is deceased, possibly as a result of sudden infant death syndrome (SIDS). After you have quickly assessed the infant and made this determination, you must communicate the condition of the baby to the mother and family. This may be difficult, and they will possibly request resuscitation attempts regardless of your findings. This becomes a judgment call, which can be clarified by utilizing online medical direction and/or standing orders. You should survey the scene and document any history of recent illness, congenital conditions, and so forth. Be supportive of family members and assist them as appropriate. Calls involving infants and children can be traumatic experiences for emergency medical providers as well. Request debriefing as necessary and follow local protocols.

Skill Drills

Skill Drill 32-1: Positioning the Airway in a Child (page 951)

1. Position the child on a **firm** surface.
2. Place a **folded** towel about 1 inch thick under the **shoulders** and **back**.
3. **Immobilize** the forehead to limit **movement** and use the head tilt-chin lift to open the airway.

Skill Drill 32-2: Inserting an Oropharyngeal Airway in a Child (page 953)

1. Determine the **appropriately sized** airway.
   Confirm the correct size **visually**, by placing it next to the patient's **face**.
2. Position the patient's **airway** with the appropriate method.
3. Open the mouth.
   Insert the airway until the **flange** rests against the **lips**.
   Reassess the airway.

Skill Drill 32-3: Inserting a Nasopharyngeal Airway in a Child (page 954)

1. Determine the correct airway size by comparing its **diameter** to the opening of the **nostril** (naris).
   Place the airway next to the patient's **face** to confirm correct **length**.
   Position the airway.
2. **Lubricate** the airway.
   Insert the **tip** into the right naris with the bevel pointing toward the **septum**.
3. Carefully move the tip forward until the **flange** rests against the **outside** of the nostril.
   Reassess the **airway**.

Skill Drill 32-4: One-rescuer BVM Ventilation on a Child (page 957)

1. Open the airway and insert the appropriate airway adjunct.
2. Hold the mask on the patient's face with a one-handed head tilt-chin lift technique (E-C grip).
   Ensure a good mask-face seal while maintaining the airway.
3. Squeeze the bag 20 times/min for a child or 30 times/min for an infant. Allow adequate time for exhalation.
4. Assess effectiveness of ventilation by watching bilateral rise and fall of the chest.

Skill Drill 32-5: Removing a Foreign Body Airway Obstruction in an Unconscious Child (page 961)

1. Position the child on a firm, flat surface.

2. Inspect the airway. Remove any visible foreign object that you can see.

3. Attempt rescue breathing. If unsuccessful, reposition the head and try again.

4. If ventilation is unsuccessful, position your hands on the abdomen above the navel and well below the chest cage. Give five abdominal thrusts.

5. Open the airway again and try to see the object.
   Only try to remove the obstruction if you can see it.
   Attempt rescue breathing. If unsuccessful, reposition the head and try again. Repeat abdominal thrusts if obstruction persists.

Skill Drill 32-6: Performing Infant Chest Compressions (page 969)

1. Position the infant on a **firm** surface while **maintaining** the airway.
   Place two **fingers** in the **middle** of the sternum just below a line between the **nipples**.

2. Use two fingers to **compress** the chest about 1/2 inch to 1 inch at a rate of **100** times/min.
   Allow the sternum to return **briefly** to its **normal** position between compressions.

Skill Drill 32-7: Performing CPR on a Child (page 970)

1. Place the child on a **firm** surface and maintain the airway with one **hand**.

2. Using two fingers of the other hand, locate the bottom of the **sternum** by tracing the lower margin of the rib cage to the notch where the ribs and sternum meet. Place the **heel** of your other hand over the lower half of the **sternum**, avoiding the **xiphoid**.

3. Compress the chest about 1 inch to 1-1/2 inches at a rate of 100/min (about 80/min with pauses for ventilations). Coordinate compressions with ventilations in a 5:1 ratio, pausing for **ventilations**.

4. Reassess for **breathing** and **pulse** after about 1 minute, and then every **few** minutes.
   If the child resumes **effective** breathing, place him or her in the **recovery** position.

Skill Drill 32-8: Immobilizing a Child (page 972)

1. Use a towel under the back, from the **shoulders** to the **hips**, to maintain the head in a **neutral** position.

2. Apply an appropriately sized **cervical collar**.

3. **Log roll** the child onto the **immobilization** device.

4. Secure the **torso** first.

5. Secure the **head**.

6. Ensure that the child is **strapped** in properly.

Skill Drill 32-10: Immobilizing an Infant Out of a Car Seat (page 974)

1. Stabilize the head in neutral position.

2. Place an immobilization device between the patient and the surface he or she is resting on.

3. Slide the infant onto the board.

4. Place a towel under the back, from the shoulders to the hips, to ensure neutral head position.

5. Secure the torso first; pad any voids.

6. Secure the head.

Chapter 33: Geriatric Emergencies

Matching

1. E (page 989)	**6.** F (page 993)
2. C (page 989)	**7.** D (page 993)
3. G (page 994)	**8.** H (page 933)
4. I (page 994)	**9.** A (page 988)
5. J (page 992)	**10.** H (page 989)

Multiple Choice

1. B (page 988)	**16.** B (page 994)
2. D (page 986)	**17.** A (page 994)
3. D (page 986)	**18.** D (page 986)
4. A (page 988)	**19.** C (page 991)
5. C (page 988)	**20.** B (page 992)
6. D (page 988)	**21.** A (page 991)
7. B (page 989)	**22.** D (page 991)
8. C (page 989)	**23.** D (page 991)
9. B (page 989)	**24.** A (page 991)
10. D (page 989)	**25.** D (page 992)
11. A (page 989)	**26.** C (page 994)
12. C (page 989)	**27.** D (page 995)
13. A (page 989)	**28.** B (page 995)
14. D (page 989)	**29.** B (page 996)
15. B (page 990)	**30.** D (page 998)

Fill-in

1. 65 (page 986)

2. mask (page 986)

3. stereotypes (page 988)

4. sweat glands (page 988)

5. Cardiac output (page 989)

6. aneurysm (page 989)

7. kyphosis (page 990)

True/False

1. F (page 989)	**5.** T (page 989)
2. T (page 988)	**6.** T (page 989)
3. T (page 988)	**7.** F (page 996)
4. F (page 988)	

Short Answer

1. –Physical
   –Psychological
   –Financial (page 996)

2. 1. Cardiac dysrhythmias/dysrhythmias/heart attack: The heart is beating too fast or too slowly, the cardiac output drops, and blood flow to the brain is interrupted. A heart attack can also cause syncope.

   2. Vascular and volume: Medication interactions can cause venous pooling, and vasodilation, widening of the blood vessel, results in a drop in blood pressure and inadequate blood flow to the brain. Another cause of syncope can be a drop in blood volume because of hidden bleeding from a condition such as an aneurysm.

   3. Neurologic: A transient ischemic attack (TIA) or "brain attack" can sometimes mimic syncope. (page 993)

3. –Repeated visits to the emergency department or clinic
   –A history of being "accident prone"
   –Soft-tissue injuries
   –Unbelievable or vague explanations of injuries
   –Psychosomatic complaints
   –Chronic pain
   –Self-destructive behavior
   –Eating and sleep disorders
   –Depression or lack of energy
   –Substance and/or sexual abuse (page 997)

4. –Dyspnea
   –Weak feeling
   –Syncope/confusion/altered mental status (page 993)

Word Fun

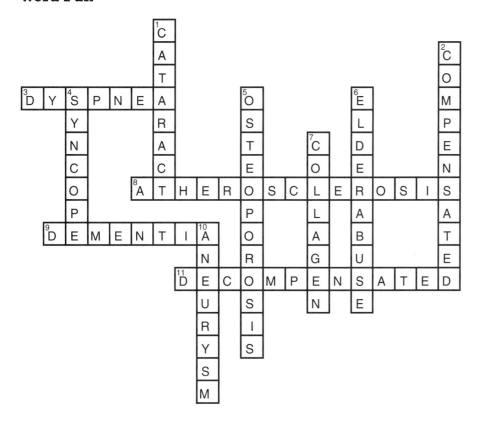

Ambulance Calls

1. –Survey the scene for any signs or clues to the patient's care.
   –Ask about patient's normal mental status.
   –Apply high-flow oxygen.
   –Obtain patient's medications to take to the hospital.
   –Place patient supine on stretcher with legs elevated.
   –Keep patient warm.
   –Rapid transport
   –Monitor vital signs en route.

2. This situation appears to be one of neglect and possible elder abuse. Perform a thorough assessment, especially if the patient is confused or is otherwise unable to express how or why she ended up on the floor. Ask for the patient's medical chart to obtain accurate information regarding her medical condition(s) and current medications. Immobilize her affected leg (and spine if needed) using the most comfortable methods possible. Geriatric patients need gentle care and many cannot tolerate conventional methods of splinting and immobilizing. Mechanisms of injury not viewed as significant in young, healthy patients can prove quite devastating or result in serious injury in older patients with frail skin and brittle bones.

3. Osteoporosis can be quite insidious in its onset. Individuals who were once relatively strong and healthy can suddenly find themselves with a fracture from something they may have done many times in the past. Postmenopausal, thin, Caucasian women are at higher risk of developing osteoporosis, and a spinal fracture in this scenario should be suspected. Perform an assessment to determine the presence of other injuries, provide full spinal immobilization, apply oxygen, and promptly transport this patient to the nearest appropriate facility. Always follow local protocols.

Chapter 34: Geriatric Assessment and Management

Matching

1. E (page 1012)
2. G (page 1015)
3. F (page 1010)
4. B (page 1010)
5. C (page 1007)
6. A (page 1015)
7. D (page 1009)
8. H (page 1015)

Multiple Choice

1. D (page 1004)
2. D (page 1016)
3. C (page 1005)
4. A (page 1006)
5. A (page 1007)
6. D (page 1008)
7. A (page 1009)
8. D (page 1010)
9. B (page 1012)
10. C (page 1013)
11. C (page 1015)
12. D (page 1016)

Fill-in

1. polypharmacy (page 1007)
2. stable (page 1009)
3. unstable (page 1009)
4. acetabulum (page 1012)
5. central cord syndrome (page 1010)
6. compression fracture (page 1010)
7. burst (page 1010)
8. seat belt fracture (page 1010)
9. septicemia (page 1015)
10. bacteremia (page 1015)

True/False

1. T (page 1015)
2. T (page 1016)
3. F (page 1004)
4. T (page 1005)
5. T (page 1006)
6. T (page 1007)
7. T (page 1007)
8. F (page 1010)
9. F (page 1012)

Short Answer

1. Apply and maintain cervical stabilization.
   Apply a cervical collar.
   Rescuers should kneel on one side of the patient.
   Rescuers roll the patient toward themselves and quickly examine the patient's back.
   Slide the backboard under the patient, and roll the patient onto the board.
   Pad the void space produced by the kyphotic spine.
   Secure the torso to the backboard with straps.
   Secure the patient's head and padding. (page 1010)
2. Assess pulse, motor, and sensory function of the extremity.
   Place the patient on a scoop stretcher or long backboard.
   Place a blanket roll between the patient's legs.
   Place blankets and pillows under the injured extremity.
   Secure both legs and the padding to the backboard with at least three cravats or straps.
   Reassess pulse, motor, and sensory function. (page 1013)
3. What is the patient's chief complaint today?
   What initial problem caused the patient to be admitted to the facility? (page 1016)

Word Fun

A crossword puzzle with the following answers:

- 1 (down): SEPTIC
- 2 (down): BACTEREMI
- 3 (across): BURST FRACTURES
- 4 (down): SYNC
- 5 (across): POLYPHARMACY
- 6 (across): ACETABULUM

Additional down entries: TEMI, REMI, P

Ambulance Calls

1. Straining or "bearing down" during a bowel movement is done by trying to forcefully exhale against a closed glottis or vocal cords. This can cause a significant decrease in heart rate that is not always well-tolerated by geriatric patients. When the Valsalva maneuver just described results in a temporary loss of consciousness, it is referred to as vasovagal syncope. Attempt to determine whether or not the patient lost consciousness before and/or after the event. As well as attempting to determine the cause of the fall, you must now care for his resultant head injury and potential spinal fractures. You should control any bleeding, provide full spinal immobilization, apply high-flow oxygen, provide prompt transport, and perform a thorough assessment and history taking to determine the presence of any other injuries or medical conditions.

2. Hip fractures are a misnomer because true "hip fractures" are in fact fractures of the femur. You should determine if the mechanism of injury or suspicion exists for possible spinal fractures. Survey the scene to determine if there was a reason for the fall or if the break was spontaneous, giving the patient the impression of "tripping" on an object. If you believe that it was a spontaneous fracture, this patient suffers from extreme osteoporosis and likely suffered other fractures during the fall. If no spinal immobilization is deemed necessary, isolated hip fracture care requires an assessment of the patient's pulse, motor, and sensation of both lower extremities. You should also determine if the affected extremity is the same or shorter than the uninjured side. It is also helpful to note if the leg is rotated inward, outward, or not at all. Immobilize the injured leg using blankets, pillows, and cravats or straps after placing the patient on a long spine board or scoop stretcher. After immobilization has occurred, reassess the pulse, motor, and sensory functions of the injured extremity. Provide reassurance for the patient because many feel that hip fractures signal the loss of their independence. Always follow local protocols.

3. Patients with kyphosis are extremely uncomfortable when immobilized on long spine boards. You should pad all voids using pillows, blankets, towels, or other appropriate forms of padding. Failure to adequately pad a patient's spine can result in increased pain and the inability of the patient to remain still. This can result in exacerbated injuries as well as a very unhappy patient. Thoracic spine injuries and injuries to the ribs can make it difficult for patients to breathe without pain. Determine if her shortness of breath is related to pain during inspiration and/or if she has a history of respiratory disease such as emphysema, chronic bronchitis, or asthma. Local weather conditions have probably contributed to her fall. Depending upon the length of exposure to the elements, she could be suffering from hypothermia as well. Geriatric patients generally do not tolerate extremes in weather; therefore avoiding extended periods of time in cold temperatures will minimize the likelihood for hypothermia.

Chapter 35: Ambulance Operations

Matching

1. D (page 1048)

2. A (page 1044)

3. E (page 1043)

4. G (page 1040)

5. F (page 1024)

6. C (page 1040)

7. B (page 1040)

Multiple Choice

1. C (page 1024)

2. A (page 1024)

3. A (page 1027)

4. B (page 1025)

5. D (page 1027)

6. D (page 1028)

7. A (page 1028)

8. D (page 1028)

9. D (page 1028)

10. B (page 1029)

11. D (page 1032)

12. A (page 1032)

13. D (page 1034)

14. D (page 1034)

15. C (page 1035)

16. C (page 1036)

17. D (page 1040)

18. B (page 1036)

19. D (page 1041)

20. B (page 1038)

21. A (page 1042)

22. C (page 1044)

23. D (page 1046)

24. B (page 1046)

25. C (page 1046)

26. C (page 1046)

27. B (page 1047)

28. D (page 1036)

29. D (page 1037)

30. C (page 1038)

31. D (page 1040)

32. D (page 1049)

Fill-in

1. jump kit (page 1032)

2. Star of Life (page 1026)

3. hearse (page 1024)

4. First responder vehicles (page 1024)

5. nine (page 1026)

6. decontaminate (page 1040)

7. airway (page 1028)

8. CPR board (page 1030)

True/False

1. T (page 1027)   **6.** T (page 1042)

2. F (page 1030)   **7.** T (page 1049)

3. T (page 1039)   **8.** F (page 1047)

4. F (page 1036)   **9.** F (page 1049)

5. F (page 1044)

Short Answer

1. Type I: Conventional, truck cab chassis with modular ambulance body that can be transferred to a newer chassis as needed

Type II: Standard van, forward-control integral cab-body ambulance

Type III: Specialty van, forward-control integral cab-body ambulance (page 1025)

2. **1.** Preparation for the call

   2. Dispatch

   3. En route to scene

   4. Arrival at scene

   5. Transfer of patient to the ambulance

   6. En route to the receiving facility (transport)

   7. At the receiving facility (delivery)

   8. En route to station

   9. Postrun (page 1026)

3. **1.** Lack of experience of the dispatcher

   2. Inadequate equipment in the ambulance

   3. Inadequate training of the EMT

   4. Inadequate driving ability

   5. Siren syndrome (page 1044)

4. **1.** To the best of your knowledge, the unit must be on a true emergency call.

   2. Both audible and visual warning devices must be used simultaneously.

   3. The unit must be operated with due regard for the safety of all others, on and off the roadway. (page 1046)

5. **1.** At the time of dispatch, select the shortest and least congested route to the scene.

   2. Avoid routes with heavy traffic congestion.

   3. Avoid one-way streets.

   4. Watch carefully for bystanders as you approach the scene.

   5. Once you arrive at the scene, park the ambulance in a safe place.

   6. Drive within the speed limit while transporting patients, except in the rare extreme emergency.

   7. Go with the flow of the traffic.

   8. Use the siren as little as possible en route.

   9. Always drive defensively.

   10. Always maintain a safe following distance.

   11. Try to maintain an open space in the lane next to you as an escape route in case the vehicle in front of you stops suddenly.

   12. Use your siren if you turn on the emergency lights, except when you are on a freeway.

   13. Always assume that other drivers will not hear the siren or see your emergency lights. (page 1042)

6. Approach from the front of the aircraft using an approach area of between nine o'clock and three o'clock as the pilot faces forward. (page 1049)

7. –A clear site that is free of loose debris, electric or telephone poles and wires, or any other hazards that might interfere with the safe operation of the helicopter

–A minimum of 100 ft. by 100 ft. is recommended for the landing zone. (page 1049)

Word Fun

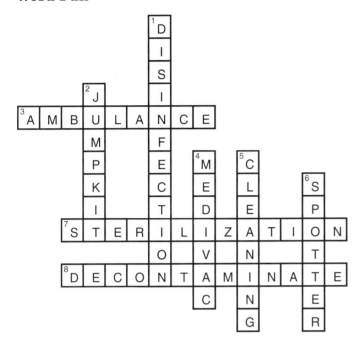

Ambulance Calls

1. Fire departments have a distinct chain of command. You should obtain permission to place yourself en route to this medical emergency from your shift captain or appropriate fire officer. Just because a call is dispatched does not mean you should automatically place yourself en route to that location. The incident commander of the confirmed structure fire may need your immediate assistance on the scene. Because you do not know the nature medical emergency at this point, it would be prudent to place that decision in appropriate hands. Always follow local protocols and chain of command.

2. Ideally, you should be very familiar with your response area, and you should take time every shift to study local roads. This can be done individually or as a group shift activity. Obviously, the larger your coverage area the more difficult it becomes to memorize addresses, especially if you are not native to the area. Regardless, you should be able to read maps quickly, and you should not rely on your memory to assist in locating a new address. To attempt to memorize all local streets is a good goal, but failing to consult with a map before leaving the station for reasons of pride is downright foolish. Ensure that each and every agency vehicle used in response to emergencies is equipped with local maps and other resources to ensure you arrive promptly at emergency scenes. Utilize your local dispatch center for directions if necessary.

3. –Park your ambulance in a safe area.
   –Ensure personal safety.
   –Either you or your partner should handle traffic control until the police arrive.
   –The person not handling traffic control should assess the patient.
   –Provide patient care while ensuring personal safety and patient safety.

Chapter 36: Gaining Access

Matching

1. E (page 1059)
2. A (page 1062)
3. D (page 1062)
4. F (page 1060)
5. B (page 1065)
6. G (page 1068)
7. C (page 1068)

Multiple Choice

1. D (page 1060)
2. B (page 1060)
3. C (page 1060)
4. A (page 1060)
5. D (page 1059)
6. A (page 1062)
7. B (page 1061)
8. D (page 1063)
9. D (page 1065)
10. C (page 1065)
11. D (page 1066)
12. B (page 1067)

Fill-in

1. Removal (page 1059)
2. safety (page 1058)
3. communication (page 1058)
4. stable (page 1061)
5. safest (page 1063)
6. harm (page 1064)
7. self-contained breathing apparatus (page 1068)

True/False

1. F (page 1060)
2. T (page 1059)
3. T (page 1058)
4. F (page 1062)
5. T (page 1061)

Short Answer

1. –Firefighters: responsible for extinguishing any fire, preventing additional ignition, ensuring that the scene is safe, and washing down spilled fuel.

   –Law enforcement: responsible for traffic control and direction, maintaining order at the scene, investigating the crash or crime scene, and establishing and maintaining lines so that bystanders are kept at a safe distance and out of the way of rescuers.

   –Rescue group: responsible for properly securing and stabilizing the vehicle, providing safe entrance and access to patients, extricating any patients, ensuring that patients are properly protected during extrication or other rescue activities, and providing adequate room so that patients can be removed properly.

   –EMS personnel: responsible for assessing and providing immediate medical care, triage and assigning priority to patients, packaging the patient, providing additional assessment and care as needed once the patient has been removed, and providing transport to the emergency department. (page 1060)

2. Is the patient in a vehicle or in some other structure?

   Is the vehicle or structure severely damaged?

   What hazards exist that pose risk to the patient and rescuers?

   In what position is the vehicle? On what type of surface? Is the vehicle stable or is it apt to roll or tip? (page 1062)

3. **1.** Provide manual stabilization to protect c-spine, as needed.

   2. Open the airway.

   3. Provide high-flow oxygen

   4. Assist or provide for adequate ventilation.

   5. Control any significant external bleeding.

   6. Treat all critical injuries. (page 1063)

4. The extent of injury and whether there is a possibility of hidden bleeding

Evaluate sensation in the trapped area to discover if an object is pressing on or impaled in the patient. (page 1063)

5. Ensure that each EMT-B can be positioned so that he/she can lift and carry at all times.

Move the patient in a series of smooth, slow, controlled steps, with stops designed between to allow for repositioning and adjustments.

Plan the exact steps and pathway that you will follow.

Choose a path that requires the least manipulation of the patient or equipment.

Make sure that sufficient personnel are available.

Make sure that you move the patient as a unit.

While moving the patient, continue to protect him/her from any hazards. (page 1064)

Word Fun

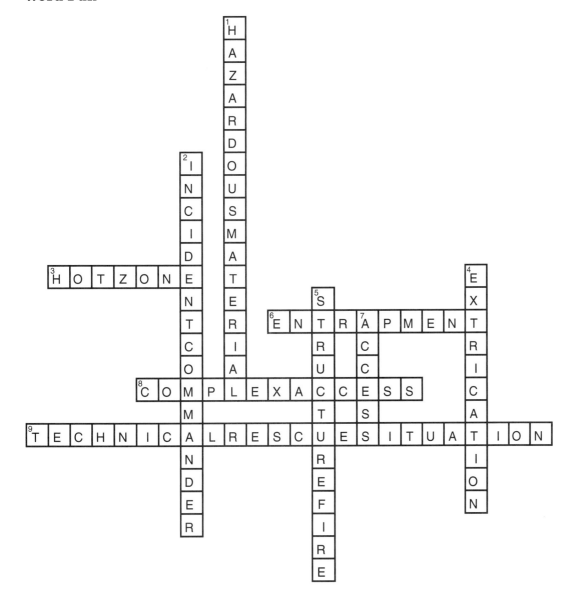

Ambulance Calls

1. You cannot assume that the man has left the premises, and you must act in the best interest of the patient. If the man is unconscious or otherwise incapacitated, time is of the essence. You should look inside the residence to see if the patient (in whole or part) is visible. Law enforcement should be immediately summoned to the scene for legal purposes if you feel that forced entry is justified. Always "try before you pry" meaning check open windows and doors to gain access, and if this is not possible, choose a small window to break rather than a door. It is less expensive to repair. Sometimes windows adjacent to doors can be broken, and access to the interior lock can be gained. You must be careful when entering, as there is a family dog that will most likely protect the property. Animal control should be requested if you feel the dog presents a safety hazard. It is prudent to err on the side that the patient needs immediate assistance rather than waiting for the third party caller to arrive with keys. Always follow local protocols.

2. Entering the water could be a death sentence for you both. If you have a cellular phone and/or department radio with you, your best course of action would be to inform incoming units of the boy's location and situation. It would be advisable to direct some responding units down stream so that if the boy should lose his grasp on the log, other responders will be available to retrieve him. If your department has areas that contain the possibility of swift water rescue (even if only seasonal), training should be conducted and appropriate helmets, throw bags and life jackets should be made available for safe response. You must assess the scene before trying to effect immediate rescue operations. Many responders have been killed by "jumping into" all types of rescues without performing a scene size-up or using the proper gear. Don't become a victim. Doing so will only make yourself part of the problem.

3. Try to learn as much about the chemical as possible by having the dispatcher contact CHEMTREC or another agency to find out about possible effects to the patient.
   Prepare necessary equipment to manage the airway and ventilation.
   Be prepared to do CPR if necessary.
   Have all equipment within reach.
   Once patient is brought to you, rapidly begin to manage the ABCs and prepare for rapid transport.

Chapter 37: Special Operations

Matching

1. J (page 1079)
2. K (page 1074)
3. L (page 1089)
4. D (page 1076)
5. H (page 1091)
6. E (page 1092)
7. B (page 1084)
8. I (page 1084)
9. A (page 1085)
10. F (page 1079)
11. G (page 1077)
12. C (page 1077)

Multiple Choice

1. D (page 1074)
2. D (page 1075)
3. C (page 1075)
4. A (page 1076)
5. D (page 1079)
6. C (page 1077)
7. D (page 1083)
8. B (page 1076)
9. D (page 1079)
10. D (page 1091)
11. B (page 1091)
12. D (page 1090)
13. A (page 1090)
14. B (page 1087)
15. D (page 1087)
16. D (page 1087)
17. D (page 1086)
18. D (page 1087)
19. B (page 1086)
20. D (page 1086)
21. A (page 1083)
22. B (page 1083)
23. D (page 1083)
24. C (page 1083)
25. A (page 1083)
26. D (page 1083)
27. A (page 1083)
28. B (page 1083)
29. D (page 1083)
30. C (page 1083)

Fill-in

1. incident command system (page 1074)
2. command post (page 1074)
3. safety officer (page 1075)
4. hazardous materials incident (page 1085)
5. extrication (page 1076)
6. disaster (page 1084)
7. Triage (page 1076)
8. contaminated (page 1091)
9. airway, breathing (page 1090)
10. Decontamination (page 1089)
11. relocate (page 1087)
12. toxic (page 1086)
13. placard (page 1086)

True/False

1. T (page 1085)
2. F (page 1088)
3. F (page 1089)
4. F (page 1092)
5. T (page 1083)
6. F (page 1083)
7. T (page 1086)
8. F (page 1089)
9. F (page 1090)
10. T (page 1076)

Short Answer

1. Level 0: Materials that would cause little, if any, health hazard if you came into contact with them
   Level 1: Materials that would cause irritation on contact, but only mild residual injury, even without treatment
   Level 2: Materials that could cause temporary damage or residual injury unless prompt medical treatment is provided
   Level 3: Materials that are extremely hazardous to health
   Level 4: Materials that are so hazardous that minimal contact will cause death (page 1089)

2. Level A: Fully encapsulated, chemical-resistant protective clothing; SCBA; special, sealed equipment
   Level B: Nonencapsulated protective clothing, or clothing designed to protect against a particular hazard; SCBA; eye protection
   Level C: Nonpermeable clothing; eye protection; facemasks
   Level D: Work uniform (page 1092)

3. 1. Command
   2. Staging
   3. Extrication
   4. Triage
   5. Treatment
   6. Supply
   7. Transportation
   8. Rehabilitation (page 1075)

4. First priority (red): Patients who need immediate care and transport
   Second priority (yellow): Patients whose treatment and transportation can be temporarily delayed
   Third priority (green): Patients whose treatment and transportation can be delayed until last
   Fourth priority (black): Patients who are already dead or have little chance for survival (page 1081)

5. (page 1088)

Class	Type
Class 1	Explosives
Class 2	Gases
Class 3	Flammable liquids
Class 4	Flammable solids
Class 5	Oxidizers
Class 6	Poisons
Class 7	Radioactive
Class 8	Corrosives
Class 9	Miscellaneous

6. The process of removing or neutralizing and properly disposing of hazardous materials from equipment, patients, and rescue personnel. The decontamination area is the designated area where contaminants are removed before an individual can go to another area. (page 1089)

Word Fun

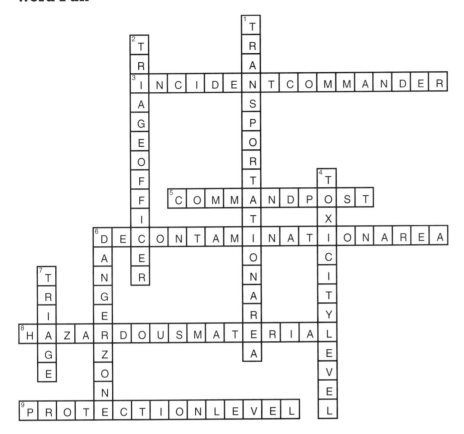

Ambulance Calls

1. –The 4-year-old should be triaged as first priority (red).
   –The 27-year-old should be triaged as third priority (green).
   –The 42-year-old should be triaged as fourth priority (black).

2. It's fortunate that this is occurring on shift change, as members from two shifts are available to respond to this mass casualty incident. Since this is a remote area, implying response times are extended, you should use this time to gather information from the crop duster pilot/responsible parties regarding the substance and notify all local hospitals. Area HazMat team members should be requested, and once the chemicals have been identified, appropriate first aid and other instructions should be relayed to the affected patients on-scene through the dispatch center. Law enforcement should be requested to cordon off the area to prevent more individuals such as co-workers and family members from entering the contaminated area. Consult HazMat team members and/or CHEMTREC for appropriate information including medical treatment, PPE and minimum distances that are required to avoid exposure to the identified substance. Obviously, do not enter the area unless you have been trained and have the proper equipment to do so.

3. The good news is that you are uphill from the possible hazardous materials. You should be uphill and upwind from contaminated areas (especially when dealing with an unidentified substance). Each chemical reacts differently to outside air, temperature and other ambient conditions. You should immediately instruct all civilians along the road to move out of the immediate area and/or instruct them to wait in a specific location if you feel that they have already been contaminated by the substance. Do not allow the driver to contaminate the passersby. Law enforcement should be immediately notified as well as the local HazMat team. Attempt to gain information regarding the shipment, keeping a safe distance (using binoculars, PA system to relay instructions, etc.) Prevent exposure to yourself and your crew and the members of the public. Always follow local protocols.

Chapter 38: Response to Terrorism and Weapons of Mass Destruction

Matching

1. I (page 1107)
2. G (page 1107)
3. E (page 1112)
4. A (page 1108)
5. J (page 1117)
6. C (page 1115)
7. B (page 1106)
8. F (page 1112)
9. D (page 1106)
10. H (page 1116)

Multiple Choice

1. D (page 1100)
2. A (page 1101)
3. B (page 1102)
4. B (page 1103)
5. A (page 1104)
6. A (page 1105)
7. D (page 1106)
8. C (page 1107)
9. A (page 1108)
10. A (page 1109)
11. A (page 1110)
12. B (page 1111)
13. A (page 1112)
14. B (page 1113)
15. D (page 1114)
16. D (page 1115)
17. C (page 1116)
18. A (page 1117)
19. A (page 1118)
20. B (page 1119)
21. B (page 1120)
22. D (page 1122)

Fill-in

1. domestic terrorism (page 1100)
2. weapon of mass destruction (page 1101)
3. State-sponsored terrorism (page 1102)
4. orange (page 1103)
5. Cross-contamination (page 1104)
6. Route of exposure (page 1106)
7. contact hazard (page 1107)
8. Nerve agents (page 1108)
9. Off-gassing (page 1109)
10. Dissemination (page 1112)
11. Virus (page 1113)
12. viral hemorrhagic fevers (page 1114)
13. Anthrax (page 1115)
14. lymph nodes (page 1116)
15. botulinum (page 1117)
16. Points of distribution (page 1119)
17. radiological dispersal device (page 1120)

True/False

1. F (page 1100)
2. T (page 1101)
3. F (page 1102)
4. T (page 1103)
5. T (page 1104)
6. F (page 1105)
7. F (page 1106)
8. F (page 1107)
9. T (page 1108)
10. F (page 1109)
11. F (page 1110)
12. T (page 1111)
13. T (page 1112)
14. F (page 1113)
15. F (page 1114)
16. T (page 1115)
17. T (page 1116)
18. F (page 1117)
19. F (page 1118)
20. F (page 1119)
21. T (page 1120)
22. T (page 1122)

Short Answer

1. What are your initial actions?
   Who should you notify, and what should you tell them?
   What type of additional resources might you require?
   How should you proceed to address the needs of the victims?
   How do you ensure your own and your partner's safety, as well as the safety of the victims?
   What is the clinical presentation of a victim exposed to a WMD?
   How are WMD patients to be assessed and treated?
   How do you avoid becoming contaminated or cross-contaminated with a WMD agent? (page 1100)

2. Vesicants
   Respiratory agents
   Nerve agents
   Metabolic agents (page 1102)

3. Type of location
   Type of call
   Number of patients
   Victim's statements
   Pre-incident indicators (page 1103)

4. Skin irritation, burning, and reddening
   Immediate intense skin pain
   Formation of large blisters
   Gray discoloration of skin
   Swollen and closed or irritated eyes
   Permanent eye injury (page 1107)

5. Shortness of breath
   Chest tightness
   Hoarseness and stridor due to upper airway constriction
   Gasping and coughing (page 1108)

6. Salivation, sweating
   Lacrimation
   Urination
   Defecation, drooling, diarrhea
   Gastric upset and cramps
   Emesis
   Muscle twitching (page 1110)

7. Shortness of breath and gasping respirations
   Tachypnea
   Flushed skin color
   Tachycardia
   Altered mental status
   Seizures
   Coma
   Apnea
   Cardiac arrest (page 1112)

8. Fever
   Chills
   Headache
   Muscle aches
   Nausea
   Vomiting
   Diarrhea
   Severe abdominal cramping
   Dehydration
   Gastrointestinal bleeding
   Necrosis of liver, spleen, kidneys, and gastrointestinal tract (page 1118)

9. Hospitals
   Colleges and universities
   Chemical and industrial sites (page 1120)

10. Time
    Distance
    Shielding (page 1122)

Word Fun

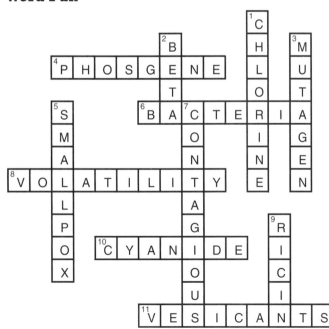

Ambulance Calls

1. There is no confirmation regarding the nature of the explosion. This could have been caused by a number of hazards, but any time there is the chance for a terrorist attack, precautions should be taken. No one should rush into the scene, because terrorists have been known to deliberately target first responders by placing secondary explosive devices. Request all available resources including local, state, and federal specialized HazMat and law enforcement agencies to assist in this call. Notify all local and regional hospitals of the situation; assess the scene from a distance. Establish command and designate a staging area for incoming units. Enter the scene only when it has been determined to be safe. Regularly scheduled mock drills to include expected agencies to respond in this type of situation can greatly improve communications and the overall effectiveness and efficiency of response.

2. The presence of numerous people with the same signs and symptoms, who were in the same location at the same time, should immediately send up red flags. These patients were exposed to contaminated food, air, or water in which they ingested some sort of toxin. Ingestion of ricin can produce these signs and symptoms and will usually be seen 4 to 8 hours after exposure. It can be difficult to initially determine what substances caused these signs and symptoms, but through careful history taking and investigation of the patients' commonalities, the exposure can be found. Unfortunately for those exposed to ricin, there is no vaccination or other specific treatment available. Only supportive measures for airway, breathing, and circulation can be applied.

3. Cyanide is colorless and has an odor similar to bitter almonds. It interferes with the body's ability to utilize oxygen and can result in headache, shortness of breath, tachypnea, altered levels of consciousness, apnea, seizures, and even death. Antidotes can be given, but are rarely carried on ambulances. Patients' clothing must be removed to avoid exposure to the cyanide because it is released as a gas from the clothing fibers. For most patients, simply removing them from the source of cyanide and providing supportive therapy for their ABCs will be all that is needed. However, those with significant exposure may require aggressive airway intervention.

Chapter 39: Advanced Airway Management

Matching

1. K (page 1132)
2. G (page 1132)
3. L (page 1132)
4. E (page 1132)
5. J (page 1132)
6. C (page 1133)
7. B (page 1132)
8. M (page 1146)
9. H (page 1135)
10. A (page 1142)
11. I (page 1137)
12. D (page 1139)
13. F (page 1139)

Multiple Choice

1. D (page 1132)
2. B (page 1132)
3. C (page 1132)
4. C (page 1132)
5. A (page 1132)
6. B (page 1132)
7. B (page 1132)
8. A (page 1132)
9. D (page 1132)
10. C (page 1133)
11. D (page 1134)
12. B (page 1134)
13. A (page 1135)
14. B (page 1135)
15. D (page 1137)
16. B (page 1137)
17. D (page 1138)
18. A (page 1139)
19. B (page 1139)
20. C (page 1141)
21. A (page 1141)
22. C (page 1141)
23. B (page 1142)
24. B (page 1142)
25. A (page 1141)
26. D (page 1138)
27. C (page 1145)
28. A (page 1145)
29. C (page 1146)
30. D (page 1150)
31. D (page 1150)
32. B (page 1137)
33. D (page 1151)
34. B (page 1152)
35. D (page 1153)
36. D (page 1154)
37. C (page 1155)
38. D (page 1156)

Labeling

The Upper and Lower Airways (page 1133)

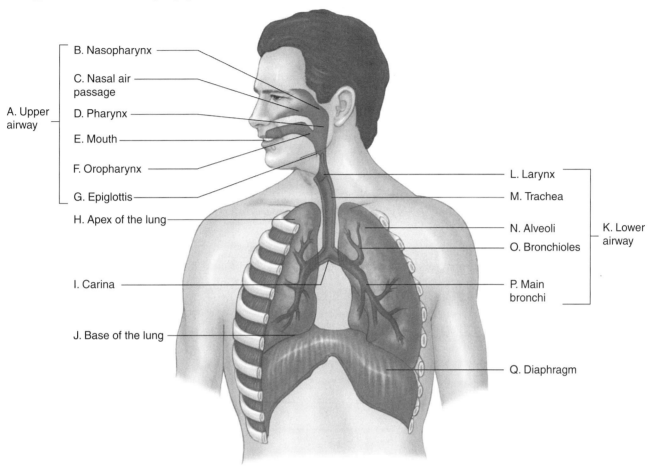

B. Nasopharynx

C. Nasal air passage

D. Pharynx

E. Mouth

F. Oropharynx

G. Epiglottis

A. Upper airway

H. Apex of the lung

I. Carina

J. Base of the lung

L. Larynx

M. Trachea

N. Alveoli

O. Bronchioles

K. Lower airway

P. Main bronchi

Q. Diaphragm

Fill-in

1. inhalation (page 1132)
2. bronchi (page 1132)
3. passive (page 1132)
4. oxygen (page 1132)
5. Carbon dioxide (page 1132)
6. 4 to 6 (page 1133)
7. bronchioles (page 1132)
8. capillaries (page 1132)

True/False

1. T (page 1140)
2. T (page 1137)
3. F (page 1140)
4. F (page 1141)
5. T (page 1142)
6. F (page 1142)

Short Answer

1. To perform the Sellick maneuver, place a thumb and index finger on either side of the midline of the cricoid cartilage. Apply firm—but not excessive—pressure, as too much pressure could collapse the larynx. Maintain this pressure until the patient is intubated. (page 1136)

2.
   1. Completely controls and protects the airway
   2. Delivers better minute volume without the difficulty of maintaining an adequate mask seal
   3. If prolonged ventilation is required, it may be left in place for a long time.
   4. Prevents gastric distention
   5. Minimizes risk of aspiration of stomach contents into the respiratory system

6. Allows for direct access to the trachea for suctioning

7. Allows for delivery of high volumes of oxygen at higher than normal pressures

8. Provides a route for administration of certain medications (page 1137)

3. **1.** Intubating the right mainstem bronchus

2. Intubating the esophagus

3. Aggravating a spinal injury

4. Taking too long to intubate

5. Patient vomiting

6. Soft-tissue trauma

7. Mechanical failure

8. Patient intolerance of ETT

9. Decrease in heart rate (page 1150)

4. **1.** Conscious or semi-conscious patients with a gag reflex

2. Children younger than age 16 years

3. Adults shorter than 5 feet tall

4. Patients who have ingested a caustic substance

5. Patients who have a known esophageal disease (page 1153)

5. Benefits: Ease of proper placement; no mask seal necessary; requires minimal skill and practice to maintain; easily used in spinal injury patients; may be inserted blindly; protects the airway from upper airway secretions; stays in place well (ETC); sturdy balloon (ETC).
Complications: Loses effectiveness (cuff malfunction); requires deeply comatose patient; requires constant balloon observation; cannot be used on patients shorter than 5' tall; requires great care in listening to breath sounds; large balloon is easily broken and tends to push the PtL out of the mouth when inflated. (page 1152)

Word Fun

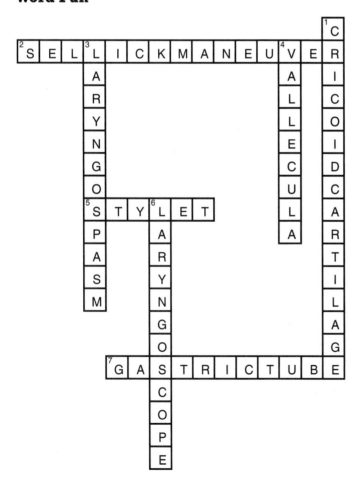

Ambulance Calls

1. If successful intubation has occurred, you will hear equal, bilateral breath sounds and no sounds over the epigastrium. This endotracheal tube should be removed, and the patient should be ventilated with high-flow oxygen via BVM device and the placement of an oral airway. Use of secondary placement devices should be utilized when assessing placement of the ET tube. Direct visualization of the ET tube passing through the cords along with the use of esophageal detector devices and/or end-tidal carbon dioxide detectors can ensure successful placement has been accomplished. If endotracheal intubation is not possible, consider the use of multilumen airways such as the Esophageal Tracheal Combitube (ETC), Pharyngeotracheal Lumen Airway (PtL) or Laryngeal Mask Airway (LMA). Always follow local protocols.

2. In this case, either nasogastric or orogastric tubes can be placed. You should measure the tube, lubricate it if necessary, place the patient in the proper position, pass the tube through the mouth or nose, confirm proper placement, aspirate gastric contents using a large syringe or suction unit and secure the tube in place. It is important to remember that this technique should be performed when other airway and cardiac needs have been addressed. Do not delay the securing of the patient's airway and/or application of the AED in the cardiac arrest patient in order to place an OG or NG tube. Also, remember to utilize the Sellick Maneuver until gastric contents have been aspirated and the abdomen is no longer distended. Always follow local protocols.

3. –Maintain c-spine control.
   –Use portable suction if needed.
   –Ventilate with BVM and 100% oxygen while c-spine and jaw thrust is maintained.
   –Insert a combitube to protect the airway (great because it is a blind insertion).
   –Continue to ventilate through combitube until patient is extricated.

Skill Drills
Skill Drill 39-1: Performing the Sellick Maneuver (page 1136)

1. Visualize the **cricoid** cartilage.
2. **Palpate** to confirm its location.
   Apply **firm** pressure on the cricoid **ring** with your thumb and index finger on either side of the **midline**. Maintain pressure until the patient is **intubated**.

Skill Drill 39-2: Performing Orotracheal Intubation (page 1148)

1. Open and clear the airway.
   Place an oropharyngeal airway, and preoxygenate with a BVM device.
2. Assemble and test intubation equipment as your partner continues to ventilate.
3. Confirm adequate preoxygenation, and remove the oral airway.
   If available, have another rescuer perform the Sellick manuever to improve visualization of the cords.
   Use the head tilt-chin lift maneuver to position a nontrauma patient for insertion of the laryngoscope.
4. In a trauma patient, maintain the cervical spine in-line and neutral as your partner lies down or straddles the patient's head to visualize the vocal cords.
5. Insert the laryngoscope from the right side of mouth, and move the tongue to the left. Lift the laryngoscope away from the posterior pharynx to visualize the vocal cords. **Do not pry or use the teeth as a fulcrum.**
   Insert the ET tube from the right side until the ET tube cuff passes between the vocal cords. Remove the laryngoscope and stylet. Hold the tube carefully until it is secured.
6. Inflate the balloon cuff, and remove the syringe as your partner prepares to ventilate.
7. Begin ventilating, and confirm placement of the ET tube by listening over the stomach and both lungs. Also confirm placement with an end-tidal carbon dioxide detector or EDD, if available.
8. Secure the tube, and continue to ventilate.
   Note and record depth of insertion (centimeter marking at the teeth), and reconfirm position after each time you move the patient.

Chapter 40: Assisting With Intravenous Therapy

Matching

1. C (page 1170)
2. G (page 1171)
3. A (page 1172)
4. H (page 1167)
5. D (page 1172)
6. B (page 1174)
7. F (page 1170)
8. E (page 1172)

Multiple Choice

1. D (page 1166)
2. B (page 1167)
3. D (page 1168)
4. A (page 1170)
5. B (page 1171)
6. D (page 1172)
7. B (page 1173)
8. C (page 1174)
9. B (page 1175)
10. C (page 1176)

Fill-in

1. administration set (page 1167)
2. Macrodrip sets (page 1168)
3. Saline locks (page 1170)
4. Jamshedi needle (page 1171)
5. phlebitis (page 1172)
6. Catheter shear (page 1174)

True/False

1. T (page 1166)
2. F (page 1167)
3. F (page 1168)
4. T (page 1170)
5. F (page 1171)
6. T (page 1172)
7. T (page 1173)
8. F (page 1174)
9. T (page 1175)
10. F (page 1176)

Short Answer

1. Follow BSI precautions.
   Obtain solution and check the bag for clarity, expiration date, and correct solution.
   Choose appropriate administration set.
   Obtain the requested catheter.
   Spike the bag.
   Remove air from the tubing.
   Prepare tape for securing tubing.
   Open alcohol prep.
   Have 4 x 4 ready for bleeding.
   Dispose of sharps.
   Hook up tubing and adjust flow. (page 1166)

2. Infiltration
   Phlebitis
   Occlusion
   Vein irritation
   Hematoma (page 1172)

3. Allergic reactions
   Air embolus
   Catheter shear
   Circulatory overload
   Vasovagal reactions (page 1173)

4. Place patient in shock position.
   Apply high-flow oxygen.
   Monitor vital signs.
   ALS provider should insert an IV catheter in case fluid resuscitation is needed. (page 1174)

5. IV fluid
   Administration set
   Height of bag
   Type of catheter
   Constricting band (page 1175)

Word Fun

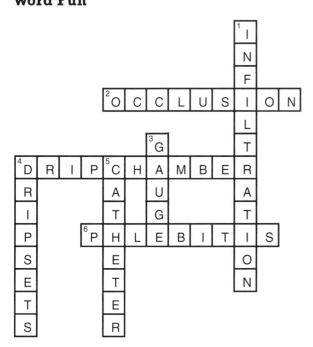

Ambulance Calls

1. You should immediately slow the IV to a TKO rate, raise the patient's head, and apply high-flow oxygen (or increase the current LPM). Notify the receiving facility of the error. Healthy adults can handle the sudden influx of intravenous fluids without detrimental effects, but individuals who have diseased or otherwise weakened hearts, lungs, or kidneys do not possess the ability to cope with the fluid overload. To avoid this occurrence, check and double check the drip chamber/flow rate to prevent accidental fluid boluses.

2. There are many things that can hinder the flow of IV fluids. One of the most obvious is failure to remove the tourniquet. Other contributing factors can include the condition of the IV fluids, the height of the bag, and perforation of the vein. Look for signs of these situations in order to determine the source of the problem. Do not automatically suggest the discontinuance of the IV, because the problem may be easily corrected.

3. Swelling around the insertion site indicates the infiltration of IV fluids into the surrounding tissues. This will also be identified with slowing or stopping of the IV fluid flow as well as pain and tightness around the IV site. When this occurs, the ALS provider must remove the IV and perform the venipuncture at another location. Direct pressure should be applied to minimize further swelling and bleeding.

Chapter 41: Assisting With Cardiac Monitoring

Matching

1. C (page 1187)

2. F (page 1188)

3. A (page 1182)

4. E (page 1187)

5. B (page 1187)

6. D (page 1188)

7. G (page 1185)

Multiple Choice

1. D (page 1182)

2. D (page 1183)

3. B (page 1184)

4. A (page 1185)

5. B (page 1187)

6. A (page 1188)

7. B (page 1189)

8. C (page 1191)

9. C (page 1192)

Fill-in

1. electrical conduction system (page 1182)

2. Sinus rhythm (page 1185)

3. Arrhythmia (page 1187)

4. Ventricular fibrillation (page 1188)

5. Asystole (page 1189)

6. limb leads (page 1191)

7. Chest leads (page 1192)

True/False

1. F (page 1182)

2. F (page 1183)

3. T (page 1185)

4. F (page 1187)

5. T (page 1188)

6. T (page 1189)

7. T (page 1191)

8. F (page 1192)

Short Answer

1. The sinoatrial node
Internodal pathways
Atrioventricular node
The bundle of His
The left bundle
The right bundle
The left anterior superior fascicle
The right posterior fascicle
The Purkinje system (page 1182)

2. Baseline period
SA node fires.
P wave forms.
QRS begins to form.
T wave forms.
The final phase (page 1185)

Word Fun

```
        T
        A
        C       E C G
        H         H
  A S Y S T O L E
        C         S
        A R R H Y T H M I A
        R         L
        D         E
  L I M B L E A D S
        A         D
                  S
```

Ambulance Calls

1. Do not be afraid to inform the paramedic that the leads have not been appropriately attached. You can save valuable time, by simply relaying what you have seen. Sometimes EMTs can feel intimidated by the presence of paramedics and become afraid to speak out when they see something that doesn't appear right. Do not underestimate your ability to help, because sometimes you may notice things that the paramedic has not.

2. This arrhythmia is sinus bradycardia. When a patient is experiencing symptomatic bradycardia, the paramedic will take steps to correct this arrhythmia. Notifying the paramedic of the slow heart rate and being familiar with basic arrhythmias such as sinus bradycardia will make you a more helpful team member.

3. In order for the 12-lead ECG machine to work properly, the patient's chest must be clean, dry, and with minimal hair in order to ensure the electrodes can adhere to the skin. This requires that the patient be wiped down to remove excessive sweat and that benzoin be used (if necessary) and chest hair be removed. Some protocols do not allow for the shaving of chest hair (due to the potential of skin abrasions and cuts and their potential impact on the use of thrombolytics). It is also important to note that brassieres of female patients must be removed. It is helpful to carry gowns on the ambulance and ask any unnecessary personnel to exit the room in order to preserve a patient's modesty. Always follow local protocols.

Appendix A: BLS Review

Matching

1. E (page A-4)
2. D (page A-12)
3. B (page A-3)
4. C (page A-5)
5. A (page A-3)

Multiple Choice

1. D (page A-3)
2. C (page A-5)
3. B (page A-5)
4. D (page A-5)
5. A (page A-6)
6. D (page A-6)
7. D (page A-6)
8. D (page A-7)
9. C (page A-8)
10. D (page A-9)
11. A (page A-10)
12. B (page A-11)
13. C (page A-17)
14. B (page A-18)
15. A (page A-20)
16. D (page A-20)
17. A (page A-21)
18. D (page A-21)
19. B (page A-28)
20. D (page A-28)
21. D (page A-28)
22. B (page A-29)
23. D (page A-11)
24. D (page A-12)
25. B (page A-13)
26. C (page A-14)

Fill-in

1. 4, 6 (page A-3)
2. barrier (page A-5)
3. ABCs (page A-6)
4. opening (page A-4)
5. Advance directives (page A-7)
6. firm (page A-8)
7. airway (page A-9)

True/False

1. T (page A-6)
2. F (page A-6)
3. T (page A-6)
4. F (page A-20)
5. F (page A-10)
6. T (page A-7)

7. T (page A-23)
8. F (page A-23)
9. F (page A-20)
10. T (page A-19)
11. F (page A-19)

Short Answer

1. 1. Rigor mortis, or stiffening of the body after death
   2. Dependent lividity (livor mortis), a discoloration of the skin due to pooling of blood
   3. Putrefaction or decomposition of the body
   4. Evidence of nonsurvivable injury, such as decapitation (page A-7)

2. (page A-4)

Procedure	Infants (younger than age 1 year)	Children (1 to 8 years)
Airway	Head tilt–chin lift; jaw thrust if spinal injury is suspected	Head tilt–chin lift; jaw thrust if spinal injury is suspected
Breathing Initial breaths	2 breaths with duration of 1 to 1½ seconds each	2 breaths with duration of 1 to 1½ seconds each
Subsequent breaths	1 breath every 3 seconds; 20 breaths/min	1 breath every 3 seconds; 20 breaths/min
Circulation Pulse check	Brachial/femoral arteries	Carotid artery
Compression area	Lower half of sternum	Lower half of sternum
Compression width	2 or 3 fingers	Heel of one hand
Compression depth	½ to 1"	1" to 1½"
Compression rate	At least 100/min	100/min
Ratio of Compressions to Ventilations	5:1 (pause for ventilation)	5:1 (pause for ventilation)
Foreign Body Obstruction	Back blows and chest thrusts	Abdominal thrusts

3. S–The patient starts breathing and has a pulse.
   T–The patient is transferred to another person who is trained in BLS or ALS, or another emergency medical responder.
   O–You are out of strength or too tired to continue.
   P–A physician who is present assumes responsibility for the patient. (page A-8)

4. To perform the head tilt-chin lift maneuver, make sure the patient is supine. Place one hand on the patient's forehead, and apply firm backward pressure with your palm to tilt the head back. Next, place the tips of your fingers of your other hand under the lower jaw near the bony part of the chin. Lift the chin forward, bringing the entire lower jaw with it, helping to tilt the head back. (page A-10)

5. To perform the jaw-thrust maneuver, kneel above the patient's head. Place your index or middle finger behind the angle of the lower jaw on both sides. Forcefully move the jaw forward, and tilt the head back. Use your thumbs to pull the patient's lower jaw down to allow breathing through the mouth and nose. (page A-11)

6. Ensure that the patient is on a firm, flat surface. Place your hands in the proper position. Lock your elbows with your arms straight and your shoulders directly over your hands. Give 15 compressions at a rate of about 100 beats/minute for an adult. Using a rocking motion, apply pressure vertically from your shoulders down through both arms to depress the sternum 1½" to 2" in the adult, then rise up gently. Count the compressions aloud. The ratio of compressions and relaxation should be 1:1. (page A-23)

7. First EMT-B moves into position to begin chest compressions after giving a breath. Second EMT-B gives the 15th compression, then moves to the patient's head. Second EMT-B checks the carotid pulse for 5 to 10 seconds. If the patient has no pulse, say, "No pulse, continue CPR." (page A-27)

8. –Standing: Stand behind the patient and wrap your arms around his or her waist. Press your fist into the patient's abdomen in a series of five quick inward and upward thrusts.

    –Supine: Straddle the hips or legs. Place the heel of one hand against the patient's abdomen and the other hand on top of the first. Press your hands into the patient's abdomen in a series of five quick inward and upward thrusts. (page A-12)

9. –Standing: Stand behind the patient and wrap your arms under the armpits and around the patient's chest. Press your fist into the patient's chest and perform backwards thrusts until the object is expelled or the patient becomes unconscious.

    –Supine: Kneel next to the patient. Place your hands as you would to deliver chest compressions. Deliver slow chest thrusts until the object is expelled. (page A-13)

10. 1. "Sandwich" the infant between your hands and arms.

     2. Deliver five quick back blows between the shoulder blades, using the heel of your hand.

     3. Turn the infant face up.

     4. Give five quick chest thrusts on the sternum at a slightly slower rate than you would give for CPR. (pages A-16)

Word Fun

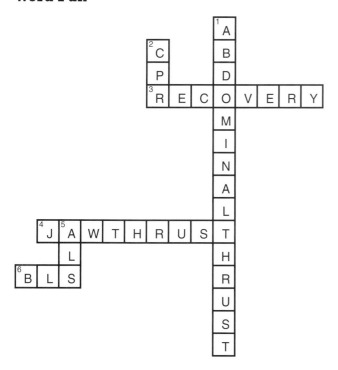

Ambulance Calls

1. –Question the family about the last time they spoke with her.
   –Explain that she has been down too long for CPR to be effective.
   –Comfort family members.
   –Notify your dispatcher to alert the supervisor and either law enforcement, the coroner, or a funeral home according to local protocols.

2. With the FDA's approval of Automated External Defibrillators for home use, it will become more common to see them being used by the lay provider. Simply purchasing an AED does not ensure appropriate usage during real life events. Training by knowledgeable, skilled instructors is needed to minimize confusion and inappropriate AED use. Remove the AED and explain to them that AED's are meant to be used only when a person is not breathing and has no pulse. Emphasize that it is appropriate to have the AED nearby in the event that a person goes into cardiorespiratory arrest, but it is not to be applied until then. After the patient has been transported to the hospital, tell the friends and family that you appreciate their willingness to be prepared for emergencies, and you would like to see them be successful in their usage of their AED. If you or your department offers CPR/AED courses, offer to train them and/or point them in the right direction to receive the appropriate training.

3. Given the scene, you must assume that there is the likelihood for trauma. This means that you must assess and maintain his airway without manipulating his spine. Use the jaw thrust maneuver and apply full c-spine precautions. Also, consider possible causes of his unconscious state, including any scene hazards and potential medical conditions.

Skill Drills

Skill Drill A-1: Positioning the Patient (page A-9)

1. Kneel beside the patient, leaving room to roll the patient toward you.
2. Grasp the patient, stabilizing the cervical spine if needed.
3. Move the head and neck as a unit with the torso as your partner pulls on the distant shoulder and hip.
4. Move the patient to a supine position with legs straight and arms at the sides.

Skill Drill A-2: Performing Chest Compressions (page A-22)

1. Slide your **index** and **middle** fingers along the rib cage to the **notch** in the **center** of the chest.
2. Push the middle finger high into the notch, and lay the index finger on the **lower portion** of the sternum.
3. Place the **heel** of the second hand on the lower half of the sternum, touching the **index finger** of your first hand.
4. Remove your first hand from the notch, and place it over the **hand** on the sternum.
5. With your arms straight, **lock** your elbows, and position your shoulders directly **over** your hands. Depress the sternum 1½ inches to 2 inches using a rhythmic motion.

Skill Drill A-3: Performing One-rescuer Adult CPR (page A-24)

1. Establish unresponsiveness, and call for help.
2. Open the airway.
3. Look, listen, and feel for breathing. If breathing is adequate, place the patient in the recovery position and monitor.
4. If not breathing, give two breaths of 2 seconds each.
5. Check for a carotid pulse.
6. If no pulse is found, apply your AED. If there is no AED, place your hands in the proper position for chest compressions. Give 15 compressions at a rate of about 100/min.
   Open the airway, and give two ventilations of 2 seconds each.
   Perform four cycles of compressions.
   Stop CPR, and check for return of the carotid pulse.
   Depending on patient condition, continue CPR, continue rescue breathing only, or place the patient in the recovery position and monitor breathing and pulse.

Skill Drill A-4: Performing Two-rescuer Adult CPR (page A-26)

1. Establish **unresponsiveness**, and take positions.
2. Open the airway.
3. Look, listen, and feel for breathing. If breathing is adequate, place the patient in the **recovery position and monitor**.
4. If not breathing, give **two** breaths of 2 seconds each.
5. Check for a **carotid** pulse.
6. If there is no pulse but an AED is available, apply it now. If no AED is available, begin **chest compressions** at about 100/min (15 compressions to **two** ventilations).
   After 1 minute, check for a **carotid** pulse. Check every few **minutes** thereafter.
   Depending on patient **condition**, continue CPR, continue rescue breathing only, or place in the recovery position and monitor.

BRUCE SPRINGSTEEN

BRUCE SPRINGSTEEN
Like a Killer in the Sun

Selected Lyrics, 1972–2017

edited by
LEONARDO COLOMBATI

translated by
FRANCESCA BOLZA

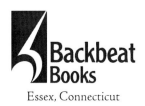

Backbeat Books

Essex, Connecticut

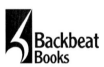

Backbeat Books

An imprint of Globe Pequot, the trade division of
The Rowman & Littlefield Publishing Group, Inc.
4501 Forbes Blvd., Ste. 200
Lanham, MD 20706
www.rowman.com

Distributed by NATIONAL BOOK NETWORK

Copyright © 2017 by Leonardo Colombati
First published in Italy in 2007 by Sironi Editore
First Backbeat paperback edition published in 2022

British Library Cataloguing in Publication Information available

Library of Congress Cataloging-in-Publication Data available

ISBN 978-1-4930-6542-4 (paperback)
ISBN 978-1-5400-0485-7 (ebook)

♾™ The paper used in this publication meets the minimum requirements of American National
Standard for Information Sciences—Permanence of Paper for Printed Library Materials, ANSI/
NISO Z39.48-1992

Being a rock star is the consolation prize.
I wanted to become a rock 'n' roller.

—Bruce Springsteen

CONTENTS

FOREWORD TO THE U.S. EDITION
by Dave Marsh

L eonardo Colombati has written a book about not one myth but many: the
myth of the rise of Bruce Springsteen, of course; the myth of America, un-
avoidably; the myths of high and low culture, mercilessly; the myth of rock 'n' roll,
necessarily; the myth of Springsteen's audience and its relationship with its icon,
intimately; the myth of what writing about rock and popular music can and
cannot be, passionately, confidently, beautifully, even as he demolishes and rebuilds
it within the first few pages of his introduction "The Great American Novel"; and,
for that matter, implicitly, the myth that there could be or should be a Great
American Novel and that if there is, that it has to be a novel.

Having written at considerable length on some of these issues myself, and
having known Leonardo for a decade or so, mostly when encamped somewhere on
the fringes of a Springsteen stage or backstage, I thought I knew what to expect,
even so soon after the publication of Springsteen's autobiography. I was dead
wrong. Leonardo's book is better, in ways that few could have predicted it was going
to be concerned with at all. Its introduction alters my way of thinking about Bruce,
about rock, about popular culture's deep connections to classical culture, and
about Springsteen's connections to American culture, especially African American
culture. Not by 180 degrees, of course, but by significant measures in each case. Its
version of Bruce's biography, which of course as his original biographer I know
thoroughly, nevertheless contains some remarkable insights. (My favorite is the
positioning of Springsteen's mythic Mary as a version of Dante's Beatrice, as an
objective and inspiration, in both spirit and flesh.)

Turned loose thereafter with the details of the biographical and artistic story,
Colombati lives up to his own standard. Most attempts to explain or analyze
Springsteen's work mainly in terms of lyrics fail because they cannot take in the
way in which his performance of those words alters, expands upon, and affirms
them. Which is to say that they waste our time by mainly explaining what is
obvious and in terms that indicate that, to them, such things are a revelation even
when to fans—deep listeners would be a preferable term—it is well known or
obvious. Often, Leonardo describes the obvious in order to move us toward a
point that is unexpectedly given a twist in a previously unheard-of direction.

To a longtime listener (let alone seeming "expert"!) this is less a shock than an affirmation: we continue to listen and re-listen to such straightforward sounds. One of the secrets of rock 'n' roll is this: the *individual* listener always finds revelations with her ears, because every performance delivers the message in a way that has everything to do with the nuances of the current placed against the backdrop of the song's own past. (And to anyone who doesn't believe that, what can one say but "oh my and a boo-hoo"?) This is why the isolated moment is as crucial as the whole construction. It is why rock is far more than its literary credibility or its often simple chords and rhythms. The secret may lie in a bass line that isn't even meant to be focused upon, which is why you missed it the first seventy-five times you heard it—or perhaps it's because the bassist himself just figured it out.

Leonardo Colombati (ever since he snuck off to his first Springsteen show) has long been a part of this process. Here he becomes the map-maker steering us into (perhaps) new dimensions, the griot insisting that participation—with the ears and the ass—not only makes the path, it is the path.

This is why a book such as this one, constantly finding riddles where there has seemed to be certainty, is so necessary, why it can shock the initiated with the realization that no one has taken the story or the incident or the line or the note this far before, or in this direction, or with the additional weight drawn from a presumably unconnected past.

To be perfectly clear: I now owe my friend Leo not just the debt of friendship but also the debt owed to someone who showed what was missing: the thing made hazy, all but invisible, until the right teller told the tale.

The premise of Bruce Springsteen's greatness has been that in order to grow, one must unlock expectations, and not only those imposed by others but the ones that have hold of us, ourselves. And so we return and return, again and again.

I do not expect to return to *Bruce Springsteen: Like a Killer in the Sun* as often as I return to "Growin' Up" or *The River* or "Queen of the Supermarket" or *Live in New York City*. But, as with those songs and albums, I know that I will return, and I am certain that I will not be alone when I do.

Dave Marsh
2017

FOREWORD TO THE ITALIAN EDITION
by Ennio Morricone

I was delighted to accept Leonardo Colombati's invitation to write an introduction to this book devoted to Bruce Springsteen. It isn't the usual hagiography praising some legendary rock star—there are no photographs of the sweaty singer raising his arms to the heavens while receiving an ovation from the thousands of ecstatic fans below the stage, and above all there is none of the sloppiness and slipshod inaccuracy that usually distinguish books about pop songs.

Throughout the twentieth century, this type of music was a bountiful source of emotions that accompanied several generations on their journey from adolescence to maturity, narrating—often far better than the other arts—the human condition in contemporary society.

This is a simple truth, long acknowledged in the United States, where pop music is considered an essential part of a single tradition in which Herman Melville and Walt Whitman, Robert Johnson and Louis Armstrong, and John Ford and Bruce Springsteen live side by side in perfect harmony. Here in Europe, on the other hand, this tradition is not accorded the same respect: the gulf created centuries ago between popular culture and—literally—"noble" culture has never been bridged. Just as, despite the numerous masterworks etched in all our memories, the cinema still struggles for acceptance simply for what it is—one art branching off the tree of narrative, visual, and musical arts—so in the field of music there is still an abyss between "cultured" and "pop" music: only music that is now considered venerable and historical or, on the contrary, experimental and elitist, is acknowledged as "real art."

I met Bruce Springsteen for the first time in Rome, in 1997, at the end of an acoustic concert he gave at the Auditorium of Santa Cecilia. He had just come out onto the stage accompanied, as he often is during his shows, by a recording of the notes of "Jill's Theme" from the music I wrote for the film *Once Upon a Time in the West*. Needless to say, I was immensely pleased. Our meeting took place backstage and was a very friendly one: Bruce hugged me and insisted on having his photograph taken with me. We had never encountered one another before and had long wanted to meet in person, particularly because both socially and politically the two of us feel like kindred spirits.

In his songs, Springsteen creates a strong sense of *pietas*—of the pain and humanity inherent in the characters he recounts. He does this not only through his music, where he uses different timbres and sounds to endow characters with a unique personality, but also through his lyrics, which are where his real power lies. Proof of this is to be found in the texts chosen and collected in this book, in the exhaustive critical review which accompanies them and highlights their literary opulence, which intertwines vastly different sources ranging from the Bible to the cinema and from the blues to current affairs, and also in the narrative power which renders the body of songs composed over thirty-five years a sort of Great American Novel. Or, to use Springsteen's own words, the screenplay for "a great film for an American drive-in." Simply reading the lyrics of "Jungleland," "Racing in the Street" and "The River" demonstrates how true this is. Springsteen's writing is cinematographic—each verse is a camera shot, each line is a scene, and each song presents to us a snapshot of the complete personality of the character taken at the decisive moment of his life.

Any composer who, like myself, has written music for the big screen, cannot feel indifference towards this cinematic style of writing: music for the cinema, if it is good, can be listened to and appreciated even without the images themselves being present. At the same time, though, Springsteen's songs—both the music and the words—might well be compared to the score of a film still to be shot: they need no images to support them because the images are created by the songs themselves. Rather than describing him as a "singer-songwriter," it would be far better to use the expression "storyteller." Springsteen, in fact, perpetuates the tradition created by bluesmen and folksingers in a way similar to the now almost extinct figure of the Italian balladeer.

Although they are very different, a certain part of my work and his shares a common basis in the simple chords we use to create structured and original melodies. The composer of instrumental music must redeem this simplicity with elaborate orchestration; the author-singer/storyteller can do so by using both voice and words, as long as the voice communicates an emotion and the words are *true*. I like Springsteen precisely because he places this need for Truth in the forefront. This is how he manages to elude passing fads and why his music runs no risk of being lost over the course of time.

INTRODUCTION

The Great American Novel

by Leonardo Colombati

PART ONE

1. Songs or Poems?

I belong to that last generation of teenagers who anxiously awaited the release of their favorite LP with a passion comparable to that with which Londoners rushed to buy copies of *Master Humphrey's Clock* to find out if poor Nelly Trent really did die in the last issue of Dickens's *The Old Curiosity Shop* a century and a half ago. Before downloading would forever change our habits and extinguish the album format, we would go to the record store, come home, shut ourselves in our bedrooms, and listen with an attention similar if not indeed superior to that we would apply to reading a book. The greatest artists of the sixties, seventies, eighties, and nineties relied on that attention. They could afford to be experimental, to indulge their creative expression to the limit. The extraordinary fact was that this was even happening in the so-called "mainstream." The Beatles were the most famous band in the world, and album after album they managed to keep that world hooked on their brilliant intuition. In 1964 girls were singing "A Hard Day's Night"; in 1966 *Revolver* ended upon the (unheard of!) notes of "Tomorrow Never Knows." In just two years a sort of Copernican revolution had occurred, and everyone could be a part of the show: the Beatles were always number one in the charts!

If you have an attentive audience, you get the chance to invent stories: for forty years rock 'n' roll has been decisive mainly because the writers were in fact story-telling; pop songs very often narrate complete tales. People like Lou Reed or Tom Waits told stories—often in the third person—of people with names and surnames, like Waldo Jeffers[1] or Susan Michelson.[2] Today, speed poses new limits to organizing texts vertically, structuring a story that develops quatrain by quatrain. Every verse, even every line must survive on its own, self-sufficiently; the first person reigns, so often barking at the moon.

This explains why an anthology of a singer-songwriter's lyrics today risks looking like an anachronism, a nostalgic operation with the potential, at best, to evoke some sort of memory in someone accustomed to hearing Paul Simon quoting Robert Frost in "The Dangling Conversation" or Bono Vox finding inspiration in Paul Celan.[3] Maybe I haven't "learned more from a three-minute record than we ever learned in school," as Springsteen sings in "No Surrender," but I would gladly pay a mind-blowing rent for a room in the Tower of Song, to spy on Leonard Cohen and Hank Williams for their secrets.

Sixty years have come and gone since April 16, 1956, when Chuck Berry sang "Roll Over, Beethoven" for the first time into a microphone, and the difference between highbrow and popular music—though never completely out of style—no longer seems relevant at this point. As children of rock 'n' roll, we know that in the past century Elvis Presley and the Velvet Underground were more decisive than Alan Berg and Karlheinz Stockhausen, and that the lyrics of many songs could easily fit within the bookshelves of literature, despite the world still being full of people who suffered from shock when the Swedish Academy awarded the Nobel Prize to Bob Dylan.[4]

"Like a Rolling Stone" . . . is it poetry? To those who asked, Bob Dylan once replied, "Poets die broke. Or drown in lakes."[5] It is however true that as a youngster Robert Zimmerman chose to call himself Dylan, a poet's name. Just to cloud the water. "Like a Rolling Stone" is a song. The fact that its author was awarded a Nobel Prize for Literature does nothing but emphasize a simple truth: the lyrics of a song are not poems, they are simply song lyrics—which in themselves form a genre in literature. Does *Hamlet* have a place in the history of literature? Does *Waiting for Godot*? Yes, they certainly do, despite the fact that they were dramas written not to be read but to be watched and listened to in a theater.[6] *Creative Evolution* and *Memoirs of the Second World War* are brilliant contributions by Henri Bergson and Winston Churchill to the world of philosophy and historiography, yet no one was shocked when Bergson and Churchill were awarded Nobel Prizes for literature, because both philosophy and historiography are recognized literary genres.

Of 120 Nobel Prizes for literature, three have been awarded to historians, eleven to playwrights, four to philosophers and one to a singer-songwriter. An honest 16 percent embracing Shaw, Sartre, Mommsen, and Beckett, and Pirandello, and Bertrand Russell. And Bob Dylan.

I know of not one single singer-songwriter with a drop of dignity to have ever equated his own song lyrics to a poem. And so it should be. Songs are NOT poems. Perhaps.

It's a minefield, of course. I know that. Springsteen got it right when he said that "talking about music is like talking about sex. Can you describe it? Are you supposed to?"[7] But what is a poem, in the end?

Straight from the roots: *poesis* in Latin from the Greek *poiesis*, an action noun from *poiein* meaning "to do," "to create." Flipping through dictionaries, one would appreciate that poetry, formally, is nothing other than composition in verse. Italian philosopher Benedetto Croce defined poetry as "cosmic intuition,"[8] the expression of a personal sentiment that reflects universal values with which all human beings can identify. In this respect, poetry is a rare, startling event and the critic's task is to pinpoint such moments even in the same opus.

We know that even good old Homer got lazy occasionally. And that some lines in the *Divine Comedy*—history's most magnificent intellectual exercise—might also warrant a Croce-like frown as actually bereft of poetry if taken out of context.

Robert Frost thought that poetry is what gets lost in translation.[9] I could go on. I have an endless supply of quotations to suit every situation, although I've yet to find one that can explain the formal difference between Coleridge's *Rime of the Ancient Mariner* and the Waterboys' "Fisherman's Blues." Is it just a matter of quality, at the end of the day? Looks that way. So we could just say that lyrics may not be very good poems, but we can't deny them poetry status.

Besides, in the Orphic myth both music and poetry rest on the lyre. And the illusion of the apparent inevitability of full circle works both ways. Dante calls the chapters of his poem "cantos," definitively complicating the dispute about whether music is the handmaiden of poetry or the other way around. German Romantics would say music has the upper hand (a deeper, more luminous code). Mallarmé disagreed and pointed to the ideal superiority of the poetic principle. Nonetheless, nobody has cracked the mystery of the son of Apollo and Calliope, who plucked such sweet melodies from the lyre that rivers stopped, stones came to life, wild animals were tamed, and trees leaned close to hear him better. On the ship built by Argos, the sweetness of Orpheus's music calmed Jason and his fifty-five companions during the most violent storms, soothing the waves of the Hellespont, off the shores of Mysia, around the island of Cyzicus, and appears to have been even more seductive than the song of the Sirens. When the Maenads ripped him to pieces and threw his limbs into the Hebrus, his head and his lyre ended up in the sea and the waves carried them to the island of Lesbos, which then became the home of lyrical poetry.

In fact, however, by concentrating on the unbridgeable distance between poetry and song—at once in honor of the lyrics' poetic self-sufficiency, already withholding inner "music" of its own, and then with particular notice to the lyrics' dependence upon melody and harmony—we have ended up underestimating the third major element of song: the performance. Through the fundamental importance of voice lies the dramatic difference between song and poetry.

How must it have been to watch Richard Burbage becoming Othello, King Lear, and Richard III on stage at the Globe? For over 400 years we have been pondering the effect, not only while *Othello*, *King Lear* and *Richard the III* are performed in theaters worldwide, with productions ranging from the sublime to the ridiculous, but also in the intimacy of our beds, a reading lamp shedding enough light for us to read any one of these tragedies, displayed with notes and commentary. Remove the set production, the actors' voices and actions from *Macbeth*, and you would be left with . . . literature.

As Bruce Springsteen's deep voice prepares to sing the second verse of "Factory," turn the volume down to zero; all you need to do is read the words on the inside of the album cover:

> Through the mansions of fear, through the mansions of pain,
> I see my daddy walking through them factory gates in the rain.

2. Spoon Rivers

The third edition of the *Norton Anthology of Poetry* contains "A wide and deep quarry of poems from the medieval period to the present day," if the preface is to be believed. The *excursus* begins with a quatrain composed by a nameless twelfth-century poet:

> Nou goth sonne under wode—
> Me reweth, Marie, thi faire rode.
> Nou goth sonne under tre—
> Me reweth, Marie, this one and the.[10]

Eight centuries later, in the grooves of a record and not in the pages of a literary anthology, another Mary and son beg for compassion:

> I come from down in the valley
> Where, mister, when you're young
> They bring you up to do
> Like your daddy done.
>
> Me and Mary we met in high school
> When she was just seventeen,
> We'd ride out of that valley
> Down to where the fields were green. . . .
>
> Then I got Mary pregnant
> And, man, that was all she wrote
> And for my nineteenth birthday
> I got a union card and a wedding coat.
>
> We went down to the courthouse
> And the judge put it all to rest,
> No wedding day smiles, no walk down the aisle,
> No flowers, no wedding dress.

In the most successful episodes, the author of "The River" echoes the epigrammatic style created by Edgar Lee Masters and used by Raymond Carver, for instance, in his *Where Water Comes Together with Other Water* poems. Springsteen often adopts the literary expedient used by the author of the *Spoon River Anthology* as he narrates the same story from two differing points of view. In *Spoon River* the tale of the McGees' matrimonial disaster is first told by Mrs. Ollie and successively by Mr. Fletcher. In the same way "The River" finds its reflection in "Spare Parts," when she remembers that "Bobby said he'd pull out . . . Bobby stayed in."

"Sinaloa Cowboys," a song that Springsteen released in 1995, shares more than one analogy with another Edgar Lee Masters poem, "'Butch' Weldy":

> After I got religion and steadied down
> They gave me a job in the canning works,
> And every morning I had to fill
> The tank in the yard with gasoline,
> That fed the blow-fires in the sheds
> To heat the soldering irons.
> And I mounted a rickety ladder to do it,
> Carrying buckets full of the stuff.
> One morning, as I stood there pouring,
> The air grew still and seemed to heave,
> And I shot up as the tank exploded,
> And down I came with both legs broken,
> And my eyes burned crisp as a couple of eggs.[11]

In "Sinaloa Cowboys," Springsteen tells the story of two Mexican brothers who manage to get to San Joaquin, in California, where they get work as farmhands and end up in a small tin shack on the edge of a ravine, cooking methamphetamine: You could spend a year in the orchards

> Or make half as much in one ten-hour shift
> Working for the men from Sinaloa, but if you slipped
> The hydriodic acid could burn right through your skin;
> They'd leave you spittin' up blood in the desert if you breathed those fumes
>   in.
> It was early one winter evening as Miguel stood watch outside
> When the shack exploded lighting up the valley night.
> Miguel carried Louis' body over his shoulder down a swale to the Creekside
> And there in the tall grass Louis Rosales died.

Miguel lifted Louis' body into his truck and then he drove
To where the morning sunlight fell on a eucalyptus grove.
There, in the dirt he dug up ten thousand dollars—all that they'd saved,
Kissed his brother's lips and placed him in his grave.

Unlike Masters, Springsteen doesn't include the moment of death in his tale. He just says, "There in the tall grass Louis Rosales died," whereas the explosion causes Butch Weldy to fall "with both legs broken, / And my eyes burned crisp as a couple of eggs." This crude and potent image is such that not even Springsteen can equal it, despite his ability to somehow anticipate the moment as he describes the effect of inhaling acid ("They'd leave you spittin' up blood in the desert"). What is certainly true is that both verses are remarkably effective. The common thread is found in such rich theoretically unpoetic detail: Masters speaks of tanks, blowtorches, warehouses, steel welding; Springsteen even includes hydriodic acid in a line.

So, is Springsteen a poet? "I'm a songwriter, I'm not a poetry man,"[12] he stated of himself. But it's a question that returns on a regular basis (just like with Dylan). By 1983, many seemed to agree with Frank McConnell's judgment that "he is a legitimate American mythologist, a storyteller of clear and authentic talent and, I would say, a major American poet."[13] A few years ago, the Weisman Art Museum organized an exhibition—*Springsteen: Troubadour of the Highway*—whose declared mission was to prove that Monmouth County, so meticulously described by Springsteen in his songs, has the same literary dignity as Faulkner's invented Yoknapatawpha County. In one article Pythia Peay went even so far as to say that "Springsteen's Asbury Park, Joyce's Dublin, and Pissarro's Paris are places each artist has immortalized, as much as the architects and engineers who built them."[14]

In September 2005, Long Branch Monmouth University organized a cycle of conferences entitled *Glory Days: A Bruce Springsteen Symposium*. One hundred and fifty professors, literary critics, journalists, and writers got up on the stage and spoke on themes like, "A Marxist Interpretation of *Darkness on the Edge of Town*," "Springsteen and Feminism," "Theology and Theory of Narration in the Works of Bruce Springsteen," "The Christocentric Imagination of Bruce Springsteen," "Steinbeck and Springsteen," "Springsteen and the Puritan Ideal of the Promised Land," "The Automobile in the Writings of Flannery O'Connor and Bruce Springsteen," "Springsteen and Sexual Identity" . . . The acts of the conference were preceded by this brief introduction:

Bruce Springsteen has produced a considerable body of original work that has impacted the direction of popular music and American culture. His influence extends from the stage into the classroom, and his works have turned up in the syllabi of courses across the United States and around the world.[15]

At this stage, one can't help but ask, in a country that has in the past two centuries expressed the likes of poets such as Whitman, Dickinson, Frost, Stevens, T.S. Eliot, and Hart Crane, and produced novelists of such magnitude as Melville, James, Fitzgerald, Faulkner, Bellow, and Roth, if it is really necessary to dig deep into popular music to find new bards. What must promptly be said is that "The River," just as all pop music, is not included in the Norton Anthology, which ends with a verse of Leslie Marmon Silko: "You see the sky now colder than the frozen river."[16] Yet under that bruised sky, along the river of American history, other voices have advanced, as Whitman said, "through all interpositions and covering and turmoils and stratagems to first principles."[17]

3. Roots

In 1619, while George Herbert versified on Redemption and Sin, Captain John Smith wrote in his far more prosaic *General History of Virginia*, "About the last of August came in a Dutch man of warre that sold us twenty negars."[18] Under the saffron skies of Georgia dawns, work songs began to ring out:

> Cotton needs a-pickin' so bad,
> Cotton needs a-pickin' so bad,
> Cotton needs a-pickin' so bad.
> Gonna pick all over this field.
>
> We planted this cotton in April
> On the full of the moon,
> We've had a hot, dry summer,
> That's why it opened so soon.[19]

Two centuries later Charles Dickens, upon visiting Philadelphia, swore he would have given anything for a bend in a road. Beneath the surface of that abrasive comment lay the genuine admiration for that extreme orthogonal order. Progress! The American machine was marching full steam ahead and there was no time to worry about slavery. As Thomas Pynchon reminds us, "Spiritual matters were not quite as immediate as material ones, like productivity! Sloth was no longer so much a Sin against God or spiritual good as against a particular sort of time, uniform, one-way, in general not reversible—that is, against clock time, which got everybody early to bed and early to rise."[20]

At the end of the Civil War, in 1865, when slavery was abolished, spirituals still echoed skywards all over the country, and guitars played twelve beats of new blues notes to accompany. However, the Academy was too busy nitpicking Wordsworth, recounting for the thousandth time in what way Coleridge dreamt of Kublai Khan, and even the author of "Song of Exposition" implored:

> Shut not your doors to me, proud libraries,
> For that which was lacking on all your well-fill'd shelves, yet needed most, I
>   bring.[21]

As though based upon some secret integration, from those days onwards popular songs began to gain space in American literature, in spite of those who continue to disregard the fact.[22] To appreciate the impact, it would suffice to listen to the album in which Springsteen pays homage to certain nineteenth- and early twentieth-century ballads, dug up before him by Peter Seeger (*We Shall Overcome: The Seeger Sessions*). Lyrics like these perhaps share a similar technical crudeness, yet surely bear an expressive force as powerful as an old-fashioned daguerreotype: *this was America!*

In "Erie Canal"[23] a man and his mule drag their barge down a canal and, when they reach a bridge to cross under, someone shouts, "Low bridge, everybody down!" because along urban paths it was commonplace to have to pass under bridges with arches barely over six feet above water. That cry, "Low bridge, everybody down!" is taken straight from real life.

A few hundred miles further south, in West Virginia, a man sings,

> Shenandoah, I love your daughter....
> I'll take her 'cross your rollin' water.[24]

A lament dating back to the country's early history, written in the first two decades of the 1800s, the song become extremely popular with sailors, who sang "Shenandoah" as they wound the capstan. In Georgia, however, black stevedores often worked for the simple promise that they would get paid the next day. So, sometimes they sang,

> I thought I heard the captain say,
> Pay me my money down.
> Tomorrow is our sailing day,
> Pay me my money down.
>
> Pay me, pay me,
> Pay me my money down,

Pay me or go to jail,
Pay me my money down.[25]

"John Henry," another song featured in *We Shall Overcome: The Seeger Sessions*, perfectly illustrates the sheer strength with which a popular song can mark the collective imagination, making a myth out of a moment forgotten by history. First known to have been transcribed in 1900, though it circulated orally years earlier, "John Henry" soon became the most famous among the "hammer songs" that gave voice to the awful conditions railroad workers endured when putting down the lines. The song tells a true story: the battle of one man against a machine during the construction of the early railroad systems in the eastern United States. Precisely at that time, steam-powered hammers began to replace traditional ones and steel-driving men such as John Henryemployed in the construction of the railway lines. So it was that John Henry bet he could compete with and beat a drill, the winner being the one to build the deepest hole in the established time. The duel occurred in a place still not conclusively identified or defined; according to some the event happened near the tunnel crossing Big Bend Mountain, West Virginia.

> John Henry driving on the right side,
> That steam drill driving on the left
> Says, "'fore I'll let your steam drill beat me down
> I'm gonna hammer myself to death, Lord, Lord,
> I'll hammer my fool self to death." . . .
>
> Now John Henry he hammered in the mountains,
> His hammer was striking fire,
> But he worked so hard he broke his heart,
> John Henry laid his hammer and died, Lord, Lord,
> John Henry laid down his hammer and died.

John Henry was a black slave from Crystal Springs, Mississippi. It seems that he really did beat the steam hammer (twenty-seven feet to twenty-one) but died of exhaustion on the spot.[26]

Popular song can not only knock down library doors, but act as inspiration (if not as a genuine source) for literature; as, for example, Colson Whitehead's *John Henry Days* bears witness:

> About 45 years ago I was in Morgan County, Kentucky. There was a bunch
> of darkeys came from Miss. to assist in driving a tunnel at the head of Big

Caney Creek for the O&K railroad. There is where I first heard this song, as they would sing it to keep time with their hammers.

Having seen your advertisement in the Chicago Defender, I am answering your request for information, concerning the Old-Time Hero of the Big Bend Tunnel Days—or Mr. John Henry . . .[27]

It's not so much a question of quality as of roots. Pop songs for America are like Dante's *Divine Comedy* and Chaucer's *Canterbury Tales* for Europeans. The "New World" was not yet conscious of having its own literature, along with a language (the Webster Dictionary dates back to 1828), when already on Revolution battlegrounds notes from fife songs like "Yankee Doodle" reverberated.

As early as 1794, North Carolina forced landowners to stop slaves "from gathering, with the purpose of drinking and singing."[28] But cotton-picking chain gangs went right on singing:

The day is done, night comes down,
Ye are long ways from home.
Oh, run, nigger, run,
Patter-roller git you.[29]

At the turn of the eighteenth century, the day after Thomas Jefferson drafted the Declaration of Independence—a manifesto defending human rights, but whose allusions to slavery were plucked from the final draft—what had not yet been set in motion was a corresponding cultural revolution, perhaps because of that effect which Noah Webster defined as mind colonization. In short, on one hand much was being done to ratify the Constitution; on the other, on a more intellectual level, one still felt irrevocably English. Some poets experimented with epic tones, such as Joel Barlow, who in his poem *The Vision of Columbus* (1787) celebrated the birth of the new republican institutions and offered prophecies regarding the opening of the Panama Canal. In reality however, such pompous and artificial poetic language, a monotonous use of the epic couplet, make these laborious compositions almost illegible. The only positive outcomes emerged from the burlesque genre, traced, for the most part, over mock epic poetry à la Pope: as is, for example, the case in John Trumbull, where rhyming couplet brazenly ridiculed New World institutions and characters. However, in order to speak of American literature, one must nevertheless await James Fenimore Cooper and Washington Irving; await Edgar Allan Poe and that five-year period called the "American Renaissance," when Hawthorne's *Scarlet Letter* (1850), Melville's *Moby Dick* (1851),

Thoreau's *Walden* (1854), and Whitman's first edition of his *Leaves of Grass* (1855) were published.[30]

It is symptomatic that mock epic was the only genre that had some vitality in American literature at the turn of the eighteenth and nineteenth centuries (see for instance, *The Hasty Pudding* by Joel Barlow, a playful celebration of the culinary delights of New England). Parody was the equivalent in music at that same time, often with denigrating intent. It is the case of blackface minstrels, who painted their faces with burnt cork and brought on stage mimicries of the African American way of life.[31]

Just as in literature the reference point for the mock epic genre was Pope,

in the history of blackface minstrelsy and thus of the minstrel show, the contribution of the English comic opera was fundamental and, starting from the latter part of the sixteenth century, actually began to feature African American slaves as characters. The actors based their representations primarily on language, using an overdramatized and freakish English which, beyond any truthfulness, had the sole objective of raising a laugh from the audience. And so the stereotype of the simple, gullible slave was born, who expressed himself in an awkward and inarticulate English, singing songs far from his original heritage.[32]

Minstrel show parodies were decidedly unpleasant: African Americans were depicted as liars, lazy, ignorant, loudmouthed, and generally drunkards; the actors sang in distorted accents accompanied by inappropriate dance steps, laughter and contempt at this point mixing indissolubly. On the other hand, however, the minstrels' musical language was a mixture of English melodies and ballads, marches and hymns, stuff certainly far from any music played by slaves. This facilitated the blending of genres, with pioneering effects on popular American song. The representation of African Americans in the minstrel shows "has often been used as instrumental to cultivate hatred and facilitate oppression. Nevertheless, it must be noted that the minstrels paved the way to ragtime and consequently to syncopated music."[33]

It remains a fact that the first highly successful piece in popular American music was "Jim Crow," written in 1828 by Thomas Dartmouth "Daddy" Rice. Dressed in rags and face painted black, Rice contorted himself in a ridiculous dance, singing, "Weel about and turn about and do jis so, / Eb'ry time I weel about and jump Jim Crow," on the notes of a melody that was part Irish tune and part English burlesque.

4. Blue Devils

Meanwhile, alongside minstrel shows, band music also began its rise and fall. It was performed by brass bands, which were military and civilian musical groups who used wind and percussion instruments. The genre reached its heyday during the Civil War when each regiment had its own brass band that marched open-column, playing "Yankee Doodle" and the "George Washington March." When the genre (above all, the instruments used to perform it) came into contact with African American music (blues and spirituals[34]), the result was jazz,[35] originating as the New Orleans black community's street marching bands.

This was the end of the nineteenth century, and this new music (in no way codified at that time and of which no recordings—obviously—or even scores exist) began to spread in southern cities, finally reaching St. Louis. It was here, in 1897, that the expression "ragtime" was first used to describe piano music with a heavily syncopated melody, played by well-educated African American musicians, who were quite often inspired by Chopin and Liszt.

On paper, the African American condition had changed at the end of the Civil War, with the abolition of slavery. Nevertheless, Yankee promises of work, housing, education, and health care were dramatically empty. Hot on the heels of long-sought freedom, a climate of disillusionment emerged and was expressed in the blues: spirituals sung by slaves beseeching their Lord to rise again and redeem them. The disappointment created "ill humor," and the expression "I'm blue" ("I'm in a bad mood") is a contracted form of "I have the blue devils." Alan Lomax wrote:

> It's dubbed "the age of anxiety," yet our age is best defined as "the century of Blues," like the melancholic musical genre born around 1900 in Mississippi Delta. Blues has always been more a way to be than a musical style. Leadbelly once told me, "When at night you're in bed and you feel uncomfortable, no matter which side you lie on, well: the blues got you."[36]

Once again, in this period of American history music seems to describe far better than literature one of the most tragic times. In fact, it was around the 1850s that the first African American poets began to appear, including George Moses Horton—born a slave in North Carolina—and James M. Whitfield, whose short poem "America" describes the country as a "land of blood, and crime, and wrong."[37] In those same years, the genre called "slave narrative" was making itself known with the sensational case of Harriet Jacobs, whose *Linda: Incidents in the Life of a Slave Girl Written by Herself* describes her seven years of voluntary imprisonment in a garret to escape the attentions of a white owner. Culture, however, remained firmly in the hands of white New England and the problems of the new working classes were also dealt with in the usual hidebound, prejudiced way even by the most courageous authors like Orestes Brownson. Each time the "savages" were mentioned it was to offer romantic praise for their "masculine" qualities.

If we want to find proof of the African American condition immediately after the abolition of slavery (in the Southern states 75 percent of the 1880 population were slaves), we need to listen to those three-line verses, where the second line just repeats the first. This went on for decades.

The tales of life on the plantations in Paul Laurence Dunbar's lyric poetry are too "European," and even Mark Twain's *Huckleberry Finn* cannot tell us of this counter-history. Neither will the work of Booker T. Washington, who in *The Story of My Life and Work*, from the early years of the twentieth century, preached black rights to a better education but neglected the issues of civil rights, segregation, and racial aggression. A case in point is the *Autobiography of an Ex-Colored Man*, published in 1912 by James Weldon Johnson, in which the story of a black man—a musician who, significantly, blends together ragtime and classical music—is narrated; because of his particularly pale skin color, the protagonist manages to pass as a white man and therefore gains acceptance in the most sophisticated milieus (a plot curiously similar to Philip Roth's novel *The Human Stain*).

Later on, in the twenties—the roaring years described by Fitzgerald—while jazz bands were blooming in clubs all over New York City, the voice of hopeless America became Blind Lemon Jefferson's in "Long Lonesome Blues" or, ten years later, in the midst of the Great Depression, Robert Johnson's in "Cross Road Blues." As everybody knows, at that crossroad in Mississippi, "poor Bob" met Satan in person, disguised as a mysterious bluesman called Ike Zinneman, and made a Faustian pact with him. Within the lyrics of the twenty-nine songs written by Robert Johnson after the fateful pact one can trace certain cardinal elements: romantic dissatisfaction (including solitude), travels, sexual metaphors (inclusive of the many euphemisms used to indicate male and female genitals), violence, irony, the world of the paranormal, the blues, alcohol. This list would be sufficient to understand how all American popular music of the twentieth century was preached by this mysterious youngster whose devil's wings flap for just enough time to allow for a chrysalis to become a butterfly. Johnson was the first to characterize the "emotionally unstable man" (and strong and independent women, such the "Little Queen of Spades"). His song lyrics overflow with bold linguistic innovation: his use of expressions like "yeah, man" and "look, daddy, so and so," which today we could easily call "hip," continue in stereotypes consistently present in rap, for instance.

The "contradiction" that traditionally developed in the call-and-response antiphony of work songs and spirituals became a "contradiction" when the various voices were fused into the single voice of the blues singer. It's as if the bluesman is talking to or questioning himself: the repetition of the first line is like pondering an idea, studying its nuances, then freezing it with the ironic closure of the final line.

With Robert Johnson and Lead Belly, rural blues became a classic, achieving definitive acceptance; and the structure survives to the present day. In 1948, however, the arrangement was revolutionized in Chicago by McKinley Morganfield, known to us as Muddy Waters, who practiced guitar by playing traditional pieces from his Mississippi Delta homeland. He then decided to record a couple of songs—"I Can't Be Satisfied" and "I Feel Like Going Home." Classic blues repertoire, but Muddy decided to plug in his guitar for some amplification and surrounded himself with musicians like Ernest "Big" Crawford on bass, Jimmy Rogers on backup (rhythm!) guitar, Otis Spann on the piano, and Little Walter on the harmonica . . . Wham! This was rhythm and blues.[38]

Muddy Waters defined a sound that had never been heard before, which became the underpinning for all twentieth-century (and twenty-first, come to that) pop music. The fusion of R&B with gospel generated soul; the combination of R&B with country & western music made rock 'n' roll.

5. Loud Farts of Eternity

In 1955 something unforeseeable happened: a conspiracy. The history of pop music burned up in a split second, out like a light. Initially it was a scream that few took notice of. Elias McDaniel—Bo Diddley to you and me—made no secret of the fact that he was the only real, original father of rock 'n' roll. The given he assumed was not objective, and this point is still hotly debated.[39]

What was that music? Surely something new, something unexpected: a rough and wild mixture of blues and country born to a dark hypnotic beat. Whether or not he was the first to play it, Chuck Berry remained without doubt something like Homer in the heroic age of rock 'n' roll; the man who had the greatest impact on the evolution of this new musical genre, the first one to write his own repertoire, the first African American to be idolized by whites, the best interpreter of the music that expressed the attitude of 1950s American youth. "Johnny B. Goode" is the quintessential rock 'n' roll song: three verses of six lines each that seem to sum up the entire meaning of rock mythology: a guitar like a gun, the dream of the boy from the sticks who wants to get rich, music that teaches more than any schoolbook ever did . . . Chuck Berry knew it all, twenty years before Bruce Springsteen.

Even before Elvis Presley, who in 1954–55 was still almost unknown. He was learning the ropes at Sun Records and growing fine; many consider that his most brilliant creative phase. One fine day, however, the rocker with the rebel tuft signed on with RCA and changed the world by placing the single "Heartbreak Hotel" / "I Was the One," released on January 27, 1956. Shocking. Before him came Bo Diddley, Bill Haley, Chuck Berry, Little Richard, and Fats Domino. But it was only when Elvis entered the world of music that everyone instantly knew that things would never be the same again and that the game of rock 'n' roll was here to stay. If others deserved the merit of having spread the seeds, he was definitely the one to have collected their fruit: the personification of a sound and an idea, the ever-changing image of the anger, dreams, and disillusions symbolic of post– Second World War teenagers. It wasn't what came out of those songs but rather the way in which he delivered them to the public, interpreting with that rich, velvety voice, shaking about in dances scandalous for the times, flirting, piercing hearts instantly with that irresistibly cheeky face. Every kid at that time empathized deeply with him; every girl dreamed of him and cried hysterically when he appeared on the *Ed Sullivan Show*. A new, mysterious and unsettling phenomenon that remains unexplainable even today.

A few years later, when Allen Ginsberg and Bob Dylan, Lou Reed, and Delmore Schwartz started strolling arm-in-arm around the Village, singer-songwriters finally stepped right into the halls of literature. A decade after Elvis shook his hips on TV, rock managed to get minds moving, too: we have contact. The Velvet Underground went further, intercepting the last remnants of pop art by working with Andy Warhol. Their mission was to be perceived as artists, not just as rockers. The result was an inimitable brew of refined lyrics and crude subjects, educated music and brash sound that a decade later would influence punk, as well as grunge in the nineties.

That was the same period when some started wondering whether it might not be true that poetry couldn't convey the rhythm or the mood of the present. That doubt is recurrent in the history of literature and often opens the way to casting aside obsolete codices. In this respect, the transition from the nineteenth to the twentieth century was assisted by real revolutions. As early as the 1850s, Whitman shocked European intellectual poetry circles by declaring that "The reader will always have his or her part to do, just as much as I have had mine."[40] The exclamatory fury of *Leaves of Grass*, the vitality and almost savage innocence of the verses, a tone that is both epic and enthusiastic, rained down not only on Tennyson-style official poets but also on the "damned," like Baudelaire or Rimbaud, with all their seditious extraneousness to the "bourgeois yes / bourgeois no" dispute. The mission of the West Hills poet was something else altogether:

One's-Self I sing, a simple separate person,
Yet utter the word Democratic, the word En-Masse.

Of physiology from top to toe I sing,
Not physiognomy alone nor brain alone is worthy for the Muse, I say the
    Form complete is worthier far.
The Female equally with the Male I sing.

Of Life immense in passion, pulse, and power,
Cheerful, for freest action form'd under the laws divine,
The Modern Man I sing.[41]

The awareness that "art can be a satisfaction and an isolation from life, which is
in itself offending"[42] matured further in the early 1900s, especially with the advent
of World War I. It "was not only a great experience for Fitzgerald, Dos Passos,
Cummings, Wilson—it was also a school of writing."[43] Seamus Heaney wrote:
"From now on, every luminous and unperturbed sureness about the consonance
of truth and beauty becomes suspicious."[44] Wilfred Owen, the young English poet
who died at the front in 1918, had already declared that Poetry did not interest
him: "My subject is War, and the pity of War. The Poetry is in the Pity."[45]

The beat poets intended to erase the line separating Art and Life. Just as pop
music starting going upstairs towards Parnassus, poets were descending that very
staircase. In his *241st Chorus* Kerouac implores Charlie Parker to forgive him for
having lost sight of true art. The admiration for music—"Music, Loud Farts of
Eternity"[46]—and jazz in particular, for its breaking with tradition and its element
of improvisation, was practically unanimous in the beat movement.[47] The natural
bop prosody that Ginsberg used became the logical American way to stream of
consciousness.

Paeans were also raised in Europe. "Why spend time with Plato when we can
glimpse another world just as easily thanks to a saxophone?"[48] wrote Cioran. While
Jean Cocteau—who had even recorded *Les Voleurs d'Enfants* in 1929, accompanied
by Dan Parrish's orchestra—went so far as to say that Louis Armstrong's "black
angel trumpet announces the end of a world."[49]

In New York at the beginning of the 1960s, folk music was also in fashion:
young poets met in coffeehouses in the Village to listen to Hank Williams wannabes.
When one such rookie, a Jewish boy named Robert Zimmerman, told his story
on stage at Gerde's Folk City, we came full circle.

When that boy from Duluth announced himself to the world under the name
of Bob Dylan, only a very few were to understand. In January 1961 he went to
visit Woody Guthrie (his God) in the hospital where he was confined. It was

apparently as a result of that encounter that Dylan reached the deep conviction that he was to unequivocally become the spiritual heir of the greatest folksinger in American history, the fighter for social justice who in the thirties and forties traveled the whole of the United States with guitar in hand, on which "This machine kills fascists" was emblazoned.

In 1963, the cover alone of The *Freewheelin' Bob Dylan* is enough to ensure its place in history: Bob and Suze Rotolo walk down the snowy streets of the Village cold and shy, and young Americans everywhere empathize instantly with these two thin figures bursting with love and awareness from every pore. But what that cover actually encompasses is not at all reassuring: the world, this time, is attacked, thrown out of bed by a guitar, a harmonica, and a voice as sharp as a razor, and is left unable to rest again. This youngster's narrative strength is still at its earliest, yet he has already won with his ability to enchant through clean metaphors in his lyrics, crowded with characters and literary bric-a-brac. Four songs above all: "Masters of War," "Girl from the North Country," "Don't Think Twice, It's All Right," and that "Blowin' in the Wind" which every one of us has sung, whistled, distorted, gotten wrong. There will be space for two more major folk albums before Newport, during a mild evening just a few steps away from the ocean, painfully finds out that a change of stylistic direction is about to happen: electrification. For now the revelation consists in showing the new American generation an angry, naive hobo, who is—let's admit it—more easily classifiable. In any case however, the change is massive.

Never before had anyone, with such brazenness and literary genius, taken it upon himself to rewrite the birth of the nation as did that know-it-all curly head through the lyrics of his songs—like "Bob Dylan's 115th Dream."

6. Revolution, Exhaustion, and Renaissance

In the ten years from 1955 to 1965, American literature produced novels like *Lolita* by Vladimir Nabokov (1955), *The Assistant* by Bernard Malamud (1957), *The Wapshot Chronicle* by John Cheever (1957), *The End of the Road* by John Barth (1958), *Crowded Sky* by Flannery O'Connor (1960), *To Kill a Mockingbird* by Harper Lee (1961), *V.* by Thomas Pynchon (1963), *Herzog* by Saul Bellow (1964), and *An American Dream* by Norman Mailer (1965). This can definitely be considered a golden age for poetry: apart from the beat group (Ferlinghetti, Ginsberg, Corso), we shouldn't overlook *A Cold Spring* by Elizabeth Bishop (1955), *Opus Posthumous* by Wallace Stevens (1957), the *Selected Poems of Delmore Schwartz* (1959), *Life Studies* by Robert Lowell, and Sylvia Plath's *Ariel* (1965).

Yet, in 1967, John Barth was already talking about the "literature of exhaustion":[50] everything was already done and the only thing left for contemporary writers was to parody their great predecessors. In that same time frame, rock 'n' roll made such a leap ahead that it seemed like light years away. From Presley, who sang that he could die without his baby,[51] we get to Dylan's "Miss Lonely," whom no one had taught how to live on the streets.[52]

These are the years in which people like Buddy Holly and Sam Cooke, Aretha Franklin and the Beach Boys, the Rolling Stones and B.B. King, the Who, the Byrds, Marvin Gaye, and Johnny Cash come smashing out of the woodwork; one after the other milestones such as Chuck Berry's *After School Session* (1957), *What'd I Say* by Ray Charles (1959), *Live at Newport* by Muddy Waters (1961), and *Otis Blue* by Otis Redding (1965) come to light, reaching an absolute climax with the release of two albums that seem to both break away from all things past yet somehow manage to piece everything until then together: *Highway 61 Revisited* by Bob Dylan (1966), and *Rubber Soul* by the Beatles (1966).[53]

Only ten years after its first cries, rock 'n' roll already seems to have pushed itself towards its own Pillars of Hercules. Elvis Presley and the British Invasion having made their grand entrance, the flower power revolution is under way: beneath the surface of its acid colors one can already catch a glimpse of a twilight. In San Francisco—where the beat generation found its so-called "renaissance"— the new hippie philosophy is gaining momentum: nonconformist, Oriental-style mysticism, drug-induced creativity, creation of primitivistic communities . . . in other words, "counterculture."

In the meantime on the East Coast, more specifically in New York, a new idea begins to circulate: music making not merely as entertainment, but rather as a cultural form. The "underground" is fundamentally anarchic from the start: it reacts to technological society with irrationalism, to the dogmatic American way of life with sarcasm, to the academies with verbal abuse. In 1967 a militant contingent to the movement would be constituted through the work of two public hustlers, Jerry Rubin and Abbie Hoffmann, the duo who coined the term *yippie* (Youth International Party). But for two years already, within the labyrinths of New York, a bohemian race had been moving in total confusion, uncultivated and impulsive, aware of its own (snobbishly) rebel spirit. The gurus were Allen Ginsberg, Julian Beck of the Living Theatre, and Andy Warhol. The latter—great interceptor of tendencies—understood that that indistinct melting pot of post-beat women and men needed a suitable soundtrack, a music that would at once both represent and stimulate the alienated mood of the New York underground scene, a phenomenon neither musical nor juvenile, but the fruit of an alternative form of culture, and as such far from the realms of business, customs and prevailing aesthetic considerations. At the Cafe Wha?, in the heart of the Village, Warhol found what he was looking for. On stage four skinny, perverse boys, all dressed in black leather, were getting kicked out by the owner for having played songs containing obscene language: "Heroin" and "Venus in Furs," the first an ode to drugs, the second to sadomasochism. The whole effect held together by piercing electric viola, intolerable guitar bursts and tribal percussion. Andy didn't miss a beat and immediately invited the four to the Factory. It was the beginning of the unique story of the Velvet Underground. *The Velvet Underground & Nico*, recorded in 1966 and released one year later with the scandalous banana drawn by Warhol on its cover, magically manages—because of its incredibly inspired lyrics and truly new sound—to perfectly capture the atmosphere of New York. The V.U. are light years away from incense, colorful clothing, and hippie utopias. This was music for intellectuals, the first expression of an artistically cultivated rock, a quantic leap forward that however performed very poorly on a commercial level. To be precise, 1961—the year in which Colonel Parker decided that Elvis was to be transformed from the king of rock to the sultan of Hollywood—saw the scepter of rock 'n' roll move overseas, into European hands. As Dave Marsh once pointed out, with one exception, the figures who unified the sixties rock scene were British. The only exception was Bob Dylan, who when passing from folk to rock 'n' roll just kept bringing it on relentlessly: *Bringing It All Back Home, Highway 61 Revisited*, and *Blonde on Blonde*. His heroic period would end in a terrible motorcycle accident, after which Dylan would dedicate himself almost entirely to the demolition of his own myth. No American group from the sixties had an artistic conception comparable to that at the base of the Who, the Stones, and the Beatles: and that was that rock must be seen as a key—perhaps *the* key—to better understanding the world. The Beach Boys and the Velvet Underground—though in diametrically opposite ways—did not search beyond form, as elegant or rough as it came.

After the great creative rush of the sixties—the Beatles disbanded, the Stones in decline, Dylan undergoing some sort of spiritual crisis—Europe became infected by progressive music just as America grew besotted by drippy soft-rock corniness. What fate would have awaited rock 'n' roll on both sides of the Atlantic had there not been a bunch of punk rockers determined that to keep the rock dream alive, it had to return to its original purity? Tommy Ramone put it this way: "By 1973, I knew that what was needed was some pure, stripped-down, no-bullshit rock 'n' roll."[54] All of a sudden an entire movement revved up, a "subculture that scornfully rejected the political idealism and Californian flower-power silliness of hippie myth."[55] And that is precisely what the Ramones and Television did, in fact, as well as the Clash and the Sex Pistols at the Hammersmith Palais in London, when singing "White Riot" and "Anarchy in the U.K." they blasted away at the soft underbelly of Britain's Bond Street, Fortnum & Mason, Buckingham Palace, and Salvation Army.

Enough with the ostentatious musical effects and technological demands of many mainstream rock bands; musical virtuosity was now looked on with suspicion: punk rock was for the people who didn't have very much skill as musicians but still felt the need to express themselves through music.[56] As it was at the very beginning. Rock 'n'roll was saving itself in a self-referential loop: punk bands were returning to the roots, listening to Bo Diddley records, drinking straight from the source of the authentic, raw, and irresistible Elvis Presley—the one of "That's All Right" and "Mystery Train"; they elected the lyrics of "Louie, Louie" as their urtext,[57] working their way backwards through the whole of the history of popular American music, eventually coming up against "ancient" Robert Johnson blues recordings.

It is thus inevitable that the New Man of rock 'n' roll was incarnated in the mid-seventies in the figure of Bruce Springsteen, a singer-songwriter whose principal merit was that of showing us the entire DNA map of American music. There is not one paradigm of modern music that he did not bend to comply with his personal narrative urgency: rockabilly, soul, rhythm and blues, punk, folk, country, pop, jazz . . . Springsteen does not change popular music, he incessantly reworks it, keeping its roots alive. And it is for this reason that, much more than any number of real or presumed innovators, he actually managed to save rock 'n' roll. He came at the right time, took the story of Rock upon himself, and made it his own. When he was recording *Born to Run*, he wanted to take the scepter that Bob Dylan had let fall. The fact that it took such a long time to finish the album can be attributed not so much to his perfectionism, but rather to a sense of awe in aiming so high up in the hierarchy of popular music. In the end, his producer Jon Landau forced him on. "Look," he told him, "you're not supposed to like it. You think Chuck Berry sits around listening to 'Maybellene'? And when he does hear it, don't you think that he wishes a few things could be changed? Now c'mon, it's time to put the record out."[58]

PART TWO

1. The Gary Cooper of Rock 'n' Roll

In the summer of 2016, half a century after his stuttering entrance into the music industry (two songs recorded under the name of the Castiles in a shopping mall in Bricktown, New Jersey), Springsteen concluded his world tour, selling over $250 million worth of tickets. And he published *Born to Run*, his autobiography, together with an anthology in which one of those two little old Castiles songs appears, "Baby I" (a naive attempt to imitate the style of the Animals). In the other one, "That's What You Got," one particular line—"I'm living the life of a lie"— introduces an underlying theme that will be consistent though subtle throughout all of his work, because even Bruce Springsteen, , the epitome of musical and moral integrity, from time to time is overwhelmed by the fear of being a fake. At twenty-three in "Growin' Up" he portrayed himself in front of a mirror "suspended in his masquerade"; at thirty-eight he feared he was just a "Brilliant Disguise"; and at sixty-six he writes of coming "from a boardwalk town where almost everything is tinged with a bit of fraud, a member in good standing amongst those who 'lie' in service of the truth . . . artists with a small 'a.'"[59]

Right from his beginnings, Springsteen runs the risk of being mistaken for the mere monument he embodies:[60] a strong-jawed, Mount Rushmore profile and an unbreakable faith in his own talent. The Boss is the perfect blend of Elvis and Dylan, come from New Jersey (America's armpit) to save the seventies from further Mellotron arabesques and Minimoog, with a stars-and-stripes ass to die for snugly fitted jeans on the cover of *Born in the U.S.A.*, the minstrel descending the Lincoln Memorial staircase to crown Obama, the knight in shining armor for the Super Bowl halftime show, the musical equivalent to fried chicken wings and the *E pluribus unum* motto engraved on the national crest. A rock-solid, unbreakable American certainty. But so much more lies beneath this masquerade. Nothing shocking, God forbid! Even if the thousands of people huddling up beneath the stage to sing "Badlands" in chorus would have trouble recognizing him as the mature man who, once disburdened of his superhero outfit, does his fifty minutes of therapy, hand-draws his own Christmas cards, laughs watching old Jerry Lewis films, has Montaigne's *Essais* and a few Russian novels on his bedside table, and is obsessed with Apollo space missions. Lately he is also haunted by ghosts disturbing his peace: the usual, incessant doubts about his self-worth and an ever-expanding anxiety—the fear of having reached the credits at the end of the show. Then again, it was Springsteen himself who explained that rock 'n' roll, in the height of its vitality, is none other than a fight against that other thing . . . death.

A few years ago he made an album, *Working on a Dream*, that could have easily been renamed *Aging*; his songs describing what it feels like to have days where "the autumn breeze drifts through the trees" ("Kingdom of Days"), those in which—as he sings in "What Love Can Do"—"the bed you lie on is nails and rust / And the love you've given's turned to ashes and dust." But his fans did not appreciate his effort. And he learned the lesson. The next album, *Wrecking Ball*, is one of the hardest and most politically explicit of his entire career. "You can never go wrong pissed off in rock 'n' roll,"[61] he said with a smile. But this thing about the passage of time—which at some point eventually ends—continues to disturb him. Not even music, the Great Exorcist, succeeds in defeating the powerful demon any longer. Because Bruce Springsteen—the Living Catalog, the king of jukeboxes, the man who took the throne by pulling an Esquire electric guitar from a stone— clearly got the fact that the rock 'n' roll dream is seductive yet dangerous[62] and that art cannot substitute for life: it can give you many things, but it gives them to "the guy with the guitar," while "the guy without the guitar is pretty much the same as he had been."[63]

This aspect, more closely, is revealing of an approach typical of the sentimental poet: problematic and self-reflective.

Frederich Schiller, whose play *The Robbers* had ladies fainting in their theater boxes a century and half before Elvis, divided poets into two categories: those who were not aware of a disconnect between themselves and the reality around them, and those who were aware of the disconnect. For the unaware, the "naive" ones (Homer, Shakespeare, and Paul McCartney), art is a form of natural expression; they are happily married to their own muse and have a sunny, pure, joyous relationship with her. For the others, the *sentimentalisch*—the poets after the fall— their relationship with Terpsichore and Calliope is always stormy and unhappy. The effect is not joy and peace, but tension, conflict with nature and society, and insatiable desire. Virgil and Ariosto belong to this second, sentimental category of poets. Bruce Springsteen certainly belongs to this group as well.

I was in Hyde Park when Springsteen grabbed the microphone and said, "I've been waiting for this moment for forty years. Ladies and gentlemen, Sir Paul McCartney!"[64] and—voilà!—there on the stage beside him appeared the great living musical genius, the Mozart of pop, the author of "Eleanor Rigby" and "Hey Jude," the coproducer of that glittering Technicolor fantasy called Pepperland where today's visitor can still find newspaper taxis, yellow submarines, egg-men and girls with kaleidoscope eyes; Schiller's ingenuous artist par excellence; the dialectic op-posite of the American guy, who would never be able to transform his own grey Forthlin Road—the Liverpool suburban street where little Paul lived—into the gleaming Penny Lane of the song by the same name. To Bruce, Freehold, Mon-mouth County, and all New Jersey were nothing more than a "death trap, a suicide trap" to escape from at 100 miles an hour in a convertible car. Springsteen recently rendered tribute to the greatness of the Fab Four,[65] though he recalled that his favorite beat group in the sixties was the Animals, who sang "We Gotta Get Out of This Place."

"The Animals were a revelation," he says, "the first records with full-blown class consciousness that I had ever heard . . . It was the first time I felt I something come across the radio that mirrored my home life, my childhood."[66]

After the Animals, Bruce would discover Bob Dylan ("He gave us the words to understand our hearts"), Roy Orbison ("The coolest uncool loser you'd ever seen"), James Brown ("There's no greater live performance than James Brown's burning ass on the Rolling Stones at the *T.A.M.I. Show*"[67]), Hank Williams ("If rock and roll was a seven-day weekend, country was Saturday night hell-raising, followed by heavy 'Sunday Morning Coming Down.' Guilt, guilt, guilt"), and Woody Guthrie ("He's the ghost in the machine—big, big ghost in the machine").[68]

Springsteen's models are all sentimental poets: they struggle to elevate reality to the ideal through rebellion, spiritual tension, and consecration of sex as the parameter of intellectual vitalism, the ethical sense of a collective purpose. In other words, they achieve this through culture in the Romantic sense of the rational path that will lead us back to Nature, and thus to our lost childhood. Only the naive, the Maccas of the world, the so-called "classics," can slip into this realm effortlessly.

Listening to a Beatles song is like stumbling onto what we most cherish: the time lost that Proust sought in his seven books. Springsteen—like Proust—can achieve a similar result only through culture. It is pop music in his case more than in any other: superficial observers like Leon Wieseltier,[69] who criticizes Springsteen for "his decision to become a spokesman for America" or even being a "Howard Zinn with a guitar,"[70] just don't get it. Springsteen is not a Pete Seeger fan because Springsteen is a radical;. Springsteen is a radical because he is a Pete Seeger fan. His discourse is something all wrapped up inside his "damned" guitar; if the linguistic codes of the blues force him to write about misfits and outlaws, as if they were the heroes or the poisoned fruit of an unjust society, so much the better. If rock 'n' roll is the language of the rebel without a cause raging over his own desperation against a backdrop of shattered sunsets and flickering neon, well, then it's worth singing about, as in "Born to Run": "I wanna die with you Wendy on the streets tonight, in an everlasting kiss . . . / 'Cause tramps like us, baby, we were born to run."

Anyone who is not aware of the self-referencing aspect we could call postmodern in Springsteen's opus might get mixed up when distilling his "messages," as in Ronald Reagan's case . . .

Bruce Springsteen, the sentimental poet. The one to bring rock 'n' roll back to its innocence and to the frenzy of Buddy Holly and Eddie Cochran's first albums, the heir to a tradition of American bards begun by Walt Whitman for the time being ends with him, the man who, "more than anyone else, owns America's heart," as Bono once said . . .[71] Bruce Springsteen—as we were saying—during his sixty-seven years of existence on this planet until now, found the time to write over 500 songs, get married twice, have three children, and bury his at first hated then dearly beloved father, a figure central to him throughout his life and work. He witnessed thirteen presidents alternate roles (from Truman to Trump); he lived through the Vietnam years, the Cold War and the nuclear nightmare, the war on petroleum and the attacks of 9/11, the wars in Iraq and the coming of an Afro American to the White House (one who declared, "I'm running for president because I can't be Bruce Springsteen"). He was fourteen years old when Oswald shot Kennedy, nineteen when Martin Luther King was killed, twenty-eight when Elvis's body was found on the carpet in Graceland. He earned an impossible amount of money, he started up and disbanded (then re-formed) a large number of groups with more or less exotic names—how can one forget Dr. Zoom and the Sonic Boom?—with whom he played starting in his mid-teens in every single bar, gym, sports arena, and stadium in America, and later abroad, from Europe to Australia, with the wild and romantic idea that music can literally save your life (an idea he himself doubted several times in his life, after having taken it for granted in his early years, as mentioned above). To whoever asks how it feels to be amongst the greatest rock stars in the world, his honest reply is, "Being a rock star is the consolation prize. I wanted to become a rock 'n' roller."[72]

Here we come across the Promised Land so often evoked in his songs: a paradise of romantic weariness, an *on the road* across landscapes—highways where Buick and Cadillacs chase each other, dark alleys and side streets make settings for hard-boiled versions of *West Side Story*, amidst broken sunsets and sobbing neon lights—constructed from set designs taken from Elia Kazan films and populated with young hooligans hanging out by diners, Brylcream-greased hair and a pack of Lucky Strikes wedged under leather biker jackets; the American Dream in which one can vaguely make out a backlit Elvis and Jimmy Dean, Brando and his band of bad guys, *Easy Rider* and *The Wild Bunch*, Roy Orbison singing for lonesome hearts and Robert Mitchum behind the wheel on *Thunder Road*, perhaps in the middle of a golden summer with a Beach Boys single sizzling away on a record player.

> Springsteen is not just another good rock singer-songwriter. He's like a flag, a monument, an anthem to everything that rock can be. To understand this, you have to have seen at least one concert. He has cut amazing records, but the real Springsteen is the one you see live on stage. The Rolling Stones were once considered the quintessential rock 'n' roll band of all time. That may have been true in the fever of the 1960s, tailing off in the 1970s. Since then, the greatest classic rock 'n' roll band in history has been Bruce Springsteen and the E Street Band. Those who love him know that with him they go to celebrate the only marvelous, liberating pagan ritual our culture has left us.[73]

The mission to keep American tradition afloat doesn't just mean songs: Springsteen lyrics often echo with big-screen references. We'll mention just a few: *Thunder Road* is a 1958 film by Arthur Ripley, in which Mitchum plays a whisky bootlegger; "Backstreets" owes its title to *Back Street*, a 1932 film starring Irene Dunne; "Darkness on the Edge of Town" calls to mind and exudes the same mood as a 1956 film, *Edge of the City*, with John Cassavetes and Sidney Poitier; numerous hints in "Local Hero" point to a Fritz Lang film, *The Woman in the Window*; *Point Blank* is a 1967 film directed by John Boorman; *All That Heaven Allows*, 1955, describes the love between a rich widow and a poor gardener (in the song "All That Heaven Will Allow" the boy has a dollar in his pocket and wears working pants); Richard Widmark and Doris Day starred in the 1958 *Tunnel of Love*, about a difficult marriage; *This Gun's for Hire*, a 1942 film with Veronica Lake, provided the refrain for "Dancing in the Dark." Not to mention films like Terrence Malick's *Badlands* and John Ford's *Grapes of Wrath*, openly providing inspiration for *Nebraska* and *The Ghost of Tom Joad*. In fact, the Oscar awarded to Springsteen in 1994 for his "Streets of Philadelphia" could also be seen as thanks from the Academy to a very successful sponsor.

Martin Scorsese said,

> There was a time in 1975 when you could hear Springsteen's songs blaring from car radios and apartment windows, and no matter how many times you listened to them, they never lost their edge: the moment in "Born to Run" when the band seems to push through to a new place, and Springsteen screams, "The highway's jammed with broken heroes on a last-chance power drive"; Randy Brecker's mournful horn over the quietly tragic "Meeting Across the River"; the soaring climax of "Jungleland."[74]

In the thirty years of his career, Springsteen has published more than 300 songs, but he reckons he has just as many still unpublished. What is even more surprising, however, is the order in which he has created this immense encyclopedia. Worth noting, and unique in the history of rock, is that each new album picks up where the last one left off, like the chapters of a novel. If "American rock overall can be seen as a long, still incomplete American epic poem,"[75] Springsteen's work must be considered as central in such a poem, in its potential to beam before and after itself. If we were to imagine such a book and structure it as Galland did in *The Thousand and One Nights*, Springsteen could perfectly interpret the role of Sheherazade. His stroke of genius was that he didn't stop the clock. Before him,

> There wasn't precedent in rock music for growing up and everything that comes with it. Partly because rock 'n' roll itself was so young, it was tradition- ally the music of youth; it was born to be wild, to rock around the clock, to rave on, to sniff glue—it was music of rebellion, not acceptance. If rock 'n' rollers didn't die before they got old, they must just become country music fans. But Springsteen's rock 'n' roll came to embrace the roots of the genre— aspects of country, R&B, folk, gospel, and the blues—in a way that went beyond his music of his appropriated onstage shtick. He blazed a trail, inten- tionally and deliberately, to bring the adult concerns of those other forms to rock 'n' roll.[76]

If Mick Jagger is still pathetically posing as a sex symbol for old folks, the twenty-four-year-old Bruce who sang "Me and Crazy Janey was makin' love in the Dirt" in "Spirit in the Night," twenty-two years later in "Living Proof" ponders, "Now, all that's sure on the boulevard is that life is just a house of cards / As fragile as each and every breath of this boy sleepin' in our bed."

Maybe the Stones were a different game forty years ago. But today . . . Jagger and Richards don't do anything beyond broadcasting how hip they are (have the Rolling Stones ever communicated anything other than their own coolness?). Springsteen tells another story. Springsteen is all the heat of rock 'n' roll *and* the Great American Novel, composed with the talent of a true writer.

Beyond the lights, the smoke, the guitar solos, and the frenzied crowd, rock 'n' roll is a mythology: the tale of Johnny B. Goode, who leaves his hometown with a guitar and goes to conquer the big city, wanting to see his name glittering at the top of the bill. As Springsteen puts, rock 'n' roll is a blues verse, where you tell the struggles and the pain of the here and now, and a gospel chorus to be sung all together to reach some form of transcendence, or at least some kind of happiness (the Promised Land?).

Inside this gigantic concrete pool of a stadium, in the middle of one of those four-hour Springsteen's shows, we can forget that nature is none other than chaos, brutality, and death and understand that beauty can save the world and that anyone can be Johnny B. Goode and shout, "It's a town full of losers and I'm pulling out of here to win."

The immense success Springsteen won throughout his career is due to the fact that he embodies two fundamental elements; firstly, he is one of the greatest performers of all time and also an exceptional writer: a unique combination of Elvis and Dylan. But the aspect that made him an all-time legend lies within his vision of rock 'n' roll as a saving grace.[77] From the melting pot of his adolescent imagination, he managed to forge a kind of mythology that combined *Rebel Without a Cause* with *Wise Blood* and "Back in the U.S.A." All this has transformed Springsteen into something more than a rock icon, something more than a showman. Maybe some kind of American archetype: "rock and roll's Gary Cooper," as it was written on the a cover of a 1985 edition of *Newsweek*.

These are all aspects that play against Springsteen, according to the Academy of Arts and Literature. The original sin is found, according to their view, in connection with the fact that his subject evolves solely within the history of rock 'n' roll. Again: "We learned more from a three-minute record than we ever learned at school," he sings in "No Surrender." Springsteen's sources certainly do not run dry in the mere figure of the American singer, instead extending to embrace literature and film. However, the undeniable center of his opus is rock itself. In this sense, driving the issue forward, Springsteen can be seen as the bishop of "the rock of exhaustion." No other artist has ever offered live on stage such a huge amount of covered material, singing a bit of everything: from Otis Redding to Woody Guthrie, from Christmas carols to Eddie Cochran's rock 'n' roll, from "Twist and Shout" to "Trapped," from Manfred Mann to the Ronettes, up until "Stayin' Alive."

This explains why to focus on the "poetics" of his songs would at once become an attempt to legitimize all popular music as well as seem like a declaration of rock 'n' roll's independence from the Norton Anthology. If Springsteen's lyrics always work even without musical support, the issue of whether or not they are poetry gets sidestepped; and this would count for an entire tradition, from "This Is Your Land" to "Smells Like Teen Spirit."

In the world of literature, thankfully, there are people who share a similar view: from Walker Percy to Stephen King, from Nick Hornby to Don DeLillo, who in the year 2000 having noted Springsteen's prolonged absence from the music industry interpreted the fact as "a local symptom of the Almighty's reluctance to appear."[78]

2. My Father's House: A Prelude

This lesser god also remodeled his humble beginnings. His Bethlehem (or if we prefer his Hoboken or Duluth) is a depressed little town in a grey county belonging to a state in which Americans set their jokes as the English set theirs in Ireland. The title of Springsteen's first album, released in 1973, is revealing: *Greetings from Asbury Park, NJ*. At that time, the geography of rock seemed like an anastatic edition of the *Navigatio Sancti Brendani*:[79] Pepperland[80] and the Yellow Brick Road,[81] Electric Ladyland[82] and Itchycoo Park.[83] Used to listening to Syd Barrett singing about a gnome named Grimble Gromble,[84] how would the rock audience react to an Italian-Irishman wondering if his bus stopped on 82nd Street?

When the *Asbury Park Evening Press* wrote on September 24, 1949, that "Mr. and Mrs. Douglas Springstein [sic], 87 Randolph Street, Freehold, are parents of a boy born yesterday at Monmouth Memorial hospital." New Jersey was deep in a serious economic crisis: in the ghettos illiteracy reached third world levels, growing hand in hand with unemployment and racial unrest, factory workers from A&M Karagheusian and Nestle frequently receiving salary cuts.

Douglas Springsteen and Adele Zirilli moved to Freehold shortly after the war, and managed to buy themselves a small house with a garden. Mrs. Springsteen, a secretary in a legal office, chose for a husband an inward-looking man, always troubled. A sense of frustration and anger brought on by a succession of failures in various job attempts as jail guard, taxi driver, and factory worker pushed him to switch off the lights at nine o'clock every night to sit in the dark with a six-pack of beer and a pack of cigarettes.

Springsteen remembers how his dad often came back from work furious and drunk. The only times father and son got close were when they took the car and—in silence—went for a drive around the block.

In "Used Cars" he sings,

> My little sister's in the front seat with an ice cream cone,
> My ma's in the back seat sittin' all alone,
> As my pa steers her slow out of the lot
> For a test drive down Michigan Avenue.

In "Mansion on the Hill" (another song from the *Nebraska* album, released in 1982), he remembers when his father took him to "those gates of hardened steel" of the "mansion on the hill," where "in the summer all the lights would shine" and "there'd be music playin' people laughin' all the time." A mansion that can easily be read as a metaphor for the realization of the American dream, a social status that the Springsteens could only covet. This piece has been seen to contain echoes descriptive of Gatsby's mansion up on the hill of West Egg,[85] which has brought us to consider an extension in the comparison between the complete works of Springsteen and F. Scott Fitzgerald, carefully evaluating in both the constant presence of the dichotomy of dream/reality.[86]

When in 1998 Douglas Springsteen died, a newspaper heading described the event, adding that "he was the most famous father in the history of rock 'n' roll." There is no need to bother with psychotherapy to appreciate that in every Springsteen song—not only those to do with his adolescence, but also the politically inclined ones, even beneath the claustrophobic atmosphere underlying his first matrimonial situation described in "Brilliant Disguise"—there is always a figure in conflict with a social role, the son in his father's house, who risks suffocation. Douglas Springsteen remains, in Bruce Springsteen's eyes, the Sun: in every one of his pieces one can find a constellation of the macrocosm created by a lyrical "self" that continues to reflect upon that teenager whose father continuously unplugged his guitar's amp and threatened to cut off his hair.

Emily Dickinson's verses resound—another child devoured by the conflict with her father,

> One need not be a Chamber—to be Haunted—
> One need not be a House—
> The Brain has Corridors—surpassing
> Material Place.[87]

In "My Father's House," from the *Nebraska* album, we can hear once again the voice of the poetess from Amherst:

> My father's house shines hard and bright,
> It stands like a beacon calling me in the night,
> Calling and calling, so cold and alone,
> Shining 'cross this dark highway where our sins lie unatoned.

It is not a gate, this time, but a door left ajar that excludes the protagonist. A woman appears in the doorway:

> I told her my story, and who I'd come for,
> She said, "I'm sorry, son, but no one by that name lives here anymore."

In "Factory," published in the *Darkness on the Edge of Town* album of 1978, other gates are described—not the ones which in "Mansion on the Hill" unforgivingly separated Doug and Bruce from social fulfillment, but the gates his father crossed every day when going to work in the factory, "through the mansions of fear, through the mansions of pain." In his autobiography, Springsteen recalls the days when he would bring his father his night-shift lunch down at the factory—something he did without a word of thanks.

> End of the day, factory whistle cries,
> Men walk through these gates with death in their eyes.[88]

One can notice a homodiegetic point of view in this foursome on childhood: the narration is in the first person, and notably from a child's point of view; the style is flat, almost as if to render the idea in black and white in memory of a difficult childhood.

At school things weren't much better: the Franciscan nuns soon converted Springsteen to committed anticlericalism; his companions soon isolated him.

Besides the Lincoln Street Institute, Freehold did not have much to offer other than the stink of sulphuric gases from the nearby factories and an undefined mass of men with gelled tufts and Irontex clothing, a rows of female laborers with scarf covered heads hiding curlers lined up outside the factories.

In an article ironically called *Bruce Springsteen and the Secret of the World*, music critic Fred Shruers sketched out this pen picture of Springsteen types hanging around Monmouth County:

> We had a word for people like Bruce: Newarkylanders. The urban canker of Newark-Elizabeth was their state capital, but they lived and played along the boardwalked Jersey shore. They wore those shoulder-strap undershirts some people called "guinea-T's"; we called them "Newarkys." They drove muscle cars and worked in garages and metal shops. They ate meatball subs made of cat parts for lunch, and after work they shouted at their moms, cruised the drive-ins, punched each other out, and balled their girlfriends in backseats.[89]

It's a mystery how all this could have become a rock 'n' roll Shangri-La in the twenty-four songs that made up Springsteen's first three albums. The only explanation of the mystery would require a psychoanalytical approach.

"In a different era she would have ended up being hung," was said with reference to Emily Dickinson. As regards Springsteen and his juvenile eccentricities—his blaring guitar during quiet nights on South Street, the many attempted escapes from home planned while listening repeatedly to "It's My Life" by the Animals, his scholastic career troubled by a degree of autism—only ten years earlier they would have probably shut him up in some institute, just as Holden Caulfield was sent to an asylum, the totalitarian kingdom of America's rule-imposing shrinks in the fifties and sixties. For much less, in Mankiewicz's film based on the dramatic story of Tennessee Williams's *Suddenly Last Summer*, Elizabeth Taylor was lined up for a lobotomy. And again in 1961, Elia Kazan punished Natalie Wood with a psychiatric clinic for her torment and unrepressed sexual impulses towards Warren Beatty in the film *Splendor in the Grass*.

Yet already by the middle of the fifties a new figure was imposing itself across Cary Grant and James Stewart's flannel-jacket-wearing males of America: in 1954 *East of Eden* came out and one year later *Rebel Without a Cause*, two films canonizing the image of the male figure as rebel misfit emerging from the slimy pond of stagnant conformism, of McCarthyism and the ever growing misinterpretation of the American dream. "Bad boys" were replacing "little men"—little father-like clones—like James Dean in his red leather jacket and Marlon Brando in black leather, who when asked by a girl what he was rebelling against answered, "Do I get to choose?"

Brando's beauty was triumphant, dangerously sexy. His T-shirt made history, first pasted to those gym-sculpted muscles (a novelty, at that time), then ripped on the immense, sweat-drenched torso, then removed altogether. In the case of James Dean, the novelty was "a crouched and huddled body that hid none of its neurotic fragility, but actually revealed with tics, giggles, lopsided gait and, every now and again, a defenceless, imploring gaze."[90]

It was precisely in 1955–56 that Norman Mailer (who had already had unbelievable success with *The Naked and the Dead*) published several articles in the *Village Voice*, a new periodical that was soon to become one of the most important mouthpieces for metropolitan counterculture. Mailer defined as hip:

> An American existentialism, profoundly different from French existentialism because Hip is based on a mysticism of the flesh, and its origins can be traced back into all the undercurrents and underworlds of American life, back into the instinctive apprehension and appreciation of existence which one finds in the Negro and the soldier, in the criminal psychopath and the dope addict and jazz musician, in the prostitute, in the actor. It is a language to describe states of being which is as yet without its philosophical dictionary.[91]

Two years later, Jack Kerouac wrote that dictionary:

> It was a rainy night. It was the myth of the rainy night. Dean was popeyed with awe. This madness would leave nowhere. I didn't know what was happening to me, and I suddenly realized it was only the tea we were smoking. Dean had bought some in New York. It made me think that everything was about to arrive—the moment when you know all and everything was decided forever.[92]

3. It's Hard to Be a Saint in the City

When *On the Road* came out, Springsteen was eight years old and his mother had only just bought him a sixty-dollar plastic guitar. Just a few months earlier Presley had been on the *Ed Sullivan Show* and Bruce, like other millions of American youngsters, had seen him on TV: "It was like Elvis came along and whispered some dream in everybody's ear, and somehow we all dreamed it."[93]

In 1964, the Beatles—again on the *Ed Sullivan Show*—would fuel more of his dreams; the following year it would be the notes of a Bob Dylan song that he captured on radio. Elvis. The Beatles. Dylan. Eric Burdon singing that he could do what he wanted with his life. Marlon Brando and his gang of bad boys. Smokey Robinson and the Drifters on the radio. Little Richard's face caked with makeup as he writhed at the piano singing "Good Golly Miss Molly." Eddie Cochran extolling the virtues of those pink peg slacks. The Ronettes, the Shirelles, and the Crystals. Mick Jagger's blatant lips on the cover of the *Aftermath* album. The promise of a golden summer that sizzles between the needle and a Beach Boys record. The Stax and the Atlantic Records stuff. Hendrix's guitar going up in flames. Dustin Hoffman down in a swimming pool dressed in a diving suit. *Bonnie and Clyde, Easy Rider*, and *The Wild Bunch* . . .

> Springsteen has taken rock forward by taking it back, keeping it young. He uses and embellishes the myths of the 1950s pop culture: his songs are populated by bad-ass loners, wiped-out heroes, bikers, hot-rodders, women of soulful mystery. Springsteen conjures up a whole half-world of shattered sunlight and fractured neon, where his characters re-enact little pageants of challenge and desperation.[94]

> [Springsteen] treats rock and roll history as our common language, our shared mythology, and thereby reinforces rock and roll's promise of community . . . His songs seem like they were filmed on location . . . Springsteen is a compulsive recorder of detail. But it's not like you'd call him a realist. Sometimes it seems as though he's looking back at the corner through a rearview mirror—the streets turned shimmery and the action blurred by the speed at which he's traveling.[95]

Using an emphatic and visionary language, a worn-out dictionary of synonyms and a kaleidoscopic mixture of images arranged in long, contorted rhyme schemes, Springsteen manages to embrace every legend in the youth culture of his time, rock 'n' roll and cinema: and so it is that the kids from the Asbury Park boardwalk, drug dealers and whores off Manhattan alleyways, are lifted upwards in the ranks to young rebel status, thus rendering the desolate panorama of New Jersey's urban sprawl a new "waterfront," a place no longer sleazy but rather exhaustingly romantic, like in the urban fantasia of "Does This Bus Stop at 82nd Street?" Springsteen orchestrates this transfiguration first of all upon himself. The shy twenty-two-year-old guitarist introduces himself in the following way at the beginning of "Growin' Up":

> I stood stone-like at midnight
> Suspended in my masquerade,
> I combed my hair till it was just right
> And commanded the night brigade.

In "It's Hard to Be a Saint in the City" this incarnation of the romantic hero goes even further:

> I had skin like leather and the diamond-hard look of a cobra,
> I was born blue and weathered but I burst just like a supernova,
> I could walk like Brando right into the sun, then dance just like a Casanova.[96]

The rhyme "cobra" / "supernova" / "Casanova" suggested a predilection of the young Springsteen for alliteration, assonance, internal rhyme, but also a strong presence of surreal images. Just listen to the first verses of the first song on Springsteen's first album, "Blinded by the Light":

> Madman drummers, bummers and Indians in the summer with a teenage diplomat,
> In the dumps with the mumps as the adolescent pumps his way into his hat.
> With a boulder on my shoulder, feelin' kinda older I tripped the merry-go-round
> With this very unpleasing sneezing and wheezing the calliope crashed to the ground.

The debt to Dylan here is obvious, as Ken Emerson remarked in *Rolling Stone*:

> *Greetings from Asbury Park, NJ*, Bruce Springsteen's uproarious debut album, sounds like "Subterranean Homesick Blues" played at 78, a typical five-minute track bursting with more words than this review. Most of it doesn't make much sense, but that is the point. Springsteen is rhyming and wailing for the sheer fun of it, and his manic exuberance more than canceled out his debts to Dylan, Van Morrison and the Band.[97]

"Blinded by the Light" and "Spirit in the Night"—both put at the head of the album—were the last tracks to be completed. President of Columbia Records Clive Davis had heard the demos, and he thought none of the tracks could be lifted as a single. That was how Springsteen came to seek out Clarence Clemons in a dive on the coast, got rid of his folksinger outfits, and plunged head-first into soul and R&B. Springsteen said:

> I wrote "Blinded by the Light" sittin' on my bed with a rhyming dictionary in one hand and a notebook in the other one. That's a song that explains why I never did any drugs. There's a line, "Some silicone sister with her manager's mister told me I got what it takes," which is possibly the first reference to a female breast implant in popular music. This song is also my only number one song. I never had another number one song except this one and it wasn't done by me. It was done by Manfred Mann, which I appreciate . . . But they changed a line. My line was, "Cut loose like a *deuce* another runner in the night." And there's "Cut loose like a *douche* another runner in the night." *Deuce* was the little Deuce Coupe. *Douche* is a feminine hygienic procedure . . . I have the feeling that that is why the song skyrocketed to number one.[98]

"Blinded by the Light" was the penance that absolved from solitude. T. S. Eliot in "East Coker" seems to be lurking in the shadows:

> So here I am, in the middle way, having had twenty years — . . .
> Trying to learn to use words, and every attempt
> Is a wholly new start, and a different kind of failure.[99]

Springsteen's transformation from caterpillar to butterfly occurs throughout the fifteen miles of highway that connect Freehold to Asbury Park, the place that will provide him with scenery, roads, people, tales. It was built in 1871 by James A. Bradley as a summer vacation spot along the Jersey Shore that could potentially compete with Long Beach and Atlantic City. By the time of Bradley's death in 1921, Asbury Park had become a pleasant resort for the middle class with splendid houses, gardens, and a breathtaking beachfront. Count Basie, Duke Ellington, and Benny Goodman enthralled tourists with their jazz bands, and when in 1957 the Garden State Parkway was inaugurated, the small town thrived with a seemingly unstoppable surge of growth. In the sixties, the Convention Hall hosted concerts by the likes of Dylan, the Beach Boys, Janis Joplin, the Doors, and the Stones. In '68 the Upstage opened, the first club in the area in which young rockers could gain experience. It was here that Bruce met Steve Van Zandt, Danny Federici, David Sancious, Vini Lopez, Garry Tallent—all people who would play with him for years thereafter. And it was there, on that stage, that the butterfly began to break into flight, taking him towards New York, a contract in the industry, fame and glory.

When in 1973 *Greetings from Asbury Park, NJ*, came out, Asbury Park was already starting its decline: in 1970 the first violent incidents between black and white communities began; the wealthier tourists abandoned these beaches, and in 1971 the Upstage closed its doors. Springsteen's postcards were already a memory of a lost past. Even so, there was no time for regrets. Eleven months after the debut album, *The Wild, the Innocent & the E Street Shuffle* came out and was remarkably jazzy: more Van Morrison[100] and less Dylan, more soul and less folk. "But it's the atmosphere of the album that will never be surpassed: the closely observed, carefree canvas it paints of a place and time when the fires of late adolescence and early adulthood still burned brightly."[101]

The Wild, the Innocent & the E Street Shuffle is Bruce Springsteen's soul album, a new *West Side Story* "inhabited by African Americans and Hispanics, which his friends Southside Johnny and Willy De Ville rooted in history, while on the West Coast it influenced Tom Waits' *Blue Valentine*."[102] If Springsteen in *Greetings from Asbury Park, NJ* was the boy from the boonies coming for a visit to the metropolis, knocked out by all the marvels, here he's torn between his roots and the city that has taken him to its heart, and which then takes center stage in *Born to Run*. The whole of it rendered with "a kind of ethical hedonism, an enlightened savagery, a wise naiveté. An American dream out of Fennimore Cooper or Mark Twain."[103]

In his first album Springsteen told about his sexual initiation at the Greasy Lake with Crazy Janey ("Spirit in the Night"). Here instead, during the ten unforgettable minutes as "New York City Serenade" unfolds, a "fish lady" is hooked up on a Manhattan sidewalk as part of one of his many trips to the Big Apple. The main character in "Kitty's Back"—probably a Bleecker Street stripper[104]—left the street "to marry some top cat", leaving her man, Catlong, sighing, "Oh, what can I do, / Oh, what can I do?" while he "lies back bent on a trash can" and "Flashing lights cut the night."

The world of Springsteen's early songs revolves around night life. The night represents rebellion and escape ("Growin' Up," "Rosalita," "Spirit in the Night," "Night," "Born to Run") but is potentially full of danger ("Incident on 57th Street," "Kitty's Back," "Jungleland"). There is always a guiding light there to make it less scary: the "stars" ("Spirit in the Night"), the "Exxon sign" ("Jungleland"), the neon lights ("Out in the Street"), the flashing lights ("Kitty's Back") . . . As Springsteen sings on "Tenth Avenue Freeze-Out," "the night is dark, but the sidewalk bright / And lined with the light of the living."

The rite of passage from one side of the Hudson River to the other—with all the social implications deriving from the small-town boy's dream of making it in the city that never sleeps—embraces a powerful metaphor in the Holland Tunnel, which two years later Springsteen will use perfectly in "Meeting Across the River" (echoing Scorsese):

> Hey, Eddie, can you lend me a few bucks
> And tonight can you get us a ride?
> Gotta make it through the tunnel,
> Got a meeting with a man on the other side.
> Hey Eddie, this guy, he's the real thing,
> So if you want to come along you gotta promise you won't say anything
> 'Cause this guy don't dance
> And the word's been passed this is our last chance.

"Incident on 57th Street"—another New York tale—is a genuine *West Side Story*, with Spanish Johnny as Tony (or Romeo) and Puerto Rican Jane as Maria (or Juliet). The main theme in "Incident" is the search for redemption. Amidst broken-down Buicks, flying P38 bullets, hatchet-swinging pimps, and "golden-heeled fairies" engaging in "a real bitch fight," the two protagonists try to live their dream of love, knowing that there will never be a happy ending for them:

> And Johnny whispered, "Good night, it's all right Jane,
> I'll meet you tomorrow night on Lover's Lane.
> We may find it out on the street tonight, baby,
> Or we may walk until the daylight, maybe."

In Springsteen's early songs there are often Hispanic characters. Apart from Spanish Johnny and Puerto Rican Jane, there is the Rosalita of the song with the same name, and the "Señorita, Spanish Rose" featuring in "Does This Bus Stop at 82nd Street?" and one of the characters in "Lost in the Flood," who, injured by a policeman, reveals his roots "screaming something in Spanish." Thirty years later in "American Skin" the same scene repeats itself, but this time as a rendition of a fact that actually happened, with Amadou Diallo, a young immigrant from Guinea, as its victim killed by four policemen and forty-one gunshots.

This attraction to Hispanic American culture—which in 1995 would be the central theme in *The Ghost of Tom Joad*—probably derives from the fact that Springsteen, Catholic on his Italian mother's side and Irish on his father's, feels a closeness to his own roots. And so it is that Hispanics join him as companions in this urban underprivileged class, and beyond a certain exotic/erotic charge held by a number of female characters, what they actually represent is the great unhappiness behind the socioeconomic situation that even Springsteen was riding in the years between the sixties and seventies.[105]

The bleak and violent reality on the streets in the early part of the seventies comes through intermittently with no frills; as in "Lost in the Flood":

> Bronx's best apostle stands with his hand on his own hardware,
> Everything stops, you hear five quick shots, the cops come up for air.
> And now the whiz-bang gang from uptown, they're shootin' up the street
> And that cat from the Bronx starts lettin' loose, but he gets blown right off
> his feet.

However, as we have said, in general street life is represented with a sort of feverish enthusiasm, never more superbly than Springsteen achieved in "Jungleland," which richly closes *Born to Run*. Here we meet two memorable characters, Magic Rat and "Barefoot girl sitting on the hood of a Dodge / Drinking warm beer in the soft summer rain," and verses that effectively underline Springsteen's voluntary adherence to the world he is describing and the distance between himself and the "poets" who

> Don't write nothing at all,
> They just stand back and let it all be
> And in the quick of the night they reach for their moment
> And try to make an honest stand,
> But they wind up wounded, not even dead,
> Tonight in Jungleland.

Revenge on the *Norton Anthology* is thus taken, in Elvis Presley's sacred name. Having reached the climax of this *American Graffiti*-like scenario where the protagonist is lost within a crowd of people (Diamond Jackie, Wild Billy, Hazy Davy, Killer Joe, Eddie, Cherry, the Rangers . . .) the lens searches for a close-up, focusing on first-time declarations of love and escape, like the one in the "4th of July, Asbury Park (Sandy)."

> The narrator of "Sandy" is an adolescent loser, the kid whose shirt gets stuck in the fun-fair ride, leaving him stranded and looking like a fool. You'd think he was ruining his chances with the girl: he can't stop telling her about his humiliations, about the girls who led him on, about the waitress that got tired of him. He can't even hand her a line without blowing it: "I promise I'll love you—forever?"[106]

But it is through *Born to Run* that Springsteen really brings home the story of two small-town kids' dream to escape with a urgency until then unheard of in any rock album.

4. Rock 'n' Roll Future

Halfway through the 1970s the American music scene had grown stale, but a new wave of singer-songwriters—of which Springsteen wasn't even the top of the class (yet)—had begun making their appearance. Even if you don't count Lou Reed and Neil Young (who were catapulted into the first half of the decade as solo artists after long periods spent in groups in the sixties), there are other voices about that sound more powerful than the kid from Freehold. In 1974, for example, there's Jackson Browne's *Late for the Sky*, whose cover (which Browne called "a Magritte in Los Angeles") hints at the tone of songs—imbued with Browne's grief over his wife's suicide and the death of a friend ("For a Dancer," "The Late Show") or anticipating anti-nuclear activism to come ("Before the Deluge")—in which Browne manages to transform his personal torments into spartan, uncluttered poetry. Springsteen himself noted how, "In seventies, post-Vietnam America, there was no album that captured the fall from Eden, the long, slow afterburn of the sixties; its heartbreak, its disappointments, its spent possibilities better than Jackson's masterpiece, *Late for the Sky*."[107]

But the real diarist of the West Coast is Tom Waits, the loser *par excellence* of American music. Resembling an on-the-skids entertainer, his jazz-blues melodies feeling like they're grasping for a handhold before soaring off to the heights of their own melancholy, over his forty-year career Waits has erected a monument to the America of the wrong side of the tracks, lower than Raymond Carver, lower even than Bukowski, offering up the flavor of a California light-years distant from the beaches, oceans, pot, and laid-back hippie bliss; the songs here are odes to diners, cheap booze, sleazy motels, and seedy dressing rooms shared with a sad stripper.

In the summer of 1974, Bob Dylan buys himself a farm northeast of Minneapolis, on the banks of the River Crow: thirty hectares of farmland he can put between himself and the world that has been wondering for a while whatever happened to the greatest American singer-songwriter. The separation from his wife Sara is now a reality, and the moment is anything but a positive one. When he picks up his guitar, though, Dylan manages as if by magic to translate his pain and exasperation into great music. Even as his heir presumptive from New Jersey is coming out with his third—and decisive—album, Dylan's *Blood on the Tracks* is being hailed as a miracle, "the truest, most honest account of a love affair from tip to stern ever put down on magnetic tape," according to Rick Moody.[108]

But for Springsteen, glory is still to come. He's part of an honest rear that numbers among its ranks other promising songwriters like Nick Drake and Elliott Murphy, but it'll take more than Jon Landau, an influential music critic from *Rolling Stone* and Springsteen's future producer, writing on May 9, 1974, after attending one of his concerts, "I saw rock and roll's future and his name is Bruce Springsteen."[109] He will have to produce the album of his consecration. And it is in that precise moment that the recording of what will become one of the most important albums in rock history begins. The sessions are exhausting and the work never seems to end, the goal being to emerge in possession of the greatest of the great records.

It is the arrival of Jon Landau that moves things on. "We went to cut the album," Springsteen recalls, "and we just began to seem to have problems. We were unable to get a satisfactory take of a single song. The piano was broken, it was making a weird sound. Things didn't sound right. And it became very frustrating. So I said, 'Mike [Appel, Springsteen's manager], we need help. We gotta have help. We're dead in our tracks right now. We need an infusion of somebody else's knowledge and energy and point of view.' This is where Jon Landau enters the picture."[110]

"When I came in," Landau remembers, "we were at the legendary 914 Studio, which had seen better days . . . I said to Bruce, 'Look, you're a first-class artist, you belong in a first-class recording studio.' So we moved to a popular studio at the time, the Record Plant."[111]

Though things were certainly better from a technical standpoint, their problems weren't over. The sound engineer was the then very young Jimmy Iovine, who still has indelible memories of those sessions: "Bruce would just pick up the guitar, look straight at the floor or at us, and say, 'Again. Again. Again.' Now, you do that for fourteen hours and you could really, really mess with somebody's mind. I had a piece of Wrigley's Spearmint gum. I took the gum out of the wrapper and I chewed on the aluminum foil. The pain was so severe that I knew it would wake me up."[112]

It took more than six months to record a single song, "Born to Run." And as Steve Van Zandt points out, "Any time you spend six months on a song there's something not exactly going right. You know, a song should take about three hours."[113] "We were recording epics at the time," recalls Bittan. "I mean, 'Jungleland' and 'Backstreets' are not easy songs to record. It's like trying to drive a Grand Prix course: every time you go around one turn, there's another."[114]

After a year and a half of work, finally the album *Born to Run* was ready. And it was a surprise. Bold, grandiose, melodramatic, powerful, the record was like a missile launched into the suffocating landscapes of 1970s rock. "With its *Jimmie Dean, Jimmie Dean* mythology, it anticipates punk and brings with it a dream of freedom that feels almost religious. Visions, grand gestures, rock 'n' roll. The dream is a day (and a night) long, just enough to drink in *Born to Run* and be blown away by it for the rest of your life."[115]

> Springsteen's singing, his words and the band's music have turned the dreams and failures two generations have dropped along the road into an epic—an epic that began when that car went over the cliff in *Rebel Without a Cause*. One feels that all it ever meant, all it ever had to say, is on this album.[116]

A record about two kids in search of something—not always together and not always in love, but always close. Two kids who don't really know what they're looking for but who are ready to go and get it in the Promised Land, while those of us who are listening and imagining

> through the eyes of Terry, Magic Rat, Mary, Bad Scooter, Wendy, Eddie, and Cherry can already see what's coming. Like in those movies where you laugh, fall in love, and feel touched all at the same time—and also feel a shiver like a premonition run down your spine. *Born to Run* is an album that makes you believe in rock 'n' roll with all your heart, with all your soul, and with all your mind.[117]

Springsteen had already tackled the theme of escape in "Rosalita (Come Out Tonight")" and in "4th of July, Asbury Park (Sandy)." His first album contained "Mary Queen of Arkansas," which sketched out the vision at the heart of the yet to come "Born to Run": the romantic search for "somewhere else." "But I know a place where we can go, Mary," the song concludes, "where I can get a good job and start all over again clean." With *Born to Run*, though, this became the point of the story itself. "Thunder Road" and the title track are not simply (probably) the two finest songs Springsteen has ever written; they also represent the culmination of everything that, over its sixty-year lifespan, rock 'n' roll has tried to say. After having sketched out the context—sometimes through humor and sometimes by means of a road epic that borders on an Ellington-esque "sentimental mood"— Springsteen was ready to make the great leap: small-town New Jersey had become too great a burden to bear for the kid who wanted to find his place in the world; innocence had been wiped away and the concrete jungle had lost all its romance in the eyes of the young storyteller. "Jersey's a dumpy joint," Springsteen said in an interview in 1974. "I mean. It's okay, it's home. But every place is a dump."[118] A few years later he added that the idea was to *escape*. He urgently needed to leave the beach of Stockton's Wing, Flamingo Lane, and the dates made under "that giant Exxon sign" behind him. It was time to say goodbye to this "death trap" and get on "Highway 9."

To translate this liberating vision into music, Springsteen was determined to find a new sound, and Dylan and Van Morrison were no longer usable as models. The first consequence of this desire for change was the reshuffle of the E Street Band. During the album's endless recording sessions, Vini Lopez gave up his place on drums first to Ernst "Boom" Carter and then, definitively, to Max Weinberg; David Sancious' jazzy piano was replaced by Roy Bittan's less-showy Fender Rhodes; old friend Miami Steve Van Zandt came on board to arrange and direct the horn section and provide (though only live) second guitar to Springsteen, who this time was less prone to long solos. Violinist Suki Lahav left her mark on the final track, "Jungleland," while Randy Brecker added embellishment to "Meeting Across the River" with his trumpet. The idea was to saturate all the spaces, creating something resembling that powerful, bombastic wall of sound invented in the sixties by Phil Spector for the girl groups he produced, with here and there some of the "softness" of the Beach Boys' *Pet Sounds*, the guitar of Duane Eddy and a pinch of Bo-beat stolen from Bo Diddley. The whole thing seasoned with a singing voice that nods explicitly to another of Bruce's idols, Roy Orbison, the writer of that "Only the Lonely" mentioned in "Thunder Road," one of the most significant lyrics in all of Springsteen's oeuvre; as Nick Hornby notes, it "knows how I feel and who I am, and that, in the end, is one of the consolations of art."[119]

The United States have invested so deeply in the American Dream because they are themselves its product. In 1630, Governor John Winthorp, while still being tossed upon the waves of the Atlantic, wrote in his journal, "Wee shall finde that the God of Israell is among us, when ten of us shall be able to resist a thousand of our enemies . . . for wee must consider that wee shall be as a citty upon a hill."[120] At the heart of the American Dream of the early Puritans was the reformulation of the covenant of God with his people—a new people in a new Promised Land. The Dream lost its mystical aura and became a political strategy a century and a half later with Thomas Jefferson and the Declaration of Independence: all men are created equal, and to all men God gave three fundamental rights—life, liberty, and the pursuit of happiness. Isn't it wonderful that there is a constitution that sings the praises of happiness? A nation that formally enshrines the aspiration to be happy is a nation moving towards the Promised Land. But it's a journey that may well end up in a dirty pool of blood, as it did for James Gatz from Minnesota, who changed his name to Jay Gatsby and in Long Island won the heart of the beautiful Daisy Buchanan.

Ten years after the publication of Fitzgerald's novel, Elvis Aaron Presley was born in Tupelo, Mississippi. It was clear to all—him included—that he had the Dream: when he was a child, he dreamed that he was the hero of comic books and films. He grew up believing in the dream and went on to live the dream. Twenty years later, when his gigantic body was found lying on the carpet after one banana-and-peanut-butter sandwich too many, everyone thought he had gone the way of Gatsby: he had brushed the dream with his fingers, and had gotten burned. But there is such majesty in the decline of Elvis, such grotesque drama, that cynically speaking, in retrospect, one couldn't ask for more from the king of rock. The star in decline is one facet of the American Dream: it reminds us all that anyone can become a star, even if only for a single hit.

"When it came to Presley," notes Gary Graff, "Springsteen was lured in by the same aspects as everyone else—the energy, the sexuality, the rebellion, and the sense of forbidden experience. But over time he became a student of the deeper implications of Presley's stardom."[121]

In the iconic cover photo of *Born to Run*, Springsteen wears a badge from the New York Elvis Presley fan club that bears Elvis's image and the inscription "ELVIS the KING" and wears a leather jacket and a tattered tank top. In his left hand he holds his beloved Esquire, and his right arm rests upon the shoulder of someone of whom only his back, one arm, and his black leather pants can be seen. But if we open the gatefold cover, we see the entire picture, including the portion that is on the back, and the unknown figure takes the shape of Clarence Clemons, wearing a big, wide-brimmed black hat and blowing into his saxophone.[122]

That photo by Eric Meola says everything about an album whose title is *Born to Run*. As Louis P. Masur rightly points out, the two men on the cover look happy, bound together by rock 'n' roll on a journey—or rather, an escape.[123] The adventure begins, and—in that black and white shot—the dream seems to be within reach. All you need to do is make a record that is as good as *After School Session*, *Highway 61 Revisited*, and *Sgt. Pepper's Lonely Hearts Club Band* . . .

5. The Hero's Journey to the Promised Land

Born to Run brings with it success, *Time* and *Newsweek* magazine covers, fame and fortune. When in "Thunder Road" Mary accepts the ride towards a romantic dream of freedom, we find ourselves up against a deep breaking point in the structure of Springsteen's work. From this point onwards, and for a long period hereafter, the author and his role face a divide. And this (temporary) separation proves to be all but simple and painless.

What essentially happens is that, as in every respectable tragedy, the hero of *Born to Run*'s desire burns so strongly as to bring upon a tremendous energy that will guide him to his own self destruction. Usually the hero has a fatal tendency to identify himself completely, allowing for just one element of interest, whether object or passion; in the case of the Springsteen epic's protagonist, it can all be summed up in the great dream of the Promised Land, expressed in both the personal sphere of interest (having a family) and the public one (getting a record deal).[124] America is the rival—the very country that inspired him to believe in that dream, to have invited him into it. But there is also a deeper interior conflict buried in the hero's soul: that damned urge to isolate himself, so typical in the American personality—as John Wayne does at the end of *The Searchers*. After all the tragic hero is always alone, and on his own must fight against the very force that will inevitably crush him.

According to Theophrastus—a disciple of Aristotle—tragedy is the catastrophe of heroic destiny. In this context, in order for the tragic effect to take place one must recognize the utmost role that *dignity* plays in the hero's downfall, while the hero, absorbed in his unresolvable conflict, deeply receiving everything within his conscience, is aware of his suffering until its bitter end. The hero in tragic drama is his own killer and, at the same time, the careful witness of his downfall. This is the reason why the great characters in ancient drama and Shakespearian tragedy always explain the motives for their actions through long and uninterrupted monologues.

The same occurs for Springsteen's hero in the second act of his drama. In the albums following *Born to Run*—we are talking about *Darkness on the Edge of Town* (1978) and *The River* (1980)—the runaway boy in search of dreams, hope, and love gets married only to find himself disenchanted and alone. And thus he starts to listen to himself. Perhaps the interlocutor he tells his story to does not even exist: some of his songs seem more like soliloquies, rather like Dostoyevsky's in *Notes from the Underground* or Trevis Bickle's *Taxi Driver*, although, unlike the nihilist from Saint Petersburg who defines himself as "less than an insect" or the insane New York taxi driver—both are swallowed up by their city's devouring slums—our hero (let us name him Scooter[125] or more simply "me") continues to flee, to follow the horizon.

In his novel *Roughing It*, Mark Twain describes how his brother was appointed Secretary of Nevada Territory:

> He was going to travel! I never had been away from home, and that word "travel" had a seductive charm for me. Pretty soon he would be hundreds and hundreds of miles away on the great plains and deserts, and among the

mountains of the Far West, and would see buffaloes and Indians, and prairie dogs, and antelopes, and have all kinds of adventures, and may be get hanged or scalped, and have ever such a fine time, and write home and tell us all about it, and be a hero."[126]

Keeping in faith to what Alexis de Tocqueville was already predicting at the beginning of the nineteenth century—according to whom "an American [. . .] changes his residence ceaselessly"[127]—some amongst the best epic poets of the New World have attempted to narrate this idea of the endless voyage: from Whitman to London, from Twain to Kerouac, from Guthrie to Dylan, up until Bruce Springsteen, a poet able to add depth to this saga of uprooting and changing place by underlining a resulting aspect. As he noted himself,

> It's in the classic American tradition. If you assume that America was founded on people who could not fit in where they were in the first place, so moved and kept moving . . . Well, that isolation is a big part of the American character. Everyone wakes up on one of those mornings when you just feel like you want to walk away and start brand new.[128]

In 1978, Springsteen wanted to see what is on the other side of the coin on which "born free" is written. We are free, surely, but we are alone, and what is worse is that the objective we had set for ourselves, which seemed reasonable, keeps shifting away from our reach. In order to voice this disappointment, a more arid style is required. The emphasis of the first three albums disappears, and the sound is reduced to the bone, becoming at once more livid and dry. Punk has brought about a new rigor within arrangements.

Darkness on the Edge of Town does not in the least resemble *Never Mind the Bollocks* or *The Clash*, but those three albums share the same signals: the journey that goes backwards, to recover rock's lost innocence. Precisely to speak of this lost innocence, the hero's journey began with mother Adele, who, acting as Ariadne, Merlin, or Obi Wan Kenobi, endowed her protected one with a line of string to show him the way out of the maze of New Jersey, the sword-steel or laser with which to defeat dragons (and certain fathers brought by life over towards "the dark side"): a Kent guitar made in Japan, which sounded awful, distorted beyond all recognition, bought for sixty-nine dollars at Caiazzo's Music Store on Center Street, in Freehold, New Jersey.

At this moment the hero decides to dive into the adventure: "The balloon goes up, the romance begins, the spaceship blasts off, the wagon train gets rolling. Dorothy sets out on the Yellow Brick Road,"[129] and there's no turning back. Very often—as Campbell analyzes thoroughly in *The Hero with a Thousand Faces*, his classic essay on the legend—this passage is rendered physically, crossing over gates, bridges, rivers. This is very much the case in Springsteen's songbook, where the narrator is about to cross Saint Mary's gate after having said farewell to his father in "Independence Day." Beyond that point lurks the unknown: Thunder Road guides us towards the "Badlands," "caught in a crossfire that I don't understand." The road to the Promised Land is long and full of danger and the hero—who proudly proclaims, "I ain't no boy, no, I'm a man"—feels as though his destiny is sliding out of his control and thinks: "If I could take one moment into my hands . . ." Similarly, the narrator of "Something in the Night" ponders:

> You're born with nothing,
> And better off that way:
> Soon as you've got something, They send
> Someone to try and take it away. . . .
>
> When we found the things we loved,
> They were crushed and dying in the dirt.

Springsteen said that he wanted his new characters to feel weathered, older, but not beaten. The songs in *Darkness* are in fact full of awareness and will.

Darkness on the Edge of Town is a black-and-white film, full of night scenes shot in sharp contrast; a *roman noir* reminiscent of James M. Cain, whom Springsteen started reading in that very period, as well as the rather harsh works written by Flannery O'Connor. The main source Springsteen taps into in order to mark this stylistic change, so noticeable in the album, is most definitely film, the Western genre primarily. In 1977, his producer and friend Jon Landau introduced him to the films of John Ford and Sergio Leone, two directors who would have a determining influence on his writings from then on. The characters portrayed in Ford films are still in essence tragic heroes (as can be seen in *The Searchers*); Leone's characters, in contrast, share with Ford's only the outfit, and not their moral values.

> Now, the progressive and gradual passage from a legendary vision to a historical one, realistic and critical of the American reality, portrayed in the western genre, peculiarly characterizes the elements which together form the essence of the *Darkness on the Edge of Town* album.[130]

This concept can be seen in the passage from the American Dream portrayed in *Born to Run* through to the American reality captured in *Darkness*.

So if the main theme running through *Born to Run* is that of an inexhaustible vital energy which runs freely expressing itself unaffected by obstacles, the main image in *Darkness on the Edge of Town* focuses on the daily struggle against a reality dominated by forces which seem to constantly move in contrast to the will of individuals going about in the attempt to attain their dreams and ideals. But in this fight the characters in the songs on this album take on the same heroic dimensions of the main characters in John Ford and Sergio Leone's films.[131]

One can consider that the theme underlying the whole album fits into the rhyming "garage" and "mirage" in "Promised Land." The search for oneself, a trip that started in such a carefree way in *Born to Run*, at this point gains in pathos, endeavor, and hard work; Springsteen above all wants to underline the faith, endurance, and stamina of these individuals, like the characters in John Ford's films, have to display in order to overcome the trials, difficulties, and disappointments that they will inevitably encounter. In fact, the protagonist in "Badlands" and "The Promised Land" makes very real acts of faith towards the ideals that propel him to embark on the journey against all odds, in this way emphasizing Ma Joad's infamous words, at the end of Ford's film:

I know. That's what makes us tough. Rich fellas come up an' they die, an' their kids ain't no good an' they die out. But we keep a-comin'. We're the people that live. They can't wipe us out; they can't lick us. We'll go on forever, Pa, 'cause we're the people.[132]

Equally, in "Badlands" we find these verses:

I believe in the love that you gave me,
I believe in the faith that could save me,
I believe in the hope and I pray that some day
It may raise me above these badlands.

Ma Joad's words were a real eye-opener for Springsteen: the characters of *Darkness*, worn out, aged, yet not defeated, find their hope in faith, a lay faith in people that Springsteen often expresses, albeit with many biblical references. Holy Scripture, together with film, is the deepest sources of inspiration. Just consider the reference to cardinal virtues in "Badlands" or these lines from "Adam Raised a Cain":

In the Bible Cain slew Abel
and East of Eden he was cast.
You're born into this life paying

for the sins of somebody else's past. . . .
You inherit the sins, you inherit the flames.

Springsteen uses biblical images in "Adam Raised a Cain" to represent the inheritance handed down from father to son.

Even the man-woman relationship—addressed in previous songs with adolescent clichés—is now viewed from a more adult, discerning perspective. The couple embracing in "Because the Night" seems a hundred years older than the main character in "Rosalita": love, at this stage, is a cry for help ("So touch me now, touch me now, touch me now . . .") and if the guy in "New York City Serenade" was trying to redeem the "fish lady" ("Shake away your street life / And hook up to the night train"), in "Candy's Room" love for sale is now seen as an antidote to solitude; when the protagonist enters the room, "she makes these hidden worlds mine." The "Iceman" character says to his girl, "Baby, this emptiness has already been judged. . . . / Better than the waiting, baby better off is the search." And he might seem to be the same guy who asked Mary to jump in the car, but

> Once they tried to steal my heart, beat it right outta my head
> But, baby, they didn't know that I was born dead.
> I am the iceman, fighting for the right to live.

Every time the hero reaches the place (often underground and mysterious, dark and lurking with danger) where he believes he will find his hidden object of desire (the Holy Grail or a painful truth), he encounters a woman who represents "the Lady of the House of Sleep,"[133] beauty personified, the height of all desires, the one who will lead him to the sublime climax of sexual adventure and who symbolically tests the hero's capacity to conquer the good side of love, which is really life itself intended and fulfilling as a defined portion of eternity. The mystic matrimony with this woman/queen symbolizes the acquisition of a determining power gained for life: the hero has taken the role of the father. All that makes up real poetry—Robert Graves wrote in his extraordinary work on the White Goddess—celebrates some particular episode or scene from this age-old story,[134] which always sees at its center one of the many impersonations of the Divine: Keats's *belle dame sans merci*; the three-sided Hecate who in Macbeth watches over the witches' brew; Acrasia, seductress of knights in Spenser's *Faerie Queene*; Leucothea, mother of all centaurs; Albina, the eldest daughter of the Danaides; the "divine face" in Apuleius's *The Golden Ass*, which appears to Lucius in the middle of the sea; Olwen, daughter of the Giant Hawthorn, hair as blond as a broom and fingers pale as forest of anemones; Athena, Osiris, Istar, Brigit, Arianrhod . . . of course as well as Delilah and Juliet, quoted in "Fire"—written by Springsteen in 1977, a piece Elvis did not have the time to record; even that Christine to whom Bruce sings "let me kiss your Spanish eyes" in "Spanish Eyes," one of the many outtakes from the *Darkness* sessions; or the girl who in "Prove It All Night" wants to buy "a gold ring and a pretty dress of blue" driving "from Monroe to Angeline"; or the immensely sensual Candy, who tells him,

> "Baby, if you wanna be wild
> You got a lot to learn,
> Close your eyes
> Let them melt,
> Let them fire,
> Let them burn . . ."

6. Rock 'n' Roll Misogyny

We have not yet reached the days in which Springsteen will begin to celebrate the joys of cunnilingus in "Red Headed Woman." But the sex scenes in the *Darkness* era are already far more torrid than the more naive and romantic ones in the first three albums.

All the girls who on September 9, 1956, tuned in to CBS to see Elvis on the *Ed Sullivan Show* understood immediately that rock 'n' roll was born to announce, firstly to America and subsequently to the rest of the world, that a sexual liberation was about to begin. When Cary Grant's flannel jackets were stored away in mothballs and replaced by red jackets like James Dean's or black leather ones like Marlon Brando's, radio waves started sending out and surfing vibes unheard of until then: in Chuck Berry's "Maybellene" the girl was the trophy for the winner of a car race; and Jerry Lee Lewis in "Whole Lotta Shakin' Goin On" furiously invites his girl to come and do some movin' around with him.

A decade later, Marvin Gaye would become the forbidden dream of the many auburn-haired readers of *Harper's Bazaar* as they sat under hairdryers at beauty salons. The man who could have any one of these women sang "I Heard It Through the Grapevine" with his heart broken in two. There is not—to this day—a female listener who does not feel the urge to take that heart up in her hands and lovingly warm it; and yet no woman would do so without a trace of doubt that beneath Marvin's desperation was none other than an astute plan to get into her pants.

As Springsteen underlines during his solo concerts on the Devils & Dust Tour, those were times in which the guys were singing way way high. A generation of young male singers who were tryin' to sound like beautiful women, you know. They were singing, "Uuh, uuuh," higher and higher . . . And I always thought they were smart, because they were singing to the woman like, "I'm ready to come up where you are, I'm ready to speak to you in your voice, you know, I'm here for you, baby, and . . . will you take off your pants?" Which is the subtext of all great popular music, not matter what it is—even the great protest music: the message underneath is always, "Will you take off your pants?" You can even use it as the last line in any good pop song, like, "It's a town full of losers and I'm pulling out of here to win . . . and will you take off your pants?"

To the occasional Springsteen fan or to those who barely recognized him under a baseball cap in "Glory Days," it would appear odd that his songs were not all about workers on the A-95 or Vietnam war veterans, but—incredibly enough— he wrote a whole lot of songs about love as well: in fact, between the eighties and nineties, he did very little other than that; although if we were to scroll through the song titles from his early years like "For You," "Sandy," and "Thunder Road," what are they if not beautiful love songs?

It is said by many that Springsteen's music—with the whole parade of cars from Camaro to Subaru—is virile music, music for *men*; and undoubtedly at his concerts the female public is but a minority. He himself jokes about it by saying that "due to what must have been some strong homoerotic undercurrent in our music" he and his E Street Band always drew "rooms full of men. And not that great-looking men, either."[135] Nevertheless, besides Jimmy the Saint, Spanish Johnny, Sonny, Little Dynamite, Wild Billy, Eddie, Magic Rat, Hazey Davy, Killer Joe, Little Gun, Johnny 99, Bill Horton, Tom Joad, Joe Roberts and his brother Frankie, in his songs we also encounter the female Kitty, Crazy Janey, Wendy, Puerto Rican Jane, Mary Lu, Candy, Diamond Jackie, Cherry, Rosalie, Sandy, Catherine LeFevre, Wanda, Sherry, Kate, Doreen, Leah, and obviously Mary.

Who are these female figures, and what do they represent? Questions that give rise to some surprising answers.

The first oddity one can detect after a look through Springsteen's lyrics is the complete lack—practically—of a physical description of his female characters. We know that "Guinnevere," sung about by Crosby, Stills & Nash, had green eyes and golden hair,[136] and the girl picked up by the guy in the Mustang in "Burma Shave" by Tom Waits had hair that spilled out like rootbeer as she took out her barrettes,[137] and that the Velvet Underground's "Femme Fatale" wears contact lenses.[138] But as for Wendy in "Born to Run"—damn it—we know nothing of what she is like!

Of Crazy Janey, the protagonist in "Spirit in the Night," we know she is an expert in things of love ("don't know what she do to you," sings Springsteen before confessing that there, at Greasy Lake, he and she made love "in the dirt"), but no information is given regarding her looks, or those of the girl in "Kitty's Back," of whom the only thing we know is that she breaks Catlong's heart. Diamond Jackie in "New York City Serenade" is defined as "so intact," at least up until she gently falls at her Billy's feet; the only thing we know about her is that she wears high heels. Here, in the same way as for the whole of Bruce's first productions, sexual intercourse is described elliptically: Jackie "falls so softly beneath him," then the camera focuses on the two of them dancing on Broadway before they forever disappear from our imagination. In "Jungleland," from behind a locked bedroom door we hear sighs of weak refusals before the "surrender."

And then there is Mary, who is something of a Beatrice to Springsteen; but even of her we are offered very little detail. The first time she appears is in "Mary Queen of Arkansas," from *Greetings from Asbury Park, NJ*, and her epiphany is, to say the least, more than a little ambiguous, seeing that Bruce tells her, "You're not man enough for me to hate you or woman enough for kissing." Hmm . . . In this piece Mary, with her "white skin so deceivin'," is described like a devil temptress, while Bruce is suffocated by her embrace and above her bed he makes out "the shadow of a noose." In short, another Crazy Jane-type, an "expert" in a rather disturbing way.

Two years later, she reappears in "Thunder Road," her dress fluttering on the porch. Something has changed. Up until that moment, the way in which Springsteen had dealt with themes about love and relationships revealed some of the damage a Catholic upbringing had upon him. Sex is seen as temptation and sin, the woman a saint or whore; love is an abstract concept, devoid of sensuality, reduced to a mere objective to reach during the escape towards a dream—the dream of *Born to Run*—which resolves itself through the (very bourgeois and un-rock-like) aspiration to settle down and have a family. In "Thunder Road" Mary is no longer the queen of Arkansas who fools men with her tricks in bed, but evolves into the woman able to redeem the sinner and crown with him the American Dream: to find the Promised Land, and essentially to aspire to happiness. Introducing Mary, this new angel with a completely Catholic name, has unleashed "ghosts in the eyes of all the boys [she] sent away." Her lovers, the ones on whom she has eloquently put a cross, are "gone with the wind"; and now the girl who wastes her "summer praying in vain for a savior" is finally *redeemed*—Springsteen uses precisely that word.

Thirty years after having written "Thunder Road," Springsteen will state that at the beginning of his career he didn't write many love songs because his father told him that they were a form of government propaganda, a fraudulent way to coax you into marriage and paying taxes.

Up until the so-called Trilogy of Love (the name given to the three albums published between 1987 and 1992), Springsteen always appeared as a slave to his slightly misogynistic view of the world. Eros, in his songs, came through in episodes of mercenary sex, as in "Candy's Room," a portrait of a prostitute in a brothel ("Strangers from the city call my baby's number and they bring her toys").

It would turn out to be providential that after a couple of false steps, Springsteen's heart would be melted not by the angelic Mary of his songs, but by the hot-blooded showgirl/singer in his E Street Band, a Jersey girl who—conducing him to therapy and giving him three children—would lead her man towards "Better Days":

> Tonight I'm layin' in your arms,
> Carvin' lucky charms
> Out of these hard luck bones.

The slightly pouty youngster who walked like "like Brando right into the sun" dancing "like a Casanova" has become a man. Thanks to a woman.

But let's not rush . . .

7. The Price You Pay

In *Darkness on the Edge of Town* our hero has been left alone, "running burned and blind" ("Something in the Night"). When he realizes that the promise has been broken and that his dreams will never come true, all that remains is desperation, as we gather from these verses in "Streets of Fire":

> I live now, only with strangers,
> I talk to only strangers,
> I walk with angels that have no place.

The attempt to recover what was lost in Independence Day fails: no one is waiting there any longer, as four years later "My Father's House" will suggest. Mary gets pregnant, there is no more work, and the marriage fails. In "The River" the protagonist says:

> Now all them things that seemed so important,
> Well, mister, they vanished right into the air.
> Now I just act like I don't remember,
> Mary acts like she don't care.

Two years earlier, in "Darkness on the Edge of Town," he'd confessed:

> I lost my money and I lost my wife,
> Them things don't seem to matter much to me now.

If anyone was in any doubt as to the fate of the two characters in "Thunder Road," just listen to "The Promise," a track written in 1976 and not published until 1999:

> Inside I felt like I was carryin' the broken spirits
> Of all the other ones who lost.
> When the promise is broken you go on living
> But it steals something from down in your soul,
> Like when the truth is spoken and it don't make no difference
> Something in your heart goes cold.

> I followed that dream through the southwestern flats
> That dead ends in two-bit bars,
> And when the promise was broken I was far away from home
> Sleepin' in the back seat of a borrowed car.

> Thunder Road, for the lost lovers and all the fixed games,
> Thunder Road, for the tires rushing by in the rain,
> Thunder Road, Billy and me we'd always say,
> Thunder Road, we were gonna take it all and throw it all away.

In "Stolen Car" we once again catch up with the boy driving a stolen car, chased down the highway by the police. Is this not perhaps the "little hometown jam" to which the protagonist alludes in "Born in the U.S.A." when he tells of how he ends up in Vietnam? If in "Born to Run" the boy promises:

> Someday, girl, I don't know when,
> We're gonna get to that place where we really want to go
> And we'll walk in the sun,
> But till then tramps like us, baby, we were born to run

Ten years later the Vietnam veteran shouts in "Born in the U.S.A.":

> Down in the shadow of the penitentiary,
> Out by the gas fires of the refinery
> I'm ten years burning down the road,
> Nowhere to run, ain't got nowhere to go

echoing Faulkner's words from *The Sound and the Fury*: "No battle is ever won . . . they are not even fought. The field only reveals to man his own folly and despair, and victory is an illusion of philosophers and fools."[139]

"What lay beyond *Darkness*: an abyss, or some sort of heroic renewal?"[140] In 1980, Springsteen tries to answer to this question with *The River* double album. He says,

> Adulthood was imminent, if it hadn't arrived already, so I knew I was gonna be following my characters over a long period of time. I thought it would be interesting and fun for my audience to have a certain sort of continuity, not explicit or literal or confined but just a loose continuity from record to record.[141]

Still in 1975, to a journalist who asked him, "Do you plan to marry? Have children?" he answered, "No, I can't do that, that's for sure."[142] But now at thirty, he starts to see things from a different point of view: "*The River*," he wrote in his autobiography, "would be my first album where love, marriage, and family would cautiously move to center stage." Although still slightly in the background. Right from the opening track, "The Ties that Bind," all that ambivalence is up front: love and family tie us to each other, the lyrics declare, but not necessarily in clear-cut ways. "When I did *The River*," Springsteen commented,

> I tried to accept the fact that the world is a paradox, and that's the way it is. And the only thing you can do with a paradox is live with it. On the album, I just said, "I don't understand all these things. I don't see where all these things fit. I don't see how all these things can work together."[143]

It's a complex album that suggests feelings of doubt and contradiction. On one hand there is the sense of belonging, the need for roots; on the other there are solitude, despair, dreams that do not come to pass. It represents for Bruce Springsteen "what *Blonde on Blonde* and *Exile on Main Street* had been for Bob Dylan and the Rolling Stones at the time. Four sides, lots of tracks, all the space required to say this was a turning point in a career but without foreseeing any painful excision."[144]

Some of the songs on the album are joyful, fun, if not exhilarating, like for instance "Cadillac Ranch," "You Can Look (But You Better Not Touch)," and "I'm a Rocker," in which Springsteen reveals his secret lethal weapon:

> I got a 007 watch and it's a one and only:
> It's got a I-Spy beeper that tells me when you're lonely.
> I got a Batmobile so I can reach ya' in a fast shake
> When your world's in crisis of an impendin' heartbreak.

Now, don't you call James Bond or Secret Agent Man,
Cause they can't do it, like I can:
I'm a rocker, baby, I'm a rocker . . .

But sometimes behind brilliant and easy arrangements, interesting stories are hidden, and not too superficially. "Sherry Darling" for example, is apparently a party song with all the right ingredients for a coy pop song: a car, a girl, the beach . . . In the meantime, however, it isn't just the girl sitting in the car:

Your Mamma's yappin' in the back seat,
Tell her to push over and move them big feet,

the narrator sings exasperatedly—and whoever has a mother-in-law cannot help but recognize this mechanism in which to identify. After which he sings,

Every Monday morning I gotta drive her down to the unemployment
agency.

"*The unemployment agency?* How often in rock does one hear talk of such things?"[145] For the first time, in *The River* Springsteen knowingly lowers his characters into a very evident social discomfort, as happens with the protagonist of the title track, who has lost his job "on account of the economy," and the female protagonist of "Jackson Cage":

Driving home she grabs something to eat
Turns a corner and drives down her street
Into a row of houses she just melts away
Like the scenery in another man's play
Into a house where the blinds are closed
To keep from seeing things she don't wanna know.

The "verdict" has already been made for this single woman living alone in the ghetto:

You can try with all your might
But you're reminded every night
That you been judged and handed life
Down in Jackson Cage.

Having decided to deal with these adult themes, Springsteen first reconsidered his style and approached country, a genre that described these same issues so exhaustively in American pop culture. He once told of a night when he was in his hotel room in New York and started singing Hank Williams' "My Bucket's Got a Hole In It."

> I drove back to New Jersey that night and sat up in my room writing "The River." I used a narrative folk voice—just a guy in a bar telling his story to the stranger on the next stool. . . .[146]

That song became a point of reference for the style of writing he would then develop in greater depth on *Nebraska* and *The Ghost of Tom Joad*.

In *The River* there's another new aspect: for the first time (with the exception of the Utah desert where "The Promised Land" is set) Springsteen doesn't describe an urban scenario: he sets his story in nature, thus imitating a classic country music pattern. True, there was the Greasy Lake episode in "Spirit in the Night," but that was just a short trip. Here, on the other hand, the river and the valley and the "green fields" are mighty symbols—the Eden where Adam and Eve lived happily until they were cast out for the sin committed. Before, when there was love, "We'd go down to the river / And into the river we'd dive"; then, when the love ends, the narrator goes back to the river "though I know the river is dry."

The sin alluded to is that of the two lovers running away from their new responsibilities: Mary's pregnant, he's out of work. They run away from one another and end up regretting it but never finding each other again: the river has run dry. Thus, in "Hungry Heart"—another bitter song that sounds like a Beach Boys' pop tune—the guy says, "Like a river that don't know where it's flowing / I took a wrong turn and I just kept going."

The same guy tries to find his way back to the love he lost in the long and passionate "Drive All Night," and he almost seems to believe his own false hopes. In "Stolen Car," after he has abandoned his wife, he says,

> And I'm driving a stolen car
> On a pitch black night,
> And I'm telling myself I'm gonna be alright,
> But I ride by night and I travel in fear
> That in this darkness I will disappear.

The images are cadenced in a slow, repetitive pace and therefore close the song on a brooding, desperate note, accentuated by the presence of keywords ("night," "fear," "darkness," "disappear") in emphatic positions at the end of the last four lines. The myth of the car speeding along America's highways (central to *Born to Run*) is definitively cracked here. Two years later, in "State Trooper," this backtracking is even more evident:

New Jersey Turnpike,
Ridin' on a wet night
'Neath the refinery's glow
Out where the great black rivers flow.

License, registration,
I ain't got none
But I got a clear conscience
'Bout the things that I done. . . .

Hey, somebody out there,
Listen to my last prayer,
Hi ho Silver-o,
Deliver me from nowhere.

With regard to *The River*, music critic Paul Nelson wrote:

> It's a contemporary, New Jersey version of *The Grapes of Wrath*, with the
> Tom Joad / Henry Fonda figure—nowadays no longer able to draw upon
> the solidarity of family—driving a stolen car through a neon Dust Bowl. . . .
> Contrary to what F. Scott Fitzgerald wrote, most American lives do have
> second acts. And . . . these postexperiential acts are usually the ones in which
> we either crack up or learn to live with our limitations and betrayals. . . . What
> makes *The River* really special is Bruce Springsteen's epic exploration of the
> second acts of American lives.[147]

8. Reason to Believe

The River ends with "Wreck on the Highway," which Springsteen himself defines
as the alpha and omega, the cornerstone of the whole album. On a rainy highway
the character witnesses a fatal accident, and while later that night he is in bed with
his lover, he realizes the fragility of life. A whole age of innocence is broken having
gained conscience that Thunder Road and the Fast Lane are one and the same.
Pandora's box has been opened, the definitive limit acknowledged. Dreams have
become illusion.

In this perspective "Wreck on the Highway" seems to represent the prologue
of that massive American Nightmare fresco that Springsteen creates (in black
and white, for the same reason that Picasso made no use of color in *Guernica*)
canceling out his own voice to reveal the voices of a vast number of misfits, losers,
and loners.

After *Born to Run*, the author and his character had begun to fatally split up: the former continued to boldly go towards the Promised Land, while the latter tended to his wounds. Further on in his musical path, Springsteen will reveal how that boy on the run won his own bets. However, the image of his dystopian self ("what would have happened if I hadn't been contracted by Columbia?") is so compelling now, so impressive is the scene before his eyes, that his little New Jersey story is no longer enough for him. He needs to go out West, to Nebraska, Texas, and California, making up new and more dramatic characters. Finally the element of ambiguity ceases to exist: this is no longer the story of Bruce Springsteen, but rather the story of the United States.

There is always a dose of ambiguity when a writer speaks of "self." The difference—also abyssal in autobiographies—between the Author's voice and that of the Narrator is very often not inferred; one can only imagine the effect in the case of songs rather than of the written book, where the voice is that which enters a home from behind a microphone across radio waves or a bunch of fiber optics. Speaking of which, Springsteen observes:

> That's something that is particular to music I think. . . . You are the writer, you are the performer, you are the singer—and if you've done your job very well and brought forth a lot of real emotion, I think it calls for the listener to take a step back and realize that they're listening to a creation of some sort, a work of imagination. That what you're doing, part of your craft is understanding—and you may be singing through the voice of another character to create that understanding.[148]

In "Wreck on the Highway," again a very thin veil separates us from tragedy: the protagonist is merely a witness, for the final time. It's rather similar to the opening lines of *Moby Dick*: "Call me Ishmael."[149] Who is this New Yorker with a biblical name, sole survivor of the Pequod shipwreck? Is it Ishmael speaking to himself, or Melville referring to us readers? Or is it Ishmael? Which voice are we listening to; who is it talking to? It is difficult to answer these questions. Surely though, if there were no one there to tell us "call me Ishmael," as though sitting on the stool next to us at the bar, we would find it pretty tricky to be taken by the story of a one-legged captain trying to capture a whale, and just that one (albeit a nice big white one) across the seven seas, and who at the end of it all actually finds him . . .

Voice is everything. The closer it gets to your ear to whisper a story, the more that story sounds convincing, credible, true. Since *Nebraska*, Springsteen has shown that he has understood it perfectly, writing songs that are little literary treasures.

It was autumn of 1981 and Springsteen was like God in the midst of the gods of rock, so screamed the headlines of London's *Times*, an artist offering the world a pure dose of superlative talent: "Iconic rocker. Archetypal American. Working-class hero. All-American sex symbol. Introspective lyricist and goofy showman . . . The man who carries the mantle of Chuck Berry, Elvis, Woody Guthrie and Bob Dylan on his shoulders."[150]

With *The River* he reached #1 on the American charts (which had not even happened with *Born to Run*),[151] while 141 concerts in front of two million spectators established his fame as extraordinary stage animal on both sides of the Atlantic; even John Lennon, shortly before his death, had noticed him proclaiming "Hungry Heart" the best rock 'n' roll single since the Beatles.[152] When Columbia found out that its golden goose had already gone back to writing songs, it was convinced that a rock album would emerge and be played on a loop on all the FM stations on short, long, and medium wave for that part of the Promised Land with net operating margins called America. But Springsteen was preparing a big surprise: in 1981, after the River Tour, he came back to New Jersey and called his guitar technician, asking him to help with some cheap and easy home recording. Toby Scott got back with a four-track Teac tape machine, which they set up in Springsteen's bedroom in Colts Neck, New Jersey. That was where he recorded *Nebraska*.

It all happened on one day, January 3, 1982, when Springsteen recorded fifteen songs one after the other:[153] just himself, his guitar, and his harmonica. The first to listen to the tape was Jon Landau, who worried greatly about the somber tone of those pieces. Yet, as Springsteen worked to adapt the songs for the E Street Band, it was precisely Jon Landau who suggested that those tapes be published as they were.[154] As the story goes, when Walter Yetnikoff, president of CBS, listened to the record's final mix, he couldn't help but be moved by it. That album was never going to smash charts, but the feeling was clearly that it was destined to become a classic, despite all the eccentricities it came with. At a time when synthesizers were uprooting guitars, and in which new wave, commercial pop, dance music, and the new romantics were all the rage—bringing a wide range of superficiality and colorfully plastic aesthetics—Springsteen offered himself to his public practically in the nude: just his voice and a guitar to tell ten intense, dark, and dramatic stories, the whole of it packaged behind a harsh cover, with a black-and-white photo promptly picked up on by David Kennedy from behind his windshield driving down a Midwest street.

Placing the needle on that vinyl, in the autumn of 1982, for a great number of people proved to be a shocking experience. A "Reason to Believe," to quote the title of the last track on the album. If Dylan had electrified songwriting with his *Bringing*

It All Back Home, transforming himself from folksinger to rocker, then Bruce Springsteen was sensationally following the opposite path, with a rough, primitive, direct, violent, and desperate album, with the "ruggedness and charm of Robert Johnson's 78s and Jackie Lomax's field recordings"[155] and lyrics ranging between nihilism and horror. No pop artist had until then traced such an unforgiving picture of his own country until then.

The importance of *Nebraska* is without doubt more literary than musical: it marks the passage to maturity in Springsteen's lyric writing, timidly approached in *The River*, finally leaving behind themes and situations revolving around the epic and the romantic. His sources are no longer so oddly sorted, and not solely musical: Guthrie, Hank Williams, the American gothic short stories of Flannery O'Connor, the noir novels of James M. Cain, the films of Terrence Malick and Charles Laughton all guided his imagination.

Dylan is still a reference point, but "While Dylan constructs his working-class characters as passive 'pawns' who are wholly manipulated by historical and social forces beyond their control, Springsteen's characters make their own history, but they do under very difficult circumstances."[156]

That is why *Nebraska*'s are tragic heroes. An external force exists—an antagonist—which suppresses them (the ones that "put the rifle" in the hand of the protagonist of "Johnny 99"), but there is an internal force as well, bringing them towards self-destruction, as becomes clear in the case of the title track's protagonist, which Springsteen wrote after having seen the film *Badlands* by Terrence Malick (1973): the true story of Charles Starkweather and Caril Fugate, who in 1958 killed ten people, living like vagabonds for eight days in the harsh lands of Nebraska and eastern Wyoming. They were caught, and he was executed the following year while she did eighteen years in prison and came out on probation in 1986. Shocked by the film, Springsteen read *Caril*, an accurate reconstruction of those events written by Ninette Beaver, and when he finished it, he was more than ready to write a song about those bloody facts:

> I saw her standin' on her front lawn
> Just twirlin' her baton.
> Me and her went for a ride, sir,
> and ten innocent people died.

> From the town of Lincoln, Nebraska
> With a sawed off 410 on my lap,
> Through to the badlands of Wyoming
> I killed everything in my path.

When the song's protagonist has to reflect upon the motives pushing him to leave such a frightening path of blood behind him, he can only say, "Well, sir, I guess there's just a meanness in this world." He doesn't blame society, or—like Johnny 99 does—the bank that "was holdin' [his] mortgage and they was takin' [his] house away," but rather the world's indistinct cruelty—which is in the end equivalent to blaming oneself.

In Malick's film the two protagonists are renamed Kit Caruthers (Martin Sheen) and Holly (Sissy Spacek). After having killed Holly's father, Kit flees with her, crossing South Dakota and Montana, leaving behind a trail of blood. The passion between them (twenty-five and fifteen years old respectively), if there ever was one, burns out rapidly. Holly assists the murders with a mixture of dismay and indifference; Kit, in turn, kills without hatred, and, as much as he acts like James Dean, boasts decent manners and conformist ideas. Malick films Kit's bloody escapades with absolutely no emotional attachment—and in so doing distances himself radically from Hollywood examples of *maudit* cinema close to him in terms of time, like *Getting Straight* (1970) and *The Strawberry Statement* (1970)—and successfully choses to situate his noir film within the unlimited confines of the badlands, thus creating the first act of a personal saga whose heart centers around the unresolvable conflict between Grace and Nature, leaving the issue of earthly suffering unanswered.

The same goes for Springsteen's more mature work. Springsteen's characters, like many of us, work hard, love their women, have a family. However, like many of us, they often ruin everything, starting with themselves. We often meet them precisely in that fatal moment in which they have wasted their last chance at salvation, when—as the author himself says—"their first dreams get killed off . . . and nothing takes its place . . . There was a Norman Mailer article that said that the one freedom that people want most is the one they can't have: the freedom from dread."[157] Springsteen's moralism—soaked through with Catholicism—breaks down into a set of questions:

> What happens when we act out of passion or cowardice, weakness or strength, love or hate, the crazed desire for redemption and transcendence? How do we deal with guilt? And what happens when all these things flow into one another, when they become part of what Springsteen calls [. . .] the Big Muddy?[158]

These issues are paralyzing and deeply frightening. In *Nebraska*, Springsteen seeks the answers on a trip at once both inside himself and *out there*, in the great natural theater of America, attempting to explore the dark territory both of his individual subconscious, and of the collective one of his country.

Flannery O'Connor wrote that the Catholic writer "will feel life from the standpoint of the central Christian mystery: that it has, for all its horror, been found by God to be worth dying for."[159] According to O'Connor, if one believes in the divinity of Christ, he must keep the world sacred while fighting to endure it. This perspective in no way reduces the writer's sphere of vision of reality; in fact it widens it. O'Connor was convinced that writers who hold the light of their Christian faith before them are the sharpest observers of the grotesque, the perverse, and the unacceptable. Her method was to "portray more the absence than the presence of grace."[160]

As we have learnt from *De Imitatione Christi*, without grace evil triumphs.[161] And evil is the red thread connecting the majority of the songs put together in *Nebraska*. The main source of inspiration for Springsteen in this respect is precisely Flannery O'Connor (as well as Walker Percy, Bobbie Ann Mason, Jim Thompson, and James M. Cain).

Springsteen appreciates O'Connor's dark spirituality and her intention of dealing with the theme of the impossibility of knowing God. "She knew original sin," Springsteen says, "knew how to give it the flesh of a story."[162] The poetic nature belonging to O'Connor, however, is filtered through Springsteen's capacity for compassion towards human destiny, even of the most unworthy kind. Where O'Connor lacks empathy and compassion for her characters' mistakes and sins, Springsteen instead displays a deep empathic feeling. O'Connor's all-knowing narrator thus finds its opposite in Springsteen's use of the first person, through which the author in a way identifies with his character.

A typical example of the first person narrative is "Highway Patrolman," where we hear, "My name is Joe Roberts," at the beginning of the piece—a technique used in the late nineteenth century in murder ballads, songs inspired by facts in the news, in which the narrator, to make them more credible, offered his own voice to the protagonist. Springsteen will comment:

> Eventually, I was using Charlie Starkweather to write about me. Take *The Executioner's Song* by Norman Mailer; you can say, "Is writing this stuff this way making the stuff itself seem fascinating and romantic?" I don't know. It's a question you ask yourself whenever you write a song.[163]

In this sense Springsteen seems to have learned from popular songs in which we see the outlaw on the one hand as a kind of hero fighting against the establishment, and on the other as the product of a degraded society that offers no hope. Let us take for instance the verse in which Charlie imagines "when the man pulls that switch, sir, and snaps my poor head back," where *poor* is taken straight from that kind of ballad illustrating a feature belonging to the outlaw, indicating a solidarity between author and public.

Springsteen, a romantic who inherits from Rousseau the idea of goodwill (evil has its roots in the social rather than the metaphysical sphere) will clarify that he and his characters are "misfits more than outlaws."[164] The misfit in "Nebraska" seems taken from the grandmother's doppelgänger, protagonist of the short story "A Good Man Is Hard to Find," for example—one of O'Connor's works which Springsteen pays particular attention to. O'Connor often resorts to these doubles who overlap, even violently, with the protagonists' figures, incarnating divine or unconscious forces which they uselessly attempt to remove or repress.

In the transposition from O'Connor's story to song, Springsteen puts aside "the character of the grandmother and the other members of the family, upon which O'Connor's irony heavily sits, focusing solely on the tragic figure, no longer ridiculous, of The Misfit, who incarnates meanness."[165] Concentrating on the only the tragic element from O'Connor's work, Springsteen can work his compassion and his sensibility.

In this view, the second song on the album in which Springsteen tells the story of a murderer and his sentence, "Johnny 99," is unmistakable:

> "Now judge, judge, I had debts no honest man could pay,
> The bank was holdin' my mortgage and they was takin' my house away.
> Now, I ain't sayin' that makes me an innocent man
> But it was more 'n all this that put that gun in my hand."

In "Johnny 99" Springsteen clearly takes the side of the accused, defining him— here as well—as *poor*, while for Judge John Brown he has reserved the epithet *mean*. Even the title is telling: the guilty is named that way because he is sentenced to ninety-nine years of prison—a number in American tradition that signifies the death sentence and can be found in a long list of songs like "99 Year Blues" by Julius Daniels and various prison penitentiary work songs, for instance "Rosie" and "Bad Man Ballad," not to mention "Poor Boy" by Woodie Guthrie, in which the protagonist is obsessed by the number ninety-nine: in fact, he plays ninety-nine dollars and loses, then kills his rival in love and gets sentenced to ninety-nine years in prison.

Guthrie's work was undoubtedly the most influential on Springsteen during the composition of *Nebraska*. More generally, Bruce must have reviewed the *Anthology of American Folk Music* at great length. Published by Folkways in 1952, the anthology contains an incredible quantity of songs recorded between 1926 and 1932. Here one can find hillbilly ballads by singers such as Dock Boggs, Dick Justice, Buell Kazee, and Bascom Lamar Lunsford; prehistoric blues tracks like those by Jim

Jackson, Blind Lemon Jefferson, and Julius Daniels; and religious songs interpreted by Ernest Phipps, Blind Willie Johnson, and the Carter Family. There is a whole world before Elvis. And for the first time Springsteen is set to discover it. Even "Open All Night"—the only rock 'n' roll on *Nebraska*—"harks back to proto-rockabillies like Harmonica Frank Floyd and Hank Mizell rather than Chuck Berry and the R&B singers who inspired Bruce's usual songs."[166] Demo or no demo, the anti-modernistic tone of the album appears intentional: Springsteen wants to describe his country's black soul, and in the United States' musical roots he finds the perfect base to start from. The road—those never-ending highways with their surrounding accessories, from motels, to roadside restaurants, signposts, and automobiles—this theater provides the context in which the vitriolic counter-history of the Golden Eighties unfolds. The romanticism associated around the image of travel—that in which *Born to Run* is permeated—has disappeared. If in 1975 the twenty-six-year-old James Dean imitator crossing "mansions of glory" in a "suicide machine" sang, "I wanna die with you Wendy on the streets tonight in an everlasting kiss," seven years later, in a much more detached fashion, he says, "I bought us two tickets on that Coast City bus. . . . / Put your makeup on, fix your hair up pretty / And meet me tonight in Atlantic City." In "Atlantic City" Springsteen sticks his nose in the middle of a gang fight, telling it to us from the point of view of a second-row delinquent, aware of the huge risks he is running: "Well, I'm tired of comin' out on the losin' end, / So, honey, last night I met this guy and I'm gonna do a little favor for him."

Flannery O'Connor said that the world of the narrative writer is full of material. For her nothing was more dangerous or anti-poetic than abstraction, whether of ideas or emotions; the main characteristic , and the most apparent, in narration— she believed—is that of facing reality through what can be seen, felt, smelled, touched, tasted.[167] Springsteen felt much the same way: "The precision of the storytelling . . . is very important. The correct detail can speak volumes about who your character is, while the wrong one can shred the credibility of your story."[168] It is not surprising that he enjoys William Price Fox's novels: "Open All Night" (on *Nebraska*) and "Darlington County" (on *Born in the U.S.A.*) were written, as explicitly admitted by their author, under the influence of *Dixiana Moon*, the picaresque novel published by Fox in 1981.[169]

Nebraska is full of revealing details drawn with the precision of a diamond tip, starting from the title track, in which Springsteen renders the brutality of capital punishment by speaking of a man who flips the switch to "snap" the convict's head. The gates of "Mansion on the Hill" are made of "hardened steel." In "Used Cars" the narrator's mother "fingers her wedding band" while her husband is dealing with the salesman—a detail telling of her mood; in the same way we understand everything from the meeting between the protagonist from "Open All Night" and the cashier Wanda from these two simple verses: "On the front seat she's sittin' in my lap, / We're wipin' our fingers on a Texaco roadmap." "Highway Patrolman" is the triumph of accuracy, right from the beginning: "My name is Joe Roberts, I work for the state, / I'm a sergeant out of Perrineville, Barracks number 8." Can't get much clearer than that . . . In fact, the song is to become the subject for *The Indian Runner*, Sean Penn's first film as a director.

Springsteen solo—the one from *Nebraska*, *The Ghost of Tom Joad*, and *Devils & Dust*, and in some way the one from *Tunnel of Love* as well—aims ambitiously at a very finely strung piece of work, which forces one to concentrate intensely on a set of precisely drawn details: the thread interlacing a story, a character's point of view, the inflections of voice . . . The sparseness of the arrangements forces the listener to focus on the substance of the songs. As happens, for instance, in "Reason to Believe" with that "effortlessly" with which Springsteen describes the indolent, natural flowing of the river's water, where two parents have come to "take away little Kyle's sin," right where an old man's funeral is taking place, the bystanders praying to God: "Lord, won't you tell us, tell us what does it mean?" Together they call upon the Lord, even the priest and groom, there on the banks of that same river, waiting in vain for the bride; but the God of *Nebraska* is far away, absent: there is just a river—unkind nature—that keeps on flowing as if nothing were wrong, and speaks, perhaps though Springsteen's words, commenting sarcastically:

> Struck me kinda funny, seem kinda funny, sir, to me,
> How at the end of every hard earned day
> People find some reason to believe.

Despite its title, *Nebraska's* closing number is there to warn us that "even that reason to believe is only there to fool us."[170]

9. The New Timer

The nihilism found in the final verses of "Reason to Believe" is the same enfolding Walker Percy's character Bickerson Bolling, protagonist in *The Moviegoer*:

> Today is my thirtieth birthday and I sit on the ocean wave in the schoolyard and wait for Kate and think of nothing. Now in the thirty-first year of my dark pilgrimage on this earth and knowing less than I ever knew before, having learned only to recognize merde when I see it, having inherited no more from my father than a good nose for merde, for every species of shit that flies—my only talent—smelling merde from every quarter, living in fact

in the very century of merde, the great shithouse of scientific humanism where needs are satisfied, everyone becomes an anyone, a warm and creative person, and prospers like a dung beetle, and one hundred percent of people are humanists and ninety-eight percent believe in God, and men are dead, dead, dead; and the malaise has settled like a fall-out and what people really fear is not that the bomb will fall but that the bomb will not fall—on my thirtieth birthday, I know nothing and there is nothing to do but fall prey to desire.[171]

"Binx" Bolling, the protagonist of Percy's novel, and the narrative voice of "Reason to Believe" share an obsession with the total lack of sense in life, after having sought faith in a world permeated only by destructive faith.

Walker Percy (winner of the 1962 National Book Award) and Bruce Springsteen never met, but there was a singular exchange of letters that involved the pair of them. Percy wrote to Springsteen on February 23, 1989, saying that he had always been an admirer of his music and of his "spiritual journey." He died in May 1990 without receiving a reply from Springsteen. Only after reading *The Moviegoer*, years later, did Springsteen put pen to paper and write to the man's widow.

In 1998, *DoubleTake* published a long Springsteen interview by Will Percy, the Alabama novelist's favorite nephew. At one point Percy asked Springsteen, "I notice that you talk about 'writing' and not 'songwriting.' Do you sit down and write lyrics and then look for music?" Springsteen replied:

When I'd write rock music, music with the whole band, it would sometimes start out purely musically, and then I'd find my way to some lyrics. I haven't written like that in a while. In much of my recent writing, the lyrics have preceded the music, though the music is always in the back of my mind. In most of the recent songs, I tell violent stories very quietly. You're hearing characters' thoughts—what they're thinking after all the events that have shaped their situation have transpired. So I try to get that internal sound, like that feeling at night when you're in bed and staring at the ceiling, reflective in some fashion. I wanted the songs to have the kind of intimacy that took you inside yourself and then back out into the world. I'll use music as a way of defining and coloring the characters, conveying the characters' rhythm of speech and pace. The music acts as a very still surface, and the lyrics create a violent emotional life over it, or under it, and I let those elements bang up against each other.

Music can seem incidental, but it ends up being very important. It allows you to suggest the passage of time in just a couple of quiet beats. Years can go by in a few bars, whereas a writer will have to come up with a clever way of saying, "And then years went by . . ." Thank God I don't have to do any of that!

> Songwriting allows you to cheat tremendously. You can present an entire life in a few minutes. And then hopefully, at the end, you reveal something about yourself and your audience and the person in the song. It has a little in common with short-story writing in that it's character-driven.[172]

This same songwriting style is also found in *Born in the U.S.A.* (1984), in which the majority of the songs are coeval to those on *Nebraska*. What's more is that even the music is the same: a rock 'n' roll that smells like old Sun records, in the heroic fifties. But those arrangements . . . Where there was once a simple acoustic guitar, now there are two electric ones; the metronome has been replaced by a snarling drum and bass section; Clarence Clemons's powerful saxophone takes the place of the ghostly harmonica; and synthesizers work incessantly under this shell, making *Born in the U.S.A.* an album perfectly in sync with its times— other than one of the most incredible bestsellers of all-time rock history. Springsteen "may shove his broody characters out the door and send them cruising down the turnpike, but he gives them music they can pound on the dashboard to."[173]

Born in the U.S.A., in a similar yet more effective way compared to the acoustic album released two years previously, manages to perfectly capture the spirit of Reagan's America, with a more muscular sound that appeals immediately to the masses, louder and more intense, yet somehow a reflection of the other side of *Nebraska*.

In fact the main characters in "Working on the Highway," of "My Hometown," and of "This Hard Land" (which does not make it onto the album and instead ends up on the *Greatest Hits* eleven years later), belong to the same category as Charles Starkweather, Joe Roberts, and Johnny 99. The worker in "Working on the Highway," as he holds "a red flag" watching the traffic passing him by "out on 95," keeps in his head "a picture of a pretty little miss" and says: "Someday, mister, I'm gonna lead a better life than this." But he ends up in jail, probably because the girl is under age:

> I wake up every morning to the work bell clang,
> Me and the warden go swinging on the Charlotte County road gang.

The New Jersey providing a background for the distressing "State Trooper" is the same one unmercifully portrayed in "My Hometown" with a touch of Zola:

> Now Main Street's whitewashed windows and vacant stores,
> Seems like there ain't nobody wants to come down here no more,
> They're closing down the textile mill across the railroad tracks,
> Foreman says, "These jobs are going, boys,
> And they ain't coming back to your hometown."

And the narrator of "This Hard Land" talks this way to his mysterious interlocutor:

> Hey there, mister, can you tell me
> What happened to the seeds I've sown?
> Can you give me a reason, sir,
> As to why they've never grown?

As Benjamin Franklin said, "Without continual growth and progress, such words as improvement, achievement, and success have no meaning."[174] Listen to what the protagonist of "Seeds"—another outtake of *Born in the U.S.A.*—says from the streets of Texas:

> Well, there's men hunkered down by the railroad tracks,
> The Elkhorn Special blowin' my hair back,
> Tents pitched on the highway in the dirty moonlight,
> And I don't know where I'm gonna sleep tonight.
>
> Parked in the lumberyard freezin' our asses off
> My kids in the back seat got a graveyard cough . . .

Eleven years later, an echo of these verses can be heard in the title track of *The Ghost of Tom Joad*: there are still "families sleeping in their cars" lining up for "hot soup on a campfire under the bridge." They look like old photographs faded sepia from an America of the thirties, even though we are smack in the middle of the nineties, the years of George Bush's New World Order, sarcastically quoted in the lyrics.

On the cover of *Born in the U.S.A.*, as Bobbie Anne Mason notes in her novel *In Country*, "Bruce Springsteen is facing the flag, as though studying it, trying to figure out its meaning."[175] As the eighties wore on, Springsteen "was simply focusing on a question that, in one form or another, his music had been asking all along: What does it mean to be born an American?"[176] The answer is a little less obvious than it may seem. "Does it mean, indeed, that we *are* living in badlands?"[177] Yes, but even when his songs are black-and-white portraits of the crude American reality, they still make use of stars-and-stripes imagery: flags, faith, home, and family. Some have even suggested that "he's got a Democratic ideology, a Republican vocabulary, and a Populist delivery system."[178]

"Born in the U.S.A." is one of the most misunderstood songs of all time—it's true. Its protagonist cries, "Nowhere to run, nowhere to go." But that chorus with clenched fist raised—"I was born in the U.S.A."—can objectively be misleading.

Yes, Springsteen is the man who—as he says himself—spent his life "judging the distance between American reality and the American dream,"[179] yet he is also the one who in "Long Walk Home" (2007) sings:

> My father said, "Son, we're lucky in this town:
> It's a beautiful place to be born,
> It just wraps its arms around you,
> Nobody crowds you, nobody goes it alone.
>
> That you know flag flying over the courthouse
> Means certain things are set in stone
> Who we are, what we'll do and what we won't.

Instead, from the *Ghost of Tom Joad*, any patriotic reference is banned. Springsteen's tone is unmistakable, as it was in *Nebraska*. The ghost of Springsteen's 1982 masterpiece haunts this new album on songs like "Highway 29" and "Straight Time." The first one "presents a road-bound couple that harkens back to the couple of 'Nebraska.'"[180] The protagonist of "Straight Time" is an ex-con who works at a rendering plant and tries to stay clean. At night, though, he has intrusive thoughts about "tripping across that thin line." Looking back on his eight years in jail, he remembers feeling beaten but then, more tragically, getting used to a life of imprisonment. In the basement there are are a "huntin' gun and a hacksaw." For the man who repeatedly says to himself, "I'm sick of doin' straight time" and to whom it "Seems you can't get any more than half free," the temptation of committing a new crime is too strong:

> Come home in the evening, can't get the smell from my hands.
> Lay my head down on the pillow and go driftin' off into foreign lands.

The first line is reminiscent of the scene in which Lady Macbeth, after having convinced her husband to kill Duncan in order to ensure the Scottish throne, uselessly attempts to wash the victim's blood off her hands:

> Out, damned spot! Out, I say!—One, two . . . What, will these hands ne'er
> be clean? . . . Here's the smell of the blood still. All the perfumes of Arabia
> will not sweeten this little hand. Oh, Oh, Oh![181]

T.S. Eliot uses it as a perfect example of an objective correlative for guilt in his essay "Hamlet and His Problems" (1919).

> Plaintive, bitter epiphanies like these are far removed from the sort of anthemic
> cries that once filled Springsteen's music, but then these are not times for

anthems ... *The Ghost of Tom Joad* is Springsteen's response to this state of affairs ... There are few escapes and almost no musical relief from the numbing circumstances of the characters' lives. You could almost say that the music gets caught in meandering motions or drifts into circles that never break.[182]

For *The Ghost of Tom Joad* Springsteen worked a great deal on the preliminaries, drawing on many sources. "Balboa Park" was inspired by an article penned by Sebastian Rotella and published in the *Los Angeles Times*,[183] and tells the story of a boy who "grew up near the Zona Norte" of Tijuana in Mexico and decides to sell himself

> Where the men in their Mercedes
> Come nightly to employ
> In the cool San Diego evening
> The services of the border boys.

"Sinaloa Cowboys" is also inspired by an article published in the *Los Angeles Times*[184] that explored the effects of the production and trafficking of methamphetamines by a group of illegal immigrants who had come to Fresno, California, from the Mexican town of Sinaloa. For "Youngstown" and "The New Timer" Springsteen acknowledged his debt to *Journey to Nowhere*, a reportage about the conditions for jobless Americans during the economic crisis of the early Reagan administration,[185] while "Galveston Bay" and "Brothers Under the Bridges" (an outtake of the album) were based on the autobiography of Alabama civil rights activist Morris Dees, *A Season for Justice*.[186]

Then of course, *The Grapes of Wrath*, both in the original Steinbeck version as well as John Ford's cinematographic one: "The Ghost of Tom Joad" and "Across the Border" are truly apocryphal representations of this dramatic tale of the Great Depression, as well as, in part, "This Hard Land," a song written in 1983, where certain verses already seem directly inspired by Steinbeck's novel, when the protagonist and his sister leave Germantown to seek fame and fortune and start traveling

> Lookin' for a place to stand
> Where the sun burst through the clouds and fall like a circle,
> A circle of fire down on this hard land.

> Now even the rain it don't come 'round,
> Don't come 'round here no more,
> And the only sound at night's the wind
> Slammin' the back porch door.

Yeah, it stirs you up like it wants to blow you down
Twistin' and churnin' up the sand,
Leavin' all them scarecrows lyin' facedown
In the dirt of this hard land.

Likewise, Steinbeck's novel says:

The dawn came, but no day. In the grey sky a red sun appeared, a dim red circle
that gave a little light, like dusk; and as that day advanced, the dusk slipped back
towards darkness, and the wind cried and whimpered over the fallen corn.[187]

Take all of *Nebraska*, half of *Born in the U.S.A.*, and the entire *The Ghost of Tom
Joad* and you get something that sounds like a modern-day *Spoon River Anthology*.
The horizon no longer stops its embrace in New York and New Jersey: now
Nebraska, Ohio, Michigan, Florida, and New Mexico provide scenarios for stories
of assassins, the unemployed, policemen, gangsters, nut cases, used car salesmen,
veterans, factory workers, fishermen, woodworkers, border patrols, shoe salesmen,
preachers, refugees, sick people . . . The first-person singular is plentiful and songs
start with formulas such as "My name is Joe Roberts" ("Highway Patrolman") or "Got
out of prison back in '86" ("Straight Time"). "Sir" or "friend" is often interjected, as if
the characters were speaking directly to the listener (or to Springsteen himself, who
may be the author but he's also the bystander to his own productions). *Laconic* may
well be the best adjective to describe the style of these songs. Springsteen explained:

When you get the music and lyrics right in these songs, your voice disappears
into the voices of those you've chosen to write about. Basically, I find the
characters and listen to them. That always leads to a series of questions
about their behavior: What should they do? What would they never do?[188]

An example of precision and eye for details may well be "The Line," where the
protagonist, who works "for the INS on the line / with California Border Patrol"
says:

Well I was good at doin' what I was told,
Kept my uniform pressed and clean.

In a seemingly small detail, a great deal of the personality of this character is
revealed, demonstrating Springsteen's skills as a short-story writer—which he certainly is. Short stories are always considered as perfection in literature. A perfection
that almost coincides with moral virtue. As Ezra Pound put it, "Fundamental
accuracy of statement is the one sole morality of writing."[189] Frank O'Connor said

that "A man can be a very great novelist as I believe Trollope was, and yet be a very inferior writer . . . I cannot think of a great storyteller who was also an inferior writer."[190] O'Connor also said that a short story is the artistic form that deals with individuals when society no longer absorbs them and they are forced to survive thanks to their inner light. In the same way, Springsteen's characters "live on islands close enough to shore to see the mainland, too far away to make the crossing light or easy."[191]

Unlike the debut songs, the characters in Springsteen's new work are perfectly aware—no one dreams of dreaming. At most, the "Youngstown" man who loses his job at the steelworks might say:

> When I die I don't want no part of heaven,
> I would not do heaven's work well.
> I pray the devil comes and takes me
> To stand in the fiery furnaces of hell.

Nothing and no one, not even God, can redeem the brutality of these lives. "The New Timer" tramp on a moving train sees

> A small house sittin' trackside
> With the glow of the Savior's beautiful light,
> A woman stood cookin' in the kitchen,
> Kid sat at the table with his old man.
> Now, I wonder, does my son miss me,
> Does he wonder where I am?

But it's just for a moment:

> Tonight I pick my campsite carefully
> Outside the Sacramento Yard,
> Gather some wood and light a fire
> In the early winter dark.
> Wind whistling cold, I pull my coat around me,
> Make some coffee and stare out into the black night.

> I lie awake, I lie awake, sir,
> With my machete by my side.
> My Jesus, your gracious love and mercy
> Tonight, I'm sorry, could not fill my heart
> Like one good rifle
> And the name of who I ought to kill.

This is probably where a more poetically mature and effective Springsteen is lurking. The influences of Steinbeck and Flannery O'Connor on the literary front, and of Ford and Malick on the—equally important—cinematographic side, left an evident impression on his writing. While the 1982 "Nebraska" is—especially in its initial verses—a true transposition of the opening sequence of Terrence Malick's *Badlands*, thirteen years later *The Grapes of Wrath* (book and film), are not just sources of inspiration, but a theme to be explored. *The Grapes of Wrath* ends with Tom Joad's mother encouraging her son to go ahead. In "The Ghost of Tom Joad" Springsteen imagines Tom's reply:

> Wherever there's a cop beatin' a guy,
> Wherever a hungry newborn baby cries,
> Where there's a fight 'gainst the blood and hatred in the air,
> Look for me, Mom, I'll be there.
> Wherever there's somebody fightin' for a place to stand
> Or decent job or a helpin' hand,
> Wherever somebody's strugglin' to be free,
> Look in their eyes, Mom, you'll see me.

As in other songs from the album, "The Ghost of Tom Joad" seems to describe the difficult times the United States experienced following the 1929 recession. In effect, Steinbeck's Tom Joad (as well as Ford's and Guthrie's) is prey to all the contradictions and difficulties of the 1930s. These sources undoubtedly underpin many verses of the song (there is a reference to the preacher, who is preacher Casey in *The Grapes of Wrath*; and Tom's words to his mother in the last strophe are echoed in those that the protagonist utters in the book's finale and in Woody Guthrie's song *Tom Joad*). But Springsteen's spark of genius was his camouflaging as a story of the past the American recession of the 1980s and 1990s, which mentions traffic police helicopters and hinges on the facts of the race riots that fueled the 1990 Los Angeles riots.

Woodie Guthrie's two-part "Tom Joad" song was part of his *Dust Bowl Ballads* album (1940), a record that influenced Springsteen strongly.[192] Oddly enough, for his ballad Guthrie used the melody of "John Hardy," an early 1900s traditional song telling the story of a miner, hanged on January 19, 1894, for killing a man during a craps game in which he lost fifty cents.[193] Folk singers often used traditional tunes, but Guthrie's appeared to be a deliberate decision, as if wishing to establish a connection between Hardy and Joad, both victims of the "system." Thus, in the shadows moving around Springsteen's "The Ghost of Tom Joad"—a 1990s song—are those of characters who had existed fifty to one hundred years before. It seems that Springsteen is saying that history doesn't change.

10. My City of Ruins

History changed America when, on the morning of September 11, 2011, two planes went smashing into Manhattan's Twin Towers while a third plane went crashing onto the Pentagon.

Whitman reacted to the assassination of Lincoln writing, "Oh Captain! My Captain!" With *The Rising* album (2002) Springsteen was proclaimed the "poet laureate" of September 11.[194] This time he did not, however, use an objective and impersonal pitch for his tale; the cold, merciless style of *Nebraska* was set aside for a more involved, heartfelt style, a sort of lay prayer in which Springsteen doesn't just want to observe and record but also tries to provide answers or at least the comfort of hope.

It was no coincidence that for *The Rising* Springsteen frequently used the blues in composing the verses and gospel for the choruses. He said himself that in most of the songs in the album, "the first verse is the blues," then,

> when the chorus hits, that's the gospel. . . . My best songs have done both of those things, blues and gospel. That's what my band, and my writing with the band, has always been about. On an album like Nebraska, you can hear the blues thing, but the band is more like Sunday church.[195] The verse is always the blues, but once you get to the chorus, it's the gospel. The verses are how the songs earn their choruses. You know, you have to earn your transcendence, you have to earn your redemption by passing through the fires of the natural world.[196]

Making his way through these patterns, Springsteen used the melancholy of blues in the verses—describing the lives of the victims of the terrorist attack—then transcended with gospel choruses and concluded by invoking faith, hope for new life, the determination to never give in. There are countless examples of the technique, for instance "Into the Fire," whose first verse describes the death of a fireman who was attempting to save someone in the World Trade Center:

> The sky was falling and streaked with blood.
> I heard you calling me,
> Then you disappeared into the dust,
> Up the stairs, into the fire.

Then, after the bluesy verse, there comes the gospel:

> May your strength give us strength,
> May your faith give us faith,
> May your hope give us hope,
> May your love give us love.

In "The Rising," a similar device is used in the first verse, as the narrator evokes his own death: "I make my way through this darkness, / I can't feel nothing but this chain that binds me"; then he cries: "Come on up for the rising, / Come on up, lay your hands in mine."

The journey, once again, is not a "free ride." How could it be? America was under attack for the first time since Pearl Harbor and *strangers* (as both Albert Camus and Billy Joel were aware) make people nervous . . . Springsteen sings "Let's Be Friends," but also "I want an eye for an eye" ("Empty Sky"), and shows the "Nothing Man" with a gun by the bed. "Lonesome Day" burst out of the gate as a statement of intent, with the singer's determination to find his way through:

> Hell's brewin' dark sun's on the rise,
> This storm'll blow through by and by.
> House is on fire, viper's in the grass,
> A little revenge and this too shall pass.

It's a theme that "reverberates throughout the record: facing unimagined crisis and what would seem to be unbearable loss, there's no way out but through."[197] After *The Rising* was released, Alan Light wrote in the *New Yorker*:

> Instead of writing the album that would undoubtedly have put him back in the spotlight—a *Born in the U.S.A.* for the new era—Springsteen came up with something riskier and more surprising, something more than the country's archetypal living rock star fulfilling his obligation as America's rock-and-roll conscience . . .[198]

The Rising has little in common with Springsteen's previous work.

> The lyrics are even more atypical than the sound. All the signature Springsteen narrative and detail has been stripped out: there is not a single Joe Roberts or Bill Horton wrestling with his conflicts, no Crazy Janey or Magic Rat, no working on the highway or racing in the street.[199]

Where the earlier Springsteen was very specific and attentive to detail, now his lyrics are at once vague, generic, and at times repetitive. He no longer focuses on individual stories that can be taken as representation of the human condition, but seems to be in search of something more universal, though less precise.

The accuracy of the narrative element is achieved only in a few lines; often, though, it seems quite the opposite, and with not altogether convincing results ("walked into the darkness of your smoky grave," from "Into the Fire," is perhaps the least pleasing line, together with "Blood on the streets, / Yeah, blood flowin' down," from "Empty Sky," and the rather horrific yet involuntarily comical image found in the first verse of "Worlds Apart": "I taste the seed upon your lips, lay my tongue upon your scars"). So much so that when the album was released, the *Village Voice's* Keith Harris complained of "the eternal vagueness of the lyrics," writing, "You can wander through *The Rising* for countless stanzas without tripping over a single concrete object."[200] In the same perspective, in a mixed review for the *Guardian*, Alexis Petridis said that the best songs of the album were highlighted by good melodies rather than lyrics, which he judged as generally "simplistic and unambiguous."[201] Hence, as Emily Dickinson was to have suggested, "Tell all the truth, but tell it slant."[202] Too often, in *The Rising* it is all too . . . straight.

For *The Rising*, some have spoken of "romantic pragmatism,"[203] a philosophy that combines the ideas of Ralph Waldo Emerson, C. S. Pierce, and John Dewey, believing that truth will be obtained by sharing an experience, intended as the link between private and public, Humanity and Nature. No epistemological difference exists between what must be and what is: reality—intended as "social experience"—is the only way to reach truth and transcend it to enrich the individual. Springsteen's album shows the possibilities of the experiential fact. The author's optimism resides in the hope that the suffering of his characters (firemen, widows, suicide terrorists) can be understood to be "real."

A salient point of the 9/11 debate is the idea that this dramatic event was a painful jab of reality in the fabled world that had been America up to that time. "*Welcome to the Desert of the Real!* proclaims the title of Slavoj Zizek's book of essays on 9/11, a phrase from the scene in the popular motion picture *Matrix* in which the hero awakens into true reality to see a desolate landscape of post-war ruins."[204] The theme of reality is central to *The Rising*. From "Into the Fire" to "My City of Ruins," Springsteen plunges his listeners into events so they can see the blood and the dust-cloaked ruins. We are in the Towers and, more significantly, in the heads of those who lost their relatives and friends in the attacks.

Don DeLillo writes that 9/11

> has no purchase on the mercies of analogy or simile. We have to take the
> shock and horror as it is. But living language is not diminished. The writer

wants to understand what this day has done to us . . . The writer begins in the towers, trying to imagine the moment, desperately. Before politics, before history and religion, there is the primal terror. People falling from the towers hand in hand. This is part of the counter-narrative, hands and spirits joining, human beauty in the crush of meshed steel . . .[205]

What Springsteen did in *The Rising* in terms of the search for truth must have met with the approval of the author of *Underworld*. But there was more—for example, when Springsteen in "Worlds Apart" sings,

> Sometimes the truth just ain't enough
> Or is it too much in times like this. . . .
> May the living let us in before the dead tear us apart.

For Springsteen the only way to sublimate an experience—even the most dramatic—is to resort to love. Truth is found in love.

11. We Are Alive

Three years after *The Rising*, Springsteen released *Devils & Dust* (2005), a semi-acoustic, somber album of narrative songs and character sketches that seemed to hark back to the thematic and sound of *The Ghost of Tom Joad*. In fact, many of the songs were written during the solo tour that followed the release of *The Ghost of Tom Joad*.[206] "I wrote a lot of music after those shows, when I'd go back to my hotel room," he says. "I still had my voice, because I hadn't sung over a rock band all night. I'd go and make up my stories."[207]

Most of these tunes were nearly finished by 1997, but Springsteen put them aside in favor of a 1999 reunion tour with the E Street Band, which led to 2002's *The Rising*. The inspiration for reviving the solo material was a new song, "Devils and Dust," that he wrote in 2003 at the start of the Iraq War:

> I've got my finger on the trigger
> But I don't know who to trust . . .

"It is basically a song about a soldier's point of view in Iraq," Springsteen says. "But it kind of opens up to a lot of other interpretations."[208]

Title track apart, as with *The Ghost of Tom Joad*, many of the songs of the album are set in the Southwest, with Spanish phrases studding the lyrics: stories of women and men, alone in their fights against their own demons. Yet there is unusual compassion, openly expressed with the frequent inclusion of modules typical of American religious music over a mainly blues, folk, and country under-pinning. The album is dominated by a sound that conjures up desert scenarios. A lot of it echoes border music typical of the area along the Mexican boundary that stretches from California as far as Texas, touching on Arizona and New Mexico. "It's a mixture that Joe Ely and Tom Russell have always used and that Dave Alvin discovered after he left the Blasters."[209]

In "Long Time Comin'"—a rock ballad with a dirty, riveting sound that bears a resemblance to some of the *Lucky Town* arrangements—the main character's cruel fate is salvaged as he waits to become a father; over a crisp R&B we hear his wish for his children:

> Well, if I had one wish in this godforsaken world, kids,
> It'd be that your mistakes would be your own,
> Yeah, your sins would be your own.

Then, with a sudden drift into gospel, he turns to his woman: "It's been a long time comin' but now it's here."

In "Jesus Was an Only Son," on the other hand, a son on the point of death speaks to his mother and kisses her hands, saying, "Still your tears." This is standard spiritual, complete with a Hammond and choir, and it bears no importance that the son is Jesus "in the hills of Nazareth / As he lay reading the Psalms of David at his mother's feet." Springsteen has always exploited biblical references, even though he is not a believer and his interest lies in the humanity of Christ. "In 'Jesus Was an Only Son' I approached the episodes of Calvary and the crucifixion from the secular side," he says. "I talked about Jesus as if he was an everyday son, and I tried to imagine the story from Mary's perspective, because for her, she was just losing her boy."[210] Introducing the song during a concert, he went so far as to say:

> The title, "Jesus Was an Only Son"—that's my main metaphor. Of course, Jesus had earthly brothers and sisters, but not on this particular day. This day, he was singular. I always figured that if you're Jesus, you gotta be think-ing, "Gee, the weather is pretty nice in Galilee this time of year, and there was that little bar . . . I could manage the place, Mary Magdalene could tend bar and we could have some kids . . . do the preaching on the weekend . . ."[211]

Other "only sons" are Rainey Williams in "Black Cowboys"—who wanders the fields "green, corn and cotton and an endless nothin' in between"—and the boxer portrayed in "The Hitter":

> Tonight in the shipyard a man draws a circle in the dirt,
> I move to the center and I take off my shirt,
> I study him for the cuts, the scars, the pain, man, no time can erase,
> I move hard to the left and I strike to the face.

The song is to be imagined as a long monologue by the boxer, who tells his mother about his life through a locked door.[212] In fact, the mother figure holds a central role in the poetry of *Devils & Dust*. Along with "Jesus Was an Only Son" and "The Hitter," a mother is present in "Long Time Comin'" (she is about to give birth) and in other two narrative songs. In "Black Cowboys" the boy loses his mother to the drugs and crime in his New York neighborhood. In "Silver Palomino"—a song dedicated to the memory of Fiona Chappel, a friend and neighbor to Bruce and Patti Springsteen and to his two children Tyler and Oliver—the "palomino" from the title is a golden horse with white tail and mane, which Springsteen describes as "she came out of the Guadalupe's on a night so cold: / Her coat was frosted diamonds in the sallow moon's glow." Guadalupe is a river that flows in Texas. Its name is taken from the Virgin of Guadalupe, who appeared to a child in Santiago Tlatelolco, Mexico, on December 9, 1531. A sanctuary was then built there dedicated, as the Madonna wished, to the Virgin of Guadalupe; a name meaning "river of light" or "river of love." The horse with the shining mane that comes out of the Guadalupe, the "river of love," in the lyrics represents the symbol of motherhood, in a complex and intriguing allegory of death.

Devils & Dust is also a skillful collision of rural genres: typical Mississippi blues four-beat bars—Sonny Terry style—and folk and country arrangements: slide guitar, banjo, violins . . . up to a "Peggy Sue" sort of rockabilly convulsion. This happens, for instance, in "All I'm Thinkin' About," a song that might easily have been penned by Buddy Holly, in which Bruce exhibits an unexpected falsetto (reminiscent of the vocal style of Skip James, Canned Heat, and Mungo Jerry). "Maria's Bed," instead, in the first part resembles one of the minor pieces in the Rolling Stones' *Beggar's Banquet*, but then bursts into a wilder rock 'n' roll, a love song that despite all the biblical references spread on the album, comes down firmly—and happily—on the secular side:

> I been up on sugar mountain, 'cross the sweet blue sea,
> I walked the valley of love and tears and mystery,
> I got run out 'a luck and gave myself up for dead,
> Then I drank the cool clear waters from Maria's bed.[213]

But are these men, who attempt to to rise up out of the dust through more or less earthly dreams of redemption, really as true and authentic as the disenchanted from *Darkness on the Edge of Town*, continuing, despite themselves, in their search for a Promised Land? Springsteen is no longer the James Dean of American music—and cannot ever be again—giving way to a more professor-like figure of rock 'n' roll who still however manages to get his uppercuts in, as for instance with "All the Way Home," where he surprises us with some tight rock, or "Leah," a jewel of a piece with a trumpet rising from a blanket full of keyboards that reminds us of several Waterboys numbers.

The Bruce Springsteen of 2005 is "as wiry and proud as Johnny Cash, Steve Earle and John Steinbeck all in one,"[214] even though his music, in these first samples of the twenty-first century, "along with other stars of rock's dominant period, has lost the attention of young Americans," Dave Marsh says. The reason is to be found in the fact that probably, hip-hop dominating today's popular music, Springsteen's records

> emphasize melody and a steady beat, not fractured harmonies and poly-rhythms. Hip-hop tore the cover off the central limitation of Western music, including rock 'n' roll: its refusal or inability to incorporate polyrhythms and its exaltation of melody and harmony over the power of beat. Bruce never had much of a black audience, although his band has always been integrated. More important, he draws on a musical history developed primarily among African Americans, he sings more often than not in a voice derived from blues, R&B, soul and gospel, and never backs away from racially charged topics. He lacks that black audience because, as a friend of mine put it, "The bottom of his music is never gonna be as interesting as the top of it," meaning his drum and bass lines stick to one rhythmic pattern per song (or section of a song).[215]

The truth is simply that in no other album released in the past decade is there such a high level of perfectionism, research, and care in songwriting details as can be appreciated in *Devils & Dust*. Where can other characters so well defined as the prostitute in "Reno" or the retiring boxer in "The Hitter" be found? Springsteen seems to be more and more tenacious in his striving to keep alive a culture that at this point is dead and buried. And one day we aficionados might give in to the temptation of putting the following words, similar to those said by the forgotten diva in *Sunset Boulevard*, right into his mouth: "I am great. It's rock that got small."

"Small" would be a good way to describe the attention span of some music critics, especially in the U.S.A., who spend so much time listening to Justin Timberlake that their ears have become as hairy as those of the infamous American werewolf in Paris. For instance, Ben Greenman, who trashed Springsteen's 2007 *Magic* album (another chapter in the Bruce Springsteen & the E Street Band saga) in the *New Yorker*, described the work as

> inert and calculated, full of stormy guitar, gelatinous keyboards, and melo-
> dramatic strings. The production seems to be hiding something—perhaps
> it's the album's generic heart. Springsteen's best albums have always had a
> thesis: youth is invincibility, the American dream is hollow, divorce can crush
> you. Magic is simply a collection of songs.[216]

Surely a surprising opinion, if one appreciates that *Magic* is in fact one of the most coherent projects in all of Springsteen's career, or more aptly, if one has patience enough to really listen to what he is singing about. The album "feels like the latest chapter in the narrative of characters whose stories Springsteen started in the 1970s and 1980s."[217]

In "Radio Nowhere"—the angry and energetic opening track—Springsteen growls "Is there anybody alive out there?" over and over.

> Springsteen isn't just pissed about the state of rock & roll radio[218]—that's like
> kicking a corpse— although he is blunt about what's missing. "A thousand
> guitars . . . pounding drums," he demands against the racing squall of his
> band. But "Radio Nowhere" is actually about how we speak and listen to
> each other through the murk . . . and how a firm beat, some Telecaster sting
> and the robust peal of Clarence Clemons' saxophone can still tell you more
> about the human condition than a thousand op-ed words.[219]

Nebraska, The Ghost of Tom Joad, and *Devils & Dust* are photographs of present-day America. The songs contained on *Magic* instead are situated in a near future—a future as black as tar, reminiscent of the nightmare anticipated by Cormac McCarthy in his novel *The Road*. Despite the album having a definite rock slant—with cheeky pop distortions, like "Livin' in the Future" and "Girls in Their Summer Clothes"—the fifteenth chapter of Springsteen's rock 'n' roll novel is ominous and outlines vaguely apocalyptic scenarios. The title-track lyrics are quite unusual:

> I got a coin in my palm,
> I can make it disappear.
> I got a card up my sleeve,
> Name it and I'll pull it out your ear. . . .
>
> Chain me in a box in the river
> And I'll rise singin' this song. . . .

I'll cut you in half
While you're smiling ear to ear.

The critic in his werewolf costume may have mistaken this for a song about prestidigitation; it's got top hats and Houdini-style shackles and padlocks, hasn't it? But if he'd read the refrain ("This is what we'll be") or lingered over some of the verses like, "And the freedom that you sought's / Drifting like a ghost amongst the trees," he'd have understood that America is the great illusionist in this case: a country that can't be trusted anymore.[220] "Magic" ends on the following notes:

On the road the sun is sinkin' low,
There's bodies hangin' in the trees.
This is what will be, this is what will be.

Springsteen's only "magic" is in his predictions. The entire album is a sort of postmodern *Arbor Mirabilis*. In "Livin' in the Future" he sings of "a letter come blowin' in on an ill wind":

Yeah, well I knew it'd come,
Still I was struck deaf and dumb. . . .

I'm rollin' through town,
A lost cowboy at sundown.

The verses are then interrupted—as disquieting as the prophecies of Nostradamus—by a refrain telling us that "None of this has happened yet."

After we have touched the subject in "Devils & Dust," the American disaster in Iraq is the scenario of three new songs. "Gypsy Biker" is the story of a family that vainly awaits the return of a boy from the war. "Devil's Arcade" is the real-time report of a soldier dying in the Persian Gulf whose last thoughts are of "a thin chain of next moments"—"a morning to order, a breakfast to make, / A bed draped in sunshine, a body that waits / For the touch of your fingers, / The end of a day"—sustained by a fellow soldier's voice saying:

Don't worry, I'm here,
Just whisper the word "tomorrow" in my ear.
A house on a quiet street, a home for the brave,[221]
The glorious kingdom of the sun on your face
Rising from a long night as dark as the grave . . .

"Last to Die" borrows the title and chorus from John Kerry's 1971 Testimony to Congress on Vietnam: "How do you ask a man to be the last man to die for a mistake?" America must face up to its sins:

> Kids asleep in the backseat,
> We're just counting the miles, you and me.
> We don't measure the blood we've drawn anymore,
> We just stack the bodies outside the door.

In *Magic*, as he'd done on *The Rising*, Springsteen abandons his trademark—the theme developed in the form of a short story. However, where in *The Rising* the lyrics were purposely generic in nature, the ones on the new album are bursting with detail, with sudden accelerations rushing ahead to capture images full of enormous plasticity. In "I'll Work for Your Love" he sings:

> Pour me a drink, Theresa, in one of those glasses you dust off
> And I'll watch the bones in your back like the stations of the cross,

while in "Girls in Their Summer Clothes" (a track that might have come straight out of *Pet Sounds*) he patchworks miniatures that together evoke the atmosphere of special September afternoons: lovers strolling hand in hand, bicycle spokes turning, footballs soaring in the air and girls "In their summer clothes / In the cool of the evening light." It seems like an idyll, but it's just a sad patch in tomorrow's nightmare:

> I was tryin' to find my way home
> But all I heard was a drone
> Bouncing off a satellite,
> Crushin' the last lone American night
> This is radio nowhere,
> Is there anybody alive out there?

The nightmare appeared to have become reality just a few months after *Magic* was released. Many economists considered the global economic downturn starting in 2007 and 2008 to have been the worst financial crisis since the Great Depression of the 1930s. When the *Wrecking Ball* album was released in 2012, it wasn't a surprise for anybody that its theme was America's Great Recession.

Although Springsteen was known to have declared, "I'm a mild-mannered rock musician of a certain age . . . my powers are limited,"[222] with *Wrecking Ball* he once again declared himself the rock 'n' roll bard of his nation, examining a society and its values in a record described as "that rare release that manages to fulfill, defy, and exceed expectations all at once."[223] Pulitzer Prize winner Leonard Pitts wrote that

> the new Bruce Springsteen album captures more raw emotional truth about
> the state of America than any politician ever could. It is Springsteen's triumph

to honor anger and lamentation, but also to look beyond them. And to remind us that, though hard times come and hard times go, hope and defiance still abide and sustain.[224]

The genesis of the record was when Springsteen wrote "We Take Care of Our Own," at the end of 2009. "The idea behind it," he says, "was that's what's *supposed* to happen, but was not happening . . ."[225] The title of the ultra-anthemic song is one easily misread in its interpretation (or rather misinterpretation). What does it mean exactly? That Americans worry about one another? On the contrary, it might come off as "we are minding our own business." However, right after that, Springsteen sings, "The road of good intentions has gone dry as a bone." "We Take Care of Our Own," as Christopher Phillips writes,

> marches in with one of Springsteen's most martial rhythms since "Badlands." And you better believe it has some of the same "trouble in the heartland" concerns, too. But then there's that chorus: rousing, uplifting, and positioning "We Take Care of Our Own" to be not only Springsteen's most misinterpreted song since the time of "Born in the U.S.A.," but misinterpreted in precisely the same way. With the imagery of flying flags, it's practically begging for it. And there are takers. Randall Roberts of the *Los Angeles Times* describes the song as an "affirmation of national glory." . . . Of course, perhaps even more than with "Born in the U.S.A.," even half-listening to the verses brings the awareness that the chorus is not as rah-rah as it sounds. This is a song of searching and not finding—searching for mercy, for love, for work, for spirit, for the American promise, and, recalling "Long Walk Home" from 2007's *Magic*, "the map that leads me home" . . . Aside from the ironic interpretation, in the society of a sub-divided America suffering from paralyzing partisanship, as well as racism, homophobia, and xenophobia . . . who exactly constitutes "our own" has become a far narrower subset that everyone who lives under that flying flag.[226]

In reality, Springsteen as an author is anything but progressive; rather, he is a radical pessimist dominated by a fixed idea: that people's destiny is foretold and cannot be escaped ("You inherit the sin, you inherit the flames," as he sings in "Adam Raised a Cain"). Hardly Woody Guthrie! His vision of history resembles something by Maistre . . . the only thing Springsteen's hero can do is live in spite of everything. "He who lives, resists," as Georges Sorel said. In the final scene in John Ford's *The Grapes of Wrath*, which Springsteen will translate into "The Ghost of Tom Joad," the outlaw's mother says, "We're people that live. Can't nobody wipe us out. Can't nobody lick us. We'll go on forever, Pa. We're the people." Yeah, they'll go on forever, but where? Where fate, and not people or free will, leads you, at least when you even just take a glance at Springsteen's songs. There is no chance of redemption on this earth, as the parable of the two lovers in "Thunder Road" demonstrates. They dreamed of escaping from this "town full of losers." In "The River" we find them already separated and unemployed and wondering, "Is a dream a lie if it can't come true, or something worse?"

All that remains is hope in *another world*. "We're Canaan bound," Springsteen sings in his 2012 "Rocky Ground." This is "a land of hope and dreams," where the three voices have already reached us from the tombstones in the country graveyard in "We Are Alive":

> And though our bodies lie alone here in the dark,
> Our spirits rise to carry the fire and light the spark,
> To stand shoulder to shoulder and heart to heart.

As he sings in "Land of Hope and Dreams," this faith will be rewarded. Dreams will no longer be frustrated and the bells of freedom shall ring. But maybe it's only rock 'n' roll . . .

Everybody knows that Springsteen is a Democrat[227] and that he has done a long series of endorsements for someone who said, "The reason I am running for president is because I can't be Bruce Springsteen."[228] But when *Wrecking Ball* came out in February 2012, Springsteen was surprisingly critical in his statements about the Obama administration;[229] even if, despite initial reluctance, Bruce came out to help the president remain in the White House, participating in seven rallies in the swing states (three in one day on the eve of Election Day). With his acoustic guitar hanging from its strap, he sang "The Promised Land" and other parts of his more political repertoire. Then Bruce and his buddy Barack slapped each other on the back, putting the future of the country in Obama's hands once again. Bruce even went in for some cool scenes, like when he walked on stage in Parma, Ohio, introduced by Bill Clinton. "I had twenty-some jobs before I got elected president, but this is the first time in my life I get to be the warm-up act for Bruce Springsteen," Clinton joked before defining the songwriter as "a guy who reflects our real American values." It was like listening to Reagan . . . However, if the compliment comes from the Democrats, Our Guy is more lenient. "For some time now, he is convinced that he really is what they write about him: a symbol. When major national events come up, such as the eve of a major election . . . he loudly makes his opinion known. Who to vote for and why: a dictate for the legions of his followers."[230]

Pulitzer winner David Remnick—the editor of the *New Yorker*—is certainly one of his followers. His extensive, wide-ranging article on Springsteen, "We Are Alive," was published in the magazine in July 2012 and was harshly criticized by Leon Wieseltier, a literary editor at the liberal magazine *New Republic*. Wieseltier defined this article as "another one of his contributions to the literature of fandom. Once again, there is a derecho of detail and the conventional view of his protagonist, the official legend, is left undisturbed. It could have been written by the record company itself."[231] Wieseltier was mainly piqued by Remnick's judgment of *Wrecking Ball*, which he defined "a musical accusation against the current recession . . . with the intent to enrich the tradition of musical progressivism." Finally, Wieseltier can do nothing more than turn on Springsteen with the stalest accusation possible: he is a rich rock star who feeds on the most hypocritical of populisms. According to Wieseltier,

> Rock 'n' roll has played also another role in American life, which is to prove that Herbert Marcuse was right. There will be no revolution in America. This society will contain its contradictions without resolving them; it will absorb the opposition and reward it; it will transform dissent into culture and commerce. Marcuse's mistake was in believing this is bad news. It is good news, because we will be spared the agony of political purifications. But it's also comic, as protest songs become entertainment for the rich and Bruce Springsteen is the idol of the elite. *The New Yorker* clinches it: he's the least dangerous man in America. "With all the unrest in the world," as Tony Curtis once said to Marilyn Monroe, "I don't think anyone should have a yacht that sleeps more than twelve."[232]

Springsteen replied,

> Well, there's an idea that [keeping in touch with the public concern] would be hard to do, but I don't think that it is; I think that you have to remain interested and awake. You have to remain alert. You have to be constantly listening—and interested in listening—to what's going on every day. As a writer, the way that I write, it's like you're hungry for food. That's the writing impulse. The writing impulse is the same as one for hunger or for sex—it's like that. It's not something that's related to your commercial fortunes. I mean, I'd do it for free. I'm glad that they're paying me, but it was something I did for free before they were paying me. And so I'm constantly looking— the writer looks for something to push up against. Tom Stoppard, the playwright, once said he was envious of Vaclav Havel because he had so much to

push up against, and he wrote so beautifully about it. I'd prefer to stay out of prison if I can, but I knew what he was talking about. You need something pushing, pushing back at you, and you tend to do your best work when there's something that you can really, really push up against. And there has been in the States over the past—certainly for me, over the past thirty years, but that's come to a head over the past four years now.[233]

Who knows how Leon Wieseltier must have taken the comment Springsteen made on January 22, 2017, in Perth, Australia, during a concert held forty-eight hours after Donald Trump took over as President of the United States?

The E Street Band is glad to be here in Western Australia. But we're a long way from home, and our hearts and spirits are with the hundreds of thousands of women and men that marched yesterday in every city in America and in Melbourne who rallied against hate and division and in support of tolerance, inclusion, reproductive rights, civil rights, racial justice, LGBTQ rights, the environment, wage equality, gender equality, healthcare, and immigrant rights. We stand with you. We are the new American resistance.

12. Lucky Town

Recently Bruce Springsteen has been spending a lot of time at the White House. There is more than one person who, half jokingly, half seriously, would like to offer him the keys to the house at 1600 Pennsylvania Avenue. "Bruce Springsteen could have won the White House had he decided to run," the *Huffington Post* wrote during the Clinton vs. Trump campaign.[234] Undoubtedly, he knows how to work the crowd, shaking dozens of hands, crowd surfing, and taking requests. In Chicago he did not bat an eyelash when someone handed him a copy of the Constitution; furthermore he's a total expert on foreign policy: his European followers are even keener than those back home, which is by far more than what Donald Trump can say for himself; they are about the same age but he is in far better shape. So much so that some of his self-styled "middle aged fans" felt the urge to write him an open letter: "Your music has been the soundtrack to our lives," the appeal reads. "You are truly a hero and an icon, and we thank you for it. That said, what the hell do you think you're doing?" ask the exhausted letter writers, referring to our hero's habit of carrying his concerts on infinitely. Admittedly, he has always been an unstoppable/tireless performer; but since he hit sixty-five years of age he does not get off stage before having played for at least three hours and fifty minutes.

Think about us, your devoted middle-aged fans. Specifically, our sciatica. And our spindly old knees. And our weak little bladders. If we leave the pit to use the bathroom after hour three it's entirely possible we'll never make it back—someone will find us after the encores, draped over the sink like a hastily discarded nylon. . . . After all, maybe we ain't that young anymore. If we were, we'd be sitting and watching Justin Bieber gurgle along to a pre-recorded track for a nice, manageable ninety minutes.[235]

"How do I do it?" Springsteen asks himself in the foreword of his autobiography; and answers by offering us a Rock 'n' Roll Survival Kit:

DNA, natural ability, study of craft, development of and devotion to an aesthetic philosophy, naked desire for . . . fame? . . . love? . . . admiration? . . . attention? . . . women? . . . sex? . . . and oh, yeah . . . a buck. Then . . . if you want to take it all the way out to the end of the night, a furious fire in the hole that just . . . don't . . . quit . . . burning. These are some of the elements that will come in handy should you come face-to-face with eighty thousand (or eighty) screaming rock 'n' roll fans who are waiting for you to do your magic trick. Waiting for you to pull something out of your hat, out of thin air, out of this world, something that before the faithful were gathered here today was just a song-fueled rumor. I am here to provide proof of life to that ever elusive, never completely believable "us." That is my magic trick.[236]

Once again this idea of a lie, of deception emerges. "It's a funny old world, mama, where a little boy's wishes come true" he sang in "The Wish," a song dedicated to his mother. From time to time, it seems as though Springsteen doesn't feel he deserves his luck, and that he lives in dread that someone will come and tell him: "Listen, Bruce, it's all been a big mistake . . ." Maybe he feels that the depression he has been intermittently suffering from during the past fifteen years[237] is a fair punishment. However, he is well aware that the work he has done on himself— although harsh—bears excellent artistic results. When speaking about his commitment he comes across straight: "There's a part of the singer going back in American history that is, of course, the canary in the coalmine," he observed. "When it gets dark, you're supposed to be singing. It's dark right now."[238] But the boldly autobiographical and disarming Springsteen nevertheless manages to make it even with a political album such as *Wrecking Ball*, for example with a song like "This Depression" that goes,

Baby, I've been low, but never this low,
I've had my faith shaken but never hopeless . . .

I haven't always been strong, but never felt so weak:
All of my prayers, gone for nothing.
I've been without love, but never forsaken:
Now the morning sun, the morning sun is breaking.

It is this more intimate and true Springsteen who says that the artist's job is to make people care about their obsessions and who, starting in 1987, in some of his albums began to recount what really happened to that boy who left New Jersey in search of the Promised Land. This is how we come to know that his real life matched—and continues to match—far better with the black-and-white of *Darkness on the Edge of Town* and *Nebraska* than with the bright red, white, and blue of the American flag within which fans and mass media had him rolled up in in the eighties, at the height of Bossmania. When he got the very fame he had so actively sought, Springsteen's initial reaction was one of refusal. By now a multimillionaire, he no longer had a house, a steady relationship, a social life. He moved from one hotel room to another, purposely closing himself as far as possible into a state of conscious isolation. Until 1986 there was not a moment of his life not spent either on tour, writing songs, or in the studio recording them. Bruce Springsteen had simply become the richest tramp on the planet. And thus, ever so subtly, the outcast and rejected end of the young hero of "Thunder Road" could be interpreted as a metaphor for the failure in the human and emotional spheres that so visibly marked Springsteen's post–*Born to Run* decade: his problematic relationship with the idea of family (the impossibility of communicating with his father, the fear of buying a house of his own, the divorce from his first wife) and his own, very personal disillusion regarding his American Dream—or rather the one Elvis suggested to him as a child; if in 1980 he was still saying, "That's what great rock is about to me, it makes the dream seem possible,"[239] twelve years later he was confessing that "Music did those things but in an abstract fashion, ultimately. It did them for the guy with the guitar, but the guy without the guitar was pretty much the same as he had been."[240] In 1987 Springsteen had directly started putting together the ends of the threads making up his own biography, and telling us the other side (the genuine one) of the boy in *Thunder Road*'s destiny. With *Tunnel of Love* he came right out into the open, confessing how despite having "the fortunes of heaven in diamonds and gold" and "a house full of Rembrandts and priceless art," what he was missing was love ("Ain't Got You"). Through his subsequent *Human Touch* and *Lucky Town* (1992) he tells us how he finally finds it.

From a purely musical point of view, the style of the songs on *Tunnel of Love* is a sharp U-turn compared to *Born in the U.S.A.*: it "wasn't a rock and roll record.

Bruce made much of the music solo, using a drum machine and playing guitar, piano, synthesizer, bass, adding the various E Street Band members for minimal overdubs."[241]

From a lyrical point of view, apart from the (very noteworthy) exceptions such as "Spare Parts" and "Cautious Man," Springsteen flees from third-person narrative storytelling and, with a disarming sincerity, says "I." "You're scraping the top of your subconscious like with a knife," he explains. "And the shavings, sometimes they turn into a song. And then occasionally, the knife plummets deeply in."[242] "Confessional poetry" comes to mind—an expression coined to describe certain American poets of the fifties and sixties (Schwartz, Lowell, Plath, Berryman, Sexton)[243] who wrote focusing on extreme moments of individual experience, the psyche, and personal trauma, including previously and occasionally still taboo matters such as mental illness, sexuality, and suicide. In the songs included in *Tunnel of Love*, Springsteen seems to remove the mask as Robert Lowell did in his *Life Studies*: his speaker is unequivocally himself.

> There are a million ways to say, "I love you" in rock & roll. Springsteen just concentrated on the simple ones and endowed them with a quiet, formidable power that made *Tunnel of Love* a sometimes rough but wholly unforgettable ride.[244]

Tunnel of Love is Springsteen's *Mon coeur mis à nu*. Quite a surprise for all those accustomed to hearing him talk about the lives of others as though he were sitting on a stool next to you in a diner (it almost feels like listening to Wyatt Earp, who in *My Darling Clementine* asked his friend if he'd ever been in love and the reply was: "Nope, been a barman all my life"). As Edgar Allan Poe wrote:

> If any ambitious man have a fancy to revolutionize, at one effort, the universal world of human thought, human opinion, and human sentiment . . . all that he has to do is to write and publish a very little book. Its title should be simple—a few plain words—"My Heart Laid Bare." . . . No man dare write it. No man ever will dare write it. No man could write, even if he dared. The paper would shrivel and blaze at every touch of the fiery pen.[245]

We know that Baudelaire took up the challenge. In *Mon coeur mis à nu* he observed that "love is a terrible game in which one of the players has to lose control of themselves."[246] Likewise, in *Tunnel of Love*, love and fear are two subjects—indissolubly intertwined—in the new thematic. In "Brilliant Disguise" the narrator addresses his woman:

I want to know if it's you I don't trust
'Cause I damn sure don't trust myself. . . .
Tonight our bed is cold,
I'm lost in the darkness of our love.
God, have mercy on the man
Who doubts what he's sure of.

Here one can clearly note how writing is used as a tool for knowledge and the transformation of traumatic personal events and as a connecting element between psychic experience and poetic expression. It seems as though Springsteen wants to bridge the gap between the poetic person and the author of the lyrics, elevating the single human being from narrator to poetic subject/object. He reaches this same objective when he abandons the first-person singular to adopt the third, as in "Cautious Man":

Bill Horton was a cautious man of the road,
He walked lookin' over his shoulder and remained faithful to its code.
When something caught his eye he'd measure his need
And then very carefully he'd proceed.

Billy met a young girl in the early days of May,
It was there in her arms he let his cautiousness slip away.
In their lovers' twilight as the evening sky grew dim
He'd lay back in her arms and laugh at what had happened to him.

On his right hand Billy tattooed the word "Love" and on his left hand was
    the word "Fear"
And in which hand he held his fate was never clear.

The antinomy between "love" and "fear" is reinforced, subtly, by that existing between "house" and "road"—the latter no longer representing the symbol of escape towards a dream, but rather incarnates the worst nightmare: Bill Horton "got dressed in the moonlight and down to the highway he strode. / When he got there he didn't find nothing but road." In the same way, the main character in "Valentine's Day" is driving his car through the night. A classic Springsteen theme is turned on its head here: the man is not fleeing from home, as in "Born to Run," but he is going home:

I'm driving a big lazy car rushin' up the highway in the dark,
I got one hand steady on the wheel and one hand's tremblin' over my heart:
It's pounding baby like it's gonna bust right on through
And it ain't gonna stop till I'm alone again with you.

He is still out there on the highway, as lonely as it might be, for reasons he can't quite explain:

> Is it the sound of the leaves left blown by the wayside
> That's got me out here on this spooky old highway tonight?
> Is it the cry of the river with the moonlight shining through?

the narrator asks himself. The road seems the epitome of inhospitality, the objecti-fication of fear: it is "dark" and "spooky," the silence broken only by "the sound of the leaves left blown by the wayside," the "timberwolf in the pines" and "the cry of the river with the moonlight shining through."[247]

This bit of doubt and fear ties into the themes expressed more overtly in some of the darker songs on *Tunnel of Love*. "What scares me is losin' you," he sings, but "the moment of truth will be when he decides whether or not he can confront this fear or whether he will run from it and wander so far down that highway that he might not ever return."[248]

The man with "Two Faces" feels trapped in this misunderstanding, and says of himself:

> Two faces have I:
> One that laughs, one that cries,
> One says hello, one says goodbye,
> One does things I don't understand,
> Makes me feel like half a man.

The key track on *Tunnel of Love* is definitely "Brilliant Disguise," a sort of psychoanalysis session undertaken in front of a mirror, as Springsteen wonders about the fidelity of his woman ("So tell me what I see when I look in your eyes, / Is that you, baby, or just a brilliant disguise?"); then he voices doubts about himself ("I damn sure don't trust myself"); lastly, he is trapped in the overall misgiving that they are both playacting ("Now you play the loving woman, I'll play the faithful man").

> Springsteen knows that he, as much as anyone, has helped to make up "love" for his generation, and that, now married and singing about marriage, he cannot lie about its status as a created thing. "Show a little faith," the twenty-five-year-old singer had demanded. As he neared forty he saw that faith can only be belief in a fiction, in the provisional selves and compacts we and others agree to make. Believing in fictions means believing, as Wallace Stevens knew, in what is "not true."[249]

Springsteen actually brings to life Baudelaire's suggestion that "woman is *natural*, which means abominable."[250] *Tunnel of Love*— this "couples" album—is a treatise on misogyny. Anyone who's ever gone through the tunnel of love in an amusement park knows that it's just as scary as the haunted house. Bruce and his beloved enter it, "Then the lights go out and it's just the three of us, / You me and all that stuff we're so scared of." Then, in "One Step Up," the man says:

> It's the same thing night on night,
> Who's wrong, baby, who's right.
> Another fight and I slam the door
> On another battle in our dirty little war.

Seems like Baudelaire's speaking again, when he declared that "the supreme delight of love is knowing you are being evil. And man and woman alike know from their birth that in evil lies all delight."[251] So in "Two Faces" Springsteen sings:

> I met a girl and we ran away,
> I swore I'd make her happy every day
> And how I made her cry.

Baudelaire was a misanthropist, often ungrateful and unbearably irritable, impatient, and fanatical. Springsteen—good for him—is a far more amenable chap. Satanism Baudelaire-style, his swearing, was all a backdoor attempt to enter Christianity, if we believe T. S. Eliot.[252] The devilish darting of our *Tunnel of Love* man isn't pseudo-Byronesque paraphernalia or Late Romantic Sabbaths, but it surely derives from a failure to see himself reflected in the female world. The man and the woman don't recognize each other. There are two lines of "Trouble in Paradise" (a track written for the *Human Touch* album) that say: "Now we share the laughing, we share the joking. / We do the sleeping with one eye open." Similarly, Baudelaire asserted that "love wants to leave itself, fuse with its victim, like the victor with the vanquished, yet preserve the privileges of the conqueror."[253] Love is a battle; the character in *Tunnel of Love* and *Human Touch* confesses he doesn't know how to fight it. The splendid Doreen with whom Bobby falls in love sobs to him: "Bobby, oh Bobby, you're such a fool! / Don't you know before you choose your wish you'd better think first / 'Cause with every wish there comes a curse?"

Bobby and Doreen, however, are exceptions to the Springsteen songbook in the eighties and nineties. As we said before, the main characters are called "me" and "you," and the third-person singular is practically banned, not so much it because it is obtusely obstinate, as per the glory of convention, in taking the carriage to five-o'clock high tea (as Paul Valery was ironical about) nor because it became suddenly unmanageable (thus the author—Joyce dixit—can do nothing other than "let it be" while he files his nails); but because, more simply, Springsteen's America has shrunk into a double bed and there's no way to slam open the door and leave strong and proud towards the sun until the war under the sheets has been lost or won, or at the very least fought until its bitter end.

One album wasn't enough. Two more were required. Five years after *Tunnel of Love*—five years in which Springsteen divorced, fell in love with his backing singer Patti Scialfa, sacked the E Street Band, moved to California, and became a father—we got *Human Touch*, which, as was to be expected, was the logical continuation of *Tunnel of Love* and made it known to us that Springsteen's new thirst was still to be quenched. In the end, the distinct impression is that we have taken part in an accelerated course in American pop music, taught by a very experienced professor who loves to linger over typical examples (Springsteen himself described the making of *Human Touch* as an exercise to get himself back into writing and recording).[254] But, in all honesty, Springsteen's first rock album without the E Street Band is probably the most mediocre in his catalog.

> At best, they were songs that transported Springsteen's new life onto CD, using the formula of crisp, trebly tunes to hook CHR (Top 20) radio.... At worst, they were minor genre: the sort of stuff he could churn out left-handed. Significantly, there were no drastic detours from E Street. *River*-era rock kept peeping through Springsteen's varnish as a Mature Artist.... The bad songs were fairly well played: the good songs were fairly badly played.[255]

Much better was *Lucky Town*, an album released at the same time as *Human Touch*, with a decidedly perverse marketing approach that caused Columbia Records executives a few headaches.

Springsteen described how, at the end of recording *Human Touch*, he wasn't completely satisfied with the result. So he got to work to find a couple of "strong" songs to add to the master. What he came up with was "Living Proof," a powerful rock track about the joys of fatherhood. The sound was nothing like the smoothness of the other songs, but instead of setting aside the new creation, he built a brand-new album around it. In *Lucky Town* he gave his fans some of the most intense compositions of the 1990s: "Better Days," the title track, "Local Hero," and "If I Should Fall Behind," which is a masterpiece of a love ballad.

In America, however, critics were poisonous. Jon Pareles in the *New York Times* observed how Springsteen was "going around in circles and beginning to seem like a man completely immersed in his own private preoccupations."[256] Sales were not very good, either. *Human Touch* and *Lucky Town* respectively made adequate second and third places in the hit parade, but were a flash in the pan. Even Bruce joked about it during a TV special, saying,

> In the crystal ball, I see romance, I see adventure, I see financial reward. I see those albums, man, I see them going back up the charts. I see them rising past that old Def Leppard, past that Kris Kross. I see them all the way up past "Weird Al" Yankovic, even. . . . Wait a minute. We're slipping. We're slipping down them charts. We're going down, down, out of sight, into the darkness . . .[257]

Looking back today, the Love Trilogy, comprising *Tunnel of Love*, *Human Touch*, and *Lucky Town*, came up trumps. Above all, Springsteen once again could be congratulated for having elaborated with the utmost sincerity the impulses reaching him from the outside world—except that this time, the outside world was behind his own front door. Thanks to these three albums, we became aware of the other turn that the "Thunder Road" kid's life might—and did—take.

13. Blood Brothers

On July 3, 1966, the Castiles held a concert inaugurating the Surf 'n' See in Sea Bright, New Jersey—a beachfront club colorfully decorated with surf memorabilia and boards—before an audience of a hundred people. Exactly fifty years later, at five o'clock on a summer afternoon in Milan, a black van dribbles its way through hot dog stands and River Tour T-shirt sellers in front of the Meazza Stadium. Perhaps someone can make out who might be behind the tinted windows; but it's too late: a heavy gate closes and Bruce Springsteen's boots set upon the burning cement in the parking lot beneath the first tower on the corner.

"Welcome back to the temple," I tell him. He responds, chuckling, by blessing me as a priest would bless his parish. He slips on an acoustic guitar, hops up the steps leading onto the stage, and faces out towards a stadium where, three hours earlier than the concert is scheduled to start, one can only see the fans who have camped out for two days and nights, securing the right to be in the pit (i.e., the area in the parterre closest to the stage; the rock equivalent of Ninth Heaven, the first mobile stage in Dante). It is just for them that he sings "Growin' Up," and leaves by saying, "See you later." And he really does go, heading back to his luxurious hotel on Lake Como, where he has spent the previous two days relaxing but evidently can't handle staying any longer without luxuriously breaking his balls. Why is it that he drove half an hour to go and another half to come back, only to step on stage for five minutes when in just three hours he'll be back on for at least four? A sign of gratitude for his most faithful fans? Perhaps. But something more personal lurks underneath, a hint of unrest. That place, so special to him . . . well, it might be the last time he gets up to play on it.

Because actually the underlying score of the River Tour 2016 was: it could be the last one. Let me be clear: nobody believes that Springsteen is retiring—"What do you want me to do, take up gardening?" he says. "Look at Tony Bennett: Tony Bennett's eighty-five and he's still singing. He still sings great. So I think you need a little bit of luck, and then you have to have something you're dying to sing about."[258] But it's one thing to idly rattle off "Fly Me to the Moon" leaned up against a piano in a theater in Las Vegas, and quite another to play your heart out for four hours nonstop, guitar around your neck, in San Siro, Wembley, Camp Nou, and at the end of it all proudly proclaim, "You've just seen . . . the heart-stopping, pants-dropping, earth-shocking, house-rocking, booty-shaking, earth-quaking, love-making, Viagra-taking, history-making—Legendary—E—Street—Band!"

How long can it last? Hmm . . . here we go again with the issue of death. "It's in most great rock music," says Springsteen. "The skulls, crossbones, death's head. It's ever-present. I hear death in all those early Elvis records, in all those early, spooky blues records. And in records made by young kids—it's in 'Thunder Road.' A sense of time and the passage of time."[259]

Around this theme of melancholy, in 2009 Springsteen released an album, *Working on a Dream*, that in a sense gave closure to the Love Trilogy. For some—possibly the very ones lamenting its lack of eclecticism—it felt like an outright provocation bordering on the outrageous. Accustomed as they are to his blue-collar hero image, they continue to want stuff that smells of gasoline and cannot accept that behind the microphone there is no longer the T-shirt-clad boy with his Esquire slung around his neck but a mature artist who, albeit very subtly, has not been ashamed for the past forty years of occasionally smelling of incense and chewing gum. It's the smell of a stingy band of the past, for example, called the Beatles.

With *Working on a Dream*, Springsteen moved away from the the track beaten by Woody Guthrie and Hank Williams and recalled some of his old-time musical favorites like Elvis and Roy Orbison, and above all Brian Wilson, John Lennon, Phil Spector, and the Ronettes. "I got re-infatuated with pop music," Springsteen said.

> There's some classic sixties pop forms. California-rock influences—*Pet Sounds* and a lot of Byrds. I wanted to take the productions that create the perfect pop universes and then subvert them with the lyrics—fill them with the hollowness and the fear, the uneasiness of these very uneasy times.[260]

Some choose to mistakenly contrast pop against rock, as though it were some-how "lighter." As if "Caroline No" were not a blade cutting straight to the heart . . . One could go on to speculate as to why Springsteen decided to use pop for his sixteenth studio recording (explicitly illustrated in "Surprise, Surprise," "This Life," the title track, and "Kingdom of Days," and in the arrangements on almost every other piece, up until the lavish pop-rock symphony of "Outlaw Pete," clearly a tribute to Ennio Morricone's soundtracks for Sergio Leone's spaghetti-Western films). According to Brian Hiatt of *Rolling Stone*, Springsteen was returning to his juvenile infatuation with pop symphonies à la Roy Orbison and Phil Spector.[261] My feeling is—apart from Springsteen salvaging a series of sounds consumed during entire sweet summer nights ages ago in Jersey—that pop was simply an instrumental choice: it is indeed the ideal music if one is inclined to write songs about clouds bunching up upon years going by (as in "This Life"). Being the great encyclopedia user that he is, Springsteen remembered certain sounds, certain arrangements, certain flavors that he had found in his youth in albums such as *Pet Sounds* and *Revolver*—clean vocal harmonies Hi-Lo style, somber harpsichord tones and electronic fantasies, trombones and bells, harmonicas and violins, vibraphones, French horns and clarinets—and attempts to revisit them all in the background of his dialogue with his loved one on the verge of sixty, like in "Kingdom of Days," where he sings,

> With you I don't hear the minutes ticking by,
> I don't feel the hours as they fly,
> I don't see the summer as it wanes:
> Just a subtle change of light upon your face.

"It's a line about time," Springsteen explains. "And I'm old enough to worry about it a little bit."[262] "This Life" starts off like a Burt Bacharach piece and ends with a programmatic *pa-pa-pa-pa* reminiscent of the Turtles and "Who Loves the Sun," a sugar-coated candy by the Velvet Underground. Just as fun, fresh, and easy as "Surprise, Surprise," a loving, tender birthday song for his wife with a perfect melody (in which one can make out "Chimes of Freedom" by Dylan and Tom Waits's "Time" echoing in the distance), a good-mood-inducing rhythm, a hint of postmodern Byrds' shiny guitars, and some riffs that seem taken from "Oh, Pretty Woman." And then of course there is the dawning of "Life Itself," in which Springsteen asks himself:

> Why do the things that we treasure most slip away in time
> Till to the music we grow deaf, to God's beauty blind?

Where has the man who wrote *Nebraska* disappeared to? David Marchese from *Spin* asked himself that very question:

> Mostly upbeat and major key, Springsteen's fifth studio album in six years plays like the sunlit counterpart to 2007's bleakly portentous *Magic*. But bliss isn't the Boss's bag. Without anything to push against, one of rock's most eloquent lyricists is in the awkward position of having little of interest to say. . . . If only all the carefully crafted music weren't continually undercut by clunky, banal lyrics. The leadoff verse of "Thunder Road" forever earned Springsteen the benefit of the doubt, but this album's glut of platitudes ("When the sun comes out tomorrow / It'll be the start of a brand new day" from "Surprise, Surprise," for instance) seems more uninspired than everyman.[263]

There's not much point in debating questions of taste, it is known. But that *Working on a Dream* is not a joyous album can definitely be said. Quite the contrary. Just listen to the closing song, "The Wrestler," about a wrestler at the end of his career (written for the film of the same name starring Mickey Rourke), which proclaims, "My only faith is in the broken bones and bruises I display," or "The Last Carnival," an elegy composed on the occasion of the death of Danny Federici, the keyboard player at Springsteen's side for forty years.

Three years later Clarence Clemons will also depart, one of the cardinal points of the E Street Band—the only family Springsteen really ever had between ages twenty and forty, the essential element in the legendary Jersey Devil, or rather the biggest live performer since James Brown. "Professor" Roy Bittan, Danny "the Phantom" Federici, "Miami" Steve Van Zandt, Garry W. Tallent, "the Mighty" Max Weinberg and . . . last but not least, "Big Man" Clarence Clemons: this was the core of one of the greatest rock 'n' roll bands of all time—until one day—October 18, 1989—Springsteen called each band member[264] to explain that after years of camaraderie he wanted to experiment with something else. In other words, he fired them. "I needed to take a break, do some other things, probably play with some other musicians, which I hadn't done in a long time . . . I just didn't know where to take the band next."[265]

The years of his divorce from the E Street Band were for Springsteen like a long trip across a desert—and not merely in the figurative sense, seeing that it coincided with the period in which he moved from the East to the West Coast with his new wife, Patti Scialfa, to set up home and family. With the Love Trilogy under his belt, Springsteen's next step was to get the E Street Band back on board. At the time it seemed almost like a losing move. By 1995, seven years had passed since Bruce and the band had played live together, and eleven since they'd been in the same recording studio (for *Tunnel of Love* the band was used sparingly and never at full complement). The idea was to make a *Greatest Hits* and include some new and unreleased tracks. It was as good a way as any to prolong the enormous and unexpected success of "Streets of Philadelphia"— which one year earlier had won the Oscar for best original soundtrack song—and attract a new generation of listeners to old hits. Springsteen felt he needed to reconnect around his history. The four unreleased tracks were the result of this first—and brief—E Street Band reunion (with Van Zandt's comeback), but "Murder Incorporated" and "This Hard Land" were two tracks written in 1983 for the *Born in the U.S.A.* album,[266] while "Secret Garden"[267] was a song written for an hypothetical addition to the Trilogy of Love, another (solo) album centering on men and women. Only "Blood Brothers" was written specifically for the anthology: nothing new from a musical perspective, but at least it was a touching x-ray of the interrupted, then resumed rapport with his old E Street Band pals.

It seemed to be a declaration of intent, the prelude to the group returning to Springsteen's music on a stable basis. But it was not to be. That same year, in fact, he released *The Ghost of Tom Joad*, another album made in (almost) total solitude. It looked like Springsteen didn't want to (or couldn't) have anything to do with rock 'n' roll anymore. The next two years of worldwide tours as a one-man band confirmed that: Springsteen seemed to have come full circle, returning to solo performances, like back in 1972 when he tested for Columbia.

Not even the 1998 release of *Tracks* appeared to be a turning point: if anything, it confirmed the fact that for Springsteen rock 'n' roll seemed to be an episode in his distant past. This box set was an anthology and, above all, it was an anthology of outtakes. What it did prove was that this was one of the most prolific and astonishing singer-songwriters. Artistes would die to have been the authors of many of the sixty-seven songs that Springsteen had dismissed over the years. For him this was an excellent exercise in re-listening to tapes, almost recovering ideas and voices from the past and getting back to making rock music.

If that was the intention, then the subsequent, riotous reunion with the E Street Band and the ensuing 1999–2000 tour can be explained both as a step in returning to his roots and the snapshot of a man who negotiated a profoundly disturbing professional crisis, took time out to recover, and was now ready to get back on the road.

From that moment onwards, the rededicated E Street Band has continued to tour the world, filling entire stadiums, to the utter joy of fans old and new:

> We stood side by side each one fightin' for the other,
> We said until we died we'd always be blood brothers.

14. The Great American Novel

In his *Bruce Springsteen's America*, Robert Coles describes Springsteen as one of those "traveling companions" William Carlos Williams was talking about: "You never know when and where the new traveling companion will show up for you . . . The singer [who becomes] your pal, your guide—even for a few minutes, your inspiring teacher who [gets] you thinking like never before."[268] Even Springsteen gets infatuated with these kinds of people:

> They were searchers—Hank Williams, Frank Sinatra, Elvis, James Brown. The people I loved—Woody Guthrie, Dylan—they were out on the frontier of the American imagination, and they were changing the course of history and our own ideas about who we were. And you can throw in Martin Luther King and Malcolm X. It was a part of what I was imagining from the very beginning, just because I got tremendous inspiration and a sense of place from the performers who had imagined it before me. It was something I wanted to take a swing at, what thrilled and excited me.[269]

He has often referred to his work as a long conversation with his audience, and it's the ability to keep that exchange going—and it is most definitely a two-way thing—that has kept him "alongside Dylan, Presley, and Johnny Cash on the Mount Rushmore of American popular music."[270]

But is Springsteen also a writer?

When entering into the merits of the question of if—and where—Springsteen's work can be considered part of the American twentieth-century's literary canon, we first need to define what we mean by "canon." Harold Bloom[271] listed twenty-six authors as the most representative of Western literature of every era. They are: Shakespeare, Dante, Chaucer, Cervantes, Molière, Montaigne, Milton, Samuel Johnson, Goethe, Wordsworth, Austen, Whitman, Dickinson, Dickens, George Eliot, Tolstoy, Ibsen, Freud, Proust, Joyce, Woolf, Kafka, Borges, Neruda, Pessoa, Beckett. According to Bloom, the works of these writers introduced new traits to literature and generated entire schools, profoundly influencing writing that came after them. Bloom's canon, however, is founded primarily on a polemical anti-historicism ("I am your true Marxist critic, following Groucho rather than Karl")[272] and thus one can only be accepted into the canon for "aesthetic" merit. That's why at the heart of the canon we find Dante and Shakespeare: because they "excel all other Western writers in cognitive acuity, linguistic energy, and power of invention."[273] Another trait that renders an opus canonical is its vitality, not just because it continues to be discussed after decades or centuries, but mainly because it forces later writers to meet it head-on (for instance, the whole chapter that Bloom dedicates to Joyce is played out in the contest between the Dubliner and Shakespeare).

The canon contains only two American poets: Walt Whitman and Emily Dickinson. Apart from them, American poetry produced fewer aspiring "sub canon" candidates than those who emerged in the field of fiction.[274] From the first part of the last century we can name a dozen: Longfellow, Masters, Pound, Eliot, Frost, Stevens, Williams, Crane, Aiken, e.e. cummings, Marianne Moore, and W.H. Auden.

Harold Bloom has done influential work in centering the American poetic tradition on an Emersonian Whitman whose major twentieth-century legatees are Stevens and Ashbery. "Much recent work attempts minor shuffling of the canonical pack but no major rewriting of the rules of the game."[275] No poetry school born in the United States after the Second World War could seem to possibly include Springsteen amongst its members—unless we take the liberty of including the lyrics of the so-called Trilogy of Love into the vast and ambiguous field of confessional poetry, to which Elizabeth Bishop, Robert Lowell, John Berryman, Ann Sexton, and Sylvia Plath belong as those poets who, by detaching themselves from modernism, were able to defeat Eliot's dogma of impersonality, making a return towards using "I." Certainly, Springsteen has nothing to do with the beat poets (Kerouac, Ginsberg, Corso, Ferlinghetti), nor with John Ashbery's postmodern complexity and opacity or James Merrill's formalistic lyric style—to quote but another few aspiring to that "sub canon."

Like all twentieth-century lyrical poetry, even the American variety "speaks through enigma and darkness," as Hugo Friedrich, the modernist theoretician, had already noted in the fifties.[276] Paradoxically—for the sake of argument—the connection binding incomprehensibility and fascination, which is at the core of modern poetry, produces what Friedrich called "dissonance": of the three possible lyrical attitudes—feel, observe, transfigure—by now this last behavior dominates poetry, as much in its view of the world as in language. As the Italian Nobel Prize poet Enrico Montale dryly remarked, "No one would write in verse if the point of poetry was to make oneself understood."[277] For modern poetry admirers, even the most uncompromising critics, outside of this "dissonance" there is a markedly scholastic and bourgeois touch—and maybe songs, too. But it is an attitude that—as Friedrich warned—demonstrates the lack of any notion with respect to three millennia of literature, as well as being puerile.

When Springsteen first looked out from his angle as songwriter, at any rate, the languages of media and the arts were rapidly dissolving into one another, pushing many to state that an irreversible crisis of literature was under way and to make a heartfelt appeal to save the novel from its own extinction,[278] questioning the function and validity of storytelling. And so we live through this clash—which often though becomes a form of contamination—between the directive of the implosion, which moves towards silence and extinction (let us consider Pynchon's *Entropy*), and the erratic and libertarian explosion of a form of literature that dives deep into the beat poets' freewheeling and into the essence of rock music, which in those years proved to be the most powerful means of expression of the emerging countercultural youth movement, anarchic, libertarian, and freakish (*Trout Fishing in America* by Richard Brautigan and *Been Down So Long It Looks Like Up to Me*, the picaresque novel written by the folksinger and poet Richard Fariña, friend of Joan Baez and Thomas Pynchon, in this context come to mind).

In the early seventies, Springsteen was exuberant, baroque, and overflowing in his style of songwriting, having come out of what Robert Lowell called the "tranquilized Fifties"[279] (referring to tranquilizer abuse, but also to the turbid and muffled conformism ruling in America at the time: "the hair-conditioned nightmare," according to Henry Miller's definition[280]) with the objective to synthesize into music the hipsters' revolution, thus creating the right scenery in which the young romantic hero can operate; constantly threatened as he is by a touch of disaster, he is yet always marching ahead faithfully towards the Promised Land.

The legend of youth, entirely excluded from the classic age until the romantic invasion and Rousseau, came to life on the seats of the Paramount Theater in New York in October of 1944, when 2,000 girls in bobby socks, bow ties, "ALCATRAZ '44" sewn on their shirt backs,[281] and photos of Frank Sinatra pinned onto pretty dresses, greeted with hysterical screams "The Voice" singing "People Will Say We're In Love," wild with desire, wiping their tears with pages ripped out of *Seventeen*[282] . . . but reached its absolute climax a decade later with the rock 'n' roll tsunami.[283] Springsteen's early songs reach back to those days in sympathy with the "Brown Eyed Handsome Man" described by Chuck Berry in *After School Session*. But this romantic age of innocence ends after the release of *Born to Run*. This is when country music—with its, directness and intensity—becomes a main musical source; the songs of Hank Williams and Roy Acuff

> resonated with Springsteen even though he may not might have expressed
> his thoughts in the same way. Williams, in particular, shared much of the
> same vocabulary: words like temptation, the Promised Land, Judgment Day,
> and heaven pepper his songs.[284]

In that same period, Springsteen began to draw inspiration from literary sources as well: Flannery O'Connor, James M. Cain, John Cheever, Sherwood Anderson, and Jim Thompson.

These authors contributed greatly to the turn my music took around 1978–82. They brought out a sense of geography and the dark strain in my writing, broadened my horizons about what might be accomplished with a pop song, and are still the cornerstone literally for what I try to accomplish today.[285]

Carver, too—with his poetry in the form of prose collected in *Fires*, *Ultramarine*, and *Where Water Comes From*, for example—resembles him a great deal, with his "dirty realism,"[286] as does Richard Ford. Many sell Carver as a minimalist writer (especially after his editor Gordon Lish instrumentally shaped his prose in that direction with an editing as heavy as a surgical amputation), but this is plain foolish; it would be like saying that Joyce is a satirical writer. Carver is a real piece of Whitman's authentic epic, and in this sense he shares more than just a distant relation to Cormac McCarthy, author of powerful western novels such as *Blood Meridian*.

If one were to put Springsteen's more mature verses into context (the one from *Nebraska*, *The Ghost of Tom Joad*, and *Devils & Dust*), it would be impossible not to notice how they move within the grooves traced by the pendulum which from Carver makes its way to McCarthy. "Cormac McCarthy's *Blood Meridian* remains a watermark in my reading," Springsteen said in a 2014 interview. "It's the combination of Faulkner and Sergio Leone's spaghetti westerns that gives the book its spark for me."[287] Laconism isn't minimalism; it's a new epic form. In this respect, verse that tends to prose, to a colloquial tone, is alienating. If we look at the first lines of "Movement," which Carver included in *Where Water Comes Together with Other Water*:

> Driving lickety-split to make the ferry!
> Snow Creek and then Dog Creek
> Fly by in the headlights.
> But the hour's all wrong—no time to think
> About the sea-run trout there.
> In the lee of the mountains
> Something on the radio about an old woman
> Who travels around inside a kettle[288]

we find that more or less the same scene—and the same feeling of disquiet—appears in Springsteen's "State Trooper."

An interesting coincidence emerges when one considers the fact that, in the same way that Carver reacted to the success of his collection of stories titled *Cathedral*—stopping writing short stories and withdrawing to Port Angeles to write poetry and meditate in a house built at the confluence of two rivers with the Juan de Fuca straits—after the success of *The River*, Springsteen suffered a profound depressive crisis and fled to a country refuge to work on something different.

Both Springsteen's mature songs and Carver's poems and short-stories— "inclined toward brevity and intensity"[289]— are focused on sadness and loss in the everyday lives of ordinary people, often lower-middle-class or isolated and marginalized people (as far as Springsteen is concerned, a garage worker, a waitress, a firefighter, a car washer, a truck driver, workers in factories, construction, refineries, gas stations . . .). From this point of view, certain similarities are also shared with Richard Ford's works of fiction, which dramatize the breakdown of such cultural institutions as marriage, family, and community: his "marginalized protagonists often typify the rootlessness and nameless longing . . . pervasive in a highly mobile, present-oriented society in which individuals, having lost a sense of the past, relentlessly pursue their own elusive identities in the here and now."[290] Springsteen likes the way Richard Ford writes about New Jersey in *The Sports-writer*, *Independence Day*, and *The Lay of the Land*. However, it is clear that one can trace influences coming from the so-called New Journalism (Capote, Mailer, Didion, Gay Talese, Tom Wolfe): a rewriting of current events through a realistic viewpoint—with, at times, a macabre touch of irony, bordering on cynicism—to an ear particularly trained to the American "sound" (well-portrayed dialogues, detailed characterizations).

Twain—through Huck Finn—was the first American writer to attempt the translation of vernacular to the printed page. Decades later, Hemingway paid homage to Twain proclaiming that "all modern American literature comes from one book by Mark Twain called *Huckleberry Finn*."[291] For decades, Hemingway's narrative was seen as the perfection of a genre aiming more than any other to achieve perfection, whereas none of his novels—excepting *The Sun Also Rises* perhaps—can be read today as anything more than mere period pieces. Frank O'Connor, who hated him, declared that Hemingway's stories illustrated "technique seeking an object,"[292] thus diminished to a lesser art. On the other hand, Wallace Stevens saw conscience replacing imagination in Hemingway's stories. A perfect example is the well-known "Hills Like White Elephants," a short story all written as a dialogue between a girl and her boyfriend while they wait for a train in a Spanish station. When the man says to her, "I'd do anything for you," she crossly replies: "Would you please please please please please please please stop talking?"[293] An unbeatable defining of detail, a guaranteed precision of effects. The girl talks: we hear her voice. Hemingway's is "redskin literature," as Philip Rahv defined that of Twain. Nor is there any better way to explain this narrative genre than comparing it with "paleface literature," like that of Henry James.[294]

There is no doubt that Springsteen's songs are "redskin poems." In *Nebraska* and *The Ghost of Tom Joad* he seems to have learned the economy of implication from Kipling, and from Hemingway the well-known "iceberg theory" revealed for the first time in *Death in the Afternoon*:

> If a writer of prose knows enough about what he is writing about he may omit things that he knows and the reader, if the writer is writing truly enough, will have a feeling of those things as strongly as though the writer had stated them. The dignity of movement of an iceberg is due to only one-eighth of it being above water.[295]

One relevant example is "Highway 29," where a shoe store salesman and a customer run away to rob a bank:

> Well, I had a gun, you know the rest:
> Money on the floorboards, shirt was covered in blood,
> And she was cryin'.

Nothing is said about the reasons for the flight or the crime; it's all left to our imagination.

Another of Hemingway's golden rules, which Fitzgerald said he took to heart, was that of using an understated ending rather than a dramatic finale. In "Highway Patrolman," the policeman chases his murderer brother as far as the Canadian border, then lets him go as he watches the car's "taillights disappear." As the man in "Downbound Train" approaches the house where he lived with his ex-wife and the song reaches its climax, the brisk pace decelerates to a slow, uneasy carpet of synthesizers and Springsteen sings:

> I rushed through the yard, I burst through the front door,
> My head pounding hard, up the stairs I climbed.
> The room was dark, our bed was empty, then I heard that long whistle whine
> And I dropped to my knees, hung my head and cried.

Then the drums come right back in, and the tempo resumes its fast pace, with a deliberately flat closing image, as if seeking to weaken the dramatic effect of the five previous verses:

> Now I swing a sledge hammer on a railroad gang
> Knocking down them cross ties, working in the rain.

Many critics have pointed out significant similarities between the poetics of Springsteen and those of Whitman—the American Homer.[296] In 1855, Whitman dreamed of inspiring a new kind of poet who would celebrate the working class and achieve the promise of American democracy, prophesying the arrival of Woody Guthrie, Bob Dylan, and Bruce Springsteen.

In one essay, Robert Coles links Springsteen to Whitman via William Carlos Williams, and not simply because all three were residents of New Jersey, but because "Springsteen and Williams are poets who continue one aspect of what *Leaves of Grass* offers—the always interested observer of a nation still restlessly in formation rather than solidly settled, fixed in its social and political way."[297] The work of these three authors underpins the vision of the United States as an evolving concept.

Whitman's problem was "naturally, ideas; he had his own ones, it happens to all of us; but obscurely and intermittently he knew that for a poet it's not such a good idea to have ideas . . . The problem for Whitman as a poet was not that of expressing his ideas but of getting rid of them."[298] Likewise, Springsteen's songs betray a similar attempt to manage without ideas, to achieve the purity of a voice that is capable of breaking itself down in the endless voice of the American people. This is the intention of the poet who writes:

> From Paumanok starting, I fly like a bird,
> Around and around to soar, to sing the idea of all,
> To the north betaking myself, to sing there arctic songs,
> To Kanada, till I absorb Kanada in myself—to Michigan then,
> To Wisconsin, Iowa, Minnesota, to sing their songs, (they are inimitable);
> Then to Ohio and Indiana to sing theirs—to Missouri and Kansas and
>   Arkansas, to sing theirs;
> To Tennessee and Kentucky—to the Carolinas and Georgia, to sing theirs,
> To Texas, and so along up toward California, to roam accepted everywhere,
> To sing first, (to the tap of the war-drum, if need be)
> The idea of all—of the western world, one and inseparable,
> And then the song of each member of These States.[299]

This is a classic example of Whitman's "titanism," which unleashed a sort of mythological projection that led the Huntington poet to be acknowledged as America's first and greatest bard. In the same way, over the last thirty years, Springsteen has embraced lands, from New Jersey to New Mexico, to establish himself as an outright "national singer." As we already pointed out, Bono has said that Bruce Springsteen, more than any other, holds the heart of America.

The assonances with Whitman do not, moreover, end here. It would be sufficient to remember the importance of the 4th of July date— "4th of July Asbury Park (Sandy)," "Independence Day"—in Springsteen's work along with the fact that the first edition of *Leaves of Grass* reads "4th (?) July, 1855," where the question mark after the date underscores the mythopoeic intentions that combined the date of the Declaration of Independence with the publication of the book that was considered the bible of American democracy for many years.

Whitman and Springsteen also share the same linguistic preoccupation. The America to which Whitman wants to give a language is a complex object and the problem is not resolved in the mere lowering of the linguistic register, in other words in a sort of philological jargon, or in the neglect of rules for the sake of populist transgression.

It is also the case in the songs in which Springsteen narrates in first person. It is sufficient to consider "This Hard Land," where the hobo fleeing from one city to another seeking fortune asks:

> Hey there, mister, can you tell me
> What happened to the seeds I've sown?
> Can you give me a reason, sir, as to why they've never grown?
> They've just blown around from town to town
> Back out on these fields
> Where they fall from my hand
> Back into the dirt of this hard land.

Here, in Springsteen as in Whitman, the "I" (or "myself" as Whitman defined it) is complex and ambiguous, dual. It embraces the voice of the narrator, of the narrating first person, and that of the "composite individual" that the author of *Leaves of Grass* yearned for.

But the most significant assonances between Springsteen and Whitman are probably when they both speak of brotherhood. In Whitman's case it is *Calamus*, the cryptically homosexual poem[300] (even if Whitman's poetics are essentially auto-erotic and there is little proof that "he had sexual relations with anyone except himself").[301] The theme of "dear love of comrades,"[302] so ambiguous in Whitman, is found in a number of Springsteen songs, in particular those in which he directly addresses one or more members of the E Street Band. One example is the finale of *Bobby Jean*:

> Maybe you'll be out there on that road somewhere,
> In some bus or train traveling along,
> In some motel room there'll be a radio playing,
> And you'll hear me sing this song.
> Well, if you do you'll know I'm thinking of you

And all the miles in between,
And I'm just calling one last time not to change your mind
But just to say I miss you baby, good luck, goodbye, Bobby Jean.

One possible reading is that it was written when Steve Van Zandt left the E Street Band (and this was explicitly confirmed by Springsteen). In fact, the words do not reveal whether the narrator is talking to a man or a woman, and even the title—"Bobby Jean"—is composed of a male and a female name.

"No Surrender" (written in the same period, during the *Born in the U.S.A.* sessions) is certainly for Steve Van Zandt as we hear: "We swore blood brothers against the wind." "Blood brothers" refers to the E Street Band and is used more precisely in the song actually entitled that way:

Now I don't know how I feel, I don't know how I feel tonight,
If I've fallen 'neath the wheel, if I've lost or I've gained sight,
I don't even know why, I don't know why I made this call
Or if any of this matters anymore after all,
But the stars are burnin' bright like some mystery uncovered,
I'll keep movin' through the dark with you in my heart, my blood brother.

Similarly, Whitman wrote:

This moment yearning and thoughtful sitting alone . . .
O I know we should be brethren and lovers,
I know I should be happy with them.[303]

The obsession with the Great American Novel has often confused critics and destroyed brilliant promise in literature. It is a dream as light as a butterfly that flies too close to the sun, risking burning its wings. Certain writers of great genius, like Melville and Pynchon, systematically did without, adopting as models—just as Joyce was doing in Europe—the myth of the great Ulysses and placing the drama outside of the United States: *Moby Dick* is a marine epic poem and *Gravity's Rainbow* ranges from London to Germany, from the Côte d'Azur to the African Continent. In most cases American novelists have tried to focus on a small slice of the country—Faulkner's Georgia, Fitzgerald's New York, Bellow's Chicago, McCarthy's West, Roth's New Jersey—leaving to others the task of going on the road and traveling coast to coast. Paradoxically, it wasn't Kerouac who managed to offer an exhaustive map of the U.S.A., but the Russian Vladimir Nabokov in *Lolita*.

If Hawthorne's *Scarlet Letter* is to be considered the American Book of Genesis—thus fire-branding the three words that underpin the foundation of the United

States: happiness, legality, and guilt—*Leaves of Grass*, *Moby Dick*, and *Lolita* are three of the four books of Exodus. The fourth may have been written by Bruce Springsteen.

For the Apocalypse we have to wait a while: several verses may already have been penned by Bradbury, Vonnegut, and DeLillo. But America is not yet at the end of its story: as a nation it is still marching towards its Promised Land.

15. Conclusion

In these early years of the twenty-first century, we find that the most powerful voices in America are muffled. Philip Roth has retired; Spielberg no longer manages to take us into the charming trauma of lost childhood; Dylan has for the past forty years been fighting a marvelous battle to demolish the spotlight the world has guardedly shone upon him, even attempting to bestow a prize on him, an immensely prestigious one, which he however has no use for. Springsteen, on the other hand, seems quite happy to accept his role of the nation's conscience: pouring out comments and statements on any "hot" current affair, both national and international; spitting out records with a Beatle-like proliferation reminiscent of their golden decade and transforming his concerts into some sort of secular masses, in which to celebrate weddings (a year ago a young couple showed up in fancy dress and asked, on stage, for his blessings) and funerals (he sang "Rebel Rebel" the night of Bowie's death and "Purple Rain" in memory of Prince), a pulpit from which to dedicate "My City of Ruins" to Central Italy's earthquake victims and from which to attack Trump for his isolationist and reactionary policies.

Maturity has given Springsteen something vaguely oracular. "That is the great fallacy," Hemingway wrote: "the wisdom of old men. They do not grow wise. They grow careful."[304]

Well, tonight Springsteen is backstage, carefully looking at the ruins on top of Rome's Palatine Hill, which at sunset is tinted pink. A tidal-like flow of human beings crowds up in the vast valley that opens out onto the feet of the imperial palaces. It is July 16, 2016, and we are in the Circus Maximus. The last date on the Italian tour. The most anticipated one, because of the location. George Travis (Bruce's tour manager since 1978) explains to me that, "For us Americans this is Ben-Hur's chariot-racing track, a legendary place. Can you imagine that in 1980 a promoter brought me here and said: 'One day Bruce will play here'?"

The string section of the Roma Sinfonietta (the orchestra that is best known for its key role in bringing to life the music of Ennio Morricone) looks out overwhelmed at the audience extending out into the horizon. Yesterday they had a rehearsal in a recording studio for what will turn out to be Springsteen's biggest surprise ever for Rome: opening the concert with "New York City Serenade" as the sun sets on the Eternal City. We all know what we are in for. And I know what everybody's feeling: they are come to realize that inside this gigantic ruin we will forget that nature is none other than chaos, brutality, and death and understand that beauty can save the world, that the music coming off the amplifiers hits you like a bullet below your breastbone—where the sound distributed by earphones in homeopathic doses will never get—and that anyone can be Johnny B. Goode and shout, "It's a town full of losers and I'm pulling out of here to win."

Lost in the crowd, as the loudspeakers spread the notes from the theme from *Once Upon a Time in the West*, I get a flashing image of what Beauty might be. Every time this man fools me. When he gets up on stage, in that specific moment, in no other place on earth does anything so significant as his show happen. You become the center of the world.

Springsteen once proclaimed, "I'll never say, 'I won't play no more gigs.' I'll keep playing until my hands get all bruised, and then some." A hundred years earlier, the "bard of America" said something similar:

> I shall go forth,
> I shall traverse the States awhile, but I cannot tell whether or how long,
> Perhaps soon some day or night while I am singing my voice will suddenly cease.[305]

This last verse echoes in my head as the concert begins. Springsteen, more anxious and fatalistic than ever, has recently stated that

> Playing a show brings a tremendous amount of euphoria, and the danger of it is, there's always that moment, comes every night, where you think, Hey, man, I'm gonna live forever! You're feeling all your power. And then you come offstage, and the main thing you realize is "Well, that's over." Mortality sets back in.[306]

I realized a couple of days ago in Milan, during the two San Siro shows, that all of a sudden, everything started taking on a different perspective. Even Springsteen ... there he was joining in with the crowd, shaking hands, holding the microphone out towards ten, twenty, thirty thousand mouths open wide in awe, and one could sense from his gaze the deep sadness that only a long farewell could signify; his eyes, small and shiny, continuously replayed on giant screens, are the eyes of a man who is suffering, because *this thing*— the essence of his life—can't last for much longer. Look at how avidly he sucks the vital energy of the kids in front row: he feels so alive! His round biceps shiny with sweat, despite an eternity of hours in the gym, are those of a man who has aged, however good his shape. My beloved vampire! Hey, Boss, you know better than all of us that life should be made up of one Bruce Springsteen and the E Street Band show per night, every night. But you recognize that you have "a finite amount of time in which I'm going to continue to do what I'm doing."[307]

It strikes me that *Wrecking Ball* ends with "We Are Alive," a song in which the dead and departed proclaim that their voices will continue to resonate. But there was also a bonus track, entitled "Swallowed Up (In the Belly of the Whale)."

> I fell asleep on a dark and starlit sea
> With nothing but the cloak of God's mercy over me.
> I come upon strange earth and a great black cave,
> I dreamt I awoke as if buried in my grave.
>
> We've been swallowed up,
> We've been swallowed up,
> Disappeared from this world,
> We've been swallowed up.
>
> The bones of sailors from the north and sailors from the east
> Lay high in a pyre in the belly of a beast,
> A beast should you wander in its path upon your ship and your flesh he'll
>   sup,
> You'll disappear from this world until you've been swallowed up.

The reference to Moby Dick is obvious: "Some of these Quakers are the most sanguinary of all sailors and whale-hunters. They are fighting Quakers; they are Quakers with a vengeance,"[308] Melville wrote. And one century later, Robert Lowell glosses:

>   They died
> When time was open-eyed,
> Wooden and childish; only bones abide
> There, in the nowhere, where their boats were found
> Sky-high, where mariners had fabled news
> Of IS, the whited monster . . .
>
>   In the sperm-whale's slick
> I see the Quakers drown and hear their cry:
> "If God himself had not been on our side,

If God himself had not been on our side,
When the Atlantic rose against us, why,
Then it had swallowed us up quick."[309]

Here there are no survivors, no one who can say, "Call me Ishmael." God does not fulfill Jonas and the great fish does not vomit him out. Just as Springsteen sings:

We trusted our skills and our good sails,
Our faith that with God the righteous in this world prevail,

But we've been swallowed up
We've been swallowed up
Disappeared from this world,
We've been swallowed up.

Mixed generations from different social classes are happily mixed under the Roman sky: the first notes of "New York City Serenade" get lost up above, where perfect is the silence, in the celestial indifference of the gods. Who are certainly appreciating.

Roy Bittan's piano intro is a blow to my tear ducts. But—shit!—to *his* as well. There it is. Because when Bruce Springsteen got onstage to find Rome at his feet out there in front of him (60,000 people waving heart banners), for a few brief instants it seemed to be too much for him, the emotional impact too great. Even now as his eyes moisten with tears I feel somehow able to step into his thoughts; and his thoughts are the following: fifty years have come and gone since recording that vinyl with the Castiles, and now look where I am, my god! So much time has passed, so many things have happened: they put me on both the covers of *Time* and *Newsweek* at the same time, I shared a stage with Chuck Berry, Bob Dylan, and Paul McCartney, I won an Oscar, I played in every gym, bar, theater, arena, and stadium in America, I traveled the world eighty times, I sold more than a billion dollars' worth of tickets, people sing my songs in Japanese pagodas and inside Antarctic igloos . . . and all this, all this has got to end, sooner or later—even this place, right here inside the millenary heart of the most beautiful city on Earth, will soon (well, not too soon: at least four hours from now!), empty out, perhaps forever. Will I see you again, girl in the front row, and you, yes, yes . . . I mean you, faithful guy, you who have looked me straight in the eye for the past weeks to understand something I would rather you didn't . . . will I ever see your sweaty, excited, moved, ecstatic faces again under my stage?

What can I say, Bruce? Only that down here with my friends—my companions in dozens of concerts, of never-ending trips to come and see you—we keep telling each other, for the past several years now, oh god, this is it, the last one, the last tour, the last show. But then you show up again. You've always come back. Maybe even this time . . . Maybe you will go on forever. In the end, this is rock 'n' roll's promise. So yes, Bruce, give me your word. Let's swear to each other, here tonight, that it will never end.

This is the secret of these shamans marching along the American highways: plough ahead, look, narrate, never judge. The reward is priceless. Whitman—this free man, this vast poet—repeats this after complaining about life, questions without replies, the sordid crowd walking at his side, and asks:

> What good amid these, O me, O life?
> *Answer.*
> That you are here—that life exists and identity,
> That the powerful play goes on, and you may contribute a verse.[310]

---

1. Waldo Jeffers is the main character in "The Gift," a song by the Velvet Underground included in their second album, *White Light/White Heat* (1967).

2. Susan Michelson is the female character in Tom Waits's "Eggs & Sausage (In a Cadillac with Susan Michelson)," included in his 1975 album *Nighthawks at the Diner*.

3. The title "A Sort of Homecoming," from U2's *The Unforgettable Fire* album (1984), was inspired by the line "Poetry is a form of homecoming," stated by the Romanian poet Paul Celan during a speech that he gave in Germany in 1960, on the occasion of receiving the Georg Buchner Prize.

4. Scottish novelist Irvine Welsh was brutal on Twitter: "I'm a Dylan fan, but this is an ill-conceived nostalgia award wrenched from the rancid prostates of senile, gibbering hippies," he wrote. He continued: "If you're a 'music' fan, look it up in the dictionary. Then 'literature.' Then compare and contrast." ("Irvine Welsh slams Nobel Prize award for Bob Dylan," *The Scotsman*, October 13, 2016). Sara Danius, Permanent Secretary of the Nobel Academy, told a news conference: "If you look far back, 5,000 years, you discover Homer and Sappho. They wrote poetic texts which were meant to be performed, and it's the same way for Bob Dylan. We still read Homer and Sappho, and we enjoy it."

5. Paul Zollo, *Songwriters on Songwriting* (New York: Da Capo Press, 2005).

6. In his banquet speech written on the occasion of the Nobel Prize award, Dylan says he is convinced that Shakespeare "thought of himself as a dramatist. The thought that he was writing literature couldn't have entered his head. His words were written for the stage. Meant to be spoken, not read. When he was writing Hamlet, I'm sure he was thinking about a lot of different things: 'Who're the right actors for these roles?' 'How should this be staged?' 'Do I really want to set this in Denmark?' His creative vision and ambitions were no doubt at the forefront of his mind, but there were also more mundane matters to consider and deal with. 'Is the financing in place?' 'Are there enough good seats for my patrons?' 'Where am I going to get a human skull?' I would bet that the farthest thing from Shakespeare's mind was the question 'Is this literature?'" (Bob Dylan, "Banquet Speech." Paper presented by the U.S. Ambassador to Sweden Azita Raji at the Nobel Banquet in Stockholm, December 10, 2016. Copyright ©2016 The Nobel Foundation).

7. Robert Wiersema, *Walk Like a Man: Coming of Age with the Music of Bruce Springsteen* (Vancouver: Greystone Books, 2011).

8. Benedetto Croce, *Estetica come scienza dell'espressione e linguistica generale. Teoria e storia* (Milano: Adelphi, 1990). Croce (1866–1952) was an Italian philosopher who served as president of PEN International, the worldwide writers' association, from 1949 until 1952.

9. "I could define poetry this way: it is that which is lost out of both prose and verse in translation." Robert Frost in *Conversations on the Craft of Poetry with Robert Frost, John Crowe Ransom, Robert Lowell, Theodore Roethke*, ed. Cleanth Brooks and Robert Penn Warren (New York: Holt, Rinehart and Winston, 1961).

10. Anonymous, "Mow Go'th Sun Under Wood," in *The Norton Anthology of Poetry* (New York: W. W. Norton & Company, 1983).

11. Edgar Lee Masters, "'Butch' Weldy," in *Spoon River Anthology* (New York: MacMillan, 1916).

12. "The Lost Interviews. 1975" excerpted in *Backstreets #57*, Winter 1997, and *Backstreets #58*, Spring 1998.

13. Frank McConnell, "A Rock Poet: From Fitzgerald to Springsteen," *Commonweal*, August 12, 1983.

14. Pythia Peay, "Soul Searching," *Washingtonian*, January–February 2001.

15. It may come as a surprise to those who still think that Springsteen's songs are just about cars and girls, or more generally that rock 'n' roll—like masturbation—is only an adolescent obsession, but recent studies published in *The Psychology of Aesthetics, Creativity & the Arts* have shown that Springsteen's music can be used to cast light on complex psychological problems, including pain and anxiety deriving from tragic events like the death of a loved one (Lorraine Mangione, "Spirit in the Night to Mary's Place: Loss, Death, and the Transformative Power of Relationships," *The Psychology of Aesthetics, Creativity & the Arts*, July 2008).

16. Leslie Marmon Silko, "How to Write a Poem About the Sky," in *The Norton Anthology of Poetry*.

17. Walt Whitman, Preface to the First Edition (1855, published by the author) of *Leaves of Grass*.

18. John Smith, *The Generall Historie of Virginia, New-England, and the Summer Isles* (London: Michael Sparkes, 1624).

19. "Cotton Needs A-Pickin'." Traditional song adapted to an old Florida tune found at the Virginia Hampton Institute and transcribed by Natalie Curtis-Burlin, performed by Charity Bailey.

20. Thomas Pynchon, "The Deadly Sins / Sloth; Nearer, My Couch, to Thee," *The New York Times*, June 6, 1993.

21. Walt Whitman, "Song of Exposition," in *Leaves of Grass* (Philadelphia: David McKay, 1900).

22. In reality, both storytelling and song form the most significant American literary corpus from the period subsequent to Columbus's discovery, along with the many travelogues.

23. Written in 1905 by Thomas S. Allen with the title "Low Bridge, Everybody Down," it was presented anonymously as if it had been written eighty years earlier for the opening of the Erie Canal, constructed from 1817 to 1825 to connect New York City with Buffalo. Pete Seeger's version can be found on the album *American Favorite Ballads, vol. 3* (1959).

24. "Shenandoah," written before 1820, dates back to early country music and was probably a work song that was adapted as a folk song. The geography of the piece is not clear, as the Shenandoah River flows through Virginia and West Virginia, about a thousand miles from the Missouri River, also referenced in the song. Others believe the text refers to Shenandoah, Iowa, just twenty miles east of the Missouri. There are many versions, by artists including Bob Dylan, Harry Belafonte, Judy Garland, Roger McGuinn, the Chieftains with Van Morrison, Emmylou Harris, and Duane Eddy. Pete Seeger's version can be found on the album *American Favorite Ballads, vol. 3* (1959).

25. "Pay Me My Money Down" was a sea song popular among stevedores in the Georgia and South Carolina ports. It was around for a long time as a calypso (as in the 1958 Kingston Trio version) and is often considered a Bahamas song. Lydia Parrish was the first to obtain rights and published the text in her *Slave Songs of the Georgia Sea Islands* (1942). Pete Seeger recorded the song with the Weavers, which can be heard on *The Weavers at Carnegie Hall* (1957).

26. Springsteen also took inspiration from "John Henry" when he wrote "The Long Goodbye," a song released in 1992 on the *Human Touch* album, where Springsteen uses the hammer to break the chain of lies that keeps him prisoner, stops him acquiring awareness of himself and defining his male identity,

knowing that "John Heny" was a prime example of working-class and proletarian culture, since it puts forward a model of humanity and virility defined in antithesis to the steam-hammer, which was threatening the human workforce at the end of the nineteenth century, when the song was composed.

27. Colson Whitehead, *John Henry Days* (New York: Doubleday, 1991).

28. Dena J. Epstein, *Sinful Tunes and Spirituals: Black Folk Music to the Civil War* (Chicago: University of Illinois Press, 1977).

29. "Run, Nigger, Run" is a folksong by an anonymous African American author, whose existence has been documented in a collection of songs, the *White's Serenaders' Song Book*, published in 1851. The quoted version is taken from John A. Lomax, *American Ballads and Folk Songs* (New York: Macmillan Company, 1934). "Pattyrollers," "paddyrollers," or "patter-rollers" were distortions of "patrollers" (taken from the French *patrouiller*) and referred to the patrol squads who kept a strict check on fugitive slaves, set up in the Southern states from the beginning of the 1700s until the end of the Civil War.

30. In 1941, literary critic Francis Otto Matthiessen called "American Renaissance" the five years between 1850 and 1855, when the best works of Emerson, Hawthorne, Melville, Thoreau, and Whitman were published. The thematic center of the American Renaissance was what Matthiessen called the "devotion" of all five of his writers to "the possibilities of democracy," in contrast to the puritan past.

31. The first to do so, imitating a black drunkard, was possibly Lewis Hallam in 1769, performing Charles Didbin's opera *The Padlock*. Later in 1799 in Boston, the singer Andrew Allen came on stage at the end of the second act of the tragedy *Oroonoko* for a musical interlude called "The Song of the Negro Boy."

32. Mariano De Simone, *"Doo-dah! Doo-dah!" Musica e musicisti nell'America dell'Ottocento* (Roma: Arcana, 2003).

33. Rudi Blesh and Janis Blesh, *They All Played Ragtime* (New York: Alfred A. Knopf, 1950).

34. In 1707, Reverend Isaac Watts published (first in London then in Boston) *Hymns and Spiritual Songs*, a book that met with huge success in all sectors of American society. Watts opposed the Calvinist tradition of singing only Old Testament psalms in church and composed hundreds of hymns emphasizing the New Testament. It's no coincidence that Watts's type of hymn singing was popular with the African American community, for whom the relationship with a divinity and more generally with what is sacred, is personalized, almost colloquial; the literary style is not really academic and institutional; conversely it is rich with fascinating imagery. In the 1800s these traits converged in the spirituals sung by the African American population and in a genre traceable to the institution of the first African American church, for which Richard Allen published an initial thirty-one hymns intended to form an independent repertoire.

35. Jazz was officially born on January 30, 1917, when the Original Dixieland Jazz Band (with a director of Italian origin, Nick La Rocca) released its first record with "Darkton Strutter's Ball" and "Indiana" on it. Nevertheless, jazz had at least half a century of "prehistoric roots" prior to this; it was an artistic way of playing music created in the United States from the encounter of African American and European music. Jazz instrumentation, melody, and harmony derived prevalently from Western musical tradition. The rhythm, phrasing, and sound formation, as well as specific blues harmony elements came from African music and the musical sensitivity of Black Africa. Jazz is the product of a white aesthetic and black poetics.

36. Alan Lomax, *Land Where the Blues Began* (New York: New Press, 2002).

37. James M. Whitfield, "America," in *America and Other Poems* (Buffalo: James S. Leavitt, 1853).

38. The term "rhythm and blues" was used for the first time in 1949 by the *Billboard* journalist Jerry Weller.

39. What was the first rock 'n' roll record? According to some the first rock 'n' roll song is "The Fat Man," recorded by Fats Domino in 1949. Others say the first was "Rocket 88," written by the eighteen-year-old Ike Turner in 1951 and recorded that same year by Jackie Brenston and his Delta Cats. As per

general convention—largely thanks to its massive success amongst the white public—it is common to refer to "Rock Around the Clock" by Bill Haley and His Comets as the first r'n'r song. It was written in 1952 by Max C. Freedman and James E. Myers and recorded by Bill Haley in April 1954; but it was only the following year, when it was added to the soundtrack of the film *Blackboard Jungle*, that it reached #1 in the charts. On July 5, 1954, the nineteen-year-old Elvis Presley recorded "That's All Right" for Sun Records as his first single (featuring "Blue Moon Kentucky" on the B-side).

40. Walt Whitman, Preface to the first edition (1855) of *Leaves of Grass*, published by the author.

41. Walt Whitman, "One's-Self I Sing," in *Leaves of Grass*.

42. Seamus Heaney, "The Interesting Case of Nero, Chekhov's Cognac and a Knocker," in *The Government of the Tongue* (London: Faber, 1988).

43. Alfred Kazin, *Bright Book of Life. American Novelists and Storytellers from Hemingway to Mailer* (London: Secker & Walburg, 1974).

44. Seamus Heaney, "The Interesting Case of Nero, Chekhov's Cognac and a Knocker."

45. Wilfred Owen, Preface to *Poems* (London: Chatto & Windus, 1920).

46. Allen Ginsberg, "Ether," in *Howl and Other Poems* (San Francisco: City Lights, 1956).

47. Miles Davis didn't thank Kerouac for this. Quite the opposite. In his autobiography he wrote, "I hate how white people always try to take credit for something after *they* discover it. Like it wasn't happening before they found out about it—which most times is always late, and they didn't have nothing to do with it happening. . . . After bebop became the rage, white music critics tried to act like they discovered it—and us—down on 52nd Street. That kind of dishonest shit makes me sick to my stomach. And when you speak out on it or don't go along with this racist bullshit, then you become a radical, a black troublemaker. Then they try to cut you out of everything" (Miles Davis and Quincy Troupe. *Miles, The Autobiography*. New York: Simon & Schuster, 1989). The attitude of the white cultural world to African American music was such that on one hand in the Roaring Twenties—mainly thanks to Francis Scott Fitzgerald—the Jazz Age legend was born, while on the other it was mainly a dishonest appropriation, an extra nuance to enrich the color scheme; jazz—jazz musicians above all—was still censured in the social context. It was the subsequent generation that recovered and updated a jazz-literature epos comparable to that of Fitzgerald. In actual fact, it was the Beat Generation authors who connected their inspiration (and their *mal de vivre*) to the bop revolution.

48. Emil Cioran, *Syllogismes de l'amertume* (Paris: Gallimard, 1952).

49. Giorgio Raimondi, *La scrittura sincopata. Jazz e letteratura nel Novecento italiano* (Milano: Bruno Mondadori, 1999). Two excellent examples of the European intelligentsia's jazz mythologization between the wars are Piet Mondrian's long essay called *Jazz and Neoplasticism* (1922) and Le Corbusier's 1937 work, *When Cathedrals Were White*. In the section on "mechanical mentality and black Americans," Le Corbusier focused on jazz, saying that "African music touched America because it was the real melody of the soul combined with a mechanical beat; it has two tempos: heart's weeping and contortion of legs, back, arms, and head. Music for an era of construction: groundbreaking. It inundated the body and heart; it inundated the U.S.A. and the world. From then on it would change all listening habits as it was so powerful, so irresistible for the mind and the body, that listeners are torn from passivity and start to dance and gesticulate, participate. It opened the sound cycle of modern times, turned over a new leaf for Conservatives." Le Corbusier, *When Cathedrals Were White* (Columbus: McGraw-Hill, 1964).

50. John Barth, "The Literature of Exhaustion," *The Atlantic Monthly*, August 1967.

51. Elvis Presley, "Heartbreak Hotel," from "Heartbreak Hotel" / "I Was the One" (1956).

52. Bob Dylan, "Like a Rolling Stone," from *Highway 61 Revisited* (1965).

53. In his autobiography, Bruce Springsteen says that the album cover of *Highway 61 Revisited* is the greatest of all time, tied with *Meet the Beatles*.

54. Tommy Ramone, "Fight Club," *Uncut*, January 2007.

55. Robert Christgau, review of "Please Kill Me: The Uncensored Oral History of Punk," *New York Times Book Review*, 1996.

56. In December 1976, the English fanzine *Sideburns* published a now-famous illustration of three chords, captioned, "This is a chord, this is another, this is a third. Now form a band."

57. Roger Sabin, *Punk Rock: So What?: The Cultural Legacy of Punk* (London: Routledge, 1999).

58. Dave Marsh, *Born to Run: The Bruce Springsteen Story* (New York: Doubleday, 1979).

59. Bruce Springsteen, *Born to Run* (London: Simon & Schuster, 2016).

60. In 1985, "Dr. Ruth" Westheimer declared that "Bruce is a national monument," as it is quoted in John Lombardi, "St. Boss—The Sanctification of Bruce Springsteen and the Rise of Mass Hip," *Esquire*, December, 1988.

61. Bruce Springsteen, international press conference at Théâtre Marigny, Paris, France, February 16, 2012. Published in *Talking About a Dream. The Essential Interviews of Bruce Springsteen*, ed. Christopher Phillips and Louis P. Masur (New York: Bloomsbury Press, 2013).

62. In 1992, Springsteen said, "I had this idea of playing out my life like it was a movie, writing the script and making all the pieces fit. And I really did that for a long time. But [. . .] it's pathetic" (James Henke, "Interview with Bruce Springsteen," *Rolling Stone*, August 6, 1992).

63. Ibid.

64. During an encore at the concert held in Hyde Park on July 14, 2012 for the Hard Rock Calling Festival, Springsteen called Paul McCartney on stage to play "I Saw Her Standing There" and "Twist and Shout" with him. After the second song, the festival organizers came on stage and turned off the amplifiers, because it was past the London curfew. Macca and the Boss were left standing there to say good bye and leave. The day after, scandal spread through media across the world. London Mayor Boris Johnson, had to apologize publicly for what happened.

65. In his autobiography, Springsteen confessed that in the mid-sixties he lived for every Beatles record release.

66. Bruce Springsteen, "Keynote Speech" (paper presented at the South by Southwest Conference, Austin, TX, March 15, 2012).

67. *T.A.M.I. Show* opened in American theaters on Christmas 1964; it is a documentary film on two concerts held in the Santa Monica Civic Auditorium on October 28 and 29, 1963. The musicians included Chuck Berry, the Beach Boys, Marvin Gaye, Smokey Robinson and the Miracles, the Supremes, and of course James Brown and the Rolling Stones at the end of the program. As Keith Richards recalls in an interview on the DVD of the film (issued in 2009), "deciding to play after James Brown and the Famous Flames was the biggest mistake of our career."

68. Bruce Springsteen, "Keynote Speech."

69. Leon Wieseltier, "A Saint in the City," *The New Republic*, August 1, 2012.

70. Howard Zinn (1922–2010), American historian active in the civil rights movement starting in the 1960s, was one of the first voices raised against the war in Vietnam. He published *A People's History of the United States* in 1980, wherein he narrated American history from the viewpoint of slaves, the dispossessed, and the working class.

71. Bono, "Bruce Springsteen's Rock & Roll Hall of Fame Induction Speech" (Waldorf Astoria, New York, March 15, 1999).

72. *Springsteen dalla A alla Z*, ed. Ermanno Labianca e Massimo Cotto (Roma: Arcana, 1999).

73. Gino Castaldo, "Provaci ancora Bruce," *La Repubblica*, April 1, 1999.

74. Martin Scorsese, foreword to *Racing in the Street: The Bruce Springsteen Reader*, ed. June Skinner Sawyers (New York: Penguin, 2004).

75. Peter Balakian, "Rock 'n' Roll," in *Sweet Nothings: An Anthology of Rock and Roll* (Bloomington: Indiana University Press 1994).

76. Christopher Phillips, "The Real World," *Backstreets* #79, Spring 2004.

77. "The first day I can remember lookin' in the mirror and standin' what I was seein' was the day I had a guitar in my hand," Springsteen told *Newsweek* in 1975 (Maureen Orth, Janet Huck, and Peter S. Greenberg, "The Making of a Rock Star," *Newsweek*, October 27, 1975).

78. Don DeLillo, quoted in Christopher Sandford, *Springsteen: Point Blank* (London: Omnibus Press, 2004).

79. *The Voyage of Saint Brendan* (Navigatio Sancti Brendani) is an anonymous work in Latin, set down in the tenth century, which narrates the tales of the fantastic travels of Brendan, a sixth-century Irish monk who according to legend set out with a group of companions in search of paradise on earth.

80. In *Yellow Submarine*—the 1968 animated film inspired by the music of the Beatles—Pepperland is a cheerful, music-loving paradise under the sea, protected by Sgt. Pepper's Lonely Hearts Club Band (the Beatles) and dominated by the titular Yellow Submarine, which rests on an Aztec-like pyramid on a hill.

81. The Yellow Brick Road's most notable portrayal is in the classic 1939 musical movie *The Wizard of Oz*, loosely based on L. Frank Baum's novel *The Marvelous Land of Oz* (1904). In 1973, Elton John published the album *Goodbye Yellow Brick Road*, which includes the famous title track.

82. *Electric Ladyland* is the title of the Jimi Hendrix Experience's third album, published in 1968.

83. "Itchycoo Park" is a psychedelic pop song recorded by the Small Faces in 1967.

84. Pink Floyd, "The Gnome," from *The Piper at the Gates of Dawn* (1967).

85. Frank McConnell, "A Rock Poet."

86. David Wyatt, *Out of the Sixties: Storytelling and the Vietnam Generation* (Cambridge: Cambridge University Press, 1993).

87. Emily Dickinson, "Poem 670," in *The Poems of Emily Dickinson*, ed. Thomas H. Johnson (Boston: Belknap Press of Harvard University Press, 1955).

88. The main source of of inspiration for "Factory"—apart from the autobiographical element—is without doubt the Animals' "We Gotta Get Out of This Place."

89. Fred Shruers, "Bruce Springsteen and the Secret of the World," *Rolling Stone*, February 5, 1981.

90. Mario Corona, "Jack Kerouac, o della contraddizione," in *Jack Kerouac: Romanzi* (Milano: Mondadori, 2001).

91. Norman Mailer, "The Hip and the Square," *Village Voice*, April 25, 1956.

92. Jack Kerouac, *On the Road* (New York: Viking Press, 1957).

93. Bruce Springsteen, quoted in Pamela Clarke Keogh, *Elvis Presley: The Man. The Life. The Legend* (New York: Atria Books, 2004).

94. Jay Cocks, "Rock's New Sensation: The Backstreets Phantom of Rock," *Time Magazine*, October 27, 1975.

95. Ariel Swartley, "The Wild, the Innocent & the E Street Shuffle," in *Stranded: Rock and Roll for a Desert Island*, ed. Greil Marcus (New York: Da Capo Press, 1996).

96. Springsteen was in favor of including "Visitation at Fort Horn" on his first album, *Greetings from Asbury Park, NJ*, instead of "It's Hard to Be a Saint in the City," but his manager, Mike Appel, pushed for the latter. "'Saint in the City' was so great," Appel recalls, "I had to convince him of that one. I had to throw a fit to get him to go with that" (Charles R. Cross, "Interview with Mike Appel," *Backstreets* #34/35, Fall 1990 / Winter 1991). Bowie recorded a version of "It's Hard to Be a Saint in the City" in 1975, but the track wasn't released until 1989, when it was included on his *Sound + Vision* box set. Producer Tony Visconti recalled how he asked Springsteen to visit Bowie in the studio in Philadelphia: "David was quite taken by meeting Bruce. We played 'Saint' to him and he kept a poker face the whole time. He said nothing when it was finished. David took him into another room for a private chat. By the time Bruce left, he was more pleasant and said his goodbyes to the rest of us. David and I never worked on 'Saint' after that, although it was finished or re-recorded eventually with someone else" (John Earls, "David Bowie Abandoned Covering Bruce Springsteen After Meeting Him," *New Musical Express*, August 19, 2016).

97. Ken Emerson, "Springsteen Goes Gritty and Serious. 'The Wild, the Innocent & the E Street Shuffle' Album Review," *Rolling Stone*, January 31, 1974.

98 .Bruce Springsteen, at the Two River Theater, Red Bank, New Jersey, April 4, 2005.

99. Thomas Stearns Eliot, "East Coker," in *Four Quartets* (New York: Harcourt, Brace & World, 1962).

100. Van Morrison's influence on Springsteen when he was composing *The Wild, the Innocent & the E Street Shuffle* is as obvious as the Irishman's irritation with his younger colleague. In a 1985 interview, Morrison said, "For years people have been saying to me, 'Have you heard this guy Springsteen? You should really check him out!' I just ignored it. Then four or five months ago I was in Amsterdam, and a friend of mine put on a video. Springsteen came on the video, and that was the first time I ever saw him, and he's definitely ripped me off. There's no doubt about that. Not only did Springsteen . . . I mean, he's even ripped my movements off as well. My seventies movements, you know what I mean?" (Stephen Davis, "Van Morrison. The Interview," *New Age*, August 1985.)

101. Parke Puterbaugh, introduction to Bruce Springsteen—*The Rolling Stone Files: The Ultimate Compendium of Interviews, Articles, Facts and Opinions from the Files of Rolling Stone* (New York: Hyperion Press, 1996).

102. Eddy Cilìa, "Nebraska," *Velvet Gallery*, June 1990.

103. Ariel Swartley, "The Wild, the Innocent & the E Street Shuffle."

104. Springsteen mentioned he got the idea for the title from a neon sign promoting the return of a popular stripper's show to a local Shore-area club. "It's a striptease number, that's what it is," he said. "A follow-up to the David Rose Orchestra. It's a strange song. Sort of big-band-y. I like it because it communicates the heat. You get the heat. That's why I want to add a trumpet player to the band, because a trumpet communicates incredible heat" ("The Lost Interviews. 1975").

105. When Springsteen sang "In Freehold"—a funny song written for the occasion—during a 1996 concert at his old school, he added a verse confessing that his first kiss was with a girl called Maria Espinoza. *The Asbury Park Press* immediately set out to trace her. They found she was still living in Freehold and was married with four children and four grandchildren. Maria said she was very surprised that Bruce even remembered her name. She said the kiss had lasted a minute, had been great—and that she'd often dreamed about it afterwards. She'd never confessed it to anyone when she was young because her parents didn't allow her to have boyfriends, and later, when Springsteen became famous, no one would have believed her anyway. Nonetheless, as the years passed, she recalled the solitary hippie who'd been the only kid with a leather jacket and long hair in those days. Maria had considered him sweet and very good-looking. Oh, and he wasn't racist. As of 1958 the Espinozas were only the second Puerto Rican family to settle in Freehold.

106. Ariel Swartley, "The Wild, the Innocent & the E Street Shuffle."

107. Bruce Springsteen, "Jackson Browne's Rock & Roll Hall of Fame Induction Speech" (Waldorf Astoria, New York, March 15, 2004).

108. Rick Moody, quoted in Benjamin Hedin, *Studio A: The Bob Dylan Reader* (New York, W. W. Norton & Company, 2004).

109. Jon Landau, "Growing Young with Rock and Roll," *The Real Paper*, May 22, 1974.

110. Bruce Springsteen, interviewed for the *Wings for Wheels* home video (2005).

111. Ibid.

112. Ibid.

113. Ibid. In 1981, Springsteen said he still didn't agree with his band-mate: "Spontaneity," he said, "is not made by fastness. Elvis, I believe, did like thirty takes of 'Hound Dog,' and you put that thing on, and it just explodes." (Bruce Springsteen, quoted in Louis P. Masur, "Tramps Like Us. The Birth of 'Born to Run,'" *Slate*, September 22, 2009).

114. Roy Bittan, quoted in Louis P. Masur, "Tramps Like Us. The Birth of 'Born to Run.'"

115. Mauro Zambellini, "Born to Run," *Il Mucchio Selvaggio*, giugno 1992.

116. Greil Marcus, "Springsteen's Thousand and One American Nights," *Rolling Stone*, October 9, 1975.

117. Massimo Cotto, "Born to Run," *Velvet Gallery*, June 1990.

118. Jerry Gilbert, "Bruce: Under the Boardwalk," *Sounds*, March 16, 1974.

119. Nick Hornby, *Songbook* (San Francisco: McSweeney's, 2002).

120. John Winthorp, quoted in Edmund Clarence Stedman and Ellen Mackay Hutchinson, *A Library of American Literature*, Vol. 1. (New York: Charles Webster, 1889).

121. Gary Graff, "Elvis Presley," in *The Ties that Bind: Bruce Springsteen A to E to Z*, ed. Gary Graff (Canton: Visible Ink Press, 2005). Springsteen has played many songs from Elvis's repertoire at his concerts: "Can't Help Falling in Love," "Heartbreak Hotel," "Hound Dog," "Mystery Train," "Good Rockin' Tonight," "Jailhouse Rock," "Burning Love" ... In the early 1980s he wrote his own version of "Follow That Dream," the title song of Presley's 1961 movie (it was released only in 1998 on the *Tracks* box set) and he recorded "Viva Las Vegas" for the 1990 benefit tribute album *The Last Temptation of Elvis*. A lot of Springsteen's songs are haunted by the ghost of Elvis:: "Johnny Bye Bye"—a B-side for the 1985 single "I'm on Fire"—is about Presley's death; "Pink Cadillac" (on the B-side of the 1984 single "Dancing in the Dark" has its roots in one of Presley's favorite rides; "57 Channels (And Nothin' On)" finds Springsteen firing a bullet at his TV screen "in the blessed name of Elvis," with a reference to legends about Presley shooting up his own TV when he wasn't happy with what was on. Then there's "Fire," a song that Springsteen wrote in the mid-1970s just for Elvis even though "there's no hard evidence to confirm the numerous reports that he had sent a demo of 'Fire' to Graceland for Presley's consideration" (Ibid.).

122. Two pairs of literary friends come to mind: Ishmael and Queequeg in *Moby Dick* and Huck and Jim in *The Adventures of Huckleberry Finn*.

123. Louis P. Masur, *Runaway Dream. Born to Run and Bruce Springsteen's American Vision* (New York: Bloomsbury Press, 2010).

124. "That's what great rock is about to me," Springsteen says. "It make the dream seem possible" (Robert Hilburn. "Out in the Streets," *Los Angeles Times*, October 1980).

125. That "Scooter" who together with "the Big Man bust this city in half" in "Tenth Avenue Freeze-Out."

126. Mark Twain, *Roughing It* (Chicago: American Publishing Company, 1872).

127. Alexis de Tocqueville, *Selected Letters on Politics and Society*. Ed. Roger Boesche (Berkley: University of California Press, 1985).

128. Bruce Springsteen, quoted in Mark Hagen. "The Midnight Cowboy," *Mojo*, January 1999.

129. Christopher Vogler, *The Writer's Journey: Mythic Structure for Writers* (Los Angeles: Michael Wiese Productions, 2007).

130. Antonella D'Amore, *Mia città di rovine. L'America di Bruce Springsteen* (Roma: Manifestolibri, 2002).

131. Ibid.

132. *The Grapes of Wrath*, directed by John Ford. 20th Century Fox, 1940.

133. The Lady of the House of Sleep is an allegory of the femme fatale, a mythic figure, and "the paragon of all paragons of beauty. The reply to all desire, the bliss-bestowing goal of every hero's earthly and unearthly quest. She is mother, sister, mistress, bride." Jospeh Campbell, *The Hero with a Thousand Faces* (New York: Pantheon Books, 1949).

134. Robert Graves, *The White Goddess* (London: Faber & Faber, 1948).

135. Bruce Springsteen, "Jackson Browne's Rock & Roll Hall of Fame Induction Speech."

136. Crosby, Stills & Nash. "Guinnevere," from *Crosby, Stills & Nash* (1969).

137. Tom Waits, "Burma Shave," from *Foreign Affairs* (1977).

138. The Velvet Underground, "Femme Fatale," from *The Velvet Underground & Nico* (1967).

139. William Faulkner, *The Sound and the Fury* (London: Jonathan Cape and Harrison Smith, 1929).

140. Mikal Gilmore, "American Skin," liner notes in *The Ties that Bind: The River Collection* box set (2016).

141. Bruce Springsteen, quoted in Mark Hagen, "Midnight Cowboy."

142. Ray Coleman, "Springsteen Crazy," *Melody Maker*, November 1975.

143. Bruce Springsteen, quoted in Dave DiMartino, "Bruce Springsteen Takes It to the River: So Don't Call Him Boss, OK?" *Creem*, January 1981.

144. Ermanno Labianca, *American Skin. Vita e musica di Bruce Springsteen* (Firenze: Giunti, 2000).

145. Alessandro Portelli. *Badlands. Springsteen e l'America: il lavoro e i sogni* (Roma: Donzelli, 2015).

146. Bruce Springsteen, *Songs* (New York: HarperEntertainment, 2003).

147. Paul Nelson, "Let Us Now Praise Famous Men," *Rolling Stone*, December 1980.

148. Bruce Springsteen, quoted in Patrick Humphries, "Springsteen," *Record Collector*, February 1999.

149. Herman Melville, *Moby-Dick; or, The Whale* (New York: Harper & Brothers, 1851).

150. June Skinner Sawyers, introduction to *Racing in the Street. The Bruce Springsteen Reader*.

151. With *The River*, Springsteen aced the annual referendum held by *The Rolling Stone*, winning seven categories on nine: best artist for critics and readers, best male vocalist and composer, best album and best single for the readers, wile the E Street Band was voted by the readers band of the year.

152. Jonathan Cott, "The Lost Lennon Tapes," *Rolling Stone*, December 8, 2010.

153. In the following order: "Bye Bye Johnny," "Starkweather (Nebraska)," "Atlantic City," "Mansion on The Hill," Born in the U.S.A., "Johnny 99," "Downbound Train," "Losin' Kind," "State Trooper," "Used Cars," "Wanda (Open All Night)," "Child Bride," "Pink Cadillac," "Highway Patrolman," and "Reason to Believe."

154. In an interview, the drummer of the E Street Band Max Weinberg reveals that Springsteen recorded all *Nebraska*'s material together with the band (Andy Greene, "Max Weinberg on His Future with Conan and Bruce," *Rolling Stone*, June 2010).

155. Luca Raimondo, "Soundcheck: 'Nebraska,'" *Follow That Dream*, June 1991.

156. Bryan K. Garman, "The Ghost of History: Bruce Springsteen, Woody Guthrie, and the Hurt Song," *Popular Music and Society*, Summer 1996.

157. Bruce Springsteen, quoted in Robert Hilburn, "Out in the Streets."

158. Cornel Bonca, "Save Me Somebody: Bruce Springsteen's Rock 'n' Roll Covenant," *Killing the Buddha*, July 29, 2001.

159. Flannery O'Connor, *Mystery & Manners: Occasional Prose*, ed. Sally and Robert Fitzgerald (New York: Farrar, Straus & Giroux, 1961).

160. Lorine M. Getz, "Nature and Grace in Flannery O'Connor's Fiction," in *Studies in Art and Religious Interpretation*, 2 (New York: Mellen, 1982).

161. "Domine Deus meus [...] opus est gratia tua et magna gratia, ut vincatur natura ad malum semper prona ab adolescentia sua" (*De Imitatione Christi*, III 55, 2).

162. Bruce Springsteen, quoted in Will Percy. "Rock and Read: Will Percy Interviews Bruce Springsteen." *Double Take*, Spring 1998.

163. Bruce Springsteen, quoted in *Springsteen dalla A alla Z*.

164. Bruce Springsteen, quoted in Neil Strauss. "Springsteen Looks Back but Keeps Walking On." *The New York Times*, May 7, 1995.

165. Antonella D'Amore, *Mia città di rovine*.

166. Dave Marsh. *Glory Days: Bruce Springsteen in the 1980s* (New York: Pantheon Books, 1987).

167. Flannery O'Connor, *Mystery & Manners*.

168. Bruce Springsteen. *Songs*.

169. Advice to a young writer from William Price Fox: "Forget punctuation and spelling. Look for the phrasing. Read Jane Austen and Flannery O'Connor. Establish character in a hurry. Show rather than tell."

Pam Kingsbury, "Humor That's Southern Fried. An Interview with William Price Fox," in *Inner Voices, Inner View: Conversations with Southern Writers* (Norwalk: Enolam Group, 2005).

170. Blue Bottazzi, "Bruce Springsteen: 'Nebraska,'" *Il Mucchio Selvaggio*, November 1982.

171. Walker Percy, *The Moviegoer* (New York: Knopf, 1961).

172. Bruce Springsteen, quoted in Will Percy, "Rock and Read."

173. Debby Bull, "Bruce Springsteen Gives the Little Guy Something to Cheer About," *Rolling Stone*, July 19–August 2, 1984.

174. Benjamin Franklin, *The Autobiography: 1706–1757*. Bedford: Applewood Books, 2008.

175. Bobbie Ann Mason, *In Country* (New York: Harper & Row, 1985). The novel tells the story of the relationship between Vietnam War veteran Emmett and his niece Samantha, whose father died in the war. In Sam's quest to learn about her father, she develops a crush on Tom, another Vietnam veteran, and she looks upon the persona of Bruce Springsteen in *Born in the U.S.A.* as a father figure.

176. Mikal Gilmore, "Bruce Springsteen: What Does It Mean, Springsteen Asked, to Be an American?" *Rolling Stone*, November 15, 1980.

177. Ibid.

178. Christopher Borick and David Rosenwasser, "Springsteen's Right Side: A Liberal Icon's Conservatorism" (paper at the Bruce Springsteen Symposium, West Long Branch, NJ, September 26, 2009).

179. Bruce Springsteen, speech at Barack Obama Presidential Rally, Madison, WI, November 5, 2012.

180. Rob Kirkpatrick, *The Words and Music of Bruce Springsteen* (Westport: Greenwood, 2007).

181. William Shakespeare, *Macbeth*, Act V, Scene I (London: Penguin, 2007).

182. Mikal Gilmore, "The Ghost of Tom Joad," *Rolling Stone*, December 17, 1995.

183. Sebastian Rotella, "Children of the Border," *Los Angeles Times*, April 3, 1993.

184. Mark Arax and Tom Gordo, "California's Illicit Farm Belt Export," *Los Angeles Times*, March 19, 1995.

185. Dale Maharidge, *Journey to Nowhere—The Saga of the New Underclass*, photography by Michael Williamson (New York: Hyperion Books, 1986).

186. Morris Dees, *A Season for Justice* (New York: Charles Scribner's Sons, 1991).

187. John Steinbeck, *The Grapes of Wrath* (New York: The Viking Press-James Lloyd, 1939).

188. Bruce Springsteen. *Songs*.

189. Ezra Pound, *ABC of Reading* (Cambridge: New Directions, 1934).

190. Frank O'Connor, quoted by Alfred Kazin, *Bright Book of Life*.

191. Ariel Swartley, "The Wild, the Innocent & the E Street Shuffle."

192. The album included "Vigilante Man" and "Ain't Got No Home," two songs Springsteen went on to record in 1988 for the Guthrie and Leadbelly tribute album *Folkways: A Vision Shared*.

193. Eva Davis was the first singer to record "John Hardy" for Columbia in 1924. Witnesses to the murder said Hardy lost twenty-five, not fifty cents.

194. Anthony O. Scott, "The Poet Laureate of 9/11: Apocalypse and Salvation on Springsteen's New Album," *Slate*, August 6, 2002.

195. Bruce Springsteen, quoted in Mark Binelli. "Bruce Springsteen's American Gospel," *Rolling Stone*, August 22, 2002.

196. Bruce Springsteen, quoted in Samuel Graydon, "America Needs Bruce Springsteen," *The Times Litlerary Supplement*, October 26, 2016.

197. Christopher Phillips, "Seachin' Through the Dust," *Backstreets* #75, Fall 2002.

198. Alan Light, "The Missing," *The New Yorker*, August 5, 2002.

199. Ibid.

200. Keith Harris, "Lift Every Voice," *The Village Voice*, August 6, 2002.

201. Alexis Petridis, "CD of the Week: Bruce Springsteen and the E Street Band," *The Guardian*, July 25, 2002.

202. Emily Dickinson, "Poem 263," in *The Poems of Emily Dickinson.*

203. Alan Light, "The Missing."

204. David Carithers, "'Come On and Rise Up:' Springsteen's Experiential Art after 9/11," *Nebula*, September 2005.

205. Don DeLillo, "In the Ruins of the Future: Reflections on Terror and Loss in the Shadow of September," *Harper's*, December 2001.

206. Two songs were actually performed on that tour: "The Hitter" and "Long Time Comin'."

207. Bruce Springsteen, quoted in Bryan Hiatt, "Springsteen Goes Back to Basics," *Rolling Stone*, April 21, 2005.

208. Ibid.

209. Ermanno Labianca and Giovanni Canitano, *Real World. Sulle strade di Bruce Springsteen* (Roma: Fazi, 2005).

210. Bruce Springsteen, introducing "Jesus Was an Only Son" at Xcel Energy Center, St. Paul, MN, May 10, 2005.

211. Bruce Springsteen, introducing "Jesus Was an Only Son" at Rose Garden Theater of The Clouds, Portland, OR, August 10, 2005.

212. "Freud is smiling in his grave somewhere," Springsteen commented introducing the song at Forest National, Brussels, Belgium, May 30, 2005.

213. "There's something humorous about 'Maria's Bed,' where he's so taken with this woman's sleeping and fucking arrangements, he could be describing the Mississippi River, or the face of God, or eternal bliss itself. When he sings, 'Then I drank the cool clear waters from Maria's bed,' my first thought was: Is it a water bed?" (Peter S. Scholtes, quoted in Christopher Phillips, "The Devil's in the Details," *Backstreets* double issue #83/84, Winter 2005/2006.)

214. Ermanno Labianca and Giovanni Canitano. *Real World.*

215. Dave Marsh. *Two Hearts.*

216. Ben Greenman, "American Sounds," *The New Yorker*, October 1, 2007.

217. Erik Flanningan, "Trust None of What You Hear," *Backstreets* #87, Spring 2008.

218. Although *Magic* debuted at #1 on the U.S. *Billboard* 200 chart, becoming Springsteen's eighth #1 album in the U.S. and selling about 335,000 copies in its first week, it received very little radio airplay.

219. David Fricke, "Bruce Springsteen: Magic," *Rolling Stone*, October 18, 2007.

220. During the speech he gave in Philadelphia on October 4, 2008, for Barack Obama's election campaign, Springsteen declared: "I've spent most of my creative life measuring the distance between that American promise and American reality. For many Americans, who are today losing their jobs, their homes, seeing their retirement funds disappear, who have no healthcare, or who have been abandoned in our inner cities, the distance between that promise and that reality has never been greater or more painful. . . . After the disastrous administration of the past eight years, we need somebody to lead us in an American reclamation project. . . . Now, I don't know about you, but I know that I want my house back, I want my America back, and I want my country back."

221. *Home of the Brave* is the title of a film directed by Irwin Winkler in 2006 that tells the story of four American soldiers in Iraq.

222. Bruce Springsteen, quoted in Josh Tyrangiel, "Born to Stump," *Time*, October 10, 2004.

223. Jim Beviglia, "Bruce Springsteen: 'Wrecking Ball,'" *American Songwriter*, March 5, 2012.

224. Leonard Pitts Jr., "Springsteen Captures the State of America," *Chicago Tribune*, March 21, 2012.

225. Bruce Springsteen, international press conference at Théâtre Marigny, Paris, France, February 16, 2012. He added that he started to write the songs for the album "when we had the huge financial crisis in the States, and there was really no accountability for years and years. People lost their homes, and I had friends who were losing their homes, and nobody went to jail. Nobody was responsible."

People lost enormous amounts of their net worth. Previous to Occupy Wall Street, there was no push-back: there was no movement, there was no voice that was saying just how outrageous—that a basic theft had occurred that struck at the heart of what the entire American idea was about."

226. Christopher Phillips, "Heck of a Job, Brucie," *Backstreets* #91, Fall/Winter 2013.

227. "I grew up in a Democratic house," Springsteen says. "The only political discussion I ever remember in my house was when I came home from school when I was little—I think someone asked me at school what we were. . . . I was probably eight or nine. And I came home and said, "Mom, what are we?" And she said, "Oh, we're Democrats. We're Democrats because they're for the working people." And that was it—that was the political discussion that went on in my house over about eighteen years" (Bruce Springsteen, quoted in Christopher Phillips, "Citizen Bruce," *Backstreets* #95, Summer/Fall 2004).

228. Barack Obama, quoted in Andy Greene, "Bruce Springsteen, Billy Joel Form Supergroup for Obama in NYC," *Rolling Stone*, October 17, 2008.

229. During the international press conference at Théâtre Marigny, Paris, France, February 16, 2012, he said, "I think he did a lot of good things. He kept GM alive, which was incredibly important to Detroit, Michigan. He got the healthcare law passed, though I wish there had been a public option and that it didn't leave citizens the victims of the insurance companies. He killed Osama bin Laden, which I think was extremely important. He brought some sanity to the top level of government. He's more friendly to corporations than I thought he would be, and there aren't as many middle-class or working-class voices heard in the administration as I thought there would be. I would have liked to see more active job creation sooner than it came, and I'd like to have seen some of these foreclosures stopped or somehow mitigated. The banks have had some kind of a settlement, a partial settlement, but really, there's a lot of people it's not going to assist. I still support the president, but there are plenty of things . . . I thought Guantánamo would have been closed by now. On the other hand, we're out of Iraq, and hopefully we'll be out of Afghanistan soon."

230. Stefano Pistolini, "Separare le carriere della politica e del rock," *IL*, October 2012.

231. Leon Wieseltier, "A Saint in the City."

232. Ibid.

233. Bruce Springsteen, International Press Conference at Théâtre Marigny, Paris, France, February 16, 2012.

234. Aristotle Tziampiris, "Why Springsteen Could Have Been President," *The Huffington Post*, August 30, 2016.

235. Peter Chianca, "Tired Fans to Bruce Springsteen: Cut It Out!" posted August 29, 2016, http://www.wickedlocal.com/

236. Bruce Springsteen. *Born to Run*.

237. In his autobiography, Springsteen wrote that he has been on antidepressants for the last twelve to fifteen years of his life, explaining that he was hit by a heavy depression shortly after his sixtieth birthday that lasted for a year and a half and devasted him. He also said that depression struck again from sixty-three to sixy-four. Springsteen remained professionally productive during these periods, however, and he says that he recorded his fine 2012 album, *Wrecking Ball*, at one of his lowest ebbs.

238. Louis P. Masur, *Runaway Dream*.

239. Bruce Springsteen, quoted in Robert Hilburn, "Out in the Streets."

240. Bruce Springsteen, quoted in James Henke, "Interview to Bruce Springsteen."

241. Dave Marsh, *Glory Days*.

242. James Henke, "The Magician's Tool," *Backstreets* #89, Summer 2010.

243. In 1959, M.L. Rosenthal first used the term 'confessional' in a review of Robert Lowell's *Life Studies* entitled "Poetry as Confession," published in *The Nation*.

244. David Fricke, "Tunnel of Love," *Rolling Stone*, December 17, 1987.

245. Edgar Allan Poe, "Marginalia," *Democratic Review*, November, 1844.

246. Charles Baudelaire, "Mon coeur mis à nu," in *Journaux intimes* (Paris: Les Éditions G. Crés et Cie, 1920).

247. The river is a typical Springsteen location, often used as a symbol of life and redemption. In "The River," the waters that flow in the valley represent the Eden from which Adam and Eve were cast out; and in "Reason to Believe," a child is baptized in the river to "take away the sin." In "This Hard Land" and "Across the Border," the Rio Bravo (or Rio Grande) is the boundary to be crossed for reaching salvation; in "If I Should Fall Behind" there's a "beautiful river" where the central character and his woman will be married; then, in "Long Time Comin'," the man performs an outright ritual of purification and rebirth by walking into the low, sandy waters of a stream, on whose banks he and his love conceive their child. Equally, in "Racing in the Street," the two lovers run to the sea—this time—to wash their sins from their hands. Conversely, on occasion the river represents the exact opposite of life and salvation. In "Spare Parts," Janey "put her baby in the river, let the river roll on"; in "State Trooper" the big black rivers flow menacingly at the sides of the highway where the night driver loses himself; in "Real World" Springsteen once again resorts to the metaphor of "black river of doubt." The river becomes a symbol of death in "Matamoros Banks" ("for two days the river keeps you down, / Then you rise to the light without a sound"); while in "Paradise" it is actually used as the metaphor for the afterlife ("I search for you on the other side / Where the river runs clean and wide").

248. Jim Beviglia, "Counting Down Bruce Springsteen: #94, 'Valentine's Day,'" *American Songwriter*, June 30, 2014.

249. David Wyatt, *Out of the Sixties*.

250. Charles Baudelaire, "Mon coeur mis à nu."

251. Ibid.

252. Thomas Stearns Eliot, "Baudelaire," in *Selected Essays 1917–1932* (London: Faber & Faber, 1951).

253. Charles Baudelaire, "Mon coeur mis à nu."

254. June Skinner Sawyers, *Tougher than the Rest. 100 Best Bruce Springsteen Songs* (New York: Omnibus Press, 2006).

255. Christopher Sandford, *Springsteen: Point Blank*.

256. Jon Pareles, "Springsteen: An Old-Fashioned Rocker in a New Era," *The New York Times*, March 29, 1992.

257. Bruce Springsteen during the Dress Rehearsal Show held on June 5, 1992, at Hollywood Center Studios #4, Hollywood, CA.

258. Bruce Springsteen, international press conference at Théâtre Marigny, Paris, France, February 16, 2012.

259. Bruce Springsteen, quoted in Mark Hagen, "Meet the New Boss," *The Observer*, January 1, 2009.

260. Springsteen, quoted in Joe Levy, "The E Street Band Chief Talks About Making His Most Romantic Record Since 'Born to Run,'" *Rolling Stone*, November 1, 2007.

261. Brian Hiatt, "Bruce's Dream. An Intimate Visit," *Rolling Stone*, January 23, 2009.

262. Mark Hagen. "Meet the New Boss."

263. David Marchese, "The Boss Finally Gets What He Wants, but What About Us?" *Spin*, January 22, 2009.

264. Steve Van Zandt had already left during the *Born in the U.S.A.* sessions, replaced by Nils Lofgren on guitar. At that same moment, Patti Scialfa entered the band as vocalist.

265. Peter Ames Carlin, *Bruce* (New York: Touchstone, 2012).

266. The first one is an outtake form those 1983 sessions. The latter was re-recorded.

267. The song gained much of its popularity after being featured on the soundtrack for the 1996 movie *Jerry Maguire*.

268. William Carlos Williams, quoted in Robert Coles, *Bruce Springsteen's America: The People Listening, A Poet Singing* (New York: Random House, 2004).

269. Bruce Springsteen, quoted in Joe Levy, "The E Street Band Chief Talks About Making His Most Romantic Record Since 'Born to Run.'"

270. Mark Hagen, "Meet the New Boss."

271. Harold Bloom, *The Western Canon: The Books and Schools of the Age* (New York: Harcourt, 1994).

272. Ibid.

273. Ibid.

274. To name but twenty: Hawthorne, Melville, Poe, Twain, James, Hemingway, Faulkner, Fitzgerald, Nabokov's American half, Mailer, Salinger, Cheever, Bellow, Capote, Gaddis, Updike, Pynchon, Philip Roth, Toni Morrison, Cormac McCarthy.

275. Timothy Morris, *Becoming Canonical in American Poetry* (Chicago: University of Illinois Press, 1995).

276. Hugo Friedrich, *The Structure of Modern Poetry: From the Mid-nineteenth to the Mid-twentieth Century* (Evanston, Northwestern University Press, 1974).

277. Eugenio Montale, quoted in Christine Ott, *Montale e la parola riflessa* (Milano: Franco Angeli, 2006).

278. Even though, to tell the truth, the American novel from 1968 to 1973 produced a very noteworthy narrative corpus. It would suffice to quote Barth's *Lost in the Funhouse* (1968), Updike's *Couples* (1968), Roth's *Portnoy's Complaint* (1969), Nabokov's *Ada* (1969), Vonnegut's *Slaughterhouse-Five* (1969), Bellow's *Mr. Sammler's Planet* (1970), Doctorow's *The Book of Daniel* (1971), and Pynchon's *Gravity's Rainbow* (1973).

279. Robert Lowell, "Memories of West Street and Lepke," in *Life Studies* (New York: Farrar, Straus & Giroux, 1959).

280. *The Air-Conditioned Nightmare* is the title of Henry Miller's 1945 novel.

281. A May 1944 issue of *Life Magazine* has an article on high school trends described the new fad of sewing "Alcatraz '44" and "Sing Sing '45" on the backs of shirts and jean jackets.

282. The story is in Jon Savage, *Teenage: The Creation of Youth Culture* (New York: Viking, 2007).

283. The phrase "rocking and rolling" originally described the movement of a ship on the ocean. In 1934, the song "Rock and Roll" by the Boswell Sisters appeared in the film *Transatlantic Merry-Go-Round*.

284. June Skinner Sawyers. *Tougher than the Rest.*

285. "Bruce Springsteen: By the Book," *The New York Times*, November 2, 2014.

286. "Dirty realism" is a term coined by Bill Buford to define a literary movement born in America between the late seventies and early eighties of the last century. "Dirty Realism is the fiction of a new generation of American authors. They write about the belly-side of contemporary life—a deserted husband, an unwed mother, a car thief, a pickpocket, a drug addict—but they write about it with a disturbing detachment, at times verging on comedy. Understated, ironic, sometimes savage, but insistently compassionate, these stories constitute a new voice in fiction" (Bill Buford, "Dirty Realism," *Granta*, Summer 1983). Labeled as "dirty realists" were, among others, Raymond Carver, Richard Ford, Cormac McCarthy, Carson McCullers, and Jayne Anne Phillips.

287. "Bruce Springsteen: By the Book."

288. Raymond Carver. "Movement," in *Where Water Comes Together with Other Water*. New York: Vintage, 1986.

289. Raymond Carver, foreword to *Where I'm Calling From: Selected Stories* (New York: Vintage, 1988).

290. Huey Guagliardo, *Perspectives on Richard Ford: Redeemed by Affection* (Jackson: University Press of Mississippi, 2000).

291. Ernest Hemingway, quoted in Chadwick Hansen, "The Character of Jim and the Ending of 'Huckleberry Finn,'" *The Massachussetts Review*. Vol. 5, No. 1, Fall 1963.

292. Frank O'Connor, quoted in Alfred Kazin, *Bright Book of Life*.

293. Ernest Hemingway, "Hills Like White Elephants," in *Men Without Women* (New York: Charles Scribner's Sons, 1927).

294. In 1939, critic Philip Rahv wrote an essay in which he divided American literature between two polar types, redskin and paleface, creating "a dissociation between energy and sensibility." The redskins were spontaneous, emotional, rebellious, the palefaces refined and intellectual. Each type had its virtues, and its faults. "At his highest level," Rahv said, "the paleface moves in an exquisite moral atmosphere; at his lowest he is genteel, snobbish, and pedantic." Rahv went on: "In giving expression to the vitality and to the aspirations of the people, the redskin is at his best; but at his worst he is a vulgar anti-intellectual, combining aggression with conformity and reverting to the crudest forms of frontier psychology." Philip Rahv, "Paleface and Redskin," in *Essays on Literature and Politics 1932–1972* (Boston: Houghton Mifflin, 1978).

295. Ernest Hemingway, *Death in the Afternoon* (New York: Charles Scribner's Sons, 1932).

296. We might mention Bryan K. Garman, *A Race of Singers: Whitman's Working Class Hero from Guthrie to Springsteen* (Chapel Hill: University of North Carolina Press, 2000).

297. Robert Coles, *Bruce Springsteen's America*.

298. Giorgio Manganelli, foreword to Walt Whitman, *Foglie d'erba* (Milano: Rizzoli, 2004).

299. Walt Whitman, "From Paumanock starting, I fly like a bird," in *Leaves of Grass*.

300. *Calamus* comprises a group of forty-five poems added to the 1860 edition of *Leaves of Grass*. Whitman describes the erect, jagged steles of the title's semi-aquatic plant with almost loving pleasure to the UK editor, W.M. Rossetti.

301. Harold Bloom, *The Western Canon*.

302. Walt Whitman, "I Hear It Was Charged Against Me," in *Leaves of Grass*.

303. Walt Whitman, "As I Ponder'd in Silence," in *Leaves of Grass*.

304. Ernest Hemingway, *A Farewell to Arms* (New York: Charles Scribner's Sons, 1929).

305. Walt Whitman, "As Time Draws Nigh," in *Leaves of Grass*.

306. Bruce Springsteen, quoted in David Kamp, "The Book of Bruce Springsteen," *Vanity Fair*, October 2016.

307. Ibid.

308. Herman Melville. *Moby-Dick*.

309. Robert Lowell. "The Quaker Graveyard in Nantucket," in *Lord Weary's Castle*. San Diego: Harcourt Brace, 1946.

310. Walt Whitman, "O Me! O Life!," in *Leaves of Grass*.

EDITOR'S NOTE
by Leonardo Colombati

The lyrics of 91 songs out of the 320 written and published by Springsteen between January 1973 and September 2017 are here presented.

The rules guiding the selection are merely subjective, as is the disposition of the text; it is neither in chronological order of composition nor of publishing, but rather follows a thematic subdivision consisting in three sections.

The first ("Jungleland") is composed of a collection of lyrics in which Springsteen tells about his childhood and youth in New Jersey, transforming his own autobiography into the story of the quest for the Promised Land: an escape in search of the American Dream of whose failures and consequences Springsteen also tells.

The second section ("This Hard Land") is composed of the lyrics belonging to the songs through which Springsteen wanted to measure the distance between the American dream and American reality, starting from the eighties and through all of the nineties, right into the twenty-first century, tragically inaugurated with the Twin Tower attack and the shock of a new Great Depression.

The third section ("Better Days") is composed of his more autobiographical works, through which Springsteen tries to portray both sides of his rise to fame, the happy and less happy aspects: the boy with high hopes who actually fulfills his dream, though here shares some of the prices he had to pay.

Presenting the American singer-songwriter's most significant lyrics in this order, I hope it will become possible to pick up on the continuous correspondence bouncing from one Springsteen album to another, and, above all, to enjoy a real story to the point of appreciating it as, though perhaps less well known, an immensely powerful Great American Novel.

♦ ♦ ♦

"They're songs," Dylan once said. "They're not written in stone. They're on plastic."[1] Considering the particular nature of the song lyrics it seems right to adopt flexible philological tools; songs are "written" for the purpose of being sung, not read: their lyrics are never definitive and chaos overrides the rules behind transcription.

Song lyrics, with their uncertain, arbitrary first lines, often resemble a jumbled mixture of "chance verses." However, this randomness is not in itself a part of the song's original structure; it is more in the superficiality of those who transcribed it time after time (perhaps using the the rule of merging short verses together just to save space on the page). When a song lyric has to be copied, sources come in the most diverse and ephemeral forms: the author's original draft; its official registration with a music publisher, if there is one; the transposition on the sleeves of the respective albums; the spread of its release on the Internet, of a purely voluntary nature; the notes jotted down on the sides of the music scores; some books having promptly printed them; the transposition of recorded sound onto the page. Apart from this last case, all other forms of transcription are precarious and unreliable, in their punctuation, their division of verses and even spelling.

Hence, for this book I have trusted above all the element of sound, convinced as I am that only through listening can one transcribe a song as closely as possible, or at least *that* song in *that* specific recording. Obviously, for one song different performances can exist, perhaps in live recordings. And in this case the adopted rule has been to choose the *editio princeps*, giving special mention to the significant variants.

Punctuation is usually banned from song lyrics printed on album librettos, a universally recognized convention with no literary or stylistic reasons backing it (as those dictating Apollinaire's same choice), but only those deriving from slovenliness and idleness. In presenting the songs, I have therefore taken the responsibility of *inventing* the punctuation; I found myself facing the possibility of opting either for an operation guaranteeing the minimum acceptable amount of commas and indents, or for a more heavy-going one, able to transform the *lyrics* into *texts*: the second option seemed to me the far more coherent choice for this project.

---

1. Bob Dylan, quoted in Paul Zollo, *Songwriters on Songwriting* (New York: Da Capo Press, 2005).

LIKE A KILLER IN THE SUN

1972–2017

by Bruce Springsteen

PROLOGUE

American Land

What is this land America so many travel there?
I'm going now while I'm still young: my darling, meet me there.
Wish me luck, my lovely, I'll send for you when I can
And we'll make our home in the American land.

Over there all the woman wear silk and satin to their knees
And children, dear, the sweets, I hear, are growing on the trees,
Gold comes rushing out the rivers straight into your hands
When you make your home in the American Land.

> There's diamonds in the sidewalks, there's gutters lined in song,
> Dear, I hear that beer flows through the faucets all night long,
> There's treasure for the taking, for any hard working man
> Who will make his home in the American land.

I docked at Ellis Island in a city of light and spire,
She met me in the valley of red-hot steel and fire,[i]
We made the steel that built the cities with the sweat of our two hands
And we made our home in the American land.

> There's diamonds in the sidewalks, there's gutters lined in song,
> Dear, I hear that beer flows through the faucets all night long,
> There's treasure for the taking, for any hard working man
> Who will make his home in the American land.

The McNicholas, the Posalskis, the Smiths, Zerillis[ii] too,
The Blacks, the Irish, the Italians, the Germans and the Jews,
Come across the water a thousand miles from home
With nothing in their bellies but the fire down below.[iii]

They died building the railroads, worked to bones and skin,
They died in the fields and factories, names scattered in the wind
They died to get here a hundred years ago, they're dyin' now
The hands that built the country were all trying to keep down.[iv]

> There's diamonds in the sidewalks, there's gutters lined in song,
> Dear, I hear that beer flows through the faucets all night long,
> There's treasure for the taking, for any hard working man
> Who will make his home in the American land.

ONE

Jungleland

Growin' Up

Used Cars

My little sister's in the front seat with an ice cream cone,
My ma's in the back seat sittin' all alone
As my pa steers her slow out of the lot
For a test drive down Michigan Avenue.[i]

Now, my ma, she fingers her wedding band
And watches the salesman stare at my old man's hands.
He's tellin' us all 'bout the break he'd give us if he could, but he just can't.
Well, if I could, I swear I know just what I'd do.

> Now, mister, the day the lottery I win
> I ain't ever gonna ride in no used car again.

Now, the neighbours come from near and far
As we pull up in our brand new used car.
I wish he'd just hit the gas and let out a cry
And tell 'em all they can kiss our asses goodbye.

My dad, he sweats the same job from mornin' to morn,
Me, I walk home on the same dirty streets where I was born.
Up the block I can hear my little sister in the front seat blowin' that horn:
The sounds echoin' all down Michigan Avenue.

Now, mister, the day my numbers comes in
> I ain't ever gonna ride in no used car again.

Mansion on the Hill

There's a place out on the edge of town, sir,
Risin' above the factories and the fields.
Now, ever since I was a child I can remember
That mansion on the hill.

In the day you can see the children playing
On the road that leads to those gates of hardened steel,
Steel gates that completely surround, sir,
The mansion on the hill.
At night my daddy'd take me and we'd ride
Through the streets of a town so silent and still,
Park on a back road along the highway side,
Look up at that mansion on the hill.

In the summer all the lights would shine,
There'd be music playin', people laughin' all the time.
Me and my sister we'd hide out in the tall corn fields,
Sit and listen to the mansion on the hill.

Tonight, down here in Linden Town[i]
I watch the cars rushin' by home from the mill.
There's a beautiful full moon rising
Above the mansion on the hill.

My Father's House

Last night I dreamed that I was a child
Out where the pines grow wild and tall,
I was trying to make it home through the forest
Before the darkness falls.

I heard the wind rustling through the trees
And ghostly voices rose from the fields.[i]
I ran with my heart pounding down that broken path
With the devil snappin' at my heels.[ii]

I broke through the trees and there in the night
My father's house stood shining hard and bright.
The branches and brambles tore my clothes, scratched my arms,
But I ran till I fell, shaking in his arms.

I awoke and I imagined the hard things that pulled us apart:
Will never again, sir, tear us from each other's hearts.
I got dressed and to that house I did ride
From out on the road, I could see its windows shining in light.

I walked up the steps and stood on the porch,
A woman I didn't recognize came and spoke to me through a chained door.
I told her my story, and who I'd come for.
She said, "I'm sorry, son, but no one by that name lives here anymore."

My father's house shines hard and bright,
It stands like a beacon calling me in the night,
Calling and calling, so cold and alone,
Shining 'cross this dark highway where our sins lie unatoned.

Growin' Up

I stood stone-like at midnight
Suspended in my masquerade,
and I combed my hair till it was just right[i]
And commanded the night brigade.

I was open to pain and crossed by the rain
And I walked on a crooked crutch.
I strolled all alone through a fallout zone
And came out with my soul untouched.

> I hid in the clouded wrath of the crowd
> But when they said, "Sit down" I stood up.
> Ooh-ooh, growin' up.

The flag of piracy flew from my mast,
My sails were set wing to wing.
I had a jukebox graduate for first mate,
She couldn't sail but she sure could sing.

I pushed B-52 and bombed 'em with the blues
With my gear set stubborn on standing,
I broke all the rules, strafed my old high school,
Never once gave thought to landing.

> I hid in the clouded wrath of the crowd
> But when they said, "Come down" I threw up.
> Ooh-ooh, growin' up.

I took month-long vacations in the stratosphere
And you know it's really hard to hold your breath.
I swear I lost everything I ever loved or feared,
I was the cosmic kid in full costume dress.

Well, my feet they finally took root in the earth
But I got me a nice little place in the stars
And I swear I found the key to the universe
In the engine of an old parked car.

> I hid in the mother breast of the crowd
> But when they said, "Pull down" I pulled up.
> Ooh-ooh, growin' up.

Spirit in the Night

Crazy Janey and her mission man
Were back in the alley tradin' hands.
'Long came Wild Billy with his friend G-man
All duded up for Saturday night.

Well, Billy slammed on his coaster brakes
And said, "Anybody wanna go on up to Greasy Lake?[i]
It's about a mile down on the dark side of route 88,
I got a bottle of rosé, so let's try it.

We'll pick up Hazy Davy and Killer Joe
And I'll take you all out to where the gypsy angels go,
They're built like light
and they dance like spirits in the night

    (All night) in the night (all night),
    Oh, you don't know what they can do to you,
    Spirits in the night
    (all night) in the night (all night),
    Stand right up now and let it shoot through you."

Now, wild young Billy was a crazy cat
And he shook some dust out of his coonskin cap.
He said, "Trust some of this it'll show you where you're at,
Or at least it'll help you really feel it."

By the time we made it up to Greasy Lake
I had my head out the window and Janey's fingers were in the cake.
I think I really dug her 'cause I was too loose to fake.
I said, "I'm hurt." She said, "Honey, let me heal it."

And we danced all night to a soul fairy band
And she kissed me just right like only a lonely angel can.
She felt so nice, just as soft as a spirit in the night

    (All night) in the night (all night),
    Janey, don't know what she do to you.
    Like a spirit in the night

(all night) all night (all night),
Stand right up and let her shoot through me.

Now, the night was bright and the stars threw light
On Billy and Davy dancin' in the moonlight.
They were down near the water in a stone mud fight,
Killer Joe gone passed out on the lawn.

Well, now Hazy Davy got really hurt;
He ran into the lake in just his socks and a shirt.
Me and Crazy Janey was makin' love in the dirt[ii]
Singin' our birthday songs.

Janey said it was time to go,
So we closed our eyes and said goodbye
To gypsy angel row, felt so right,
Together we moved like spirits in the night,

(All night) in the night (all night),
oh, you don't know what they can do to you,
Spirits in the night,
(all night) all night (all night),
Stand right up and let her shoot through you.

Incident on 57th Street[i]

Spanish Johnny[ii] drove in
From the underworld last night
With bruised arms and broken rhythm in a beat-up old Buick,
But dressed just like dynamite.
He tried sellin' his heart to the hard girls
Over on Easy Street,[iii]
But they sighed, "Johnny it falls apart so easy
And you know hearts these days are cheap."

And the pimps swung their axes
And said, "Johnny, you're a cheater."
Well, the pimps swung their axes
And said, "Johnny, you're a liar."
And from out of the shadows came a young girl's voice
Said, "Johnny, don't cry."

Puerto Rican Jane,[iv]
Oh, won't you tell me what's your name?
I want to drive you down to the other side of town where paradise ain't so
    crowded.
There'll be action goin' down on Shanty Lane[v] tonight,
All them golden-heeled fairies in a real bitch fight.
Pull .38s and kiss the girls good night.

> Oh, good night, it's alright Jane,
> Now, let them black boys in to light the soul flame,
> We may find it out on the street tonight, baby,
> Or we may walk until the daylight, maybe.

Well, like a cool Romeo he made his moves,
Oh, she looked so fine!
Like a late Juliet she knew he'd never be true
But then she didn't really mind.
Upstairs a band was playin',
Singer was singin' something about goin' home.
She whispered, "Spanish Johnny, you can leave me tonight
But just don't leave me alone."

And Johnny cried, "Puerto Rican Jane,
Word is down the cops have found the vein.
Oh, them barefoot boys left their homes for the woods,
Them little barefoot street boys they say homes ain't no good,
They left the corners, threw away all their switchblade knives
And kissed each other good-bye."

Johnny was sittin' on the fire escape
Watchin' the kids playin' down the street.
He called down, "Hey little heroes, summer's long,
But I guess it ain't very sweet around here anymore."
Janey sleeps in sheets damp with sweat,
Johnny sits up alone and watches her dream on,
And the sister prays for lost then breaks down in the chapel
After everyone's gone.

Jane moves over to share her pillow
But opens her eyes to see Johnny up and putting his clothes on.
She says, "Those romantic young boys,
All they ever want to do is fight."
Those romantic young boys,
They're callin' through the window,
"Hey Spanish Johnny,
You want to make a little easy money tonight?"

   And Johnny whispered, "Good night, it's all right Jane,
   I'll meet you tomorrow night on Lover's Lane.
   We may find it out on the street tonight, baby,
   Or we may walk until the daylight, maybe."

New York City Serenade

Billy, he's down by the railroad tracks[i]
Sittin' low in the back seat of his Cadillac.
Diamond Jackie, she's so intact
As she falls so softly beneath him.

Jackie's heels are stacked,
Billy's got cleats on his boots,[ii]
Together they're gonna boogaloo[iii] down Broadway
And come back home with the loot.

It's midnight in Manhattan,
This is no time to get cute,
It's a mad dog's promenade.
So walk tall or, baby, don't walk at all.

Fish lady, oh fish lady,[iv]
She baits them tenement walls,
She won't take corner boys,
They ain't got no money and they're so easy.

I said, "Hey, baby, won't you take my hand and walk with me down Broadway?
Well, mama, take my arm and move with me down Broadway.
I'm a young man, I talk it real loud,
Yeah, babe I walk it real proud for you.

So shake away your street life,
Shake away your city life,
Hook up to the train,
And hook up to the night train."

But I know that she won't take the train,
No she won't take the train,
But I know that she won't take the train,
No she won't take the train,
But I know that she won't take the train,
No she won't take the train,
But I know that she won't take the train,
No she won't take the train . . .

She's afraid them tracks are gonna slow her down
And when she turns this boy'll be gone.
So long,
sometimes you just gotta walk on, walk on . . .

Hey vibes man, hey jazz man,
play me your serenade,
Any deeper blue
and you're playin' in your grave.[v]

Save your notes, don't spend 'em on the blues boy,
Save your notes, don't spend 'em on the darlin' yearlin' sharp boy.
Straight for the church note ringin',
vibes man sting a trash can.

Listen to your junk man,
Listen to your junk man,
Listen to your junk man:
He's singin',
He's singin',
He's singin',
All dressed up in satin,
Walkin' past the alley . . .

Meeting Across the River

Hey, Eddie, can you lend me a few bucks
And tonight can you get us a ride?
Gotta make it through the tunnel,[i]
Got a meeting with a man on the other side.
Hey Eddie, this guy, he's the real thing,
So if you want to come along
You gotta promise you won't say anything
'Cause this guy don't dance
And the word's been passed this is our last chance.

We gotta stay cool tonight, Eddie,
'Cause man, we got ourselves out on that line
And if we blow this one
They ain't gonna be looking for just me this time.
And all we gotta do is hold up our end,
Here stuff this in your pocket,
It'll look like you're carrying a friend.
And remember, just don't smile,
Change your shirt, 'cause tonight we got style.

Well, Cherry says she's gonna walk
'Cause she found out I took her radio and hocked it.
But Eddie, man, she don't understand
That two grand's practically sitting here in my pocket.
And tonight's gonna be everything that I said
And when I walk through that door
I'm just gonna throw that money on the bed.
She'll see this time I wasn't just talking
Then I'm gonna go out walking.[ii]

Hey Eddie, can you catch us a ride?

Jungleland

The rangers had a homecoming
In Harlem late last night
And the Magic Rat drove his sleek machine
Over the Jersey state line.
Barefoot girl sitting on the hood of a Dodge
Drinking warm beer in the soft summer rain.
The Rat pulls into town, rolls up his pants,
Together they take a stab at romance
And disappear down Flamingo Lane.[i]

Well, the Maximum Lawmen run down Flamingo
Chasing the Rat and the barefoot girl
And the kids round here look just like shadows,
Always quiet, holding hands.
From the churches to the jails
Tonight all is silence in the world
As we take our stand
Down in Jungleland.

The midnight gang's assembled
And picked a rendezvous for the night,
They'll meet 'neath that giant Exxon sign[ii]
That brings this fair city light.
Man, there's an opera[iii] out on the Turnpike,
There's a ballet being fought out in the alley
Until the local cops, Cherry Tops
Rips this holy night.

The street's alive as secret debts are paid,
Contacts made, they vanished unseen,
Kids flash guitars just like switchblades
Hustling for the record machine.
The hungry and the hunted
Explode into rock 'n' roll bands[iv]
That face off against each other out in the street
Down in Jungleland.

In the parking lot the visionaries
Dress in the latest rage,
Inside the backstreet girls are dancing
To the records that the dj plays.
Lonely-hearted lovers struggle in dark corners,
Desperate as the night moves on.
Just a look and a whisper, and they're gone.

Beneath the city two hearts beat,
Soul engines running through a night so tender,
In a bedroom locked, in whispers of soft
Refusal and then surrender.
In the tunnels uptown
The Rat's own dream guns him down
As shots echo down them hallways in the night.
No one watches when the ambulance pulls away
Or as the girl shuts out the bedroom light.

Outside the street's on fire in a real death waltz
Between flesh and what's fantasy
And the poets down here don't write nothing at all,
They just stand back and let it all be.[v]
And in the quick of the night
They reach for their moment and try to make an honest stand
But they wind up wounded, not even dead,
Tonight in Jungleland.[vi]

A Runaway American Dream

Rosalita (Come Out Tonight)

Spread out now, Rosie,[i] doctor come cut loose her mama's reins,[ii]
You know playin' blindman's bluff is a little baby's game.
You pick up Little Dynamite, I'm gonna pick up Little Gun
And together we're gonna go out tonight and make that highway run.[iii]
You don't have to call me lieutenant, Rosie, and I don't want to be your son,
The only lover I'm gonna need is your soft sweet little girl's tongue,[iv]
Ah, Rosie you're the one.

Dynamite's in the belfry playin' with the bats,
Little Gun's downtown in front of Woolworth's[v] tryin' out his attitude on all the
    cats,
Papa's on the corner waitin' for the bus,
Mama she's home in the window waitin' up for us.
She'll be there in that chair when they wrestle her upstairs, 'cause y'know we ain't
    gonna come.
I ain't here for business, I'm only here for fun
And Rosie you're the one.

    Rosalita, jump a little lighter,
    Señorita, come sit by my fire,
    I just want to be your love, ain't no lie,
    Rosie, you're my stone desire.

Jack the Rabbit and Weak Knees Willie, you know, they're gonna be there,
Ah, Sloppy Sue and Big Bones Billie, they'll be comin' up for air.
We're gonna play some pool, skip some school, act real cool, stay out all night, it's
    gonna feel all right.
So, Rosie, come out tonight, baby, come out tonight,
Windows are for cheaters, chimneys for the poor,
Closets are for hangers, winners use the door,
So use it, Rosie, that's what it's there for.

    Rosalita, jump a little lighter,
    Señorita, come sit by my fire,
    I just want to be your love, ain't no lie,
    Rosie, you're my stone desire.

Now, I know your mama she don't like me 'cause I play in a rock 'n' roll band
And I know your daddy he don't dig me, but he never did understand.
Papa lowered the boom, he locked you in your room, I'm comin' to lend a hand,
I'm comin' to liberate you, confiscate you, I want to be your man.
Someday we'll look back on this and it will all seem funny . . .
But now you're sad, your mama's mad, and your papa says he knows that I don't
    have any money.
Tell him this is last chance to get his daughter in a fine romance
Because a record company, Rosie, just gave me a big advance!

My tires were slashed and I almost crashed, but the Lord had mercy,
My machine she's a dud, I'm stuck in the mud somewhere in the swamps of
    Jersey.
Hold on tight, stay up all night, 'cause Rosie I'm comin' on strong,
By the time we meet the morning light I will hold you in my arms.
I know a pretty little place in Southern California down San Diego way,
There's a little café where they play guitars all night and day,
You can hear them in the back room strummin',
So hold tight, baby, 'cause don't you know daddy's comin'.

    Rosalita, jump a little lighter,
    Señorita, come sit by my fire,
    I just want to be your love, ain't no lie,
    Rosie, you're my stone desire.

4th of July, Asbury Park (Sandy)

Sandy, the fireworks are hailin' over Little Eden tonight
Forcin' a light into all those stoned-out faces left stranded on this warm July.[i]
Down in town the Circuit's[ii] full with switchblade lovers, so fast, so shiny, so
    sharp
As the wizards play down on Pinball Way on the boardwalk[iii] way past dark,
And the boys from the Casino[iv] dance with their shirts open like Latin lovers on
    the shore
Chasin' all them silly New York virgins by the score.

    Sandy, the aurora is risin' behind us.
    This pier lights our carnival life forever.
    Love me tonight for I may never see you again,
    Hey Sandy girl, my my baby.

Now the greasers, they tramp the streets or get busted for sleeping on the beach
    all night,
Them boys in their high heels, ah Sandy, their skins is so white.
And me, I just got tired of hangin' in them dusty arcades bangin' them pleasure
    machines,
Chasin' the factory girls underneath the boardwalk where they all promise to
    unsnap their jeans.[v]
And you know that tilt-a-whirl down on the south beach drag? I got on it last
    night and my shirt got caught
And they kept me spinnin' I didn't think I'd ever get off.

    Oh Sandy, the aurora is risin' behind us.
    This pier lights our carnival life on the water.
    Runnin', laughin' 'neath the boardwalk at night with the boss's daughter.
    I remember, Sandy girl, my my my baby.

Sandy, that waitress I was seeing lost her desire for me.
I spoke with her last night, she said she won't set herself on fire for me any
    more.
She worked that joint under the boardwalk, she was always the girl you saw
    boppin' down the beach with the radio.
The kids say last night she was dressed like a star in one of them cheap little
    seaside bars, and I saw her parked with lover boy out on the Kokomo.[vi]

Did you hear the cops finally busted Madame Marie[vii] for tellin' fortunes better
  than they do?
For me this boardwalk life is through, babe, you ought to quit this scene too.

  Sandy, the aurora is rising behind us.
  This pier lights our carnival life forever.
  Oh, love me tonight and I promise I'll love you forever.
  Oh, I mean it, Sandy, girl . . .

Backstreets

One soft infested summer me and Terry[i] became friends
Trying in vain to breathe the fire we was born in,
Catching rides to the outskirts, tying faith between our teeth,
Sleeping in that old abandoned beach house, getting wasted in the heat

    And hiding on the backstreets,
    Hiding on the backstreets
    With a love so hard and filled with defeat,
    Running for our lives at night on them backstreets.

Slow dancing in the dark on the beach at Stockton's Wing[ii]
Where desperate lovers park we sat with the last of the Duke Street Kings,[iii]
Huddled in our cars, waiting for the bells that ring,
In the deep heart of the night to set us loose from everything,

    To go running on the backstreets,
    Running on the backstreets.
    We swore we'd live forever
    On the backstreets we take it together.

Endless juke joints and Valentino drag
Where dancers scraped the tears up off the street dressed down in rags,
Running into the darkness, some hurt bad, some really dying,
At night sometimes it seemed you could hear the whole damn city crying.[iv]
Blame it on the lies that killed us, blame it on the truth that ran us down,
You can blame it all on me, Terry, it don't matter to me now.
When the breakdown hit at midnight there was nothing left to say
But I hated him and I hated you when you went away.

Laying here in the dark, you're like an angel on my chest,
Just another tramp of hearts crying tears of faithlessness.
Remember all the movies, Terry, we'd go see
Trying to learn how to walk like heroes we thought we had to be?[v]
And after all this time to find we're just like all the rest
Stranded in the park and forced to confess

    To hiding on the backstreets,
    Hiding on the backstreets.

We swore forever friends
On the backstreets until the end.

Hiding on the backstreets, hiding on the backstreets,
Hiding on the backstreets, hiding on the backstreets,
Hiding on the backstreets, hiding on the backstreets,
Hiding on the backstreets, hiding on the backstreets,
Hiding on the backstreets, hiding on the backstreets,
Hiding on the backstreets, hiding on the backstreets,
Hiding on the backstreets, hiding on the backstreets,
Hiding on the backstreets, hiding on the backstreets,
Hiding on the backstreets, hiding on the backstreets,
It's alright to go hiding on the backstreets tonight,
Hiding on the backstreets, hiding on the backstreets,
Hiding on the backstreets, hiding on the backstreets,
Hiding on the backstreets, hiding on the backstreets,
Hiding on the backstreets . . .

Born to Run

In the day we sweat it out in the streets of a runaway American Dream,
At night we ride through mansions of glory in suicide machines,
Sprung from cages out on Highway 9,[i]
Chrome wheeled, fuel injected and steppin' out over the line.
Baby, this town rips the bones from your back,
It's a death trap, it's a suicide rap,
We gotta get out while we're young
'Cause tramps like us, baby, we were born to run.

Wendy, let me in, I wanna be your friend, I want to guard your dreams and
    visions,
Just wrap your legs 'round these velvet rims and strap your hands across my
    engines,
Together we could break this trap,
We'll run till we drop, baby we'll never go back.
Will you walk with me out on the wire?
'Cause, baby, I'm just a scared and lonely rider
But I gotta find out how it feels,
I want to know if love is wild, girl, I want to know if love is real.

Beyond the Palace[ii] hemi-powered drones[iii] scream down the boulevard,
The girls comb their hair in rearview mirrors and the boys try to look so hard.
The amusement park rises bold and stark, kids are huddled on the beach in a
    mist.
I wanna die with you, Wendy, on the streets tonight in an everlasting kiss.

The highway's jammed with broken heroes on a last chance power drive,
Everybody's out on the run tonight but there's no place left to hide.
Together, Wendy, we'll live with the sadness,
I'll love you with all the madness in my soul.
Someday girl, I don't know when, we're gonna get to that place where we really
    want to go and we'll walk in the sun[iv]
But till then tramps like us, baby, we were born to run,
Ah honey, tramps like us, baby, we were born to run,
Come on, Wendy, tramps like us, baby, we were born to run.

Independence Day

Well, papa go to bed now, it's getting late,
Nothing we can say is gonna change anything now.
I'll be leaving in the morning from St. Mary's Gate,
We wouldn't change this thing even if we could somehow.

'Cause the darkness of this house has got the best of us,
There's a darkness in this town that's got us too,
But they can't touch me now and you can't touch me now:
They ain't gonna do to me what I watched them do to you.

So say goodbye, it's Independence Day,
It's Independence Day all down the line
Just say goodbye, it's Independence Day,
It's Independence Day this time.

Now I don't know what it always was with us:
We chose the words and, yeah, we drew the lines.
There was just no way this house could hold the two of us
—I guess that we were just too much of the same kind.

Well, say goodbye, it's Independence Day,
It's Independence Day, all boys must run away.
So say goodbye, it's Independence Day:
All men must make their way come Independence Day.

Now the rooms are all empty down at Frankie's joint
And the highway she's deserted clear down to Breaker's Point.
There's a lot of people leaving town now, leaving their friends, their homes:
At night they walk that dark and dusty highway all alone.
Well, Papa go to bed now, it's getting late,
Nothing we can say can change anything now,
Because there's just different people coming down here now and they see things
in different ways
And soon everything we've known will just be swept away

So say goodbye, it's Independence Day.
Papa, now I know the things you wanted that you could not say.
But won't you just say goodbye, it's Independence Day:
I swear I never meant to take those things away.

Thunder Road

The screen door slams, Mary's dress waves,
Like a vision she dances across the porch as the radio plays
Roy Orbison singing for the lonely,[i]
Hey that's me and I want you only,
Don't turn me home again, I just can't face myself alone again.

Don't run back inside, darling, you know just what I'm here for,
So you're scared and you're thinking that maybe we ain't that young anymore.[ii]
Show a little faith, there's magic in the night,
You ain't a beauty but, hey, you're alright,
Oh, and that's alright with me.

You can hide 'neath your covers and study your pain,
Make crosses from your lovers, throw roses in the rain,
Waste your summer praying in vain
For a savior to rise from these streets.[iii]

Well, now I'm no hero, that's understood,
All the redemption I can offer, girl, is beneath this dirty hood
With a chance to make it good somehow,
Hey, what else can we do now

Except roll down the window and let the wind blow back your hair?
Well, the night's busting open, these two lanes will take us anywhere.
We got one last chance to make it real,
To trade in these wings on some wheels.
Climb in back, heaven's waiting on down the tracks.

Oh, come take my hand,
Riding out tonight to case the Promised Land,
Oh Thunder Road, oh Thunder Road, oh Thunder Road[iv]
Lying out there like a killer in the sun,
Hey, I know it's late we can make it if we run.
Oh Thunder Road, sit tight take hold, Thunder Road.

Well, I got this guitar and I learned how to make it talk,
And my car's out back if you're ready to take that long walk
From your front porch to my front seat,

The door's open but the ride it ain't free
And I know you're lonely for words that I ain't spoken
But tonight we'll be free, all the promises'll be broken.

There were ghosts in the eyes of all the boys you sent away,
They haunt this dusty beach road
In the skeleton frames of burned out Chevrolets,
They scream your name at night in the street,
Your graduation gown lies in rags at their feet,

And in the lonely cool before dawn
You hear their engines roaring on,
But when you get to the porch they're gone on the wind,
So Mary climb in,
It's a town full of losers and I'm pulling out of here to win.[v]

Where Our Sins Lie
Unatoned

.

Badlands

Lights out tonight, trouble in the heartland.
Got a head-on collision smashin' in my guts, man,
I'm caught in a crossfire that I don't understand.
But there's one thing I know for sure, girl:

I don't give a damn for the same old played-out scenes,
I don't give a damn for just the in-betweens,
Honey, I want the heart, I want the soul, I want control right now.
You better listen to me, baby:

Talk about a dream, try to make it real,
You wake up in the night with a fear so real,
Spend your life waiting for a moment that just don't come.
Well, don't waste your time waiting.

> Badlands,[i] you gotta live it everyday,
> Let the broken hearts stand as the price you've gotta pay.
> We'll keep pushin' till it's understood
> And these badlands start treating us good.

Workin' in the fields till you get your back burned,
Workin' 'neath the wheel till you get your facts learned,
Baby, I got my facts learned real good right now.
You better get it straight, darling:

Poor man wanna be rich, rich man wanna be king
And a king ain't satisfied till he rules everything.
I wanna go out tonight,
I wanna find out what I got.

I believe in the love that you gave me,
I believe in the faith that can save me,
I believe in the hope and I pray
That some day it may raise me above these

> Badlands, you gotta live it everyday,
> Let the broken hearts stand as the price you've gotta pay.
> We'll keep pushin' till it's understood
> And these badlands start treating us good.

For the ones who had a notion, a notion deep inside
That it ain't no sin to be glad you're alive,
I wanna find one face that ain't looking through me,
I wanna find one place, I wanna spit in the face of these

Badlands, you gotta live it everyday,
Let the broken hearts stand as the price you've gotta pay.
We'll keep pushin' till it's understood
And these badlands start treating us good.

Adam Raised a Cain

In the summer that I was baptized
My father held me to his side
As they put me to the water,
He said how on that day I cried.[i]

We were prisoners of love, a love in chains,
He was standin' in the door,
I was standin' in the rain
With the same hot blood burning in our veins.

> Adam raised a Cain,
> Adam raised a Cain,
> Adam raised a Cain,
> Adam raised a Cain.

All of the old faces
Ask you why you're back,
They fit you with position
And the keys to your daddy's Cadillac.

In the darkness of your room
Your mother calls you by your true name,
You remember the faces, the places, the names,
You know it's never over, it's relentless as the rain.[ii]

> Adam raised a Cain,
> Adam raised a Cain,
> Adam raised a Cain,
> Adam raised a Cain.

In the Bible Cain slew Abel
And East of Eden, mama, he was cast.
You're born into this life paying
For the sins of somebody else's past.

Daddy worked his whole life for nothing but the pain,
Now he walks these empty rooms
Looking for something to blame.[iii]
You inherit the sins, you inherit the flames.

Adam raised a Cain,
Adam raised a Cain,
Adam raised a Cain,
Adam raised a Cain.

Lost but not forgotten,
From the dark heart of a dream

Adam raised a Cain,
Adam raised a Cain,
Adam raised a Cain,
Adam raised a Cain . . .

The Promised Land

On a rattlesnake speedway in the Utah desert[i]
I pick up my money and head back into town,
Driving cross the Waynesboro County[ii] line
I got the radio on and I'm just killing time
Working all day in my daddy's garage,
Driving all night chasing some mirage,
Pretty soon, little girl, I'm gonna take charge.

> The dogs on Main Street howl 'cause they understand.
> If I could take one moment into my hands . . .
> Mister, I ain't a boy, no, I'm a man
> And I believe in a promised land.[iii]

I've done my best to live the right way,
I get up every morning and go to work each day.
But your eyes go blind and your blood runs cold:
Sometimes I feel so weak I just want to explode,
Explode and tear this whole town apart,
Take a knife and cut this pain from my heart,
Find somebody itching for something to start.

> The dogs on Main Street howl 'cause they understand.
> If I could reach one moment into my hands . . .
> Mister, I ain't a boy, no, I'm a man
> And I believe in a promised land.

There's a dark cloud rising from the desert floor,
I packed my bags and I'm heading straight into the storm.
Gonna be a twister to blow everything down
That ain't got the faith to stand its ground.
Blow away the dreams that tear you apart,
Blow away the dreams that break your heart,
Blow away the lies that leave you nothing
But lost and brokenhearted.

> The dogs on Main Street howl 'cause they understand.
> If I could take one moment into my hands . . .
> Mister, I ain't a boy, no, I'm a man
> And I believe in a promised land.

Come On (Let's Go Tonight)

Put on your black dress, baby, and put your hair up right:
There's a party way down in Factory Town tonight.
I'll be going down there: if you need a ride,
Come on, come on, let's go tonight.

How many men fail, their dreams denied,
They walk through these streets with death in their eyes.[i]
Now the man on the radio says, "Elvis Presley died."
Come on, come on, let's go tonight.

Well, now some came to witness, now some came to weep,
Drawn by death's strange glory, they stood in the street,
Drawn together forever in the promise of an endless sleep.
Come on, come on, let's go tonight.

Because the Night

Take me now, baby, here as I am,
Pull me close, try and understand,
I work all day out in the hot sun,
I break my back till the mornin' comes.[i]

Come on now, try and understand
The way I feel when I'm in your hands,
Take me now as the sun descends,[ii]
They can't hurt you now,
They can't hurt you now,
They can't hurt you now . . .

    Because the night belongs to lovers,
    Because the night belongs to us,
    Because the night belongs to lovers,
    Because the night belongs to us.

What I got I have earned,
What I'm not, baby, I have learned.
Desire and hunger is the fire I breathe,
Just stay in my bed till the morning comes.[iii]

Come on now, try and understand
The way I feel when I'm in your hands.[iv]
Take me now as the sun descends,
They can't hurt you now,
They can't hurt you now,
They can't hurt you now . . .

    Because the night belongs to lovers,
    Because the night belongs to us,
    Because the night belongs to lovers,
    Because the night belongs to us.

Your love seeds with doubt
The vicious circle turns and burns without,
Though I cannot live, forgive me now,

The time has come to take this moment and
They can't hurt you now,
They can't hurt you now . . .[v]

> Because the night belongs to lovers,
> Because the night belongs to us . . .
> Because the night belongs to lovers,
> Because the night belongs to us . . .

Iceman

Sleepy town, ain't got the guts to budge.
Baby, this emptiness has already been judged,
I wanna go out tonight, I wanna find out what I got.[i]

You're a strange part of me, you're a preacher's girl,
And I don't want no piece of this mechanical world,
Got my arms open wide and my blood is running hot.

We'll take the midnight road right to the devil's door
And even the white angels of Eden with their flamin' swords
Won't be able to stop us from hitting town in this dirty old Ford.

Well, it don't take no nerve when you got nothing to guard,
I got tombstones in my eyes and I'm running real hard,
My baby was a lover and the world just blew her away.

Once they tried to steal my heart, beat it right outta my head
But, baby, they didn't know that I was born dead.
I am the iceman, fighting for the right to live.

I say, better than the glory roads of heaven,
Better off riding hellbound in the dirt,
Better than the bright lines of the freeway,
Better than the shadows of your daddy's church,
Better than the waiting, baby, better off is the search.

Racing in the Street

I got a sixty-nine Chevy with a 396,
Fuelie heads and a Hurst on the floor.[i]
She's waiting tonight down in the parking lot
Outside the Seven-Eleven store.

Me and my partner Sonny built her straight out of scratch,
He rides with me from town to town.
We only run for the money, got no strings attached,
We shut 'em up and then we shut 'em down.

> Tonight, tonight the strip's just right,
> I wanna blow 'em off in my first heat.
> Summer's here and the time is right
> for goin' racin' in the street.

We take all the action we can meet
And we cover all the northeast state,
When the strip shuts down we run 'em in the street
From the fire roads to the interstate.

Some guys, they just give up living
And start dying little by little, piece by piece,
Some guys come home from work
And wash up and go racin' in the street.

> Tonight, tonight the strip's just right,
> I wanna blow 'em all out of their seats,
> Calling out around the world,
> We're going racin' in the street.

I met her on the strip three years ago
In a Camaro[ii] with this dude from LA,
I blew that Camaro off my back
And drove that little girl away.

But now there's wrinkles around my baby's eyes
And she cries herself to sleep at night,
When I come home the house is dark
She sighs, "Baby, did you make it all right?"

She sits on the porch of her daddy's house
But all her pretty dreams are torn,
She stares off alone into the night
With the eyes of one who hates for just being born.

For all the shut down strangers and hot rod angels
Rumbling through this promised land
Tonight my baby and me we're gonna ride to the sea
And wash these sins off our hands.

> Tonight, tonight the highway's bright,
> out of our way mister you best keep
> 'Cause summer's here and the time is right
> for goin' racin' in the street.[iii]

Heart of Darkness

The Promise

Johnny works in a factory
And Billy works downtown,
Terry works in a rock and roll band
Lookin' for that million-dollar sound.
I got a little job down in Darlington[i]
But some nights I don't go,
Some nights I go to the drive-in
Or some nights I stay home.

I followed that dream
Just like those guys do up on the screen
And I drive a Challenger[ii] down Route 9
Through the dead ends and all the bad scenes,
And when the promise was broken,
I cashed in a few of my dreams.

Well, now I built that Challenger by myself,
But I needed money and so I sold it,
I lived a secret I should'a kept to myself,
But I got drunk one night and I told it.
All my life I fought that fight,
The fight that no man can ever win,
Every day it just gets harder to live
This dream I'm believin' in.

Thunder Road,
Oh baby, you were so right.
Thunder Road,
There's something dyin' on the highway tonight.

I won big once and I hit the coast
Yeah, but I paid the cost,[iii]
Inside I felt like I was carryin'
The broken spirits of all the other ones who lost.
When the promise is broken you go on living
But it steals something from down in your soul.
When the truth is spoken and it don't make no difference,
Something in your heart growns cold.

I followed that dream
Through the southwestern tracks
That dead ends in two-bit bars,
And when the promise was broken
I was far away from home,
Sleepin' in the back seat of a borrowed car.[iv]

    Thunder Road,
    This is for the lost lovers and all the fixed games.
    Thunder Road,
    This for the tires rushing by in the rain.

    Thunder Road,
    Me and Billy we'd always say.
    Thunder Road,
    We were gonna take it all and throw it all away.

Darkness on the Edge of Town

They're still racing out at the Trestles,[i]
But that blood it never burned in her veins.
Now I hear she's got a house up in Fairview[ii]
And a style she's trying to maintain.
Well if she wants to see me
You can tell her that I'm easily found,
Tell her there's a spot out 'neath Abram's Bridge[iii]
And tell her there's a darkness on the edge of town,
There's a darkness on the edge of town.

Everybody's got a secret Sonny,
Something that they just can't face,
Some folks spend their whole lives trying to keep it,
They carry it with them every step that they take
Till some day they just cut it loose,
Cut it loose or let it drag 'em down
Where no one asks any questions
Or looks too long in your face,
In the darkness on the edge of town,
In the darkness on the edge of town.

Some folks are born into a good life,
Other folks get it anyway anyhow.
I lost my money and I lost my wife,
Them things don't seem to matter much to me now.
Tonight I'll be on that hill 'cause I can't stop,
I'll be on that hill with everything I got,
Lives on the line where dreams are found and lost,
I'll be there on time and I'll pay the cost
For wanting things that can only be found
In the darkness on the edge of town,
In the darkness on the edge of town.[iv]

The River

I come from down in the valley
Where, mister, when you're young
They bring you up to do
Like your daddy done.
Me and Mary we met in high school
When she was just seventeen,
We'd ride out of that valley
Down to where the fields were green.

> We'd go down to the river
> And into the river we'd dive,
> Oh down to the river we'd ride.

Then I got Mary pregnant
And, man, that was all she wrote,
And for my nineteenth birthday
I got a union card and a wedding coat.
We went down to the courthouse
And the judge put it all to rest,
No wedding day smiles, no walk down the aisle,
No flowers, no wedding dress.

> That night we went down to the river
> And into the river we'd dive,
> Oh down to the river we did ride.

I got a job working construction
For the Johnstown Company,[i]
But lately there ain't been much work
On account of the economy.[ii]
Now all them things that seemed so important,
Well, mister, they vanished right into the air.
Now I just act like I don't remember,
Mary acts like she don't care.

But I remember us riding in my brother's car,
Her body tan and wet down at the reservoir.

At night on them banks I'd lie awake
And pull her close just to feel each breath she'd take.
Now those memories come back to haunt me,
They haunt me like a curse.
Is a dream a lie if it don't come true
Or is it something worse

   That sends me down to the river,
   Though I know the river is dry,
   That sends me down to the river tonight.

   Down to the river
   My baby and I,
   Oh down to the river we ride.

Stolen Car

I met a little girl and I settled down
In a little house out on the edge of town.
We got married and swore we'd never part,
Then little by little we drifted from each other's heart.[i]

At first I thought it was just restlessness
That would fade as time went by and our love grew deep.
In the end it was something more, I guess,
That tore us apart and made us weep.

And I'm driving a stolen car
Down on Eldridge Avenue,[ii]
Each night I wait to get caught
But I never do.

She asked if I remembered the letters I wrote
When our love was young and bold.
She said last night she read those letters
And they made her feel one hundred years old.

And I'm driving a stolen car
On a pitch black night
And I'm telling myself I'm gonna be alright,
But I ride by night and I travel in fear
That in this darkness I will disappear.[iii]

TWO

This Hard Land

Deliver Me from Nowhere

Wreck on the Highway

Last night I was out driving
Coming home at the end of the working day.
I was riding alone through the drizzling rain
On a deserted stretch of a county two-lane
When I came upon a wreck on the highway.

There was blood and glass all over
And there was nobody there but me.
As the rain tumbled down hard and cold
I seen a young man lying by the side of the road,
He cried, "Mister, won't you help me please?"

An ambulance finally came and took him to Riverside.[i]
I watched as they drove him away
And I thought of a girlfriend or a young wife
And a state trooper knocking in the middle of the night
To say your baby died in a wreck on the highway.

Sometimes I sit up in the darkness
And I watch my baby as she sleeps,
Then I climb in bed and I hold her tight.
I just lay there awake in the middle of the night
Thinking 'bout the wreck on the highway.

Nebraska

I saw her standin' on her front lawn
Just twirlin' her baton.[i]
Me and her went for a ride, sir,
and ten innocent people died.[ii]

From the town of Lincoln, Nebraska[iii]
With a sawed off 410 on my lap,
Through to the badlands of Wyoming
I killed everything in my path.

I can't say that I'm sorry
For the things that we done.
At least for a little while, sir,
Me and her we had us some fun.[iv]

The jury brought in a guilty verdict
And the judge, he sentenced me to death.
Midnight in a prison storeroom
With leather straps across my chest.

Sheriff, when the man pulls that switch, sir,
And snaps my poor head back,
You make sure my pretty baby
Is sittin' right there on my lap.[v]

They declared me unfit to live,
Said into that great void my soul'd be hurled.
They wanted to know why I did what I did,
Well, sir, I guess there's just a meanness in this world.[vi]

Atlantic City

Well, they blew up the chicken man[i] in Philly last night,
Now they blew up his house too.
Down on the boardwalk they're getting' ready for a fight,
Gonna see what them racket boys can do.

Now there's trouble busin' in from outta state
And the D.A. can't get no relief.
Gonna be a rumble out on the promenade
And the gamblin' commission's hangin' on by the skin of its teeth.

> Everything dies, baby, that's a fact,
> But maybe everything that dies someday comes back.
> Put your makeup on, fix your hair up pretty
> And meet me tonight in Atlantic City.[ii]

Well, I got a job and tried to put my money away
But I got debts that no honest man can pay,
So I drew what I had from the Central Trust[iii]
And I bought us two tickets on that Coast City bus.[iv]

> Everything dies, baby, that's a fact,
> But maybe everything that dies someday comes back.
> Put your makeup on, fix your hair up pretty
> And meet me tonight in Atlantic City.

Now our luck may have died and our love may be cold
But with you forever I'll stay.
We're goin' out where the sand's turnin' to gold,
So put on your stockings, baby, 'cause the night's getting cold.

> And maybe everything dies, baby, that's a fact,
> But maybe everything that dies someday comes back.

Now I been lookin' for a job, but it's hard to find,
Down here it's just winners and losers and don't get caught on the wrong side of
    that line.
Well, I'm tired of comin' out on the losin' end,
So, honey, last night I met this guy and I'm gonna do a little favor for him.

Everything dies, baby, that's a fact,
But maybe everything that dies someday comes back.
Put your hair nice, and set up pretty
And meet me tonight in Atlantic City.

Johnny 99

Well, they closed down the auto plant in Mahwah[i] late that month,
Ralph went out lookin' for a job but he couldn't find none,
He came home too drunk from mixin' Tanqueray[ii] and wine,
He got a gun, shot a night clerk, now they call'm Johnny 99.[iii]

Down in the part of town where when you hit a red light you don't stop
Johnny's wavin' his gun around and threatenin' to blow his top,
When an off-duty cop snuck up on him from behind,
Out in front of the Club Tip Top they slapped the cuffs on Johnny 99.

The city supplied a public defender but the judge was Mean John Brown,[iv]
He came into the courtroom and stared young Johnny down,
"Well, the evidence is clear, gonna let the sentence, son, fit the crime:
Prison for 98 and a year and we'll call it even Johnny 99."

A fistfight broke out in the courtroom, they had to drag Johnny's girl away,
His mama stood up and shouted, "Judge don't take my boy this way."
"Well, son, you got a statement you'd like to make
Before the bailiff comes to forever take you away?"[v]

"Now judge, judge, I had debts no honest man could pay,[vi]
The bank was holdin' my mortgage and they was takin' my house away.
Now, I ain't sayin' that makes me an innocent man
But it was more 'n all this that put that gun in my hand.

"Well, your honor, I do believe I'd be better off dead
And if you can take a man's life for the thoughts that's in his head,
Then won't you sit back in that chair and think it over, judge, one more time
And let 'em shave off my hair and put me on that execution line?"[vii]

Highway Patrolman

My name is Joe Roberts, I work for the State,
I'm a sergeant out of Perrineville,[i] barracks number 8.
I always done an honest job, as honest as I could,
I got a brother named Frankie, and Frankie ain't no good.

Now, ever since we was young kids, it's been the same come down:
I get a call on the shortwave,[ii] Frankie's in trouble downtown.
Well, if it was any other man I'd put him straight away,
But when it's your brother sometimes you look the other way.

> Me and Frankie laughin' and drinkin',
> Nothin' feels better than blood on blood.
> Takin' turns dancin' with Maria[iii]
> As the band played "Night of the Johnstown Flood."[iv]
> I catch him when he's strayin' like any brother would.
> Man turns his back on his family, well, he just ain't no good.

Well, Frankie went in the army back in 1965,
I got a farm deferment, settled down, took Maria for my wife.
But them wheat prices kept on droppin' till it was like we were getting' robbed.
Frankie came home in '68, and me, I took this job.

> Yeah, we're laughin' and drinkin',
> Nothin' feels better than blood on blood.
> Takin' turns dancin' with Maria
> As the band played "Night of the Johnstown Flood."
> I catch him when he's strayin', teach him how to walk that line.
> Man turns his back on his family, he ain't no friend of mine.

Well, the night was like any other, I got a call 'bout quarter to nine.
There was trouble in a roadhouse, out on the Michigan line,
There was a kid lyin' on the floor, lookin' bad, bleedin' hard from his head,
There was a girl cryin' at a table, and it was Frank, they said.

Well, I went out and I jumped in my car and I hit the lights,
I must of done one hundred and ten through Michigan County[v] that night.
It was out at the crossroads, down round Willow Bank,
Seen a Buick with Ohio plates: behind the wheel was Frank.

I chased him through them county roads
Till a sign said "Canadian border 5 miles from here."
I pulled over the side of the highway
And watched his taillights disappear.

Me and Frankie laughin' and drinkin',
Nothin' feels better than blood on blood.
Takin' turns dancin' with Maria
As the band played "Night of the Johnstown Flood."
I catch him when he's strayin' like any brother would.
Man turns his back on his family, well, he just ain't no good.

State Trooper

New Jersey Turnpike,[i]
Ridin' on a wet night
'Neath the refinery's glow,
Out where the great black rivers flow.

License, registration . . .
I ain't got none,
But I got a clear conscience
'Bout the things that I done.

> Mister State Trooper,
> Please don't stop me,
> Please don't stop me,
> Please don't stop me . . .

Maybe you got a kid,
Maybe you got a pretty wife,
The only thing that I got's
Been both'rin' me my whole life.

> Mister State Trooper,
> Please don't stop me,
> Please don't you stop me,
> Please don't you stop me . . .

In the wee wee hours
Your mind gets hazy,[ii]
Radio relay towers[iii]
Lead me to my baby.

Radio's jammed up
With talk show stations,
It's just talk, talk, talk, talk,
Till you lose your patience.

> Mister State Trooper,
> Please don't you stop me . . .

Hey, somebody out there,
Listen to my last prayer,
Hi ho Silver-o,[iv]
Deliver me from nowhere.[v]

Open All Night

Well, I had the carburetor, baby, cleaned and checked,
With her line blown out she's hummin' like a turbojet,
Propped her up in the backyard on concrete blocks
For a new clutch plate and a new set of shocks.
Took her down to the carwash, check the plugs and points.
Well, I'm goin' out tonight. I'm gonna rock that joint.

Early north Jersey industrial skyline,
I'm a all-set cobra jet creepin' through the nightime,
Gotta find a gas station, gotta find a payphone,
This turnpike sure is spooky at night when you're all alone.
Gotta hit the gas, baby, I'm running late,
This New Jersey in the mornin' like a lunar landscape.

Now, the boss don't dig me, so he put me on the nightshift.
It takes me two hours to get back to where my baby lives,[i]
In the wee wee hours your mind gets hazy,
Radio relay towers, won't you lead me to my baby?
Underneath the overpass, trooper hits his party light switch,
Goodnight, good luck, one two power shift.

I met Wanda when she was employed
Behind the counter at route 60 Bob's Big Boy
Fried chicken[ii] on the front seat, she's sittin' in my lap,
We're wipin' our fingers on a Texaco roadmap.
I remember Wanda up on scrap metal hill
With them big brown eyes that make your heart stand still.

Well, at five a.m. oil pressure's sinkin' fast,
I make a pit stop, wipe the windshield, check the gas.
Gotta call my baby on the telephone,
Let her know that her daddy's comin' on home.
Sit tight, little mama, I'm comin' 'round,
I got three more hours, but I'm coverin' ground.

Your eyes get itchy in the wee wee hours,
Sun's just a red ball risin' over them refinery towers,
Radio's jammed up with gospel stations,
Lost souls callin' long distance salvation.
Hey, mister deejay, woncha hear my last prayer:
Hey ho, rock and roll, deliver me from nowhere.

Reason to Believe

Seen a man standin' over a dead dog by the highway in a ditch,
He's lookin' down kinda puzzled pokin' that dog with a stick.
Got his car door flung open, he's standin' out on Highway 31
Like if he stood there long enough that dog'd get up and run.[i]
Struck me kinda funny, seem kinda funny, sir, to me,
Still at the end of every hard earned day people find some reason to believe.

Now, Mary Lou loved Johnny[ii] with a love mean and true,
She said, "Baby, I'll work for you every day and bring my money home to you."
One day he up and left her and ever since that
She waits down at the end of that dirt road for young Johnny to come back.
Struck me kinda funny, funny, yeah, indeed,
How at the end of every hard earned day people find some reason to believe.

Take a baby to the river, Kyle William they called him,
Wash the baby in the water, take away little Kyle's sin.
In a whitewash shotgun shack, an old man passes away,
Take his body to the graveyard and over him they pray,
"Lord, won't you tell us, tell us what does it mean?
At the end of every hard earned day people find some reason to believe.

Congregation gathers down by the riverside,
Preacher stands with his Bible, groom stands waitin' for his bride.
Congregation gone and the sun sets behind a weepin' willow tree,
Groom stands alone and watches the river rush on so effortlessly,[iii]
Wonderin' where can his baby be.
Still at the end of every hard earned day people find some reason to believe.[iv]

This Hard Land

Hey there, mister, can you tell me
What happened to the seeds I've sown?
Can you give me a reason, sir,
As to why they've never grown?[i]
They've just blown around from town to town,
Back on to these fields,
Where they fall from, from my hand,
Back into the dirt of this hard land.

Well, me and my sister
From Germantown[ii] we did ride,
We made our bed, sir,
From the rock on the mountainside.
We've been blowin' around from town to town
Lookin' for a place to land
Where the sun burst through the clouds and fall like a circle,
A circle of fire down on this hard land.

Now even the rain it don't come 'round,
Don't come 'round here no more
And the only sound at night's the wind
Slammin' the back porch door.
Yeah, it stirs you up like it wants to blow you down,
Twistin' and churnin' up the sand,
Leavin' all them scarecrows lyin' facedown
Into the dirt of this hard land.

From a building up on the hill
I can hear a tape deck blastin' "Home on the Range,"[iii]
I can hear them Bar-M choppers[iv]
Sweepin' low across the plains.
It's me and you Frank, we're lookin' for lost cattle,
Hooves twistin' and churnin' up the sand,
We're ridin' in the whirlwind searchin' for lost treasure
Way down south of the Rio Grande,[v]
We're ridin' 'cross that river in the moonlight
Up onto the banks of this hard land.

Hey, Frank, won't you pack your bags
And meet me tonight down at Liberty Hall?[vi]
Just one kiss from you, my brother,
And we'll ride until we fall,
We'll sleep in the fields, we'll sleep by the rivers
and in the morning we'll make a plan.
Well, if you can't make it, stay hard, stay hungry, stay alive if you can,
And meet me in a dream of this hard land.

Born in the U.S.A.

Born down in a dead man's town,
The first kick I took was when I hit the ground.
You end up like a dog that's been beat too much
Till you spend half your life just covering up.

> Born in the U.S.A.,
> I was born in the U.S.A.,
> I was born in the U.S.A.,
> Born in the U.S.A.

Got in a little hometown jam
So they put a rifle in my hand,
Sent me off to a foreign land
To go and kill the yellow man.

> Born in the U.S.A.,
> I was born in the U.S.A.,
> I was born in the U.S.A.,
> Born in the U.S.A.

Come back home to the refinery,
Hiring man says, "Son, if it was up to me . . ."
Went down to see my V.A. man,
He said, "Son, don't you understand?"

I had a brother at Khe Sahn[i] fighting off the Viet Cong,
They're still there, he's all gone.
He had a woman he loved in Saigon,
I got a picture of him in her arms now.

Down in the shadow of the penitentiary,
Out by the gas fires of the refinery,
I'm ten years burning down the road,
Nowhere to run ain't got nowhere to go.

Born in the U.S.A.,
I was born in the U.S.A.,
Born in the U.S.A.,
I'm a long gone daddy in the U.S.A.[ii]

Born in the U.S.A.,
Born in the U.S.A.,
Born in the U.S.A.,
I'm a cool rocking daddy in the U.S.A.

Downbound Train

I had a job, I had a girl,
I had something going, mister, in this world.
I got laid off down at the lumber yard,
Our love went bad, times got hard.
Now I work down at the carwash[i]
where all it ever does is rain.
Don't you feel like you're a rider
On a downbound train?[ii]

She just said, "Joe, I gotta go,
We had it once we ain't got it any more."
She packed her bags, left me behind,
She bought a ticket on the Central Line.[iii]
Nights as I sleep, I hear that whistle whining,
I feel her kiss in the misty rain
And I feel like I'm a rider
On a downbound train.

Last night I heard your voice,
You were crying, crying, you were so alone.
You said your love had never died,
You were waiting for me at home.
Put on my jacket, I ran through the woods,
I ran till I thought my chest would explode.
There in the clearing, beyond the highway,
In the moonlight, our wedding house shone.

I rushed through the yard,
I burst through the front door,
My head pounding hard,
Up the stairs I climbed.
The room was dark, our bed was empty,
Then I heard that long whistle whine
And I dropped to my knees,
Hung my head and cried.

Now I swing a sledge hammer on a railroad gang,
Knocking down them cross ties, working in the rain.
Now don't it feel like you're a rider
on a downbound train?

Car Wash

Well, my name is Catherine LeFevre,
I work at the Astrowash on Sunset and Vine,[i]
I drop my kids at school in the morning
And I pick them up at Mary's just 'fore suppertime.

> Well, I work down at the car wash
> For a dollar and a dime
> And mister, I hate my boss.
> It's at the car wash I'm doing my time.

Pick up my water bottle and my towel, sir
And I take 'em one by one,
From Mercedes to VW's,
I do 'em all and I don't favor none.

> Well, I work down at the car wash
> For a dollar and a dime
> And mister, I hate my boss.
> It's at the car wash I'm doing my time.

Well, someday I'll sing in a nightclub,
I'll get a million-dollar break,
A handsome man will come here with a contract in his hand
And say, "Catherine, this has all been some mistake."

> Well, I work down at the car wash
> For a dollar and a dime
> And mister, I hate my boss.
> It's at the car wash I'm doing my time.

Spare Parts

Bobby said he'd pull out, Bobby stayed in,
Janey had a baby, it wasn't any sin.
They were set to marry on a summer day,
Bobby got scared and he ran away.

Jane moved in with her ma out on Shawnee Lake,[i]
She sighed, "Ma, sometimes my whole life feels like one big mistake."
She settled in in a back room, time passed on,
Later that winter a son came along.

    Spare parts and broken hearts
    Keep the world turnin' around.

Now, Janey walked that baby across the floor night after night,
But she was a young girl and she missed the party lights.
Meanwhile in South Texas in a dirty oil patch
Bobby heard 'bout his son bein' born and swore he wasn't ever goin' back.

    Spare parts and broken hearts
    Keep the world turnin' around.

Janey heard about a woman over in Calverton,[ii]
Put her baby in the river, let the river roll on.
She looked at her boy in the crib where he lay,
Got down on her knees, cried till she prayed.[iii]

Mist was on the water, low run the tide,
Janey held her son down at the riverside,
Waist deep in water, how bright the sun shone,
She lifted him in her arms and carried him home.

As he lay sleeping in her bed Janey took a look around at everything,
Went to a drawer in her bureau and got out her old engagement ring,
Took out her wedding dress, tied that ring up in its sash,
Went straight down to the pawn shop man and walked out with some good cold
    cash.

    Spare parts and broken hearts
    Keep the world turnin' around . . .

Cautious Man

Bill Horton was a cautious man of the road,
He walked lookin' over his shoulder and remained faithful to its code.
When something caught his eye he'd measure his need
And then very carefully he'd proceed.

Billy met a young girl in the early days of May:
It was there in her arms he let his cautiousness slip away.
In their lovers' twilight, as the evening sky grew dim,
He'd lay back in her arms and laugh at what had happened to him.

On his right hand Billy tattooed the word LOVE and on his left hand was the
    word FEAR,[i]
And in which hand he held his fate was never clear.
Come Indian summer, he took his young lover for his bride
And with his own hands built a great house down by the riverside.

Now Billy was an honest man, he wanted to do what was right,
He worked hard to fill their lives with happy days and loving nights.
Alone on his knees in the darkness for steadiness he'd pray
For he knew in a restless heart the seed of betrayal lay.

One night Billy awoke from a terrible dream callin' his wife's name,
She lay breathing beside him in a peaceful sleep, a thousand miles away.
He got dressed in the moonlight and down to the highway he strode;
When he got there he didn't find nothing but road.

Billy felt a coldness rise up inside him that he couldn't name,
Just as the words tattooed 'cross his knuckles, he knew would always remain.
At their bedside he brushed the hair from his wife's face as the moon shone on
    her skin so white
Filling their room with the beauty of God's fallen light.

The Grapes of Wrath

Streets of Philadelphia

I was bruised and battered and I couldn't tell what I felt,
I was unrecognizable to myself.
Saw my reflection in a window, I didn't know my own face.
Oh brother, are you gonna leave me wasting away
On the streets of Philadelphia?

I walked the avenue till my legs felt like stone,
I heard the voices of friends vanished and gone.
At night I could hear the blood in my veins
Just as black and whispering as the rain
On the streets of Philadelphia.

Ain't no angel gonna greet me,
It's just you and I, my friend
And my clothes don't fit me no more.
I walked a thousand miles
Just to slip this skin.

The night has fallen, I'm lyin' awake,
I can feel myself fading away.
So receive me brother with your faithless kiss
or will we leave each other alone like this
On the streets of Philadelphia.

Black Cowboys

Last Rainey Williams' playground was the Mott Haven[i] streets
Where he ran past melted candles and flower wreaths,
Names and photos of young black faces,
Whose death and blood consecrated these places.

Rainey's mother said, "Rainey stay at my side,
For you are my blessing, you are my pride.
It's your love here that keeps my soul alive.
I want you to come home from school and stay inside."

Rainey'd do his work and put his books away.
There was a channel showed a western movie everyday.
Lynette brought him home books on the black cowboys of the Oklahoma
        range[ii]
And the Seminole scouts who fought the tribes of the Great Plains.[iii]

Summer come and the days grew long.
Rainey always had his mother's smile to depend on.
Along a street of stray bullets he made his way,
To the warmth of her arms at the end of each day.

Come the fall, the rain flooded these homes,
Here in Ezekiel's valley of dry bones,[iv]
It fell hard and dark to the ground,
It fell without a sound.

Lynette took up with a man whose business was the boulevard,
Whose smile was fixed in a face that was never off guard.
In the pipes 'neath the kitchen sink his secrets he kept.
In the day, behind drawn curtains, in Lynette's bedroom he slept.

Then she got lost in the days.
The smile Rainey depended on dusted away,
The arms that held him were no more his home.
He lay at night, his head pressed to her chest listening to the ghost in her
        bones.

In the kitchen Rainey slipped his hand between the pipes,
From a brown bag pulled five hundred dollar bills and stuck it in his coat side,
stood in the dark at his mother's bed,
brushed her hair and kissed her eyes.

In the twilight Rainey walked to the station along streets of stone.
Through Pennsylvania and Ohio his train drifted on,
Through the small towns of Indiana the big train crept,
As he lay his head back on the seat and slept.

He awoke and the towns gave way to muddy fields of green,
Corn and cotton and an endless nothin' in between.
Over the rutted hills of Oklahoma the red sun slipped and was gone.
The moon rose and stripped the earth to its bone.[v]

Youngstown

Here in northeast Ohio
Back in eighteen-o-three
James and Danny Heaton[i] found the ore
That was linin' Yellow Creek.

They built a blast furnace
Here along the shore
And they made the cannon balls
That helped the union win the war.

> Here in Youngstown,
> Here in Youngstown,
> My sweet Jenny,[ii] I'm sinkin' down,
> Here, darlin', in Youngstown.

Well, my daddy worked the furnaces,
Kept 'em hotter than hell,
I come home from 'Nam, worked my way to scarfer,
A job that'd suit the devil as well.

Taconite, coke and limestone
Fed my children and made my pay,
Then smokestacks reachin' like the arms of God
Into a beautiful sky of soot and clay.

> Here in Youngstown,
> Here in Youngstown,
> My sweet Jenny, I'm sinkin' down,
> Here, darlin', in Youngstown.

Well, my daddy come on the Ohio works
When he come home from World War Two.
Now the yard's just scrap and rubble,
He said, "Them big boys did what Hitler couldn't do.

These mills they built the tanks and bombs
That won this country's wars.
We sent our sons to Korea and Vietnam,
Now we're wondering what they were dyin' for."

Here in Youngstown,
Here in Youngstown,
My sweet Jenny, I'm sinkin' down,
Here, darlin', in Youngstown.

From the Monongahela Valley[iii]
To the Mesabi iron range[iv]
To the coal mines of Appalachia[v]
The story's always the same:

Seven hundred tons of metal a day.
Now, sir, you tell me the world's changed,
Once I made you rich enough,
Rich enough to forget my name.

In Youngstown,
In Youngstown,
My sweet Jenny, I'm sinkin' down,
Here, darlin', in Youngstown.

When I die, I don't want no part of heaven,
I would not do heaven's work well,
I pray the devil comes and takes me
To stand in the fiery furnaces of hell.

The Hitter

Come to the door, Ma, and unlock the chain.
I was just passin' through and got caught in the rain.
There's nothing that I want, nothin' that you need say,
Just let me lie down for a while and I'll be on my way.

I was no more than a kid when you put me on the Southern Queen.[i]
With the police on my back I fled to New Orleans.
I fought in the dockyards and with the the money I made
I knew the fight was my home and any blood was my trade.

Baton Rouge, Ponchatoula and Lafayette Town,
Well, they paid me their money, Ma, I knocked the men down.
I did what I did, it come easily.
Restraint and mercy, Ma, were always strangers to me.

I fought champion Jack Thompson[ii] in a field full of mud.
Rain poured through the tent to the canvas and mixed with our blood.
In the twelfth, I slipped my tongue over my broken jaw,
I stood over him and I pounded his bloody body into the floor.

Well, the bell rang and rang and still I kept on
till I felt my glove leather slip 'tween his skin and bone.

Then the women and the money came fast and the days I lost track.
The women red, the money green, but the numbers were black.
I fought for the men in their silk suits to lay down their bets.
Well, I took my good share, Ma, I have no regrets.

I took the fix at the state armory with Big John McDowell.[iii]
From high in the rafters I watched myself fall;
As they raised his arm, my stomach twisted, and the sky it went black,
I stuffed my bag with their good money and never looked back.

Understand, in the end, Ma, every man plays the game:
If you know me one different then speak out his name.

Ma, if my voice now you don't recognize[iv]
Then just open the door and look into your dark eyes.

I ask of you nothin', not a kiss, not a smile.
Just open the door and let me lie down for a while.

Now the gray rain is fallin' and my ring fightin's done.
So in the work fields and alleys, I take them who'll come.
If you're a better man than me, then just step to the line,
Show me your money and speak out your crime.

There's nothin' I want, Ma, nothin' that you need say.
Just let me lie down for a while and I'll be on my way.

Tonight in the shipyard[v] a man draws a circle in the dirt.
I move to the center and take off my shirt,
I study him for the cuts, the scars, the pain, man, no time can erase,
I move hard to the left and I strike to the face.

The Ghost of Tom Joad

Men walkin' 'long the railroad tracks
Goin' someplace there's no goin' back,
Highway patrol choppers comin' up over the ridge,[i]
Hot soup on a campfire under the bridge.

Shelter line stretchin' round the corner,
Welcome to the new world order,[ii]
Families sleepin' in their cars in the southwest,
No home, no job, no peace, no rest.

    The highway is alive tonight[iii]
    But nobody's kiddin' nobody about where it goes.
    I'm sittin' down here in the campfire light
    Searchin' for the ghost of Tom Joad.

He pulls a prayer book out of his sleeping bag,
Preacher[iv] lights up a butt and takes a drag,
Waitin' for when the last shall be first and the first shall be last,[v]
In a cardboard box 'neath the underpass.

Got a one-way ticket to the promised land,
You got a hole in your belly and gun in your hand,
Sleeping on a pillow of solid rock,
Bathin' in the city aqueduct.

The highway is alive tonight
But where it's headed everybody knows.
I'm sittin' down here in the campfire light
Waitin' on the ghost of Tom Joad.

Now Tom said, "Mom, wherever there's a cop beatin' a guy,
Wherever a hungry newborn baby cries,
Where there's a fight 'gainst the blood and hatred in the air,
Look for me, Mom, I'll be there.

"Wherever there's somebody fightin' for a place to stand
Or decent job or a helpin' hand,

Wherever somebody's strugglin' to be free,
Look in their eyes, Mom, you'll see me."[vi]

The highway is alive tonight
But nobody's kiddin' nobody about where it goes.
I'm sittin' downhere in the campfire light
With the ghost of old Tom Joad.

The New Timer[i]

He rode the rails since the great depression,
Fifty years out on the skids
He said, "You don't cross nobody,
You'll be all right out here, kid."[ii]

Left my family in Pennsylvania,
Searchin' for work I hit the road.
I met Frank in east Texas, in a freight yard
Blown through with snow.[iii]

From New Mexico to Colorado,
California to the sea,
Frank he showed me the ropes, sir,
Just till I could get back on my feet.

I hoed sugar beets outside of Firebaugh,[iv]
I picked the peaches from the Marysville[v] trees,
They bunked us in a barn just like animals,
Me and a hundred others just like me.

We split up come the springtime.
I never seen Frank again,
'Cept one rainy night he blew by me on grainer,
Shouted my name and disappeared in the rain and the wind.

They found him shot dead outside Stockton,[vi]
His body lyin' on a muddy hill,
Nothin' taken, nothin' stolen,
Somebody killed him just to kill.

Late that summer I was rollin' through the plains of Texas.
A vision passed before my eyes:
A small house sittin' trackside
With the glow of the Savior's beautiful light.

A woman stood cookin' in the kitchen,
Kid sat at the table with his old man.
Now I wonder, does my son miss me,
Does he wonder where I am?

Tonight I pick my campsite carefully
Outside the Sacramento[vii] Yard,
Gather some wood and light a fire
In the early winter dark.

Wind whistlin' cold, I pull my coat around me,
Make some coffee and stare out into the black night.
I lie awake, I lie awake, sir,
With my machete by my side.

My Jesus, your gracious love and mercy,
Tonight, I'm sorry, could not fill my heart
Like one good rifle
And the name of who I ought to kill.

Highway 29

I slipped on her shoe,
She was a perfect size seven.
I said, "There's no smokin' in the store, ma'am."
She crossed her legs and then

We made some small talk—
That's where it should have stopped.
She slipped me a number,
I put it in my pocket,

My hand slipped up her skirt,
Everything slipped my mind
In that little roadhouse
On highway 29.[i]

It was a small town bank,
It was a mess.
Well, I had a gun,
you know the rest.

Money on the floorboards,
Shirt was covered in blood and she was cryin'.
Her and me we headed south
On highway 29.

In a little desert motel
The air it was hot and clean.
I slept the sleep of the dead,
I didn't dream.

I woke in the morning,
Washed my face in the sink.
We headed into the Sierra Madres[ii]
'Cross the borderline.

The winter sun
Shot through the black trees.
I told myself it was all something in her,
But as we drove I knew it was something in me,

Something had been comin'
For a long long time
And something that was here with me now
On highway 29.

The road was filled with broken glass
And gasoline.
She wasn't sayin' nothin':
It was just a dream.

The wind come silent through the windshield,
All I could see was snow and sky and pines.
I closed my eyes and I was runnin',
I was runnin', then I was flyin' . . .

The Line

I got my discharge from Fort Irwin,[i]
Took a place on the San Diego County line,
Felt funny bein' a civilian again,
It'd been some time.
My wife had died a year ago,
I was still tryin' to find my way back whole,
Went to work for the INS on the line
With the California Border Patrol.[ii]

Bobby Ramirez was a ten-year veteran,
We became friends,
His family was from Guanajuato,[iii]
So the job it was different for him.
He said, "They risk death in the deserts and mountains,
Pay all they got to the smugglers' rings,
We send 'em home and they come right back again.
Carl, hunger is a powerful thing."

Well, I was good at doin' what I was told,
Kept my uniform pressed and clean,
At night I chased their shadows
Through the *arroyos*[iv] and ravines.
Drug runners, farmers with their families,
Young women with little children by their sides
Come night we'd wait out in the canyons
And try to keep 'em from crossin' the line.

Well, the first time that I saw her,
She was in the holdin' pen:
Our eyes met and she looked away,
Then she looked back again.
Her hair was black as coal,
Her eyes reminded me of what I'd lost.
She had a young child cryin' in her arms and I asked,
"Señora, is there anything I can do?"

There's a bar in Tijuana[v] where me and Bobby drink alongside
The same people we'd sent back the day before.
We met there, she said her name was Louisa,
She was from Sonora[vi] and had just come north.
We danced and I held her in my arms
And I knew what I would do.
She said she had some family in Madera County;[vii]
If she, her child and her younger brother could just get through . . .

At night they come across the levy
In the searchlights' dusty glow;
We'd rush 'em in our Broncos
And force 'em back down into the river below.
She climbed into my truck,
She leaned towards me and we kissed.
As we drove her brother's shirt slipped open
And I saw the tape across his chest.

We were just about on the highway
When Bobby's jeep come up in the dust on my right
I pulled over and let my engine run
And stepped out into his lights.
I felt myself movin',
Felt my gun restin' 'neath my hand,
We stood there starin' at each other
As off through the *arroyo* she ran.

Bobby Ramirez he never said nothin'.
Six months later I left the line,
I drifted to the central valley
And took what work I could find.
At night I searched the local bars
And the migrant towns
Lookin' for my Louisa
With the black hair fallin' down.

Reno[i]

She took off her stockings,
I held them to my face.
She had your ankles,
I felt filled with grace.
"Two hundred dollars straight in,
Two-fifty up the ass," she smiled and said.
She unbuckled my belt, pulled back her hair,
And sat in front me on the bed.

She said, "Honey, how's that feel,
Do you want me to go slow?"
My eyes drifted out the window,
Down the road below.
I felt my stomach tighten,
The sun bloodied the sky
And sliced through the hotel blinds,
I closed my eyes.

Sunlight on the Amatitlan,[ii]
Sunlight streaming thru your hair.
In the Valle de Dos Rios,[iii]
Smell of mock orange filled the air.
We rode with the *vaqueros*
Down into cool rivers of green.
I was sure the work and that smile comin' out 'neath your hat
Was all I'd ever need

Somehow all you ever need's,
Never really quite enough, you know.
You and I, Maria, we learned so.

She slipped me out of her mouth,
"You're ready," she said.
She took off her bra and panties, wet her finger,
Slipped it inside her and crawled over me on the bed.
She poured me another whisky,

Said, "Here's to the best you ever had,"
We laughed and made the toast.
It wasn't the best I ever had, not even close.

Across the Border

Tonight my bag is packed,
Tomorrow I'll walk these tracks
That will lead me across the border.

Tomorrow my love and I
Will sleep 'neath auburn skies
Somewhere across the border.

We'll leave behind, my dear,
The pain and sadness we found here
And we'll drink from the Bravo's muddy waters,

Where the sky grows grey and white
We'll meet on the other side,
There, across the border.

For you I'll build a house
High up on a grassy hill,
Somewhere across the border.

Where pain and memory,
Pain and memory have been stilled,
There, across the border,

And sweet blossoms fills the air,
Pastures of gold and green
Roll down into cool clear waters,

And in your arms 'neath the open skies,
I'll kiss the sorrow from your eyes,
There, across the border.

Tonight we'll sing the songs,
I'll dream of you my *corazón*
And tomorrow my heart will be strong,

And may the saints' blessing and grace
Carry me safely into your arms,
There, across the border.

For what are we
Without hope in our hearts
That someday we'll drink from God's blessed waters

And eat the fruit from the vine?
I know love and fortune will be mine
Somewhere across the border.

Matamoros Banks

For two days the river keeps you down,
Then you rise to the light without a sound
Past the playgrounds and empty switching yards.
The turtles eat the skin from your eyes, so they lay open to the stars.

Your clothes give away to the current and river stone
Till every trace of who you ever were is gone,
And the thing of the earth they make their claim
That the things of heaven may do the same.

    Goodbye, my darling,
    For your love I give God thanks.
    Meet me on the Matamoros,
    Meet me on the Matamoros,
    Meet me on the Matamoros banks.[i]

Over rivers of stone and ancient ocean beds
I walk on twine and tire tread.
My pockets full of dust, my mouth filled with cool stone,
The pale moon opens the earth to its bones.

    I long, my darling, for your kiss,
    For your sweet love I give God thanks,
    The touch of your loving fingertips.
    Meet me on the Matamoros,
    Meet me on the Matamoros,
    Meet me on the Matamoros banks.

Your sweet memory comes on the evenin' wind.
I sleep and dream of holding you in my arms again.
The lights of Brownsville, across the river shine,
A shout rings out and into the silty red river I dive.

    I long, my darling, for your kiss,
    For your sweet love I give God thanks,
    A touch of your loving fingertips.
    Meet me on the Matamoros,
    Meet me on the Matamoros,
    Meet me on the Matamoros banks.

Jesus Was an Only Son

Jesus was an only son
As he walked up Calvary Hill,
His mother Mary walking beside him
In the path where his blood spilled.

Jesus was an only son
In the hills of Nazareth,
As he lay reading the Psalms of David
At his mother's feet.

A mother prays, "Sleep tight, my child, sleep well,
For I'll be at your side
That no shadow, no darkness, no tolling bell,
Shall pierce your dreams this night."

In the garden at Gethsemane
He prayed for the life he'd never live,
He beseeched his Heavenly Father to remove
The cup of death from his lips.

Now there's a loss that can never be replaced,
A destination that can never be reached,
A light you'll never find in another's face,
A sea whose distance cannot be breached.

Well, Jesus kissed his mother's hands,
Whispered, "Mother, still your tears,
For remember the soul of the universe[i]
Willed a world and it appeared."

The Last Lone American Night

The Rising

Can't see nothin' in front of me,
Can't see nothin' coming up behind,
I make my way through this darkness,
I can't feel nothing but this chain that binds me.[i]

Lost track of how far I've gone,
How far I've gone, how high I've climbed,
On my back's a sixty-pound stone,[ii]
On my shoulder a half-mile line.[iii]

    Come on up for the rising,
    Come on up, lay your hands in mine,
    Come on up for the rising,
    Come on up for the rising tonight.

Left the house this morning,
Bells ringing filled the air,
Wearin' the cross of my calling[iv]
On wheels of fire I come rollin' down here.

    Come on up for the rising,
    Come on up, lay your hands in mine,
    Come on up for the rising,
    Come on up for the rising tonight.

Spirits above and behind me,
Faces gone, black eyes burnin' bright;
May their precious blood forever bind me,
Lord, as I stand before your fiery light.

I see you, Mary, in the garden,
In the garden of a thousand sighs,
There's holy pictures of our children
Dancin' in a sky filled with light.

May I feel your arms around me,
May I feel your blood mix with mine,
A dream of life comes to me
Like a catfish dancin' on the end of the line.[v]

Sky of blackness and sorrow,
Sky of love, sky of tears,
Sky of glory and sadness,
Sky of mercy, sky of fear,

Sky of memory and shadow,
Your burnin' wind fills my arms tonight,
Sky of longing and emptiness,
Sky of fullness, sky of blessed life.

Come on up for the rising,
Come on up, lay your hands in mine,
Come on up for the rising,
Come on up for the rising tonight.

You're Missing

Shirts in the closet, shoes in the hall,
Mama's in the kitchen, baby and all.
Everything is everything,
Everything is everything,
But you're missing.[i]

Coffee cup's on the counter, jacket's on the chair,
Paper's on the doorstep, you're not there.
Everything is everything,[ii]
Everything is everything,
But you're missing.

Pictures on the nightstand, TV's on in the den,
Your house is waiting, your house is waiting,
For you to walk in,
For you to walk in,
But you're missing.

You're missing when I shut out the lights,
You're missing when I close my eyes,
You're missing when I see the sun rise,
You're missing . . .

Children are asking if it's alright,
Will you be in our arms tonight?

Morning is morning, the evening falls,
I have too much room in my bed, too many phone calls.
How's everything, everything?
Everything, everything,
Bu you're missing.

God's drifting in heaven,
Devil's in the mailbox.[iii]
I got dust on my shoes,
Nothing but teardrops.

Nothing Man[i]

I don't remember how I felt, I never thought I'd live
To read about myself in my hometown paper.
How my brave young life was forever changed
In a misty cloud of pink vapor.[ii]

> Darlin', give me your kiss,
> Only understand,
> I am the nothing man.

Around here everybody acts the same,
Around here everybody acts like nothing's changed.
Friday night club meets at Al's Barbecue,
The sky is still the same unbelievable blue.

> Darlin', give me your kiss,
> Come and take my hand,
> I am the nothing man.

You can call me Joe, buy me a drink and shake my hand.
You want courage, I'll show you courage you can understand.
Pearl and silver[iii] restin' on my night table,
It's just me, Lord, pray I'm able.

> Darlin', with this kiss
> Say you understand,
> I am the nothing man.

My City of Ruins

There's a blood red circle
On the cold dark ground
And the rain is falling down.
The church door's thrown open,
I can hear the organ's song,
But the congregation's gone.
My city of ruins . . .
My city of ruins . . .

Now the sweet bells of mercy
Drift through the evening trees,
Young men on the corner like scattered leaves.
The boarded up windows,
The empty streets
While my brother's down on his knees.
My city of ruins . . .
My city of ruins . . .

    Come on, rise up!
    Come on, rise up!
    Come on, rise up!
    Come on, rise up!
    Come on, rise up!
    Come on, rise up!
    Come on, rise up!

Now there's tears on the pillow,
Darlin', where we slept,
And you took my heart when you left.
Without your sweet kiss,
My soul is lost, my friend.
Tell me how do I begin again?
My city's in ruins . . .
My city's in ruins . . .

Now with these hands,
With these hands,

With these hands,
With these hands,
I pray, Lord,
With these hands,
I pray for the strength, Lord,
With these hands,
I pray for the faith, Lord,
With these hands,
I pray for your love, Lord,
With these hands,
I pray for the strength, Lord,
With these hands,
I pray for your love, Lord,
With these hands,
I pray for the faith, Lord,
With these hands,
I pray for the strength, Lord.
With these hands,
Come on . . . Come on . . .

    Come on, rise up!
    Come on, rise up!
    Come on, rise up!
    Come on, rise up!
    Come on, rise up!
    Come on, rise up!
    Come on, rise up!
    Come on, rise up!
    Come on, rise up!
    Come on, rise up!
    Come on, rise up!

Radio Nowhere

I was tryin' to find my way home
But all I heard was a drone
Bouncing off a satellite,
Crushin' the last lone American night.

   This is radio nowhere,
   Is there anybody alive out there?[i]
   This is radio nowhere,
   Is there anybody alive out there?

I was spinnin' 'round a dead dial,
Just another lost number in a file,
Dancin' down a dark hole,
Just searchin' for a world with some soul.

   This is radio nowhere,
   Is there anybody alive out there?
   This is radio nowhere,
   Is there anybody alive out there?
   Is there anybody alive out there?

I just want to hear some rhythm . . .
I just want to hear some rhythm . . .
I just want to hear some rhythm . . .
I just want to hear some rhythm . . .

I want a thousand guitars,
I want pounding drums,
I want a million different voices
Speaking in tongues.

   This is radio nowhere,
   Is there anybody alive out there?
   This is radio nowhere,
   Is there anybody alive out there?
   Is there anybody alive out there?

I was driving through the misty rain,
Yeah, searchin' for a mystery train[ii]
Boppin' through the wild blue,
Tryin' to make a connection with you.

    This is radio nowhere,
    Is there anybody alive out there?
    This is radio nowhere,
    Is there anybody alive out there?
    Is there anybody alive out there?

I just want to feel some rhythm . . .
I just want to feel some rhythm . . .
I just want to feel some rhythm . . .
I just want to feel your rhythm . . .
I just want to feel your rhythm . . .
I just want to feel your rhythm . . .
I just want to feel your rhythm . . .
I just want to feel your rhythm . . .

Hunter of Invisible Game

I hauled myself up out of the ditch
And built me an ark out of gopher wood and pitch,
Sat down by the roadside and waited on the rain.
I am the hunter of invisible game.

Well, I woke last night to the heavy clicking and clack
And a scarecrow on fire along the railroad tracks:
There were empty cities and burning plains.
I am the hunter of invisible game.

We all come up a little short and we go down hard;
These days I spend my time skipping through the dark.
Through the empires of dust I chant your name:
I am the hunter of invisible game.

Through the bone yard rattle and black smoke we rolled on,
Down into the valley where the beast has his throne.
There I sing my song and I sharpen my blade:
I am the hunter of invisible game.

Strength is vanity and time is illusion.
I feel you breathing—the rest is confusion.
Your skin touches mine; what else to explain?
I am the hunter of invisible game

Now, pray for yourself and that you may not fall
When the hour of deliverance comes on us all,
When our hope and faith and courage and trust
Can rise or vanish like dust into dust.

Now there's a kingdom of love waiting to be reclaimed.
I am the hunter of invisible game,
I am the hunter of invisible game,
I am the hunter of invisible game.

Magic

I got a coin in my palm,
I can make it disappear.
I got a card up my sleeve,
Name it and I'll pull it out your ear.
I got a rabbit in the hat,
If you want to come and see,
This is what will be,
This is what will be.

I got shackles on my wrist,
Soon I'll slip 'em and be gone.
Chain me in a box in the river
And I'll rise singin' this song.
Trust none of what you hear
And less of what you see.
This is what will be,
This is what will be.

I got a shiny saw blade,
All I need's a volunteer.
I'll cut you in half
While you're smilin' ear to ear
And the freedom that you sought's
Driftin' like a ghost amongst the trees.
This is what will be,
This is what will be.

Now there's a fire down below
But it's coming up here,
So leave everything you know,
Carry only what you fear.
On the road the sun is sinkin' low,
There's bodies hanging in the trees.
This is what will be,
This is what will be.

Devils & Dust

I got my finger on the trigger
But I don't know who to trust.
When I look into your eyes
There's just devils and dust.
We're a long, long way from home, Bobbie[i]
Home's a long, long way from us.
I feel a dirty wind blowing,[ii]
Devils and dust.

    I got God on my side,[iii]
    And I'm just trying to survive.
    What if what you do to survive
    Kills the things you love?[iv]
    Fear's a powerful thing,
    It can turn your heart black, you can trust,
    It'll take your God filled soul
    And fill it with devils and dust.

Well, I dreamed of you last night
In a field of blood and stone,
The blood began to dry,
The smell began to rise.
Well, I dreamed of you last night,
In a field of mud and bone,
Your blood began to dry,
The smell began to rise.

    I got God on our side,
    And I'm just trying to survive.
    What if what you do to survive
    Kills the things you love?
    Fear's a powerful thing,
    It can turn your heart black, you can trust,
    It'll take your God filled soul
    And fill it with devils and dust.

Now every woman and every man
They want to take a righteous stand,
Find the love that God wills
And the faith that He commands.
I've got my finger on the trigger
And tonight faith just ain't enough.
When I look inside my heart
There's just devils and dust.

> I got God on my side,
> And I'm just trying to survive.
> What if what you do to survive
> Kills the things you love?
> Fear's a powerful thing,
> It can turn your heart black, you can trust,
> It'll take your God filled soul
> And fill it with devils and dust.

Devil's Arcade

Remember the morning we dug up your gun
The worms in the barrel, the hanging sun,
Those first nervous evenings of perfume and gin,
The lost smell on your breath as I helped you get it in,
The rush of your lips, the feel of your name,
The beat in your heart, the devil's arcade.

You said heroes are needed, so heroes get made.
Somebody made a bet, somebody paid.
The cool desert morning and nothing to save,
Just metal and plastic where your body caved,
The slow games of poker with Lieutenant Ray,
In the ward with the blue walls, a sea with no name
Where you lie adrift with the heroes of the devil's arcade.

You sleep and dream of your buddies Charlie and Jim
And wake with the thick desert dust on your skin.

A voice says, "Don't worry, I'm here.
Just whisper the word 'tomorrow' in my ear."
A house on a quiet street, a home for the brave,[l]
The glorious kingdom of the sun on your face
Rising from a long night as dark as the grave,
On a thin chain of next moments and something like faith,
On a morning to order a breakfast to make,
A bed draped in sunshine, a body that waits
For the touch of your fingers, the end of the day,
The beat of your heart,
The beat of your heart
The beat of your heart,
The beat of your heart
The beat of your heart,
The beat of her heart,
The beat of your heart,
The slow burning away
Of the bitter fires of the devil's arcade.

The Wall

Cigarettes and a bottle of beer—this poem that I wrote for you,
This black stone[i] and these hard tears are all I got left now of you.
I remember you in your Marine uniform laughing, laughing at your ship out
    party,
I read Robert McNamara says he's sorry.[ii]

Your high boots and striped T-shirt, ah, Billy you looked so bad.
Yeah, you and your rock 'n' roll band, you were the best thing this shit town ever
    had.
Now the men that put you here eat with their families in rich dining halls,
And apology and forgiveness got no place here at all, here at the wall.

Well, I'm sorry I missed you last year, I couldn't find no one to drive me.
If your eyes could cut through that black stone, tell me, would they recognize me?
For the living time it must be served as the day goes on
Cigarettes and a bottle of beer, skin on black stone.

On the ground dog tags and wreaths of flowers, with the ribbons red as the
    blood,
Red as the blood you spilled in the Central Highlands mud.
Limousines rush down Pennsylvania Avenue, rustling the leaves as they fall,
And apology and forgiveness got no place here at all, here at the wall.

Outlaw Pete

He was born a little baby on the Appalachian Trail,
At six months old he'd done three months in jail,
He robbed a bank in his diapers and his little bare baby feet,
All he said was, "Folks, my name is Outlaw Pete.

> "I'm Outlaw Pete!
> I'm Outlaw Pete!
> Can you hear me?"

At twenty-five a Mustang pony he did steal
And he rode her 'round and 'round on heaven's wheel.
"Father Jesus, I'm an outlaw, killer and a thief,
And I slow down only to sow my grief .

> "I'm Outlaw Pete!
> I'm Outlaw Pete!
> Can you hear me?"

He cut his trail of tears across the countryside
And where he went, women wept and men died.

One night he awoke from a vision of his own death,
Saddled his pony and rode out deep into the West,
Married a Navajo girl and settled down on the res,
And as the snow fell he held their beautiful daughter to his chest.

> "I'm Outlaw Pete!
> I'm Outlaw Pete!
> Can you hear me?
> Can you hear me?
> Can you hear me?"

Out of the East on an Irish stallion came bounty hunter Dan,
His heart quickened and burdened by the need to get his man.
He found Pete peacefully fishing by the river, pulled his gun and got the drop,
He said, "Pete, you think you've changed, but you have not."

He cocked his pistol, pulled the trigger and shouted, "Let it start!"
Pete drew a knife from his boot and pierced Dan through the heart.

Dan smiled as he lay in his own blood dying in the sun,
Whispered in Pete's ear, "We cannot undo these things we've done.

"You're Outlaw Pete!
You're Outlaw Pete!
Can you hear me?
Can you hear me?
Can you hear me?"

For forty days and nights Pete rode and did not stop
Till he sat high upon an icy mountaintop.
He watched a hawk on a desert updraft, slip and slide,
Moved to the edge and dug his spurs deep into his pony's side.

Some say Pete and his pony vanished over the edge,
And some say they remain frozen high upon that icy ledge.
The young Navajo girl washes in the river, her skin so fair
And braids a piece of Pete's buckskin chaps into her hair.

"Outlaw Pete!
Outlaw Pete!
Can you hear me?
Can you hear me?
Can you hear me?
Can you hear me?
Can you hear me?
Can you hear me?
Can you hear me?
Can you hear me?
Can you hear me?
Can you hear me?
Can you hear me?
Can you hear me?"

The Wrestler

Have you ever seen a one-trick pony[i] in the field so happy and free?
If you've ever seen a one-trick pony then you've seen me.
Have you ever seen a one-legged dog[ii] makin' his way down the street?
If you've ever seen a one-legged dog then you've seen me.

Then you've seen me, I come and stand at every door,
Then you've seen me, I always leave with less than I had before,
Then you've seen me, bet I can make you smile when the blood it hits the floor.
Tell me, friend, can you ask for anything more?
Tell me, can you ask for anything more?

Have you ever seen a scarecrow filled with nothing but dust and weeds?
If you've ever seen that scarecrow then you've seen me.
Have you ever seen a one-armed man punchin' at nothing but the breeze?
If you've ever seen a one-armed man then you've seen me.

Then you've seen me, I come and stand at every door,
Then you've seen me, I always leave with less than I had before,
Then you've seen me, bet I can make you smile when the blood it hits the floor.
Tell me, friend, can you ask for anything more?
Tell me, can you ask for anything more?

These things that have comforted me, I drive away,
This place that is my home, I cannot stay.
My only faith is in the broken bones and bruises I display.

Have you ever seen a one-legged man tryin' to dance his way free?
If you've ever seen a one-legged man then you've seen me

We Are Alive

We Take Care of Our Own

I've been knocking on the door that holds the throne,[i]
I've been looking for the map that leads me home,
I've been stumbling on good hearts turned to stone,
The road of good intentions has gone dry as a bone.[ii]

>   We take care of our own,
>   We take care of our own,
>   Wherever this flag's flown,
>   We take care of our own.[iii]

From Chicago to New Orleans,[iv] from the muscle to the bone,
From the shotgun shack[v] to the Superdome,[vi]
There ain't no help, the cavalry's stayed home,[vii]
There ain't no one hearing the bugle blown.

>   We take care of our own,
>   We take care of our own,
>   Wherever this flag's flown,
>   We take care of our own.

Where are the eyes, the eyes with the will to see?
Where are the hearts that run over with mercy?
Where's the love that has not forsaken me?
Where's the work that'll set my hands, my soul free?

Where's the Spirit that'll reign, reign over me?
Where's the promise from sea to shining sea?[viii]
Where's the promise from sea to shining sea?
Wherever this flag is flown, wherever this flag is flown . . .

>   We take care of our own,
>   We take care of our own,
>   Wherever this flag is flown,
>   We take care of our own.

Easy Money

You put on your coat, I'll put on my hat,
You put out the dog, I'll put out the cat,
You put on your red dress for me tonight, honey:
We're going on the town now looking for easy money.

There's nothing to it, mister, you won't hear a sound
When your whole world comes tumbling down,
And all them fat cats they just think it's funny.
I'm going on the town now looking for easy money.

I got a Smith & Wesson .38,
I got a hellfire burning and I got me a taste.
Got me a date on the far shore where it's bright and sunny:
I'm going on the town tonight looking for easy money.

You put on your coat, I'll put on my hat,
You put out the dog, I'll put out the cat,
You put on your red dress—you're looking real good, honey:
We're going on the town now looking for easy money . . .

Jack of All Trades

I'll mow your lawn, clean the leaves out your drain,
I'll mend your roof to keep out the rain,
I'll take the work that God provides:
I'm a Jack of all trades, honey, we'll be alright.

I'll hammer the nails and I'll set the stone,
I'll harvest your crops when they're ripe and grown.
I'll pull that engine apart and patch her up till she's running right:
I'm a Jack of all trades, we'll be alright.

The hurricane blows, brings a hard rain;
When the blue sky breaks, it feels like the world's gonna change.
We'll start caring for each other, like Jesus said that we might.
I'm a Jack of all trades, we'll be alright.

The banker man grows fat, the working man grows thin:
It's all happened before and it'll happen again,
It'll happen again, yeah, they'll bet your life.
I'm a Jack of all trades, darling, we'll be alright.

Now, sometimes tomorrow comes soaked in treasure and blood;
Here we stood the drought, now we'll stand the flood.
There's a new world coming, I can see the light.
I'm a Jack of all trades, we'll be alright.

So you use what you've got and you learn to make do:
You take the old, you make it new.
If I had me a gun, I'd find the bastards and shoot 'em on sight.
I'm a Jack of all trades, we'll be alright.

Death to My Hometown

Well, no cannonballs did fly,
No rifles cut us down
No bombs fell from the sky,
No blood soaked the ground,
No powder flash blinded the eye,
No deathly thunder sounded,
But just as sure as the hand of God,
They brought death to my hometown,
They brought death to my hometown, boys!

No shells ripped the evening sky,
No cities burning down,
No army stormed the shores for which we'd die,
No dictators were crowned.
I awoke from a quiet night,
I never heard a sound;
The marauders raided in the dark
And brought death to my hometown, boys,
Death to my hometown!

They destroyed our families, factories,
And they took our homes,
They left our bodies on the plains,
The vultures picked our bones.

So listen up, my sonny boy,
Be ready for when they come,
For they'll be returning
Sure as the rising sun.
Now, get yourself a song to sing
And sing it till you're done,
Yeah, sing it hard and sing it well,
Send the robber barons straight to hell,
The greedy thieves who came around
And ate the flesh of everything they found,
Whose crimes have gone unpunished now,
Who walk the streets as free men now . . .

Ah, they brought death to our hometown, boys,
Death to our hometown, boys,
Death to our hometown, boys,
Death to our hometown, whoa!

Rocky Ground

We've been traveling over rocky ground, rocky ground,
We've been traveling over rocky ground, rocky ground,
We've been traveling over rocky ground, rocky ground,
We've been traveling over rocky ground, rocky ground.[i]

Rise up shepherd, rise up![ii]
Your flock has roamed far from the hill,
The stars have faded, the sky is still,
The angels are shouting, "Glory hallelujah!"

We've been traveling over rocky ground, rocky ground,
We've been traveling over rocky ground, rocky ground.

Forty days and nights of rain washed this land.[iii]
Jesus said the money changers in this temple will not stand.[iv]
Find your flock, get them to higher ground:
The floodwater's rising, we're Canaan bound.[v]

We've been traveling over rocky ground, rocky ground,
We've been traveling over rocky ground, rocky ground.

Tend to your flock or they will stray.
We'll be called for our service come judgment day.
Before we cross that river wide
The blood on our hands will come back on us twice.[vi]

Rise up shepherd, rise up!
Your flock has roamed far from the hill,
The stars have faded, the sky is still,
Sun's in the heavens and a new day is rising.

You use your muscle and your mind and you pray your best
That your best is good enough, the Lord will do the rest.
You raise your children and you teach them to walk straight and sure,
You pray that hard times, hard times come no more.
You try to sleep, you toss and turn, the bottom's dropping out;
Where you once had faith now there's only doubt.
You pray for guidance only silence now meets your prayers.
The morning breaks, you awake, but no one's there.

We've been traveling over rocky ground, rocky ground,
We've been traveling over rocky ground, rocky ground . . .

There's a new day coming,
A new day's coming,
A new day's coming . . .

We've been traveling over rocky ground, rocky ground,
We've been traveling over rocky ground, rocky ground
We've been traveling over rocky ground, rocky ground,
We've been traveling over rocky ground, rocky ground . . .

Land of Hope and Dreams

This train—I'm running this train . . .
Don't you wanna ride this train, this train, this train . . .

Grab your ticket and your suitcase:
Thunder's rollin' down this track.
Well, you don't know where you're goin' now,
But you know you won't be back.
Well, darlin' if you're weary
Lay your head upon my chest;
We'll take what we can carry,
Yeah, and we'll leave the rest.
Big wheels roll through fields where sunlight streams:
Meet me in a land of hope and dreams.

Well, I will provide for you
And I'll stand by your side;
You'll need a good companion now
For this part of the ride.
Leave behind your sorrows,
Let this day be the last:
Tomorrow there'll be sunshine
And all this darkness past.
Big wheels roll through fields where sunlight streams:
Oh, meet me in a land of hope and dreams.

This train carries saints and sinners,
This train carries losers and winners,
This train carries whores and gamblers,
This train carries lost souls.

I said this train—dreams will not be thwarted,
This train—faith will be rewarded,
This train—hear the steel wheels singing,
This train—bells of freedom ringing.

Yes, this train carries saints and sinners,
This train carries losers and winners,

This train carries whores and gamblers,
This train carries lost souls.

I said, this train carries broken-hearted,
This train—thieves and sweet souls departed,
This train carries fools and kings thrown,
This train—all aboard!

I said, now this train—dreams will not be thwarted,
This train—faith will be rewarded,
This train—the steel wheels singing,
This train—bells of freedom ringing.[i]

Come on this train!
People get ready!
You don't need no ticket.
All you gotta do is
Just get onboard,
Onboard this train . . .[ii]

This train, now . . .

People get ready!
You don't need no ticket,
You don't need no ticket,
You just get onboard,
You just thank the Lord . . .

People get ready . . .

We Are Alive

There's a cross up yonder on Calvary Hill,
There's a slip of blood on a silver knife,
There's a graveyard kid down below
Where at night the dead come to life.
Well, above the stars they crackle and fire;
A dead man's moon throws seven rings.
We'd put our ears to the cold grave stones.
This is the song they'd sing:

> "We are alive—and though our bodies lie alone here in the dark
> Our spirits rise to carry the fire and light the spark,
> To stand shoulder to shoulder and heart to heart."

A voice cried, "I was killed in Maryland in 1877[i]
When the railroad workers made their stand."
"Well, I was killed in 1963,
One Sunday morning in Birmingham."[ii]
"I died last year crossing the southern desert,
My children left behind in San Pablo."
"Well, they've left our bodies here to rot.
Oh, please let them know

> "We are alive—And though we lie alone here in the dark
> Our souls will rise to carry the fire and light the spark,
> To fight shoulder to shoulder and heart to heart."

Let your mind rest easy, sleep well, my friend;
It's only our bodies that betray us in the end.

Well I awoke last night in the dark and dreamy deep;
From my head to my feet my body'd gone stone cold,
There were worms crawling all around me,
My fingers scratchin' at an earth black and six foot low.
Alone in the blackness of my grave,
Alone I'd been left to die.
Then I heard voices calling all 'round me;
The earth rose above me, my eyes filled with sky.

"We are alive—and though our bodies lie alone here in the dark
Our souls and spirits rise to carry the fire and light the spark,
To fight shoulder to shoulder and heart to heart ..."

THREE
Better Days

Glory Days

Dancing in the Dark

I get up in the evening and I ain't got nothing to say,[i]
I come home in the morning, I go to bed feeling the same way.
I ain't nothing but tired, man, I'm just tired and bored with myself,
Hey there baby, I could use just a little help.

> You can't start a fire,
> You can't start a fire without a spark.
> This gun's for hire[ii]
> Even if we're just dancing in the dark.

Message keeps getting clearer, radio's on and I'm moving 'round the place;
I check my look in the mirror, I wanna change my clothes, my hair, my face.
Man, I ain't getting nowhere: I'm just living in a dump like this.
There's something happening somewhere, baby, I just know that there is.

> You can't start a fire,
> You can't start a fire without a spark.
> This gun's for hire
> Even if we're just dancing in the dark.

You sit around getting older,
There's a joke here somewhere and it's on me.
I'll shake this world off my shoulders,
Come on baby this laugh's on me.

Stay on the streets of this town and they'll be carving you up alright.
They say you gotta stay hungry: hey baby, I'm just about starving tonight.
I'm dying for some action, I'm sick of sitting 'round here trying to write this book,
I need a love reaction: come on now, baby, gimme just one look.

> You can't start a fire
> Sitting 'round crying over a broken heart.
> This gun's for hire
> Even if we're just dancing in the dark.

> You can't start a fire
> Worrying about your little world falling apart.
> This gun's for hire
> Even if we're just dancing in the dark . . .

Glory Days

I had a friend was a big baseball player
Back in high school;
He could throw that speedball by you,
Make you look like a fool boy.
Saw him the other night at this roadside bar:
I was walking in, he was walking out;
We went back inside sat down had a few drinks,
But all he kept talking about was[i]

> Glory days, well, they'll pass you by,
> Glory days—In the wink of a young girl's eye,
> Glory days, glory days.

Well, there's a girl that lives up the block:
Back in school she could turn all the boy's heads.
Sometimes on a Friday I'll stop by and have a few drinks
After she put her kids to bed.
Her and her husband Bobby well they split up,
I guess it's two years gone by now.
We just sit around talking about the old times;
she says when she feels like crying she starts laughing thinking about

> Glory days, well, they'll pass you by,
> Glory days—In the wink of a young girl's eye,
> Glory days, glory days.[ii]

Now, I think I'm going down to the well tonight
And I'm going to drink till I get my fill.
And I hope when I get old I don't sit around thinking about it,
But I probably will.
Yeah, just sitting back, trying to recapture
A little of the glory of.
Well, time slips away and leaves you with nothing, mister,
But boring stories of

> Glory days, well, they'll pass you by,
> Glory days—In the wink of a young girl's eye,
> Glory days, glory days.

No Surrender

We busted out of class: had to get away from those fools.
We learned more from a three minute record, baby, than we ever learned in
    school.
Tonight I hear the neighborhood drummer sound,
I can feel my heart begin to pound.
You say you're tired and you just want to close your eyes
And follow your dreams down.

    Well, we made a promise we swore we'd always remember:
    No retreat, baby, no surrender.
    Like soldiers in the winter's night with a vow to defend:
    No retreat, baby, no surrender.

Now, young faces grow sad and old, and hearts of fire grow cold.
We swore blood brothers against the wind . . .
I'm ready to grow young again
And hear your sister's voice calling us home across the open yards.
Well, maybe we could cut someplace of our own
With these drums and these guitars.

    Well, we made a promise we swore we'd always remember:
    No retreat, baby, no surrender.
    Blood brothers in the stormy night with a vow to defend:
    No retreat, baby, no surrender.

Now on the street tonight the lights grow dim,
The walls of my room are closing in;
There's a war outside still raging:
You say it ain't ours anymore to win.
I want to sleep beneath peaceful skies in my lover's bed
With a wide open country in my eyes
And these romantic dreams in my head.

    Well, we made a promise we swore we'd always remember:
    No retreat, baby, no surrender.
    Blood brothers in the stormy night with a vow to defend:
    No retreat, baby, no surrender . . .

Bobby Jean

Well, I came by your house the other day:
Your mother said you went away,
She said there was nothing
That I could have done,
There was nothing nobody could say.
Now, me and you we've known each other
Ever since we were sixteen;
I wished I would have known,
I wished I could have called you
Just to say goodbye, Bobby Jean.

Now, you hung with me when all the others
Turned away, turned up their nose;
We liked the same music,
We liked the same bands,
We liked the same clothes.
Yeah, we told each other that we were the wildest,
the wildest things we'd ever seen.
Now, I wished you would have told me,
I wished I could have talked to you
Just to say goodbye Bobby Jean.

Now, we went walking in the rain
Talking about the pain from the world we hid.
Now, there ain't nobody, nowhere, nohow
Gonna ever understand me the way you did.

Well, maybe you'll be out there on that road somewhere,
In some bus or train travelling along;
In some motel room
There'll be a radio playing
And you'll hear me sing this song.
Well, if you do, you'll know I'm thinking of you
And all the miles in between,
And I'm just calling one last time,
Not to change your mind,
but just to say I miss you baby good luck, goodbye,
Bobby Jean.

Blood Brothers

We played king of the mountain out on the end,
The world come chargin' up the hill, and we were women and men.
Now there's so much that time, time and memory fade away:
We got our own roads to ride and chances we gotta take;
We stood side by side each one fightin' for the other.
We said until we died we'd always be blood brothers.

Now the hardness of this world slowly grinds your dreams away
Makin' a fool's joke out of the promises we make;
And what once seemed black and white turns to so many shades of gray:
We lose ourselves in work to do, work to do and bills to pay.
And it's a ride, ride, ride, and there ain't much cover
With no one runnin' by your side, my blood brother,

On through the houses of the dead past those fallen in their tracks,
Always movin' ahead, and never lookin' back.

Now, I don't know how I feel, I don't know how I feel tonight,
If I've fallen 'neath the wheel, if I've lost or I've gained sight;
I don't even know why, I don't know why I made this call
Or if any of this matters anymore after all . . .
But the stars are burnin' bright like some mystery uncovered:
I'll keep movin' through the dark with you in my heart, my blood brother.

The Last Carnival

Sundown, sundown:
They're taking all the tents down.
Where have you gone, my handsome Billy?

Sundown, sundown:
The carnival train's leavin' town.
Where are you now, my darlin' Billy?

We won't be dancing together on the high wire,
Facing the lions with you at my side anymore,
We won't be breathin' the smoke and the fire
On the midway.

Hangin' from the trapeze my wrists waitin' for your wrists:
Two daredevils high up on the wall of death.
You throwin' the knife that lands inches from my heart
—Sundown.

Moonrise, moonrise:
The light that was in your eyes
has gone away.

Daybreak, daybreak:
The thing in you that made me ache
has gone to stay.

We'll be riding the train without you, tonight,
The train that keeps on movin'—its black smoke scorching the evening sky;
A million stars shining above us like every soul livin' and dead
Has been gathered together by a God to sing a hymn over your bones.

Sundown, sundown:
Empty are the fairgrounds.
Where are you now, my handsome Billy?

Real World

Tunnel of Love

Fat man sitting on a little stool
Takes the money from my hand while his eyes take a walk all over you,
Hands me the ticket, smiles and whispers good luck.
Cuddle up angel, cuddle up my little dove:
We'll ride down, baby, into this tunnel of love

I can feel the soft silk of your blouse
And them soft thrills in our little fun house;
Then the lights go out and it's just the three of us:
You me and all that stuff we're so scared of.
Gotta ride down, baby, into this tunnel of love.

There's a crazy mirror showing us both in 5-D:
I'm laughing at you you're laughing at me.
There's a room of shadows that gets so dark, brother;
It's easy for two people to lose each other in this tunnel of love.

It ought to be easy, ought to be simple enough:
Man meets woman and they fall in love.
But this house is haunted and the ride gets rough,
And you've got to learn to live with what you can't rise above
If you want to ride on down in through this tunnel of love.

The Honeymooners

Two kids get married—same old thing:
Folks congratulate you, church bells ring,
Who's got the ring, who's gonna pay the priest,
Get your mama in the paper, picture or two at least . . .

And at the reception all the old records play,
"Where you gonna live, are you gonna take her away?"
In a corner my new nephew's showin' me his knife;
"You swore that you'd love her for the rest of your life."

Went to kiss you at the altar: we bumped heads.
Honeymoon night we figured we best shake on it instead.
Dressed kinda funny, laughin' we hop in bed:
"You can swear it on your feet, you can swear it on your head."

Come mornin', my new family's sitting on the front porch swing,
Smilin' kinda funny, nobody says a thing.
My new brother-in-law's throwin' a football, he tosses me a pass;
We all sit down on the front stoop—everybody happy at last.

One Step Up

Woke up this morning: my house was cold.
Checked out the furnace: she wasn't burnin'.
Went out and hopped in my old Ford
Hit the engine but she ain't turnin'.
We've given each other some hard lessons lately,
But we ain't learnin'.
We're the same sad story, that's a fact
—One step up and two steps back.

Bird on a wire outside my motel room,
But he ain't singin'.
Girl in white outside a church in June,
But the church bells they ain't ringing.
I'm sittin' here in this bar tonight,
But all I'm thinkin' is
I'm the same old story, same old act
—One step up and two steps back.

It's the same thing night on night:
Who's wrong, baby, who's right . . .
Another fight and I slam the door
On another battle in our dirty little war.
When I look at myself I don't see
The man I wanted to be;
Somewhere along the line I slipped off track:
I'm caught movin' one step up and two steps back.

There's a girl across the bar:
I get the message she's sendin'.
Mmm . . . she ain't lookin' too married
And me, well, honey, I'm pretending.
Last night I dreamed I held you in my arms:
The music was never-ending.
We danced as the evening sky faded to black
—One step up and two steps back.

Brilliant Disguise

I hold you in my arms as the band plays.
What are those words whispered, baby, just as you turn away?
I saw you last night out on the edge of town,
I wanna read your mind to know just what I've got in this new thing I've found.
So, tell me what I see when I look in your eyes:
Is that you baby or just a brilliant disguise?

I heard somebody call your name from underneath our willow,
I saw something tucked in shame underneath your pillow.
Well, I've tried so hard, baby, but I just can't see
What a woman like you is doing with me.
So, tell me who I see when I look in your eyes:
Is that you baby or just a brilliant disguise?

Now, look at me, baby, struggling to do everything right,
And then it all falls apart when out go the lights.
I'm just a lonely pilgrim, I walk this world in wealth;
I want to know if it's you I don't trust, 'cause I damn sure don't trust myself.

Now you play the loving woman, I'll play the faithful man,
But just don't look too close into the palm of my hand.
We stood at the altar, the gypsy swore our future was right;
But come the wee wee hours . . . well, maybe, baby, the gypsy lied.
So when you look at me you better look hard and look twice:
Is that me baby or just a brilliant disguise?

Tonight our bed is cold: I'm lost in the darkness of our love.
God have mercy on the man who doubts what he's sure of.

Tougher than the Rest

Well, it's Saturday night: you're all dressed up in blue.
I been watching you awhile, maybe you been watching me too.
So somebody ran out, left somebody's heart in a mess;
Well, if you're looking for love, honey, I'm tougher than the rest.

Some girls they want a handsome Dan or some good-lookin' Joe,
On their arm some girls like a sweet-talkin' Romeo,
Well, 'round here, baby, I learned you get what you can get,
So, if you're rough enough for love, honey, I'm tougher than the rest.

The road is dark and it's a thin thin line,
But I want you to know I'll walk it for you any time.
Maybe your other boyfriends couldn't pass the test;
Well, if you're rough and ready for love, honey, I'm tougher than the rest.

Well, it ain't no secret I've been around a time or two;
Well, I don't know, baby, maybe you've been around, too.
Well, there's another dance: all you gotta do is say yes,
And if you're rough and ready for love, honey, I'm tougher than the rest,
If you're rough enough for love, baby, I'm tougher than the rest.

The Wish

Dirty old street all slushed up in the rain and snow,
Little boy and his ma shivering outside a rundown music store window.
That night on top of the Christmas tree shines one beautiful star
And lying underneath a brand-new Japanese guitar.[i]

I remember in the morning, ma, hearing your alarm clock ring:
I'd lie in bed and listen to you getting ready for work, the sound of your makeup
    case on the sink
And the ladies at the office, all lipstick, perfume and rustlin' skirts,[ii]
And how proud and happy you always looked walking home from work.

If pa's eyes were windows into a world so deadly and true
You couldn't stop me from looking, but you kept me from crawlin' through.
And if it's a funny old world, mama, where a little boy's wishes come true
Well, I got a few in my pocket and a special one just for you.

It ain't no phone call on Sunday, flowers or a mother's day card,
It ain't no house on a hill with a garden and a nice little yard;
I got my hot rod down on Bond Street,[iii] I'm older but you'll know me in a
    glance:
We'll find us a little rock 'n' roll bar and, baby, we'll go out and dance.

Well, it was me in my Beatle boots, you in pink curlers and matador pants
Pullin' me up on the couch to do the twist for my uncles and aunts.
Well, I found a girl of my own now, ma: I popped the question on your birthday.
She stood waiting on the front porch while you were telling me to get out there
    and say what it was that I had to say

Last night we all sat around laughing at the things that guitar brought us,
And I lay awake thinking 'bout the other things it's brought us.
Well, tonight I'm takin' requests here in the kitchen—this one's for you, ma, let
    me come right out and say it;
It's overdue, but baby, if you're looking for a sad song, well I ain't gonna play it.

With Every Wish

Ol' catfish in the lake—we called him Big Jim:
When I was a kid my only wish was to get my line in him.
Skipped church one Sunday rowed out and throw'd in my line;
Jim took that hook pole and me right over the side.
Went driftin' down past old tires and rusty cans of beer;
The angel of the lake whispered in my ear,
"Before you choose your wish, son, you better think first:
With every wish there comes a curse."

I fell in love with beautiful Doreen:
She was the prettiest thing this old town'd ever seen.
I courted her and I made her mine,
But I grew jealous whenever another man'd come walkin' down the line.
And my jealousy made me treat her mean and cruel;
She sighed, "Bobby oh Bobby you're such a fool!
Don't you know before you choose your wish you'd better think first
'Cause with every wish there comes a curse?"

These days I sit around and laugh at the many rivers I've crossed,
But on the far banks there's always another forest where a man can get lost.
Well, there in the high trees love's bluebird glides
Guiding us 'cross to another river on the other side,
And there someone is waitin' with a look in her eyes,
And though my heart's grown weary and more than a little bit shy
Tonight I'll drink from her waters to quench my thirst
And leave the angels to worry with every wish . . .

Real World

Mister Trouble come walkin' this way;
Year gone by feels like one long day,
But I'm alive and I'm feelin' all right.
Well, I run that hard road outta heartbreak city,
Built a roadside carnival out of hurt and self-pity:
It was all wrong . . . Well, now I'm moving on.

> Ain't no church bells ringing, ain't no flags unfurled:
> It's just me and you and the love we're bringing
> Into the real world,
> Into the real world.

I built a shrine in my heart: it wasn't pretty to see,
Made out of fool's gold memory and tears cried.
Now I'm headin' over the rise,
I'm searchin' for one clear moment of love and truth;
I still got a little faith, but what I need is some proof tonight:
I'm lookin' for it in your eyes.

> Ain't no church bells ringing, ain't no flags unfurled:
> It's just me and you and the love we're bringing
> Into the real world,
> Into the real world.

Well, tonight I just wanna shout!
I feel my soul waist deep and sinkin' into this black river of doubt.
I just wanna rise and walk along the riverside
And when the morning comes, baby, I don't wanna hide:
I'll stand right at your side with my arms open wide.

Well, tonight I just wanna shout!
I feel my soul waist deep and sinkin' into this black river of doubt.
I just wanna rise and walk along the riverside,
'Til the morning comes I'll stand right by your side.

I wanna find some answers, I wanna ask for some help;
I'm tired of running scared. Baby, let's get our bags packed:
We'll take it here to hell and heaven and back.

And if love is hopeless—hopeless at best—
Come on, put on your party dress: it's ours tonight
And we're goin' with the tumblin' dice.

> Ain't no church bells ringing, ain't no flags unfurled:
> It's just me and you and the love we're bringing
> Into the real world,
> Into the real world.

Better Days

Well, my soul checked out missing as I sat listening
To the hours and minutes tickin' away,
Yeah, just sittin' around waitin' for my life to begin
While it was all just slippin' away.
I'm tired of waitin' for tomorrow to come
Or that train to come roarin' 'round the bend:
I got a new suit of clothes and a pretty red rose
And a woman I can call my friend.

These are better days, baby,
Yeah, there's better days shining through,
These are better days, baby,
Better days with a girl like you.

Well, I took a piss at fortune's sweet kiss:
It's like eatin' caviar and dirt.
It's a sad funny ending to find yourself pretending
A rich man in a poor man's shirt.
Now, my ass was draggin' when from a passin' gypsy wagon
Your heart like a diamond shone.
Tonight I'm layin' in your arms carvin' lucky charms
Out of these hard luck bones.

These are better days, baby,
These are better days, it's true.
These are better days,
There's better days shining through.

Now a life of leisure and a pirate's treasure
Don't make much for tragedy,
But it's a sad man my friend who's livin' in his own skin
And can't stand the company.
Every fool's got a reason to feelin' sorry for himself
And turn his heart to stone.
Tonight this fool's halfway to heaven and just a mile outta hell
And I feel like I'm comin' home.

These are better days, baby,
Yeah, there's better days shining through,
These are better days, baby,
Better days with a girl like you.

These are better days, baby,
These are better days, it's true.
These are better days,
There's better days shining through.

If I Should Fall Behind

We said we'd walk together, baby, come what may,
That come the twilight should we lose our way,
If as we're walkin' a hand should slip free
I'll wait for you
And should I fall behind wait for me.

We swore we'd travel, darlin', side by side,
We'd help each other stay in stride;
But each lover's steps fall so differently.
But I'll wait for you
And if I should fall behind wait for me.

Now, everyone dreams of a love lasting and true,
But you and I know what this world can do.
So let's make our steps clear that the other may see,
And I'll wait for you
And if I should fall behind wait for me.

Now, there's a beautiful river in the valley ahead:
There, 'neath the oak's bough soon we will be wed.
Should we lose each other in the shadow of the evening trees
I'll wait for you
And should I fall behind wait for me.

Living Proof

Well, now on a summer night
In a dusky room
Come a little piece of the Lord's undying light
Crying like he swallowed the fiery moon;
In his mother's arms
It was all the beauty I could take
Like the missing words to some prayer
that I could never make.

In a world so hard and dirty,
So fouled and confused,
Searching for a little bit of God's mercy
I found living proof.

Well, I put my heart and soul,
I put 'em high upon a shelf
Right next to the faith,
The faith that I'd lost in myself.
I went down into the desert city
Just tryin' so hard to shed my skin;
I crawled deep into some kind of darkness
Lookin' to burn out every trace of who I'd been.

You do some sad, sad things, baby.
When it's you you're tryin' to lose;
You do some sad and hurtful things
—I've seen living proof.

You shot through my anger and rage
To show me my prison was just an open cage:
There were no keys, no guards,
Just one frightened man and some old shadows for bars.

Well, now all that's sure on the boulevard
Is that life is just a house of cards
As fragile as each and every breath
Of this boy sleepin' in our bed.

Tonight let's lie beneath the eaves
—Just a close band of happy thieves.
And when that train comes we'll get on board
And steal what we can from the treasures of the Lord.

It's been a long, long drought, baby.
Tonight the rain's pourin' down on our roof.
Looking for a little bit of God's mercy
I found living proof.

Long Time Comin'

Out where the creek turns shallow and sandy
And the moon comes skimmin' away the stars
The wind in the mesquite comes rushin' over the hilltops
Straight into my arms,
Straight into my arms.

I'm riding hard carryin' a catch of roses
And a fresh map that I made;
Tonight I'm gonna get birth naked and bury my old soul
And dance on its grave,
And dance on its grave.

    It's been a long time comin', my dear,
    It's been a long time comin', but now it's here.

Well, my daddy he was just a stranger,
Lived in a hotel downtown;
When I was a kid he was just somebody,
Somebody I'd see around,
Somebody I'd see around.

Now, down below and pullin' on my shirt
I got some kids of my own;
Well, if I had one wish in this god forsaken world, kids,
It'd be that your mistakes would be your own,
Yeah, your sins would be your own.

    It's been a long time comin', my dear,
    It's been a long time comin', but now it's here.

Out, 'neath the arms of Cassiopeia
Where the sword of Orion sweeps
It's me and you, Rosie,[i] cracklin' like crossed wires
And you breathin' in your sleep,
You breathin' in your sleep.

Well, there's just a spark of campfire burning,
Two kids in a sleeping bag beside.

I reach 'neath your shirt, lay my hands across your belly
And feel another one kickin' inside:
I ain't gonna fuck it up this time.

    It's been a long time comin', my dear,
    It's been a long time comin', but now it's here.

EPILOGUE

Long Walk Home

Last night I stood at your doorstep
Trying to figure out what went wrong;
You just slipped somethin' into my palm,
Then you were gone.

I could smell the same deep green of summer,
Above me the same night sky was glowin';
In the distance I could see the town
Where I was born.

> It's gonna be a long walk home,
> Hey, pretty darling, don't wait up for me,
> Gonna be a long walk home,
> A long walk home.

In town I passed Sal's grocery,
The barbershop on South Street,
I looked into their faces:
They were all rank strangers to me.

The veterans' hall high up on the hill
Stood silent and alone,
The diner was shuttered and boarded
With a sign that just said "GONE."

> It's gonna be a long walk home,
> Hey, pretty darling, don't wait up for me,
> Gonna be a long walk home,
> Hey, pretty darling, don't wait up for me,
> Gonna be a long walk home,
> It's gonna be a long walk home.

Here everybody has a neighbor,
Everybody has a friend,
Everybody has a reason to begin again.

My father said, "Son, we're lucky in this town,
It's a beautiful place to be born,

It just wraps its arms around you:
Nobody crowds you, nobody goes it alone.

That you know, flag flying over the courthouse
Means certain things are set in stone:
Who we are, what we'll do
And what we won't."

> It's gonna be a long walk home,
> Hey, pretty darling, don't wait up for me,
> Gonna be a long walk home,
> Hey, pretty darling, don't wait up for me,
> Gonna be a long walk home,
> It's gonna be a long walk home . . .

NOTES TO THE LYRICS

by Leonardo Colombati

Prologue

"American Land"

©2006 Bruce Springsteen (GMR)

Released on: *We Shall Overcome: The Seeger Sessions—American Land Edition* album (2006) live at Madison Square Garden, New York, NY, June 22, 2006 | *Live in Dublin* album (2007) live at Point Theatre, Dublin, November 18, 2006 | *London Calling: Live in Hyde Park* home video (2010) recorded live at Hyde Park, London, June 28, 2009 | *Wrecking Ball* album (2012)

Live premiere: 06/22/2006—Madison Square Garden, New York, NY

"American Land" is based on a poem written around 1900 by a Slovak steelworker named Andrei Kodaly. The lyrics were inspired by an incident in a Bessemer mill in McKeesport, Pennsylvania. A Slovak friend and coworker of Kovaly had saved enough money to enable his family to come over from Slovakia. While his wife and children were on the way to America, he lost his life on the job. In 1947, after finishing a concert for the International Workers' Union near Pittsburgh, Pete Seeger met Kovaly, who reportedly sang the song to him. Seeger translated the poem into English, put it to music (giving it a vaguely Eastern European flavor) and recorded it with the title "He Lies in the American Land," including it on his *American Industrial Ballads* album (1957). Springsteen's version partially welcomes just the first two stanzas, to then move away from the original. Even the music is totally different from that composed by Seeger: Springsteen in fact arranges his "American Land" around a more Celtic key, perhaps drawing inspiration from the traditional Scottish piece "Gallant Forty-Two."

[i] The line "She met me in the valley of red-hot steel and fire" is present in the lyrics printed on the album booklet *We Shall Overcome—American Land Edition*, even if in the live recording Springsteen sings "I wandered through the valley of red-hot steel and fire."

[ii] The Zerillis quoted in the lyrics are the family of Springsteen's mother, Adele, whose father, Antonio, came to America around the turn of the century from Vico Equense, in Southern Italy, at the age of twelve.

[iii] The lines "Come across the water a thousand miles from home / With nothing in their bellies but the fire down below" are present on the lyrics printed on the album booklet *We Shall Overcome—American Land Edition*, even though in the live recording Springsteen sings: "the Puerto Ricans, illegals, the Asians, Arabs miles from home / come across the water with a fire down below."

[iv] This verse is adopted in its entirety from Woody Guthrie's "Deportee (Plane Wreck at Los Gatos)." Guthrie wrote the lyrics in 1948, detailing the crash of a plane near Los Gatos Canyon, in California. He was inspired to write the song by what he considered the racist mistreatment of the passengers before and after the accident (the crash resulted in the deaths of thirty-two people, four Americans and twenty-eight migrant farm workers who were being deported from California back to Mexico). A decade later, Guthrie's poem was set to music by Martin Hoffman. Shortly afterward, Pete Seeger began performing the song at concerts. Bruce Springsteen himself recorded "Deportee (Plane Wreck at Los Gatos)" for the tribute album 'Til We Outnumber 'Em: The Songs of Woody Guthrie (2000).

ONE

Jungleland

Growin' Up

"Used cars," "Mansion on the Hill," and "My Father's House"—three songs taken from the *Nebraska* album of 1982—speak of Springsteen's childhood, with particular attention to his relationship with his father. Springsteen recalls that his family lived with his grandparents until he was six. "There was something about the walls, the lack of decoration, the almost painful plainness."[1]

"Growin' Up"—from the *Greetings from Asbury Park, NJ* album of 1973—represents the hinge between childhood and adolescence. The discovery of rock 'n' roll is the event that will symbolically mark this passage. "The first day I can remember looking in a mirror and being able to stand what I was seeing was the day I had a guitar in my hand,"[2] Springsteen said.

The section closes with a group of songs in which Springsteen describes both the romantic and violent sides of his young provincial heroes, back and forth between New Jersey and a New York populated by jazz players, fancied-up drug dealers, pimps and whores (the "South Side sisters" in "It's Hard to Be a Saint in the City," the stripteaser in "Kitty's Back," and the "fish-lady" in "Incident on 57th Street"). It is like a *bildungsroman* that develops, firstly, around an ever more cinematographic style of writing. Even the title of Springsteen's second album comes from *The Wild and the Innocent*, a 1959 Audie Murphy Western about a pair of frontier teenagers whose first journey to the big city nearly corrupts them both. "There were just a lot of characters around; everybody had nicknames. A lot of street life, and the boardwalk," Bruce says. "I was drawing a lot from where I came from. I'm going to make this gumbo, and what's my life? . . . Well, New Jersey."[3]

As Bruce strained toward some kind of glorious future, his life still took place in a dying city, Asbury Park. The only way out came from his guitar. "Had no dough, nowhere to go, nothing to do," he recalls. "Didn't know many people. It was cold and I wrote a lot. And I got to feeling guilty if I didn't. Terrible guilt feelings. Like it was masturbation. That bad!"[4] It didn't take long for girls to notice and come round to this introverted guitarist. "Bruce would cut out from South Street and spend whole evenings wedged in a phone box, where, he said, 'I used to stand and call my girl and get her to call me back, and then talk to her all night.'"[5] A year or two later, he would chase "the factory girls underneath the boardwalk where they promise to unsnap their jeans," as he sings in "4th of July, Asbury Park (Sandy)."

However, Asbury Park continued to feel tight to him. "He had 'stuff to say,' and needed a bigger stage than Jersey from which to say it."[6] He needed the Big Apple.

"Used Cars"

©1982 Bruce Springsteen (GMR)

Released on: *Nebraska* album (1982)

Live premiere: 06/29/1984—St. Paul Civic Center, St. Paul, MN

"Used Cars," written in the autumn of 1981 and published one year later on *Nebraska*, is in memory of Springsteen's father, Douglas, and of his childhood spent in a 1950s American suburb. Introducing it during a concert in Philadelphia in 2005, its author describes how they "had about every, every kind of used car imaginable. We had one that didn't even have a working muffler; so that was the one where if my pop would spot a police car, he'd turn the engine off real quickly till it went by. Then we had the used car that didn't go in reverse. I always remember we'd pull it in a parking place and me and him pushing it, pushing it out, pushing it back, back out to get it out. Never went in reverse. Then we had, of course, the no-heater, but that was small potatoes. Then we had the great no-starter; my room was right over the backyard and I'd hear my poor old, old dad out there in the morning on the ice-cold ground, underneath the hood trying to get the thing going. Now there are no more used cars; those are gone; they are now 'pre-owned.' I don't know what happened to the word 'used'; I mean, was it like a bad word or . . . ? Why did it get thrown out? I mean, 'pre-owned' is pretty stupid!"

After the Born in the U.S.A. Tour, "Used Cars" was performed only once (in Freehold, 1996) until 2005 when Springsteen sporadically proposed it again during the acoustic tour following *Devils & Dust*. On June 10, 2009, it was played at Ypsilanti in Michigan, during one of the election rallies Springsteen did for Barack Obama's election campaign.

[i] Michigan Avenue is in Brick Town, Monmouth County, twenty-five miles from Freehold, NJ, Springsteen's natal city.

"Mansion on the Hill"

©1982 Bruce Springsteen (GMR)

Released on: *Nebraska* album (1982) | *Live in New York City* album & home video (2001) recorded live at Madison Square Garden, New York, NY, June 29, 2000

Live premiere: 06/29/1984—St. Paul Civic Center, St. Paul, MN

This was the first song Springsteen finished writing for *Nebraska* (1982), tied to childhood memories of his paternal figure. During a concert at the Shoreline Amphitheatre in 1986, Springsteen told the audience that the song is about when he was a kid and his father used to drive them out to this old house on the outside of town. "He used to drive out of town and look at this big white house. It became a kind of touchstone for me. Now, when I dream, sometimes I'm on the outside looking in—and sometimes I'm the man on the inside."

The song owes much, right from its title, to "A Mansion on the Hill" by Hank Williams, where the woman who lives in the house on the hill leaves the narrator, declaring her desire to live alone and without love. It is typical of the romantic relationship disturbed by class differences. Springsteen's lyrics are also embedded with class issues. Around 1970 Springsteen took his girlfriend out to a family meeting at his grandfather Zerilli's house, which the pair referred to as "the house on the hill." Bruce's grandfather Anthony (Antonio) Alexander Andrei Zerilli served three years in the navy, spent three years in Sing Sing, and made some money; his modest farmhouse was a mansion on a hill to young Bruce.

Johnny Cash covered this on the 2000 album *Badlands: A Tribute to Bruce Springsteen's Nebraska*.

[i] Linden Town is in New Jersey, on the New Jersey Turnpike. Factory workers could be the ones leaving from the General Motors factory assembly line or the Phillips Bayway refinery.

"My Father's House"

©1982 Bruce Springsteen (GMR)

Released on: *Nebraska* album (1982)

Live premiere: 07/26/1984—Exhibition Grandstand Stadium, Toronto, Canada

This was the last song Springsteen finished for *Nebraska* (1982). At a concert in Los Angeles in 1990, Springsteen introduced the song with this story: "I had this habit for a long time: I used to get in my car and drive back through my old neighborhood in the town I grew up in. I'd always drive past the old houses that I used to live in, sometimes late at night. I got so I would do it really regularly—two, three, four times a week for years. I eventually got to wondering, 'What the hell am I doing?' So, I went to see the psychiatrist. I said, 'Doc, for years I've been getting in my car and driving past my old houses late at night. What am I doing?' He said, 'I want you to tell me what you think you're doing.' I go, 'That's what I'm paying you for.' He said, 'Well, something bad happened and you're going back thinking you can make it right again. Something went wrong and you keep going back to see if you can fix it or somehow make it right.' I sat there, and I said, 'That is what I'm doing.' He said, 'Well, you can't.'"

The theme of the son returning to his father's home is an evident reference to the evangelic parable of the prodigal son, even though in "My Father's House" the father is no longer there to wait for his son where sins "lie unatoned." Noted first among Springsteen's inspirations must be "Precious Memories," a gospel hymn written by J.B.F. Wright in 1925 and recorded by a number of artists—Johnny Cash, Aretha Franklin, and Bob Dylan to name but a few:

> Precious memories, how they linger,
> How they ever flood my soul . . .
> And old home scenes of my childhood,
> In fond memory appears.
> As I travel on life's pathway,
> Know not what the years may hold.

Springsteen recorded his version of the song during the *Nebraska* rehearsals. A further source could be "I'm on My Way Back to the Old Home" by Bill Monroe. "My Father's House" is included in the *Chapter and Verse* anthology (2016).

[i] The lines "I heard the wind rustling through the trees / and ghostly voices rose from the fields" are reminiscent of a Flannery O'Connor short story, "The Turkey," in which a child, robbed of the wild turkey he had found, runs across the woods towards home: "He could hear the wind blowing through the tree tops like a long, satisfied pull of air."[7]

[ii] In "devil snappin' at my heels," there is yet another reference to Flannery O'Connor's "The Turkey" when we read that while running the boy "felt certain that Something Terrible was running after him with stiff arms and fingers ready to grab him."[8] But one can also make out an echo of "Hellhounds on My Trail" recorded by Robert Johnson in 1937.

"Growin' Up"

©1972 Bruce Springsteen (GMR)

Released on: *Greetings from Asbury Park, NJ* album (1973) | *Live/1975–85* box set (1986) recoded live at the Roxy Theatre, Los Angeles, CA, July 7, 1978 | *In Concert/MTV Plugged* home video (1992) recorded live at Warner Hollywood Studios, Los Angeles, CA, September 22, 1992 | *Tracks* box set

(1998) May 3, 1972 demo version | *Live in Dublin* album & home video (2007) recorded live at the Depot Theater, Dublin, November 17, 2006

Live premiere: 12/07/1972—Kenny's Castaways, New York, NY

According to Sony's database of Springsteen recording sessions, "Growin' Up" was cut on June 7, 1972 (the first studio session for the *Greetings from Asbury Park, NJ* album), and on June 27, 1972, at 914 Sound Studios in Blauvelt, New York. The song was written in 1971 and shares similar music with "Eloise," an unreleased demo.

A solo demo of "Growin' Up" was performed during Springsteen's first formal studio audition for CBS Records on March 5, 1972. It features Springsteen solo on vocals and acoustic guitar. Springsteen recalls he was twenty-two when he walked into John Hammond's office and had the audition. After he had played a couple of songs, Hammond said that he had to be on Columbia Records, but he needed to see him play live. "The kid absolutely knocked me out," he told *Newsweek* in 1975. "I only hear somebody really good once every ten years, and not only was Bruce the best, he was a lot better than Dylan when I first heard him."[9]

The live version released in the *Live/1975–85* box set, cut at the Roxy in Los Angeles in 1978, includes a spoken intermezzo: "I think, I ain't sure, but I think my mother and father and my sister, they're here again tonight. Hey, are you guys out there? You're over there? For six years, they've been following me around California, trying to get me to come back home. Hey, Ma! Give it up, Ma! Give me a break! You know, they're still trying to get me to go back to college. Every time I come in the house, 'You know, it's not too late, you can still go back to college,' they tell me. I say, 'All right, all right, Ma.' But it's funny, 'cause when I was growin' up, there were two things that were unpopular in my house. One was me, and the other one was my guitar. And my father, he used to sit in the kitchen. And we had this grate, like the heat's supposed to come through, except it wasn't hooked up to any, any like, heating ducts. It was just open, straight down to the kitchen. And there was a gas stove right underneath it. And when I used to start playing, he used to turn on the gas jets and try to smoke me out of my room. I'd end up out on the, out on the roof or something, you know. And he used to always refer to this guitar, you know, never Fender guitar, Gibson guitar: it was always the 'goddamned guitar,' you know. Whenever he stuck his head into my door, that's all I'd hear: 'Turn down the goddamned guitar.' He used to try to get me to be a lawyer. And it was funny 'cause I was in a motorcycle accident when I was seventeen. And like, this cat just, you know, ran head-on into me and then got out and yelled at me for ruining his Cadillac. And we had like a suit, a legal suit. And my father took me down to this lawyer in town. He said, 'Oh man, I gotta defend this?' I looked about, just about exactly the same way I look right now. And we were going to court, right? The day of the suit. Like I go, 'I'm like, in the right! I just got hit, and my leg's messed up.' And I remember my lawyer telling me, 'If I was the judge, I'd find you guilty!' I don't know for what. For being, just for being there, I guess, you know. But anyway, my father always said, 'You know, you should be a lawyer. You know, you get, get a little something for yourself.' Then my mother, she used to say, 'No, no, no, no. He should be an author. He should write books. You know, you should . . . That's a good life, you can get a little something for yourself.' Well, like, what they didn't understand was that I wanted everything. And so you guys, you, one of you guys wanted a lawyer, and the other one wanted an author. Well, tonight, you are both just gonna have to settle for rock 'n' roll!"

David Bowie recorded a version of "Growin' Up" in the early stages of the *Diamond Dogs* sessions with Ronnie Wood on lead guitar. In 1990 this was released as a bonus track on the reissue of his *Pin Ups* album, and in 2004 it appeared on the bonus disc of the thirtieth anniversary edition of *Diamond Dogs*.

[i] When he admits to combing his hair "till it was just right," it conjures up "the image of Rod Stewart's rock classic 'Every Picture Tells a Story,' released two years earlier, wherein the protagonist of Stewart's randy tale combs his air 'a thousand ways' and ends up looking just the same."[10]

"Spirit in the Night"
©1972 Bruce Springsteen (GMR)

Released on: *Greetings from Asbury Park, NJ* album (1973) | *Live/1975–85* box set (1986) recorded live at the Roxy Theatre, Los Angeles, CA, July 7, 1978 | *Live in Barcelona* home video (2003) recorded live at Palau Sant Jordi, Barcelona, October 16, 2002 | *Wings for Wheels: The Making of Born to Run* home video (2005) recorded live at the Ahmanson Theatre, Los Angeles, CA, May 1, 1973 | *Hammersmith Odeon London '75* album & home video (2005) recorded live at The Hammersmith Odeon, London, November 18, 1975 | *The Promise: The Darkness on the Edge of Town Story* box set (2010) recorded live at Sam Houston Coliseum, Houston, TX, July 15, 1978

Live premiere: 01/31/1973—Max's Kansas City, New York, NY

At the end of the *Greetings from Asbury Park, NJ* sessions, the president of Columbia Records, Clive Davis, was still not quite satisfied and said there were no singles. Springsteen went back home and wrote "Spirit in the Night" and "Blinded by the

Light." For those songs he needed a sax player and called Clarence Clemons. The song was composed in August 1972 and completed by early September. It was also released as a single with "For You" on the B-side. In his autobiography, Springsteen recalls when he heard the song blasting from the radio of a car while he was standing on a street corner before a college gig in Connecticut, suddenly feeling part of the mystery train of popular music.

"Spirit in the Night" was a #40 U.S. hit for Manfred Mann's Earth Band when they covered it in 1975. It was released on their *Nightingales & Bombers* album.

[i] Although Greasy Lake is a mythical place, former E Street Band drummer Vini Lopez has stated that it is actually a composite of two locations that band members used to visit. One was Lake Carasaljo, near the intersection of U.S. Route 9 and New Jersey Route 88 in Lakewood, New Jersey. The other was a swampy lake near Garden State Parkway exit 88. "Lopez says band members got off the Garden State at that exit, drove west on Highway 70 less than a quarter of a mile, then turned north onto an undeveloped road and reached a lovers' lane complete with swamps and a lake. The lake is clearly visible on a United States Geological Survey map of the Lakewood area dated 1970–71. The lake is now gone, a victim of the Lakewood Industrial Park development near the Lakewood airport."[11] Some have claimed that Greasy Lake is a lake near Howell, New Jersey. It gets its name from the idea that homeless people living around the lake used it for bathing. The homeless people were known as "gypsy angels" or "spirits in the night." *Greasy Lake & Other Stories* is a collection of short stories by T.C. Boyle published in 1985. The collection reflects the fears, anxieties, and issues of America in the 1960s, especially in regard to the fear of a nuclear holocaust. The title story of this collection was inspired by Bruce Springsteen's song. The "Greasy Lake" characters are three wanna-be-bad teenagers: "We wore torn-up leather jackets, slouched around with toothpicks in our mouths, sniffed glue and ether," the narrator says. The lake, "so stripped of vegetation it looked as if the Air Force had strafed it," has turned into a lagoon of refuse with broken bottles lining its banks.[12]

[ii] Wild Billy, Crazy Janey, and Hazy Davy existed in real life [for Wild Billy and Crazy Janey, see note 1 to "Rosalita" (Come Out Tonight)"]. Hazy Davy was the nickname that Springsteen gave to David Hazlett, the drummer in Mercy Flight, a college rock band that existed between 1969 and 1973 in Richmond, Virginia. The band opened for Bruce Springsteen's Steel Mill several times. In September 1970, Springsteen asked David Hazlett to substitute for Vini Lopez in Steel Mill for the upcoming September 11 show at Clearwater Swim Club in Atlantic Highlands, New Jersey. At the time, Lopez was stuck in Richmond prison for about a month

sorting out some legal difficulties (marijuana possession). Hazlett packed up and left for the Jersey shore, and he started rehearsing with Steel Mill at Carl "Tinker" West's Challenger Eastern Surfboards factory in Wanamassa, New Jersey. "It was a time of peace, love, and Vietnam. For most people music was a way of gathering" Hazlett recalls. "Brucey was about the best at bringing the crowds from a roar to a whisper in seconds; he always had the ability to do this . . . My name is David Hazlett and he always called me Hazy. I've also been called Purple Haze: it's just a nickname depending on the era I guess . . . I'm not sure if that night I crawled into Greasy Lake with just my socks and a shirt. I must have drunk too much rosé . . . I'm glad someone remembers; thanks, Brucey."[13]

[iii] Despite what David Hazlett remembers, during a 1974 interview on a Richmond, Virginia, radio station, Springsteen mentioned that in late 1971 one of the albums he was listening to a lot was the Band's then-new *Cahoots* album, and that one of the Robbie Robertson songs on that album, "The Moon Struck One" had a character called Little John that in a roundabout way became the Hazy Davy character in "Spirit in the Night." He also mentioned that he sort of borrowed one of Robertson's verses and scrambled it up a bit and used it in his song: "Little John was stung by a snake over by the lake / And it looked like he's really, really hurt, he was lyin' in the dirt."

"Incident on 57th Street"
©1973 Bruce Springsteen (GMR)

Released on: *The Wild, the Innocent & the E Street Shuffle* album (1973) | "Fire"/ "Incident on 57th Street" single (1986) recorded live at Nassau Coliseum, Uniondale, NY, December 28, 1980 | *Live in Barcelona* home video (2003) recorded live at Palau Sant Jordi, Barcelona, October 16, 2002

Live premiere: 01/19/1974—Kent State University, Kent, OH

The song was released on *The Wild, the Innocent & the E Street Shuffle* album (1973) and played live for the first time on January 19, 1974, at Kent State University, in Kent, Ohio.

"Incident on 57th Street" is a "virtual mini-opera about Johnny, a 'romantic young boy' torn between Jane and the bright knives out on the street. Springsteen never resolves the conflict (if he ever does his music will probably become less interesting). Instead he milks it for all it's worth, wrapping up all the song's movements and juxtapositions with his unabashedly melodramatic and loonily sotted Sloppy Joe voice."[14] When introducing the song during the show in Rome on June

6, 2005, Springsteen said: "When I was young, I didn't write any love songs, so I hid my love songs in other songs. My father told me that love songs were government propaganda: they were meant to just get you married and have children and pay taxes . . ."

"Sprawling, methodical, impassioned, and manipulative," Ariel Swartley wrote in an essay on the various pleasures of listening to Springsteen's second album, "Incident on 57th Street" "teeters on the edge of melodrama and slips into rapture . . . 'Good night, it's all right, Jane.' Springsteen's final choruses are incantations. Benedictions. Acts of surrender. He's caught up in his own spells."[15] "Incident on 57th Street" is "the moment when Springsteen the writer came into his own."[16] Dave Marsh calls it one of the "few precious moments in rock when you can hear a musician overcoming both his own limits and the restrictions of the form."[17]

According to Clarence Clemons, the introduction to "Jungleland" evolved from the piano and violin introduction to the version of "Incident on 57th Street" that Springsteen had been playing live.[18]

[i] 57th Street is one of New York's major thoroughfares, which runs as a two-way street East–West in midtown Manhattan.

[ii] Someone suggested that Spanish Johnny comes to midtown Manhattan after getting beat up while trying to work as a male escort.[19] Although rejected by everyone else, he finds redemption when Jane sympathizes with him. They sleep together, but when his old companions call to him asking him to join them in making "some easy money," he leaves Jane to join them.

[iii] Springsteen himself has suggested that the lyrics of "Jungleland" (1975) may tell what happened after "Incident on 57th Street," with Spanish Johnny becoming "Jungleland"'s Magic Rat.[20]

[iv] "Incident on 57th Street" is set in New York City, and the story of Spanish Johnny and Puerto Rican Jane has parallels to Leonard Bernstein's *West Side Story* in telling a *Romeo and Juliet*–like story with Latin American characters set in New York. Johnny is explicitly referred to as "a cool Romeo" and Jane as "a late Juliet."

[v] Shanty Lane doesn't exist.

"New York City Serenade"
©1973 Bruce Springsteen (GMR)

Released on: *The Wild, the Innocent & the E Street Shuffle* album (1973)

Live premiere: 07/18/1973—Max's Kansas City, New York, NY

Although Springsteen claimed to have written it "pretty quick, in a day or so,"[21] "New York City Serenade"—one of his lengthiest studio tracks, clocking at 9:55—has quite a long story. In fact, it was created by merging an early 1972 song entitled "Vibes Man" and an early 1973 one called "New York Song," both unreleased. The new composition was recorded during the early part of the second phase of *The Wild, the Innocent, & the E Street Shuffle* recording sessions that took place from June 28 to September 25, 1973. By that time, David Sancious was included as the pianist of the band, together with other three niche session contributors: Suki Lahav (vocals), Richard Blackwell (congas, percussion), and Albee Tellone (baritone sax). A string section was not used on the studio recording of the song; instead, Sancious used a Mellotron.

According to Albee Tellone, the "New York City Serenade" famous piano intro was put together by Sancious as a classic piece influenced by jazz and blues, since he had both a classical upbringing and a blues sensibility. "'New York City Serenade' gets that beat, it gets that groove going," Springsteen says. "It just goes on forever, it's one of those songs that hooks up with a rhythm and goes on and on into the night. That song's really special to me."[22] The song was his romantic story of New York City, a place that had been his getaway from small-town New Jersey.

After having been occasionally performed from July 1973 onwards, "New York City Serenade" wasn't played for twenty-five years following its last inclusion in the setlist on August 10, 1975 at the Allen Theatre in Cleveland, Ohio. Springsteen proposed it once again, surprisingly, on August 9, 1999, at the Continental Airlines Arena in East Rutherford, New Jersey, and four more times during the Reunion Tour. The song will also be performed once again during the Rising Tour of 2003, and once during the Working on a Dream Tour in 2009. During the Wrecking Ball Tour, Springsteen preformed "New York City Serenade" at the Capannelle Hippodrome in Rome, accompanied by the Roma Sinfonietta's string section, Ennio Morricone's orchestra. This live version was released on the *Ippodromo delle Capannelle, Rome 2013* official live download in 2015. Also in Rome, at the Circus Maximus, on July 16, 2016, before an audience of 60,000 people, Springsteen opened his show with "New York City Serenade," accompanied, once again, by the Roma Sinfonietta.

[i] In "New York Song"—one of several prototypes for "New York City Serenade"—there is a "Blackie" and not a "Billy" "down by the railroad track."

[ii] The lyric "Billy's got cleats on his boots" is similar to one used in "Jesse," an unreleased song written by Springsteen, who recorded it in mid-1972: "You got cleats on your boots / And a woman who shoots / Every time you shuffle out the stage door."

[iii] Boogaloo is a genre of Latin music and dance that was popular in the United States in the 1960s. Although it came to prominence after the bossa nova and was influenced by the new drumbeat of modern samba, boogaloo originated in New York City, mainly among teenage Puerto Ricans.

[iv] As per prototype, the "fish lady" has the "Street Queen" from a track with the same name composed in 1972 by Springsteen and never published: "She got high class, / She rides around in a cut-down Chevy machine. / Her eyes are plate glass, / Oh and legs like a limousine. / She comes stocked with sass, / And pride ain't there to be mean. / She's the baddest thing this town's ever seen. / Oh, street queen." Another reference is "Marie" (the title of another 1972 unreleased song), "the queen of all the stallions" who "skins me alive, carves her initials in my side."

[v] The verse is taken from the "Vibes Man," a song never published: "Vibes man in the alley, / Play me your spitball serenade / Any deeper blue / and you'll be playing in your grave, / Save your notes, / Spend them on your blues, boy . . ."

"Meeting Across the River"

©1975 Bruce Springsteen (GMR)

Released on: *Born to Run* album (1975)

Live premiere: 09/26/1975—Hancher Auditorium, Iowa City, IA

Recorded on May 28, 1975 a the Record Plant, "Meeting Across the River" is included in the *Born to Run* album (1975), featuring Randy Brecker on trumpet and Richard Davis on upright bass: along with Roy Bittan on the piano, they give a jazz-inspired poignancy to the song that suggests a film noir feel.

Original pressings of *Born to Run* billed the song as "The Heist," suggesting what the man across the river was employing the narrator and Eddie for.

> The stroke that hinted at Springsteen's narrative gift was that he chose to write the lyric as just one side of a conversation. "Hey Eddie, can you lend me a few bucks / And tonight can you get us a ride?" asks first-person un-named. From those opening lines all his fears, failures, and serial delusions of grandeur hang out there in empty air, unanswered and exposed, until this poor dope who's "planning" a stick-up without a car or a gun has finished his fantasy about impressing his wife.[23]

"I had that little piano riff," Springsteen recalls, "and I'm not exactly sure where the lyric came from. I don't know, there was something North Jersey in it; I can't quite explain . . . There was that New York–New Jersey, big-time/small-time thing, you know? It's funny, because back then, when you lived in New Jersey, you could've been a million miles from New York City and yet it was always there. By that time, I think we'd been counted out, and it probably had something to do with that, a feeling I had about myself maybe, that you'd been underestimated. Most of the folks that go into my business have had the experience of someone counting them out, or of being underestimated, of someone judging your life as being without great value. So that song grew out of, 'Hey, that guy's sort of a small-time player, but he's still got his sights set on what's across that river.' I suppose that was where the emotions of it came from."[24]

The song led to the creation in 2005 of a book titled *Meeting Across the River: Stories Inspired by the Haunting Bruce Springsteen Song*: a collection of twenty-one fictional short stories by various authors edited by Jessica Kaye and Richard Brewer.

The first live performance of the song was on September 26, 1975, at the Hancher Auditorium of University of Iowa. Played only nine times during the Born to Run Tour and only five on the Darkness Tour, "Meeting Across the River" disappeared from the setlists for twenty years, until Springsteen played it again on May 21, 1999, at Earls Court, in London.

[i] The tunnel is the Holland Tunnel, under the Hudson River between Jersey City and Manhattan.

[ii] The last lines of the songs resemble one scene of *The Killing*, the 1956 noir movie directed by Stanley Kubrick. One of the members of the gang that is planning one last heist before settling down tells his wife, Sherry, about the impending robbery. Sherry is bitter because he hasn't delivered on the promises of wealth he once made her, so he hopes telling her about the robbery will placate and impress her.

"Jungleland"
©1975 Bruce Springsteen (GMR)

Released on: *Born to Run* album (1975) | *Live in New York City* album & home video (2001) recorded live at Madison Square Garden, New York, NY, June 29, 2000 | *Hammersmith Odeon London '75* album & home video (2005) recorded live at The Hammersmith Odeon, London, November 18, 1975 | *The 25th Anniversary Rock & Roll Hall of Fame Concerts* box set (2010) recorded live at Madison Square Garden, NY, October 29, 2009 | *London Calling: Live in Hyde Park* home video (2010) recorded live at Hyde Park, London, June 28, 2009 | *The Promise: The Darkness on the Edge of Town Story* box set (2010) recorded live at Sam Houston Coliseum, Houston, TX, July 15, 1978 | *The Ties that Bind: The River Collection* box set (2015) recorded live at Arizona State University, Tempe, AZ, November 5, 1980

Live premiere: 07/13/1974—The Bottom Line, New York, NY

"Jungleland" is an almost ten-minute-long closing song on Springsteen's 1975 album *Born to Run*. It contains one of the most recognizable sax solos in rock 'n' roll; and it also features short-term E Streeter Suki Lahav, who performs the delicate violin introduction accompanied by Roy Bittan on piano. A 1974 document indicates that "Jungleland" was a candidate for the title of the album, as were several phrases taken from the lyrics: "The Hungry and the Hunted," "From the Churches to the Jails," and "Between Flesh and Fantasy."

"Jungleland" is "a ride through terror, it resolves itself finally as a ride into delight."[25] The chosen word by critics and fans to describe it is "epic." "'Jungleland' *is* an epic. Yes, it's long, but that's not the reason it deserves the appellation. It's epic because it creates an entire world in a relatively short time, and yet it still leaves enough open space to fire the imagination. It's epic in musical scope, an endlessly inventive arrangement that showcases every one of the members of the E Street band while also stressing their whole-is-better-than-the-parts aesthetic. Most of all, it's an epic for its fearlessness, the way that Springsteen attempts something on such a grand scale and knocks every bit of it out of the park."[26]

An initial recording of the song was made at 914 Sound Studios in Blauvelt, New Jersey, without the presence of Steve Van Zandt, Suki Lahav, and producer Jon Landau. Bruce continued to tinker with and refine the song over the course of the next few months. The definitive version was recorded in April 1975 at the Record Plant studios in New York City and mixed in July.

The post-apocalyptic horror/fantasy novel *The Stand* by Stephen King opens with three epigraphs, one of which is a section of lyrics from the song.

Following the death of Clarence Clemons in 2011, the song was not played until July 28, 2012, when during the second of two shows in Gothenburg, Sweden, in a hugely emotional moment Big Man's nephew Jake Clemons performed the signature saxophone solo, occupying Clarence's usual spot on the stage.

On December 17, 2007, at the Palais Omnisports in Paris, Springsteen dedicated "Jungleland" to the editor of this book.

[i] "Flamingo Lane" was a local name for a brief stretch of First Avenue, in Asbury Park, New Jersey, which the Flamingo Motel overlooks. It's pink. It's seedy. It's on "the circuit" at the corner of First Avenue and Kinglsey Street. And from all accounts, the Flamingo Motel has quite a history. Southside Johnny once said that

he used to take girls there all the time, adding that "some other guy from Asbury Park . . . who would remain nameless took girls there, too."[27]

[ii] The Exxon sign is supposed to be a sign for an Esso station which was previously found on Cookman Avenue, Asbury Park, next to Dogan's Pub, a few short steps away from the Palace. The sign was torn down in 2002 during renovation work on the Asbury Park perimeter.

[iii] The piece is the Garden State Arts Center, in Telegraph Hill Park, at exit 116 of Garden State Parkway.

[iv] "This is where Springsteen begins to draw parallels between the heightened fantasy world he has created with the fantasy world of rock 'n' roll that he lives every day . . . Bruce realized that without his talent he could have been one of the live fast / die young characters populating his songs. As if to punctuate this point, he lets loose a furious guitar solo heading into the bridge."[28]

[v] "Springsteen doesn't write rock opera; he lives it."[29]

[vi] Lyrics end here, but Springsteen starts using guttural cries in which "you can hear Go-Cart Mozart's insane ramblings, the Ragamuffin Gunner's jaded fatalism, Crazy Janey's healing sweet nothings, Zero and Blind Terry's ghostly laughter, Madame Marie's foreboding warnings, Spanish Johnny's tragically romantic serenade to Puerto Rican Jane. They all, all denizens of 'Jungleland,' come out to join the Rat and the barefoot girl for one final bow, and the curtain closes."[30]

A Runaway American Dream

The six songs making up this section focus on the boy who up until now we have seen lost amongst the other characters of "Spirit of the Night" and "Jungleland." In "4th of July, Asbury Park (Sandy)" and "Backstreets," the Jersey Shore begins reconfigure itself no longer as the theater for new "rebels without a cause," but rather a place to flee from if dreams are to be sought after and achieved. This boy's dream is to reach fame and fortune with his music, as we learn in "Rosalita" (Come Out Tonight)," his musical, humoristic autobiography. The farewell to the paternal home is consumed and in "Thunder Road" the boy is finally "pulling out of here to win."

"Rosalita" is the first song in which Springsteen speaks of two young lovers running away together by car. "Born to Run" and "Thunder Road" refine this theme. "This is funny," Springsteen recalled during a show held on July 7, 1978 at the Roxy Theatre in Los Angeles, CA, "'cause, when I get out, I got out with my girlfriend, I take her around in my car and we drive around anytime the car place down and she says, 'Hey, you're the guy, you write the songs about the cars all the time, you guy you fix the car.' I got at the hood, and it's like *Alice in Wonderland*, so, 'Hey, where this go?' I don't know about that stuff, but I think I understand the spiritual and religious significance of 396. So I write these song anyways, anytime."

"*Born to Run* was about searching for that place. It was a moment when I was young and that's what I was doing. I was very untethered and you had a rough map and you were about to set out in search of your frontier—personally and emotionally—and everything was very, very wide open. And that's how the record felt, just wide open, full of possibilities, full of fear, you know, but that's life."[31]

Springsteen's major flaw as a composer at the time was his pompous declaration of greatness, achieved by romanticizing American themes with a majestic sound. "The music, it was romantic," he told in an TV interview with Elvis Costello, "because I grew up on the great romanticism of the Drifters and Spector records and Benny King and that generation of beautiful romance that was in those songs."[32]

"Rosalita (Come Out Tonight)"
©1973 Bruce Springsteen (GMR)

Released on: *The Wild, the Innocent & the E Street Shuffle* album (1973) | *Live/1975–85* box set (1986) recorded live at the Roxy Theatre, Los Angeles, CA, July 7, 1978 | *Hammersmith Odeon London '75* album & home video (2005) recorded live at the Hammersmith Odeon, London, November 18, 1975 | *London Calling: Live in Hyde Park* home video (2010) recorded live at Hyde Park, London, June 28, 2009 | *The Promise: The Darkness on the Edge of*

Town Story box set (2010) recorded live at Arizona Veterans Memorial Coliseum, Phoenix, AZ, July 8, 1978 | *The Promise: The Darkness on the Edge of Town Story* box set (2010) recorded live at Sam Houston Coliseum, Houston, TX, July 15, 1978 | *The Ties that Bind: The River Collection* box set (2015) recorded live at Arizona State University, Tempe, AZ, November 5, 1980

Live premiere: 02/14/1973—Virginia Commonwealth University, Richmond, VA

Written in August 1972 and completed during the summer of 1973 in his apartment on 1703 Webb Street, in Asbury Park, "Rosalita (Come Out Tonight)" was published on *The Wild, the Innocent & the E Street Shuffle*.

In his autobiography Springsteen wrote that when he was young he had a girlfriend whose mother had threatened to get a court injunction against him due to his humble beginnings. He wrote "Rosalita" as a proud response to her.

Never released as a single in the U.S. and generally unknown upon its initial album release, as Springsteen gained commercial success "Rosalita" became one of his most popular airplay tracks. Novelist George P. Pelecanos has called it "one of the great rock 'n' roll performances, and as close to a perfect song as anyone's ever recorded."[33] The song is one of the Rock & Roll Hall of Fame's 500 Songs That Shaped Rock and Roll.

"Rosalita"—with some different lyrics—is known to have been performed at least four times during what is considered the Greetings from Asbury Park, NJ Tour (October 1972 to September 1973). The first live performance, on February 14, 1973 at Virginia Commonwealth University in Richmond, Virginia, featured the Beach Boys' "Fun Fun Fun" in the midsection. Following the March 17, 1973 show at Oliver's in Boston, Massachusetts, Springsteen was interviewed backstage and mentioned incorporating new material into the shows, specifically "Rosalita." Beginning with the three-night residency at Joe's Place in Cambridge, Massachusetts, in January 1974 "Rosalita" closed the main sets of all Springsteen shows until, on October 19, 1984, during the Born in the U.S.A. Tour, it was dropped from the show. Springsteen biographer Dave Marsh said this was done to "disrupt the ritual expectations of the fanatic fans . . . establishing through a burst of creativity just who was boss."[34] From that night, "Rosalita" made few, precious debuts (one under the pouring rain in closing a show in Milan in June of 2003, with Jon Landau onstage playing guitar) up until the Magic Tour of 2007–08, during which the song began to be played much more frequently.

In 1984, many years after the song's initial release, MTV began showing a music video for the song. The video was a straight concert performance (from a

Darkness Tour performance on July 8, 1978 at the Arizona Veterans Memorial Coliseum in Phoenix, Arizona) that included band introductions and numerous adoring women rushing the stage.

[i] Thirty-five years after the publication of *The Wild, the Innocent & the E Street Shuffle*, it became finally possible to give Rosalita a surname. Just out of high school, Diane Lozito met Bruce Springsteen in summer 1971 at a show on the Jersey Shore. Her boyfriend, a law student named Bill Cahill (the "Wild Billy" on "Spirit in the Night"), took her to the Upstage Club in Asbury Park; he knew the guitar player, Springsteen. They became friends and she kept running into him throughout the summer. "Billy and his friends were major party boys," Lozito recalled in an interview with Peter Knobler. "But Bruce didn't drink or get high. One night at the beach, when Billy and the others were drinking, Bruce and I tucked around a rock and started kissing. Then I said, 'It's time to go'—because I was so scared of getting busted by Billy. That was a nice night. Light coming off the ocean, nothing like it." Springsteen carried a notebook and was always jotting things down. "The next day he showed me the line, 'She kissed me just right, like only a lonely angel can.'" That was "Spirit in the Night." As Knobler wrote, soon Billy was out of the picture, Lozito and Springsteen talked about moving in together, and she took him to meet her mother. Lozito watched as Springsteen wrote in his book: "I know your mama, she don't like me 'cause I play in a rock and roll band." "OK, your dad," Springsteen said, "he's a musician. He's gotta love me. Ask him." But Lozito's father told her, "All musicians are bums." Springsteen and Lozito moved in together a year later over her parents' objections and he wrote the classics that turned up on his first three albums. "I'd ask, 'Why isn't my name in those songs?'" Lozito says. "He'd tell me, 'It's boring having a whole album about the same girl. And nothing rhymes with Diane.'" Eventually Springsteen met the rest of Lozito's family, including her grandmother, Rose Lozito. In that part of Jersey, it's pronounced Lazita. Rose Lazita. "He wrote 'Rosalita' in bits and pieces and didn't have a title for it," she says. "My mom is Rita Lozito. Then he met my grandma. So I assume that's where he put it together."[35] The couple split in 1975.

Diane Lozito is also the real Sandy in "4th of July, Asbury Park (Sandy)," she's the girl in "Thundercrak," she's the Crazy Janey in "Spirit in the Night," she's the Terry in "Backstreets," and "Bobby Jean" is probably also about her. Today Lozito lives in Oregon, where she works as a estate broker.

[ii] In the first version of the song, the one performed for the first time live on February 4, 1973, at Virginia Commonwealth University in Richmond, the lyrics read: "Spread out now, Rosie, / doctor come cut loose her chiffon reins."

[iii] In the first version of the song, the one performed for the first time live February 4, 1973, at Virginia Commonwealth University in Richmond, the lyrics read: "The only lover I'm ever gonna need / Is your soft sweet samurai tongue."

[iv] "Run" can be intended as a noun, as well as a verb, leaving us open to two different interpretations.

[v] Woolworth's was a department store at the time situated on Cookman Avenue in Asbury Park, a place well known to Bruce seeing that between 1968 and 1970 he often played next door at the Upstage Club.

"4th of July, Asbury Park (Sandy)"
©1973 Bruce Springsteen (GMR)

Released on: *The Wild, the Innocent & the E Street Shuffle* album (1973) | *Live/1975–85* box set (1986) recorded live at Nassau Coliseum, Uniondale, NY, December 31, 1980 | *Hammersmith Odeon London '75* album & home video (2005) recorded live at the Hammersmith Odeon, London, November 18, 1975

"4th of July, Asbury Park (Sandy)" is one of the seven songs on *The Wild, the Innocent & the E Street Shuffle* album (1973). When he wrote it, Springsteen was living with his girlfriend five minutes from Asbury Park, in Bradley Beach. "Sandy" was a composite of some of the girls he had been dating in that period. He used the boardwalk as a metaphor for the end of a summer romance and the changes he was experiencing in his own life. The Sandy of the song may be none other than Diane Lozito, Springsteen's girlfriend between summer 1971 and early 1975 [see note 1 to "Rosalita"].

Springsteen had hired a children's church choir to sing on the studio recording of the song, "but they didn't show," Lahav told the *Jerusalem Post* in 2007. "And I was around. And I had this high, pure, clear voice. So that was my first time."[36] Lahav's voice was recorded and overdubbed repeatedly to give the choir-like effect that Springsteen wanted. Vini Lopez explained in 2007 that he and Clarence Clemons tried to sound like Lahav when singing backing vocals on the song live. "Not easy," he recalled.

The song was heavily identified with Danny Federici's accordion part, which is the main musical element. On March 20, 2008, at Conseco Fieldhouse in Indianapolis, Indiana, during the Magic Tour, the song was performed in an album-style full-band arrangement and featured Danny Federici on accordion. Federici, who was already ill, showed up unannounced at this show and played on a number of songs, including this one. This was his last performance on stage before he died. The live version of "4th of July, Asbury Park (Sandy)" taken at that show was released on the *Magic Tour Highlights* digital EP in 2008.

A version of the song recorded by the Hollies charted in North America and became a hit in Europe in 1975. It was included in their album *Another Night*.

[i] Since the concert held on October 31, 1973 at the Main Point in Bryn Mawr, Pennsylvania, Springsteen always sings, "this fourth of July" instead of "this warm July."

[ii] Kingsley Street and Ocean Avenue were known as the Circuit, because they formed a long ring in front of the beach at Asbury Park. During the 1960s and early 1970s, it was the place to be, as hot cars cruised by the Stone Pony, the Wonder Bar, and the Xanadu.

[iii] In 1917 Asbury Park, a renowned beach place, was struck by fire, destroying a number of hotels and large part of the boardwalk (a wooden walkway running parallel to the coast) originally built by the city's founder, James Bradley. For the reconstruction the architects Warren and Wetmore (famous for New York's Grand Central Station) were contracted, and they drew plans for the Casino and the Convention Hall, two areas partially developed on stilts and placed at the ends of the boardwalk.

[iv] The Casino was built in 1929. One wing, the grand hall, was dedicated to concerts; the other held a beautiful carousel and various amusements. Contrary to what one may infer from the name, it never had anything to do with casinos or gambling. It saw its moment of glory in the thirties and forties of the last century, and was at any rate one of the main attractions the coast offered until the early seventies. Then from the eighties it started an irreversible decline. Its dismantling began in 1982. In 1986 a violent hurricane caused many buildings to collapse and the palace fell into its deep ruin (as can also be seen in the images of the "Tunnel of Love" video). From 1997 to 2000 it was partially reopened as Skatepark Casino, with a skateboard ramp.

[v] Another famous son of Asbury Park is Stephen Crane (1871–1900), recognized primarily for his Civil War novel *The Red Badge of Courage*, which has become an American classic. Between July 2 and September 11, 1892, Crane published at least ten news reports on Asbury Park affairs in the *New York Tribune*. A storm of controversy erupted over a report he wrote on the Junior Order of United American Mechanics. The report juxtaposes the "bronzed, slope-shouldered, uncouth" marching men "begrimed with dust" and the spectators dressed in "summer

gowns, lace parasols, tennis trousers, straw hats, and indifferent smiles . . . Such an assemblage of the spraddle-legged men of the middle class, whose hands were bent and shoulders stooped from delving and constructing, had never appeared to an Asbury Park summer crowd, and the latter was vaguely amused."[37] Crane was considered one of the local riffraff. Basically, he was a kind of prototype of Springsteen's tramps. In his book on Asbury Park, journalist and poet Daniel Wolff points out that Crane's short story "The Pace of Youth" is a literary precursor of sorts to "4th of July, Asbury Park (Sandy)." Written in 1893 and published two years later in the New York *Press*, the story is about a summer romance along the Shore between the daughter of the town's leading businessman and a guy who works at Stimson's Mammoth Merry-Go-Round.[38]

[vi] Springsteen rewrote the third verse of "4th of July, Asbury Park (Sandy)" before a radio performance broadcast on April 19, 1974, on Boston's WBCN-FM; the song was played in an acoustic arrangement with Bruce Springsteen on guitar and Danny Federici on accordion, just like during the Greetings from Asbury Park, NJ Tour: "Now, Sandy, the angels have lost their desire for us. / I spoke with 'em last night, they said they won't set themselves on fire for us anymore, / But still when the weather gets hot, they ride that crazy road down from heaven, on their Harleys they come and they go. / You could see 'em dressed like stars in all the cheap little seashore bars out parked with their babies, out on the Kokomo." From that point on, Springsteen always sang this new stanza when live.

[vii] The Madame Marie mentioned in the song is Marie Castello, a real-life fortune-teller who worked on the Asbury Park boardwalk starting in 1932 and was still working there when she passed away in 2008. She was the longest-running tenant on the Asbury Park boardwalk, where she operated from a small one-room concrete structure called the Temple of Knowledge: a kind of cube-shaped cabin, with walls once painted white (later revarnished in blue), upon which eyes, stars, and planets were drawn. Anyone passing through Asbury Park couldn't help but notice that enormous woman lying on a long chair outside her Temple, up until it was closed in 1988. It reopened for a day on the 4th of July, 2004, which must have had a lot to do with a wave of nostalgia. But on the July 4, 2007, the stand opened once again, this time to receive clients two hours a day every Saturday and Sunday during summer. The rates rose from five to thirty-five dollars. During her only interview given in September of 2007, Marie declared having closed her business for a period due to business not being so good at the time. According to Stephen Castello, contrarily to what Springsteen sings, his mother was never arrested. In an interview with Ed Bradley for *60 Minutes*, Springsteen states that he called on

Madame Marie at least once: "She said I would become rich and famous. But then she probably said the same thing to every guitarist." Marie Castello died on June 27, 2008, at the age of ninety-three. Springsteen offered his condolences and memories of her on his website, saying: "Back in the day when I was a fixture on the Asbury Park boardwalk, I'd often stop and talk to Madame Marie as she sat on her folding chair outside the Temple of Knowledge. I'd sit across from her on the metal guard rail bordering the beach, and watch as she led the day trippers into the small back room where she would unlock a few of the mysteries of their future. She always told me mine looked pretty good—she was right. The world has lost enough mystery as it is—we need our fortunetellers." Madame Marie's business was inherited by her granddaughter Sally.

"Backstreets"

©1975 Bruce Springsteen (GMR)

Released on: *Born to Run* album (1975) | *Live/1975–85* box set (1986) recorded live at the Roxy Theatre, Los Angeles, CA, July 7, 1978 | *Live in New York City* home video (2001) recorded live at Madison Square Garden, New York, NY, June 29, 2000 | *Hammersmith Odeon London '75* album & home video (2005) recorded live at the Hammersmith Odeon, London, November 18, 1975 | *The Promise: The Darkness on the Edge of Town Story* box set (2010) recorded live at Sam Houston Coliseum, Houston, TX, July 15, 1978 | *The Ties that Bind: The River Collection* box set (2015) recorded live at Arizona State University, Tempe, AZ, November 5, 1980

Live premiere: 08/08/1975—Civic Theatre, Akron, OH

According to Sony's database of Bruce Springsteen's recording sessions, "Backstreets" was recorded in five different studio sessions between April and July 1975 at the Record Plant in New York City, and released on the *Born to Run* album (1975).

Greil Marcus wrote that the song "begins with music so stately, so heartbreaking, that it might be the prelude to a rock 'n' roll version of *The Iliad*."[39]

On the *Born to Run* album, the song was already six and a half minutes long, but in 1976, 1977, and 1978, the live performances of the song were extended with an interlude that is commonly known as the "Sad Eyes" interlude, a title probably assigned to it by bootleggers: it is a mostly soft-piano-based monologue toward the end of the song that gradually rises in tempo before it suddenly stops and the "Hiding on the backstreets" coda kicks back in full band. The "Sad Eyes" interlude disappeared with the end of the Darkness on the Edge of Town Tour, evolving through those three years to later be used as the basis for part of "Drive All Night."

[i] "Backstreets" has been also interpreted as a narrative about a homosexual relationship, since the name Terry is sexually ambiguous—even if it is highly likely that the character is female. It has also been said to potentially represent a platonic but intense friendship between two men that has faded. However, listening to any of the numerous bootleg versions of "Backstreets" from the Darkness on the Edge of Town Tour, Terry is repeatedly referred to as "she" and "little girl," confirming that Terry is indeed a woman. Another interpretation is that it is about Springsteen's relationship with his former girlfriend Diane Lozito. In his autobiography, Springsteen states that "Backstreets" is about a broken friendship.

[ii] Stockton Wing Beach refers to a place near Richard Stockton College, a university campus situated in southeast New Jersey.

[iii] Fictitious name.

[iv] An alternative studio take of "Backstreets" recorded sometime between May and July 1975 at the Record Plant in New York City had a different verse: "Endless juke joints and Valentino drag, / Watching the heroes in the funhouse ripping off the fags, / The teenage ice exploded in crazy sets of fights / Running off down the boardwalk, turning in the night."

[v] Springsteen had not read Walker Percy's *The Moviegoer* (1961) yet—a novel he came to love deeply, in which for the protagonist, the movie lover Binx, only film in its ambiguous form can redeem the aseptic and monotonous "new South" in which he lives, is a sort of guarantee that Binx himself will call "certified." A certain neighborhood in New Orleans, for instance, gains consistency only when Binx sees it reproduced on screen in a film by Elia Kazan starring Richard Widmark.

"Born to Run"

©1975 Bruce Springsteen (GMR)

Released on: *Born to Run* album (1975) | *Live/1975–85* box set (1986) recorded live at Giants Stadium, East Rutherford, NJ, August 19, 1985 | *Chimes of Freedom* EP (1988) recorded live at Memorial Sports Arena, Los Angeles, CA, April 27, 1988 | *Live in New York City* album & home video (2001) recorded live at Madison Square Garden, New York, NY, June 29, 2000 | *Live in Barcelona* home video (2003) recorded live at Palau Sant Jordi, Barcelona, October 16, 2002 | *Hammersmith Odeon London '75* album & home video (2005) recorded live at the Hammersmith Odeon, London, November 18, 1975 | *The 25th Anniversary Rock & Roll Hall of Fame Concerts* box set (2010) feat. Billy Joel, recorded live at Madison Square Garden, NY, October 29, 2009 | *London*

Calling: Live in Hyde Park home video (2010) recorded live at Hyde Park, London, June 28, 2009 | *The Promise: The Darkness on the Edge of Town Story* box set (2010) recorded live at Arizona Veterans Memorial Coliseum, Phoenix, AZ, July 8, 1978 | *The Promise: The Darkness on the Edge of Town Story* box set (2010) recorded live at Sam Houston Coliseum, Houston, TX, July 15, 1978 | *The Ties that Bind: The River Collection* box set (2015) recorded live at Arizona State University, Tempe, AZ, November 5, 1980

Live premiere: 05/09/1974—Harvard Square Theater, Cambridge, MA

Greil Marcus called the opening guitar riff on "Born to Run" "the finest compression of the rock 'n' roll thrill since the opening of 'Layla.'" [40] "Few intros send as exhilarating a rush of blood to the head and loins as 'Born to Run,'" the title track of Bruce Springsteen's third album, released in 1975. "Hungry hints of Bruce's all-American influences Kerouac (*On the Road*) and Whitman ('Song of the Open Road') hover on the horizon. 'Born to Run' prompts people to act on their impractical desires—leave town, drive all night, hit the city, ask Wendy out, lean forward to kiss Wendy once she's out with you. It's about youth. It suggests you must pursue your dreams, which, in truth, is possibly the most invidious and suspect of pop culture's panaceas. If you pursue your dreams and don't find them, where does that leave you? It leaves you as a character from *The River* or *Tunnel of Love*, a character too tired and bruised to even dream. The criminal alternative, however, is never to feel what this record feels—never to feel young, gifted, good-looking and overconfident. To be running from, not running to 'that place where we really wanna go'—heaven, paradise, wherever." [41]

Rolling Stone magazine ranked "Born to Run" #21 on their list of the 500 Greatest Songs of All Time and is included in the Rock & Roll Hall of Fame's 500 Songs That Shaped Rock and Roll. In 1980, the New Jersey legislature named it the state's Unofficial Youth Rock Anthem. It was named the #1 Springsteen song of all time in a 2003 poll by *Uncut* magazine.

Springsteen wrote it sitting on the edge of his bed in a cottage he'd newly rented at 7½ West End Court in West Long Branch, New Jersey. In those days he was repeatedly listening to Roy Orbison, Phil Spector, and Duane Eddy. It was early 1974 when the words "born to run" hit him. At first he thought it was the name of a movie or a slogan on a wall. He liked the phrase because it suggested a cinematic drama that he was seeking.

Recorded during the summer of 1974 at 914 Studio in Blauvelt, New York, under the production of Mike Appel—Springsteen's manager at the time—it was the only track recorded in the 1974 sessions to end up on the *Born to Run* album the following year.

The lyrics of the song in the spring 1974 live versions were dramatically different from the final ones, so much so that the song's meaning shifts. After "runaway American dream," Springsteen sings, "At night we stop and tremble in the heat / With murder in our dreams." The song is darker. He is not singing to Wendy, whose name does not appear. Springsteen was working the themes of loneliness and violence to the extreme. After "boys try to look so hard," he sings, "Like animals pacing in a dark black cage / Senses on overload, / They're gonna end this night in a senseless fight / And then watch the world explode." The "broken heroes" of this early version of "Born to Run" have "a loneliness in their eyes," and instead of loving "with all the madness in my soul," the narrator seeks to "drive through this madness burstin' off the radio." "Sometime between July and the end of the summer, Springsteen transformed 'Born to Run.' He told one writer, 'I'm still fiddling with the words for the new single, but I think it will be good.' The notes of alienation, loneliness, and violence yielded to love, companionship, and redemption."[42]

Frankie Goes to Hollywood covered this song in their debut album *Welcome to the Pleasuredome* in 1984.

[i] Highway 9 is actually Route 9, a major north–south artery through the lower half of New Jersey, running through Freehold, following the shore past Atlantic City and ending near Cape May. On "Zero and Blind Terry"—an outtake from *The Wild, the Innocent & the E Street Shuffle* later included in the *Tracks* box set—Springsteen correctly named it Route 9.

[ii] On the south part of Kingsley Street, between Lake Avenue and Cookman Avenue, in Asbury Park there is a memorial cemetery that extends across nearly seven square miles. Until May 2004, there was a building in its place, probably the most famous and remarkable in all of coastal New Jersey. For a hundred years, within the wooden walls of the Palace people had fun and dreamed just as Springsteen did during the years of his youth. The building of the Palace began on February 20, 1888, under the direction of Ernest S. Schnitzler: he had planned a phantasmagorical amusement area at whose center he installed a grand carousel with seventy horses. In 1895 the Ferris wheel was built, sixty-five feet tall. In 1920 Schnitzler sold the Palace to August Williams, who in 1929 opened the Casino right next door. In the thirties the Fun House was built inside, with its house of horror and hall of mirrors, the building surrounded by pinball machines; then in 1945, a wax museum was also set up, with some of the statues—amongst which was Benito Mussolini—hung upside down. In 1956 the Palace expanded another three square miles and a series of neon light figures were installed; the painter Leslie W. Thomas painted a series of murals, one of which looked out onto Cookman Avenue, portraying the face of

a clown: almost sixteen feet tall, it was reminiscent of the figure commissioned by the entrepreneur George C. Tilyou for the entrance of Steeplechase Park in Coney Island. This the reason why the big face on the Palace wall came to be called "Tillie": it was in fact a stylized portrait of Tilyou. As years went by, Tillie became the unofficial symbol of Asbury Park. In 1970 Asbury Park was shocked by four days of racial clashes: the beginning of a definitive decline. As it was to be also for the Palace. In 1972, a concentrated mass of medical waste and garbage, extending fifty miles in length, was purposely discharged in the ocean to then wash up on the Jersey Shore, causing massive damage to the area's tourism industry and a 55 percent fall in the Palace's annual turnover. The following year was the crisis of fecal bacteria: Asbury Park emptied out entirely. The new owners of the Palace went bankrupt and on November 27, 1988, with no warning, it was closed. It decayed for a decade, abandoned to time and vandals. In 2002, a group of New York investors bought it and signed an agreement for its renovation with the Asbury Park City Council. An offer to buy it from "Save Tillie" (the organization born in defense of the architectural, historic, and artistic heritage of the city) was rejected. "Save Tillie" only managed to save about a hundred of original artifacts from the Palace, and the part of the wall on which Tillie was painted was removed from the wall in May 2004. A few days later, the Palace began its complete demolition.

[iii] A "hemi" is the 426 Hemi engine made famous by Chrysler muscle cars. "Drones" in this context are automatons, the young men driving their cars up and down the strip without a thought to the future.

[iv] Journalist David Kamp gave Springsteen an amateur-psychoanalytic theory of "Born to Run": "I told him that the pact the song's narrator makes with Wendy—'We can live with the sadness, I'll love you with all the madness in my soul'—jumped out at me, now that I'd read the book, as the pact that Doug Springsteen made with Adele. Springsteen smiled. 'That was their pact,' he said. I'm thinking of two people who had moved, relatively recently at the time you wrote the song, from New Jersey to California. 'Yeah, my folks. I think that was the place I envisioned, was West. Where do people run? They run West. That's kind of where I imagined the characters going.' 'So,' I asked, 'is the song the internal monologue of Doug Springsteen?' 'I wouldn't go that far,' Springsteen said. 'I never connected this song particularly with my father. I mean, I think it pertains as far as feeling trapped internally. He did. Which is why they ended up leaving for California when their kids were so young. We were nineteen, seventeen, and at a very critical moment in our lives. In my sister's life, particularly. She just had a baby! So they had to go.' Springsteen seemed to be warming, ever so slightly, to my premise. 'In a funny

way,' he said, 'my parents actually lived this song at that particular time.' 'That's what I'm saying,' I responded. 'I'm wondering if—' '—later on, it clicked in my head?' he said, finishing my thought. 'I don't know where things come from. At the end of the day, you don't know where everything comes from. It's very possible.'"[43]

"Independence Day"

©1980 Bruce Springsteen (GMR)

Released on: *The River* album (1980) | *Live/1975–85* box set (1986) recorded live at Brendan Byrne Arena, East Rutherford, NJ, July 6, 1981 | *The Ties that Bind: The River Collection* box set (2015) recorded live at Arizona State University, Tempe, AZ, November 5, 1980

Live premiere: 07/07/1978—The Roxy, Los Angeles, CA

Douglas Springsteen quit school at eighteen, went to war two years later, served as a truck driver at the Battle of the Bulge, and went back to Freehold in 1945. In 1947 he married Adele Zerilli and landed a job—the first of many—on the factory floor of the Ford auto plant in nearby Edison. His relationship with his eldest son, Bruce, was difficult. Steve Van Zandt recalls that Springsteen's father was "scary" and best avoided. In fact, he seems to have been bipolar, and he was capable of terrible rages, often aimed at his son.

During a show at the Palladium, in New York City, in November 1976, Springsteen laid things out in the starkest terms: "My father, he worked a lot of different places. He worked in a rug mill for a while, he drove a cab for a while, and he was a guard down at the jail for a while. I can remember when he worked down there, he used to always come home real pissed off, drunk, sit in the kitchen. At night, nine o'clock, he used to shut off all the lights, every light in the house, and he used to get real pissed off if me or my sister turned any of them on. And he'd sit in the kitchen with a six-pack, a cigarette . . . He'd make me sit down at that table in the dark. In the wintertime, he used to turn on the gas stove and close all the doors, so it got real hot in there. And I remember just sitting in the dark . . . No matter how long I sat there, I could never ever see his face. We'd start talking about nothing much, how I was doing. Pretty soon, he asked me what I thought I was doing with myself. And we'd always end up screaming at each other. My mother, she'd always end up running in from the front room crying, and trying to pull him off me, try to keep us from fighting with each other . . . I'd always end up running out the back door and pulling away from him. Pulling away from him, running down the driveway screaming at him, telling him, telling him, telling him, how it was my life and I was going to do what I wanted to do." Over the years, the relationship between the two would become more stable. "My dad was very non-verbal—you couldn't really have a conversation with him," Springsteen told David Remnick. "I had to make my peace with that, but I had to have a conversation with him, because I needed to have one. It ain't the best way to go about it, but that was the only way I could, so I did, and eventually he did respond. He might not have liked the songs, but I think he liked that they existed. It meant that he mattered. He'd get asked, 'What are your favorite songs?' And he'd say, 'The ones that are about me.'"[44]

One of the cornerstone tracks on *The River* double album of 1980, "Independence Day" was ready to be included on *Darkness on the Edge of Town*, but didn't make it because "Factory" was preferred to it, a song also centered on the father-son relationship.

"Thunder Road"
©1975 Bruce Springsteen (GMR)

Released on: *Born to Run* album (1975) | *Live/1975–85* box set (1986) recorded live at the Roxy Theatre, Los Angeles, CA, October 18, 1975 | *In Concert/ MTV Plugged* album & home video (1993) recorded live at Warner Hollywood Studios, Los Angeles, CA, September 22, 1992 | *Hungry Heart* EP (1995) recorded live at Sony Music Studios, April 5, 1995 | *Live in New York City* home video (2001) recorded live at Madison Square Garden, New York, NY, June 29, 2000 | *Live in Barcelona* home video (2003) recorded live at Palau Sant Jordi, Barcelona, October 16, 2002 | *Hammersmith Odeon London '75* album & home video (2005) recorded live at the Hammersmith Odeon, London, November 18, 1975 | *VH1 Storytellers: Bruce Springsteen* home video (2005) recorded live at Two River Theater, Red Bank, NJ, April 4, 2005 | *London Calling: Live in Hyde Park* home video (2010) recorded live at Hyde Park, London, June 28, 2009 | *The Promise: The Darkness on the Edge of Town Story* box set (2010) recorded live at Sam Houston Coliseum, Houston, TX, July 15, 1978 | *The Ties that Bind: The River Collection* box set (2015) recorded live at Arizona State University, Tempe, AZ, November 5, 1980

Live premiere: 02/05/1975—The Main Point, Bryn Mawr, PA

"Thunder Road" underwent considerable evolution as it was written. An early version titled "Wings for Wheels" was written at the end of 1974: the female character's name wasn't Mary but Angelina, and then Chrissie and Christina.

"I had a little old Aeolian piano sitting in the front of my living room," Springsteen recalls, "and I knew I was interested in writing on the piano at that time, partly because I was interested in those thematic movements. . . . There is something about the melody of "Thunder Road" that just suggests 'new day,' it suggests morning, it suggests something opening up."[45]

The full-band version of "Thunder Road" that opens the *Born to Run* album was recorded at the Record Plant in New York City, in March and April 1975. It was more than seven minutes long, but producer Jon Landau suggested shrinking it to about four, and moving Clarence Clemons's saxophone solo from the middle of the song to the end.

[i] Springsteen makes reference to the song "Only the Lonely," written by Joe Melson and Roy Orbison, then brought to success by the latter in 1960. During the recording of *Born to Run*, Springsteen listened to Roy Orbison continuously.

[ii] Springsteen recently recalled that the song was written immediately after the Vietnam War, when everybody felt not young anymore.

[iii] Jay Cocks—Martin Scorsese's *Gangs of New York* screen-writer—states that the young protagonist of the film, Jack Amsterdam (played by Leonardo DiCaprio) was born from this verse in "Thunder Road." Scorsese explains his intention to attribute to Amsterdam "the passion, the frustration, the contradictions, and the dreams of an Irishman arriving to America."[46]

[iv] Forty-two American cities (including Vineland, New Jersey) have a street named "Thunder Road." During a show in Passaic on September 19, 1978, Springsteen prefaced the performance of "Thunder Road" with a lengthy spoken introduction: "There was this Robert Mitchum movie. And it was about these moonshine runners down south. And I never saw the movie, I only saw the poster in the lobby at the theater. And I took the title and I wrote this song, but I didn't think that there was ever a place that was like what I wrote in this song. And we were out in the desert over the summertime driving to Nevada and we came upon this house on the side of the road, this Indian had built. It had a big picture of Geronimo out front with 'Landlord,' said 'Landlord' over the top, and a big sign said, 'This is the land of peace, love, justice, and no mercy.' And it pointed down this little dirt road that said 'Thunder Road.'" In fact, *Thunder Road* is the title of a film starring Robert Mitchum (1958). His character, Luke Doolin, is a liquor smuggler fighting with the State Treasury Department and big-city crime. "The Ballad of Thunder Road" featured on the soundtrack, written and performed by Mitchum himself, topped the charts for twenty weeks.

[v] The original version of "Wings for Wheels" concluded with, "This is a town full of losers, and baby I was born to win," instead of the studio version's ending.

Where Our Sins Lie Unatoned

This section is made up of songs coming from the 1977–78 *Darkness on the Edge of Town* album sessions. The post–*Born to Run* era was tarnished by a growing estrangement between Springsteen and his manager Mike Appel, with Jon Landau's increased involvement, much to Appel's dissatisfaction, till the situation came to a head in July 1976, when Springsteen sued Appel for mismanagement. As a result of this lawsuit—and Appel's countersuit—Springsteen received an injunction preventing him from entering a recording studio without his ex-manager. Springsteen was unable to record new material until both parties agreed to settle their differences out of court on May 1977. During this period, Springsteen was writing furiously, and the songs that appeared on *Darkness on the Edge of Town* were only the tip of the iceberg.

Apart from the ten songs that ended up on the 1978 album, among the others there were the four outtakes later published on the 1998 *Tracks* box set—"Give the Girl a Kiss," "Iceman," "Hearts of Stone," and "Don't Look Back"—plus the twenty-one unreleased songs later published on *The Promise* with modern vocals and additional instrumentation recorded in 2010, including "Fire" (released as a single in 1978 by the Pointer Sisters), "Because the Night" (cowritten with Patti Smith and released by her as a single in 1978), and "The Promise" (re-recorded by Springsteen solo at the piano for the 1999 anthology *18 Tracks*).

"However frustrating the layoff of 1976–77 proved, it gave Springsteen an opportunity to assess himself and the position he found himself in. Catapulted to the top after *Born to Run*, the year gave him time to gain a perspective on himself and his career. As an artist, it gave him the opportunity to chart the changes his country was undergoing—how the characters in his songs were coping with maturity and recession; how dreams were stifled, but never died."[47]

What happens to the boy in "Born to Run" when he starts comparing his dreams to reality? Inevitably he begins to perceive that reality is dramatically different. "Badlands" and "Adam Raised a Cain" are furious realizations that "might be understood even without lyrics. The sound is pounding and rentless; the guitar screams, the organ howls, the vocals roar, the drums crash . . . You could say that this music is about survival. 'When Bruce Springsteen sings on his new album, that's not about *fun*,' said Pete Townshend, 'that's fucking *triumph*, man.'"[48] The young guy of "Thunder Road" still "believes in his promised land despite a lack of evidence."[49]

In the 2010 documentary *The Promise: The Making of Darkness on the Edge of Town*, Springsteen said "The Promised Land" is about "how we honor the community and the place we came from." Ultimately, Springsteen suggested that the message of the song is the need to lose one's illusions of a life without limitations while holding onto a sense of the possibilities in life.

Starting from *Darkness on the Edge of Town* onwards, Springsteen shows more attention in portraying man-woman relationships. The late-adolescent character of "Spirit in the Night" and "Rosalita" and the romantic one of "Incident on 57th Street" gives way to a more mature and tormented narrative. The man in *Darkness*—and later in *The River*—fights against solitude and alienation from the world in which he is living, and the woman, in this sense, can be a seen as a safe haven as well as the mirror of his own fear. In "Because the Night" and "Candy's Room" the protagonist seeks his redemption in love; but if in the first song the man asks the woman to keep him by her side in the bedroom, in the second Candy's room turns into a prison. And yet Candy is no longer the redeeming prostitute—as is the "fish lady" in "New York City Serenade"—when the priestess of the initiation rite brings the man to the coveted hidden worlds, which will prove equivalent to the discovery of the most intimate and private part of the female soul.

With "Iceman," Springsteen returns to the classic theme of love on the run, but this time—contrarily to "Thunder Road"—hope is not the result of a naive dream, but rather emerges from the pain of admitting its unreality. "Sherry Darling" in this context is illuminating, a song written during the *Darkness* sessions that will be published on the successive album *The River*: underneath the light lyrics lies the denial of "Thunder Road"'s theme: the man and woman running away from the town full of losers are still in the car, but in the back seat is her mother, who gets taken to the job agency, and the free ride will never be free again.

The section closes with "Racing in the Street," a true bridge to mark the gap between the Springsteen before and after *Darkness on the Edge of Town*. The song could be read as a possible realization of the potential inherent in "Thunder Road"; that song is a declaration of what the protagonist and his girlfriend are going to do, while "Racing in the Street" is the reality of how they might end up. Most importantly, "Racing in the Street" is the first song in which Springsteen introduces the suffering woman. Rock has always had songs where women are won and lost as trophies in contests, but Springsteen treats that theme with much more compassion than is usual in the genre.[50] While romanticization of the ordinary, anonymous Americans found in "Racing in the Street" is common in rock, Springsteen's detailed depiction of them in this song shows real understanding and compassion, perhaps due to his having lived among them.[51]

"Badlands"

©1978 Bruce Springsteen (GMR)

Released on: *Darkness on the Edge of Town* album (1978) | *Live/1975–85* box set (1986) recorded live at Arizona State University, Tempe, AZ, November 5, 1980 | *Live in New York City* home video (2001) recorded live at Madison Square Garden, New York, NY, June 29, 2000 | *Live in Barcelona* home video (2003) recorded live at Palau Sant Jordi, Barcelona, October 16, 2002 | *Hammersmith Odeon London '75* album & home video (2005) recorded live at the Hammersmith Odeon, London, November 18, 1975 | *London Calling: Live in Hyde Park* home video (2010) recorded live at Hyde Park, London, June 28, 2009 | *The Promise: The Darkness on the Edge of Town Story* box set (2010) recorded live at Arizona Veterans Memorial Coliseum, Phoenix, AZ, July 8, 1978 | *The Promise: The Darkness on the Edge of Town Story* box set (2010) recorded live at Sam Houston Coliseum, Houston, TX, July 15, 1978 | *The Promise: The Darkness on the Edge of Town* Story box set (2010) recorded live at the Paramount Theatre, Asbury Park, NJ, 2009 | *The Ties that Bind: The River Collection* box set (2015) recorded live at Arizona State University, Tempe, AZ, November 5, 1980

Live premiere: 05/23/1978—Shea Theater, Buffalo, NY

According to Springsteen, he came up with the title "Badlands" before he started writing the song. He felt it was a great title but that it would be easy to blow it by not writing a worthy song for it.

On March 15, 2012, in a keynote speech to an audience at the South by Southwest music festival, Springsteen discussed at length the Animals' influence on his music, praising their harsh, propulsive sound and lyrical content. Saying that his album *Darkness on the Edge of Town* was "filled with Animals," Springsteen played the opening riffs to "Don't Let Me Be Misunderstood" and his own "Badlands" back to back, then said, "Listen up, youngsters! This is how successful theft is accomplished!"

"Badlands" is also the first song in which one can appreciate the influence of *The Grapes of Wrath*, directed by John Ford, and *Badlands*, directed by Terrence Malick.

A first version of "Badlands" was recorded by Bruce Springsteen and the E Street Band in August 1977 at the Atlantic Studios in New York City, with very different lyrics: "Here on the street I'm a-getting pushed 'round / Here on the street, I'm a-here getting put down. / What do you want with me? You're looking at me right now / And I'm talkin' to you, baby . . ."

During the River Tour (1980–81) pianist Roy Bittan used to play some notes of Ennio Morricone's theme from *Once Upon a Time in the West* as a prelude to the song. The version on the *Live/1975–85* box set was recorded in Arizona the night after Ronald Reagan was elected president. Bruce introduced the song by saying, "I don't know what you guys thought of what happened last night, but I thought it was pretty terrifying."

[i] "Badlands are a type of dry terrain where softer sedimentary rocks and clay-rich soils have been extensively eroded by wind and water."[52] They are characterized by canyons, ravines, and gullies. Some of the best-known badland formations can be found at Makoshika State Park in Montana and Badlands National Park in South Dakota. Another popular area of badland formations is Toadstool Geological Park in the Oglala National Grassland of northwestern Nebraska. A small badland called Hell's Half-Acre is present in Wyoming.

"Adam Raised a Cain"
©1978 Bruce Springsteen (GMR)

Released on: *Darkness on the Edge of Town* album (1978) | *Live/1975–85* box set (1986) recorded live at the Roxy Theatre, Los Angeles, CA, July 7, 1978 | *The Promise: The Darkness on the Edge of Town Story* box set (2010) recorded live at Sam Houston Coliseum, Houston, TX, July 15, 1978 | *The Promise: The Darkness on the Edge of Town Story* box set (2010) recorded live at the Paramount Theatre, Asbury Park, NJ, 2009

Live premiere: 05/23/1978—Shea Theater, Buffalo, NY

"Adam Raised a Cain" is inspired by the film *East of Eden* (from John Steinbeck's 1955 novel), in which the troubled son, Cal Trask—played by James Dean—struggles with his father, Adam Trask.

The image of a father who spends a whole life of hard work and pain uselessly seeking someone to blame clearly evokes God's condemnation of Adam: "Cursed is the ground because of you; through painful toil you will eat food from it all the days of your life" (Genesis: 3:15–17).

Doug Springsteen died in 1998, at seventy-three, after years of illness, including a stroke and heart disease. "I was lucky that modern medicine gave him another ten years of life," Springsteen said. "T-Bone Burnett said that rock and roll is all about 'Daaaaddy!' It's one embarrassing scream of 'Daaaaddy!' It's just fathers and sons, and you're out there proving something to somebody in the most intense way possible. It's, like, 'Hey, I was worth a little more attention than I got! You blew that one, big guy!'"[53]

In the 2010 documentary *The Promise: The Making of Darkness on the Edge of Town*, sound mixer Chuck Plotkin described Springsteen's instructions for how the jarring assault of this song should sound next to the more melodic tunes on *Darkness*. Springsteen told Plotkin to think of a movie showing two lovers having a picnic, when the scene suddenly cuts to a dead body. This song, the singer explained, is that body.

[i] An earlier version of the song, recorded in August 1977 at Atlantic Studios in New York City, had "Later as I grew older, tell me how on that day I cried."

[ii] An earlier version of the song, recorded in August 1977 at Atlantic Studios in New York City, had "She knows you didn't come back, it's all a little game, / You remember the faces, you remember the names."

[iii] An earlier version of the song, recorded in August 1977 at Atlantic Studios in New York City, had "Now he haunts these empty rooms, rattling these chains."

"The Promised Land"
©1978 Bruce Springsteen (GMR)

Released on: *Darkness on the Edge of Town* album (1978) | *Live/1975–85* box set (1986) recorded live at the Coliseum, Los Angeles, CA, September 30, 1985 | *Live in Barcelona* home video (2003) recorded live at Palau Sant Jordi, Barcelona, October 16, 2002 | *London Calling: Live in Hyde Park* home video (2010) recorded live at Hyde Park, London, June 28, 2009 | *The Promise: The Darkness on the Edge of Town Story* box set (2010) recorded live at Arizona Veterans Memorial Coliseum, Phoenix, AZ, July 8, 1978 | *The Promise: The Darkness on the Edge of Town Story* box set (2010) recorded live at Sam Houston Coliseum, Houston, TX, July 15, 1978 | *The Promise: The Darkness on the Edge of Town Story* box set (2010) recorded live at the Paramount Theatre, Asbury Park, NJ, 2009 | *The Ties that Bind: The River Collection* box set (2015) recorded live at Arizona State University, Tempe, AZ, November 5, 1980

Live premiere: 05/23/1978—Shea Theater, Buffalo, NY

"The Promised Land" is the third single from the *Darkness on the Edge of Town* album after "Prove It All Night" and "Badlands."

"The distinctly non-Jersey imagery of this song—tornadoes, a 'rattlesnake speedway in the Utah desert'—was inspired by a road trip Springsteen took as he worked on *Darkness on the Edge of Town*. The simple, straightforward music, meanwhile, is one of the best examples of Springsteen stripping down in the aftermath of the wall-of-sound grandeur of *Born to Run*: 'I remember him telling me he really wanted to downsize the scale, that big sound,' producer Jon Landau said years later, describing the transition out of the highly orchestrated *Born to Run*. Bittan's spare but expansive piano and Weinberg's driving beat fit lyrics that balance images of isolation and frustration with a hunger for independence within a larger community.'It really begins our folk-based rock,' Springsteen said of 'The Promised Land.' 'It goes back to blues and folk, and folk structures—I was not trying to be really melodic, because that immediately pulls you into the pop world. I was trying to create this mixture, this sort of rock-folk music that stretches back all the way, in some ways, to Woodie Guthrie and country music and up through the Animals.'"54

The thematic cornerstone of the entire *Darkness on the Edge of Town* album—commitment—is summed up in this song. "In the face of all the betrayals," Springsteen said, "in the face of all the imperfections that surround you in whatever kind of life you lead, it's the characters' refusal to let go of their own humanity, to let go their own belief in the other side."55

[i] After his parents moved to California in 1969, Springsteen drove across the country several times to visit them. He usually took the US 80 from Salt Lake City to Nevada, a highway close to the Bonnerville Salt Flats, the Utah desert's most famous road.

[ii] No Waynesboro County exists in the United States. Five cities called Waynesboro exist, none of which are in Utah, where a Wayne County does.

[iii] "The Promised Land" is also the title of a Chuck Berry song. He wrote it in jail, when he had been sentenced to three years in prison for having transported a fourteen-year girl across state lines. Berry's "Promised Land" is about a man who leaves his home in Virginia, bound for the promises of California: "Tell the folks back home this is the promised land callin' / And the poor boy's on the line." The song was included in Berry's *St. Louis to Liverpool* album (1964).

"Come On (Let's Go Tonight)"
©2010 Bruce Springsteen (GMR)

Released on: *The Promise* album (2010)

Live premiere: 12/07/2010—The Casino, Asbury Park, NJ

Prior to the release of *The Promise* in 2010, one unofficial studio take of "Come on (Let's Go Tonight)" had been circulating on bootlegs. It was recorded in June 1977 at Atlantic Studios in New York City, and features some different lyrics, not referencing Elvis Presley (who would die few weeks later) and sharing some lines—and the same melody—with "Factory."

There is also a home demo, recorded around late March or early April 1981 at Springsteen's home in Colts Neck, New Jersey. It features some different lyrics and would soon evolve into "Johnny Bye-Bye."

The studio version of "Come on (Let's Go Tonight)," referencing the death of Presley, was recorded at the end of August 1977. In the 2010 version, David Lindley—a multi-instrumentalist known for his work with Jackson Browne—plays the violin.

The Promise is a collection of twenty-two previously unreleased songs from the *Darkness on the Edge of Town* recording sessions. Depending on their level of completion back in 1977–1978, some were only remastered, some were overdubbed with 2010 vocals or music, and some were completely re-recorded in 2010.

[i] The line will become, "Men walk through these gates with death in their eyes" on "Factory," one of the songs of *Darkness on the Edge of Town*.

"Because the Night"
©1978 Bruce Springsteen, Patti Smith (GMR)

Released on: *Live/1975–85* box set (1986) recorded live at Nassau Coliseum, Uniondale, NY, December 28, 1980 | *The Promise: The Darkness on the Edge of Town Story* box set (2010) recorded live at Sam Houston Coliseum, Houston, TX, July 15, 1978

Live premiere: 12/30/1977—CBGB Theater, New York, NY (with Patti Smith)

In 1977, Springsteen was at Atlantic Studios in New York City, working on the songs for his fourth album (*Darkness on the Edge of Town*), when Patti Smith, recording in the same studio, heard from producer Jimmy Iovine about a track that Bruce was trying to complete: he was not satisfied with it and later declared he already knew he wasn't going to finish it since it was "another love song."[56] Iovine, who was working with both musicians, brought Smith a demo of the song, and Smith added her own lyrics, recording it for her album *Easter* (1978), and scoring her first and biggest hit single. "Bruce did the hook, Patti the words, and we [the Smith band] gave it the cannon-blast beat," said Smith's guitarist Lenny Kaye.[57]

It appears that, when Springsteen gave "Because the Night" to Patti Smith, he had the music and the chorus written, but not the verses.[58] She wrote the words in one night, making the song more of a passionate lust story, with the pre-chorus of "Touch me now" at the end of the song. When Springsteen performed the song, his lyrics were more comforting to the girl, as he took the persona of a workingman ("I work all day out in the hot sun") tempering her fears with his love, telling her,

"They can't hurt you now." The different versions provide an interesting contrast, as they show the perspectives of each side of the couple depicted in the song.

Springsteen's excellent 1978 studio version wasn't officially released until *The Promise*, more than thirty years later.

"Because the Night" debuted live on December 30, 1977, at CBGB's in New York City, when Springsteen joined the Patti Smith Group dueting with Patti. The E Street Band played the song for the first time on May 30, 1978, at the Music Hall in Boston, Massachusetts. "Because the Night" was largely played (seventy-six times) during the Darkness Tour in 1978, becoming one of the highlights of Springsteen's live shows since then.

The lyrics here reproduced are relative to the first recording of Springsteen's track to end up on a record: we are talking therefore about the "Because the Night" version performed live at the Nassau Coliseum in Uniondale, New York, on December 28, 1980, during the River Tour.

[i] Both Patti Smith and Bruce Springsteen's studio versions have, "Desirous hunger is the fire I breathe, / Love is a banquet on which we feed."

[ii] Both Patti Smith and Bruce Springsteen's studio versions have, "Take my hand come undercover."

[iii] Both Patti Smith and Bruce Springsteen's studio versions have, "Have I doubt when I'm alone, / Love is a ring, the telephone, / Love is an angel disguised as lust / Here in our bed till the morning comes."

[iv] Patti Smith's version has, "With love we sleep with doubt, / The vicious circle turns and burns without. / You I cannot live, forgive, / the yearning burning I believe it's time, too real to feel. / So touch me now, / Touch me now, touch me now." Bruce Springsteen's studio version has, "With love we sleep with doubt, / The vicious circle turns and burns without. / You I cannot live, forgive now, / The time has come to take the moment and / They can't hurt you now, / They can't hurt you now."

"Iceman"

©1998 Bruce Springsteen (GMR)

Released on: *Tracks* box set (1998)

Live premiere: 05/17/2005—Tower Theater, Philadelphia, PA

Recorded on October 27, 1977 during the *Darkness on the Edge of Town* sessions, "Iceman" was published only twenty-one years later on the *Tracks* box set.

When he heard a tape containing the song, Springsteen was surprised because he had forgotten he had even written it. He has played it live only three times to date: the first time in 2005, at the Tower Theater in Philadelphia; the second time in 2014, at Time Warner Cable Arena in Charlotte, North Carolina; and the last one in 2016, at the Accorhotels Arena in Paris

[i] Springsteen will use this line on "Badlands."

"Racing in the Street"
©1978 Bruce Springsteen (GMR)

Released on: *Darkness on the Edge of Town* album (1978) | *Live/1975–85* box set (1986) recorded live at Brendan Byrne Arena, East Rutherfrod, NJ, December 27, 1980 | *The Promise* album (2010) | *The Promise: The Darkness on the Edge of Town Story* box set (2010) recorded live at the Sam Houston Coliseum, Houston, TX, July 15, 1978 | *The Promise: The Darkness on the Edge of Town Story* box set (2010) recorded live at the Paramount Theatre, Asbury Park, NJ, 2009

Live premiere: 05/23/1978—Shea Theater, Buffalo, NY

A first version of "Racing in the Street"—with slightly different lyrics from the definitive take that would be published on the *Darkness on the Edge of Town* album—was recorded at Atlantic Studios, in New York City, in the fall of 1977. Springsteen revealed that the song was inspired by some talks he had in an Asbury Park bar with his friend Matt, in 1976. He wanted his street racers to carry the years between the car songs of the 1960s and 1978 America. In fact, the instrumental break after the second verse and chorus is an allusion to the Beach Boys' 1964 song "Don't Worry Baby," itself about the emotional aspects of drag racing. Greil Marcus sees "Racing in the Street" as picking up the characters of various Beach Boys songs fifteen years later in their lives, never finding anywhere else the freedom they had found in their cars and driving forever towards a dead end that they could see but could neither wish away nor reach.[59] Structurally, the song is also influenced by Van Morrison's "Tupelo Honey," and the organ refrain references "It's My Life," a song by the Animals that Springsteen has revered since adolescence.

On August 9, 1978, at the Agora in Cleveland, Springsteen introduced "Racing in the Street" with these words: "Back in Asbury Park there's these two roads, there's Kingsley Avenue [actually Kingsley Street] and Ocean Avenue, and they form a sort of an oval. And on Friday night they burn about half the gas in the United States in between stoplights down there. But outside of town, there's this little fire road, and that's where they go racing in the street."

On April 25, 2005, at the Fox Theatre in Detroit, Michigan, Springsteen began talking about having seen Monte Hellman's 1971 road movie *Two-Lane Blacktop*, starring James Taylor and Dennis Wilson as two lost souls whose lives are about nothing more than driving their '55 Chevy from race to race. Springsteen told the audience that he'd written the following song before he had seen the film but later was struck by how similar it was in its theme. The protagonists of *Two-Lane Blacktop*—known only as The Driver and The Mechanic—compete in drag races, pick up a female hitchhiker known only as The Girl, and eventually face a challenger referred to only by name of the factory-fresh muscle car he drives: GTO. "Springsteen's description of Candy from 'Candy's Room'—whose 'sadness hidden in that pretty face' could make her a dead ringer for The Girl—as more obvious candidates like 'Racing in the Street,' whose opening lines sound like they could be spoken by The Driver: 'I got a '69 Chevy with a 396 / Fuelie heads and a Hurst on the floor.'"[60]

A 1978 previously unreleased studio version of "Racing in the Street" is now in *The Promise* double-album (2010).

[i] Car enthusiasts have debated whether 1969 Chevrolet models could be ordered, customized, or built to the exact specifications given in the song of a 396-cubic-inch Chevrolet big-block engine with Fuelie heads and a Hurst Performance shifter. Chevrolet 396cu big block engines were in fact incompatible with "Fuelie heads," which were designed for the small block engines (327/350cu) only. The first version of the song had a different start: "I got a 32 Ford, she's a 318 / Fuelie heads and a Hurst on the floor."

[ii] The Chevrolet Camaro is a muscle car that first went on sale on 1967.

[iii] The first version of the song had "Come on out now little one and we'll go dying in the street."

Heart of Darkness

"So Mary climb in: it's a town full of losers and I'm pulling out of here to win." What happened to those two guys? The four songs included in this section tell how bitter was the end of their story, "A story of ambition and loss as ill-starred (and deeply American) as *Citizen Kane*."[61]

"The Promise"
©1999 Bruce Springsteen (GMR)

Released on: *18 Tracks* anthology (1999) | *The Promise* album (2010) | *The Promise: The Darkness on the Edge of Town Story* box set (2010) recorded in New York, NY, 1978

Live premiere: 08/03/1976—Monmouth Arts Center, Red Bank, NJ

For long time "The Promise" has been the Holy Grail for Springsteen's die-hard fans, since the song was played live occasionally between 1976 and 1978, and surfaced on some legendary bootlegs.

"The Promise" debuted live on August 3, 1976, at the Monmouth Arts Center in Red Bank, New Jersey, during what was later known as the "Lawsuit Tour." Fans and critics have speculated over whether the song is about the infamous legal fight between Springsteen and his ex-manager Mike Appel that kept the former from the recording studio (the lawsuit began that July, a few weeks before the live premiere of the song). When he heard the song for the first time in South Bend, Indiana (on October 9, 1976, at the University of Notre Dame), the *Chicago Reader* critic John Milward was moved to write, "The song's metaphor is 'The Challenger,' a race car that the singer has built by hand 'to carry the broken dreams of all those who have lost.' But the real twist comes during the song's bridge, when he sings the words 'thunder road' and immediately transforms his car into his rock and roll dreams. In 'The Promise,' Springsteen mythologizes himself and compares his struggle to be true to his art to the desperate struggle of the young racer. He sings in 'Thunder Road' that 'tonight's the night all the promises will be broken,' but the dream etched in 'The Promise' and put into perspective by Springsteen's own experience is clearly a romantic notion that is not easily shattered. Despite a landscape filled with losers—the singer eventually sells his car when he needs money—it's clear that in Springsteen's heart the Challenger's potential will never die."[62]

Dave Marsh writes in his Springsteen biography that "'The Promise' is rather about the price everyone pays for success—and the dangers of settling for anything less."[63]

In "The Promise" all the youthful visions of "Thunder Road" "have been stolen, battered, and left for the dead on the side of the road."[64] Played one after the other, the two songs form a full story, a play of mirrors inside an already highly self-referential opera like Springsteen's, and a source of deep emotion rarely found in rock 'n' roll. In the 2010 documentary *The Promise: The Making of Darkness on the Edge of Town*, Springsteen said that it's "a song about fighting and not winning," and in the handwritten lyrics notebook that was reproduced in the box set, he listed it as "The Promise (Return to Th. Rd.)" in one place. A few years earlier, when he played two benefit solo acoustic shows for *DoubleTake* magazine, on February 2003 at the Somerville Theatre in Somerville, Massachusetts, he said that when he wrote the song, he "was reflecting on sort of the flip side of 'Thunder Road.'"

Springsteen played "The Promise" nineteen times in 1976–77 concerts, while the song's lyrics and arrangement were still a work in progress. When he finally reached a settlement in his yearlong litigation with Mike Appel and was able to go into a studio and record, "The Promise" was one of the songs he made a demo of that same evening. A version of the song cut on June 30, 1977, at Atlantic Studios in New York, was included in 2010 on *The Promise* double album, which features unreleased tracks from the *Darkness on the Edge of Town* sessions. The song was also recorded on January 12, 1978, at the Record Plant Studios in New York. Both versions were recorded with full-band arrangement.

Originally considering the song for the *Darkness on the Edge of Town* album, as evidenced in several handwritten lists of candidate tracks for Springsteen's fourth studio album, but fearing that the song would be read as his reaction to the lawsuit, causing a misinterpretation of the message he meant to convey, Springsteen held it back and replaced it with "Racing in the Street." He played it twenty times during the Darkness on the Edge of Town Tour in 1978: on the tour's opening night it was played in the full E Street Band arrangement that would not be used again until 2010, while on the remaining dates it was played in a solo piano arrangement.

Finally, in 1999, "The Promise" was officially released for the first time, on the *18 Tracks* anthology. The studio version cut in 1977–78 didn't convince Springsteen. So, one day, he took a seat at the studio's piano and looked up at Toby Scott: "'Toby, turn the thing on.' Two takes later he stood up. 'Okay, that's good. Put it on the record.'"[65] The lyrics included in this book refer to this particular version of "The Promise."

The song was played live on March 19, 1999, at the Convention Hall in Asbury Park, after a twenty-one-year hiatus.

[i] The small city of Darlington is the county seat of Darlington County, in the northeastern part of South Carolina. Springsteen's song "Darlington County" is on the *Born in the U.S.A.* album (1984).

[ii] The Challenger was Dodge's answer to the Mustang and the Camaro. The second-generation Challenger was introduced in fall 1969. Chrysler intended the new Dodge as "the most potent pony car ever." Challenger also shared the name of the surfboards that Tinker West made in the factory where Springsteen had lived and worked while he was with Steel Mill.

[iii] The 1977 studio version now on *The Promise* double album (2010) had "But somehow I paid the big cost."

[iv] The 1977 studio version now on *The Promise* double album (2010) omitted this verse.

"Darkness on the Edge of Town"

©1978 Bruce Springsteen (GMR)

Released on: *Darkness on the Edge of Town* album (1978) | *Live/1975–85* box set (1986) recorded live at Nassau Coliseum, Uniondale, NY, December 29,1980 | *In Concert/MTV Plugged* album & home video (1993) recorded live at Warner Hollywood Studios, Los Angeles, CA, September 22, 1992 | "The Ghost of Tom Joad" single (1996) recorded live at the Tower Theater, Philadelphia, PA, December 9, 1995 | *Live in New York City* home video (2001) recorded live at Madison Square Garden, New York, NY, June 29, 2000 | *Live in Barcelona* home video (2003) recorded live at Palau Sant Jordi, Barcelona, October 16, 2002 | *The Promise: The Darkness on the Edge of Town Story* box set (2010) recorded live at Sam Houston Coliseum, Houston, TX, July 15, 1978 | *The Promise: The Darkness on the Edge of Town Story* box set (2010) recorded live at the Paramount Theatre, Asbury Park, NJ, 2009

Live premiere: 05/23/1978—Shea Theater, Buffalo, NY

Born to Run was a romantic story about escape. *Darkness on the Edge of Town*'s album-closing title track is the bitter end to that fairytale. The narrator has lost his wife, his money, and his hope for a better life, but he remains defiant: "Tonight I'll be on that hill 'cause I can't stop." Steve Van Zandt said it highlights the feel of the whole album. "'It looks heroic, sometimes it feels heroic, but it's actually an obsession, a compulsion,' he says. 'The song just sums up that record very accurately, in terms of the stories now, we're gonna not necessarily have a happy ending. You still have the cinematic thing going on, but it's smaller. The cameras are zooming in. It's more of an independent film now.'"[66]

A first version of "Darkness on the Edge of Town" was recorded in June 1977 at Atlantic Studios in New York City. A second version was recorded on March 10, 1978 the Record Plant Studios in New York City and appeared as the title track on Springsteen's fourth album—an album that, at one point, was going to be called *American Madness*, after a 1932 Frank Capra movie about life in America during the Depression.

[i] The 1977 version of the song had "Well, they're still racing out at the speedway."

[ii] Fairview is a suburban Bergen County, New Jersey, town that is named for its view of the Hackensack River valley.

[iii] There doesn't appear to really be an Abram's Bridge.

[iv] "I think that for me there was always something about the last verse in 'Darkness'; the character comes forward and asserts his will: 'Tonight I'll *be*, tonight I will be.' And for me . . . that last moment of survival, where his will is the only promise he has, that's all he can give out. And at the same time, that last verse always reminds me of the artist's promise to his audience, and the challenge that he throws out to his audience, which is: if I'm going there, you're coming with me. So I still sing that one with gusto."[67]

"The River"

©1979 Bruce Springsteen (GMR)

Released on: *The River* album (1980) | *Live/1975–85* box set (1986) recorded live at the Coliseum, Los Angeles, CA, September 30, 1985 | *Live in New York City* album & home video (2001) recorded live at Madison Square Garden, New York, NY, June 29, 2000 | *¡Released!—The Human Rights Concerts 1986–1998* home video (2013) feat. Sting, recorded live at River Plate Stadium, Buenos Aires, Argentina, 10/14/1988 | *The Ties that Bind: The River Collection* box set (2015) recorded live at Arizona State University, Tempe, AZ, November 5, 1980

Live premiere: 09/21/1979—Madison Square Garden, New York, NY

A solo demo of a song called "Oh Angelyne" was recorded at Springsteen's home in Holmdel, New Jersey, probably in May 1979. The song eventually evolved into "The River," recorded with the E Street Band at the Power Station, in New York on August 26 and 29, 1979. Further work was undertaken on January 21 and April 12 and 24, 1980. The song was first played live on September 21 and 22, 1979, on the occasion of the Madison Square Garden MUSE benefit concerts also known as No Nukes. Outstanding video footage of "The River"'s premiere on the first night was included in the 1980 theatrical movie release *No Nukes* (later available on home video, and also on the official Springsteen's *Video Anthology* DVD).

Springsteen explained that the song was inspired by country music, and by Hank Williams in particular ("My Bucket's Got a Hole in It"). He used a narrative folk voice—just a guy in a bar telling his story to the stranger on the next stool. The song is based on the crisis of the construction industry in late 1970s New Jersey.

The imagery of the chorus and the end of the song were inspired by lines from another Hank Williams's song, "Long Gone Lonesome Blues," a #1 hit on the country & western chart in 1950.

"The River" is also a description of Springsteen's sister Ginny's life since her accidental pregnancy at eighteen, her early marriage, and her husband's job loss. When his sister first heard it at the first MUSE benefit concert, she went backstage, saying, "That's my life." Springsteen recalls that as being the best review he ever got. Ginny recalls that hearing the song live at the Madison Square Garden was unnerving. She didn't like it at first—though later she came to acknowledge it as her favorite song. Today, Ginny and Mickey are still happily married. But in the impoverishment of the couples' ménage from "The River" it is surely not difficult to note the development of the bond between the two kids from "Thunder Road": are not the two Maries, protagonists on both tracks, possibly the same person?

[i] The first version of "The River"—when its title still was "Oh Angelyne"—had "I worked construction with the Jenkins Company."

[ii] It would suffice to arm the narrator with one simple word—"economy"—in order to evoke a whole mentality. "It is as though for his character the economy were an abstract and impersonal force, inevitable like the weather, a polysyllabic word in a language made up of monosyllables, and thus arcane, mysterious, difficult—even more so by the contrast with its colloquial tone, almost in the vernacular, of the words preceding it, 'ain't,' 'on account of': it is the representation of the squashing relationship between the single workman and the market forces which to him seem inevitable, inscrutable, unavoidable."[68]

"Stolen Car"

©1980 Bruce Springsteen (GMR)

Released on: *The River* album (1980) | *Tracks* box set (1998) alternate version

Live premiere: 10/03/1980—Crisler Arena, Ann Arbor, MI

A first version of the song was recorded on June 20 and 21, 1979. It's the one sometimes referred to as the "Son you may kiss the bride" version, which had additional verses and an instrumentation not as dark as in the version released on *The River*; it was included in the *Tracks* box set only in 1998. The version released on *The River* was recorded at the Power Station in New York, NY, in January 21, 1980.

"Stolen Car" was the predecessor for some of the music Springsteen would be writing in the future, the archetype for the male role in his later songs about men and women.

Often played during the 1980–81 The River Tour, "Stolen Car" was played only five times during the 1984–85 Born in the U.S.A. Tour and disappeared from the setlists until February 19, 2003, when Springsteen played it at the Somerville Theatre, in Somerville, Massachusetts, in the first of a two-night benefit stand for *Doubletake* magazine. After that, it was played only five more times before it was occasionally revived during the 2016 The River World Tour.

The song was featured in the film *Cop Land* with the main character (Sylvester Stallone) playing it on his record player. Same with "Drive All Night," which also happens to be on *The River*.

[i] The "Son you may kiss the bride" version of the song had a different verse: "Well, I found me a little girl and I settled down / In a pretty little house in a pretty little town. / We got married and promised never to part, / Then, I fell a victim to the hungry heart." This version of "Stolen Car" was written quickly and first recorded the day after "Hungry Heart," which is a song about a man who can't abide his family life anymore. Music critic Clinton Heylin has suggested that it may have begun as a continuation of that song, as "Stolen Car" originally used similar language to explain the marriage failure.[69]

[ii] There's an Eldridge Avenue in the New Monmouth section of Middletown Township, about twenty miles north of Asbury Park. The "Son you may kiss the bride" version of the song had "Stanton light"—on Stanton Place, crossing the main road from Belmar to Asbury Park—instead of "Eldridge Avenue." Steel Mill played at the Clearwater Swim Club in Middletown on September 11, 1970—a gig, now steeped in folklore, that turned into a melee when the music didn't stop, as ordered, at ten p.m. Police, who had made a number of drug-related arrests during the concert, jumped onto the stage as the band played beyond the prescribed time, which then escalated the event into a near-riot. During the ensuing mayhem, some sound equipment fell onto the local chief of police (who was very slightly injured). Danny Federici (future keyboardist of the E Street Band) earned his famous

nickname of "the Phantom" by disappearing from the melee with lightning speed. Springsteen spoke about the events at Clearwater Swim Club during his eulogy to Danny Federici in 2008.

[iii] The "Son you may kiss the bride" version of the song had extra verses at the end of the song:

> There's a river runs by that little town
> Down into the sea.
> It was there in the shade I laid my body down
> As she flowed by so effortlessly.
>
> There's a party out on County Line
> And there'll be dancing down at Seven Trees.
> From the banks I can see those party lights shine
> Maybe she's there, maybe she's waiting for me.
>
> Last night I dreamed I made the call.
> I promised to come home forever more.
> Once again we stood on the wedding steps at Victory Hall
> And walked arm in arm through the chapel door.
>
> I remember how good I felt inside
> When the preacher said, "Son, you may kiss the bride."
> But as I leaned over to touch those pretty lips
> I felt it all slip away through my fingertips.
>
> And I'm driving a stolen car running on borrowed time.
> And I don't even know why.
> Just driving a stolen car through the pitch-black night.
> No one sees me as I ride by,
> Nobody even sees me as I ride by.

In the final verse, the song's protagonist dreams of his wedding day and the joy and hope he felt, but as he dreams of kissing his bride at the end of the ceremony he feels everything slip away again. A subtle difference between this version and the *River* version is that whereas on the *River* version the singer fears he will disappear into the night, in this version he already has, like a ghost. The lyrics of this version also include river imagery used in some other songs on *The River*, including the title track and "Hungry Heart." In this version of the song, the singer—or his ghost—surrenders to the river similarly to the boy in Flannery O'Connor's story "The River," whose "fury and fear left him"[70] as he drowned in the river he was intending to baptize himself in. Clinton Heylin referred to Springsteen replacing this version with the version released on *The River* as "an act of self-sabotage."[71]

TWO

This Hard Land

Deliver Me from Nowhere

At the core of this section are the narrative songs that Springsteen wrote and recorded for the *Nebraska* and *Born in the U.S.A.* albums between 1982 and 1984.

When *Nebraska* was released, *Time* described it as "an acoustic bypass through the American heartland . . . like a Library of Congress field recording made out behind some shutdown auto plant."[72] In a little over forty minutes Springsteen scratched away the gold dust gilding the patriotic eighties (the "Reaganomic" years—cuts on social spending, job loss, increase in public spending on arms—and in war against the "Evil Empire"[73]), confirming himself in "the most complete and probably the most convincing statement of resistance and refusal that Ronald Reagan's U.S.A. has yet elicited from any artist or any politician."[74]

From a stylistic point of view, all the songs on *Nebraska* are written in the first person, with the exclusion of "Johnny 99." To sound realistic, Springsteen "sings in colloquialisms, drops the endings to his words, relies on such slang words as 'ain't,' and often uses improper verb tenses."[75] But it's the point of view that matters the most. Apart from the three autobiographical songs ("Used Cars," "Mansion on the Hill," and "My Father's House," already included in the first section of this book), the voice that tells his own story is sometimes that of the typical "unreliable narrator."[76] That's the case in "Nebraska," where the narrator's mental illness brings him to believe that the serial murders he committed are amusing and justifiable for the mere fact that "there's just a meanness in this world." Here, the character's unreliability is similar to that found in *The Adventures of Huckleberry Finn*, where Huck's innocence leads him to make overly charitable judgments about the characters in the novel. Same with the gangster-narrator of "Atlantic City," whose world of values brings him to believe that right and wrong do not exist, only a fine line dividing "winners and losers." The ability to put oneself in someone else's shoes, to speak in the voice of another person who has his own, singular view of life, allows Springsteen to create well-rounded characters, similar to Patrick Bateman in *American Psycho* ("Nebraska"), or Franz Kafka's self-alienating narrators ("State Trooper"). An extreme example is the narrator of "Working on the Highway"—a song written during the sessions for *Nebraska* and later included on *Born in the U.S.A.*—who is the equivalent of Nabokov's Humbert Humbert in *Lolita*: how old is the "pretty little miss" that the narrator practically kidnaps and takes to

Florida to marry Springsteen doesn't say, but it is significant that the original title of the song was "Child Bride."

Nebraska is not a rock album. Springsteen consciously makes reference to the lesson learned in the *Anthology of American Folk Music*, a fundamental anthology of popular music published by Folkways in 1952, in which recordings from Dick Justice, Blind Lemon Jefferson, Dock Boggs, and Yank Rachele, among others, made between 1926 and 1932, are collected. Sources of inspiration other than folk, blues, and hillbilly music most definitely come from Hank Williams, Johnny Cash, and Jimmy Rodgers' country music. And then of course Woody Guthrie.

From this point of view, *Born in the U.S.A.* is a million miles away, with its thunderous electric guitars and synthesizers. And yet, "underneath the layer of the album's mostly streamlined and charts-friendly pop," it's easy to detect "narratives that could be heard as continuing *Nebraska's* intervention in the official story of the United States."[77] "A tale of outright devastation; a tale of an American whose birthrights have been torn from his grasp, and paid off with indelible memories of violence and ruin."[78] Surely the incredible popularity of the album, the "Dancing in the Dark" super-pop video, the American flag on the cover, Springsteen's body-builder muscles and his clenched fist raised in the air to sing, "I was born in the U.S.A." are all factors contributing to the fact that the album was read superficially by many, not realizing that the songs spoke the same language as those in *Nebraska*. The famous Annie Leibovitz cover photograph shows Springsteen in a worn pair of Levi's, posed before a waving American flag and with a baseball cap stuffed into his pocket. Springsteen's body apparently signified "a vibrant, working-class, white male heterosexuality" in a historical moment in which "Michael Jackson's sexual identity was unclear, Prince's eroticism baldly crossed gender boundaries, and Madonna turned feminity into a series of disposable images."[79] His image, even before the chorus of "Born in the U.S.A.," was subject to political misunderstandings, leading to "the conservative conviction that the icon Springsteen represented a Republican version of America."[80] But the lyrics of the four songs taken from the *Born in the U.S.A.* sessions that are included in this section of the book ("This Hard Land," Born in the U.S.A., "Downbound Train," and "Car Wash") are here to testify that we are still in the *Nebraska* territory.

The section is opened by "Wreck on the Highway," a song taken from *The River* that Springsteen himself indicates as seminal for his subsequent work (i.e., the narrative songs in *Nebraska* and *Born in the U.S.A.*), and it is closed by two songs from *Tunnel of Love* that come from that same tree: "Spare Parts" and "Cautious Man."

Wreck on the Highway

©1980 Bruce Springsteen (GMR)

Released on *The River* album (1980)

Live premiere: 10/03/1980—Crisler Arena, Ann Arbor, MI

Placed at the end of *The River*, "Wreck on the Highway" reveals the composing style that Springsteen will improve in *Nebraska*. Despite his rarely presenting it live (between the 1980–81 and the 2016–17 River Tours it was played only eleven times), Springsteen calls it the alpha and the omega, the cornerstone of *The River*. "I wrote that song real fast, in one night," Springsteen recalls. "We came in and played a few takes of it and that's pretty much what's on the album, I think. That's an automatic song, a song that you don't really think about, or work on. You just look back and it sorta surprise you."[81]

The main character of the song, facing his own mortality, feels that the age of innocence is over and that Thunder Road and the Fast Lane are not the same thing. To Dave Marsh, the singer in "Wreck on the Highway" may well have been the hero from other songs on *The River*, including the title track and "Stolen Car," or even the heroes from earlier Springsteen albums such as *Born to Run* and *Darkness on the Edge of Town*, but that regardless he sees and speaks and sings for all of them. Pandora's vase has been opened, the definitive limit acknowledged. All dreams have become mere illusions. In this sense "Wreck on the Highway" works perfectly as a prologue to that grand fresco portraying the America of the defeated which Springsteen composes withdrawing his own voice and eyes, revealing instead his subjects' voices and eyes. There's still a veil in "Wreck on the Highway" that separate us from the drama: the protagonist is only a witness—for the last time.

The title and theme of the song were borrowed from "Wreck on the Highway," a country song written by Dorsey Dixon in late 1937 after a serious road accident near Rockingham, North Carolina, and originally recorded in 1938 by Dixon under the title "Didn't Hear Nobody Pray." The song was eventually recorded by Chicago radio duo Karl and Harty in 1940 and by Roy Acuff in 1942 under the title "Wreck on the Highway." The version sung by Acuff—known as the king of country music—is the one that gave the song its popularity.

When Springsteen was writing the songs for *The River*, country music had already become his primary source of inspiration. It is interesting to note how the man who in the seventies was saluted as "the future of rock 'n' roll" is now a symbolic fencepost in modern country. Kenny Chesney has covered two of his songs—"I'm on Fire" and "One Step Up"—and always refers to Springsteen as one of his heroes; Eric Church's "Springsteen" was a Top 10 hit in 2012; young country star Kip Moore has been praised as a "hillbilly Springsteen" for his gritty story songs and blue-collar viewpoint; the lyrics of Rodney Atkins' 2009 hit "It's America" ranked Springsteen songs alongside Chevrolet and NASA moon flights as symbols of U.S. patriotism, while Pat Green's "Feels Just Like It Should" finds a couple singing "Born to Run" while cruising down the highway in a convertible; and Josh Abbott Band's song "I'll Sing About Mine" takes issue with the trend, lamenting that songs about "the Dairy Queen, pickup trucks and Springsteen / Make the place I love sound like a bad cartoon." What seems to connect Springsteen to country music themes is that "his catalog is deep in story songs about working-class people struggling to make it in the suburbs. The suburbs are now the core geographic location for country's core audience. 'It's blue-collared working-man music,' [Eric] Church says of Springsteen. 'He sings about the plight of the people working in the factories, the people who are downtrodden.' . . . In that regard, there's a direct correlation between Springsteen and Merle Haggard, whose straightforward language as a songwriter built his reputation as the poet of the common man. Where Haggard scoffed at 'your so-called Social Security' in 'Big City' and struggled with unemployment in 'If We Make It Through December,' Springsteen addressed boarded-up family stores in 'My Hometown' and a construction worker's economic pain in 'The River.'"[82]

[i] The Riverside Medical Center is probably the Riverview Medical Center in Red Bank, New Jersey. Since 1996 it has been part of the Meridian Health Care System.

Nebraska

©1982 Bruce Springsteen (GMR)

Released on *Nebraska* album (1982) | *Live/1975–85* box set (1986) recorded live at Brendan Byrne Arena, East Rutherford, NJ, August 6, 1984 | *VH1 Storytellers: Bruce Springsteen* home video (2005) recorded live at Two River Theater, Red Bank, NJ, April 4, 2005

Live premiere: 01/07/1984—Civic Center, St. Paul, MN

In 1981 Springsteen saw Terrence Malick's movie *Badlands* (1973) on television. The story, though fictional, was loosely based on the real-life murder spree of Charles Starkweather and Caril Fugate. The couple (seventeen and fourteen years old) murdered eleven people in Nebraska and Wyoming in two months, between December 1957 and January 1958. Starkweather was executed seventeen months after the events, and Fugate served seventeen years in prison before her release in 1976. *Badlands* is set in 1959 and is narrated by the impressionable fifteen-year-old Holly Sargis (Sissy Spacek), a teenage girl living in a dead-end South Dakota town called Fort Dupree. One day she meets the twenty-five-year-old garbage collector Kit Carruthers (Martin Sheen), a disturbed, troubled greaser who resembles James Dean, an actor Holly admires. Kit charms Holly, and she slowly falls in love with him, even if her father disapproves of the relationship: that's why Kit comes to Holly's house and shoots her father dead. The couple goes on the run together, making their way towards the badlands of Montana . . .

Impressed by the movie, Springsteen researched the Starkweather killings, including interviewing Ninette Beaver, who had written a book about it: *Caril*.[83] The result was "Nebraska," a song written from Starkweather's perspective. The story unfolds without judgment. Although the narrator describes the murders and his trial and impending execution, he sings in a flat, unemotional voice, which makes the events described seem all the more chilling. Cinema once agian inspired this stylistic choice: not only Malick's *Badlands*, but also Ulu Grosbard's *True Confessions* (1981), starring Robert De Niro and Robert Duvall. "There was a stillness on the surface of those pictures," Springsteen said, "while underneath lay a world of moral ambiguity and violence."[84]

Is it appropriate to write in the voice of a killer, as Bruce Springsteen did in "Nebraska?" When asked, Bob Dylan answered,

> It's not inappropriate to put yourself in somebody else's place. That's a quite common thing to do. Folksingers used to do that all the time, and I've done a bit of that, too. "House of the Rising Sun" is written from a woman's point of view, and up until Eric Burdon did it, men used to sing it from a woman's point of view . . . Why not write a song for the guy who killed all the people at the McDonald's out in San Diego? I'm sure he's got a voice, too. And if he talked from the grave I'm sure he could get a lot of people to feel sorry for him, to sympathize with him . . . I don't know what Bruce's intentions were . . . I grew up in the same area as Charlie Starkweather and I remember that happening. That affected everybody out there. And everybody pretty much kept their mouth shut about it. Because he did have a sort of a James Dean quality to him. He was in the papers a lot. I must have been about seventeen or eighteen when that happened. I don't recall how most people felt about it. Nobody glorified him, though.[85]

Fourteen years after the publishing of *Nebraska*, Springsteen released another song about a capital punishment: the Oscar-nominated "Dead Man Walkin'," opener of the soundtrack for Tim Robbins' 1995 motion picture *Dead Man Walking*, starring Sean Penn and Susan Sarandon. Springsteen sings in narrative style in the voice of a death-row inmate similar to Sean Penn's film character. Robbins told the *Los Angeles Times*, "Bruce Springsteen's 'Nebraska' is a big inspiration." The song was first released on the film's soundtrack album, and on single in early 1996.

[i] These first two verses exactly describe the first shot in Malick's film *Badlands*.

[ii] "Nebraska" is sung as a first-person narrative by Charles Starkweather, who along with his teenage girlfriend Caril Fugate murdered eleven people over an eight-day period. Springsteen sings of ten deaths, as Starkweather had already killed one man prior to their meeting.

[iii] Charles Starkweather was born in Lincoln, Nebraska, in 1938, the third of seven children of Guy and Helen Starkweather—a respectable family of working-class background.

[iv] In a letter to his parentsfrom his prison cell, Charles Starkweather wrote, "But dad I'm not real sorry for what I did cause for the first time me and Caril have [sic] some fun." In *Badlands*, Kit—the character based on Starkweather and played by Martin Sheen—says, "I can't deny we had fun, though."

[v] Music critic Paul Nelson noted that this image perhaps "finds its origin in Fritz Lang's 1937 nod to Bonnie and Clyde, *You Only Live Once*: Henry Fonda, on his way to the electric chair, says [to a prison guard], 'You can sit on my lap when they throw the switch.'"[86] In real life Starkweather did his best to take Fugate down with him, although she escaped execution.

[vi] Starkweather was not known to have attributed his actions to "a meanness in this world." In the Flannery O'Connor short story "A Good Man Is Hard to Find," the violent character known as The Misfit, shows no remorse for the crimes he has committed and discusses it before shooting his next victim, a chatty grandmother, three times in the chest: "'Jesus was the only One that ever raised the dead,' The Misfit continued, 'and He shouldn't have done it. He shown everything off balance. If He did what He said, then it's nothing for you to do but throw away everything and follow Him, and if He didn't, then it's nothing for you to do but enjoy the few minutes you got left the best way you can—by killing somebody or burning down his house or doing some other meanness to him. No pleasure but meanness,' he said and his voice had become almost a snarl."[87]

Atlantic City

©1982 Bruce Springsteen (GMR)

Released on *Nebraska* album (1982) | *In Concert/MTV Plugged* album & home video (1993) recorded live at Warner Hollywood Studios, Los Angeles, CA, September 22, 1992 | *Live in New York City* album and home video (2001) recorded live at Madison Square Garden, New York, NY, June 29, 2000 | *Live in Dublin* album and home video (2007) recorded live at the Depot, Dublin, Ireland, November 19, 2006

Live premiere: 06/29/1984—Civic Center, St. Paul, MN

In late March or early April 1981, Springsteen wrote a song called "Fistful of Dollars"—inspired by Sergio Leone's 1964 spaghetti western with the same title, starring Clint Eastwood—during a break of the River Tour. The song eventually evolved into "Atlantic City," which Springsteen recorded—as all the other songs on *Nebraska*—solo in a spare room of his home in Colts Neck, New Jersey, with a TEAC TASCAM four-track cassette recorder. Legend dictates that the bulk of the songs were recorded in one all-day/night session on January 3, 1982. Springsteen himself has said it took three days, although he later said it took no more than a few weeks.[88]

In a letter to Jon Landau, Springsteen noted that "this song should probably be done with whole band + really rockin' out." As such, it was also recorded with the band at the Power Station in April 1982 during the so-called "Electric Nebraska" sessions. But this version was never released. Full-band live versions of "Atlantic City" appear on *In Concert/MTV Plugged* (1993), *Live in New York City* (2000), and *Live in Dublin* (2007).

"Atlantic City" was Springsteen's first video, even if he doesn't appear in the footage. In keeping with the bleakness of the subject matter, it was shot using black-and-white footage of Atlantic City from inside a moving car. The only instruction he gave to the director was that its images should in no way resemble those of the song.

Many artists made their cover of "Atlantic City," including the Band for their *Jericho* album (1983).

[i] Philip Testa (1924–1981), also known as the Chicken Man (because of his pockmarked face and the involvement in a poultry business), was the second-in-command of Angelo Bruno—the boss of the Philadelphia mob—who was shot-gunned to death on March 21, 1980. It is believed that the killing was ordered by Antonio "Tony Bananas," whose body was found stuffed in a body bag in the trunk of

a car in New York City few weeks later. The Chicken Man led the family for one year as the boss, until he was killed by the blast of a nail bomb allegedly ordered by his underboss Pete Casella. The bomb exploded under his front porch; the house was ravaged and witnesses claimed that pieces of Testa's body were scattered blocks away.

[ii] The title and many of the images of Springsteen's "Atlantic City" are shared with a 1981 Louis Malle movie starring Burt Lancaster and Susan Sarandon. Sally (Sarandon) is a young waitress in an Atlantic City casino who has dreams of becoming a blackjack dealer in Monte Carlo. Sally's estranged husband Dave returns to her one day with the intention of selling a large amount of cocaine that he stole in Philadelphia and meets Lou (Lancaster), an aging former gangster who lives in Sally's apartment building and runs numbers. Dave convinces Lou to sell the cocaine for him, but as Lou sells the first batch, Dave is attacked and killed by the mobsters from whom he stole the drugs. Lou is left with the remaining cocaine and continues to sell to impress Sally, whom he has long pined for, with money. Sally and Lou make love one day, but she returns to her apartment to find it trashed; she has been tracked down by Dave's killers, who beat her to find out if she has the drugs. They leave, but Lou laments not being able to protect her. Sally is fired from the casino when her late husband's criminal record is discovered. Lou sells the remainder of the cocaine, while both Sally and the mobsters discover Lou's affiliation with Dave. The mobsters corner them one night, but are killed when Lou produces a gun and shoots them. He and Sally then steal their car and leave the city. That night, from a hotel outside Atlantic City, they watch the TV news reporting on the killing. A police sketch of the suspect is shown. It looks nothing like Lou. Lou is overjoyed with relief and pride. He confesses to Sally that this was the first time he had ever killed anyone. At a motel during the night, Lou takes the phone to the bathroom to call Grace and brag about the killings. Sally also wakes and steals the money with the intention of sneaking off; Lou witnesses this, allowing her to leave and giving her the car keys so she can escape to France rather than go to Miami with Lou. Lou returns to Atlantic City to be with Grace and continues selling a portion of the cocaine that he had stashed away.

[iii] Central Jersey Bank & Trust headquarters were on Route 9 in Freehold, New Jersey.

[iv] The Coast City bus belongs to Coast City Coaches, with an office in the bus depot on Salt Lake Avenue, Asbury Park.

Johnny 99

©1982 Bruce Springsteen (GMR)

Released on *Nebraska* album (1982) | *Live/1975–85* box set (1986) recorded live at Brendan Byrne Arena, East Rutherford, NJ, August 6, 1984

Live premiere: 08/19/1985—Giants Stadium, East Rutherford, NJ

Two acoustic home demo takes of "Johnny 99" were recorded at Springsteen's home studio in Colts Neck, New Jersey, following the end of the River Tour, sometime between mid-September and December 1981. The take included in the *Nebraska* album was cut in January 1982. As for the other sixteen songs[89] that he put on cassette in that period, Springsteen's intention was to create a batch of multi-channel, professional-sounding, finished solo demos to demonstrate to the E Street Band at sessions for the follow-up to the *River* album. It was during the E Street Band sessions in late March and early April of 1982 that Bruce first attempted to record full-band arrangements of the demos. However, it soon became apparent to him that a majority of those songs did not work well with full-band arrangements. "'Johnny 99'—I thought, 'Oh, that'd be great if we could do a rock version.' But when you did that, the song disappeared. A lot of its contents was in its style, in the treatment of it. It needed that kinda austere, echoey sound, just one guitar—one guy telling his story. That's what made the record work, the sound of real conversation."[90]

During a September 22, 1984, concert in Pittsburgh, Springsteen used the introduction to "Johnny 99" to respond to President Ronald Reagan referencing the message of hope in Bruce Springsteen's songs, stating, "The President was mentioning my name the other day, and I kinda got to wondering what his favorite album musta been. I don't think it was the *Nebraska* album. I don't think he's been listening to this one."

Other artists have recorded "Johnny 99." Most famously, Johnny Cash recorded it along with another *Nebraska* song, "Highway Patrolman," for an album that Cash entitled *Johnny 99* (1983). The song has also been recorded by Los Lobos for *Badlands: A Tribute to Bruce Springsteen's Nebraska* (2000), and by John Hiatt, who wrote in the liner notes of the album One Step Up / Two Steps Back: The Songs of Bruce Springsteen (1997) , "This song has it all . . . crime, punishment, drama, mama, and a one-way ticket to hell."

In fact, "Johnny 99" is another song that, like *Nebraska*, ends (perhaps) on death row. In 1970 Springsteen—at the time with Steel Mill—had already written "He's Guilty (The Judge Song)," with the following lines:

Well, the judge and the jury came into the court room
At about 9:30 the 23rd of June.
"Now, we're here to try this boy for his crimes,
to see if we set him free or make him serve his time."
Jury all got up in the chairs,
"He's guilty, he's guilty, send that boy to jail."

The song was finally published in 2016, in the *Chapter and Verse* anthology.

[i] Ford Motor Company operated an assembly plant in Mahwah, New Jersey, starting in 1955. The plant produced six million cars in the twenty-five years it operated before the last car rolled off the line on June 20, 1980. At the time of its completion, it was the largest motor vehicle assembly plant in the United States. Nearly 250,000 autoworkers lost their jobs.

[ii] Tanqueray is a brand of gin that originated in England and is now produced in Scotland. Its largest market is North America, where it is the highest-selling gin import.

[iii] Johnny 99 is the nickname pinned onto Ralph after his crime, because he is sentenced to ninety-nine years of prison. In many popular folk and blues songs the ninety-nine-year sentence was a synonym for a life sentence. In Julius Daniels's "99 Year Blues" (1927) a young black man who is arrested for basically being poor and black is sentenced to serve ninety-nine years in "Joe Brown's coal mine." In Woody Guthrie's "Poor Boy" (1944) the narrator is literally persecuted by the number ninety-nine: he will lose at cards and will be sentenced to ninety-nine years of prison for murder.

[iv] For the judge's name, John Brown, Springsteen perhaps found inspiration in the Joe Brown quoted in Julius Daniels's "99 Year Blues." A sheriff—not a judge—named John Brown is on Bob Marley & the Wailers' "I Shot the Sheriff (1973) and covered by Eric Clapton in 1974. Springsteen, who has always been a Bob Marley fan, furthermore shared the bill with Marley at Max's Kansas City in New York during six memorable nights in July 1973, just as *Burnin'*—the album containing "I Shot the Sheriff"—was coming out.

[v] The earliest demo of the song had,

"Well Johnny, Johnny, we're ready to put you away.
Is there anything, son, that you want to say?
From here on after we can only hear you, buddy, when you shout,
You're going deep down, deep in some hole and you ain't ever gonna come back out."

[vi] The protagonist in "Johnny 99" notes that he has "debts no honest man could pay," repeating a line used by the protagonist in "Atlantic City."

[vii] The earliest demo of the song had an extra verse:

"It's only two hundred dollars that was all I was asking for,
Judge, just two hundred and I would have been on my way out the door.
He reached beneath the counter and I saw something shiny in his hand.
He started . . . he spewed blood like a fountain, and I dropped my gun and run."

Highway Patrolman

©1982 Bruce Springsteen (GMR)

Released on *Nebraska* album (1982) | *Live in Dublin* album and home video (2007) recorded live at the Depot, Dublin, Ireland, November 19, 2006

Live premiere: 06/29/1984—Civic Center, St. Paul, MN

Originally entitled "Deputy," like the rest of the album "Highway Patrolman" was recorded on Springsteen's four-track cassette recorder with the intention of performing it later on the album with his full band; however, it was felt that the demo version was superior to the eventual "band cut," so the song was released on the album in its original form. "I just kinda sat there," Springsteen recalls. "You can hear the chair creaking on "Highway Patrolman."[91]

This is one of the best set of lyrics ever written by Springsteen, with an almost cinematographic touch, so much so that in 1991 Sean Penn (a great admirer of Springsteen who at one time dated Bruce's sister Pamela) would pick up on the story of Frankie and Joe Roberts in the film marking his debut as a director, *The Indian Runner*, starring David Morse (as Joe Roberts) and Viggo Mortensen (as his brother Frankie). The film was shot partially in Nebraska; Joe wears the uniform of a Cass Country sheriff's deputy.

Johnny Cash recorded a version of the song for his *Johnny 99* album (1983).

[i] The story is set in an area where one can drive into Canada; however, the only American city called Perrineville is in New Jersey, only fifteen miles from Freehold. But there is, at least, an unincorporated community called Perronville in Harris, Michigan.

[ii] The "Highway Patrolman" lyrics printed on the *Nebraska* album inner sleeve have "I get a call over the radio," the same as the lyrics shown on Springsteen's official website. But Springsteen clearly sings, "I get a call on the shortwave," as he

does on the live version included in *Live in Dublin*. In Springsteen's *Songs*, there's another transcription, "I get a call over the shortwave."

[iii] The story of brothers Joe and Frankie may appear simple: Joe is a "good" policeman who doesn't arrest his "bad" brother because of the ties that bind them. In reality, as Peter Gambaccini observed,[92] Frankie is in fact a bad guy, but life challenged him harshly; he served in Vietnam while his brother was discharged in order to take care of the family farm and eventually had the chance to marry that Maria with whom the brothers were "takin' turns dancin'," Is that an allusion to the fact that maybe Maria "danced" with Frankie before she did it with Joe? If this is the case, we can say that the issue of who is in debt to whom has never been treated as brilliantly as in "Highway Patrolman."

[iv] There had never been song called "Night of the Johnstown Flood" until 2010—twenty eight years after *Nebraska* was published—when a bluegrass group called Rock Creek Jug Band gave the title to one of the songs for their album *Simpler Times*. The Johnstown Flood occurred on May 31, 1889, after the catastrophic failure of the South Fork Dam on the Little Conemaugh River, fourteen miles upstream of Johnstown, Pennsylvania. The dam broke after several days of extremely heavy rainfall, releasing twenty million tons (eighteen million cubic meters) of water from the reservoir known as Lake Conemaugh. The flood killed 2,209 people and caused $17 million in damage (about $450 million in 2017 dollars). Johnstown rapidly recovered from the disaster and soon became a flourishing industrial town. The immediate post–World War II years mark Johnstown's peak as a steel maker and fabricator. At its peak, steel provided Johnstowners with more than 13,000 full-time, well-paying jobs. However, increased domestic and foreign competition, coupled with Johnstown's relative distance from its primary iron source in the western Great Lakes, led to a steady decline in profitability. Extensive damage from another big flood in 1977 was heavy and there was talk of the steel companies pulling out, as Springsteen tells in "The River."

[v] While the lyrics state, "I musta done a hundred and ten through Michigan County that night," in actuality there is no Michigan County anywhere in the United States.

State Trooper

©1982 Bruce Springsteen (GMR)

Released on *Nebraska* album (1982)

Live premiere: 09/08/1984—Civic Center, Hartford, CT

Recorded in just a single take at Springsteen's home studio in Colts Neck, New Jersey, on January 3, 1982, "State Trooper" draws heavily on New York synth-punk duo Suicide's 1977 song "Frankie Teardrop" for inspiration. Springsteen plays the same droning chords on the acoustic guitar over and over as his character slowly loses his mind, then lets out an unhinged scream as the song fades. Considering this edgy little number, Springsteen wrote to Landau that he didn't even know if it was really a song or not.

[i] The New Jersey Turnpike is a toll road that stretches for 122 miles from Ridgfield Park, near the southern border of the state, to the George Washington Bridge in Fort Lee, New Jersey. The exit for Freehold, exit 8, at the sixty-seventh mile, connects with Route 33. Chuck Berry's 1956 song "You Can't Catch Me" features the lyrics "New Jersey Turnpike in the wee wee hours, / I was rolling slowly 'cause of drizzlin' showers." Simon & Garfunkel's song "America" (1968) contains the line "Counting the cars on the New Jersey Turnpike." Belgian indie-rock band dEUS's song "Theme from Turnpike" (1996) is a direct homage to Springsteen: "New Jersey Turnpike riding on a wet night." The song was used for the closing credits in one of the episodes of *The Sopranos*. Much of the opening credits of the famous television series (in which Steve Van Zandt from the E Street Band played the role of Silvio Dante) consists of shots of or from the New Jersey Turnpike.

[ii] This line also appears on "Open All Night."

[iii] The AM radio tower at mile 109 on the New Jersey Turnpike was demolished in the mid-1980s.

[iv] Each time he mounted Silver, his magnificent white stallion, the Lone Ranger yelled the customary "Hi-yo, *Silver*! Away!" and then galloped away while someone inevitably asked with astonishment who that masked rider was. The Texan ranger character and his Indian assistant, Tonto, fought against injustice in the old West, debuting on radio in 1933 and rapidly becoming an indestructible icon in American culture. The show *The Lone Ranger*—with Brace Beemer lending his voice to the hero—gained such great success that in 1949 it moved to the small screen for eight seasons, with Clayton Moore as the protagonist in the big white hat and black mask. Then came the various films, comics, and cartoons.

[v] It is a crucial line that also appears on "Open All Night" and "Living on the Edge of the World" (an earlier version of the song that appears on *Tracks*). As Springsteen said, "If you have a good line, you don't like to throw it away—you don't write that many."[93]

Open All Night

©1982 Bruce Springsteen (GMR)

Released on *Nebraska* album (1982) | *Live in Dublin* album and home video (2007) recorded live at the Depot, Dublin, Ireland, November 19, 2006

Live premiere: 10/03/1982—The Stone Pony, Asbury Park, NJ

Of the ten songs on *Nebraska*, "Open All Night" is the only one to feature an electric guitar. It's also one of the first songs to have been written: Springsteen played a snippet of it in the middle of "Ramrod" during the November 28, 1980, concert at the Madison Square Garden in New York City.

An early demo version of the song was recorded in Springsteen's home studio in Colts Neck, New Jersey, sometime between late March and early 1981. The lyrics were very different from the final version. There was also a verse, later used in "This Hard Land," that said,

> Mister, can you tell me what happened to the seeds
> What happened to the seeds I've sown?
> Yeah, where they fall from my hand
> And they fell on the ground of this hard land?

As regards the composition of the song, Springsteen said: "I got into this writer, William Price Fox, who wrote *Dixiana Moon* and a lot of short stories. He's just great with detail. In "Open All Night" I remember he had some short story that inspired me. I forgot what it was. But I was just interested in maintaining a real line through the thing."[94]

Springsteen played the whole song for the first time on October 3, 1982, at the Stone Pony in Asbury Park, New Jersey, during a gig with Cats on a Smooth Surface. During a show on August 26, 1984, in Landover, Maryland, he introduced the song with a funny story:

> This is a song about the golden roadway of the east, the New Jersey Turnpike. I used to work up in New York City all the time, so I'd always have to drive home late at night, and my girlfriend lived farther down in South Jersey. I used to kind of like the ride: I'd get out there around three thirty, just start driving, the window down a little bit . . .
>
> I never had too much trouble on the turnpike, but if you get off at exit 8, that's the Freehold exit, you've got to ride through Hightstown down 33 to the shore. Out in Hightstown, those guys, they don't have nothing to do but sit around and wait for you all night long. So, I was driving home one night, I was thinking about seeing my girlfriend, thinking about raiding her

refrigerator, seeing my girl and making a peanut butter and jelly sandwich, seeing my girl and making a ham and cheese sandwich, and raiding the refrigerator, and going back in the refrigerator again . . . Now, I know I wasn't speeding, but I must've been going suspiciously slow because all of a sudden, I seen them red lights, I get pulled over, and he comes up and says, "License and registration, please."

Now, I didn't have any. See, I always forget my wallet—one of them people who always leaves their wallet home. So I give my name and he goes back and sits in the patrol car, and he calls me back in about five minutes and kind of looks at me and he says, "Hey, uh . . . Are you . . . Are you that rock 'n' roll singer?"

So I said, "Yeah! yeah," you know, "That's me! That's me."

He said, "Did you . . . you the guy that . . . You wrote that 'Born to Run' song?"

I said, "Yeah, yeah, that's me! Yeah, I wrote that one! That's me . . ."

He said, 'Yeah, well you know,' he says, "I got some of your albums at home."

I said, "Yeah?"

He said, "Yeah, and son, you're in a lot of trouble."

So, they took me in and impounded my truck. But the weirdest thing about it was I had to go to traffic court. And when you go to traffic court, there's generally three pleas that you can plead. One is innocent, which hardly nobody pleads that. The other one is "guilty," which not many people plead that. But the one that almost everybody pleads is "guilty with an explanation." If you sit in traffic court all night, you figure out that the whole world is guilty with an explanation. And what that means is that—you really did what they said you did, but now you've got about five minutes to bullshit your way out of it.

So, like I'm sitting there, and somebody—some guy recognizes me and he comes over, and he's one of them people who when they sit down, they sit so close to you that you got to, like, lean away . . . He was drunk. And he gets up before me, and he was caught doing sixty on a residential side street, and his explanation was that he was drunk and thought he was on the main highway.

So anyway, my turn came up, and I got up. And they got a little microphone and . . . you know, you got to stand there, and everybody's looking at you, and you feel like a complete jerk. And I said, "Well, Judge, now, let me start at the beginning . . . Well, I had the carburator, baby, cleaned and checked . . .

"Open All Night" was released as a single (with "The Big Payback" on the B-side) for the European market. For the Session Band Tour of 2006, the song was transformed into an eight-minute show-stopping rave-up whose lyrics were rapped against a big band swing arrangement and a pseudo–Andrews Sisters female backing vocal trio. This is the version that appears on the *Live in Dublin* album and home video.

[i] The lyrics printed on the *Nebraska* album inner sleeve have "It's an all-night run to get back to where my baby lives," same as the lyrics shown on Springsteen's official website and on Bruce Springsteen's *Songs*. But Springsteen clearly sings, "It takes me two hours to get back to where my baby lives," as he does on the live version included in *Live in Dublin*.

[ii] Bob's Big Boy is a fast-food chain founded in 1936, famous for its Big Boy hamburger. There is a Bob's Big Boy Family Restaurant on the Garden State Parkway, in South Amboy, New Jersey. In the earliest version of "Open All Night," the girl (not called Wanda yet) was "counter girl at the Exit 24 HoJo."

Reason to Believe

©1982 Bruce Springsteen (GMR)

Released on *Nebraska* album (1982) | *Live/1975–85* box set (1986) recorded live at Giants Stadium, East Rutherford, NJ, August 19, 1985

Live premiere: 06/29/1984—Civic Center, St. Paul, MN

At the bottom of the bleak darkness of *Nebraska* finally comes a hint of daylight. Or does it? Is "Reason to Believe" an optimistic song? Could we really find some reason to believe "at the end of every hard-earned day"? The narrator seems to be left in astonished wonderment—but maybe it's only dark sarcasm. One thing is sure: "Reason to Believe" is the most provocative, open-ended song Bruce Springsteen has ever written.

The startling, stripped-down version that appears on *Nebraska* was recorded in January 1982. The song was also recorded with the band at the Power Station in April 1982 during the so-called "Electric Nebraska" sessions. A full-band version with the E Street Band can be heard on the *Live/1975–85* box set. For the Devils & Dust Solo and Acoustic Tour of 2005, Springsteen gave a shake-you-up, wake-you-up performance of the song, with a harmonica, a bullet-mic, 215 stomps on the floor and a "gotta-shout-to-be-heard blues voice that conjures up a whole mess of darkness and pain."[95]

[i] U.S. Route 31—also known as Highway 31— is a long north–south highway connecting southern Alabama to Northern Michigan. Nebraska Highway 31 stretches from near Louisville to Kennard at an intersection with U.S. Highway 30. But Springsteen said that the first verse of the song (with the dog hit by the

car) was inspired by his own experience driving down Highway 33 on his way to Millstone, a township in Monmouth County, New Jersey.

[ii] Is this guy Ralph also known as Johnny 99? And Mary Lou . . . could she possibly be the one who gave her name to an outtake from the *River* sessions that will be eventually included in the *Tracks* box set? ("Mary Lou" was an early version of "Be True," released as the B-side of the "Fade Away" single of 1981). There is also a Steel Mill song called "Marie Louise Watson," written by Springsteen in 1970, also known as "Black Widow Spider."

[iii] The word "effortlessly" was already on "Stolen Car." The unstoppable stream of the river is already in the sound of the four-syllable word "which shoots out from a forest of monosyllables."[96]

[iv] "Reason to Believe" closes *Nebraska*—Springsteen's darker, soul-searching journey—and should give an indication of what he found at the end of the road. But the song is enigmatic and the interpretations are starkly divided. Proponents of the pessimistic reading of "Reason to Believe" say that the unexplained death and rejected love in the four verses indicate that the chorus of the song ("Struck me kinda funny, seem kinda funny, sir, to me, / Still at the end of every hard-earned day people find some reason to believe") is a dark joke. Dave Marsh says that the song "stares down all of Bruce's rock 'n' roll idealism and mocks its certainty . . . If this stuff really strikes him funny, it's a cheerless joke. . . . Because in earlier songs Springsteen often found reason for optimism in the most terrible circumstances, many listeners took the chorus to be an affirmation. But 'Reason to Believe' said yes to nothing. It stared straight into the void about which Springsteen-as-Starkweather spoke and found there exactly what was expected: nothing at all."[97] The optimistic reading of "Reason to Believe" takes the chorus at its word and believes "that it is an affirmation of mankind's relentless ability to find hope where there seems to be none. True, the four images in the song are dark and bleak, but they still embody faith . . . No one in this song has given up or accepted the nihilistic conclusion that life is pointless. The characters in this song still have clear dreams and desires."[98]

This Hard Land

©1995 Bruce Springsteen (GMR)

Released on *Greatest Hits* anthology (1995) | *Tracks* box set (1998) | "Dead Man Walkin'" single (1996) recorded live at the Tower Theater, Philadelphia, PA, December 9, 1995

Live premiere: 03/23/1993—Count Basie Theater, Red Bank, NJ

"This Hard Land"—a mix of stark Dust Bowl folk and swirling Jersey Shore barroom rock—was originally recorded on May 11, 13, and 14, 1982, at the Power Station in New York City, during the *Born in the U.S.A.* sessions. Despite the fact that it's one of the best songs Springsteen wrote in the 1980s, it didn't find its place on his 1984 blockbuster album.

The song was re-recorded in 1995 by Springsteen and the reunited E Street band and included on the *Greatest Hits* compilation album. But the best version still remains the one recorded back in 1982, which was included on the *Tracks* box set in 1998.

"'This Hard Land' is a Western movie in five minutes, a story of friendship and brotherhood told through the life of a brother and a sister in the south-west of the U.S; you can see the dust, feel the saddle, hear the floorboards creaking underfoot. It was written for *Born in the U.S.A.*, wouldn't have been out of place on *Nebraska*, and finally emerged live onstage in 1993. It's almost country but not quite; it's almost rock but not quite that either. No matter how you want to label it, it's an absolutely beautiful, rollicking, wide-open song with a gorgeously narrated story."[99]

"We recorded about eighty songs for *Born in the U.S.A.* Some of them are great," said E Street Band drummer Max Weinberg. "'This Hard Land,' which didn't make it on the record, is just fantastic. That's probably my favorite song we've done."[100]

"'This Hard Land' has always been one of my favorites, and I don't understand how I could let it be unreleased for so long," Springsteen said to Sweden's *Pop* magazine in 1998. "I really wanted to write music about *you*, and *your* friends, so that you really could feel it when you stood there among thousands of others in the audience. When people think back on their closest friends, the friends they had when they grew up, those friendships always go hand in hand with the music and all the strong feelings that the music brought, feelings which were even stronger if you shared them with somebody. It was an essential part of what rock 'n' roll was about and I really tried to write songs that captured that. 'This Hard Land' was one of those."[101]

[i] In the first verse, Springsteen puts the listener in a place: that "you" is each of us listeners, maybe on the stool next to the narrator's in a midwestern bar. At any rate, the tone, the use of that "mister" instead of "buddy," makes one think that the narrator poses that question to a person of a higher social and intellectual standing than himself. That "you," then, becomes a pointed finger up against our indifference to social distress. But, in the end, as Springsteen says, "This Hard Land" traces the

search for home against the restlessness and isolation that is at the heart of the American character.

[ii] "This Hard Land's" geography is problematic. The protagonist, who probably arrives in Texas (if one takes the few clues dispersed within the lyrics as being true), says he is coming from Germantown. Several cities in the United States share this name. The most probable are the Germantown in Tennessee and the one in Kentucky.

[iii] "Home on the Range" is a classic western song that in 1947 became the state song of Kansas. The lyrics were originally written by Dr. Brewster M. Highley in a poem entitled "My Western Home" in the early 1870s. The music was later written by Daniel E. Kelley, a carpenter and friend of Higley, in 1878. The song was eventually adopted by ranchers and cowboys, and spread across the United States in various forms. The most popular version of the song was recorded by Bing Crosby in 1933.

[iv] What are "Bar-M choppers"? Some suggested that the chopper Springsteen is referring to is the typical motorcycle with the frame cut to rake out the front wheel—like the Harleys in Easy Rider—and that the Bar-M is the shape of the chrome piping used to extend the wheel. But the majority of the annotators believes that what he is referring to are helicopters used by a large cattle ranch called "Bar-M" to herd stray cattle. Using choppers for cattle herding has been around since the late 1950s, and many ranches are named "Bar-XXX" or "Lazy-XXX," etc. The names refer to the cattle brands they use. For instance, a Bar-M brand would be one with a solid line over, or under, a capital "M." The Lazy-M ranch would use a sideways "M."

[v] The Rio Grande river forms part of the Mexico–United State border. In Mexico, it is known as the Rio Bravo.

[vi] Springsteen played at the Liberty Hall in Houston, Texas, on October 7, 1974.

Born in the U.S.A.

©1984 Bruce Springsteen (GMR)

Released on *Born in the U.S.A.* album 1984 | *Live/1975–85* box set (1986) recorded live at the Coliseum, Los Angeles, CA, September 30, 1985 | *Tracks* box set (1998) demo version | *Live in New York City* album & home video (2001) recorded live at Madison Square Garden, New York, NY, June 29,

2000 | *Live in Barcelona* home video (2003) recorded live at Palau Sant Jordi, Barcelona, October 16, 2002 | *Get Up! Stand Up!—Highlights from the Human Rights Concerts 1986–1998* album (2013) recorded live at the River Plate Stadium, Buenos Aires, Argentina, 10/14/1988 | *¡Released!—The Human Rights Concerts 1986–1998* home video (2013) recorded live at the River Plate Stadium, Buenos Aires, Argentina, 10/14/1988

Live premiere: 06/08/1984—The Stone Pony, Asbury Park, NJ

To bring this track back into context—tearing it out of the catalog of hymns to put it back into that of protest songs—proved to be a real challenge for Springsteen. In 1981 director Paul Schrader sent Springsteen a a script called *Born in the U.S.A.*—a film about some fictional musicians. He wanted Springsteen to come up with some music for the film. One day, while he was writing a new song called "Vietnam," he looked over and sang off the top of Schrader's cover page, "I was born in the U.S.A." He recorded the song for *Nebraska* but didn't use it. Six months later he cut it with the band and that version became the title song for his next record. He later gave Schrader a song called "Light of Day," and the film was released under that title.

The solo acoustic demo of "Born in the U.S.A." was recorded in late December 1981 or early January 1982 at Thrill Hill Recording (Springsteen's home studio) in Colts Neck, New Jersey, and was included on the *Nebraska* demo tape that Springsteen sent to Jon Landau (this version surfaced on the *Tracks* box set in 1998). The full-band version that opens the *Born in the U.S.A.* album was recorded in just four takes at the Power Station on April 27–28 and May 3, 1982. Springsteen said that the sound of "Born in the U.S.A." was martial, but "the lyrics dealt with the problems Vietnam vets faced when they came back home after fighting in 'the only war that America had ever lost.'"[102] If you want to understand the song, you must consider both lyrics and music. But music is stronger; primarily an emotional language: "Whatever you've written lyrically almost comes in second to what the listener is feeling," Springsteen noticed. "I guess the same fate awaited Woody Guthrie's 'This Land Is Your Land' around the campfire. But that didn't make me feel any better."[103]

What had happened? It was the summer of 1984 when "Bossmania" exploded all across the United States, as a result of the release of the album *Born in the U.S.A.* and its relevant tour. During the performance of that song, which was continuously played on the radio (it was also released as a single and went on *Billboard*'s Top 10), every evening ten, twenty, a hundred American flags appeared out of the blue, its chorus screamed by the public with raised fists—and as if that weren't enough, even by President Reagan, who was running his re-election campaign. Somebody in his organization thought that Springsteen might endorse Reagan (not knowing Springsteen at all . . .) and made inquiries to Springsteen's management that were politely rebuffed. Nevertheless, on September 19, 1984, at a campaign stop in Hammonton, New Jersey, Reagan added the following to his speech: "America's future rests in a thousand dreams inside your hearts; it rests in the message of hope in songs so many young Americans admire: New Jersey's own Bruce Springsteen. And helping you make those dreams come true is what this job of mine is all about."

During a September 21 concert in Pittsburgh, Pennsylvania, Springsteen responded by introducing "Johnny 99" as follows: "The President was mentioning my name the other day, and I kinda got to wondering what his favorite album musta been. I don't think it was the *Nebraska* album. I don't think he's been listening to this one."

But the "damage was done and "Born in the U.S.A." became a hymn: millions of Americans and Europeans listened to it over and over again, day and night, in their cars, workplaces, kitchens, bedrooms—but they don't listen to it, as if they had all fallen victim to superficiality's spell. The attempt to reappropriate his song began on October 13, 1986, when Springsteen presented himself on stage for the Bridge Benefit organized by Neil Young in Mountainview, California. He pulled up a chair and strummed a red-trimmed acoustic guitar. "This is a song about a snake that comes around to eat its own tail,"[104] he said, and began a version of the song unlike anything heard before. But undoubtedly the best version is the one included on *Live in New York City*, where Springsteen's fierce singing emerges from a frightening guitar lick that evokes oriental sensations, and after sixteen years "Born in the U.S.A." finally shows itself as it is: a song about a Vietnam War veteran.

Springsteen declared that the song is probably one of his five or six best ones.[105] Stephen King agrees. He put the first line of the song, "Born down in a dead man's town," as the epigraph of his 1986 horror novel *It*. In 1978 he used lines from "Jungleland" as the epigraph of his postapocalyptic novel *The Stand*.

[i] The Battle of Khe Sanh was conducted in South Vietnam between January 21 and July 9, 1968, when the North Vietnamese Army launched a full-scale attack on American forces. A massive aerial bombardment campaign was launched by the U.S. Air Force to support the Marine base: over 100,000 tons of bombs were dropped. On July 9, 1968, the flag of the Viet Cong was set up at Khe Sanh airfield. It was the first time in the war that the Americans abandoned a major combat base because of enemy pressure.

[ii] Springsteen quotes Hank Williams's "I'm a Long Gone Daddy" (1948).

Downbound Train

©1984 Bruce Springsteen (GMR)

Released on *Born in the U.S.A.* album (1984)

Live premiere: 07/02/1984—Civic Center, St. Paul, MN

Springsteen wrote "Downbound Train" and recorded it, including one of the three takes that he made on the *Nebraska* demo tape that he sent to Jon Landau, in late December 1981 or early January 1982 at his home studio in Colts Neck, New Jersey. In his notes to Landau he describes the song as an "uptempo rocker for full effect / needs band / could be exciting." In all likelihood, he never seriously considered the song for release in its solo iteration. As such, it was recorded with the band at the Power Station in April and May of 1982 during sessions for *Born in the U.S.A.* The slowed-down version he eventually went with brings out the desolation in the lyrics about a guy bouncing from job to job as he watches his life fall apart.

[i] The image of the "downbound train" is proablably taken from "The Hell-Bound Train," a J. W. Pruitt song written around 1910 and found by Alan Lomax.

[ii] Talking about the *Born in the U.S.A.* album, one of the characaters of Bobbie Ann Mason's novel *In Country* says, "I like the song about the car wash—where it rains all the time and he lost his job and his girlfriend. That's the saddest song. That song really scares me."[106]

Car Wash

©1998 Bruce Springsteen (GMR)

Released on *Tracks* box set (1998)

Live premiere: 06/13/1999—B. Placher Stadion. Leipzig, Germany

"Car Wash" was recorded at the Hit Factory in New York on May 31, 1983, during the *Born in the U.S.A.* sessions, but it was released only fifteen years later on the *Tracks* box set. It is another song set in a car wash—like "Downbound Train"—and one of the few in Springsteen's canon sung from a woman's point of view (together with "A Good Man Is Hard to Find" and "Spare Parts"). Actually, it is Springsteen's first known composition with a female narrator, opening with the same "My name is" statement previously employed on "Highway Patrolman" and the *Nebraska* outtake "Losin' Kind."

Springsteen has played "Car Wash" live only once to date: it happened in Leipzig, Germany, in 1999.

[i] "Springsteen's early '83 stint living in Los Angeles is reflected in the "Car Wash" lyrics, which specifically mention the "Astrowash on Sunset and Vine." For the record, "Astro" is a popular prefix for businesses in L.A. Bruce could have set his story at Astro Burger on Santa Monica Boulevard, Astro Liquor on Avalon Blvd., or Astro Pharmacy on Hollywood Blvd."[107]

Spare Parts

©1987 Bruce Springsteen (GMR)

Released on *Tunnel of Love* album (1987) | "Spare Parts" single (1988) recorded live at Bramall Lane Stadium, Sheffield, England, July 9, 1988

Live premiere: 02/25/1988—Centrum, Worchester, MA

Following the release of the *Live/1975–85* box set, Springsteen began a new series of solo-based home studio sessions on January 20, 1987, that would form the foundation of the material issued on the *Tunnel of Love* album. He cut three songs on the very first day of recording: "Walk Like a Man," "When You Need Me," and "Spare Parts." For the latter, Springsteen played several instruments and was backed by Garry Tallent (bass), Danny Federici (organ), Max Weinberg (percussion) and James Wood (harmonica).

"Spare Parts" recalls a sixteenth-century ballad from Scotland, "Mary Hamilton," in which the mother ties her infant up in her apron and throws it out to sea, sighing, "Sink ye, swim ye, bonny wee babe, / Ye'll get no more of me." The song was included in *The English and Scottish Popular Ballads* anthologized by Francis James Child during the second half of the nineteenth century. In all versions of the song, Mary Hamilton is a personal attendant to the Queen of Scotland who becomes pregnant by the Queen's husband, which results in the birth of a baby. Mary kills the infant—in some versions by casting it out to sea or drowning it. The crime is seen and she is convicted. The ballad recounts Mary's thoughts about her life and her impending death in a first-person narrative.

On May 16, 1988, at Madison Square Garden in New York City, Springsteen introduced the song by saying:

> There was this fella and this girl. They met in a little shot-and-beer bar down along the coast on the weekend. He was a house painter, kind of young and a little on the wild side, wasn't saving his money or anything. And she was a little older and she was looking for somebody to love her. They met on a Friday or Saturday night and they started to go out. There were a lot of things about him that she liked, he was kind of sweet-tempered guy,

you know, real, real gentle, telling jokes all the time . . . And they moved in together, they got a little garage apartment about two blocks in off the beach in the wintertime, and things were going real nice . . . and . . . she got pregnant, and they were making plans to be married. He saved his money for the first time and he went down and got her a ring, brought it home, surprised her; and she went down and picked out a dress . . . And then something happened. I guess he got a little scared, maybe he was a little young or something, and he took off on her, but she never really let him go, she kept him in her mind and she kept him in her heart every night and every day. When she got in bed at night, she thought of him and saw his face; and the only problem was that he wasn´t ever coming back. And the world took that dream and broke her heart with every day, because there comes a time when you gotta take that past and you gotta put it away. So this is a song about a woman struggling to understand the value of her own individual existence, and the value of the life of her child, trying to put down that past, those old dreams that are tying her down, and find something new and beautiful and meaningful now.

"Spare Parts" was included in Springsteen's 1987 *Tunnel of Love* album, and it was released also as a single worldwide (with the exception of the U.S.) in 1988 with a live version of the song on the B-side, recorded at Sheffield, England, on July 9, 1988. The live footage was used for the official video.

[i] Shawnee Lake is located in County Morris, in New Jersey, near the Mahlon Dickerson city park.

[ii] Calverton is a town on the Peconic River, in the eastern end of Long Island, New York. The story that Janey has been hearing about a mother in Calverton is mysterious. According to Jim Cullen, "the place name 'Calverton' evokes Calvary, the site of Christ's crucifixion, and underlines the agonizing quality of Janey's struggle."[108]

[iii] "Now a man of the tribe of Levi married a Levite woman, and she became pregnant and gave birth to a son. When she saw that he was a fine child, she hid him for three months. But when she could hide him no longer, she got a papyrus basket for him and coated it with tar and pitch. Then she placed the child in it and put it among the reeds along the bank of the Nile." (Exodus, 2:1–3)

Cautious Man

©1987 Bruce Springsteen (GMR)

Released on *Tunnel of Love* album (1987)

Live premiere: 02/25/1988—Centrum, Worchester, MA

"Cautious Man" is the only character piece on *Tunnel of Love* along with "Spare Parts"; but is so thinly veiled, it's as if only the names have been changed —their real names being Bruce and Julianne. When he recorded the solo version that ended up on the *Tunnel of Love* album, sometime between January and May 1987, Springsteen's marriage with actress Julianne Phillips was on its last legs.

Very few performances of this song are known. "Spare Parts" was played only once during the 1988 Tunnel of Love Express Tour and eight times during the 2005 Devils & Dust Solo and Acoustic Tour. In Los Angeles, on February 5, 2005, Springsteen dedicated "Cautious Man" to Sean Penn, who was in the audience: "I felt like I'm on the brink for a long time; and those were the kinds of characters that interested me: on the brink of learning something, not sure exactly what . . . I'm gonna do this for my friend, Sean, another . . . brinksman."

[i] Springsteen has admitted lifting the idea of the LOVE and FEAR tattoo from the 1955 film *The Night of the Hunter*, directed by Charles Laughton and starring Robert Mitchum, which was selected by *Cahiers du cinéma* in 2008 as the second-best film of all time behind *Citizen Kane*. The protagonist, Reverend Harry Powell, is a self-anointed preacher with a penchant for switchblade knives, a misogynist who is both attracted to and repulsed by women. He travels rural roads, preaching in small towns, and rationalizes his serial murders by telling himself that he is punishing sinful women and gaining money to preach God's word. The letters "L-O-V-E" are tattooed on the fingers of his right hand, and the letters "H-A-T-E" on those of his left hand. Powell uses them as symbols in impromptu sermons.

The Grapes of Wrath

The Ghost of Tom Joad is the second part of that black-and-white film which Springsteen started recording in 1982 with *Nebraska*. Like *Nebraska* it is an acoustic album (even though this time there is participation, here and there, from a few musicians other than Bruce); and, like *Nebraska*, it seems the musical equivalent of a short story collection. When it was released in 1995, *Rolling Stone* critic Mikal Gilmore called it "among the bravest work that anyone has given us this decade."[109]

Following in the footsteps of traditional balladry, a somber Springsteen tells the stories of desperate men and women from to New York City to California, way down to the Mexican border, and even beyond that. "I had an interest in writing about the country—all of it," he said.[110] "As we tuck our children into bed at night, this is an America many of us fail to see, but it is a part of the country we live in, an increasing part. I believe a place and a people are judged not just by their accomplishments, but also by their compassion and sense of justice. In future, that's the frontier where we will all be tested. How well we do will be the America we leave behind for our children and grandchildren."[111]

Five songs included in this section come from *The Ghost of Tom Joad* and the other five from *Devils & Dust*, an album released in 2005 that included songs written during the *Ghost of Tom Joad* sessions and the acoustic tour in 1995–97. It's a trip across the United States, from East to West: from New York to Pennsylvania ("Streets of Philadelphia"), Ohio ("Youngstown"), Indiana and Louisiana ("The Hitter"), Oklahoma ("Black Cowboys" and "The Ghost of Tom Joad"), Texas ("The New Timer"), Nevada ("Reno"), California ("Highway 29"), the California/Mexico border ("The Line"), and the Texas/Mexico border ("Across the Border" and "Matamoros Banks").

Streets of Philadelphia

©1993 Bruce Springsteen (GMR)

Released on *Philadelphia—Music from the Motion Picture* soundtrack album (1993) | *Hungry Heart* EP (1995) recorded live at Sony Music Studios, April 5, 1995

Live premiere: 01/27/1994—Universal Amphitheatre, Los Angeles, CA

In early 1993, director Jonathan Demme asked Springsteen to write a song for his in-progress film *Philadelphia*. The movie was about a gay man's struggle with AIDS, starring Tom Hanks, Antonio Banderas, and Denzel Washington. Springsteen had already written a partial lyric about the death from sarcoma of a close friend.

He completed the song around June 1993 and recorded with him supplying almost all of the instrumentation (on vocals, guitar, bass, synthesizer, and drum machine), with bass and background vocals by Tommy Sims. It was used in the film during the opening sequence, and was also included in the film's soundtrack album, issued on December 30, 1993. Released as a single in February 1994, the song was a hit in many countries, particularly Canada, France, Germany, Ireland, and Norway, where it topped the singles charts. It peaked at #2 in the United Kingdom, becoming Springsteen's highest charting hit there.

The song was a critical triumph and went on to win the Academy Award for Best Original Song and four Grammy Awards, including Song of the Year; Best Rock Song; Best Rock Vocal Performance, Solo; and Best Song Written Specifically for a Motion Picture or Television.

Giving his Academy Award acceptance speech on March 21, 1994, Springsteen said, "This is the first song I ever wrote for a motion picture, so I guess it's all downhill from here . . ."

In 2013 Sir Elton John performed the song at the National Academy of Recording Arts and Sciences tribute concert honoring Bruce Springsteen as the 2013 MusiCares Person of the Year.

Black Cowboys

©2005 Bruce Springsteen (GMR)

Released on *Devils & Dust* album (2005)

Live premiere: 03/10/2005—Paramount Theatre, Asbury Park, NJ

One of the songs possibly written during the 1995–97 solo tour of *The Ghost of Tom Joad*, "Black Cowboys" was inspired by Jonathan Kozol's 1995 book *Amazing Grace: The Lives of Children and the Conscience of a Nation*, which focused specifically on the Mott Haven neighborhood of New York City, described as ravaged by drugs, violence, hunger, and AIDS.

"Springsteen crafts a story blending the feelings of sadness and abandonment of a young black boy from the Mott Haven neighborhood in the Bronx whose mother has taken up with a drug dealer with the boy's ideations of life as one of the black cowboys on the Oklahoma range. It is a piece of history he learned about from movies and books his mother once brought home for him."[112]

Introducing the song during a concert in Detroit, Michigan, on April 25, 2005, Springsteen said, "I kind of combined my love of westerns—it's a thing where you still pick up the papers every week and somebody, in our inner cities, is innocently shot. And I came across the photos of those street-side memorials with the flowers and pictures of somebody who died on that spot and I wrote this particular song." Springsteen added, "I always felt deeply American, and I believe that we carry all of American geography within us. . . . Musicians, writers, and filmmakers are drawn, by aesthetic or commercial or deep psychological reasons, to choose a certain type of geography that they go into and explore. Whether it's Martin Scorsese with Little Italy or John Cheever with the suburbs of Long Island, they create these worlds that are half-real and half-fantasy."[113]

Despite its AABBCCDD rhyme scheme, the lyric was printed in the disc booklet as prose.

[i] Squeezed in between the Harlem River and Yankee Stadium, Mott Haven is New York's poorest neighborhood. Two-thirds of the residents are Hispanic and one-third are African American. It was named Mott Haven after Jordan Mott, owner of Mott Iron Works, bought the original property from Gouverneur Morris II in 1849. Morris was asked if he minded if the area was called Mott Haven, a name it had quickly acquired. "I don't care . . . while [Mott] is about it, he might as well change the Harlem River to the Jordan."

[ii] Contrary to what the homogenous imagery depicted by Hollywood and history books would lead you to believe, in the 1870s and 1880s approximately 25 percent of the 35,000 cowboys on the Western Frontier were black.[114] In particular, African Americans had an important role in the cowboy culture of the Great Plains. In fact, many, if not most, of the Texas and Indian Territory outfits that participated on the long overland drives to the Kansas railheads employed African Americans whose skills (working cattle, caring for horses, working as blacksmiths or cooks) were essential to the operation. When African American cowboys entered the Great Plains after the Civil War to work on the long overland drives that linked Texas to the Kansas railheads, they were merely continuing a centuries-old pattern rooted in the American South, Mexico, the Caribbean, southern Iberia, and perhaps even West Africa. In fact, Terry Jordan, a geographer who has thoroughly studied the diffusion and material culture of cattle ranching, notes that African slaves were the *vaqueros* for the herds in southwestern Spain by the sixteenth century.[115]

[iii] Seminole Scouts—also known as Seminole Negro or Indian Scouts—were employed by the United States Army between 1870 and 1914. Despite the name, the unit included both Black Seminoles and some native Seminoles. However, because most of the Seminole scouts were of African descent, they were often attached to the Buffalo Soldier regiments, to guide the troops through hostile territory. The majority of their service was in the 1870s, in which they played a significant role in ending the Texas-Indian Wars. They were disbanded in 1914.

[iv] A reference to Ezekiel 37:1–7: "The hand of the Lord was on me, and he brought me out by the Spirit of the Lord and set me in the middle of a valley; it was full of bones. He led me back and forth among them, and I saw a great many bones on the floor of the valley, bones that were very dry . . . Then he said to me, "Prophesy to these bones and say to them, 'Dry bones, hear the word of the Lord! This is what the Sovereign Lord says to these bones: I will make breath enter you, and you will come to life.' . . . So I prophesied as I was commanded. And as I was prophesying, there was a noise, a rattling sound, and the bones came together, bone to bone.'"

[v] This image is also in the last line of "Matamoros Banks": "The pale moon opens the earth to its bones."

Youngstown

©1995 Bruce Springsteen (GMR)

Released on *The Ghost of Tom Joad* album (1995) | *Live in New York City* album & home video (2001) recorded live at Madison Square Garden, New York, NY, June 29, 2000 | *London Calling: Live in Hyde Park* home video (2010) recorded live at Hyde Park, London, June 28, 2009

Live premiere: 11/21/1995—State Theatre New Jersey, New Brunswick, NJ

Recorded between April and June 1995 at Thrill Hill West (Springsteen's Los Angeles home studio), the song tells the tale of the rise and fall of Youngstown, Ohio, over several generations, from the discovery of iron ore nearby in 1803 through the decline of the steel industry in the area in the 1970s.

Introducing the song in Chicago on March 12, 1995, Springsteen said, "I think I had ten songs on *The Ghost of Tom Joad* record and I was wandering around downstairs one night when I couldn't sleep, and I went into my living room and pulled a book off the shelf. It was a book called *Journey to Nowhere*, and the text was written by a fellow named Dale Maharidge and the photos by Michael Williamson; they were two reporters who hopped a train in St. Louis, I think, and they rode it west out through to California and up north into Oregon in the mid-1980s, sort of chronicling what they were seeing going on out on the road. . . . I guess there was a chapter on Youngstown, Ohio, in the book. I remember I read the book, I read it all in one sitting and I lay in bed and . . . I've had a fortunate life, but it was real easy to imagine what if your craft, like the one thing you do all of a sudden you couldn't do any more, something that you've put thirty years of your life in, forty years of your life, something that was who you were, that was what you did, that was what kept your head high and was what fed your children . . .

what if you came home all of a sudden, you stopped getting your kids fed, getting them the kind of medical care they need . . . People who built the buildings that we live in, who built the bridges that we cross, the very infrastructure of the country that we take for granted . . ."

Writing for the *New York Times Magazine*, author Nicholas Dawidoff said that "Youngstown" was the best song on the album and was an example of the "best of his songs [which] have all the tension and complexity of great short fiction."[116]

"Youngstown" was heavily rearranged into a hard rock number for the Reunion Tour of 1999, with the last two minutes taken over by Nils Lofgren's guitar solo, which features several tempo changes and crescendos before culminating in the guitarist spinning in circles on the stage.

[i] In 1802, the Heaton brothers James, Isaac, and Daniel settled in the Mahoning Valley, Ohio, and built the first iron-producing blast furnace west of the Allegheny, in the Youngstown area. Each of the brothers built his own furnace, forming the center of the greatest industrial activity in the Mahoning Valley. Its weekly output of iron ranged from two to three tons. During the Napoleonic Wars, demand for iron and iron products was very high, and the furnaces of the Mahoning Valley prospered. By the mid-nineteenth century, Youngstown was the site of several iron industrial plants, and because of easy rail connections to adjacent states, the iron industry continued to expand despite the depletion of local natural resources. Between the 1920s and the 1960s, Youngstown was known as an important industrial hub that featured the massive furnaces and foundries of such companies as Republic Steel and U.S. Steel. When economic changes forced the closure of plants throughout the 1970s, the city was left with few substantial economic alternatives. The September 19, 1977, announcement of the closure of a large portion of Youngstown Sheet and Tube, an event still referred to as "Black Monday," is widely regarded as the death knell of the old area steel industry in Youngstown. In the wake of the steel plant shutdowns, the community lost an estimated 40,000 manufacturing jobs.

[ii] The Jeanette furnace—which the workers referred to as "Jenny"—was a blast furnace that once stood along the Mahoning River at the Brier Hill Plant of the Youngstown Sheet and Tube Company (YS&T). Built at a cost of $3 million, it was lighted on September 20, 1918, by its namesake, Mary Jeanette Thomas, daughter of W. A. Thomas, who was the president of Brier Hill Steel. The furnace produced more than eleven million tons of steel in its lifetime until the Brier Hill Plant was shut down in September 1977. It was one of the oldest blast furnaces in the United States, and the last of its kind in Youngstown.

[iii] Located six miles upstream from Pittsburgh on the Monongahela River, Homestead, Pennsylvania, was the site of one of the bitterest labor struggles of the nineteenth century. The home of the Carnegie Steel Company, which employed 3,800 skilled and unskilled workers, Homestead was the center of the nation's burgeoning steel industry. In 1892, in a bid to break an emerging union of skilled workers, the Amagamated Association of Iron and Steel Workers, Henry Clay Frick, the head of the steel works, proposed cutting skilled workers wages. When negotiations broke down, he locked out the steelworkers, built a three-mile-long wooden fence, topped with barbed wire, around the plant, and brought in two barges carrying 300 Pinkerton guards to protect the plant. As the Pinkerton agents arrived on the morning of July 6, a fierce day-long battle erupted between the Pinkertons and the steelworkers involving rifles and even a Civil War cannon. When the Pinkertons surrendered, three agents and seven workers were dead. Pennsylvania's governor brought in 4,000 state militiamen to quell the violence. When Frick was seriously wounded in an assassination attempt two weeks after the battle with the Pinkertons, public opinion shifted against the union. The Homestead strike lasted five months and was a victory for the company. It blacklisted many union leaders from the steel industry for life, and replaced many skilled workers with unskilled workers. The steel industry remained largely without unions until the Great Depression of the 1930s.

[iv] Discovered in 1866, the Mesabi Iron Range, located in northeast Minnesota, is the chief iron ore mining district in the United States. Several large-scale strikes took place on the Mesabi Iron Range during the early 1900s. The mines produced the majority of iron need by the United States in the Second World War.

The Hitter

©2005 Bruce Springsteen (GMR)

Released on *Devils & Dust* album (2005)

Live premiere: 11/13/1996—Landmark Theatre, Syracuse, NY

"We carry the seeds of our own destruction. And I guess that's what this song is about. You know. God set us up so that we build with this hand, and we burn with this one."[117]

Springsteen debuted this song on the the Ghost of Tom Joad Tour of 1996, nine years before its inclusion on the *Devils & Dust* album. It was just a few days after Mike Tyson lost the WBA Heavyweight Championship to Evander Holyfield, and Bruce introduced the song by asking, "Anybody see the fight the other night? That was something," he laughed, "Oops—Big Mike went down!"

The core recording of "The Hitter"—which may date from 1997–98—is Springsteen solo, on all instruments (vocals, guitar, keyboards, and percussion). The strings (Nashville String Machine) and horns (Brice Andrus, Donald Strand, Susan Welty, and Thomas Witte) were recorded and added in 2004.

"The song features a title character as nasty and unredeemable as perhaps any in the Springsteen catalog, a statement made truer when you include only those whom Bruce inhabits in their respective songs in the first person. 'The Hitter' is reminiscent of something Randy Newman would have written in his heyday, a portrait of an unlikable, moral-free character whose powerful story still deserves to be told . . . This is a song that's not for the timid of spirit. But it is songwriting of the highest order nonetheless. That's because Springsteen manages to elicit, if not sympathy, at least some understanding for 'The Hitter,' which is more mercy than the character would ever show to his unfortunate opponents."[118]

The song has striking similarities to the 1959 Marlon Brando film *The Fugitive Kid*. In this adaptation of Tennessee Williams's *Orpheus Descending*, directed by Sidney Lumet, Brando plays Valentine "Snakeskin" Xavier, a drifter in trouble with the law. He's a guitar player, not a boxer, but he plays many of the same Louisiana towns mentioned in "The Hitter," and there's a scene early in the film when Val stands on a doorstep in the pouring rain, begging through the chain to come in and lie down for a while.

In 2008, Tom Jones turned Springsteen's spare, reflective folk ballad into a smoldering soul number, complete with weeping horns, making "The Hitter" feel less like a lament and more like a matter of life and death. Jones's version was included on his *24 Hours* album.

[i] Numerous vessels had that name. In the 1941 film *The Lady Eve, Southern Queen* is the name of a ship ridden by Henry Ford, fresh from his portrayal of Tom Joad in 1940's *The Grapes of Wrath*.

[ii] Jack Thompson (1904–1946), also known as "The Frisco Flash," was the world welterweight champion in 1930 and 1931. But there was also a William "Jack" Abednego Thompson (1811–1880), an English bare-knuckle boxer who was considered the "champion of champions" of his times. His outspoken character (he would make up rhymes about his opponents during the fights) and record in the ring attracted a massive fan base, including Sir Arthur Conan Doyle, who wrote a verse to the fighter, titled "Bendigo's Sermon":

> You didn't know of Bendigo?
> Well, that knocks me out!
> Who's your board schoolteacher?

What's he been about?
Chock-a-block with fairy tales;
Full of useless cram,
And never heard of Bendigo
The Pride of Nottingham.[119]

[iii] Big John McDowell seems to be Springsteen's creation.

[iv] The 1996 live version had "It's my face you don't recognize."

[v] The 1996 live version had "Stockyard."

The Ghost of Tom Joad

©1995 Bruce Springsteen (GMR)

Released on *The Ghost of Tom Joad* album (1995) | *Sowing the Seeds* anthology (2007) | *The 25th Anniversary Rock & Roll Hall of Fame Concerts* box set (2009) recorded live at Madison Square Garden, New York, NY, October 29, 2009 | *High Hopes* album (2014) feat. Tom Morello

Live premiere: 10/28/1995—Shoreline Amphitheatre, Mountain View, CA

Written as a rock song for the *Greatest Hits* project, but abandoned when Springsteen couldn't find an arrangement, "The Ghost of Tom Joad" was re-shaped as an acoustic song and recorded on May 23, 1995, at Thrill Hill West (Springsteen's Los Angeles home studio). Springsteen handles guitar and vocals and his four-man backing band on this recording is Danny Federici (keyboards), Garry Tallent (bass), Marty Rifkin (pedal steel, dobro), and Gary Mallaber (drums). After working with the E Street Band in New York, Springsteen went back to California and started recording at home. The first songs he penned were "Straight Time," "Highway 29," and "The Ghost of Tom Joad." He also had a notebook filled with unfinished song ideas. Once he cut "Tom Joad," he got the feeling he had a record: an acoustic album with elements picked up from the themes he had worked on in the past.

The song takes inspiration from John Ford's 1940 film adaptation of John Steinbeck's 1939 classic novel *The Grapes of Wrath*, starring Henry Fonda as Tom Joad. The film tells the story of the Joads, an Oklahoma family, who, after losing their farm during the Great Depression in the 1930s, become migrant workers and begin an arduous journey across the United States as they travel to California in search of work and opportunities for the family members.

In a 1995 interview, Springsteen explained that it was the film more than the book that made an impact on him.

That picture, I guess I saw in the late seventies and it had a really deep effect on me. I think I'd read some John Steinbeck, probably earlier than that—in high school, and there was something about the film that sort of crystallized the story for me. And it always stayed with me after that; for some reason there was something in that picture that always resonated throughout almost all of my other work. It was just an image that popped out as I was sitting around on the couch messing around with the guitar.[120]

The song also takes inspiration from Woody Guthrie's 1940 song "Tom Joad," which explores the novel's protagonist's life.[121]

"The Ghost of Tom Joad" was recorded by Tom Morello's Rage Against the Machine and released as a free single in 1997. Springsteen made a rock arrangement of the song that was premiered live on April 7, 2008, in Anaheim, California, performed with Morello sharing lead vocals (it's on the *Magic Tour Highlights* digital EP). Springsteen then recorded the rock arrangement in the studio with the E Street Band and Morello in 2013 and issued it on the *High Hopes* album in 2014. Pete Seeger recorded the song with Springsteen adding a counterpoint vocal in the compilation Sowing the Seeds celebrating Appleseed Recordings' tenth anniversary.

[i] Springsteen's song is set in the 1980s and 1990s, with contemporary times being likened to Dust Bowl images.

[ii] This is a sarcastic reference to President George Bush's September 11, 1990, "Toward a New World Order" speech to a joint session of Congress—a "rationalization for imperial ambitions"[122] in the Middle East following the first Gulf War.

[iii] This line was previously used in "Seaside Bar Song," an outtake from the 1973 album sessions for *The Wild, the Innocent & the E Street Shuffle* that was then released on the *Tracks* box set in 1998.

[iv] In *The Grapes of Wrath*, Jim Casy is a former preacher who has lost his faith—a friend of Tom Joad from their childhood. He travels with the Joads on Route 66, reaching a peach orchard in California. There, Casy becomes a labor organizer and tries to recruit for a labor union; he is involved in a strike that eventually turns violent. When Tom Joad witnesses Casy's fatal beating, he kills the attacker and flees as a fugitive.

[v] Ironic reference to Matthew 20:16.

[vi] This is an extensive paraphrase of Tom Joad's famous speech in Steinbeck's novel, when he bids his mother farewell and promises to work for the oppressed—affirming Whitman's idea of the individual as a manifestation of the collective soul (or as Emerson termed it, the Over-Soul):

I'll be all aroun' in the dark. I'll be ever'where—wherever you look. Wherever they's a fight so hungry people can eat, I'll be there. Wherever they's a cop beatin' up a guy, I'll be there. If Casy knowed, why, I'll be in the way guys yell when they're mad an'—I'll be in the way kids laugh when they're hungry an' they know supper's ready. An' when our folks eat the stuff they raise an' live in the houses they build—why, I'll be there.[123]

Nunnally Johnson's screenplay for the movie directed by John Ford quotes from Steinbeck almost directly. The references at the end of *The Ghost of Tom Joad*'s credits list "John Ford's *The Grapes of Wrath*, written by Nunnally Johnson, based on the novel by John Steinbeck, a Twentieth Century-Fox film." But there is also a second source: Woody Guthrie's "Tom Joad."

The New Timer

©1995 Bruce Springsteen (GMR)

Released on *The Ghost of Tom Joad* album (1995)

Live premiere: 11/30/1995—Berkeley Community Theatre, Berkeley, CA

Released on the *Ghost of Tom Joad* album, "The New Timer" is "as riveting and authentic a piece of Depression-era folk storytelling as any artist recorded in the latter half of the twentieth century."[124] In his foreword to the 1996 edition of Maharidge and Williamson's *Journey to Nowhere*, Springsteen revealed that he drew inspiration from that book to write the song.

The the protagonist is modeled upon the character of Don, a young manager who goes bankrupt due to the economic crisis of the eighties, losing his job, wealth, and house, even his wife, who leaves him, taking their three children with her. Don decided to tell his story to the writers of the book, alternating the narration with the story of Thomas Jefferson "Alabama" Glenn, an elderly hobo they meet in Sacramento, California, who chooses the street during the Great Depression. Springsteen binds the two stories together, drawing inspiration from the figure of "Alabama" for his character Frank, the old hobo who becomes mentor to the protagonist of the song.

Surely Springsteen also took inspiration from the song "Pastures of Plenty" by Woody Guthrie (1941). Even "Around a Western Water Tank," a hobo song found and arranged by Alan Lomax, probably inspired Springsteen's story.

[i] Maharidge defines "new timer" as a "new breed of street person, forced to the bottom by economic hardship."[125]

[ii] These two lines quote the first of Alabama's rules of survival in *Journey to Nowhere*.

[iii] In *Journey to Nowhere*, Don, on the train from Kansas City to Pueblo, sees snowflakes and swirls of snow falling upon him.

[iv] Quote from "Pasture of Plenty" by Woodie Guthrie. Firebaugh, California, is situated on the River San Joaquin.

[v] Marysville, California, north of Sacramento, is the city in whose hinterland Steinbeck sets the last chapters of *The Grapes of Wrath*.

[vi] Stockton, in the San Joaquin Valley, is connected to San Francisco via a canal sixty miles long. It saw its best days during the Gold Rush, in the middle of the nineteenth century. Frank's death scene is traced around the (true) story of Alabama in *Journey to Nowhere*, when the authors of the book find his corpse.

[vii] Sacramento, California's capital, was literally invaded by hundreds of jobless people ("the newtimers") because of the great economic crisis of 1982.

Highway 29

©1995 Bruce Springsteen (GMR)

Released on *The Ghost of Tom Joad* album (1995)

Live premiere: 11/21/1995—State Theater, New Brunswick, NJ

"Highway 29" was recorded between March and June 1995 at Thrill Hill Recording (Springsteen's home studio) in Beverly Hills, California. It was one of the first songs written for *The Ghost of Tom Joad* album. The shoe salesman's escape with his client, the trail of blood they leave behind them, are reminiscent of themes already used in "Nebraska." But above all, the story narrated in "Highway 29" is remarkably similar to an outtake of the *Nebraska* album called "Losin' Kind," where a driver called Frank Davis meets a girl outside a bar in Wilsonville, out on Highway 17:

> Well, we drove around in my Buick, getting drunk and having fun.
> We ended up at this Best Western out on Highway 101,
> It was around 3 a.m. We went out to this empty little roadside bar;
> It was there the cash register was open, it was there I hit that guy too hard.
> But I knew when I hit him for the second time
> That one attracts the other when you're the losin' kind.

[i] Highway 29 is a part of the Nevada Highway, which crosses the Nevada–California border, where the Amargosa Desert lies.

[ii] The Sierra Madre mountain chain at the border between the United States and Mexico was home to the legendary Pancho Villa.

The Line

©1995 Bruce Springsteen (GMR)

Released on *The Ghost of Tom Joad* album (1995)

Live premiere: 11/21/1995—State Theater, New Brunswick, NJ

"California was Mexico until 1948," Springsteen said talking about "The Line," probably the finest of the *Ghost of Tom Joad* narrative songs. "Mexican writer Carlos Fuentes says that the border is more like a scar than a borderline," he added. "This song is about a young guy trying to figure out where that line really is."[126]

Introducing "The Line" during a concert in New York City, on December 17, 1995, Springsteen said,

> When I was a kid, I was always watching all the old Westerns; and everybody was always sort of fascinated by the outlaw, you know, but I was, I was interested in the sheriff. I always thought, "Man, that´s a tough job," like Henry Fonda in *My Darling Clementine* or Gary Cooper in *High Noon*: they were the people that interested me, So, this is a song set at the San Diego border station where there's a lot of young guys that get out of the army and they end up working for the INS and the border patrol, and it's a very confusing job; it's very difficult to know where the line really is.

[i] Fort Irwin is a major training area for the United States military located in the Mojave Desert, in northern San Bernardino County, California.

[ii] California Border Patrol is part of USBP (United States Border Patrol), the federal agency of INS (Immigration and Naturalization Service). Since March 2003, USBP has been a component of the U.S. Department of Homeland Security.

[iii] Guanajuato is a state in North-Central Mexico.

[iv] Arroyos are canals used in crop irrigation.

[v] Tijuana, Mexico, is only fifteen miles from San Diego, on the Gold Coast of Baja California.

[vi] Sonora is a state located in Northwest Mexico that shares the U.S.–Mexico border with Arizona and New Mexico. Illegal crossings take place through tunnels, hidden cars and trucks, or, most commonly, simply passing through a gap in the fence, especially in the more remote areas.

[vii] Madera County is at the center of California, in the eastern San Joaquin Valley and the central Sierra Nevada.

Reno

©2005 Bruce Springsteen (GMR)

Released on *Devils & Dust* album (2005)

Live premiere: 04/22/2005—Paramount Theatre, Asbury Park, NJ

The core recording of "Reno"—which may date from 1997–98—is Springsteen solo, on all instruments (vocals, guitar, keyboards, and tambourine). The strings (Nashville String Machine) and horns (Brice Andrus, Donald Strand, Susan Welty, and Thomas Witte) were recorded and added in 2004.

The song was released on *Devils & Dust*, and because Springsteen sings about having anal sex with a prostitute the album was slapped with a "parental advisory" sticker in the States. Moreover, Starbucks, which had been considered a possible retail outlet for the album, declined to sell copies of *Devils & Dust* because of "Reno." At a concert at the Tower Theater in Philadelphia, Springsteen introduced the song by joking that the album would be available "at Dunkin' Donuts and Krispy Kreme stores everywhere." Introducing the song in Dallas, on April 28, 2005, Springsteen said, "If there's any little kids here, it might be a nice time to check out some of those fine T-shirts we have out there, some very nice merchandise for those little kiddies . . . This is a love song; it's also about not being able to handle the real thing, so you settle for something else that doesn't work out that good either."

The name of the singer's lost love is Maria, connecting this song to "Maria's Bed" (another track from *Devils & Dust*) and "Highway Patrolman" (from *Nebraska*). But "it's a Louisa that might have the most connection with this song. In 'The Line,' after our narrator Carl loses his beloved Louisa, we're left with him drifting, from town to town and bar to bar, hoping to catch a glimpse of her. It's worth nothing that, without exception, every time Springsteen performed 'The Line' on the Devils & Dust Tour . . . he followed it immediately with 'Reno.' It might as well be Carl in that room."[127]

[i] Reno, Nevada—known as "The Biggest Little City in the World"—is famous for its casinos. The state of Nevada is the only jurisdiction in the United States where prostitution is permitted.

[ii] While a liner note on the *Devils & Dust* booklet says the Amatitlan is a "Central Mexican River," the lyric would actually seem to refer a Central American lake: Lake Amatitlan is located just south of Guatemala City.

[iii] The only Valle de Dos Rios is in southern Spain.

Across the Border

©1995 Bruce Springsteen (GMR)

Released on *The Ghost of Tom Joad* album (1995)

Live premiere: 11/21/1995—State Theater, New Brunswick, NJ

Recorded between April and June 1995 at Thrill Hill West (Springsteen's Los Angeles home studio), "Across the Border," evoking the spirit of Psalm 23, is Springsteen's answer to Tom Joad's famous final speech in *The Grapes of Wrath*. Introducing the song at the Berkeley Theatre, Springsteen said,

> When I was a kid I grew up in a house where there wasn't a lot of culture. I don't think we knew exactly what the word meant; there wasn´t a lot of books or there wasn't any discussions about art. Matter of fact we were all highly suspicious of black-and-white movies at the time . . . When I was twenty-six, a close friend of mine showed me John Ford's *Grapes of Wrath*, and it was a picture that resonated throughout the whole rest of my life and I keep going back to it. I remember when I saw it, I remember thinking that night, "Yeah, that´s what I wanna do." It´s a lovely film, and there's this scene towards the end—it was always my favorite part—where Tom Joad has killed a security guard who killed his friend and he's gonna have to leave his family and they've traveled so far and they've suffered so much and he knows his mother has lost so much and that now she's gonna have to lose her son . . . And it's set up first by this dance scene, which Ford does in a lot of his pictures, but this scene is particularly lovely because it's in the midst of a lot of suffering: there's this scene of community that holds out the possibility of beauty in the world, which is something, I think, we all chase after 'cause in beauty there's hope and in hope there's some type of divine love . . . And this scene is very beautiful, and at the end of it, Tom—the dance is over—goes into the tent where his mother is sleeping in this camp and he touches her very gently and he says, "Ma, I have to go, I have to go now," and she gets up and they step outside under these dark trees and they sit and now she says, "Tommy, I knew this day was gonna come, but how am I gonna know where you are? How am I gonna know if you're alive?" And he says, "Well, Ma, all I know is I gotta go out and I gotta scratch around and I gotta see what's wrong and then I gotta see if there's some way that I can make it right," and he says, "You'll know how I am because I'll be in the dark all around you at night when you lie sleeping, I'll be in guys' voices when they're yelling 'cause they're mad, and I'll be in children's voices when they're coming

in at night for their supper and they know that there's food on the table and that they're gonna be safe, because maybe they got it wrong and maybe we're not all individual souls, maybe we're just some small, small piece of some big soul," and he disappears, he disappears into the darkness, and the next scene is the Joads heading north to look for more work and the father says, "You know, Ma, Tommy's gone, what are we gonna do ?" and she says, "Well, we're just gonna keep on going."

In 1997, Springsteen received a signed copy of *The Grapes of Wrath* from Steinbeck's widow.

"The song was religious in nature," Springsteen explained, "in the sense that it was about going someplace where love exists: a place where you can live and feel good, and where you can have a chance at making something and building something for yourself."[128]

On January 22, "Across the Border" was played in its full-band album arrangement at Sony Music Studios in New York City during the taping for the *Where It's At: The Rolling Stone State of the Union* documentary, celebrating *Rolling Stone* magazine's thirtieth anniversary. Springsteen was backed by musicians from the *Ghost of Tom Joad* album sessions: Danny Federici on accordion, Jim Hanson on bass, Marty Rifkin on pedal steel guitar, and Gary Mallaber on drums. *Where It's At: The Rolling Stone State of the Union* premiered on ABC on May 21,1998, and was later aired on MTV and VH-1.

Matamoros Banks

©2005 Bruce Springsteen (GMR)

Released on *Devils & Dust* album (2005)

Live premiere: 04/21/2005—Paramount Theatre, Asbury Park, NJ

Introducing the song at a show in Akron, Ohio, on September 25, 1996, Springsteen said, "I was at the end of the *Tom Joad* record and I needed a few songs and I think I wrote 'Across the Border,' and I had that down at the end of the record. I played it through and listened to it, and I said, 'Yeah, that's good—but that's the dream. That's the *that thing* that keeps people moving along for some reason. I felt like I needed something else, something that wasn't so much of a dream."

"Matamoros Banks," recorded by Springsteen solo in 1997 (strings by the Nashville String Machine were recorded in 2004 then added onto the core recording), is actually a sequel to "Across the Border," "a good reminder that the narrator of 'Across the Border' never actually makes the trip in that song."[129]

In the *Devils & Dust* booklet, the lyrics of the songs are preceded by a brief introduction: "Each year many die crossing the deserts, mountains, and rivers of our southern border in search of a better life. Here I follow the journey backwards, from the body at the river bottom, to the man walking across the desert towards the banks of the Rio Grande."

"I wrote this song backwards," he explained during a show at East Rutherford, New York, on May 19, 2005. "First verse: body at the bottom of the river; second verse: walks across the desert; third verse: comes to the banks of the Matamoros side." (The chronological order of the verses, rather than 3-2-1, is actually 3-1-2.)

[i] Matamoros is a small Mexican town on the Rio Bravo (which is called the Rio Grande in America), a river originating in Colorado's Rocky Mountains that crosses New Mexico, marking the border between Texas and the Mexican states of Chiuaua, Coahuila, and Tamaulipas, and after 3,000 miles flows into the Gulf of Mexico. Its course divides twin cities such as El Paso, Texas, and Ciudad Juarez (Chiuaua), then Laredo and Nuevo Laredo, and finally Brownsville and Matamoros, by which point the river becomes nothing but a muddy stream. Here hundreds of thousands of Mexicans come with the hope of finding work: Nuevo Laredo has become a slum where more than three hundred thousand Mexicans live. To avoid dying of hunger, there is often only one solution: bust the American border, work for six months or a year in Texas, accepting any condition, to then come back and build a brick house for one's wife and children.

Jesus Was an Only Son
©2005 Bruce Springsteen (GMR)

Released on *Devils & Dust* album (2005) | *VH1 Storytellers: Bruce Springsteen* home video (2005) recorded live at Two River Theater, Red Bank, NJ, April 4, 2005

Live premiere: 04/04/2005—Two River Theater, Red Bank, NJ

"I was raised Catholic," Bruce said talking about this song, "so Jesus was my de facto homeboy."[130] In an interview with the *New York Times* he added, "Catholic school, Catholic school, Catholic school. You're indoctrinated. It's a none-too-subtle form of brainwashing, and of course, it works very well. I'm not a churchgoer, but I realized, as time passed, that my music is filled with Catholic imagery."[131]

[i] "The soul of the universe" is an image that is very distant from the Christian message: in the Bible (to which the lyrics make reference) not the slightest connection is made. In fact, the source would seem to be, once again, Steinbeck's *The Grapes*

of Wrath, as Tom Joad bids goodbye to Ma Joad in Chapter 28, relating to her a bit of Jim Casy's wisdom: "Says one time he went out in the wilderness to find his own soul, an' he foun' he didn't have no soul that was his'n. Says he foun' he jus' got a little piece of a great big soul. Says a wilderness ain't no good, 'cause his little piece of a soul wasn't no good 'less it was with the rest, an' was whole."[132]

The Last Lone American Night

When on September 11, 2001, two airplanes went smashing into the Twin Towers, *Time* wrote that America needed to feel Springsteen's presence. Some time later, the *New York Times* confirmed: "Most pop stars seemed irrelevant immediately after Sept. 11. Mr. Springsteen, who has spent most of his career singing about American dreams and disappointments, did not."[133] Nine months had passed since the Al Qaeda attacks on the World Trade Center and the Pentagon, and Springsteen—as he stated himself— felt obliged to give something to the people who had been hit by that tragedy, and in particular to the families of the 158 members of the Monmouth County community— the New Jersey County where he was born and lives—who had lost their lives in the Twin Towers. It seems that he got the inspiration for an album inspired by that new Pearl Harbor when, as Bruce left a Sea Bright parking lot a few days after the attack, a man drove by and shouted out the window, "We need you—*now!*"[134]

Scott Calef noted that "*The Rising* helped us collectively make sense of the numbingly unfathomable events of that day by reducing them to a personal scale," and as a healing album, it "helped us to understand, gave us hope that we as a people could again 'rise up.' It helped us to look forward and not just back and showed us something important about ourselves and each other."[135]

Christopher Phillips wrote, "*For all the poets down here that don't write nothin' at all*, Bruce Springsteen took a look around his neighborhood, picked up a pen and a guitar, and went to work. In the blink of an eye and in the midst of a world crisis, he completed his first album of new material since 1995, and in doing so reaffirmed the possibilities of modern rock."[136]

At the dawn of the twenty-first century, man suddenly found himself contemplating the idea that Armageddon was not so far off. Using multiple viewpoints— widows, widowers, victims, perpetrators, first responders—in songs such "Nothing Man," "You're Missing," "The Rising," and "My City of Ruins," Springsteen synthesized the emotions underlying his characters to paint a broad picture of this frightened and fragile world.

Five years later, with *Magic* Springsteen expressed disillusionment with the state of American society and pointed his finger up directly towards the White House and its fortieth tenant, George W. Bush. "Radio Nowhere" sounds like a post-apocalyptic cry, like "Hunter of Invisible Game," a song written that same period: "There were empty cities and burning plains, / . . . Down into the valley where the beast has his throne." "Magic" is a bluffing portrait of how politics seem to have become like a new form of magic ("It's a song I wrote about how we live sort of in this Orwellian moment when what's true can be made to seem like a lie and what's a lie can be made to seem true," he said);[137] "Devil's Arcade"—which in this section is put together, in coherence with its themes, with "Devils and Dust"—expresses beyond the shadow of a doubt Springsteen's position on Bush's administration and American foreign policy, and especially his attitude towards their intervention in Iraq. "Devils & Dust" shows an American soldier with his finger on the trigger: he was sent to a foreign land to fight a war not belonging to him—as many times before. "Devil's Arcade" exposes the wounds that soldier takes home with him. "The Wall"—a song written in 1998 and published only in 2014 on the album *High Hopes*—is the touching memory of a longtime friend of Springsteen's who doesn't ever get home from war (in Vietnam) again.

Introducing "Livin' in the Future"—another song from *Magic*—at the Brendan Byrne Arena in East Rutherford, New Jersey, on October 9, 2007, Springsteen said that, despite its title, the song was "about what's happening now, about how along with all the things we love about America—cheeseburgers, Max's Hot Dogs at the Jersey Shore, the Bill of Rights, Clarence 'Big Man' Clemons—we've had to add to the American picture rendition, illegal wiretapping, no right to habeas corpus, rolling back of our civil liberties, attacks on the Constitution . . . These are things that aren't just un-American, they're anti-American."

The epic nature of Springsteen's first albums has become the cold, hard history of an unrecognizable country. Only the antiheroes in "Outlaw Pete" and "The Wrestler" are there to move us: survivors of a past that has become a burden, in search of (the final) refuge in which to stop and remove themselves from a future that doesn't belong to them.

The Rising
©2002 Bruce Springsteen (GMR)

Released on *The Rising* album (2002) | "Lonesome Day" single (2002) recorded live at Hayden Planetarium, New York, NY | *Live in Barcelona* home video (2003) recorded live at Palau Sant Jordi, Barcelona, October 16, 2002 | *London Calling: Live in Hyde Park* home video (2010) recorded live at Hyde Park, London, June 28, 2009

Live premiere: 07/25/2002—Convention Hall, Asbury Park, NJ

Following the tragic events of September 11, 2001, Springsteen wrote a number of new songs that were influenced by the disaster. A new series of studio sessions with the E Street Band took place in Atlanta from late January to mid-March 2002. It is known that a total of seventeen songs were recorded during the sessions—fifteen on the album plus "Harry's Place" and "Down in the Hole," both of which would eventually be issued on 2014's *High Hopes*.

The title track—an anthemic song told from the perspective of a rescue worker—was one of the last songs written for the album. "I was tryin' to describe the most powerful images on the 11th," Springsteen said. "People coming down [inside the World Trade Center] talked about the emergency workers ascending. I felt left with that image at the end of the day—those guys were going up the stairs, they could be ascending a smoky staircase or they could be in the afterlife."[138]

"The Rising" is, "in a word, cathartic; it is a salve to tortured souls in a troubled world."[139]

[i] Springsteen considers "The Rising" a bookend to "Into the Fire," the other firefighter song on *The Rising*:

> The sky was falling and streaked with blood.
> I heard you calling me, then you disappeared into the dust,
> Up the stairs, into the fire,
> Up the stairs, into the fire.
> I need your kiss, but love and duty called you someplace higher,
> Somewhere up the stairs into the fire.

[ii] "The 'sixty-pound stone' Bruce refers to is an air cylinder and harness that is part of a self-contained breathing apparatus (SCBA)."[140]

[iii] Springsteen is referring to the hose usually carried into a building on the firefighters' shoulders in a line.

[iv] Springsteen is referring to the international insignia of the fire service, the Cross Pattee-Nowy.

[v] "That was a funny line—the catfish line popped out of my head, 'cause I fish out here once in a while and there's that moment when *bing*! y'know, you're suspended between life and death, incredible life and a moment of death."[141]

You're Missing

©2002 Bruce Springsteen (GMR)

Released on *The Rising* album (2002)

Live premiere: 07/25/2002—Convention Hall, Asbury Park, NJ

"You're Missing" was written, along with "Into the Fire," between September 11 and the September 21 telethon in which Springsteen participated. According to

Rolling Stone, it was "built around a melody Springsteen worked up one night while messing around on the piano with Patti and the kids."[142]

When producer Brendan O'Brien met Springsteen in New Jersey, a demo for this song became their first collaboration. "'At one point,' Springsteen recalls, 'Brendan said, "Well, I think we should find another chord for this spot." I said, "Find another chord?! Wait a minute, now! Hold on, hold on!"' He laughs. "'Those are the chords!" But then I'm thinking that my job now as the producee, is to say yes. So I said OK, we changed it, and it sounded good. Once I got comfortable with that, it was like, "Go, man, go." By the end of the day, we had a real nice demo.'"[143]

[i] The verse seems to be refashioned from another Springsteen song with a very similar title, "Missing," used in the 1995 Sean Penn film *The Crossing Guard*.

[ii] The use of tautology (everything is everything, morning is morning) is characteristic of the whole album's style, in which issues seems to revolve around themselves through the use of many repetitions ("an eye for an eye," "the blood of my blood" in "Empty Sky," "may your strength give us strength, may your love brings us love" in "Into the Fire," "let's let love give what it gives" in "Words Apart") and of pleonasms ("a tear from your eye" in "Waitin' on a Sunny Day" and "a kiss from your lips" in Empty Sky").

[iii] The line evokes the anthrax scare of late 2001.

Nothing Man

©2002 Bruce Springsteen (GMR)

Released on *The Rising* album (2002)

Live premiere: 09/30/2003—Xcel Energy Center, St. Paul, MN

"Nothing Man" was the oldest song on *The Rising*. Springsteen penned it in 1994: it "had been born of the same feeling of isolation that had yielded 'Streets of Philadelphia' and 'Missing,' could with a little retooling be turned into a song about a first responder with post-traumatic stress disorder."[144]

Who's this "nothing man"? Dave Marsh wrote that the song "portrays the disintegration of a former hero—he might be a firefighter who survived the towers' collapse, he might be a Vietnam vet, he might be one of Timothy McVeigh's comrades from the Gulf War . . ."[145] Springsteen said,

> You'd think it was written along with the new songs I had written . . . I think it was originally written as a soldier's song when I wrote it many, many years ago. It was someone who survived a very catastrophic and transforming

experience, returning home and going back to his family and his neighborhood, where others haven't had that experience. It was that one line, "the sky's still the same unbelievable blue." Well, how can that be? How can things remain unchanged, because I've changed so much?[146]

[i] The song shares its title with *The Nothing Man*, a novel written by Jim Thompson, whom Springsteen admires a lot.

[ii] The pink vapor that changed the character's life is a detail that—assuming Springsteen retouched the original lyrics from 1994—could have been taken from a front-page *Wall Street Journal* article by John Bussey, published the day after 9/11, where the author described bodies falling from the World Trade Center: "After the 80-floor drop, the impact left small puffs of pink and red vapor drifting at ground level."[147]

[iii] "Pearl and silver" is clearly a gun. Taking the subject of the song as a guy with post-traumatic stress syndrome and/or survivor's guilt so bad that he contemplates suicide, it is not clear if the "nothing man" prays to be able to pull the trigger or to have the strength to keep from doing it. Christpher Phillips believes that the narrator is "on a path that can lead from isolation to self-destruction. But he asks for understanding, and prays for strength."[148]

My City of Ruins
©2001 Bruce Springsteen (GMR)

Released on *America: A Tribute to Heroes* album (2001) recorded live at Sony Music Studios, New York, NY, September 21, 2001 | *The Rising* album (2002) | *Live in Barcelona* home video (2003) recorded live at Palau Sant Jordi, Barcelona, October 16, 2002

Live premiere: 12/17/2000—Convention Hall, Asbury Park, NJ

"My City of Ruins" was written by Springsteen in November 2000 and premiered live on December 17, 2000, at a benefit gig in Asbury Park. It was a cry of pain that well described the current state of Asbury Park—its deterioration and the absence of people in the area.

The song took on a new meaning soon after the 9/11 attacks, when Springsteen played it on September 21, 2001, during the *America: A Tribute to Heroes* telethon: with only a guitar and a harmonica, Springsteen opened the program, introducing the number as "a prayer for our fallen brothers and sisters" and modifying a few phrases in the song, while he was joined on stage by Patti Scialfa, Steve Van Zandt, Soozie Tyrell, Clarence Clemons, Lisa Lowell, Dee Holmes, and Layonne Holmes on backing vocals.[149] This live recording was included as the first track on the subsequent album released of the telethon performances.

"It's a gospel song," Springsteen said. "It's like a lot of my things, like 'The Promised Land' or 'Land of Hopes and Dreams'... they're fundamentally gospel-rooted, or blues-and-gospel-rooted. It seemed like that element was going to be a significant element of the record in some fashion."[150]

Radio Nowhere
©2007 Bruce Springsteen (GMR)

Released on *Magic* album (2007) | *London Calling: Live in Hyde Park* home video (2010) recorded live at Hyde Park, London, June 28, 2009

Live premiere: 09/24/2007—Convention Hall, Asbury Park, NJ

In December 2006 producer Brendan O'Brien visited Springsteen at Bruce's Colts Neck, New Jersey, home to listen to a large batch of songs Bruce had written over what is likely to have been several years. From this meeting a subgroup of songs were preselected as being most suitable for an E Street Band–style album. Studio sessions began in Atlanta in February 2007, initially with just Springsteen and O'Brien. E Street Band members started to become involved in late February and finished recordings by early May. The *Magic* album was ready, and "Radio Nowhere" was chosen as its first single. O'Brien told *Rolling Stone* that the version of the song recorded for *Magic* was barely changed from the version Springsteen had played him at his house the previous year. "It's a pretty straight-ahead rocker," O'Brien described it. "The most straightforward song I've heard him do in years."[151]

"It's an end-of-the-world scenario—he's seeing the apocalypse," Springsteen explained. "All communications are down. That's my business, that's what it's all about—trying to connect to you. It comes down to trying to make people happy, feel less lonely, but also being a conduit for a dialogue about the events of the day, the issues that impact people's lives, personal and social and political and religious."[152]

"Radio Nowhere" was released as a free limited-timespan digital single on August 28, 2007. It was awarded Best Solo Rock Vocal Performance and Best Rock Song at the Grammy Awards of 2008. At the MTV Europe Music Awards 2007 in Munich, Germany, when asked by Foo Fighters frontman Dave Grohl which song he wished he had written, R.E.M.'s Michael Stipe cited "Radio Nowhere."

[i] This line has been a staple exhortation of Springsteen live shows. He has been yelling it out for years—notably during the 1999–2000 E Street Reunion

Tour—as the show enters its final stretch and he wants to rally the crowd one more time. It is also arguably the central question running through his entire body of work, reflecting the primal importance that he gives to the connective power of rock 'n' roll.

[ii] A reference to Elvis Presley's "Mystery Train."

Hunter of Invisible Game
©2014 Bruce Springsteen (GMR)

Released on *High Hopes* album (2014)

Live premiere: 02/12/2014—Entertaiment Center, Adelaide, Australia

This acoustic waltz finds Springsteen singing about a hunter traveling through a wasteland. In a March 2014 interview for *Rolling Stone*, Springsteen told Sean Sennett,

> I wrote [the title] down years ago, and I don't remember a lot about it except I said, "That's a nice title." I wrote it down and it sat there. Then I did more reading of other things. And I started to get into this sort of post-apocalyptic idea. The idea of these travelers in the wasteland, and what's the guy trying to do? He's trying to hold onto their humanness, their humanity in all of this ruin. That was the idea. That's who this guy is, the guy who is hunting out remnants of what makes the spirit. It was one of those songs that came together a certain way and I didn't think much about it when I wrote it. I put it away. Now it's probably one of my favorite things on the record.[153]

The record is *High Hopes*, published in 2014. The song was recorded between 2004 and 2008 with producer Brendan O'Brien (but with a later overdub of Tom Morello's guitar). *High Hopes* producer Ron Aniello told *Rolling Stone* that the editing Springsteen and he did on the song "was very light." He added: "With respect to Brendan, that's his production, and I didn't want to meddle too much. We touched it up and Bruce might have changed a lyric or two. I actually can't remember, but for the most part those were [sic] the Brendan O'Brien stuff."[154]

To my ears, "Hunter of Invisible Game" together with "Radio Nowhere" and "Last to Die" was inspired by the reading of the 2006 Cormac McCarthy's post-apocalyptic novel *The Road*—the tale of a journey taken by a father and his young son across a landscape blasted by an unspecified cataclysm that has destroyed most of civilization and, in the intervening years, almost all life on Earth. Springsteen had definitely read and liked the novel, which was awarded the Pulitzer Prize for fiction. Interviewed by the *New York Times* about his literary tastes, in 2014

Springsteen listed Philip Roth, Cormac McCarthy, and Richard Ford as his current favorites, adding that Cormac McCarthy's *Blood Meridian* remained a watermark in his reading, and revealing that the last book that had made him cry was Cormac McCarthy's *The Road*.[155]

Springsteen codirected a ten-minute film based on the song title with his long-time video collaborator, Thom Zimny.

Magic

©2007 Bruce Springsteen (GMR)

Released on *Magic* album (2007)

Live premiere: 09/25/2007—Convention Hall, Asbury Park, NJ

Springsteen explained, "The song 'Magic' is about living in a time when anything that is true can be made to seem like a lie, and anything that is a lie can be made to seem true. There are people that have taken that as their credo. The classic quote was from one of the Bushies in the *New York Times*: 'We make our own reality. You guys report it, we make it.' I may loathe that statement—the unbelievable stupidity and arrogance of it—more than I loathe 'Bring it on' and 'Mission accomplished.' That song, it's all about illusion. That's the heart of my record right there."[156]

Introducing the song during a concert held in Washington, D.C. on November 11, 2007, Springsteen said, "This is the title song from our smash LP. It's about living through a time when the truth gets twisted into lies and lies get twisted into the truth and the wheel of history spins round and round. So, hey, this is where it happens! We are here in the city of magic . . . but it's not really about magic, this song, it's really about tricks . . ."

Devils & Dust

©2005 Bruce Springsteen (GMR)

Released on *Devils & Dust* album (2005) | *VH1 Storytellers: Bruce Springsteen* home video (2005) recorded live at Two River Theater, Red Bank, NJ, April 4, 2005

Live premiere: 09/25/2007—Convention Hall, Asbury Park, NJ

"Devils & Dust" is the only song on Springsteen's 2005 album of the same title positively verified to have been composed after 2001. It was played for the first time on April 11, 2003, during a soundcheck at the Pacific Coliseum in Vancouver, Canada, on the Rising Tour. The song was played in a country-style, full-band arrangement and featured many different lyrics from the album version; but it was not played on the regular show.

"Devils & Dust" was used as the 2005 album's overture: "It works as a metaphor for all the music underneath it," Springsteen said, "the individual stories of people wrestling with their own demons."[157]

The particular demon of the song's character is war. "Devils & Dust," as Springsteen explained, "is basically a song about a soldier's point of view in Iraq."[158] In fact, the song was written in reaction to the "Enduring Freedom" mission, wherein 160,000 troops were sent into Iraq on March 2003 in order "to disarm Iraq of weapons of mass destruction, to end Saddam Hussein's support for terrorism, and to free Iraqi people," according to U.S. President George W. Bush and UK Prime Minister Tony Blair.

Springsteen had already written about a soldier in Iraq in "Souls of the Departed," a song included on his 1992 *Lucky Town* album that referenced the first Gulf War:

> On the road to Basra stood young Lieutenant Jimmy Bly
> Detailed to go through the clothes of the soldiers who died.
> At night in dreams he sees their souls rise
> Like dark geese into the Oklahoma skies.

On May 10, 2004, Springsteen sang it in a duet with Neil Young at the Xcel Energy Center in St. Paul, during the Vote for Change Tour in support of John Kerry's presidential election campaign, publicly reinforcing his position regarding American military intervention in Iraq.

"I don't try to get real polemical about it or anything," Springsteen said. "That seems the wrong way to go about it. I just try to present the human issues and what we're risking. That's my interest when I go to write something like 'Devils & Dust.'"[159]

[i] Bobbie is Bob Dylan, as some other allusion in the song seem to confirm. The first version of the song—the one played at the soundcheck in Vancouver in 2003—had "We're a long, long way from home, baby."

[ii] Springsteen alludes to Dylan's "Blowin' in the Wind," from the *Freewheelin' Bob Dylan* album of 1963.

[iii] Springsteen alludes to Dylan's "With God on Our Side," an antiwar song from 1964's *The Times They Are A-Changin'* that ends, "If God's on our side, he'll stop the next war." Like Dylan's song, Springsteen's touches upon the irony of the idea of having God on one's side, particularly as a justification for violence and war.

Devil's Arcade

©2007 Bruce Springsteen (GMR)

Released on *Magic* album (2007)

Live premiere: 09/24/2007—Convention Hall, Asbury Park, NJ

The story in "Devil's Arcade" is about an Iraq war casualty. It can be seen as a sequel to the story in "Devils & Dust." The song has puzzled people over what Springsteen is actually singing about. There are few doubts that it looks at how an injured soldier, coming back from a war, deals with the more intimate aspects of home life. He has maybe lost the use of his limbs, he has been dug up from the sand and after a spell in hospital has been sent home.

The first verse is written from the point of view of the soldier's girlfriend after he has returned injured from Iraq (talking specifically about them making love again; there is no other way to interpret "The lost smell on your breath as I helped you get it in"). The second verse is about the soldier's description of his time at war and then in a military hospital. The final verse is about the life after war for a damaged soldier and his girlfriend trying to resume their love, but the experiences of the soldier casts a long shadow.

Some of the most upsetting images from this war are the ones of soldiers returning home. "Devil's Arcade" provides a glimpse into a world rarely shown in the media, and the images are tough.

[i] *Home of the Brave* is the title of a film directed by Irwin Winkler (2006) about four American soldiers in Iraq.

The Wall

©2014 Bruce Springsteen (GMR)

Released on *High Hopes* album (2014)

Live premiere: 02/19/2003—Somerville Theatre, Somerville, MA

"The Wall" was written between December 1997 and January 1998. The lyrics were written by Springsteen after he and Patti Scialfa visited the Vietnam Veterans Memorial in Washington on December 7, 1997. They were in the capital city to attend the Kennedy Center Honors ceremony, and while there they went to see the Memorial. "So we went," Springsteen recalls, "and we're there in the day and I found Walter [Cichon]'s name. I'm not sure if I found Bart Haynes. Bart Haynes was the drummer in the Castiles and he was our first friend that was killed overseas, and then Walter."[160]

Walter Cichon was the lead singer of the Motifs, a mid-1960s British Invasion–inspired New Jersey shore band that eventually released a single, "Molly," in 1965, becoming a major inspiration to other kids forming bands during that period. Sadly, Walter Cichon, the Motifs' dynamic lead singer, was drafted in 1967 and killed in Vietnam on March 30, 1968. He was twenty-two.

"The Wall" premiered live at the Somerville Theatre in Somerville, Massachusetts, on February 19, 2003. And it was played twice during 2005's Devils & Dust Tour Solo and Acoustic Tour. Recording sessions for *High Hopes* date from the late '90s (perhaps from sessions for *Tracks*) with the E Street Band, including Danny Federici. In 2014, producer Ron Aniello added his parts on synths and accordion and Curt Ramm's cornet. Springsteen wrote about the song in the liner notes:

> "The Wall" is something I'd played on stage a few times and remains very close to my heart. The title and idea were Joe Grushecky's; then the song appeared after Patti and I made a visit to the Vietnam Veterans Memorial in Washington. It was inspired by my memories of Walter Cichon. Walter was one of the great early Jersey Shore rockers, who along with his brother Ray (one of my early guitar mentors) led the Motifs. The Motifs were a local rock band who were always a head above everybody else. Raw, sexy, and rebellious, they were the heroes you aspired to be. But these were heroes you could touch, speak to, and go to with your musical inquiries. Cool, but always accessible, they were an inspiration to me, and many young working musicians in 1960s central New Jersey. Though my character in "The Wall" is a Marine, Walter was actually in the Army, A Company, Third Battalion, Eighth Infantry. He was the first person I ever stood in the presence of who was filled with the mystique of the true rock star. Walter went missing in action in Vietnam in March 1968. He still performs somewhat regularly in my mind, the way he stood, dressed, held the tambourine, the casual cool, the freeness. The man who by his attitude, his walk, said, "You can defy all this, all of what's here, all of what you've been taught, taught to fear, to love, and you'll still be all right." His was a terrible loss to us, his loved ones and the local music scene. I still miss him.

[i] Springsteen refers to the black stone used to make Washington, D.C.'s Memorial Wall.

[ii] Bruce Springsteen and Patti Scialfa were sitting not far from Robert McNamara at the 1997 Kennedy Center Honors ceremony. "There was this unusual experience that night of sitting a few tables away from Robert McNamara," Springsteen later said. McNamara, name-checked in the song, was the U.S. Secretary

of Defense from 1961 to 1968, during which time he played a large role in escalating the United States involvement in the Vietnam War.

Outlaw Pete

©2009 Bruce Springsteen (GMR)

Released on *Working on a Dream* album (2009)

Live premiere: 03/23/2009—Convention Hall, Asbury Park, NJ

Springsteen told me that "Outlaw Pete" was "a little homage" to Ennio Morricone (not so little: the song last more than eight minutes). "I had a cowboy song and I said, 'I got to dress this up with a little bit of Ennio Morricone's style.' Ennio is one of the greatest composers for film in the world."

The song is about a bank-robbing baby whose exploits become a meditation on sin, fate, and free will. According to Springsteen, it's "essentially the story of a man trying to outlive and outlast his sins."[161] He explained about this fable concerning a character who can't escape his past:

> The past is never the past. It is always present. And you better reckon with it in your life and in your daily experience, or it will get you. It will get you really bad. It will come and it will devour you, it will remove you from the present. It will steal your future and this happens every day . . . So the song is about this happening to this character. He moves ahead. He tries to make the right moves. He awakes from a vision of his death, and realizes: life is finite. Time is with me always. And I'm frightened. And he rides west, where he settles down. But the past comes back in the form of this bounty hunter, whose mind is also quickened and burdened by the need to get his man. And these possessed creatures meet along the shores of this river where the bounty hunter of course is killed, and his last words are: "We can't undo the things we've done." In other words, your past is your past. You carry it with you always. These are your sins. You carry them with you always. You better learn how to live with them, learn the story that they're telling you. Because they're whispering your future in your ear, and if you don't listen, it will be contaminated by the toxicity of your past.[162]

The song was adapted into a book by Springsteen and illustrator Frank Caruso and published on November 4, 2014. Memories of the 1950 children's book *Brave Cowboy Bill*, which Springsteen's mother read to him as a child, inspired the tale of a cowboy who "cut his trail of tears across the countryside." "Like Tom Sawyer, Huck Finn, Dorothy Gale, and for me, even Popeye, Outlaw Pete cuts deep into the folklore of our country," says Caruso, "and weaves its way into the fabric of great American literary characters."[163]

The Wrestler

©2008 Bruce Springsteen (GMR)

Released on *Working on a Dream* album (2009)

Live premiere: 03/23/2009—Convention Hall, Asbury Park, NJ

"The Wrestler" was written by Springsteen as the title song of the Darren Aronofsky film starring Mickey Rourke. The actor says that Springsteen penned the song after he had written a letter to him. Said Rourke, "The only reason I wrote Bruce Springsteen a letter was because after about six days, I knew something magical was happening on the movie. [. . .] I told him, 'We have no money, but we did it in New Jersey.'" Springsteen called Rourke some time later after reading the script and told him, "I wrote you a little something." The actor told that after he first heard the song, "I had to listen to it like 100 times. He really got it . . . The song sums up the whole character. He did me such an honor and such a favor."[164]

Springsteen recalls having written the song while he was touring Europe. He said that he was grounding the song from his own experience, referring to someone who is no longer able to live a normal life and is unable "to stand the things that nurture you. Because much of our life is spent running. We're running, we're on the run; one of my specialties."[165]

The song was cut just in time to be added on the closing titles of *The Wrestler* for its premiere in August 2008 at the 65th Venice International Film Festival. In December 2008 it received a nomination for the Golden Globe Award for Best Original Song and won the award during the 66th Golden Globe Awards on January 11, 2009.

In January 2009, "The Wrestler" was added as a bonus track on Springsteen's *Working on a Dream* album.

[i] A "one-trick pony" is one that is skilled in only one area, or one that has success only once. *One-Trick Pony* is also a 1980 film written by and starring Paul Simon, who plays Jonah Levin, a once-popular folk-rock musician who hasn't had a hit in ten years and now opens for other bands, trying to record a new album but facing an indifferent record-company executive who's pressuring him to create a hit record with the help of a trendy producer (Lou Reed).

[ii] Darren Aronofsky—who directed *The Wrestler*—was so confused about the "one-legged dog" line that he confronted Springsteen about the idea. He says,

"When we made *The Wrestler* I got to hang out a little bit with him and there's that line in the song . . . When we were mixing the song Bruce wasn't around and we were like, 'What the hell's a one-legged dog walking down the street?' I could picture a three-legged dog or two-legged dog. So the night he won a Golden Globe for the song, I had a couple of drinks in me and I was sitting next to him and I was like, 'With all humility and honor to who you are, what the hell is a one-legged dog walkin' down the street?' He said, 'Art often comes out of the mistakes and that's when the poetry comes alive and you have to welcome them.'"[166]

We Are Alive

In 2012, Springsteen released his seventeenth studio album, *Wrecking Ball*—his "angriest yet," as the *Hollywood Reporter* called it.[167]

From a musical point of view, the album is very rock 'n' roll, but with unexpected textures—loops, electronic percussion, an amazing sweep of influences and rhythms, from hip-hop to Irish folk rhythms, with touches of gospel and jazz. Upon listening to the first song, "We Take Care of Our Own," one can come to think one is dealing with the ideal successor of *Magic* and *Working on a Dream*; however, the four following songs take us in the vicinity of *We Shall Overcome: The Seeger Sessions*. For his indictment of Wall Street greed and corruption and the devastation it has wrought, Springsteen chooses the sepia-colored approach, in this way creating an ideal—and distressing—link between 2012 and 1929. He explained,

> I use a lot of folk music. There's some Civil War music. There's gospel music. There are '30s horns in "Jack of all Trades." That's the way I used the music—the idea was that the music was going to contextualize historically that this has happened before: it happened in the 1970s, it happened in the '30s, it happened in the 1800s . . . it's cyclical.[168]

"Easy Money," a country-folk song with bluegrass tones, brings us back to the age of the Dust Bowls of the thirties and of Woody Guthrie's *Dust Bowl Ballads*: crucial songs (adored by Springsteen) like "I Ain't Got No Home," "Vigilante Man," "Tom Joad," and "Refugee." With "Jack of All Trades" the scene does not change: on the notes of a slow, quaint waltz reminding us of "Unchained Melody," Springsteen tells the story of the "ordinary man," making his way in times of recession, as is perfectly evoked by the wind instruments' interlude in funeral marching band style. Here is a "jack of all trades, master of none"—as the proverb goes—whose work misadventures resemble the ones lived by Springsteen's father. And yet this man never gives up and continues to believe that everything will be all right. In him we sense no resignation; perhaps there is anger, a loud kind of anger that comes across in the verse "If I had me a gun, I'd find the bastards and shoot 'em on sight." Who are the bastards? The answer comes easily: they are the "fat cats," the rich people against whom the protagonist of "Easy Money" throws himself in anger, who really has nothing better to do than to retrace, after a fashion, in small scale the criminal element; the money speculators are up there having fun on Banker's Hill in "Shackled and Drawn" while the poor people are dragged along in chains; they are the money changers Jesus chases out of the temple, as Springsteen recalls in "Rocky Ground."

Hence, the enemy—in '29 and still today—are the Wall Street sharks. They are the predators who in "Death to My Hometown" raided the city at night, spreading death everywhere. The same enemies galvanized Occupy Wall Street, the peaceful protest movement that in those days fought against economic and social disparity. "Occupy Wall Street changed the national conversation,"[169] Springsteen said.

"In the U.S.A. there's a populist anti-capitalism available, a tradition of the artist as the common man (rarely woman), pitching rural truth against urban deceit, pioneer values against bureaucratic routines. This tradition (Mark Twain to Woody Guthrie, Kerouac to Creedence Clearwater Revival) lies behind Springsteen's message and his image."[170] Taking stock of reality, Springsteen—as he has done so many times in the past—tries to explore the shadows, the dark side of the country's collective subconscious. Yet this makes up only the first part of his album. He himself clarifies that the second focal point on the record is the search for something that keeps us going forward: what he defines as a "new day."

"Rocky Ground" is perhaps the most surprising song on the album, mainly due to its rap interlude sung by Michele Moore and to the sampling of old extracts recorded in Mississippi by Alan Lomax. It sounds like a postmodern gospel song in which dawn is proclaimed after a new great flood, borrowing from the Old Testament (with more or less faithful quotations from Isaiah and the books of Genesis and Exodus) and the Gospel according to Mark. Once again, Springsteen displays a tendency towards the ideal of the Promised Land, the new land of milk and honey in which the American Dream can come true. Yet, contrarily to what actually happened, for instance in "Thunder Road" and "Born to Run," where the Promised Land was a tangible dream (and it all boiled down to the escape of a boy and his "belle" from the hard American suburb), now one looks towards the Land of Canaan as both a trip inside oneself and a transcendental passage, as "Land of Hope and Dreams" confirms, inclusive of the final quote in "People Get Ready" by Curtis Mayfield: the train that requires no ticket and will take us all— saints and sinners—to "fields covered in light" is a decidedly evident allegory to the celestial world (indeed the piece is dedicated to Clarence Clemons, whose saxophone is here heard for the last time).

"We Are Alive" closes the album: a *Spoon River Anthology* mariachi style lasting six minutes (with a trumpet riff borrowed from Johnny Cash's "Ring of Fire"), where from the cold tombstones aglow in the moonlight, the voices of those who died for freedom can be heard—strikers, Ku Klux Klan victims, illegal immigrants— which takes us to the ultimate message, the revelation: their souls rise up "To carry the fire and light the spark, / To fight shoulder to shoulder and heart to heart." Herein lies the essense of Springsteenian faith: despite the humiliation and violence suffered, his characters never lose the strength to seek a new beginning, eternally, without ever feeling defeated; just as Ma Joad said in *The Grapes of Wrath*: "We keep a-comin'. We're the people that live. They can't lick us. We'll go on forever, Pa, 'cause we're the people.'"[171]

We Take Care of Our Own

©2012 Bruce Springsteen (GMR)

Released on *Wrecking Ball* album (2012)

Live premiere: 02/12/2012—Staples Center, Los Angeles, CA

"We Take Care of Our Own" is the first song written for *Wrecking Ball*—around 2009 or 2010—and the first single from the album, released digitally on January 19, 2012.

Springsteen said, "'We Take Care of Our Own,' it asks the question that the rest of [*Wrecking Ball* does]. Which is, of course: Do we? Do we take care of our own? And we often don't. We don't provide an equal playing field for our citizens. And at the same time, [the song] doesn't cede what would be patriotism or images like the flag to just the right. I claim those, as I've done in a lot of my work throughout the years."[172]

The song made its live debut on February 12, 2012, at the Grammy Awards ceremony.

[i] According to some, the throne referred to here is the White House, in that the people knocked at President Obama's door and got no reply. In the past, Springsteen committed himself to play for Obama's presidential campaign. And their friendship continued throughout the years: Springsteen played in all secrecy at Obama's farewell party held at the White House the day after Trump's election. Yet, when *Wrecking Ball* was released, Springsteen's view on the first four years of the first Afro American President's administration was not so sweet:

> I think he did a lot of good things: he kept GM alive, which was incredibly important to Detroit, Michigan. He got the healthcare law passed, though I wish there had been a public option and that it didn't leave citizens the victims of the insurance companies. He killed Osama bin Laden, which I think was extremely important. He brought some sanity to the top level of government. He's more friendly to corporations than I thought he would be,

and there aren't as many middle-class or working-class voices heard in the administration as I thought there would be. I would have liked to see more active job creation sooner than it came, and I'd like to have seen some of these foreclosures stopped or somehow mitigated. The banks have had some kind of a settlement, a partial settlement, but really, there's a lot of people it's not going to assist. I still support the president, but there are plenty of things—I thought Guantánamo would have been closed by now. On the other hand, we're out of Iraq, and hopefully we'll be out of Afghanistan soon.[173]

It must, however, be said that "We Take Care of Our Own" was played throughout Barack Obama's 2012 presidential campaign and after his victory speech at his headquarters in Chicago. Sales of the song rose 409 percent following Obama's speech at the Democratic National Convention. There is thus a second interpretation. According to Alessandro Portelli, "The song starts with the singer who is 'knocking on the door that holds the throne'— what throne, if not that of a God who doesn't respond?"[174] The echo of Dylan's "Knocking on Heaven's Door" also suggests that the door being knocked upon is in fact a more transcendental one.

[ii] A striking reference to the proverb "The road to hell is paved with good intentions." A further warning to Obama?

[iii] The meaning of the title has already been discussed in the introduction. Springsteen said, "We've destroyed the idea of an equal playing field . . . If you were born at the top, your chances for progress were great, and if you were born struggling, more often than not that's where you were going to remain. So that's a big promise that's been broken."[175]

[iv] Springsteen vertically divides the United States tracing a line from north to south, from Chicago to New Orleans. The first is Obama's natal city; the second in 2005 is the stage on which Hurricane Katrina plays its tragedy.

[v] A shotgun shack is a narrow rectangular house, usually no more than about twelve feet wide, with rooms arranged one behind the other and doors at each end of the house. It was the most popular style of house in the southern United States from the end of the American Civil War (1861–65) through the 1920s. The term "shotgun" is a reference to the idea that if all the doors are opened, a shotgun blast fired into the house from the front doorway will fly cleanly to the other end and out at the back.

[vi] The reference is to the Louisiana Superdome, the New Orleans Saints' football stadium, used in 2005 as shelter for the homeless after Hurricane Katrina.

[vii] The highlighted lyrics on the track's video quote "Calvary" and not "cavalry" — a typing mistake amended in the lyrics reproduced on Springsteen's official site. The reference to cavalry fits better with the reference to trumpets in the following verse: a bugle is in fact a trumpet used in the army. It must be noted however that it really does sound like Bruce is singing "Calvary." Did Springsteen want to swap his political standpoint for a more ideological one? Was he perhaps intending to say that the sacrifice of Calvary is not enough to save us if we don't save ourselves?

[viii] Springsteen here quotes a verse from "America the Beautiful" ("America! America! / God shed His grace on thee, / And crown thy good with brotherhood / From sea to shining sea!"), one of the most renowned patriotic songs, whose text was first written in 1895 by Katharine Lee Bates, with music composed by Samuel A. Ward. The hymn was first published in 1910.

Easy Money

©2012 Bruce Springsteen (GMR)

Released on *Wrecking Ball* album (2012)

Live premiere: 03/18/2012—Philips Arena, Atlanta, GA

"Easy Money" was written and recorded around February 2011. Before *Wrecking Ball*, Springsteen wrote a new song for another album he was working on. He recalls,

> After the crash of 2008, I was furious at what had been done by a handful of trading companies on Wall Street. *Wrecking Ball* was a shot of anger at the injustice that continues on and has widened with deregulation, dysfunctional regulatory agencies, and capitalism gone wild at the expense of hardworking Americans.[176]

[i] The term "fat cat"—used to describe a rich, greedy person who "lives easy" off the work of others—was first used in the 1920s. The term's coinage for political purposes has been attributed to Frank Kent, a writer for the *Baltimore Sun* whose essay "Fat Cats and Free Rides" explained, "A Fat Cat is a man of large means and no political experience who having reached middle age, and success in business, and finding no further thrill . . . of satisfaction in the mere piling up of more millions, develops a yearning for some sort of public honor and is willing to pay for it. The machine has what it seeks, public honor, and he has the money the machine

needs."[177] In his 1973 song "Down and Out in New York City," James Brown refers to "All the fat cats, in the bad hats."

Jack of All Trades

©2012 Bruce Springsteen (GMR)

Released on *Wrecking Ball* album (2012)

Live premiere: 03/02/2012—NBC Studio 6B, New York, NY

Like most of the songs on *Wrecking Ball*, "Jack of All Trades"—despite its slow waltz arrangement with a piano motif that explicitly references the Righteous Brothers' "Unchained Melody"—is about the Great Recession's disproportionate impact on the working class and the looting of our economies and lives by banks brazenly gorging on our money.

"Why would we who love Springsteen's music and share his rage?" asked English journalist Ed Vulliamy from the pages of the *Guardian*. The answer is that all the other superstars who have played at his level have eventually

> bloated away from serious commitment. Perky Sir Paul McCartney rounds off the jubilee for Her Majesty's whooping, servile subjects. Sir Mick Jagger showed a sign of rigor mortis by refusing to serenade the burghers of Davos, but struts and frets his years upon the world's stages to little cogent effect. Of the young ones, Coldplay filled the Emirates Stadium with even less political content than Arsenal . . . Across the Irish Sea, U2 traded "Sunday Bloody Sunday" for one of the great tax avoidance scandals in showbiz . . . Springsteen stands alone for sheer stature, durability, and profile. His adrenalin-pumping shows are woven into American life, yet subvert its capitalist fundamentals, that innate American principle of screw-thy-neighbor, in favor of what he insists to be "real" America—working class, militant, street-savvy, tough but romantic, nomadic but with roots—compiled into what feels like a single epic but vernacular rock-opera lasting four decades. Springsteen does this because he believes in what he says.[178]

The brokenhearted "Jack of All Trades" picks up at the end with a searing guitar solo by Tom Morello. "When the song finally gets to what it's been slowly building to for the five minutes prior, it's with a note of resignation that what rings out is not the cathartic sax solo that would have occupied that space on any other Springsteen record, but a limp Tom Morello guitar solo as he dispenses with his best Brian May impression. It's a Clemons-shaped void that no amount of distorted guitar can fill."[179]

Death to My Hometown

©2012 Bruce Springsteen (GMR)

Released on *Wrecking Ball* album (2012)

Live premiere: 03/02/2012—NBC Studio 6B, New York, NY

"It sounds like an Irish rebel song, but it's all about what happened four years ago," Springsteen said to Jon Stewart in 2012 about the fiery third single from *Wrecking Ball*, a devastating indictment of a society that no longer cares about the working class. The Celtic-fueled song finds the narrator describing the way the recession is destroying all he has ever known.

The studio version samples "The Last Words of Copernicus" from the 1869 *Sacred Harp*, by Sarah Lancaster of Buena Vista, Georgia. The source for the sample is Alan Lomax's recording of the 1959 United Sacred Harp Musical Association convention at Corinth Baptist Church in Fyffe, Alabama, which was reissued in 1997 by Rounder Records. You can hear the sample in the musical intro to the song and in the musical breaks after every repetition of the song's chorus. What you hear is mostly the song's alto line at the start of the fugue, which was added to the song by S. M. Denson in 1911 (it was a three-liner in the 1869 book). It appears this alto was adapted from the alto written by James Landrum White for his 1909 fifth edition of *The Sacred Harp*. "Lancaster chose to set her tune to the first two stanzas of a 1755 hymn text by Philip Doddridge. The title of Doddridge's hymn was 'God the everlasting Light of the Saints Above.' It was based on Isaiah 60:20. Sarah Lancaster associated these words with the sixteenth-century astronomer Nicolaus Copernicus in titling her composition."[180]

Rocky Ground

©2012 Bruce Springsteen (GMR)

Released on *Wrecking Ball* album (2012)

Live premiere: 03/09/2012—Apollo Theater, New York, NY

"Rocky Ground" is the second single from the *Wrecking Ball* album and was released exclusively in select stores as a limited-edition 7-inch 45-rpm vinyl single as a part of Record Store Day on April 21, 2012. This bold melding of church hymn, plain-folks lament, and hip-hop protest was put at #7 on *Rolling Stone*'s "50 Best Songs of 2012" list.

The track also features the voice of gospel singer Michelle Moore, who provides backing vocals and also delivers a brief rap towards the song's end. Springsteen has stated that he originally attempted to do the rapping himself but was not satisfied with the sound. According to producer Ron Aniello, they considered several people for the part. Aniello even considered getting famous gospel singers like Al Green or Mavis Staples.

The studio version of "Rocky Ground" uses excerpts of the traditional gospel song "I'm a Soldier in the Army of the Lord," performed by the Congregation of the Church of God in Christ and recorded by Alan Lomax in July 1942 in Clarksdale, Mississippi. It can now be found on Lomax's collection *The Land Where The Blues Began*, released on Rounder Records in 2002.

[i] The term "rocky ground" is taken from the biblical parable of the sower: "And as he sowed, some seed fell on the path, and the birds came and ate it up. Other seed fell on rocky ground, where it did not have much soil, and it sprang up quickly, since it had no depth of soil. And when the sun rose, it was scorched; and since it had no root, it withered away" (Mark 4:4–6).

[ii] "Rise Up, Shepherd, and Follow" is a spiritual published for the first time in 1867 under the title "A Christmas Plantation Song" in *Slave Songs of the United States*, a collection of songs sung by Georgia and South Carolina plantation slaves during the American Civil War. The track was also added to Alan Lomax's collection *The Folk Songs of North America* (1975) and made popular by Dorothy Maynor (1910–1996), a soprano, founder of the Harlem School of Music in New York. The singing is structured using the typical call-and-response model:

> There's a star in the East on Christmas morn.
> Rise up shepherd and follow.
> It'll show you the place where the child is born.
> Rise up shepherd and follow.
> Leave your sheep and leave your lambs.
> Rise up shepherd and follow . . .

[iii] "In the six hundredth year of Noah's life, in the second month, on the seventeenth day of the month, on that day all the fountains of the great deep burst forth, and the windows of the heavens were opened. And rain fell upon the earth forty days and forty nights" (Genesis 7:11–12).

[iv] "On reaching Jerusalem, Jesus entered the temple courts and began driving out those who were buying and selling there. He overturned the tables of the money changers and the benches of those selling doves, and would not allow anyone to carry merchandise through the temple courts" (Mark 11:15–16).

[v] This is the land that God promised to Abraham and his people: "The Lord said, 'I have indeed seen the misery of my people in Egypt. I have heard them crying out because of their slave drivers, and I am concerned about their suffering. So I have come down to rescue them from the hand of the Egyptians and to bring them up out of that land into a good and spacious land, a land flowing with milk and honey—the home of the Canaanites, Hittites, Amorites, Perizzites, Hivites and Jebusites'" (Exodus 3:7–8).

[vi] "For your hands are defiled with blood and your fingers with iniquity; your lips have spoken lies; your tongue mutters wickedness" (Isaiah 59:3).

Land of Hope and Dreams

©2001 Bruce Springsteen (GMR)

Released on *Wrecking Ball* album (2012)

Live premiere: 03/19/1999—Convention Hall, Asbury Park, NJ

"Land of Hope and Dreams" was written in 1998 or early 1999, and debuted live with the E Street Band on March 19, 1999, in Asbury Park, New Jersey. The song came during the close of a decade in which Springsteen had parted ways with the E Street Band, gotten married again and had children, and had released very little new music in a rock vein. He later said, "I was having a hard time locating my rock voice. I knew I didn't want it to be what it was, but I didn't know . . . I'd made some records over the past years, I made one in '94 that I didn't release. Then I made a series of demos, kind of in search of that voice. And I was having a hard time finding it. And there was a point I said: 'Well, gee, maybe I just don't do that now. Maybe that's something that I did.'" But after writing "Land of Hope and Dreams," he felt it was "as good as any songs like this that I've ever written. It was like, there's that voice I was looking for."[181] In Springsteen's intentions, the song sums up much of what he wanted his band to be about and renewed their pledge to their audience. Introducing it at the first concert of the 1999 Reunion Tour in Barcelona, he said, "This is the rededication of our band, the rebirth of our band."

A live version of "Land of Hope and Dreams" is on the *Live in New York City* album of 2001. A studio version was recorded in the latter half of 2011 for *Wrecking Ball*, after the passing of the E Street Band saxophonist Clarence Clemons. The song was reworked with electronic drums and a gospel choir. Producer Ron Aniello also had a couple of recorded Clemons saxophone performances of "Land of Hope and Dreams." They were in a different key and a different tempo, so he

tweaked them on the computer, but didn't reveal the result to Springsteen because of what he was going through after the passing of his friend. Later, when
they were mixing the song, Springsteen said that he wished they had Clarence
performing on it, so Aniello told him about the saxophone recording he was
working on. He added it to the track and it was a special moment for Springsteen
when he heard it. "When the solo section hit, Clarence's sax filled the room. I
cried."[182]

For "Land of Hope and Dreams" Springsteen adapted the mandolin solo from
Joe Grushecky's "Labor of Love" virtually note by note. That song was included in
Grushecky's 1995 album *American Babylon*, which Springsteen played on.

A recording of the song was played after President Barack Obama's farewell
address in 2017.

In the live performance of this song on January 27, 2017, at the Perth Arena,
Springsteen added the line "this train carries immigrants." Not many days had
gone by since President Donald Trump had announced that he was reviewing his
stance on immigration from Muslim countries.

[i] The refrain is a deliberate inversion of the traditional American gospel song
"This Train Is Bound for Glory," recorded in the 1920s and often associated with
Woody Guthrie as the inspiration for his 1943 autobiography *Bound for Glory*—
even if in Dave Marsh's opinion, Springsteen's song was based more off of Sister
Rosetta Tharpe's rendition.[183] In Springsteen's take, all are welcome on the train—
not just "the righteous and the holy" of the original, but "saints and sinners," "losers
and winners," "whores and gamblers."

[ii] The studio version of "Land of Hope and Dreams" ends with lines from
"People Get Ready" performed by the Victorious Gospel Choir. The song was
written by Curtis Mayfield and originally released by the Impressions on their
1965 album *People Get Ready*.

We Are Alive
©2012 Bruce Springsteen (GMR)

Released on *Wrecking Ball* album (2012)

Live premiere: 03/09/2012—Apollo Theater, New York , NY

Springsteen closes his seventeenth album, *Wrecking Ball*, with this campfire song for
the oppressed and downtrodden, who having passed away have risen again, their
faith rewarded. "Those spirits don't go away. They haunt, they rabble-rouse, from
beyond the grave. They have not been and can never be silenced."[184]

"We Are Alive" is a six-minute sort of mariachi *Spoon River Anthology* that borrows its horn riff from Johnny Cash's "Ring of Fire" and its imagery—again—from the Bible. Springsteen joked about the fact that he almost can't help including references from the scriptures into his songs almost unbidden: "It's like Al Pacino in *The Godfather*: I try to get out but they pull you back in! Once a Catholic, always a Catholic."[185] The song echoes a verse from the Acts of the Apostles: "All the believers were one in heart and mind. No one claimed that any of their possessions was their own, but they shared everything they had" (Acts 4:32).

Springsteen returns towards a "Christian socialism," recalling the experience of Christ's Resurrection and taking inspiration from the very step in which Luke intends to underline the intrinsic bond between the Gospel's proclamation and the life of sharing of the community. In this respect, "We Are Alive" may sound like a consolation prize; in reality it gives closure to the entire Springsteenian message around the theme of the Promise. Take it or leave it.

[i] The Great Railroad Strike began on July 14, 1877, in Martinsburg, West Virginia, after the Baltimore & Ohio Railroad cut wages for the third time in a year. This strike finally ended some forty-five days later, after it was put down by local and state militias and federal troops. Because of economic problems and pressure on wages by the railroads, workers in numerous other cities, in New York, Pennsylvania, and Maryland, into Illinois and Missouri, also went out on strike. An estimated 100 people were killed in the unrest across the country.

[ii] On September 15, 1963, four members of the Ku Klux Klan planted at least fifteen sticks of dynamite attached to a timing device beneath the front steps of the 16th Street Baptist Church in Birmingham, Alabama, killing four girls and injuring twenty-two others. Described by Martin Luther King as "one of the most vicious and tragic crimes ever perpetrated against humanity," the bombing marked a turning point in the United States during the Civil Rights Movement and contributed to support for passage of the Civil Rights Act of 1964. Although the FBI had concluded in 1965 that the 16th Street Baptist Church bombing had been committed by four known Ku Klux Klansmen and segregationists—Thomas Edwin Blanton Jr., Herman Frank Cash, Robert Edward Chambliss, and Bobby Frank Cherry—no prosecutions ensued until 1977, when Robert Chambliss was tried and convicted of the first-degree murder of one of the victims, eleven-year-old Carol Denise McNair. Thomas Blanton and Bobby Cherry were each convicted of four counts of murder and

sentenced to life imprisonment in 2001 and 2002 respectively,[186] whereas Herman Cash, who died in 1994, was never charged for his alleged involvement in the bombing.

THREE

Better Days

Glory Days

In 1984–85, the *Born in the U.S.A.* album and tour, together with his participation in U.S.A. for Africa's "We Are the World" charity single project, gave Springsteen an enormous amount of popularity, ten years after *Born to Run*. "The genie was out of the bottle." Garry Tallent says.[187] In fact, Bruce had become a true American icon.

Springsteen has always expressed some mixed feelings about the *Born in the U.S.A.* album, believing that *Nebraska* contains some of his strongest writing, while *Born in the U.S.A.* did not necessarily follow suit. The title track "more or less stood by itself," he declared. "The rest of the album contains a group of songs about which I've always had some ambivalence."[188] Even so, and despite expressing the "grab-bag nature" of the album, he acknowledged its powerful effect on his career: *Born in the U.S.A.* changed his life and gave him his largest audience, forcing him to question the way he presented his music.

The plain truth is that his career—from the explosion of the "Born to Run" phenomenon to *The River* at the top of the charts, up until the mass hysteria surrounding *Born in the U.S.A.*—proceeded smoothly, and Springsteen never stopped to look at the effects on his personal life. "Off the road, life was a puzzle," he recalls in his autobiography. Without the nightly hit of adrenaline the show provided him with, he was at loose ends.

Some songs on *Born in the U.S.A.* gave some indication that this autobiography was not particularly triumphant: "Dancing in the Dark" for example is a tale of frustration and isolation set in recording studios and hotel rooms. "Glory Days" is another song about rock 'n' roll's promise, but "isn't really optimistic," as Dave Marsh noted; "behind its glee are some sad stories—the baseball pitcher who never topped his high school heroics, the good ol' girl whose marriage fell apart, the rock and roll singer who's embarrassed by his own fixation on the past. All are wasting away for the same reason, which isn't that they're living in the past but that they're missing the moment."[189]

During the *Born in the U.S.A.* recording sessions, Springsteen cut a semiserious pop-culture commentary wrapped in an appealing, old-fashioned rocker entitled "TV Movie":

I woke up last night shaking from a dream,
For in that dream I died.

My wife rolled over and told me
That my life would be immortalized,
Not in some major motion picture
Or great American novel, you see,
No, they're gonna make a TV movie out of me.

Well, now, it's one-two-three—you take the money,
Yeah, it's as easy as A B C,
Yeah, they're gonna make a TV movie out of me.

"TV Movie" was "a joke, but it had some ironic undertones," Springsteen says.[190] The song—which remained unreleased until it got on the *Tracks* box set—highlights his unrest regarding his growing popularity. In 1984, at thirty-five years of age, he had no house, no wife, no kids. His only "family" was the E Street Band—which had even lost one of it cornerstones: Steve Van Zandt, Springsteen's lifelong friend and companion, had left the band to attempt a solo career; and Bruce gave him a good farewell in "No Surrender" and "Bobby Jean."

Five years later, in 1989, he said goodbye to his past, storing the band away in mothballs until in "Blood Brothers" he would nostalgically recall the ties that bind him to his old fellows and the desire to pick up upon the interrupted path. Henceforth, the rededicated E Street Band would not even be stopped by the death of Danny Federici (which would lead Springsteen to write "The Last Carnival") and of Clarence Clemons.

During the days of *Darkness on the Edge of Town*, Springsteen asked himself, "What do you do if your dreams comes true? What then?" The triumphal whoop of "Rosalita" ("The record company, Rosie, just gave me a big advance") had soon become a *cri de coeur*. He'd seen the dark side. As Springsteen told Dave Marsh, "I got out there—hey, the wind's whipping through your hair, you feel real good, you're the guy with the golden guitar or whatever, and all of a sudden you feel that sense of dread that's overwhelming."[191]

What had happened to the romantic dreamer from "Thunder Road"? Had he achieved his dreams? The answer is yes. But there is always a price to pay.

Dancing in the Dark
©1984 Bruce Springsteen (GMR)

Released on *Born in the U.S.A.* album (1984) | *London Calling: Live in Hyde Park* home video (2010) recorded live at Hyde Park, London, June 28, 2009

Live premiere: 06/08/1984—The Stone Pony, Asbury Park, NJ

"Dancing in the Dark" was the last song on *Born in the U.S.A.* to be recorded. It was written after Jon Landau convinced Springsteen that the album needed a single. According to Dave Marsh, Springsteen was not impressed with Landau's approach. "Look," he snarled, "I've written seventy songs. You want another one, you write it."[192] Despite this reaction, Bruce sat in his hotel room and wrote the song in a single night. It sums up his state of mind and his feeling of isolation after the success of *The River*. The song is "a marching song against boredom, a battle cry against loneliness, and an accounting of the price the loner pays."[193] Six takes were cut at the Hit Factory on February 14, 1984.

To test the song out, Springsteen took an acetate copy to Asbury Park's Club Xanadu. When the dance floor overflowed, he handed the disc to the DJ and explained what it was. When the DJ faded out the other song and turned up the volume on "Dancing in the Dark," the dance floor seemed to explode.

Released as a single prior to the album's release, "Dancing in the Dark" spent four weeks at #2 on the *Billboard* Hot 100 (Springsteen's highest-charting song to date)[194] and eventually sold over three million copies worldwide. It was also the first of a record-tying seven Top 10 hit singles to be released from *Born in the U.S.A.*: "Cover Me" (#7), "Born in the U.S.A." (#9), "I'm on Fire" (#6), "Glory Days" (#5), "I'm Goin' Down'" (#9), and "My Hometown" (#6).

In a first-for-Springsteen effort to gain dance and club play for his music, Arthur Baker created the 12-inch Blaster Mix of "Dancing in the Dark," wherein he reworked the album version. The remix was released on July 2, 1984. The result generated a lot of media buzz for Springsteen, as well as actual club play; the remix went to #7 on the *Billboard* Hot Dance Music / Club Play chart, and had the most sales of any 12-inch single in the United States in 1984.

"Dancing in the Dark" also won Springsteen his first Grammy Award, picking up the prize for Best Rock Vocal Performance in 1985. In the 1984 *Rolling Stone* readers poll, "Dancing in the Dark" was voted single of the year. The track is listed as one of the Rock and Roll Hall of Fame's 500 Songs That Shaped Rock and Roll.

Directed by Brian De Palma, the video of "Dancing in the Dark" was shot at the Civic Center in Saint Paul, Minnesota, on June 28 and 29, 1984. The first night was a pure video-shot; the second was on the opening date of the Born in the U.S.A. Tour. Bruce Springsteen and the E Street Band performed the song twice during that show to allow Brian De Palma to get all the footage he needed. Springsteen is not playing a guitar, allowing him to invite a young woman from the audience, performed by Courtney Cox, to dance along with him on the stage at the end. In September 1985, the video won the MTV Video Music Award for Best Stage Performance.

[i] In "Angel from Montgomery," country singer John Prine asks, "How the hell can a person go to work in the morning and come home in the evening and have nothing to say?" The song originally appeared on his self-titled 1971 album *John Prine*. Bonnie Raitt recorded it for her *Streetlights* album of 1974.

[ii] *This Gun for Hire* is a 1942 film noir starring Veronica Lake and Robert Preston, directed by Frank Tuttle and based on the 1936 novel by Graham Greene.

Glory Days

©1984 Bruce Springsteen (GMR)

Released on *Born in the U.S.A.* album (1984) | *In Concert/MTV Plugged* album & home video (1993) recorded live at Warner Hollywood Studios, Los Angeles, CA, September 22, 1992

Live premiere: 06/08/1984—The Stone Pony, Asbury Park, NJ

"Glory Days" was recorded in April–May 1982 during the first wave of *Born in the U.S.A.* sessions. It was also released as the fifth single from the album, peaking at #5 on the *Billboard* Hot 100 pop single charts in the summer of 1985.

Introducing the song on October 25, 1984, at the Los Angeles Sports Arena, Springsteen said,

> This is a song about history . . . Now, I don't mean history like what the Greeks were doing or what Pythagoras was thinking or who Sophocles was fooling around with. I'm talking about personal history, I'm talking about the *National Enquirer* kind of stuff: you're getting the dirt now, I'm in a confessional mood, you see? Now, what this is kind of about is that usually when I get home, there's nothing on TV but *The Twilight Zone*. The strange thing about it is it's usually only on the TV in my room . . . There was this one actor on this one *Twilight Zone*: he was old and he wanted to be young again 'cause he thought when he was young he had all that fun, he had all the girls and all the good jobs and he was feeling old, feeling like a drag; and so, of course, the man slips into the Twilight Zone, but when he goes back there, he finds out that everybody that he thought was being nice to him was treating him like a dog and that his girlfriend was running around with these other guys and in the end he wants to come back and be the age that he is. And the reason I bring this up is because is that always happens to me—like I go out and somebody's always coming up to me and saying, "Bruce, remember me, man, we used to have all that

fun in high school? We were going out with all the girls and having a great time; we didn't have any responsibilities, we didn't have any cares in the whole world . . ." I always sit there going, "All right, all right . . ." but then when I think about it, I realize that I HATED high school, I couldn't wait to get out of high school, I'm glad right now that I don't have to go back to high school when fall comes around! In high school I was only interested in two things: one of them was the guitar, and the other one . . . Now, the guitar's the one that I became proficient at, but the other one . . . I'm still looking for some volunteers who wanna practice, practice, practice . . . Anyway, this is about how all things must pass. Ain't it right, Big Man? The Big Man says it's so: he's got the wisdom of the ages, he's gotta be right. It ain't nothing but glory days . . .

[i] The lyrics to the first verse are autobiographical, being "a recount of an encounter Springsteen had with former Little League baseball teammate Joe DePugh in the summer of 1973."[195]

[ii] There is an unofficial studio version of "Glory Days"—an alternate mix of the album version—with an extra verse following the second chorus:

> My old man worked twenty years on the line,
> And they let him go.
> Now everywhere he goes out looking for work,
> They just tell him that he's too old.
> I was nine years old when he was working
> At the Metuchen Ford plant assembly line,
> Now he just sits on a stool down at the Legion Hall,
> But I can tell what's on his mind . . .

Reportedly Springsteen decided to cut this verse because he realized that it did not fit with the song's story line.

No Surrender
©1984 Bruce Springsteen (GMR)

Released on *Born in the U.S.A.* album (1984) | *Live/1975–85* box set (1986) recorded live at Brendan Byrne Arena, East Rutherford, NJ, August 6, 1984 | *London Calling: Live in Hyde Park* home video (2010) recorded live at Hyde Park, London, June 28, 2009

Live premiere: 06/08/1984—The Stone Pony, Asbury Park, NJ

Springsteen considered leaving "No Surrender" off the *Born in the U.S.A.* album, explaining that "you don't hold out and triumph all the time in life. . . .You compromise, you suffer defeat; you slip into life's gray areas."[196] It was Steve Van Zandt who convinced Springsteen otherwise, arguing that the portrait of friendship and the song's expression of the inspirational power of rock music was an important part of the picture.

On July 9, 1984, during a show in Cleveland, Springsteen would dedicate the song to his friend: "There's this song by Big Country called 'In a Big Country,' and it had a great line that said, 'In a big country, a dream will stay with you.' This is for Little Steven, wherever he may be."

During the Born in the U.S.A. Tour, "No Surrender" was rarely played: instead of having a full-band version the song was a slow acoustic guitar and harmonica version, which can be heard on the *Live/1975–85* box set. A full-band version of the song, performed with Brian Fallon of the Gaslight Anthem as special guest, is on the London *Calling: Live in Hyde Park* home video.

Bobby Jean

©1984 Bruce Springsteen (GMR)

Released on *Born in the U.S.A.* album (1984) | *Live/1975–85* box set (1986) recorded live at Giants Stadium, East Rutherford, NJ, August 21, 1985 | *London Calling: Live in Hyde Park* home video (2010) recorded live at Hyde Park, London, June 28, 2009

Live premiere: 06/08/1984—The Stone Pony, Asbury Park, NJ

"Bobby Jean" was Springsteen's answer to Steve Van Zandt's decision to leave the E Street Band. During the 1982 sessions for *Born in the U.S.A.* Van Zandt formed his own band, the Disciples of Soul, and recorded his first solo album, *Men Without Women*, followed by *Voice of America* two years later. According to Peter Ames Carlin, the distance between Van Zandt and Springsteen had grown increasingly obvious, and Van Zandt was upset over his loss of influence. For a long time, the balance between Springsteen's manager and producer Landau and Van Zandt had been tense, but productively so. Jon represented "the career, the business, the narrative end," the guitarist says, while he himself represented "rock 'n' roll, the street, where it was coming from. A healthy balance, and it proved to be quite successful . . . At a certain point, I needed my role to expand," he explains. Instead, the pendulum swung the opposite direction. "All of a sudden I could tell he wasn't hearing me. I'm not getting through. That was new to me, and I wasn't comfortable with it."[197]

Blood Brothers

©1995 Bruce Springsteen (GMR)

Released on *Greatest Hits* anthology (1995) | *Blood Brothers* EP & home video (1996)

Live premiere: 04/05/1995—Sony Music Studios, New York, NY

After sixteen years of work together and a friendship, eight albums and a stratospheric number of shows played, Bruce Springsteen and the E Street Band split up in 1989: Springsteen wanted to innovate his sound and hence decided to disband. Six years later, the band came together again to record a few tracks to put at the end of the *Greatest Hits* collection. "'Blood Brothers' was about trying to understand the meaning of friendship as you grow older," Springsteen told Neil Strauss. "I guess I wrote it the night before I went in the studio with the band, and I was trying to sort out what I was doing and what those relationships meant to me now and what those types of friendships mean as a person moves through life."[198]

In January 1995, Springsteen assembled the entire E Street Band (plus alumnus Little Steven) together in New York for about ten days of studio sessions. Although Springsteen had utilized individual band members in the studio since 1987, this was seemingly the first time the E Street Band had worked together in the studio since March 1984. Four different complete studio takes of "Blood Brothers" have circulated among collectors, all of which were recorded during the January 1995 sessions in New York; a rock version was included on the *Blood Brothers* EP.

"Blood Brothers" has been performed only five times live. At Orlando's Amway Arena, on April 23, 2008, Bruce and the band chose it to open the show in a new arrangement while accompanying images of Danny Federici, who had passed away the previous week, were projected onscreen.

The Last Carnival

©2009 Bruce Springsteen (GMR)

Released on *Working on a Dream* album (2009)

Live premiere: —

Springsteen wrote this song about the death of Daniel Federici, his organ player and E Street Band stalwart. He explained that it started out as a way of making sense of Federici's passing: "He was a part of that sound of the boardwalk the band grew up with and that's something that's going to be missing now."[199]

Federici died on April 17, 2008, having suffered for three years with melanoma. Federici's son, Jason, plays the accordion on this track.

Springsteen wrote it resuscitating Wild Billy and his circus nearly forty years later. In fact, "The Last Carnival" is a sort of sequel to "Wild Billy's Circus Song," the mood sketch of carnival life included on *The Wild, the Innocent & the E Street Shuffle* in 1973:

> The machinist climbs his ferris wheel like a brave
> And the fire eater's lyin' in a pool of sweat, victim of the heatwave.
> Behind the tent the hired hand tightens his legs on the sword swallower's blade,
> And circus town's on the shortwave.

Suddenly, "the metaphor that Springsteen maybe hinted at a bit too vaguely in the original song becomes achingly clear. The band *is* the circus, and Springsteen and the rest, devastated as they might be, now they have to move on without their friend."[200]

> And the circus boss leans over, whispers into the little boy's ear,
> "Hey son, you want to try the big top?"
> All aboard, Nebraska's our next stop.

As the sole survivor of the two daredevils' team, Bruce climbs alone onto the steaming train, pausing for one last glance into the gloom rising in the fields behind.

Real World

Jon Pareles of the *New York Times* described *Tunnel of Love* saying that now Springsteen was "confronting another illusion: the myth of love as a perfect bliss and panacea."[201] In the sleeve notes to his 1987 record Springsteen wrote, "Thanks Julie," but listening to the songs it seemed evident that all was not well with the marriage with Julianne Phillips. More than a trip in the tunnel of love, the album seems like a hopeless race in a haunted house.

"Before *Tunnel of Love*, Springsteen had mostly eschewed writing love songs," Sarfraz Manzoor wrote in the *Guardian*. "His songs were more likely to deal with losing your job than losing your heart. Love, when it appeared, was largely infatuation and painted in the primary colors of youthful yearning. 'We'll live with the sadness and I'll love you with all madness in my soul,' he sings on the title track of *Born to Run*. In his early records Springsteen implied that happiness was a girl, a guy, and a car; on *Tunnel of Love* he began to wonder what if the car was heading in the wrong direction."[202]

Springsteen had married Phillips in May 1985; the couple filed for divorce less than a year after the release of the album. Bruce had begun an affair with his backup singer Patti Scialfa. The two first lived in New Jersey and later in New York for a short time before moving to Los Angeles, where they started a family. On July 25, 1990, Scialfa gave birth to the couple's first child, Evan James. Bruce and Patti married on June 8, 1991, and they had a second child, Jessica Rae, in 1991, and a third one, Samuel Ryan, in 1994. The family returned to New Jersey in the early 1990s, where they still live.

The songs composed by Springsteen in the two years spanning 1990–91 and later included on the *Human Touch* and *Lucky Town* albums reflect his new sentimental situation and continue the "therapy sessions" initiated with *Tunnel of Love*. Once again with all honesty, Springsteen tells about the high and low points of his private life, the difficulties of a blossoming love story that fights against the ghosts of depression, the personal and conjugal peace of mind finally attained, and the joys of fatherhood.

In the so-called "Love Trilogy" the joys and dramas are no longer lived on the road but "under the covers." Several fans, at the time the three said albums were published, were confused when they heard Springsteen singing, for example, in "57 Channels (And Nothin' On)":

> I bought a bourgeois house in the Hollywood hills
> With a truckload of hundred thousand dollar bills . . .

or in "Local Hero" saying he saw his own face "staring out of a black velvet painting / From the window of the five and dime . . . / Between the Doberman and Bruce

Lee." Even his old accomplice Steve Van Zandt expressed his doubts—to use an euphemism—when he first heard a piece like "Ain't Got You," with those lyrics telling of a fellow who gets "paid a king's ransom for doin' what comes naturally," who's got "the fortunes of heaven" and a "house full of Rembrandt and priceless art." Stevie recognized the self-mockery but didn't care. He was aghast. "We had one of our biggest fights of our lives," Van Zandt recalled in an interview with the *New Yorker*'s editor, Dave Remnick. "I'm, like, 'What the fuck is this?' And he's, like, 'Well, what do you mean, it's the truth. It's just who I am, it's my life.' And I'm, like, 'This is bullshit. People don't need you talking about your life. Nobody gives a *shit* about *your* life. They need you for *their* lives. *That's your thing.* Giving some logic and reason and sympathy and passion to this cold, fragmented, confusing world—that's your gift. Explaining their lives to them. *Their* lives, not yours.'" [203]

But Van Zandt proved to be wrong. Springsteen, telling us of his life, has managed to tell us our own as well.

Tunnel of Love

©1987 Bruce Springsteen (GMR)

Released on *Tunnel of Love* album (1987)

Live premiere: 02/25/1988—The Centrum, Worcester, MA

The title track of Springsteen's eighth studio album was recorded sometime between January and May 1987 at Thrill Hill East (his New Jersey home studio). On this song, Springsteen plays several instruments and is backed by Roy Bittan on synthesizers, Nils Lofgren on lead guitar, and Max Weinberg on drums. Springsteen's future wife, Patti Scialfa, provides backing vocals. Effects on the song include the sounds of a family riding a roller coaster in Point Pleasant, New Jersey, recorded by Toby Scott and an assistant who spent the majority of a summer's day recruiting and coaching the park's customers to direct their reactions to the microphones at the coaster's final turn. The Schiffer family named in the song's credits were the park's owners and operators.

"Tunnel of Love" was released as the second single from the album, reaching #9 on the *Billboard* Hot 100 charts.

The Honeymooners

©1998 Bruce Springsteen (GMR)

Released on *Tracks* box set (1998)

Live premiere: —

Recorded on February 22, 1987 (the same day as "The Wish"), at Thrill Hill Recording, Rumson, New Jersey, during the *Tunnel of Love* sessions, "The Honeymooners" will be released only eleven year later on the *Tracks* box set. Its story is basically twenty-four hours in the life of a young man getting married, moving from ceremony to reception to honeymoon night to morning after with the new in-laws. Springsteen said, "Of course it's a true story. But it's not necessarily autobiographical. Not necessarily."[204] Bruce Springsteen and Julianne Phillips were married in Lake Oswego, Oregon, on May 13, 1985, surrounded by intense media attention. "I remember the night that I got married," Springsteen recalls. "I was standing at the altar by myself, and I was waiting for my wife, and I can remember standing there thinking, 'Man, I have everything. I got it all.' And you have those moments. But you end up with a lot more than you expected."[205]

If there was any doubt that Springsteen recorded *Tunnel of Love* at home, it is dispelled at about 1:52 of "The Honeymooners," when the sounds of a barking dog and a car going by can clearly be heard.

One Step Up

©1987 Bruce Springsteen (GMR)

Released on *Tunnel of Love* album (1987)

Live premiere: 02/25/1988—The Centrum, Worcester. MA

Unlike much of the *Tunnel of Love* album, "One Step Up" was not recorded in Springsteen's home studio, but at A&M Studios in Los Angeles between May and August 1987. Springsteen plays all instruments, and future wife Patti Scialfa provides backing vocals.

"One Step Up" was released in February 1988 as *Tunnel of Love*'s third single, reaching #13 on the *Billboard* Hot 100 chart.

In 2002, country singer Kenny Chesney covered this on his *No Shirt, No Shoes, No Problems* album. When he sent his version to Springsteen, Bruce sent him back a note telling Chesney he had done a great job with it, bringing a lot of sensitivity to the lyrics.

Brilliant Disguise

©1987 Bruce Springsteen (GMR)

Released on *Tunnel of Love* album (1987) | *VH1 Storytellers: Bruce Springsteen* home video (2005) recorded live at Two River Theater, Red Bank, NJ, April 4, 2005

Live premiere: 02/25/1988—The Centrum, Worcester, MA

"Brilliant Disguise" was released as the first single from the *Tunnel of Love* album, reaching the #5 position on the *Billboard* Hot 100 chart.

Director Meiert Avis made a beautiful video of the song, shot in black and white. The setting is the kitchen of a modest home, Springsteen sits uncomfortably on the edge of a chair, facing the camera; he plays his guitar as he sings (live) the lyrics about what it means to try to trust someone, looking straight into the camera, never flinching as it slowly pans in, ending with an extreme close-up.

"The song is asking: who's on this side of the bed? . . . You gotta stop dropping your masks," Springsteen said.[206] On his 2005 *Storytellers* appearance, he explained how he used to enjoy going to strip clubs around the time he wrote this song, and then he brought out his wife Patti Scialfa to sing it with him. Said Bruce: "I guess it sounds like a song of betrayal—who's that person sleeping next to me, who am I? Do I know enough about myself to be honest with that person? But a funny thing happens: songs shift their meanings when you sing them, they shift their meanings in time, they shift their meanings with who you sing them with. When you sing this song with someone you love, it turns into something else."

Tougher than the Rest

©1987 Bruce Springsteen (GMR)

Released on *Tunnel of Love* album (1987) | *Chimes of Freedom* EP (1988) recorded live at Memorial Sports Arena, Los Angeles, CA, on April 27, 1988

Live premiere: 02/25/1988—The Centrum, Worcester, MA

Like much of the *Tunnel of Love* album, "Tougher than the Rest" was recorded in Springsteen's Thrill Hill East home studio between January and May 1987. Springsteen played several instruments, backed by Danny Federici on organ and Max Weinberg on percussion. Night after night on the 1988 Tunnel of Love Express Tour, this subtle ballad made for a singularly intimate duet between Springsteen and his future wife, Patti Scialfa.

"Tougher than the Rest" was also released as a single in some countries—but not in the U.S. —reaching the Top 20 in the United Kingdom. A live—and slower—version of the song, recorded on April 27, 1988, at Los Angeles Memorial Sports Arena, was released on the *Chimes of Freedom* EP in 1988. It's the same cut used for the music video, which features live concert footage interspersed with vignettes of couples (gay, lesbian, and heterosexual) made at venues on the Tunnel of Love Express Tour.

"This song is unusual in that it applies this macho way of talking to something sensitive," says Win Butler of Arcade Fire. "But it's even better hearing Patti sing it live with Bruce."[207]

The Wish

©1998 Bruce Springsteen (GMR)

Released on *Tracks* box set (1998)

Live premiere: 11/17/1990—Shrine Auditorium, Los Angeles, CA

Recorded on February 22, 1987, at Thrill Hill East home studio, "The Wish" debuted at the Christic Institute benefit concert in Los Angeles, November 17, 1990, preceded by a long, touching introduction about what it means, psychologically, to write a song about your mother. Bruce resurrected "The Wish" for eighteen performances on the Ghost of Tom Joad Tour. Introducing it during a show in Copenhagen's Falkoner-Teotret in Denmark, he said,

> I wrote it a long time ago, 'bout ten years ago, but I never do it. And the reason that I haven't done it would be because it was a song I wrote about my mother. I ain't always writing about my father, and you know . . . it's nice and macho. In rock 'n' roll it's okay to write about your father. It's been done! But, gee, I'd written about him a long time, I figured people may have been sick of that by now . . . But writing about your mother is a tricky thing, because in rock you can write about fucking your mother. That's all right. I mean, that's been done. But, generally, the singing about your mother is confined to country music. They do it very well. Or to gospel music. A lot of good mother singers in gospel music. On the other hand, the greatest mother lover of all time—Elvis Presley—was a rock singer. But he didn't sing a song about his mother, except that first demo that he made; and they never put that out. So, you see, I'm treading on thin ice here. But it takes a man to sing about his mother . . ."

The studio version of the song was finally released on the *Tracks* box set in 1998.

[i] In December 1954, Adele took out a personal loan for sixty dollars and bought Bruce a Japanese-made "Kent" electric guitar and amplifier package as a Christmas present at Caiazzo's Music Store on Central Street. Interviewed by Charlie Rose in 1998, Springsteen recalled, "It was a very divining moment, standing in front of the music store, with someone who's going to do everything she can to give you what you needed that night, that day, and having the faith that you were going to make sense of it—or not: that it was just what you needed and desired at the moment. It was a great sacrifice on her part. It was sixty dollars, but that was finance company money."

[ii] The ladies "all lipstick, perfume and rustlin' skirts" who work with Springsteen's mother shared office space at the Lawyers Title insurance Company, 31 West Main Street in Freehold, New Jersey.

[iii] Bond Street is a small residential street in West Freehold. The lyrics printed in the *Tracks* booklet say "hatred." But when you listen to the song, "hatred" becomes "hotrod," which "makes a lot of sense, since Bruce is rumored to have rented garage space there at one time for part of his car collection."[208]

With Every Wish

©1992 Bruce Springsteen (GMR)

Released on *Human Touch* album (1992)

Live premiere: 06/15/1992—Globe Arena, Stockholm, Sweden

Springsteen did virtually no songwriting between 1988 and mid-1989. His decision to start a family with Patti Scialfa seems to have coincided with his decision to put the E Street Band into semipermanent retirement. He started to write again in fall 1989, and one of the first songs he penned was "With Every Wish," which was recorded later that same year. Springsteen plays guitar, Roy Bittan plays keyboards, Douglas Lunn is on bass, Kurt Wortman plays drums, and Mark Isham plays trumpet.

The song was released in 1992 on the *Human Touch* album, and played only six times to date (all during the 1992–1993 World Tour).

Real World

©1992 Bruce Springsteen, Roy Bittan (GMR)

Released on *Human Touch* album (1992)

Live premiere: 11/16/1990—Shrine Auditorium, Los Angeles, CA

In 1990, Roy Bittan gave Springsteen a tape with one of his own compositions on it. Springsteen created this splendid ballad from it and performed it for the first time at the Christic Institute benefit concert in Los Angeles, November 18, 1990, solo on piano.

The full-band version that would then be included on the *Human Touch* album was recorded in December 1989 at Soundworks West, Los Angeles. Springsteen handles lead guitar and vocals, and his four-man backing band on this recording is Randy Jackson (bass), Roy Bittan (keyboards), Jeff Porcaro (drums), and Tim Pierce (rhythm guitar). Background vocals are courtesy of Bobby King. But this studio version does not pay proper homage to this as one of Springsteen's best songs of the nineties. The fan-favorite long-lost piano version of "Real World" resurfaced during the 1995 Devils & Dust Solo and Acoustic Tour.

Better Days

©1992 Bruce Springsteen, Roy Bittan (GMR)

Released on *Lucky Town* album (1992) | *In Concert/MTV Plugged* album & home video (1992) recorded live at Warner Hollywood Studios, Los Angeles, CA, September 22, 1992

Live premiere: 11/16/1990—Shrine Auditorium, Los Angeles, CA

"Better Days" was released as the first single from the *Lucky Town* album on March 21, 1992, reaching #16 on the *Billboard* Hot 100. It opens the album "with a burst of energy and an irresistible optimism that makes it almost impossible to dislike . . . It's not often that a happy state of mind translates into a good song but the rousing 'Better Days' fall into that fortunate category."[209]

If I Should Fall Behind

©1992 Bruce Springsteen, Roy Bittan (GMR)

Released on *Lucky Town* album (1992) | *In Concert/MTV Plugged* album & home video (1992) recorded live at Warner Hollywood Studios, Los Angeles, CA, September 22, 1992 | *Live in New York City* album & home video (2001) recorded live at Madison Square Garden, New York, NY, June 29, 2000 | *Live in Dublin* album and home video (2007) recorded live at the Depot, Dublin, Ireland, November 19, 2006

Live premiere: 06/15/1992—Globe Arena, Stockholm, Sweden

Recorded sometime from July to December 1991 at Thrill Hill West, (Springsteen's Los Angeles home studio), "If I Should Fall Behind" is a tender letter of devotion to wife Scialfa, as they navigated a new life (the couple had their first child in 1990 and were married in 1991). As Springsteen told a 1992 crowd in California, "This is my best song about making even small connections."

The song was regularly performed on the 1999 E Street Band Reunion tour: Springsteen, Little Steven Van Zandt, Clarence Clemons, and Patti Scialfa took turns singing. A "waltz" rendition is on *Live in Dublin*.

Living Proof

©1992 Bruce Springsteen, Roy Bittan (GMR)

Released on *Lucky Town* album (1992) | *In Concert/MTV Plugged* album & home video (1992) recorded live at Warner Hollywood Studios, Los Angeles, CA, September 22, 1992

Live premiere: 05/09/1992—Studio 8, GE Building, Rockefeller Center, New York, NY

"Living Proof" is the first song that Springsteen wrote for the *Lucky Town* album. At the end of the *Human Touch* album he still felt the need for another song and wrote "Living Proof," about fatherhood. Children are the "living proof" of our belief in one another, that love is real.

Springsteen premiered the song during his *Saturday Night Live* appearance in 1992.

Long Time Comin'

©2005 Bruce Springsteen, Roy Bittan (GMR)

Released on *Devils & Dust* album (2005)

Live premiere: 10/16/1996—Paramount Theater, Denver, CO

Springsteen said that he considers "Long Time Comin'" a sort of conclusion of "My Father's House," which is "probably the best song I've written about my dad," he wrote in his autobiography.[210]

Written for *The Ghost of Tom Joad* and finished in 1996 while on the Solo Acoustic Tour, the song was released on the *Devils & Dust* album of 2005. The recording is a hybrid of two sessions quite some years apart. The basic track (Springsteen, Danny Federici, Marty Rifkin, Soozie Tyrell, and Patti Scialfa) dates from 1997 or 1998. The bass guitar (Brendan O'Brien) and drums (Steve Jordan) were added to the mix in 2004.

"Long Time Comin'" is one of the few optimistic songs in Springsteen's canon. "I don't write too many happy songs," Springsteen said, introducing it in Paris on May 25, 1997; "because I found that the public in general doesn't like 'em, number one; and two, they come back and they bite you in the ass later, you know. You're real happy about something, and you'll see it comes back and gets you. 'Take that, Mr. Happy Song Writer!' That does happen. But this one I wrote in spite of myself."

[i] Is it the "little girl" from "Rosalita" all grown up?

Epilogue

Long Walk Home

©2007 Bruce Springsteen (GMR)

Released on: *Magic* album (2007)

Live premiere: 11/11/2006—Wembley Arena, London, England

Premiered live as "Gonna Be a Long Walk Home" at Wembley Arena in November 2006 during the Seeger Sessions Tour, "Long Walk Home" was released one year later on the *Magic* album, and it was #8 on *Rolling Stone*'s list of the 100 Best Songs of 2007.

The song reflects a turbulent time in America, marked by economic decline, constitutional decay, and endless foreign wars. It's no accident that this is the song Springsteen quoted when he endorsed Barack Obama for president in 2008. "He speaks to the America I've envisioned in my music for the past 35 years," Springsteen said. "A place where 'nobody crowds you, and nobody goes it alone.'"[211]

"There's a line from 'Long Walk Home,'" Springsteen said, "that has tremendous power. A father tells his son that the flag flying above the courthouse means 'certain things are set in stone . . . what we'll do and what we won't.' But we live in a moment where those things aren't set in stone. No, because those things have been chipped away at horrendously. Who would have ever thought we'd live in a country with no right to habeas corpus? That's Orwellian. That's what political hysteria is about and how effective it is. I felt it in myself. You get frightened for your family, for your home. And you realize how countries can move way off course, very far from democratic ideals. Add another terrorist attack or two, and the country can turn into a pretty scary place. Philip Roth caught it in *The Plot Against America*: It happens in a very American way—the flag is flying over civil liberties as they crumble. It was a fascinating insight."[212]

---

1. Bruce Springsteen. *Songs.*

2. Bruce Springsteen, quoted in Dave Marsh, *Born to Run.*

3. Peter Carlin. *Bruce.*

4. Christopher Sandford. *Springsteen: Point Blank.*

5. Ibid.

6. Ibid.

7. Flannery O'Connor, "The Turkey," in *The Complete Stories* (New York: Farrar, Straus and Giroux, 1989).

8. Ibid.

9. Maureen Orth, Janet Huck, and Peter S. Greenberg, "The Making of a Rock Star."

10. June Skinner Sawyers. *Tougher than the Rest.*

11. Bob Crane, *A Place to Stand. A Guide to Bruce Springsteen's Sense of Place* (Baltimore: Palace Book, 2002).

12. T.C. Boyle, *Greasy Lake and Other Stories* (New York: Viking Penguin, 1985).

13. Torsten Mörke, "Interview with David Hazlett" posted November 2000, http://www.castiles.net/.

14. Ken Emerson, "Springsteen Goes Gritty and Serious."

15. Ariel Swartley, "The Wild, the Innocent & the E Street Shuffle."

16. Patrick Humphries, *The Complete Guide to the Music of Bruce Springsteen* (New York: Omnibus Press, 1996).

17. Dave Marsh. *Born to Run.*

18. Clarence Clemons and Don Reo, *Big Man: Real Life & Tall Tales* (New York: Grand Central Publishing, 2009).

19. Robert Kirkpatrick, *The Words and Music of Bruce Springsteen.*

20. Dave Marsh. *Born to Run.*

21. "The Lost Interviews. 1975."

22. "The Lost Interviews. 1975."

23. Phil Sutcliffe, "You Talking to Me?" *Mojo*, January 2006.

24. Brian Hiatt, "Bruce Springsteen on Making 'Born to Run': 'We Went to Extremes,'" *Rolling Stone*, August 25, 2015.

25. Greil Marcus, "Springsteen's Thousand and One American Nights.'Born to Run' Album Review," *Rolling Stone*, October 9, 1975.

26. Jim Beviglia, "The 10 Best Bruce Springsteen Songs of All Time: Bowing Out as an HBO Documentary Beckons," posted August 8, 2010, http://houston.culturemap.com/

27. Bob Crane, *A Place to Stand.*

28. Jim Beviglia, "The 10 Best Bruce Springsteen Songs of All Time."

29. Dave Marsh, "Bruce Springsteen: A Rock Star Is Born," *Rolling Stone*, September 25, 1975.

30. Jim Beviglia, "The 10 best Bruce Springsteen songs of all time."

31. Brian Hiatt, "Bruce Springsteen on Making 'Born to Run.'"

32. Bruce Springsteen interviewed by Elvis Costello on Spectacle television show, September 25, 2009 and October 27, 2010, now in *Talk About a Dream. The Essential Interviews of Bruce Springsteen.*

33. "Bruce Springsteen's 40 Greatest Songs," *Uncut*, February 17, 2015.

34. Dave Marsh. *Glory Days.*

35. Peter Knobler, "I Was the Girl in the Song," *More*, April 2008.

36. David Horovitz, "Bruce Springsteen's Kibbutz Violinist," *The Jerusalem Post*, October 22, 2007.

37. Stephen Crane, "Parades and Entertainments," *The New York Tribune*, August 21, 1892.

38. Daniel Wolff, *4th of July, Asbury Park: A History of the Promised Land* (New York: Bloomsbury, 2006).

39. Greil Marcus, "Springsteen's Thousand and One American Nights."

40. Ibid.

41. Chris Roberts, "Born to Run," in "Bruce Springsteen's 40 Greatest Songs."

42. Louis P. Masur, "Tramps Like Us."

43. David Kamp, "The Book of Bruce Springsteen."

44. Bruce Springsteen quoted in David Remnick, "We Are Alive," *The New Yorker*, July 30, 2012.

45. Brian Hiatt, "Bruce Springsteen on Making 'Born to Run.'"

46. Antonio Monda, *La magnifica illusione. Un viaggio nel cinema americano* (Roma: Fazi, 2007).

47. *Patrick* Humphries and Chris Hunt, *Bruce Springsteen: Blinded by the Light* (London: Plexus, 1985).

48. Dave Marsh. *Born to Run.*

49. Robert Kirkpatrick, *The Words and Music of Bruce Springsteen.*

50. Jim Cullen, *Born in the U.S.A.: Bruce Springsteen and the American Tradition* (Middletown: Wesleyan University Press, 2005).

51. Dave Marsh. *Born to Run.*

52. "Badlands," in *Chambers's Encyclopaedia*, Vol. 2 (London: George Newnes, 1961).

53. Bruce Springsteen, quoted in David Remnick, "We Are Alive."

54. "100 Greatest Bruce Springsteen Songs of All Time." *Rolling Stone*, January 16, 2014.

55. Bruce Springsteen, quoted in Dave Marsh, "Bruce Springsteen Raises Cain," *Rolling Stone*, August 24, 1978.

56. Clinton Heylin, *Springsteen Song by Song: A Critical Look* (New York: Viking Books, 2012).

57. Lenny Kaye, quoted in "100 Greatest Bruce Springsteen Songs of All Time."

58. James E. Perone, *The Album: A Guide to Pop Music's Most Provocative, Influential, and Important Creations*, Volume 1 (Santa Barbara: Praeger, 2012).

59. Greil Marcus, *In the Fascist Bathroom: Punk in Pop Music, 1977–1992* (Cambridge: Harvard University Press, 1999).

60. Keith Phipps, "The Restless Dreams and Lonely Highways of Two-Lane Blacktop," *The Dissolve*, May 26, 2015.

61. Mikal Gilmore, "Bruce Springsteen's America," In *Night Beat: A Shadow History of Rock & Roll* (New York: Anchor, 1998).

62. John Milward, quoted in Dave Marsh. *Born to Run.*

63. Ibid.

64. Peter Ames Carlin. *Bruce.*

65. Ibid.

66. "100 Greatest Bruce Springsteen Songs of All Time."

67. Bruce Springsteen, quoted in Caryn Rose, "Somerville Nights," *Backstreets* #76, Winter/Spring 2003.

68. Alessandro Portelli, *Badlands.*

69. Clinton Heylin, *E Street Shuffle: The Glory Days of Bruce Springsteen and the E Street Band* (London: Constable, 2012).

70. Flannery O'Connor, "The River," In *A Good Man Is Hard to Find* (San Diego: Harcourt, Brace and Company, 1955).

71. Clinton Heylin, *E Street Shuffle.*

72. Rob Kirkpatrick, *Magic in the Night.*

73. The phrase "evil empire" was first applied to the Soviet Union in 1983 by Ronald Reagan.

74. Greil Marcus, *In the Fascist Bathroom.*

75. Bryan K. Garman, "The Ghost of History."

76. An unreliable narrator is a narrator whose credibility has been seriously compromised. The term was coined in 1961 by literary critic Wayne C. Booth, who distinguished between a reliable and unreliable narrator on the grounds of whether the narrator's speech violates or conforms with general norms and values. He writes, 'I have called a narrator *reliable* when he speaks for or acts in accordance with the norms of the work (which is to say the implied author's norms), *unreliable* when he does not.' Wayne C. Booth, *The Rhetoric of Fiction* (Chicago: University of Chicago Press, 1961). Discernible types of unreliable narrators are the picaro (a narrator who is characterized by exaggeration and bragging); the madman (a narrator who is either only experiencing mental defense mechanisms, such as posttraumatic dissociation and self-alienation, or severe mental illness, such as schizophrenia or paranoia); the clown (a narrator who does not take narrations seriously and consciously plays with conventions, truth, and the reader's expectations); the naïf (a narrator whose perception is immature or limited through his or her point of view); and the liar (a mature narrator of sound cognition who deliberately misrepresents themselves, often to obscure their unseemly or discreditable past conduct).

77. Greil Marcus, *In the Fascist Bathroom*.

78. Mikal Gilmore, "Bruce Springsteen's America."

79. Jim Cullen. *Born in the U.S.A.*

80. Klaus D. Heissenberger, "An All-American Body? Bruce Springsteen's Working-Class Masculinity in the 1980s," in *The EmBodyment of American Culture*, ed. Heinz Tschachler, Maureen Devine, and Michael Draxlbauer (Münster: LIT Verlag, 2003).

81. Bruce Springsteen, quoted in Dave Marsh, "Springsteen," *Musician*, February 1981.

82. Tom Roland, "Bruce Springsteen's Enduring Effect on the Country Charts Influences Two Top 10 Singles," *Billboard*, May 8, 2012.

83. "Honest to God, I know I should know who you are, but I'm just drawing a blank," Beaver told him on the phone. They talked for an half an hour about Starkweather and Fugate. Playing Lincoln in 1984, Springsteen dedicated the song to Beaver, who attended as his guest.

84. Bruce Springsteen, *Songs*.

85. Bob Dylan, quoted in Bill Flanagan, *Written in My Soul: Conversations With Rock's Great Songwriters* (Chicago: Contemporary Books, 1987).

86. Paul Nelson, "Bruce Springsteen: 'Nebraska,'" *Musician*, November 1982.

87. Flannery O'Connor, "A Good Man Is Hard to Find," In *A Good Man Is Hard to Find*.

88. Bruce Springsteen, *Songs*.

89. In January 1982, Springsteen sent a cassette comprised of fourteen demos to Jon Landau, along with what is almost certainly a live recording, not a studio demo, of a fifteenth song, "Johnny Bye Bye," often played in 1981 during the River Tour. "Nebraska," "Atlantic City," "Mansion on the Hill," "Johnny 99," "Highway Patrolman," "State Trooper," "Used Cars," "Open All Night," and "Reason to Believe" were published on the *Nebraska* album in the stripped-down versions that Landau heard on the cassette. "Vietnam" (the future "Born in the U.S.A"), "Downbound Train," and "Child Bride" (the future "Working on the Highway") were recorded by the E Street Band and published on the *Born in the U.S.A.* album. "Pink Cadillac" and "Johnny Bye Bye" were recorded by the E Street Band and published respectively on the "Dancing in the Dark" and "I'm on Fire" singles. "Losin' Kind" was never released. Two or three months later, with a few of these fifteen songs by then earmarked for coverage by the E Street Band, Springsteen recorded two additional songs ("My Father's House" and "The Big Payback") at home on the same equipment, thus making a total of seventeen different songs.

90. Bruce Springsteen, quoted in Roger Cott and Patrick Humphries, "American Heartbeat: The Bruce Springsteen Interview," *Hot Press*, November 2, 1984.

91. Bruce Springsteen, quoted in Dave Marsh, *Glory Days*.

92. Peter Gambaccini, *Bruce Springsteen* (London: Omnibus Press, 1981).

93. Bruce Springsteen, quoted in Mark Hagen, "Midnight Cowboy."

94. Bruce Springsteen, quoted in *Talk About a Dream. The Essential Interviews of Bruce Springsteen.* Ed. Christopher Phillips and Louis P. Masur. New York: Bloomsbury Press, 2013.

95. Andrew E. Massimino, "And the Next Day . . ." *Backstreets* #83/84, Winter 2005/2006.

96. Alessandro Portelli, *Badlands*.

97. Dave Marsh. *Glory Days*.

98. Melissa Milazzo, "Bruce Springsteen: Reason to Believe," posted May 10, 2010, http://melissamilazzo.wordpress.com/

99. Caryn Rose, "10 of the Best: Bruce Springsteen," *The Guardian*, March 19, 2014.

100. Max Weinberg interviewed by *Backstreets* in 1984, quoted in "100 Greatest Bruce Springsteen Songs of All Time."

101. Bruce Springsteen interviewed by *Pop* in 1998, quoted in Erik Flannigan and Christopher Phillips, "'Tracks:' The Backstreets Liner Notes," *Backstreets* #61, Winter 1998.

102. Bruce Springsteen. *Songs*.

103. Ibid.

104. Bruce Springsteen, quoted in Dave Marsh, *Glory Days*.

105. June Skinner Sawyers. *Tougher than the Rest*.

106. Bobbie Ann Mason, *In Country*.

107. Erik Flannigan and Christopher Phillips, "'Tracks.'"

108. Jim Cullen, *Born in the U.S.A.*

109. Mikal Gilmore, "'The Ghost of Tom Joad.'"

110. Springsteen interviewed by Nicholas Dawidoff for *The New York Times* in 1997, quoted in Marya Morris, "Geography and Place. From 'My Hometown' to 'This Hard Land': Bruce Springsteen's Use of Geography, Landscapes, and Places to Depict the American Experience," *Interdisciplinary Literary Studies*, Vol. 9, No. 1, Glory Days: A Bruce Springsteen Celebration, Penn State University Press, Fall 2007.

111. Bruce Springsteen, introduction to Dale Maharidge, *Journey to Nowhere—The Saga of the New Underclass*.

112. Marya Morris, "Geography and Place."

113. Bruce Springsteen, quoted in Robert Everett-Green, "Springsteen Is No Less than Storyteller-in-Chief for His Generation," *Toronto Globe and Mail*, July 16, 2005.

114. Abby Ronner, "Giddy Out: Will New York's federation of Black Cowboys Be Sent Packing?" *The Village Voice*, April 20, 2016.

115. Terry G. Jordan, *North American Cattle Ranching Frontiers: Origins, Diffusion, and Differentiation* (Albuquerque: University of New Mexico Press, 1993).

116. Nicholas Dawidoff, "The Pop Populist," *The New York Time Magazine*, January 26, 1997.

117. Bruce Springsteen, quoted in Christopher Phillips, "With These Hands," *Backstreets* #83/84, Winter 2005/2006.

118. Jim Beviglia, *Counting Down Bruce Springsteen: His 100 Finest Songs* (Lanham: Rownman & Littlefield, 2014).

119. Arthur Conan Doyle, "Bendigo's Sermon." In *Songs of the Road* (London: Smith, Elder & Co., 1911).

120. Bruce Springsteen, interviewed by Bob Costas for Columbia Radio Hour, November 1995. Now in *Talk About a Dream*.

121. "Tom Joad" is divided into two parts and was originally released in 1940 on Guthrie's *Dust Bowl Ballads Volume 1*. Springsteen played it a few times in 1996 and 1997.

122. "George Bush Meet Woodrow Wilson," *New York Times*, November 20, 1990.

123. John Steinbeck, *The Grapes of Wrath*.

124. Marya Morris, "Geography and Place."

125. Dale Maharidge, *Journey to Nowhere—The Saga of the New Underclass*.

126. Bruce Springsteen, quoted in David Masciotra, *Working on a Dream: The Progressive Political Vision of Bruce Springsteen* (New York: Continuum, 2010).

127. Christopher Phillips, "With These Hands."

128. Bruce Springsteen, quoted in Caryn Rose. "Somerville Nights."

129. Christopher Phillips. "The Devil's in the Details," *Backstreets* #83/84, Winter 2005/2006.

130. Bruce Springsteen, quoted in Christopher Phillips, "The Devil's in the Details."

131. Bruce Springsteen, quoted in Jon Pareles, "Bruce Almighty." *The New York Times*, April 24, 2005.

132. John Steinbeck, *The Grapes of Wrath*.

133. Jon Pareles, "Music; His Kind of Heroes, His Kind of Songs," *The New York Times*, July 14, 2002.

134. Susan Hamburger, "'Bruce, We Need You Now': Bruce Springsteen's Response to 9/11 with 'The Rising" (Paper read at the South Atlantic Modern Language Association meeting, Durham, NC, November 9, 2012).

135. Scott Calef, "A Little of That Human Touch: Knowledge and Empathy in the Music of Bruce Springsteen," in *Bruce Springsteen and Philosophy: Darkness on the Edge of Truth*. Popular Culture and Philosophy, Vol. 32, ed. Randall E. Auxier and Doug Anderson (Chicago: Open Court, 2008).

136. Christopher Phillips. "Searchin' Through the Dust."

137. Bruce Springsteen, introducing "Magic" at Civic Center, Hartford, Connecticut, October 2, 2007.

138. Bruce Springsteen, quoted in Andrew E. Massimino and Christopher Phillips. "Beyond the Songs." *Backstreets* #75, Fall 2002.

139. June Skinner Sawyers. *Tougher than the Rest*.

140. Philip Hausler, "Wheels of Fire," *Backstreets* #75, Fall 2002.

141. Bruce Springsteen, quoted in Adam Sweeting, "Into the Fire." *Uncut*, September 2002.

142. Mark Binelli, "Bruce Springsteen's American Gospel."

143. Ibid.

144. Marc Dolan, *Bruce Springsteen and the Promise of Rock 'n' Roll* (New York: W.W. Norton and Company, 2012).

145. Dave Marsh, *Two Hearts*.

146. Bruce Springsteen, quoted in Andrew E. Massimino and Christopher Phillips, "Beyond the Songs."

147. John Bussey, "The Eye of the Storm: One Man's Journey Through Desperation and Chaos," *The Wall Street Journal*, September 12, 2001.

148. Christopher Phillips, "Searchin' Through the Dust."

149. In 2004, *Rolling Stone* magazine selected this concert as one of the 50 Moments that Changed Rock 'n' Roll.

150. Bruce Springsteen, quoted in Adam Sweeting, "Into the Fire."

151. Brendan O'Brien, quoted in Joe Levy, "Bruce Springsteen's Restless Heart: The Rolling Stone Interview," *Rolling Stone*, October 17, 2007.

152. Ibid.

153. Bruce Springsteen, quoted in Sean Sennett, "Bruce Springsteen Q&A: On Top Down Under," *Rolling Stone*, March 11, 2014.

154. Ron Aniello, quoted in Andy Greene, "Bruce Springsteen Producer Breaks Down 'High Hopes': Exclusive," *Rolling Stone*, December 30, 2013.

155. Bruce Springsteen, quoted in "Bruce Springsteen: By the Book."

156. Brendan O'Brien, quoted in Joe Levy. "Bruce Springsteen's Restless Heart."

157. Bruce Springsteen, quoted in Christopher Phillips. "The Devil's in the Details."

158. Bruce Springsteen, quoted in Brian Hiatt, "Springsteen Goes Back to Basics."

159. Bruce Springsteen quoted in Renée Montagne. "Springsteen discusses his latest release, Part 1." National public Radio's *Morning Edition*, April 26, 2005.

160. Bruce Springsteen interviewed on December 19, 2013 during Dave Marsh's *Live From E Street Nation* show on Sirius XM's E Street Radio channel. The interview premiered on January 10, 2014.

161. Bruce Springsteen, quoted in Elysa Gardner, "Illustrator Draws on the Boss for 'Outlaw Pete' book," *USA Today*, November 3, 2014.

162. Bruce Springsteen, quoted in Mark Hagen, "Meet the New Boss." *The Guardian*, January 18, 2009.

163. Frank Caruso, quoted in Elysa Gardner, "Illustrator Draws on the Boss for 'Outlaw Pete' book."

164. Mickey Rourke, quoted in Edward Douglas, "Mickey Rourke Piledrives The Wrestler," Coming Soon, December 17, 2008.

165. Bruce Springsteen, quoted in Mark Hagen. "Meet the New Boss."

166. Darren Aronowsky, quoted in "Aronofsky Quizzed Springsteen over One-legged Dog Line," *IMDb*, November 26, 2010.

167. Tim Appelo, "Bruce Springsteen's New Album Is His 'Angriest' Yet," *Hollywood Reporter*, January 13, 2012.

168. Bruce Springsteen, International Press Conference at Théâtre Marigny, Paris, France, February 16, 2012.

169. Bruce Springsteen, quoted in Benjamin Hart, "Bruce Springsteen Talks Occupy Movement, New Album," *The Huffington Post*, February 18, 2012.

170. Simon Firth, "The Real Thing—Bruce Springsteen," in *Music for Pleasure: Essays in the Sociology of Pop* (New York: Routledge, 1988).

171. John Steinbeck, *The Grapes of Wrath*.

172. Bruce Springsteen, International Press Conference at Théâtre Marigny, Paris, France, February 16, 2012.

173. Ibid.

174. Alessandro Portelli, *Badlands*.

175. Bruce Springsteen, at the International Press Conference in Paris, Théâtre Marigny, February 16, 2012.

176. Bruce Springsteen. *Born to Run.*

177. Frank Kent, quoted in David G. Farber, *Sloan Rules: Alfred P. Sloan and the Triumph of General Motors* (Chicago: University of Chicago Press, 2012).

178. Ed Vulliamy, "Bruce Springsteen: Last of the Protest Singers," *The Guardian*, June 9, 2012.

179. Bob Russell, "Bruce Springsteen: 'Wrecking Ball,'" *Pop Culture Ponderings*, April 9, 2012.

180. Jesse P. Karlsberg and John Plunkett, "Bruce Springsteen's sacred Harp Sample," posted March 28, 2012, http://originalsacredharp.com/

181. Bruce Springsteen, quoted in Jon Pareles, "Music; His Kind of Heroes, His Kind of Songs."

182. Bruce Springsteen, quoted in "Bruce Springsteen: 'I Cried When I Heard Clarence Clemons on "Wrecking Ball,"' *New Musical Express*, March 14, 2012.

183. Dave Marsh, *Bruce Springsteen on Tour: 1968–2005* (New York: Bloomsbury, 2006).

184. Bruce Springsteen. *Born to Run.*

185. Bruce Springsteen, International Press Conference in Paris, Théâtre Marigny, February 16, 2012.

186. Jay Reeves, "Case closed; Cherry Guilty," *Times Daily*, May 23, 2002.

187. Garry Tallent, quoted in Peter Ames Carlin, *Bruce*.

188. Bruce Springsteen, quoted in Larry Rodgers, "Bruce Springsteen, Born in the U.S.A., 25 Years Old Today," *The Arizona Republic*, June 4, 2009.

189. Dave Marsh. *Glory Days*.

190. Bruce Springsteen, quoted in Erik Flannigan and Christopher Phillips, "'Tracks.'"

191. Bruce Springsteen, quoted in Dave Marsh. *Glory Days*.

192. Ibid.

193. Ibid.

194. It was kept off the #1 spot by Duran Duran's "The Reflex" and Prince's ""When Doves Cry."

195. Kevin Coyne, "Story Behind the Glory," *Cape Cod Times*, July 10, 2011.

196. Bruce Springsteen, quoted in Larry Rodgers, "Bruce Springsteen, Born in the U.S.A., 25 Years Old Today."

197. Peter Ames Carlin. *Bruce*.

198. Bruce Springsteen, quoted in Neil Strauss, "Human Touch," *Guitar World*, October 1995.

199. Bruce Springsteen quoted in Mark Hagen, "Meet the New Boss."

200. Jim Beviglia, "Counting Down Bruce Springsteen: #48, 'The Last Carnival,'" *American Songwriter*, June 30, 2014.

201. John Pareles, "Springsteen Looks at Love," *The New York Times*, October 4, 1987.

202. Sarfraz Manzoor, "My Favourite Album: 'Tunnel of Love' by Bruce Springsteen," *The Guardian*, August 31, 2011.

203. David Remnick. "We Are Alive."

204. Bruce Springsteen, quoted in Erik Flannigan and Christopher Phillips, "'Tracks'"

205. Ibid.

206. Bruce Springsteen quoted in Caryn Rose, "Somerville Nights."

207. Win Butler, quoted in "100 Greatest Bruce Springsteen Songs of All Time."

208. Bob Crane, *A Place to Stand.*

209. June Skinner Sawyers. *Tougher than the Rest.*

210. Bruce Springsteen. *Born to Run.*

211. Bruce Springsteen in a letter to fans published on his official website in 2008.

212. Bruce Springsteen, quoted in Joe Levy, "The E Street Band Chief Talks About Making His Most Romantic Record Since 'Born to Run.'"

APPENDIX

by Leonardo Colombati

Biography

1949

On September 23, Bruce Frederick Springsteen is born at Long Branch Hospital, New Jersey, first child of Douglas Springsteen and Adele Zerilli. That very evening, President Truman announces that a "nuclear detonation" has occurred in the USSR.

Bruce's father, Doug, is of Dutch and Irish ancestry. He quit his studies at Freehold Regional School after his freshman year in 1941, taking a job in Freehold's Karagheusian rug mill until June 1943, when at eighteen he joined the army and was sent to Europe in the midst of the war. "He served as a truck driver at the Battle of the Bulge, saw what little of the world he was going to see and returned home," Springsteen wrote in his autobiography. Back in Freehold, he began to work on the factory floor of Ford auto plant in nearby Edison.

Bruce's mother, Adele, is of Italian ancestry. She has a full-time job as a secretary for a real estate lawyerwhen she marries Doug Springsteen on February 22, 1947, and moves to 87 Randolph Street—the house of Doug's parents, Fred and Alice—in Freehold.

1950

On December 8, Virginia ("Ginny") Springsteen is born. Bruce's sister will be portrayed in "The River."

1952

Bruce's maternal grandmother, Adelina, sings "Pony Boy" to Bruce in the crib (he will record the song and release it on his 1992 *Human Touch* album). Aged three, he listens to the country & western hits from Nashville: Gene Autry, Roy Rogers, and his favorite, Hank Williams.

1954

The family moves out of Bruce's grandmother house to a small, half-shotgun-style house at 39½ Institute Street. Bruce feels his grandparents' place to be his true home. The new house instead is a mess, with no hot running water, where family relationships lack stability. Bruce's grandmother is devoted to him, and his mother is loyal to her brooding and unstable husband, but rules are nonexistent. Bruce stays up until three in the morning and sleeps until three in the afternoon. He eats when and whatever he wants. Bruce would later recall that in that house he was a "timid little tyrant."

His father Doug has just taken work at the county jail. He comes back home at night and get drunk sitting at the kitchen table in the dark with a cigarette in his mouth, often depressed and harshly judgmental. Much later, he will be diagnosed with paranoid schizophrenia.

1955

Bruce begins school life as a first grader at St. Rose of Lima Catholic School.

1957

Bruce's parents let him stay up late to watch the last of the three famous Elvis Presley TV appearances on the *Ed Sullivan Show*. The January 6 performance is the infamous "from the waist-up only" broadcast. As Springsteen recalls, "Seventy million Americans that night were exposed to this hip-shaking human earthquake." The seven-year-old boy tells his parents he wants a guitar like Elvis's, and within a few weeks his mother rents a small, semi-toy acoustic (no amp) from Diehl's Music on South Street in Freehold. However, other than posing in the mirror, Bruce loses interest in trying to learn how to play, finding it too difficult.

1962

In February, Adele Springsteen gives birth to her and Douglas's third child, a daughter they name Pamela. The family moves to a white house at 68 South Street.

Fred Springsteen dies and the widowed Alice—Bruce's grandmother—moves in with her son's family, while the bulldozer knocks down their family house on Randolph Street. Bruce's beloved place, his sanctuary, is condemned to be turned into a parking lot. He later confesses that he didn't return there for many years, because he realized that it was the place he loved the most.

On June 29, Bruce's mother, Adele, takes him and his sister Ginny to see their first concert, a Chubby Checker matinee.

1963

Having saved up some money doing odd jobs, Bruce purchases a secondhand acoustic guitar (no amp) for eighteen dollars at Freehold's Western Auto Appliance Store. Bruce's first cousin Frank Bruno provides some introductory lessons. The first song he learns is "Greensleeves."

In May, Bruce graduates from St. Rose of Lima and tell his parents he does not wish to attend a Catholic high school. In September, he begins his freshman year at Freehold Regional High School and turns fourteen years old.

His relationship with his father is far from good, and is destined to worsen in the ensuing years.

1964

On February 9, Bruce, along with over seventy-three million other Americans, watches the Beatles' debut live appearance on American television on *The Ed Sullivan Show*. This, along with subsequent TV appearances during 1964 of other "British Invasion" bands—such as the Dave Clark Five, the Rolling Stones, the Kinks, and especially the Animals—has a profound, inspirational impact on Bruce. He begins to spend much of his time listening to records and practicing his acoustic guitar. The first rock 'n' roll song he learns is the Beatles' version of "Twist and Shout."

In December, Bruce's mother, knowing of his strong wish to have an electric guitar, takes out a personal loan for sixty dollars and buys Bruce a Japanese-made "Kent" electric guitar and amplifier package as a Christmas present at Caiazzo's Music Store on Central Street. "It sounded awful, distorted beyond recognition," Springsteen recalls in his autobiography. But, as he told *Newsweek* writer Maureen Orth in the famous 1975 cover story, "The first day I can remember lookin' in the mirror and standin' what I was seein' was the day I had a guitar in my hand."

1965

Together with a guy named Donnie Powell, who plays the drums, Bruce forms a duo called the Merchants and starts to play in Donnie's living room while his parents are out. A few other neighborhood kids soon come in and form a band now called the Rogues: with Bruce there are a guy called Jay, with a Gibson guitar and a real amp; another guy called Jimmy McGuire on the bass guitar; and Craig Caprioni on vocals. The band practices in the basement of 68 Barkalow Avenue—Craig Caprioni's house—and has their first show at the Freehold Elks Club in front of about seventy-five locals, ending with with the band's "secret weapon": Bruce singing "Twist and Shout."

In the meantime, Bruce's classmate George Theiss at Freehold Regional High School has formed a band called the Five Diamonds, soon abandoning them to form the Sierras along with Vinnie Roslin on bass, Mike DeLouise on guitar, and Bart Haynes on drums. The thirty-two-year-old Gordon "Tex" Vinyard opens his house to the Sierras and proposes himself as their manager. Bass player Frank Marziotti is added to the band, whose name has changed to the Castiles.

In June, Springsteen knocks at Tex Vinyard's door, asking for an audition as the guitarist of George Theiss's band. He plays some chords, and Vinyard tells him to come back with some more songs, which he does, showing up the following night with five songs, Vinyard says, "that would blow your ears off." Bruce tells him that he just learned them just by listening to them on the radio.

After visiting and performing alone for Tex Vinyard, Springsteen is invited for a tryout rehearsal with the four already hired members (George Theiss, Frank Marziotti, Bart Haynes, and singer Danny Hyland) present. Everyone is impressed and Springsteen is given the job, thus completing the formal band lineup. They will spend the next six weeks or so rehearsing and developing a repertoire before performing publicly.

The first Castiles gig is in August at the Angle-Inn Trailer Park on Route 33, just east of the Shore Drive-In. The group's growing repertoire includes songs by the Rolling Stones ("The Last Time"), the Kinks ("All Day and All of the Night"), the Who (an instrumental version of "My Generation"), the Beatles ("Twist and Shout"), and Them ("Mystic Eyes"), but also such numbers as Ray Charles's "What'd I Say," Glenn Miller's "In the Mood," and Henry Mancini's "Moon River." By the time of this show original member Danny Hyland has been replaced by Richie Goldstein, who leaves after few shows, replaced by Paul Popkin. At this point the band consists of George Theiss (guitar and vocals), Bruce Springsteen (guitar and vocals), Frank Marziotti (bass), Paul Popkin (vocals and tambourine), and Bart Haynes (drums).

In July, Bruce attends a concert of a band called the Mates held at the Clearwater Pool in Middletown, New Jersey, making friends with the guitarist, Steve Van Zandt.

In October, the Castiles play at a wedding party in Monmouth County, New Jersey. New songs are included in the setlist, like Sonny & Cher's "I Got You Babe," the Yardbirds' "For Your Love," the Shadows' "Walk Don't Run," the Beatles' "Money (That's What I Want)," and the Rolling Stones' "Tell Me." There is also an original song, "Sidewalk," cowritten by Bruce—one of his earliest creations.

1966

In January, the Castiles' drummer, Bart Haynes, gives up the sticks for good and joins the Marines. He will be killed in action by mortar fire in Vietnam. Vinnie "Skeebots" Mannello replaces him.

On April 22, the Castiles participate in a "Battle of the Bands" orchestrated by promoter Norman Seldin, featuring twenty-five local groups, at Matawan-Keyport Roller Drome in Matawan, New Jersey. Springsteen, Vini Lopez (future E Street

Band drummer) and Vinnie Roslin (future Steel Mill bass guitarist) meet for the first time at this event.

In May, Frank Marziotti leaves the band, replaced by new bass player Curt Fluhr. A few days later, on May 18, the Castiles record two songs at Mr. Music Inc. Studio in Bricktown, New Jersey. Seven or eight acetate test pressings of the studio takes of "Baby I" and "That's What You Get"—both written by Springsteen and Theiss—are made (at least four of which survived). "Baby I" will be officially released on September 23, 2016, on *Chapter & Verse*, the companion album to Springsteen's autobiography *Born to Run*.

On Juy 3, Springsteen attends at a Rolling Stones concert at Asbury Park's Convention Hall.

In September, organist Bobby Alfano joins the Castiles. In December, the band plays some gigs at Café Wha? in New York City.

1967

The Castiles play more than thirty shows at Café Wha?

On June 19, Springsteen graduates. He walks into Freehold Regional to collect his cap only to be told that he will be barred from the auditorium unless he gets his shoulder-length hair cut. He turns around and marches out the front door to catch a bus up to the Greenwich Village in New York.

In late July, Springsteen crushes his leg and suffers a concussion after being T-boned on his small Yamaha motorcycle by a Cadillac as he is on his way home to South Street. He is unconscious for thirty minutes while the ambulance drives him to the hospital in Neptune. Back home, while he is recovering in bed, his father brings the barber to crop his hair. After the motorcycle wreck, Bruce will walk with a slight drag.

On September 16, the Castiles are the main act for the grand opening night at the Left Foot, an "over thirteen, under eighteen" club located in the recreation center of St Peter's Episcopal Church at 37 Throckmorton Street. This is the only concert by the Castiles of which we have a complete (bootleg) recording. Bruce handles the lead vocals on almost all songs, including Jimi Hendrix's "Fire," "Hey Joe," and "Purple Haze," Sam & Dave's "Hold On, I'm Comin'," Moby Grape's "Omaha," and Willie Dixon's "You Can't Judge a Book by the Cover." Theiss sings on "Eleanor Rigby," the Kinks' "See My Friends," and the Blues Project's haunting "Steve's Song." The band also plays three original songs: "Sidewalk" and "Look into My Window," written by Springsteen and Theiss, and "Mr. Jones," written by Springsteen. A recording of "You Can't Judge a Book by the Cover" will be officially released on September 23, 2016, on *Chapter & Verse*.

His father's drinking problem worsens, while Bruce begins to attend a liberal arts course at the Ocean County College in Toms River in October.

1968

In January the Castiles shows continue at Cafe Wha? in New York, while Bruce is midway through his first year in college focusing his studies on English and earning good marks in his writing classes.

On February 19, Tom and Margaret Potter open the Upstage, a club on Cookman Avenue in Asbury Park. Bruce and his friends are already clients at the neighboring restaurant, the Green Mermaid, and that evening they play at the club's opening. The Upstage, open from eight at night till five in the morning, becomes the meeting spot for every musician on the Jersey Shore. The first weekend he is there, Bruce meets Danny Federici and Vini Lopez. A few weeks later he makes friends with Garry Tallent and Southside Johnny.

On March 10, the Castiles perform at the grand opening of the Hullaballoo franchise's Freehold location. "At the Hullabaloo you play fifty-five minutes on and five minutes off, all night long," Springsteen recalls. During one of those five-minute breaks, he again meets Steve Van Zandt, who is there as the front man of another band called the Shadows. This time something lights a spark and the two become friends, creating an all-rock 'n' roll world of their own.

In May, Springsteen gives the first of several solo performances at the Off Broad Street Coffee House, just opened to cater to the burgeoning singer-songwriter music scene taking hold at the time. These performances include an array of folk-oriented songs Bruce has written from late 1967 to mid-1968, material that doesn't fit into the rock setlists performed by the Castiles, bearing some similarity to the 1967–68 material of Tim Buckley, Leonard Cohen, and Donovan. Among these songs are "Clouds," "Slum Sentiments," "Sunline," "Death of a Good Man," "Inside the Castle Walls," "Alone," "For Never Asking," "The Virgin Flower," "A Winter's Revelation," and "The War Song."

On August 10, the Castiles play their last gig at Le Teendezvous, in New Shrewbury, New Jersey. Castiles founder George Theiss subsequently will join the already established local band Rusty Chain, while Bob Alfano and Vinnie Mannello will form Sunny Jim. Both Curt Flhur and Paul Popkin decide to forgo musical careers.

Influenced by hard-rocking psychedelic blues trios such as Cream and the Jimi Hendrix Experience, Springsteen forms the band Earth with bassist John Graham and drummer Michael Burke. In September, Earth plays at Bruce's college. The setlist includes the Jimi Hendrix Experience's "Fire," "Foxy Lady," and "Purple

Haze"; Cream's "Crossroads," "Politician," "Spoonful," "Swlabr," "Toad," and "Sunshine of Your Love"; "Traffic's "Dear Mr. Fantasy"; Steppenwolf's "Born to Be Wild"; Ten Years After's "Help Me"; the Moody Blues' "Another Morning"; the Yardbirds' "Smokestack Lightning"; the Doors' "Back Door Man"; and some traditional blues like "Slow Blues in G," "Fast Blues Break in G," and "Sitting on Top of the World."

Two Springsteen poems—"My Lady" and "Earth Children Turn Their New Eyes Upward"—are published in *Seascapes*, his school's literary yearbook. But during that fall, Springsteen drops out of college.

1969

Earth splits up on February 14, after a short, six-month existence.

February 22, at the Upstage, is the beginning of a new band called Child. They are Bruce Springsteen (vocals and guitar), Danny Federici (organ), Vinnie Roslin (bass), and Vini Lopez (drums). A few days later, Child conducts its first rehearsal at Carl "Tinker" West's Challenger Eastern Surfboards factory in Wanamassa, New Jersey. Tinker—a legendary surfboard designer/shaper with San Diego–based Challenger West Surfboards—came to the Jersey shore in 1966 and set up a concert promotion business called Blah Productions. Interested in new artists, Tinker becomes Child's manager and sound engineer, allowing the band to rehearse in his factory.

Child starts to play in various clubs on the Shore. Springsteen writes new songs for the band, including "Jennifer," "Sister Theresa," "Garden State Parkway Blues," "Resurrection," "The War Is Over," and "KT-88." On July 20, the band plays at the Pandemonium, in Wanamassa, the night that man first walks on the moon. Numerous TV monitors are installed inside the club for the occasion, creating a major distraction during Child's performance that upsets some of the band members—especially the always nervous Vini "Mad Dog" Lopez; an ensuing argument over the issue takes place between Lopez and the club's manager. Mad Dog becomes more and more aggressive with the audience, asking to turn "the fucking TV" off. The result is that the band is fired on the spot.

In summer, Springsteen is bused to a conscription exam in Trenton, and is rejected as "unfit" due to his motorbike wreck. When he goes home to South Street and admits he failed the induction, Doug says simply, "Good."

Most extraordinarily, Adele goes along with Doug's plan to pull up stakes and move with Bruce's seven-year-old sister, Pam, from their native Freehold to the promised land of California, with all of their belongings packed atop an AMC Rambler. By this point, the mental illness that runs in his family has befallen Doug, leading to bouts of paranoia and tears, and he is eager to start his life anew—even if it means leaving behind Bruce (who is not yet twenty) and his other daughter, Virginia, who is not only a mere eighteen but also a new wife and mother, having married the young man, Mickey Shave, who got her pregnant in her senior year of high school. (The Shaves are still happily married.)

Together with Vini Lopez and Danny Federici, Bruce takes over the rent for the house on South Street: his family home is instantly transformed into a hippie frat house. The three mates last only one month before they are thrown out by the landlord. Upon leaving Freehold, they take up residence a few block off the ocean in Bradley Beach.

In November, Springsteen learns that another progressive rock band from Long Island, New York, is not only using the name Child but has also just released an album under that name. Consequently, the band decides to change its name from Child to Steel Mill.

In December, Tinker West puts Steel Mill in his station wagon and leads them to California, where they have a paying New Year's Eve gig at the Esalen Insitute in the mountains of Big Sur—a hippie paradise inhabited by "spiritual seekers that believe they are being amoebas, going through phagocytosis," as Lopez recalls.

1970

In January and February Steel Mill is in California playing another gig at Esalen Institute, two gigs in Kentfield, and eight in San Francisco, three of which are at the legendary Fillmore West. Owner Bill Graham has seen one of Steel Mill's four performances at the Matrix and subsequently contacted the group, hiring them as a last-minute substitute for another act that canceled. Steel Mill impresses Graham, who invites them to make a studio demo session and offers the band a contract, which they reject due to its poor terms and conditions. In the second night at Fillmore West there is another up-and-coming young band, Maryland-based Grin, led by Nils Lofgren. It's the first time that Springsteen meets his future guitarist.

The setlists of these Californian gigs contain only songs penned by Springsteen, like the explosive "The Wind and the Rain" and a group of antiwar songs like "We'll All Man the Guns," "The War Is Over," "The War Song," and "America Under Fire" with a climactic coda of "America the Beautiful" including a sarcastic recital of the the Mickey Mouse Club theme song chorus. Epic songs, like the sprawling "Garden State Parkway Blues," often stretch to thirty minutes in performance. On February 22, Steel Mill makes a formal recording of three Springsteen compositions—"He's Guilty (The Judge Song)," "Goin' Back to Georgia," and "The Train Song"—at the Pacific Recording Studio in San Mateo, California, not too far from Doug and Adele Springsteen's home. Springsteen pays them a visit and stays over for a few days. One of the songs recorded in California, "He's Guilty (The Judge Song)," will be officially issued in September 2016 on *Chapter and Verse*.

The band drives nonstop for three days from California to Richmond, Virginia to make it on time to a gig at the Center. It's Vinnie Roslin's final performance as a member of Steel Mill. His place is taken by Steve Van Zandt, who debuts as Free Mill's bassist on March 27 at Richmond's Hullabaloo.

On August 14, Steel Mill plays its most famous concert under the stars at the 7th and Marshall Street Parking Deck in Richmond, headlining and closing a triple bill gig with blues band Mario & the Stingers and Mercy Flight. An audience tape of the gig will circulate for many years: the recorded twelve-song, 110-minute setlist—opened by "Dancing in the Streets" and closed by a ten-minute rendition of "Good Lovin' Woman"—is not the complete show. A day or so after this show Springsteen meets privately with Mercy Flight's lead singer Robbin Thompson and offers him a position in Steel Mill. Thompson accepts it.

On August 29, Steel Mill is among the twenty artists performing at Nashville's Centennial Park Band Shell for the third annual Nashville Music Festival, whose headliner is Springsteen's beloved Roy Orbison. The weather is lovely and the crowd is about 50,000, the largest audience Springsteen would play in front of until the 1980s. Springsteen will recall this show in his speech inducting Orbison into the Rock & Roll Hall of Fame in 1987.

On September 9, at the Clearwater Swim Club in Atlantic Highlands, New Jersey, Steel Mill plays a gig now steeped in folklore. In the band's lineup for this show is drummer Dave Hazlett, filling in for the absent Vini Lopez, who is stuck in Richmond due to a marijuana bust on a communal property where his girlfriend lives. Steel Mill wants to use its earnings from this show to help defray Vini's legal costs. Due to a number of complaints from nearby residents, town officials have lowered the curfew time for the concert from eleven o'clock to ten o'clock, and called for a much stronger police presence. Several audience arrests for marijuana possession raise tensions in the crowd. Then when ten o'clock comes around the police switch off the power to the instruments, escalating the event into a near-riot. During the ensuing mayhem, some sound equipment falls onto the local Chief of Police, and Danny Federici earns his famous nickname of "the Phantom" by disappearing from the melee with lightning speed. Charging him with assault on a police officer and resisting arrest, the police begin to search for him. Danny eventually will turn himself in and will be released on bail in November 1970.

On October 11, in Richmond, Steel Mill opens for Ike and Tina Turner. In the meantime Bruce's rock-burned ears yearn for new music. He's picked up on the FM radio stations and become enraptured first by Van Morrison's new His

Band and the Street Choir, then by Joe Cocker's *Mad Dogs & Englishmen*. As Springsteen recalls, he was interested in returning to his soul roots, and asked Mad Dog and Steve if they were willing to move forward with him into something completely different.

1971

Springsteen decides that Steel Mill is over. The band plays a gig on January 18 at South Amboy's D'Scene, another two at the Upstage, and then quit.

On March 18, Springsteen is billed as the headliner at a Jewish community-sponsored dance orchestrated by the Young Hebrew Association and held at Deal's Recreation Center in Deal, New Jersey. For the gig, he utilizes a four-piece backing band consisting of Lopez and Van Zandt, plus two new members: David Sancious on keyboards and Garry Tallent on bass. Patti Scialfa—at the time still in high school—attends the show and meets Bruce for the first time. They get married eighteen years later. For the time being, Bruce is seeing a girl by the name of Pam Bracken.

Bruce Springsteen & the Friendly Enemies (the temporary name chosen for the band) continue to play concerts and take members on board, until they become a small army. For a few shows to be held in May at the Sunshine Inn in Asbury Park, the band is re-baptized Dr. Zoom and the Sonic Boom. The members are Bruce Springsteen (vocals, guitar), Steve Van Zandt (guitar), David Sancious (keyboards), Garry Tallent (bass), Vini Lopez (drums), Southside Johnny (harmonica, vocals), Bobby Williams (drums), Albee Tellone (tenor saxophone), and Bobby Feigenbaum (alto saxophone). There is also an eight-member backing vocal troupe nicknamed "The Zoomettes," plus Big Danny Gallagher handling the onstage props. This situationist lark also features a board game set up on stage.

On July 10, the Bruce Springsteen Band makes its debut, which essentially has the same formation as Dr. Zoom and the Sonic Boom minus Southside Johnny, the Zoomettes and various improvised guests. Alongside Springsteen, Van Zandt, Lopez, Sancious, and Tallent, we find Bobby Feigenbaum on the sax, Harvey Cherlin on trumpet, and a vocal duo formed by Delores Holmes and Barbara Dinkins. To this nine-member formation, Tinker West is added on the congas.

In August, Bruce meets a girl named Diane Lozito, who works in a little stand on the Asbury boardwalk. Lozito will be portrayed in several of Springsteen's songs, such as "Rosalita (Come Out Tonight)," "She's the One," and "Backstreets."

On September 4, at a show at the Student Prince in Asbury Park, Bruce meets Clarence Clemons, who is playing with Norman Seldin & the Joyful Noyze at the nearby Wonder Bar. The story of how Big Man first met the Boss has entered into the E Street Band mythology. Clemons recalled that it was truly a rainy, windy night, and when he opened the door of the Student Prince the whole thing flew off its hinges and blew away down the street. The band was onstage, staring at him framed in the doorway, when he asked if he could play with them. Asked directly, Springsteen confirmed this version.

On September 11, at the Sunshine Inn in Asbury Park, the Bruce Springsteen Band opens for Peter Frampton's Humble Pie, who at the end of the show ask Springsteen and Co. to open for their national tour. Frampton offers to organize an audition for the band with A&M Records, but Tinker West inexplicably refuses the offer.

On October 30, the Bruce Springsteen Band plays the Upstage the night the club will close for good. Tinker West feels that he can't manage Springsteen's career anymore, but he believes in his twenty-two-year old client, and therefore plans a meeting with a pair of aspiring producers in New York City named Mike Appel and Jim Cretecos. An audition is set for November and is a smash. Bruce sings "Song to the Orphans" and a surreal ballad called "Baby Doll" "as if his life depended on it," Appel told Dave Marsh years later. Springsteen and Appel shake hands. Bruce is going to California for the holidays and will concentrate on writing some new songs; Appel will wait for him.

In December Springsteen leaves for San Mateo to visit his family, warning his band members that he doesn't know when he'll return and inviting them to feel free from any engagements. In the end, Springsteen will stay in California only for a month, returning to New Jersey with a load of new songs including "You Can't Change," "Like a Stranger," Cowboys of the Sea," "Southern Sun," "Down to Mexico," and "Magic Kind of Loving."

1972

On February 14, Springsteen plays eight songs to Appel and Cretecos in Appel's New York office. Among the new compositions there are "Arabian Night," "It's Hard to Be a Saint in the City," "The Angel," and "For You." A few days after this performance, Springsteen signs a long-term management contract with Laurel Canyon—Appel and Cretecos's company.

The Bruce Springsteen Band continues to play along the Jersey Shore until the fateful date: Mike Appel has managed to schedule a private audition in front of the legendary John Hammond, the man who discovered Count Basie, Billie Holiday. and Aretha Franklin, and signed Pete Seeger, Bob Dylan, and Leonard Cohen to Columbia Records. The meeting is set up for May 2 in Hammond's New York office in the A&R department at Columbia Records. Bruce's set begins with "It's

Hard to Be a Saint in the City," after which Hammond says, "You've got to be on Columbia Records." Springsteen also plays "Growin' Up," "Mary Queen of Arkansas," and "If I Was the Priest." When Bruce has finished, Hammond says that he needs to see how Bruce interacts with a live audience; so Appel immediately goes about organizing a brief performance at the Gaslight Au-Go-Go on Bleecker Street for that same evening.

On June 9, Springsteen signs with Columbia Records. For the first album, Columbia commits to paying an advance of $25,000 and allows for a budget of $40,000 for recording expenses. The next day, Bruce calls his parents and tells them the good news. Bruce's sister Pamela recalls that Doug Springteen "was pretty excited" and that he said, "From now on, I'm never going to tell anyone what they should or shouldn't do with their lives."

A few days later, on June 17, Springsteen makes a guest appearance with Norman Seldin & the Joyful Noyze at the Shipbottom Lounge in Point Pleasant, New Jersey. Clarence Clemons is the saxophonist of the band; this is believed to have been the first time Bruce and the Big Man have played together since Clarence's now famous Student Prince walk-in jam with Springsteen in September 1971.

Around this time, Bruce comes across what is to become one of the most recognizable instruments in the history of rock 'n' roll at a guitar shop owned by New Jersey–based luthier Phil Petillo: the now iconic 1950s Fender Esquire that has remained close to Springsteen's side throughout his rise to the apex of superstardom, having been played both in the studio and on stages around the world. It's the one on the cover of albums like *Born to Run*, *Human Touch*, and *Wrecking Ball*—the one that Bruce was playing during the Super Bowl halftime show in 2009. Boasting a Telecaster body and Esquire neck, the guitar had already undergone significant modifications by the time it landed in Springsteen's hands (for $180!). After Springsteen bought it, Petillo added hot-wound single-coil pickups and his patented Petillo Precision Frets, in addition to a titanium six-saddle bridge.

The recording of Springsteen's debut album, *Greetings from Asbury Park, NJ*, begins in early July with full-band sessions held at 914 Sound Studios in Blauvelt, New York. Appel and Cretecos run the control room as producers. The musicians are David Sancious (piano), Gary Tallent (bass), and Vini Lopez (drums). Surprisingly, Steve Van Zandt is not among the musicians involved by Springsteen in the recording of his first album. Appel and Hammond are not convinced that using multiple guitars, especially electric ones, is really necessary; so Steve is left out: for more than two years he will lay his guitar aside and work construction, running a jackhammer and playing football on the weekends. Recording sessions span a four-month period, from early June to late October 1972. Clarence Clemons is called to play the saxophone on "Blinded by the Light" and "Spirit in the Night"—two songs just written by Bruce.

Tony Scaduto's biography of Dylan is one of the first books that Springsteen has ever read. His admiration for the author of "Like a Rolling Stone" is great; although Bruce starts to fear that the buzz Columbia is creating about him as the "new Dylan" could backfire on him.

1973

Greetings from Asbury Park, NJ is released on January 5, 1973, together with the "Blinded by the Light" / "The Angel" single. *Rolling Stone* music critic Lester Bangs hails Springsteen as a daring new artist who sets himself apart from his contemporaries. Despite the good reviews, the album only reaches #60 in the charts, selling just 25,000 copies. But Springsteen builds his reputation on a series of amazing concerts, which will win him the nickname of the Jersey Devil. He usually starts with one of his solo acoustic songs or comes out with Garry Tallent and his tuba to make the warped calliope sound for "Circus Song" (soon to evolve into "Wild Billy's Circus Story"). Then he calls for the rest of the band—which is not yet called the E Street Band—whose lineup consists of Danny Federici, Garry Tallent, Vini Lopez and Clarence Clemons. A few new songs are played, like "Thundercrack," "Bishop Danced," "Zero and Blind Terry," "Seaside Bar Song," and "Santa Ana." None of them will make it onto Springsteen's second album; they will be released only in 1998 on the *Tracks* box set.

In the first months of the year, Bruce and his band open for some legendary artists such as Lou Reed, Stevie Wonder, Paul Butterfield, the Beach Boys, and the Eagles. David Bowie shows up to see Springsteen in action at Max's Kansas City in New York. In a *Musician* magazine interview in 1987 Bowie commented on Bruce's performance on that night: "I hated him as a solo . . . As soon as the band came on it was like a different person and he was marvelous . . ."[1] In June, Bowie would be the first artist to record (though not release) a Springsteen composition ("Growin' Up").

On April 28 at the Cole Field House of the University of Maryland the triple bill consists of Chuck Berry headlining, Jerry Lee Lewis second billed and Bruce Springsteen opening. Berry's backing band having mysteriously disappeared, Bruce volunteers his band's services for free, and they improvise as best they can in front of a crowd of 15,000.

From June 1 to 3, Bruce Springsteen and his band open for Chicago's shows: in Philadelphia and New York they get booed. In July the recordings that will unleash *The Wild, the Innocent & the E Street Shuffle* begin. On those same days

Bruce and the boys play Max's Kansas City, sharing the bill with another promising band: Bob Marley & the Wailers. The audience is made up of, among others, Alice Cooper, Lou Reed, Patti Smith, and Garland Jeffreys.

Springsteen's second album is released on November 11 and sells better than *Greetings*, but doesn't meet Columbia's expectations. Inside the label, there is much talk about dropping Bruce. The Wild Tour has already started in Hampden Sydney, Virginia, on September 28.

1974

On February 12, prior to the start of a show in Lexington, Kentucky, there is an argument between road manager Steve Appel (manager Mike Appel's brother) and Vini Lopez. Springsteen, after discussing the incident with Mike Appel by phone following the show, asks Lopez to submit his resignation. His place will be taken by Ernst "Boom" Carter, a childhood friend of David Sancious.

In the meantime, the relationship between Bruce and Diane Lozito is coming to an end. After a series of arguments, fights, and breakups she moves secretly to Nantucket, while Bruce writes his version of their story on "Backstreets," a lover's tale of romance, obsession, and promises broken.

On April 10, Springsteen plays at Charlie's Place in Cambridge, Massachusetts. This is when he meets his future manager-producer Jon Landau for the first time. One month later, on May 9, Landau comes back to see Bruce and the E Street Band at Cambridge's Harvard Square Theater: they are playing two shows there, a double bill, opening for headliner Bonnie Raitt. This is one of most famous Springsteen gigs yet, opened by a thirteen-minute-long version of "New York City Serenade," with a terrific setlist including a rare performance of "The Fever," a unique cover of the blues classic "I Sold My Heart to the Junkman," and the premiere of a still unreleased "Born to Run." At the end of the show, Landau writes his review for *Real Paper* with the famous line "I saw rock and roll's future and its name is Bruce Springsteen." The MC's use of the name "the E Street Band" in his introduction (which can be heard in various bootlegs) is the earliest appearance of that name on any show, or any audio or promotional material, yet unearthed. The name had been conjured up only a few weeks earlier, in honor of the street in Belmar, New Jersey, where David Sancious's mother lived and allowed the guys to rehearse in her garage. The house was at 1107 E Street.

In May, Springsteen starts recording sessions at 914 Sound Studios. The first song he has composed for his third album is "Born to Run," written at his rented cottage at 7½ West End Court in West Long Branch. The first version (a full-band instrumental take) is cut on May 21; the definitive take is recorded on August 6.

Ernst "Boom" Carter is on drums—his only appearance on a Springsteen recorded song.

Two days later, Bruce Springsteen and the E Street Band play at the Monmouth Arts Center in Red Bank, New Jersey, opening the show with "New York City Serenade"—the last one with the famous intro played by David Sancious, who has already come to Bruce with the dismaying news that he has been offered a solo deal with Columbia's sister label, Epic, and wants to take Boom Carter with him. The split is friendly. Appel places a notice in the Musicians Needed section of the *Village Voice's* classified ads, seeking a drummer ("No Jr. Ginger Bakers's" [sic]) and a pianist ("Classical to Jerry Lee Lewis"), along with a trumpet player ("Jazz, R&B, & Latin") and a violinist. "All must sing. Male or Female. Bruce Springsteen and the E Street Band. Columbia Records." After a series of tryout sessions held at 914 Sound Studios during the third week of August, pianist Roy Bittan and drummer Max Weinberg are selected as the two new members of the E Street Band. With the new lineup settled the group spends about ten hours per day for the next two weeks in rehearsal. The live debut for Bittan and Weinberg is at the Main Point in Bryn Mawr, Pennsylvania, on September 19.

On October 4, Bruce Springsteen and the E Street Band play at Lincoln Center's Avery Fisher Hall in New York City. This is the debut of Israeli violinist Suki Lahav and the night of the first performance of "She's the One." A few days later, Springsteen and the band play at the Capitol Theatre in Passaic, New Jersey. They are billed as the opening act for John Sebastian; but when Sebastian watches Bruce's soundcheck he says, "There is not a chance in the fucking world that I'm following this!" The result is that Springsteen will close the show.

At the end of November, Springsteen visits David Bowie at Sigma Sound Studios in Philadelphia. Bowie has recently recorded a cover of "It's Hard to Be a Saint in the City," but apparently it isn't finished yet, so Bruce doesn't get to hear it (it will remain in the vaults until the early 1990s, when Bowie finally releases it). Later that same day (November 25) Springsteen attends Bowie's evening concert at the Philadelphia Spectrum. The two men's mutual admiration will be constant from then on.

Springsteen is again at 914 Sound Studios for new recording sessions. "Jungleland"—whose first version was cut in August—still needs further recordings. Definitive takes of "A Love So Fine," "A Night Like This," "Walking in the Street," "Janey Needs a Shooter," and "Angel's Song" won't be used for the forthcoming album.

On December 14, Springsteen attends a Billy Joel concert in New Brunswick, New Jersey, in the small gymnasium of Rutgers University, which was affectionately nicknamed "the Barn." During the show Joel dedicates the song "The Entertainer" to Springsteen; then, for the third encore, Bruce joins him for an impromptu version of "Twist and Shout."

1975

In the first months of the year, the band performs nonstop in numerous clubs on the West Coast. The February 5 show at the Main Point in Bryn Mawr, Pennsylvania, is broadcast by WMMR-FM. The eighteen-song setlist includes spellbinding renditions of "Incident on 57th Street," "New York City Serenade," and "For You" (in the solo piano arrangement), the earliest known performance of "Thunder Road" (with work-in-progress title "Wings for Wheels"), plus a wild version of Chuck Berry's "Back in the U.S.A." and a long "Rosalita" that includes a snippet of the "Theme from Shaft" in the midsection. The entire performance will be issued in the 1990 bootleg *The Saint, the Incident & the Main Point Shuffle*.

On March 9, Suki Lahav plays with the E Street Band for the last time at the final gig of the Wild & Innocent Tour, in Washington, D.C., although she participates in the *Born to Run* studio sessions that follow this tour. Suki will move to Israel permanently later in 1975.

Recording sessions—now conducted at the Record Plant—start in March and continue through July. Jon Landau has taken the lead on the production, while Jimmy Iovine substitutes for Suki's husband, Louis Lahav, as the recording engineer. The recording process seems never-ending. Finally, in a three-day, seventy-two-hour sprint, working in three studios simultaneously, Springsteen and Clemons manage to finish the "Jungleland" sax solo, phrase by phrase, in one, while they mix "Thunder Road" in another, singing "Backstreets" in a third as the band rehearses in another spare room. The record will be ready on the very same day the Born to Run Tour begins.

It's July 20 when Springsteen begins the tour in Providence, Rhode Island, the night "Miami" Steve Van Zandt debuts as the guitarist of the E Street Band. The historical lineup of the band—Bittan, Federici, Van Zandt, Tallent, Clemons, Weinberg—has taken shape and will remain unchanged until 1984.

The day before, Bruce had listened to an acetate pressing of the master recording of *Born to Run* with the entire band and his new girlfriend, Karen Darvin. The album is not released yet when on August 13 Springsteen and the band open a historic five-night (ten-show) residency at the Bottom Line in New York City with an astonishing "Thunder Road" played by Bruce alone on the piano. Celebrities have come in flocks, including Robert De Niro, who takes special note of Bruce's pre-encore "Are you talkin' to *me*?" routine (which the actor later transmutes into a creepy highlight of his performance as a psychotic in 1976's *Taxi Driver*), along with director Martin Scorsese.

Columbia releases *Born to Run* on August 25. The album vaults into the Top 10 in its second week on the charts and soon goes gold, reaching its peak position of #3. On October 27, *Time* and *Newsweek* magazines put Springsteen on the cover in the same week. In a rave review for *Rolling Stone*, Greil Marcus writes that Springsteen enhances romanticized American themes with his majestic sound, ideal style of rock 'n' roll, evocative lyrics, and an impassioned delivery that defines what is a "magnificent" album: "It is the drama that counts; the stories Springsteen is telling are nothing new, though no one has ever told them better or made them matter more."[2] Lester Bangs writes: "In a time of squalor and belittled desire, Springsteen's music is majestic and passionate with no apologies."[3]

In October Springsteen opens a four-night stand at the Roxy in Los Angeles. *Le tout* Hollywood is at the club: Robert De Niro, Jack Nicholson, Warren Beatty, and music's elite, too: Phil Spector, David Bowie, Jackson Browne, Neil Diamond, George Harrison . . .

With a five-day break in the West Coast leg of the tour, on October 23, Bruce flies to New York to attend a surprise, sixty-first birthday party for Gerde's Folk City owner Mike Porco—who hired Bob Dylan for his first New York club gigs in 1961. Dylan turns up with Joan Baez and other members of his soon-to-tour Rolling Thunder Revue. This is the first time Springsteen and Dylan meet.

On November 18, Bruce Springsteen and the E Street Band play at Hammersmith Odeon in London. It's their first ever appearance outside the U.S.A. and is quite turbulent. Before the show, in fact, Springsteen has torn "Finally London is ready for Bruce Springsteen & the E Street Band" promotional posters from the walls and given orders that the buttons with "I have seen the future of rock 'n' roll at the Hammersmith Odeon" printed on them not be given out—furious with the hype and publicity. The controversy clearly affects the performance, as the *Hammersmith Odeon London 75* DVD shows. The European mini-tour continues in Stockholm and Amsterdam, going back to London for a second gig.

Upon his return to the United States, relations between Springsteen and Mike Appel begin to falter. Bruce's manager submits a management contract to Danny Federici and to Clarence Clemons. Both sign, but when the other members of the band convince the two that they have signed a phony contract, Bruce asks Appel to dismiss it. He does so, but the band still feels duped. Appel, thereafter, is more and more jealous of the influence of Jon Landau on Bruce and does everything to keep Landau out of the way.

Bruce Springsteen and the E Street Band celebrate New Year's Eve with a show at Tower Theater in Philadelphia. The entire concert is professionally recorded (along with several other shows in December) under the guidance of Jimmy Iovine as part of a plan to release a live album. It is Appel's idea, but Springsteen is not convinced, and wants to get back to the recording studio.

1976

The first three months of the year are dedicated to rest—and to the new squabbles between Springsteen and Appel. The latter would like Springsteen to play arenas: the Born to Run Tour, despite its great success, was not profitable because playing in small theaters doesn't cover the costs of a crew of twenty people. But Bruce is opposed, and turns down a $500,000 offer to play at the JFK Stadium in Philadelphia before 100,000 spectators. Meanwhile, Appel arranges for CBS to advance Laurel Canyon (his management company) $500,000 against future Springsteen earnings and offers to renegotiate the contracts with Springsteen—including giving Springsteen half the stock of all Laurel Canyon companies. Springsteen replies that he wants to pursue the relationship with Laurel Canyon on the basis of a handshake, but when he comes into possession of the contract between Columbia and Laurel Canyon he discovers that the latter is guaranteed forty cents per album, while he and Appel get only ten. Moreover, Springsteen doesn't control his own song publishing rights under the contract: Laurel Canyon holds them, and can grant or refuse right to use the material to whomever it chooses, whatever Springsteen's wishes. And so Bruce asks Jon Landau for his opinion, and Landau suggests a legal office and an auditor.

The second leg of the Born to Run Tour—soon nicknamed by the road crew as the "Chicken Scratch Tour" because of the high proportion of secondary market, southern state locations—starts in Columbia, South Carolina, on March 25, ending at the Halsey Field House in Annapolis, Maryland, on May 28.

In the meantime, on May 14, Laurel Canyon sends Springsteen a check for $67,000 that is meant to represent everything he is owed for the period spanning from March 1972 to March 1976. But the auditor chosen by Springsteen discovers that the proceeds belonging to Springsteen for that period add up to $2 million. In the auditor's report it is written that records showed that Laurel Canyon had "conducted Springsteen's business in a slipshod, wasteful and neglectful manner." In his reply dated July 2, Appel communicates to Springsteen that he will not allow Jon Landau to produce the fourth LP. On July 27, Springsteen files suit in federal court in Manhattan, alleging fraud, undue influence, and breach of trust. Two days later, Appel files suit in New York Supreme Court, asking the court to bar Springsteen and Landau from entering a recording studio together. Judge Armold Fein grants Appel's injunction, effectively barring Bruce and Landau from recording together. This marks the beginning of a long legal battle that will decidedly influence Bruce's career. "Mike Appel thought he would be Colonel Parker and I'd be Elvis," Springsteen would later say. "Only he wasn't the Colonel, and I wasn't Elvis."[4]

To distract himself, Springsteen makes some unlisted performances. On May 30, he's at Southside Johnny & the Asbury Jukes' first concert with major public exposure at the Stone Pony in Asbury Park, celebrating the recent release of Southside's debut album, *I Don't Want to Go Home*. The producer of the album, Steve Van Zandt, is onstage playing rhythm guitar for most of the show. And what a lineup of guests it is: Lee Dorsey, Clarence Clemons, Max Weinberg, Ronnie Spector, and Bruce Springsteen, who joins for one song, the closing "Having a Party." On June 7, Springsteen plays at *Crawdaddy's* tenth-anniversary party in New York; writer William Borroughs is there and reports that Bruce, "at twenty-six, is heading for Grand Old Manhood."[5]

Springsteen also spends time with his new girlfriend, a college graduate from Little Silver, New Jersey, named Joy Hannan. Bruce has recently rented a farm off Telegraph Hill in Holmdel, New Jersey.

The "Lawsuit Tour"—so called due to the legal dispute between Bruce and Appel—starts on August 1 from Red Bank, New Jersey, with the debut of the Miami Horns. The show features the premiere of "Rendezvous" and "Something in the Night." Two days later, Bruce plays "The Promise" for the first time—a song clearly inspired by Appel's "betrayal." On October 28, Springsteen plays the first show of a six-night stand at New York City's Palladium. The third night marks the only guest appearance by Patti Smith at a Springsteen concert, on a customized, one-off arrangement of "Rosalita." The final show at the Palladium is one of the best Springsteen gigs of all time. Stunning covers of the Animals' "It's My Life" (Carl D'Errico, cowriter of the song, is in the audience) and "We Gotta Get Out of This Place" are also featured, and Ronnie Spector guests on three of her most famous Ronettes-era hits ("Baby, I Love You," "Walking in the Rain," and "Be My Baby"), all given inspired arrangements by the E Street Band.

In November 1976, the Bottom Line hosts a very special show: a mixture of spoken word, poems, and songs featuring the Patti Smith Group, Bruce Springsteen, and former Velvet Underground member John Cale. Patti and Bruce improvise two semi-spoken-word pieces with Patti on vocals and Bruce on piano; the full Patti Smith Group joins on the Velvet Underground's "We're Gonna Have a Real Good Time Together," which features John Cale and Bruce on piano. He then returns later in the show to play guitar on several more songs, among them "My Generation" and "Gloria."

1977

March 25 concludes the Lawsuit Tour: at the Music Hall in Boston, Springsteen gifts us with one of his best concerts, reproduced in the bootleg *Forced to Confess*.

On May 28, at three in the morning, Mike Appel and Bruce Springsteen finally reach an out-of-court agreement that will never come out in public. It seems that in return for setting Springsteen free, Appel has received $800,000 and 50 percent of the publishing rights to all the songs that Springsteen has recorded up till then. With his lawsuit with Mike Appel settled only about eighteen hours beforehand, an upbeat Springsteen and Steve Van Zandt drive to Philadelphia to attend an Elvis Presley concert. It's Van Zandt's first Presley show. Bruce has seen Presley in concert once before (at one of the four Madison Square Garden shows of June 8–11, 1972). Although Springsteen is a big enough star at this point to have been given VIP treatment if he'd sought it, Bruce and Steve attend the show merely as members of the public. This is one of the last performances of drug-affected Presley. In a late 1970s interview Springsteen commented that he and Van Zandt drove back to New Jersey without saying a word to one another, such was their disappointment with the performance. However, he would later say that he enjoyed the show tremendously.

Just four days after settling the lawsuit, recording sessions for what would become *Darkness on the Edge of Town* begin, on June 1. That first night Springsteen lays down at least eight songs, including a take of "Something in the Night" that actually makes the final album. The sessions at Atlantic Studios are only two or three weeks old when problems surface. Bruce doesn't like the sound he is getting from the studio, and Atlantic doesn't offer a particularly comfortable or livable environment for the musicians. So operations shift to the nearby Record Plant. According to recording engineer Jimmy Iovine, the Atlantic and Record Plant sessions yielded about thirty completed tracks available for inclusion on the *Darkness* album. As of 2017, thirty-two songs have been officially released (the ten on the original album, four on the *Tracks* box set of 1998, and eighteen on *The Promise* double-album of 2010). "Drive All Night," "Independence Day," and "Point Blank" will be picked up upon again in 1980 for *The River*, while "Because the Night," written with Patti Smith, will be recorded by the latter and published successfully in 1978. The two sing the track together on December 30 at CBGB's in New York, during one of Patti's shows.

In October, in the meantime, Bruce drops in on a session for Lou Reed's work-in-progress album at the Record Plant, and records a spoken narrative that forms a brief part of Reed's eleven-minute song "Street Hassle." In the last line of the narrative Bruce states, "Tramps like us, we were born to pay." It's not known if the inclusion of this line was Bruce or Reed's idea. The recording will be released on Reed's *Street Hassle* album in March 1978.

Springsteen, having left Karen Darvin (she will later marry Todd Rundgren), starts seeing a seventeen-year-old high-school girl named Joy Hannah. But it doesn't last. Towards the end of the year, he will form a stable couple with the photographer Lynn Goldsmith.

1978

The *Darkness on the Edge of Town* mixing sessions begin in early January and drag on until late March. The album is not published yet when, on May 23, the Darkness Tour kicks off from Buffalo. When *Darkness on the Edge of Town* is finally released on June 6, reviews are overwhelmingly positive. In an article for *Rolling Stone*, Dave Marsh views it as a landmark record because of the clarity of its production, Springsteen's unique guitar playing, and the programming, which he says connected the characters and themes in a subtle yet cohesive manner. The album reaches #5 on *Billboard*'s chart and is elected album of the year by *New Musical Express* in the UK.

Some of the best shows in Springsteen's career take place one after the other during these months, like the one held on September 19 at the Capitol Theatre in Passaic, broadcast on WNEW-FM, which will give birth to *Pièce de Résistance*, perhaps the most famous bootleg in the history of rock 'n' roll together with Dylan's *Great White Wonder*. Another landmark show is on December 15 at the Winterland in San Francisco. *Los Angeles Times* critic Robert Hilburn, who goes to see Springsteen in Tucson, Arizona, that winter, writes that "listening to the eloquence of his songs made me forget about doubts and think about my own dreams again."[6]

The Darkness Tour ends with legendary concerts in Cleveland on New Year's Eve and New Year's Day. Over its 150 nights, Bruce Springsteen and the E Street Band played to more than a million fans.

1979

On January 11, Springsteen and his band celebrate Clarence Clemons's thirty-seventh birthday with a private show at the Lock Stock & Barrell in Fair Haven, New Jersey. Bruce, meanwhile, has split up from Lynn Goldsmith and is already seeing the actress Joyce Hyser. They live together in Homdel for the first part of 1979. During this period, he keeps a low profile, focusing his attention on composing new material for his next album.

Recording sessions for what will become *The River* begin in late March at the Power Station in New York City. A new song called "Roulette" is recorded on April 3, just days after the March 28 Three Mile Island nuclear accident that inspired the lyrics. But few days later, the actor Robin Williams arrives at Springsteen's home for a visit as Bruce and Joyce Hyser are riding a motocross bike. As Bruce goes to greet his friend, he loses control of the bike and ends up against a tree, resulting in a serious knee injury that forces him into a three-week period of convalescence. By Easter, Springsteen and Hyser have already split. Soon Bruce will start a brief relationship with Joyce Moore, a Monmouth College senior.

On September 21, Bruce Springsteen and the E Street Band close the first of the two MUSE (Musicians United for Safe Energy) benefit concerts at Madison Square Garden in New York City, also known as "No Nukes." Jackson Browne; Tom Petty; the Doobie Brothers; Crosby, Stills & Nash; James Taylor; Carly Simon; Bonnie Raitt; Chaka Khan; Ry Cooder; John Hall; and Graham Nash are on the bill. Springsteen's twelve-song set includes the premiere of "The River." During the last encore on the second night, Lynn Goldsmith is taking photos, which Bruce thinks she has agreed not to do. He drags her up on stage, announces her as "my ex-girlfriend," and then has her escorted away.

On October 4, Springsteen signs off a sequence of ten songs for his new album, provisionally entitled *The Ties that Bind*. The songs are "The Ties that Bind," "Cindy," "Hungry Heart," "Stolen Car," and "Be True" on side one; "The River," "You Can Look (But You Better Not Touch)," "The Price You Pay," "I Wanna Marry You," and "Loose Ends" on side two. Wheels are put in motion to produce artwork for the cover. But, before long, Springsteen has a change of heart about the album concept, deciding the material is too slight. The single album is shelved, and Springsteen begins a new series of studio sessions.

1980

In January, recording sessions continue at the Power Station, with a lot of new songs recorded by Springsteen and the band: "Meet Me in the City," "Jackson Cage," "I Wanna Be With You," "Ramrod," "Bring On the Night," "Stolen Car," "Dollhouse," "Restless Nights," Where the Bands Are," "Crush on You," "Independence Day," "Take 'Em as They Come" . . . One day Bruce drops by the studio next door to chat and jam a bit with industrial/experimental outfit Suicide (Alan Vega and Martin Rev), who are recording their second album. In a 1984 interview with *Rolling Stone* magazine Springsteen later mentions Suicide's "Frankie Teardrop" as one of the most amazing songs he ever heard. Suicide's song "Dream Baby Dream" would be covered by Springsteen during his 2005 solo tour and a studio recording officially released on 2014's *High Hopes*.

On January 9, at the Fast Lane in Asbury Park, Springsteen joins Atlantic City Expressway—fronted by Jon Bon Jovi—on stage to play "The Promised Land."

Come springtime Springsteen keeps popping out new songs: "I'm a Rocker," "Wreck on the Highway," "Cadillac Ranch," "Two Hearts," "Held Up Without a Gun," "Sherry Darling," "Drive All Night," "Fade Away," "Out in the Street" . . . Columbia starts having to accept the idea of publishing a double album to take the place of the now shipwrecked *The Ties that Bind*. Springsteen will later state that he eventually realized that he wasn't making a record, he was embarking on an odyssey.

In July, Bruce Springsteen and the E Street Band undertake recording sessions for Gary U.S. Bonds in the immediate aftermath of the final sessions for the album that comes to be called *The River*. Bruce contributes guitar and vocals, and coproduces (with Van Zandt) four tracks—"This Little Girl," "Dedication," "Your Love," and "Jole Blon"—the first three of which are Bruce compositions. The recordings will be released on Bonds' album *Dedication* in April 1981.

On October 3, in Ann Arbor, Michigan, the River Tour begins with Springsteen shouting "Born to Run" (and forgetting some words . . .). The title track of the forthcoming double album is introduced by Roy Bittan playing the theme from *Once Upon a Time in the West* on piano. Two weeks later, *The River* is published: four sides, twenty songs, "a rock 'n' roll milestone," as *Rolling Stone* critic Paul Nelson wrote in his review;[7] while *Melody Maker* contributor Paolo Hewitt compared listening to *The River* to "taking a trip through the rock 'n' roll heartland as you've never experienced it. It's a walk down all the streets, all the places, all the people and all the souls that rock has ever visited, excited, cried for and loved."[8] The album is Springsteen's first to go #1 on the *Billboard* 200, spending four weeks at the top of the chart and selling over 1.6 million copies in the U.S. between its release and Christmas. "Hungry Heart" is released as the album's first single and reaches #5 on the pop singles chart. In his last interview ever, only a few hours prior to his murder on December 8, 1980, Jon Lennon declares that "Hungry Heart" is his favorite song on the radio.

On December 28, at the Nassau Coliseum in Uniondale, New Jersey, Springsteen performs "This Land Is Your Land" by Woody Guthrie, whose biography, written by Joe Klein, he has recently read. Again at the Nassau Coliseum, Bruce celebrates New Year's offering the crowd a setlist of thirty-eight songs for a total of four hours and ten minutes of music.

1981

In February the second single taken from *The River*, "Fade Away" / "Be True," is published and makes it to the Top 20.

On April 7 in Hamburg, Springsteen's first real European tour begins: thirty-three concerts in twenty-one cities in ten countries (Germany, France, Switzerland, Spain, Belgium, Holland, Denmark, Sweden, Norway, and England). On May 11, in Newcastle, Bruce plays for the first time in England since 1975; dates follow in Manchester, Edinburgh, Stafford, Brighton, Birmingham, and London, where he sells out Wembley Arena six nights running. Keith Richards and Mick Jagger from the Rolling Stones, the Sex Pistols, Elvis Costello, Pete Townshend of the Who, and Bono from U2 all visit him backstage. *The Times* prints its first page stating that Springsteen has become at this stage, "God amongst the gods."

Back in the U.S.A., on June 22 Springsteen attends Max Weinberg's wedding and plays some songs at the reception together with the other members of the band. During a short break of the River Tour, Bruce begins the recording of some new material—solo on acoustic guitar. A song entitled "Fist Full of Dollars" will later evolve into "Atlantic City." Other new compositions are "Come On (Let's Go Tonight)," "Open All Night," and "Robert Ford and Jesse James." They are not professionally made recordings; Springsteen only uses a common, run-of-the-mill cassette recorder.

On July 2 his show inaugurates the Brendan Byrne Arena, a 20,000-seat venue built next to Giants Stadium in East Rutherford, New Jersey, in an area known as the Meadowlands. With six sold-out concerts, Springsteen baptizes the stage he will from now on come to consider home. During the show on July 3, the spectators are offered for the first time a copy of Tom Waits's "Jersey Girl," which Waits and Springsteen will sing together in Los Angeles on August 24 in a historic duet destined never to be repeated.

The River Tour ends at the Riverfront Coliseum in Cincinnati, Ohio, on September 14. In 141 concerts Bruce Springsteen and the E Street Band have played in front of close to two million people.

Bruce spends his thirty-first birthday in Honolulu, Hawaii, where he is Clarence Clemons's best man at his wedding with Christina Sandgren. Back to the East Coast, he continues to record solo at his new house in Colts Neck, New Jersey. The songs are written quickly and recorded in three or four takes, just as demos. He watches John Houston's *Wise Blood* and Terrence Malick's *Badlands*, and has a couple of telephone conversations with the latter. "I wanted black bedtime stories," he says.

In November, Springsteen visits studio sessions being conducted at the Power Station by Steve Van Zandt for his work-in-progress debut solo album and provides harmony vocals on "Men Without Women," "Angel Eyes," and "Until the

Good Is Gone." They will be included on Little Steven's *Men Without Women* album, released in October 1982.

1982

Legend dictates that the bulk of the songs that will end up on the *Nebraska* album were recorded by Springsteen solo on a TEAC TASCAM four-track cassette recorder in one all-day/night session on January 3. Springsteen himself has said it took three days, although he later said it took "no more than a few weeks" in *Songs*. Fourteen songs are recorded: apart from the ten that will be included on *Nebraska*, there are "The Big Payback," "Born in the U.S.A.," "Losin' Kind," "Child Bride" (a first version of "Working on the Highway"), "Downbound Train," and "Pink Cadillac." Bruce's intention is to create a batch of finished solo demos to demonstrate to the E Street Band at sessions for the follow-up to *The River* due to start in New York City in February. For this reason, he brings the cassette with some notes to Jon Landau.

Early in March, Springsteen and Roy Bittan fly to Los Angeles to participate in a Quincy Jones–produced recording session for Donna Summer's album-in-progress. After initially considering "Cover Me" for donation, Bruce gives the Queen of Disco the stylistically similar "Protection," which will be released in August on Summer's self-titled album.

It is during the E Street Band sessions in late March and early April that Bruce first attempts to record full-band arrangements of the demos that he has made on his own at Colts Neck. However, it soon becomes apparent to him that a majority of these songs do not lend themselves well to these full-band arrangements. In April Bruce hands his recording engineer Toby Scott the original solo demo tape, asking if Scott can just master off the tape. It takes Scott a few weeks to get back to Bruce with a definitive answer . . . but the answer is "Yes."

In the meantime, Springsteen makes a series of semi-clandestine appearances in clubs around the coast. He will play three times, between April and June, at the Big Man's West in Red Bank—Clarence's new club— with Clarence Clemons & the Red Bank Rockers. In the same club he will accompany Beaver Brown, a semi-famous Rhode Island club band, for a further eight evenings. But the most curious friendship is that between Bruce and the Cats on a Smooth Surface, a group headed by guitarist and singer Bobby Bandiera (who at the end of the eighties will become part of the Asbury Jukes led by Southside Johnny). The Cats play at the Stone Pony in Asbury Park, and Bruce watches a couple of their shows before getting up onstage on May 2 to perform "Long Tall Sally" and "Twist and Shout" with them. After that first evening twelve more will follow, from May till October, always at the Stone Pony. Initially, Bruce joins the group around two thirty in the morning, when no more than thirty spectators are still there. But after three or four shows, the word has spread and the club starts drawing in up to 800 people per night.

In 1982, Springsteen's only official live appearance is on June 12, when he takes part in the "Rally for Disarmament" organized by Jackson Browne at Central Park, in New York. In front of 700,000 spectators Bruce accompanies Browne in "Running on Empty" and performs an acoustic version of "The Promised Land."

The final—and radical—decision to release the solo demo tapes of ten songs as his next official album takes place in May. The E Street Band sessions come to a halt and Springsteen focuses his attention for the next couple of months on over-seeing the final preparations of *Nebraska*. However, mixing of the band material continues through June, alongside the *Nebraska* tracks. In fact, they toy with the idea of a double record, with the acoustic *Nebraska* and the electric *Born in the U.S.A.* in one package, but the tone of the music proves too different.

A sequence for the band album is compiled, as follows: "Born in the U.S.A.," "Murder Incorporated," "Downbound Train," "I'm Goin' Down," "Glory Days," and "My Love Will Not Let You Down" on side one; "Working on the Highway," "Darlington County," "Frankie," "I'm on Fire," and "This Hard Land" on side two. But the time is not yet ripe.

This summer also sees the effective departure of Steve Van Zandt as a member of the E Street Band (although a formal announcement isn't made until May 1984). Van Zandt puts together his band (the Disciples of Soul) in June 1982, and the group makes its live debut in July. At the same time, he changes his stage name from "Miami Steve" to "Little Steven" to reflect his change of status to a full-time solo artist.

Nebraska—Springsteen's solo and acoustic album—is released on October 4 and surprisingly reaches #3 on the charts. No tour is foreseen to promote the album.

During these months Springsteen goes through a very hard depressive phase. "I thought, 'This can't be happening to me. *I'm the guy with the guitar*,"[9] he later tells Dave Marsh. He decides to rest for a few weeks in California, where he has a house, and one day drops in to Clover Studios in Los Angeles to visit Chuck Plotkin and Toby Scott, who are the respective producer and recording engineer for Bette Midler's album-in-progress *No Frills*. Springsteen donates his unreleased and never-performed song "Pink Cadillac" to the Midler project. After hearing the Midler studio version, however, he will not allow her to use it on the album, and *No Frills* is released without it in July 1983.

Back to the East Coast, one day in October, Springsteen goes to the Stone Pony to attend a concert of Cats on a Smooth Surface. Backstage, he makes out a familiar figure dressed in jeans and cowboy boots. It is a woman he has already met in the past. Her name is Patti Scialfa.

On December 31, the wedding reception for Steve Van Zandt and his bride Maureen Santoro in New York City is a rock 'n' roll parade. Percy Sledge sings "When a Man Loves a Woman" as the bride and groom walk down the aisle. The ceremony is performed by the Reverend Richard Penniman—a.k.a. Little Richard. Music is supplied by Little Milton and the wedding band from *The Godfather*, who are joined by best man Bruce and various other guests, including Gary U.S. Bonds, Southside Johnny, and the E Street Band.

1983

In January, together with his friend Matty Delia, Springsteen rides across the U.S.A. in his navy Camaro, stubbornly sticking to the worst neon-lit motels, playing in some bars on the road and eventually hitting California. In the garage of his house in Los Angeles he has a full twenty-four-track studio, and over the next month he cuts some new songs: "Shut Out the Light," "Sugarland," "Follow That Dream," and "Car Wash." But the depression keeps grabbing hold of him. Landau suggests that he seek professional support, and finds him a therapist in Los Angeles.

Back on the East Coast, Springsteen buys a villa in Rumson, New Jersey, on the southern bank of the Navesink River and just a mile from the ocean. He begins therapy with Dr. Wayne Myers in New York City (which he will continue until Dr. Myers's passing in 2008) and an almost vegetarian diet. He still plays softball most summer afternoons, but he has now started to run six miles a day as well. Soon he will be pumping iron. And, as early as May 1983, *Rolling Stone* notes, "Springsteen's muscles have swelled to Popeye size." "I had a body that just kind of popped in six months," he told David Kamp in a 2016 interview for *Vanity Fair*. "I found that I simply enjoyed the exercise," he said. "It was perfectly Sisyphean for my personality—lifting something heavy up and putting it down in the same spot for no particularly good reason. I've always felt a lot in common with Sisyphus. I'm always rolling that rock, man. One way or another, I'm always rolling that rock."[10]

A new round of recording with the E Street Band begins at the Hit Factory in New York in May. It's their first studio get-together in nearly a year. Steve Van Zandt, who is busy recording his second solo album and touring with his own group, is not present during much of this round. New songs are recorded, such as "Light of Day," "None but the Brave," "My Hometown," "TV Movie," "Stand on It," and "Janey Don't You Lose Heart." But from all of that material, nothing seems to fit together to make a coherent album. "It just wasn't a record; it just didn't sound like one," Springsteen recalls. On the one side, he has material he recorded alone in his Los Angeles garage; on the other, the rock 'n' roll songs recorded in New York with the band. The difference in sound quality between the home recording and the studio stuff is too wide. Just as soon as he realizes that the album he wants to make is a rock 'n' roll one, things begin to unblock. In September he writes "Bobby Jean" and "No Surrender" in a stream of energy, two songs that speak of his friendship with Steve; the spell is broken.

1984

"Dancing in the Dark" is the last song on *Born in the U.S.A.* to be recorded, after Jon Landau convinces Bruce that the album needs a single. Having written more than seventy songs for the album, Springsteen tells Landau that he has no intention of writing another one. But that same night, sitting in his hotel room, he writes the song on the spur of the moment. The song is recorded on February 14.

Four days later, a private jam session featuring Springsteen and guitarist Nils Lofgren takes place at Springsteen's residence in Rumson. Lofgren has recounted that Springsteen had just finished the *Born in the U.S.A.* record and played it to him in the car. When they got to Bruce's home, while watching MTV together, they heard the news that Little Steven had left the group and that his replacement was going to be someone from New Jersey. Lofgren took that opportunity to say to Springsteen that he would love to be auditioned if the band were to need a new guitarist. Three months later, Lofgren would become a new E Street Band member.

On May 9, the "Dancing in the Dark" / "Pink Cadillac" single is released, spending four weeks at #2 on the *Billboard* Hot 100 and eventually selling over one million singles in the U.S. alone. On June 6, the release of *Born in the U.S.A.* follows. Springsteen's seventh LP reaches #1 on U.S. and UK charts, becoming his most commercially successful album and one of the highest-selling records ever, having sold more than 30 million copies worldwide. Annie Leibovitz's cover photo for *Born in the U.S.A.* suddenly becomes an American pop icon, while throughout the entire country "Bossmania" is spreading.

The Born in the U.S.A. Tour takes off from the St. Paul Civic Center in St. Paul, Minnesota, on June 29—three days before Patti Scialfa joins the E Street Band. It's the live debut for Nils Lofgren as well. "Dancing in the Dark" is played twice for the video shoot, directed by Brian De Palma. Pulled out of the audience during the shoot to dance with Bruce is actress Courtney Cox, later to become a household name as Monica in *Friends*.

On July 31, "Cover Me" / "Jersey Girl" is the second single released from the *Born in the U.S.A.* album. It peaks at #7 on the *Billboard* Hot 100 singles charts. Five days later, Bruce Springsteen and the E Street Band play the first of ten sold-out shows at the Meadowlands Arena in New Jersey. On the last night, Steve Van Zandt guests on "Two Hearts" and "Drift Away."

In September, during a brief break from the tour, Bruce attends a Michael Jackson concert at JFK Stadium in Philadelphia. Afterwards, Bruce and Michael meet each other for the very first time in the reception room of Michael's suite in Philadelphia.

On September 19, in Hammonton, New Jersey, President Ronald Reagan tells an enthusiastic crowd, "America's future rests in the message of hope in the songs of a man so many young Americans admire, New Jersey's Bruce Springsteen." Two day later, at Pittsburgh's Civic Arena, speaking before "Johnny 99," Bruce responds, "Well, the President was mentioning my name in his speech the other day, and I kind of got to wondering what his favorite album of mine must've been . . . I don't think it was the *Nebraska* album; I don't think he's been listening to this one."

The third single from the *Born in the U.S.A.* album, "Born in the U.S.A." / "Shut Out the Light," comes out on October 30, peaking at #9 on the *Billboard* Hot 100 singles charts. It's just one day after Springsteen's first encounter with actress Julianne Phillips backstage at the Los Angeles Sports Arena. The two immediately start a steady relationship.

1985

The first leg of the Born in the U.S.A. Tour ends with two shows at the Carrier Dome in Syracuse, New York, on January 26 and 27. The next day, Springsteen is at A&M Studios in Los Angeles, for the recording of "We Are the World," the charity single written by Michael Jackson and Lionel Richie and produced by Quincy Jones. The supergroup of singers called U.S.A. for Africa includes Stevie Wonder, Paul Simon, Tina Turner, Billy Joel, Diana Ross, Dionne Warwick, Al Jarreau, Cyndi Lauper, and Bob Dylan, among others. Bruce's vocal performance is a standout.

On February 23, Springsteen and Madonna join Prince on stage at Inglewood's Forum during his Purple Rain Tour and play "Baby I'm a Star," "Purple Rain," and "America" with him. Just few days before, the third single taken from *Born in the U.S.A.*, "I'm on Fire" / "Johnny Bye Bye," is published, peaking at #6 on the *Billboard* Hot 100 pop singles chart.

On February 28, Bruce attends the 27th Grammy Awards ceremony at the Shrine Auditorium in Los Angeles, together with his mother and his soon-to-be-wife,

Julianne Phillips. He wins a Grammy for "Dancing in the Dark" in the category of Best Rock Vocal Performance.

In March, Springsteen is busy on his first tour in Australia and Japan: fourteen dates for a total of over 300,000 spectators. On March 22, at Sydney's Entertainment Center, he duets with Neil Young on "1969."

Upon returning to the United States, Springsteen marries Julianne Phillips on May 13, on Lake Oswego in Oregon. Steve Van Zandt and Clarence Clemons are Bruce's best men. Following the reception the honeymooners spend a week in Hawaii.

On May 31, the fifth single released from the *Born in the U.S.A.* album, "Glory Days" / "Stand on It," peaks at #5 on the *Billboard* Hot 100 pop singles charts. The next day, a massive European leg of the Born in the U.S.A. Tour begins from the small village of Slane in County Meath, about thirty miles north of Dublin, Ireland. In a picturesque outdoor setting Bruce Springsteen and the E Street Band play in front of 100,000 people, including Ron Wood, Eric Clapton, Pete Townshend, Bono, and Elvis Costello. The European Tour will reach eleven more cities, for a total of eighteen concerts and over 1.1 million spectators. To celebrate the 4th of July, in the first of three dates at Wembley Arena in London, Springsteen opens with "Independence Day" one of the best shows of the tour, which in August moves back to America, while the sixth single is released: "I'm Goin' Down" / "Janey Don't You Lose Heart" peaks at #9 on the *Billboard* Hot 100 pop singles charts.

On October 2, at the Los Angeles Coliseum, on the notes of "Glory Days," the curtain comes down on one of the most gigantic tours of all time: 158 concerts in sixty-six cities for a total of 4.8 million spectators. To fully close the circle, the last single is also finally ready, "My Hometown" / "Santa Claus Is Coming to Town." With this seventh single to make it to the Top 10, *Born in the U.S.A.* sets an unprecedented record.

The next day, Bruce and Julianne return home to their cottage in LA. The aftermath of the Born in the U.S.A. Tour is a strange time: Springsteen understands that he will never be up so high in the mainstream pop firmament again. It is the end of something.

1986

Springsteen spends much of the first half of 1986 listening, along with Jon Landau and Chuck Plotkin, to 200 hours of live recordings from the last ten years of concerts. The idea is to make a live album.

In the meantime, his marriage with Julianne is already suffering a crisis. "I was sliding back toward the chasm where rage, fear, distrust, insecurity and a family-patented misogyny made war with my better angels," Springsteen recalls. "In the dead of night, my contended sleep would occasionally be disturbed by the dreaded ticking, emanating as from the belly of Hook's alligator, of my 'clock.'"[11]

Springsteen's only 1986 appearance on a stage is at the Shoreline Amphitheatre in Mountain View, California, for the first Bridge School Benefit concert organized by Neil Young for assisting children with severe physical impairments and complex communication needs. Bruce plays an acoustic show accompanied by Nils Lofgren (guitar) and Danny Federici (accordion).

On November 10, Columbia releases Springsteen's long-awaited and highly anticipated live album, entitled *Bruce Springsteen & the E Street Band Live/1975–85*, a box set with either five vinyl records, three cassettes, or three CDs containing forty tracks recorded at various concerts between 1975 and 1985, for a total of 216 minutes of music. The album generated advance orders of more than 1.5 million copies, making it the largest dollar-volume pre-order in the history of the record business at the time. Record stores around the country found fans waiting in line on Monday morning before opening, and one New York store reportedly sold the album right off the back of the delivery truck. The album debuted at #1 on the *Billboard* album chart, a then-rare occurrence that hadn't happened in ten years since Stevie Wonder's *Songs in the Key of Life* in 1976 (and never before to a live album). It also became the first five-record set to reach the Top 10 and the first to sell over a million copies.

1987

In January Springsteen is elected, for the third time in a row, artist of the year by *Rolling Stone* magazine. On January 21, he gives a moving induction speech for Roy Orbison at the second annual Rock and Roll Hall of Fame ceremony, held at the Waldorf Astoria in New York City, and then duets with him on "Oh, Pretty Woman." He has just begun a new series of solo-based home studio sessions that will form the foundation of his new album; on the day of the ceremony he has already cut three songs on that first day of recording at Thrill Hill East (his New Jersey home studio): "Walk Like a Man," "Spare Parts," and "When You Need Me." The second day of sessions four days later is even more successful, with five songs recorded. All the material is cut with just Springsteen on acoustic guitar to a rhythm track. Like *Nebraska*, it is another "homemade" record.

In February Springsteen joins Steve Van Zandt at Shakedown Studios in New York City for his Van Zandt's self-produced third solo album-in-progress. Bruce provides background vocals on "Native American," which will be released on the album, *Freedom—No Compromise* in May.

In September, Bruce is DannyFederici's best man at his marriage to bride Kathlyn Helmeid. The E Street Band plays a rousing set at the reception in Janesville, Wisconsin.

Between May and July, Springsteen records at A&M Studios in Los Angeles. He makes much of the music solo, using a drum machine and playing guitar, piano, synthesizer, and bass. Then, back on the East Coast, he brings specific E Street Band members into the Hit Factory in New York City to embellish or add parts. Lyrics, for the first time, aren't centered around the man on the "road" but around the questions and concerns of the man in the "house," as Springsteen explains in his autobiography.

On September 25, Springsteen guests with U2 at JFK Stadium in Philadelphia, singing with Bono on "Stand by Me."

On October 3, the "Brilliant Disguise"/ "Lucky Man" single anticipates the release of the long-awaited new album, reaching the #5 position on the *Billboard* Hot 100 chart and #1 on Mainstream Rock Tracks. *Tunnel of Love*—Springsteen's eighth studio album—is released six day later and goes straight to #1, going triple platinum in the U.S. The album is a disappointment to anyone expecting a follow-up to *Born in the U.S.A.*: musically, *Tunnel of Love* is far from the bombastic style of its predecessor. As for the lyrics, only two songs ("Spare Parts" and "Cautious Man") are character pieces. The others are chapters in the autobiographical novel of Springsteen's marriage crisis. "The battleground has moved from the streets to the sheets, but the battle hasn't changed significantly," *Rolling Stone* magazine's Steve Pond wrote.[12] "You really shouldn't be allowed to hear this record until you've been married for a few years," Steven Hyden wrote in a 2014 article for *Grantland*, "though at that point it might strike a little too close to home. If Ingmar Bergman had been born in Freehold and cut his artistic teeth at the Stone Pony, he would've made this record in place of *Scenes from a Marriage* . . . The songs are about men and women who flirt, have sex, fall in love, get married, get bored, have sex with other people, and wind up stuck in the middle of that dark night from the second disc of *The River*."[13]

On October 22, Springsteen attends John Hammond's funeral, the man who signed him onto Columbia, singing Bob Dylan's "Forever Young."

On October 30, Springsteen joins Roy Orbison for the filming of *Roy Orbison & Friends: A Black & White Night*. The film is shot in the Cocoanut Grove, a nightclub in Los Angeles. Bruce plays guitar and shares vocals with Roy on "Dream Baby (How Long Must I Dream)," and plays guitar on the rest of the seventeen songs, sitting on a chair behind Orbison on the stage. The lineup includes Jackson Browne, Elvis Costello, T-Bone Burnett, J.D. Souther, Jennifer Warnes, k.d. lang,

Bonnie Raitt, and Tom Waits. The backing group is the TCB Band, who accompanied Elvis Presley between 1969 and 1977.

"Tunnel of Love" / "Two for the Road" is the second single released from the album, reaching #9 on the *Billboard* Hot 100 chart.

On December 13, Springsteen takes part in an all-star benefit for homeless children, backing Dion on "A Teenager in Love" along with Paul Simon, Rubén Blades, Lou Reed, James Taylor, and Billy Joel. He also plays "Born to Run" solo acoustic and "Glory Days" with Paul Simon and Billy Joel, backed by David Letterman's house band. The Chuck Berry classic "Rock and Roll Music" closes the show, featuring all of the evening's performers, with Bruce, Billy Joel, James Taylor, and Paul Simon taking verses.

1988

On January 20, at the Waldorf Astoria in New York City, Springsteen attends with then-wife Julianne Phillips the third annual Rock & Roll Hall of Fame induction ceremony with Bob Dylan, the Beatles, and the Beach Boys, who are the evening's key Hall of Fame inductees. It's the last time that Springsteen and Phillips are seen in public together. During an unforgettable night, he gives the induction speech for Dylan and performs in various supporting roles on "Twist and Shout," "I Saw Her Standing There," "Born on the Bayou," "(I Can't Get No) Satisfaction," "Like a Rolling Stone," and "All Along the Watchtower," in an unprecedented jam session including Ben E. King, Jeff Beck, George Harrison, Mick Jagger, John Fogerty, Billy Joel, Bob Dylan, Elton John, Yoko Ono, the Beach Boys, Little Richard, Ringo Starr, and Paul Simon among others.

On February 25, the Tunnel of Love Express Tour begins from the Centrum in Worcester, Massachusetts. The show seems to be designed to disorient Springsteen's audiences. The stage backdrop is a tapestry of Adam and Eve in the Garden of Eden. A theatrical entrance begins the show, set up to mimic fairgoers entering a carnival ride, with Springsteen assistant Terry Magovern playing a ticket-taker at the gate near an ominous and foreshadowing sign that says, "This is a dark ride." Roy Bittan is already on synthesizer as an extended intro to "Tunnel of Love" is played. Band members enter the stage two by two, taking tickets from Magovern, each more sharply dressed than for previous tours: Max Weinberg and Danny Federici, Garry Tallent and Nils Lofgren, the Miami Horns. Next comes Patti Scialfa in a tight miniskirt and big hair, carrying a bunch of balloons. Penultimately, Clarence Clemons enters with a single rose between his teeth. Springsteen appears last, dressed in trousers, a jacket, and a white shirt, tossing roses into the pit. The band's traditional positions on stage are flipped, with Clemons on the right, Bittan on the left, and so on; onstage spontaneity is kept to a minimum. The setlist is unusually static, and many of Springsteen's most popular concert numbers are omitted altogether. Instead, the shows feature Springsteen B-sides and outtakes as well as renditions of obscure genre songs by others.

The fourth single from the *Tunnel of Love* album, "One Step Up" / "Roulette," reaches #13 on the *Billboard* Hot 100 chart.

The European leg of the Tunnel of Love Express Tour begins in June, in Turin, Italy, in front of a crowd of 70,000. In Rome, the night before the two shows programmed at Stadio Flaminio, Springsteen plays "I'm on Fire," "The River," and "Dancing in the Dark" on the Spanish Steps with street musicians, on a borrowed guitar, in front of an audience of fifteen. During his stay in Rome, Bruce is portrayed in intimate poses with Patti Scialfa by Italian paparazzi. "When I look at her," Springsteen wrote in 2016, "I see and feel my best self." On June 18, the day before the concert at the Hippodrome de Vincennes, Springsteen and Clemons make a guest appearance in Paris at the S.O.S. Racism Concert. "The Promised Land" and "My Hometown" are followed by fantastic solo performances of "Blowin' in the Wind" and "Bad Moon Rising."

The most moving moment of the tour happens on July 19, when Bruce Springsteen and the E Street Band play at Radrennbahn Weissensee, a large cycling track located in East Berlin, in front of 220,000 East German fans. State television and radio record the show and censor it before airing it. Bruce then finds out that promoters have printed "Concert for Nicaragua" on the tickets, which upsets him and prompts him to give his infamous German-language speech prior to "Chimes of Freedom" (a few minutes before the concert, Bruce had the words translated and written down in phonetic spelling by his personal German driver, George Kerwinski) about "not being here for or against any certain government, but to play rock 'n' roll for you, East Berliners, in the hope that one day all barriers will be torn down." The speech originally included the word "walls" instead of "barriers," but this was changed at the proverbial last minute because Jon Landau considered the evocation of the Berlin Wall too blatant. Kerwinski had to literally climb onstage during the show and tell Bruce to say "barrier." Of course, the entire speech was censored in the original East German television and radio broadcasts anyway.

The Tunnel of Love Express Tour closes at Nou Camp in Barcelona after sixty-eight concerts attended by over two million people.

Soon afterward, the *Chimes of Freedom* EP is released, with live recordings of "Tougher than the Rest," "Be True," "Born to Run" (acoustic), and "Chimes of Freedom" by Dylan, whose proceeds go to Amnesty International. For this same organization a tour is set up—Human Rights Now!—that sees Springsteen, Sting,

Peter Gabriel, Tracy Chapman and Youssou N'Dour on the same stage. On September 2, the first concert is held at the Wembley Stadium in London. The tour then touches Italy, France, Hungary, Costa Rica, Canada, the United States, Japan, India, Greece, Zimbabwe, Ivory Coast, and Brazil, to finish on October 15 at the River Plate Stadium in Buenos Aires, after twenty concerts before 1.3 million spectators. Clemons has said that the tour for Amnesty International was his favorite, because it was the first time he ever saw so many black people at Bruce's concerts.

1989

On July 8, Springsteen participates in the annual Rock & Roll Hall of Fame ceremony at the Waldorf-Astoria in New York, in which Phil Spector, Dion, and the Rolling Stones are inducted. Bruce, presenting himself in the company of Patti Scialfa, gets onstage and dedicates an acoustic version of "Cryin'" to Roy Orbison, who has recently passed away; then duets with Mick Jagger in "It's Only Rock 'n' Roll."

Under the terms of the divorce of March 30, Springsteen pays Julianne Phillips $20 million. Meanwhile, there are rumors that Robert Stigwood offered him $10 million to play Che, opposite Meryl Streep, in *Evita*, and that he refused.

The *Video Anthology/1978–88* is published. Springsteen records a brilliant version of "Viva Las Vegas" that is included in Presley tribute album *The Last Temptation of Elvis*, and on June 30, in Atlantic City, he joins Jackson Browne on stage and with him sings "Stay," "Sweet Little Sixteen," and "Running on Empty." On August 11 at the Garden State Arts Center in Holmdel, New Jersey, he joins Ringo Starr and his All-Starr Band to perform "Get Back," "Long Tall Sally," "Photograph," and "With a Little Help from My Friends."

For his fortieth birthday, he plays for a small party invited to McLoone's in Sea Bright, accompanied by the complete E Street Band, including Little Steven joins. They play "Around and Around," "Sweet Little Sixteen," "Stand by Me," "What'd I Say," "Glory Days," "Havin' a Party," and "Twist and Shout." Halfway through the show, Springsteen tells the small crowd, "I may be old, but damn, I'm still handsome!" and dances with his mother. This is the last de facto E Street gig for a long time. In fact, Bruce has decided to break up the band, and on October 18, he calls them up one by one, breaking the news. In his memoir, *Big Man*, Clarence Clemons wrote that he and Nils Lofgren were in Japan with Ringo Starr as members of Ringo's All-Starr Band when the call came. "Ringo and I were drinking tea in a Japanese suite when the phone rang and the world changed," Clemons recalled. "I took the phone. 'Hey, Daddy-o,' I said. 'What's going on? How are you, man?'" What he heard was shocking. "'No shit?' I said eventually. 'I mean, I don't know what to say, Bruce.' . . . I hung up the phone and took a deep breath. I let it out slowly and sat back in the chair. I turned to Ringo. 'He's breaking up the band,' I said. 'For real?' said Ringo . . . 'Having been through this kind of breakup myself, you may have heard about it, I can tell you that life does go on.'"[14]

Springsteen would later admit that, even if it hurt, after sixteen years the band needed a break.

In December, he buys a villa in Beverly Hills for $14 million and moves there with Patti, who is pregnant. In Los Angeles he starts recording songs for a new album: "With Every Wish," "Trouble in Paradise," "Real World," "Roll of the Dice," "Soul Driver" . . . With him is a small group of session men: Randy Jackson (bass), Roy Bittan (keyboards), and Jeff Porcaro (drums).

1990

Recordings for the new album continue, with backing vocals by Bobby King and Sam Moore.

On February 12, Springsteen attends a private dinner-concert held on the beautiful estate of movie producer and investor Ted Field, for a fundraiser for the Rainforest Foundation's fight to preserve the Amazon ecosystem, billed as "An Evening in Brazil." About 800 guests attend (the cream of Hollywood), each donating $5,000 a head for the privilege to hear an all-star band including Sting (the organizer), Paul Simon, Don Henley, Bruce Hornsby, Herbie Hancock, Brandford Marsalis and Paulinho Da Costa.

On March 1, during a Tom Petty concert at the Inglewood Forum in California, Bob Dylan and Springsteen get onstage to sing with Creedence Clearwater Revival's "Travelin' Band."

On July 25, at Cedars-Sinai Medical Center in Los Angeles, Patti Scialfa gives birth to Evan James Springsteen.

On November 16 and 17, Springsteen plays two acoustic concerts at Los Angeles's Shrine Auditorium to benefit the Christic Institute. It's the first time after nearly twenty years that Bruce has performed solo for a whole concert. The performances are stunning, including world premieres of "Red Headed Woman," "57 Channels (And Nothin' On)," "When the Lights Go Out," and "Real World." This last one, performed by Bruce on the piano, is one of the most inspired performances of his career. For encores Bonnie Raitt and Jackson Browne join in on Dylan's "Highway 61 Revisited" and "Across the Borderline."

1991

On January 16, Springsteen attends the sixth Annual Rock & Roll Hall of Fame Awards at the Waldorf Astoria in New York City, with the Impressions, Wilson

Pickett, the Byrds, and Ike & Tina Turner as the evening's key inductees. Bruce does not give an induction speech but takes the stage alongside Jackson Browne, Don Henley, and Chaka Khan to perform "People Get Ready" and then participates in the closing jam, trading lead vocals with John Fogerty on "In the Midnight Hour," backed by the Byrds, John Lee Hooker, Patti Smith, Robert Cray, and Bonnie Raitt, among others.

In February recordings finish for what will then become the album *Human Touch*.

Bruce and Patti get married on June 8 on their own property in Beverly Hills. Among the ninety guests are the complete E Street Band, Jon Landau, Jackson Browne, Bonnie Raitt, John Fogerty, and Sting. During the ceremony, they play a new song Bruce has written specifically for that day, "If I Should Fall Behind." The couple have their honeymoon "fifties-style" in a little log cabin in Yosemite Park.

Although Springsteen has completed the *Human Touch* album sessions by early 1991 and has more than enough material to release the hoped-for spring album, he chooses to hold off and opts instead to write more songs during the summer of 1991. The *Lucky Town* recording sessions begin in September at Bruce's Los Angeles home studio and are then augmented at A&M Studios later during the year.

On December 30 Jessica Rae is born, Bruce and Patti's second child.

1992

On March 27, *Human Touch* and *Lucky Town* are jointly released, and respectively reach second and third places in the American charts. *Human Touch*'s release is met with a generally mixed critical reception. Better reviews greet *Lucky Town*, even if most critics write that the aims of the two albums would have been better realized by a single, more carefully shaped collection. Years later, Bruce will comment: "I tried writing happy songs in the early 1990s and it didn't work; the public didn't like it."

On May 9, Springsteen appears for the first time ever on TV on *Saturday Night Live*, playing "Lucky Town," "57 Channels (And Nothin' On)," and "Living Proof" with the core of his new tour band: Shane Fontayne (guitar), Tommy Sims (bass), Roy Bittan (keyboards), Zack Alford (drums), and Bobby King (backing vocals).

One June 5, at the Hollywood Center Studios #4, Springsteen does a "Dress Rehearsal Concert" with the new band, with the newly hired Crystal Taliefero (guitar, vocals) and four female backing singers. Steve Van Zandt joins Bruce on stage for "Glory Days" and "Bobby Jean."

On June 15 at the Globe Arena in Stockholm, the 1992–93 tour begins, Springsteen's first without the E Street Band. On July 23, after fifteen dates in

Europe, the American leg kicks off with a record-breaking eleven-night stand at the Brendan Byrne Arena in East Rutherford, New Jersey. Forty-nine shows are to follow (the last taking place on December 17 in Lexington, Kentucky).

1993

On January 6, at St. Bartholomew's Church in New York City, Springsteen sings "If I Should Fall Behind" at the funeral of Kristen Ann Carr, daughter of Springsteen's co-manager Barbara Carr and stepdaughter of Dave Marsh. Kristen was diagnosed with sarcoma at the age of nineteen and told that her future was uncertain: sarcoma did not respond well to the usual treatments for cancer, and little to no progress had been made in finding treatments that would work. Kristen's response was, "Okay, let's change that." She began brainstorming about raising funds against sarcoma alternately from a bed at Memorial Sloan-Kettering Cancer Center and from her off-campus apartment at New York University, where she was an honor student in journalism. Before she died at the age of twenty-one, she instructed her family to continue the mission that she had started. The Kristen Ann Carr Fund was established that same year. Springsteen would help the foundation by participating to various benefit events over the years.

On January 12, he gives the induction speech for Creedence Clearwater Revival to the Rock & Roll Hall of Fame, also backing John Fogerty on "Who'll Stop the Rain," "Green River," and "Born in the Bayou."

In March, he takes part in the recording sessions for Patti Scialfa's debut album, providing guitar and harmony vocals on "Talk to Me Like the Rain" and background vocals on "Big Black Heaven." Both recordings will be issued on Scialfa's *Rumble Doll* album in July 1993.

On March 23, Springsteen plays a benefit show at the Count Basie Theatre in New Jersey, offering a fantastic setlist. He opens with a trio of solo acoustic songs: "Does This Bus Stop at 82nd Street?" (last played in 1975), Woody Guthrie's "Ain't Got No Home" (only played once before), and "This Hard Land" (a *Born in the U.S.A.* outtake never played before). The band comes in then for a set full of surprises, like the first known live performance of "Viva Las Vegas," the live premiere of "When You're Alone," the first performance of "Blinded by the Light" in seventeen years, and Springsteen's only performance ever of Billy Ray Cyrus's "Achy Breaky Heart." E Street mate Max Weinberg guests on "Glory Days."

The European leg of the World Tour starts from Glasgow on March 31. Bruce Springsteen and his new band would fill stadiums playing thirty shows in Scotland, Ireland, England, France, Spain, Portugal, Italy, Switzerland, Belgium, the Netherlands, Germany, Sweden, Denmark, and Norway. The World Tour ends with the last concert in Oslo's Valle Hovin Stadion, after 101 shows in 62 different cities with a total attendance of 2 million people.

Back in the U.S.A., on June 24 Springsteen plays a "Concert to Fight Hunger" at Brendan Byrne Arena in East Rutherford, New Jersey, to benefit World Hunger Year, the Food & Hunger Hotline, and the Community Food Bank of New Jersey. The show is opened by a duet with Joe Ely on "Ain't Got No Home." Max Weinberg plays on "Jersey Girl." Steve Van Zandt & the Miami Horns play with Bruce on "Glory Days," "It's Been a Long time," "Havin' a Party," and "It's All Right," and they are joined by Clarence Clemons in the midst of "Tenth Avenue Freeze-Out," striding out of the shadows just as Bruce gets to the part about the Big Man joining the band, for an ovation from the crowd of 19,000. "I've never heard a reaction that intense before," guitarist Shane Fontayne would comment.

The day after the Meadowlands show, Springsteen makes a surprise appearance on *Late Night with David Letterman* on June 25, playing "Glory Days" backed by Letterman's in-house band. The show is Letterman's last on NBC before he moves to present the *Late Show* on CBS.

On June 26, Springsteen plays a benefit concert for the Kristen Ann Carr Fund at Madison Square Garden in New York City. Terence Trent D'Arby joins him on "Many Rivers to Cross," "I Have Faith in These Desolate Times," "Jole Blon," and "Jumpin' Jack Flash." The event exceeds all expectations and allows the newly formed KACF to begin funding the training of sarcoma experts almost immediately.

In early 1993 director Jonathan Demme approached Springsteen about writing a song for his film-in-progress, *Philadelphia*. Springsteen was non-committal to the project but told Demme he would try and come up with something appropriate for the film. Following the conclusion of the 1992–93 World Tour in support of *Human Touch* and *Lucky Town* in June–July Springsteen retreats to his home studio and comes up with "Streets of Philadelphia." A first version is recorded during August 1993 at Thrill Hill West (Bruce's California home studio) and features only Springsteen on vocals, guitar, bass, synthesizer, and drum machine. Later that same month, background vocals by Tommy Sims are added. The song is issued on December 30 as part of the *Philadelphia* soundtrack CD.

1994

On January 5 Sam Ryan Springsteen is born, third child to Bruce and Patti.

On March 21, at the 66th Academy Awards, Bruce wins an Oscar for "Streets of Philadelphia" in the Best Original Song category, receiving the prize from the hands of Whitney Houston (it's the first time that the Best Song Oscar has gone to a rocker). The song is a critical triumph and wins four Grammy Awards, including Song of the Year, Best Rock Song, Best Rock Vocal Performance, and Best Song Written Specifically for a Motion Picture.

"Street of Philadelphia" is released as a single in February, blowing up into a worldwide smash, crowning the charts in eight countries, and peaking at #9 on *Billboard's* Hot 100 singles list.

With "Streets of Philadelphia" on the charts, Springsteen returns to his studio in Los Angeles for an album that—as he tells the German magazine *Bravo*—he hopes to have out by the end of the year. In April he records some synthesizer-based songs, with occasional help from Roy Bittan (keyboards), Tommy Sims (bass), and Zach Alford (drums). But all of these songs remain unheard and/or unknown, making this period somewhat of a mystery, even today.

On April 30, he participates in a private party in West Hollywood, California, to launch the new club House of Blues, and sings "Sex Machine" with James Brown and a backing vocal group consisting of Dan Aykroyd, Magic Johnson, Wesley Snipes, and Woody Harrelson. Danny Federici is in the house band on keyboards.

But the strangest gig of the year is the one at the Hollywood Palladium, on May 29, when Bruce participates as the guest star at an American Booksellers Association Convention and is jokingly introduced as "a guy who isn't up to our musical standards, but we'll let him play anyhow," before he joins on stage the Rock Bottom Remainders, a rather tongue-in-cheek band name for an amateur outfit consisting of bestselling authors like Stephen King, Dave Marsh, Ken Follett and *The Simpsons'* creator, Matt Groening. Together they play "Gloria."

On October 20, Springsteen and Neil Young guest at a Bob Dylan concert at the Roseland Ballroom in New York City, both playing guitar on "Rainy Day Women #12 & 35" and "Highway 61 Revisited."

Springsteen visits Patti Smith after her husband's death. According to Lenny Kaye, "Bruce took Patti's young kid Jackson out for a bike ride, and was generally cool."

Between October and December he records seven or eight new songs utilizing a three-man backup band consisting of Shane Fontayne (guitar), Tommy Sims (bass), and Zach Alford (drums). None of this material has yet leaked out. These sessions seem to have given way to a surprise resolution to reconvene the E Street Band in conjunction with a related decision to release a *Greatest Hits* anthology: Springsteen feels that he needs to reconnect with his history.

1995

Along with the decision to put out an oldies set, Jon Landau has the idea of reviving the E Street Band. Springsteen agrees immediately. The calls to the band go out on January 5. When Clemons gets it at his house in San Francisco, he flies back to New York so quickly he doesn't have time to cancel the party his friends have planned for him. On the 9th, all the members (including Steve Van Zandt) gather at the Factory for the first E Street Band session in eleven years. Some new songs are recorded—"Secret Garden," "Blood Brothers," "Without You," Back in Your Arms," "Waiting on the End of the World"—together with a new version of "This Hard Land," a *Born in the U.S.A.* outtake, and the cover of the Havalinas' "High Hopes."

Greatest Hits is released on February 28, 1995. It contains fourteen oldies, plus a 1982 version of "Murder Incorporated" (a song that had never surfaced before), and three songs just recorded with the E Street Band: "Secret Garden," "Blood Brothers," and "This Hard Land." The compilation is commercially successful, hitting the peaks of the U.S. and UK album charts (for the first time since *Tunnel of Love*).

Bruce Springsteen and the E Street Band reconvene at Tramps, a club off Gramercy Park in Manhattan, where Jonathan Demme will shoot a live video for the hits package's lead single, "Murder Incorporated." It's the band's first gig together since October 15, 1988. They play for two hours.

The mini-reunion continues on April 5, when Springsteen and the band appear on the *Late Show with David Letterman* playing "Murder Incorporated" and "Secret Garden." That same night they move to the Sony Music Studio soundstage, where they tape a whole concert: a shortened hour-long version is broadcast on television around the world. Live versions of "Streets of Philadelphia," "Murder Incorporated," and "Thunder Road" are officially released on the *Hungry Heart Berlin '95* CD single, which also contains a "Hungry Heart" take recorded during a performance that Springsteen gives on July 9 at Café Eckstein in Berlin with Wolfgang Niedecken and His Leopardefellband.

On September 5, Cleveland's Rock & Roll Hall of Fame Museum celebrates its official opening with a huge concert at the Municipal Stadium, which lasts seven hours and ends at two in the morning. Among the artists in the lineup are Bob Dylan, Chuck Berry, Jerry Lee Lewis, Aretha Franklin, Johnny Cash, James Brown, Little Richard, Lou Reed, Jackson Browne, and Bruce Springsteen and the E Street Band, who open the show playing "Johnny B. Goode" with Chuck Berry, accompany Jerry Lee Lewis in "Great Balls of Fire" and "Whole Lotta Shakin' Goin' On," and perform "Shake, Rattle and Roll," "She's the One," and "Darkness on the Edge of Town" on their set before bringing Dylan onstage for the historic duet "Forever Young."

Springsteen's studio sessions and live appearances with the E Street Band seem to trigger a burst of songwriting activity in the months that follow. Back home in Los Angeles, Bruce pulls out his motorcycle and heads off for one of his regulars trip into the desert with his friend Matty Delia. On the occasion of this short trip, Springsteen comes into contact with stories of ordinary madness along the coast between Mexico and the United States and starts to think about writing on the subject. Once he cuts "The Ghost of Tom Joad" he feels he has the right tone for the record that he wants to make: a follow-up to *Nebraska* with stories set in the mid-nineties and in the land of his current residence, California. The result is *The Ghost of Tom Joad*, released on November 21. The album consists of seven solo tracks and five tracks recorded with the help of Danny Federici (accordion, keyboards), Garry Tallent (bass), Soozie Tyrell (violin), Marty Rifkin (pedal steel guitar), and Gary Mallaber (drums). *The Ghost of Tom Joad* receives mostly favorable reviews. However, due to its folkish nature—very far from the expected E Street Band rock 'n' roll comeback— it reached only #11 on the *Billboard* 200, breaking a string of eight consecutive Top 5 studio albums in the U.S. for Springsteen.

On November 19, Springsteen takes part in Frank Sinatra's eightieth birthday tribute concert at the Shrine Auditorium in Los Angeles—together with Tony Bennett, Little Richard, Bono, and others—and gives a great spoken introduction about Sinatra and his influence on him and everybody else from New Jersey, before playing an acoustic "Angel Eyes."

Three days later, the Ghost of Tom Joad Solo Acoustic Tour kicks off from the Count Basie Theatre in Red Bank, New Jersey. At theaters seating up to 5,000 people, Springsteen is alone on stage, singing and playing acoustic guitar for two and a half hours. Bruce will play 127 shows over the next eighteen months, completing the tour in May 1997.

1996

The soundtrack to Tim Robbins's new film, *Dead Man Walking*, comes out. For the occasion Springsteen composed a song with the same name.

The first American leg of the Solo Acoustic Tour continues until January 28. Then Springsteen moves to Europe, where he plays until the beginning of August (also making his debut at the Royal Albert Hall in London). On April 10, in Rome, before the concert, he meets with Italian composer Ennio Morricone—one of his favorites.

In May, Bruce and Patti move their family from California back to New Jersey, setting up in a farmhouse just east of Freehold.

The fall American leg of the Solo Acoustic Tour kicks off in Pittsburgh in September. The October 26 concert at the Event Center Arena of the San Jose State University is part of a seminar entitled *Souls of the People: Steinbeck* and organized by the John Steinbeck Research Center. Consequently, the show features an extra-long introduction to "Across the Border" in which Bruce speaks about—and reads extensively from—Steinbeck's *Grapes of Wrath*.

On November 8, the concert in the gymnasium of St. Rose of Lima School in Freehold, New Jersey, is a unique homecoming: alumnus Springsteen's first known performance at his primary school since 1965, when Bruce (as a member of the Castiles) played CYO dances there. He dedicates "This Hard Land" to Castiles manager Tex Vinyard's wife, Marion (in the audience), and plays some songs together with Soozie Tyrell and Patti Scialfa, before ending the concert with a little comedy piece written for the occasion—"In Freehold."

The three-night stand at the Paramount Theatre in Asbury Park on November 21, 24, and 25 is full of surprises and special guests, like Danny Federici and Vini Lopez (the latter on stage with Springsteen after 22 years).

1997

In the first two months of the year, Springsteen brings his Solo Acoustic Tour to Japan (four shows) and Australia (ten shows). The tour ends in Paris on May 26.

On May 5, he receives the Polar Music Prize from King Carl XVI Gustaf of Sweden during a ceremony in Stockholm.

Back in the U.S.A., for his forty-seventh birthday he organizes a private "Fiesta" theme party in a field on his and Patti's Colts Neck farm, with the New York City roots/bluegrass outfit the Gotham Playboys providing the music. Bruce has heard about the band from Soozie Tyrell and allegedly joins in on some songs during the party. A few weeks later, Springsteen hires several members of the group (Jeremy Chatzky, Sam Bardfeld, Larry Eagle, Mark Clifford, and Charles Giordano) to back him during a November 2 recording session at Bruce's home studio undertaken for the purpose of contributing a song for a planned spring 1998 Pete Seeger charity album. This group will eventually become the Sessions Band.

On December 12, at the JFK Center for Performing Arts in Washington, D.C., with Bob Dylan one of the honorees of the annual Kennedy Center Honors, Springsteen performs "The Times They Are A-Changin.'"

1998

In February, Springsteen tells Toby Scott (his audio archivist and recording engineer) his intention to put all the unreleased tracks recorded over the past twenty-five years in a box set. They have at least 350 unused songs dating from 1972 and 1997. Scott starts to work, gathering the potential material from Springsteen's massive audio library (located, along with Sony's sound archives, in the high-tech Iron Mountain facility near Buffalo, New York), while Bruce's New Jersey home studio (Thrill Hill East) serves as the main operational center for all *Tracks* project activities.

On April 26, after a long period of illness, Douglas Springsteen dies at the the age of seventy-three. Bruce's father is buried at the St. Rose of Lima Cemetery, in Freehold, New Jersey. His widow, Adele, moves back to New Jersey.

By late June the number of evaluated songs for the *Tracks* box set is down to about 128. It is narrowed down yet again during July to about one hundred songs. A commercial decision is then made later in the summer to reduce the size of the release to a four-CD (sixty-six-track) package.

Tracks is released on November 9. The box set mostly consists of never-before-released songs recorded during the sessions for Springsteen's many albums, but also includes a number of single B-sides, as well as demos and alternate versions of already-released material. Despite stellar reviews, the initial sales are well below expectations.

A few days later, Bruce calls Roy Bittan to gauge his interest in an E Street Band reunion tour. The answer is positive. But Bruce is still worried it would be a nostalgic exercise. In the beginning, he suggests that Landau book only ten shows because he isn't sure of the chemistry. Some of the band members are not even invited directly by him, but by one of the accountants in his financial manager's office. Tallent, for one, feels more than a little slighted, and initially says, "Thanks, but no thanks."

Talks of an agreement between Springsteen's management and band members start. Since 1975, Springsteen has been officially 100 percent owner of the "E Street Band" brand. Up until the (temporary) breakup in 1989, the band members were on the Boss's payroll and had no rights on any percentage of proceeds earned through ticket sales and merchandising. Not to mention albums. Except for *Live/1975–85*, all records are in Bruce Springsteen's name and never in Bruce Springsteen and the E Street Band's. Thus a new agreement is signed, whose details are not shared in the public domain. It is only stated that the E Street Band is made up of Bruce, Roy Bittan, Danny Federici, Steve Van Zandt, Nils Lofgren, Garry Tallent, Patti Scialfa, Clarence Clemons, and Max Weinberg; that none of the above can be fired; and that the members equally share all proceeds from concerts (royalties on ticket sales and merchandising), except Springsteen, who gets a bigger share. By virtue of this agreement, Soozie Tyrell, joining the group in 2002, will never be officially accredited as a member of the E Street Band, and neither will Charles Giordano and Jake Clemons, who will be called on to replace Federici and Clemons after their deaths.

Having cleared up the legal issues, on December 8, with an official statement the imminent reunion of the E Street Band is announced (inclusive of Steve Van Zandt) for a world tour. Two days later, Springsteen appears unexpectedly in Paris during a show supporting Amnesty International in which Peter Gabriel, Alanis Morissette, Radiohead, Youssou N'Dour, and Tracy Chapman participate, and performs solo "The Ghost of Tom Joad," "Born in the U.S.A.," "Working on the Highway," and "No Surrender."

1999

Partly as a consequence of the slow sales of the *Tracks* box set, it is decided in January to release an abbreviated single CD version titled *18 Tracks*, containing fifteen recordings already issued on *Tracks*, plus three previously unreleased songs ("The Fever," "Trouble River," and "The Promise").

When the E Street Band meets up for rehearsals in the first days of March at Asbury Park's Convention Hall, Bruce's doubts remain, because the old connections aren't yet there. On the fifth day of rehearsals Bruce decides that what is missing is . . . the audience. Therefore, they let in about twenty-five people who had been hanging out in the front of the theater to hear the band play "The Promised Land," "Tougher than the Rest," "She's the One," "Backstreets," and "Bobby Jean." Everything becomes electric suddenly.

The first official occasion for the reunited E Street Band is the Rock & Roll Hall of Fame Ceremony held on March 15 at the Waldorf Astoria, where Springsteen is scheduled to be inducted. After a spectacular induction speech made by Bono, Bruce and the band come up on stage playing "The Promised Land," "Backstreets," "Tenth Avenue Freeze-Out," and "In the Midnight Hour" in a duet with Wilson Pickett and with Billy Joel on keyboards. Later Bruce joins an all-star jam session with, among others, Bono, Joel, Paul McCartney, Robbie Robertson, Dion, Eric Clapton, Lauryn Hill, Bonnie Raitt, Melissa Etheridge, Chris Isaak, the Staple Singers, and D'Angelo.

The Reunion Tour kicks off from Barcelona on April 9 and, after thirty-six sold-out shows in Europe, hits the States in May with a record fifteen-show stand at the old Meadowlands Arena in New Jersey, with a total attendance of 300,000. The new song "Land of Hope and Dreams," played throughout the tour, is always preceded by Bruce telling the audience that he's come to "resuscitate you, regenerate you, reconfiscate you, reindoctrinate you, resexualate you, rededicate you, reliberate you with the power and the promise . . . with the majesty, the mystery, and the ministry of ROCK 'N' ROLL!"

2000

Springsteen makes his first-ever appearance in a feature film (i.e., excluding documentaries and music films/videos), playing himself during a two-minute dream sequence for the movie *High Fidelity*. In the film Bruce performs a blues riff on guitar while talking to the film's dreaming lead character (John Cusack), who ends the conversation with Bruce by saying "Good luck, goodbye" (a spoof of the final line in Springsteen's song "Bobby Jean").

The American leg of the Reunion Tour goes on. On June 4, Springsteen plays a new song, titled "American Skin (41 Shots)," during a concert in Atlanta, Georgia. It is inspired by the recent shooting of Amadou Diallo, a twenty-three-year-old immigrant from Guinea who was killed by four New York City plainclothes policemen. The four officers fired a combined total of forty-one shots, nineteen of which struck Diallo, outside his apartment in Bronx. The post-shooting investigation found no weapons on Diallo's body, contrary to what the policemen had declared; the item he had pulled out of his jacket was not a gun, but a rectangular black wallet. They were charged with second-degree murder. On February 25, 2000, a jury in Albany acquitted the officers of all charges. The song—especially the line "You can get killed just for living in your American skin"—is criticized by Police Commissioner Howard Safir and Patrick J. Lynch, the president of the Patrolmen's Benevolent Association, who urge New York City officers to boycott Springsteen's concerts at Madison Square Garden—where Bruce plays it again.

The ten-night stand at Madison Square Garden is the final act of the Reunion Tour. Bruce Springsteen and the E Street Band played 133 shows in sixty-two cities, selling more than 2.7 million tickets.

In November, Bruce plays with Joe Grushecky and the Houserockers at the Light of Day benefit for the Parkinson's Disease Foundation, organized at the Stone Pony by Bob Benjamin. One month later, he plays two Christmas shows at the Convention Hall in Asbury Park with a lot of friends on stage (the E Streeters plus Bobby Bandiera, Jimmy Vivino, Lisa Lowell, and Southside Johnny). A new song titled "My City of Ruins" is dedicated to Asbury Park.

2001

On March 27, Sony releases *Live in New York City*, a double album recorded at concerts on June 29 and July 1 at Madison Square Garden, that reaches #5 on the *Billboard* 200 and #1 on the *Billboard* Internet Album Charts and is also released in home video.

During the first half of the year, Bruce does some rare guest appearances on stage while also carrying on some recording sessions with the E Street Band— their first together since 1995.

On September 11, 2001, the twin towers of the World Trade Center in New York and part of the Pentagon in Washington are attacked and destroyed by Al

Qaeda terrorists. Many innocent people lose their lives in the blackest day of American history since the Japanese attack on Pearl Harbor. Ten days after the massacre, Springsteen opens the *America: A Tribute to Heroes* national telethon from the Sony Music Studios in New York City with the song he played recently for another city, "My City of Ruins." Bruce plays acoustic guitar and harmonica, joined by Steve Van Zandt, Patti Scialfa, Clarence Clemons, Soozie Tyrell, Lisa Lowell, Dee Holmes, and Layonne Holmes on backing vocals.

Rolling Stone polls its readers: to start again after September 11, which artist would best represent America? Springsteen receives the greatest number of votes (38 percent), followed by Dylan (24 percent). On the day of the 9/11 tragedy, Springsteen is going to pick up his children from school when a car drives by and from the rolled-down window a voice shouts out to him, "Bruce, we need you."

2002

On January 12, a sixtieth birthday party for Clarence Clemons is organized at the B.B. King Dance and Nite Club in the Foxwoods Resort Casino of Mashantucket, Connecticut. Springsteen plays "Raise Your Hand," "Pink Cadillac," and "Mustang Sally" before B.B. King himself presents the cake, joining Bruce on "Glory Days."

Following the tragic events of September 11, 2001, Springsteen has written a number of new songs influenced by the disaster. A new series of studio sessions with the E Street Band takes place at Southern Tracks Studios in Atlanta from late January to mid-March with Brendan O'Brien as producer. It's the first time since 1973 that someone other than Springsteen or Landau is sitting in the control room.

On May 23, together with former Castiles member George Theiss, Springsteen attends the inauguration of Vinyard Park, between Jackson Street and Central Street in Freehold, dedicated to his old patrons Tex and Marion Vinyard.

On July 30 Columbia releases *The Rising*—the twelfth studio album by Bruce Springsteen, and his first with the E Street Band in eighteen years. Based on Springsteen's reflections during the aftermath of the 9/11 attacks, the album receives widespread acclaim from critics. Thom Jurek of *AllMusic* calls the record "one of the very best examples in recent history of how popular art can evoke a time period and all of its confusing and often contradictory notions, feelings and impulses,"[15] while *Uncut* magazine considers *The Rising* "a brave and beautiful album of humanity, hurt and hope from the songwriter best qualified to speak to and for his country. . . . A towering achievement."[16] The album debuts at #1 on the *Billboard* 200 chart, peaking at #1 in England, Belgium, Canada, Denmark, Finland, Germany, Italy, the Netherlands, Spain, and France as well.

The Rising Tour kicks off from the Continental Airlines Arena in East Ruther-ford, New Jersey, on August 7. Soozie Tyrell on violin is added to the band.

2003

The Rising wins three Grammy Awards: Best Rock Album, Best Rock Song ("The Rising"), and Best Male Rock Vocal Performance.

The Rising Tour continues in America and Australia before it gets to Europe for twenty-four shows in big stadiums, opening in Rotterdam and closing at S. Siro Stadium in Milan under heavy rain (Springsteen told me that he considers this as one of his "top, top five shows ever"). In summer, the tour comes back to the U.S.: from mid-July through early October, Bruce Springsteen and the E Street Band play thirty-three dates in stadiums, starting with what would become an unprecedented ten-night stand in New Jersey's Giants Stadium, selling all the 566,560 tickets available—a ticket-selling feat that no other musical act can come close to. Overall, the tour grossed $221.5 million over its two years.

Live in Barcelona—a full concert home video of the October 16, 2002, perfor-mance at Palau Sant Jordi—is released in November, the same day of the release of *The Essential Bruce Springsteen*, a three-disc compilation album also including previously unreleased cuts ("From Small Things," "None but the Brave, "County Fair"), B-sides ("The Big Payback," "Held Up Without a Gun"), contributions to soundtracks ("Missing," "Lift Me Up," "Dead Man Walking"), and other rarities.

2004

In January, Springsteen provides guitar and keyboards to recordings of "You Can't Go Back," "Rose," and "Love (Stand Up"), three of Patti Scialfa's songs that would be released in July on Scialfa's album *23rd Street Lullaby*.

Rolling Stone magazine ranks their "Fifty Greatest Artists of All Time" as "The Immortals." In the top three slots: the Beatles, Bob Dylan, and Elvis Presley. Springsteen is at #23.

In February, with "Disorder in the House" (a track written in memory of Warren Zevon, who died in late 2003), Springsteen is awarded his eleventh Grammy. A few weeks later, he inducts Jackson Browne into the Rock & Roll Hall of Fame at a ceremony in New York City. In his speech, Bruce recalls first seeing Browne at the Bitter End in the early seventies after he played his own set at Max's Kansas City. He also notes that the audiences the two drew were a little different. "Jackson Browne was a bona fide rock 'n' roll sex star," said Springsteen. "Now, being a little competitive, I also noticed that while the E Street Band and I were sweatin' our asses off for hours just to put some fannies in the seats, that obviously due to what must have been some strong homoerotic undercurrent in our music, we were drawing rooms filled with men. Not that great-lookin' men, either. Meanwhile, Jackson is drawing more women than an Indigo Girls show!"

On September 16, thirty-six years after their split, the Castiles get aired for the first time on radio. A few weeks earlier the Reverend Fred Coleman had found some cassettes containing recordings from two shows the band had played in 1967 at the Left Foot in Freehold. Extracts of the shows are sent on air by National Public Radio in addition to interviews held by George Theiss and Bob Alfano.

In October Springsteen land the E Street Band take part in the Vote for Change Tour, in support of Democrat John Kerry's campaign for the presidency. R.E.M., John Fogerty, Bright Eyes, Pearl Jam, Dave Matthews Band, John Mellencamp, Jackson Browne, and others all work together to create the mood. The duets with Michael Stipe on "Because the Night" and "Man on the Moon," and with Eddie Vedder on "Better Man" and "No Surrender," are unforgettable.

2005

On March 14, Springsteen inducts Rock & Roll Hall of Fame nominees U2 and joins them for "I Still Haven't Found What I'm Looking For."

On March 19, Springsteen is at Thrill Hill East, recording with the musicians used for the 1997 recording of "We Shall Overcome" and other two traditional songs ("My Oklahoma Home" and "Jesse James"). His intention is to make an album of folk songs made popular by Pete Seeger. In this second "Seeger Session," eight other tracks are recorded: "Old Dan Tucker," "Mrs. McGrath," "Erie Canal," "O Mary Don't You Weep," "John Henry," "Shenandoah," "Froggie Went A-Courtin'" and "Pay Me My Money Down." The band—soon renamed the Sessions Band— is made of Frank Bruno (guitar), Mark Clifford (banjo), Jeremy Chatzky (bass), Charles Giordano (accordion, organ), Sam Barfield (violin), Soozie Tyrell (violin), Ed Manion (sax), Art Baron (tuba), Richie Rosenberg (trombone), Mark Pender (trumpet), Patti Scialfa (vocals), and Larry Eagle (drums).

On April 4, Springsteen plays (alone at the guitar and piano) at the Rechnitz Theater in Red Bank, New Jersey, for the taping of the *Storytellers* series for VH1. The performance will be officially released on DVD in September 2005.

Devils & Dust, Bruce's thirteenth studio album and his third acoustic one (after *Nebraska* and *The Ghost of Tom Joad*) is released on April 25, debuting at #1 on the *Billboard* 200 album chart.

The Devils & Dust Solo and Acoustic Tour kicks off from Detroit on April 25, featuring Springsteen performing alone on stage on a variety of instruments: guitar, harmonica, piano, electric piano, pump organ, dobro, autoharp, ukulele, banjo, stomping board. The stage set is sparse, with a few instrument stations laid out, a carpet and lamp, two reddish chandeliers, and darkish, subdued stage lighting. After fourteen shows, the tour goes to Europe for nineteen dates, and then back to the U.S. until the closing gig in Trenton on November 22.

One week before the end of the tour, Columbia releases the *Born to Run 30th Anniversary Edition* box set. The package includes a remastered CD version of the original album; *Wings for Wheels*, a lengthy documentary on the making of the album, with bonus film of three songs recorded live on May 1, 1973, at the Ahmanson Theatre in Los Angeles; and the DVD *Bruce Springsteen & the E Street Band Hammersmith Odeon, London '75*, a full-length concert film recorded on November 18, 1975, during the brief European leg of the Born to Run tour.

After lengthy negotiations, meanwhile, Springsteen signs a new deal with Sony BMG bringing in $101 million. During the ten years of the contract, Springsteen must put out five or six albums containing uncut versions, plus a series of box set anthologies and live recordings. According to the German magazine *Der Spiegel*, Bertelsmann AG pushed for Sony Corp to sack Andrew Lack, chief executive of 50–50 joint venture Sony BMG, after he signed the contract with Springsteen, Bertelsmann fearing that Springsteen could not bring in as much as Lack agreed to pay him. Lack would be appointed chairman of Sony BMG in 2006.

2006

On January 7, Bruce attends the sixtieth birthday party of Jann Wenner (founder of *Rolling Stone* magazine) at Le Bernardin on West 51st Street in New York City. In lieu of a toast Bruce performs a song that he wrote for the occasion. Additional performances are offered by Bette Midler, John Mellencamp, and David Bowie. Other guests on hand are John Kerry, Uma Thurman, Caroline Kennedy, Al Gore, Tom Wolfe, Larry David, Robin Williams, Richard Gere, Robbie Robertson, Michael Douglas, and Atlantic Records founder Ahmet Ertegun.

The third and final "Seeger Session" is held at Rumson on January 21. Lisa Lowell (vocals) is added to the band. New songs are recorded, including "Eyes on the Prize," "Jacob's Ladder," "Buffalo Gals," "How Can I Keep from Singing?," "Bring 'Em Home," and "American Land."

On February 8, at the Staples Center in Los Angeles, Springsteen receives a Grammy Award for Best Solo Rock Vocal for "Devils & Dust" and performs the song solo, returning to the stage to perform "In the Midnight Hour" as a finale in tribute to Wilson Pickett, who passed away in January. With Bruce on stage are Sam Moore, Elvis Costello, the Edge, Bonnie Raitt, Dr. John, and Irma Thomas.

In February, Springsteen contributes vocals and guitar to "Code of Silence," "A Good Life," and "Is She the One"—three songs for Joe Grushecky's third solo album, *A Good Life*, which will be released in August.

We Shall Overcome: The Seeger Sessions—the first Springsteen album with songs not written by him—is released on April 26, receiving widespread acclaim. Pete Seeger himself is pleased by the result, saying, "It was a great honor. [Springsteen]'s an extraordinary person, as well as an extraordinary singer." The album quickly hits #1 in England, Italy, Norway, and Sweden and sets itself in the Top 5 on the American charts.

The Bruce Springsteen with the Seeger Sessions Band Tour—billed as "an all-new evening of gospel, folk, and blues"—kicks off on April 30 from New Orleans's Fairgrounds, where Springsteen and his band are the headliners at the New Orleans Jazz & Heritage Festival. The show—a great mixture of songs from the *We Shall Overcome* album and revisited Springsteen classics such as "Johnny 99," "Open All Night," and "My City of Ruins"—is joyful, emotional, and very well received by the audience, closed by a slow, touching rendition of "When the Saints Go Marchin' In."

The tour continues with seventeen American shows and thirty-seven European ones. The tour version of the Sessions Band is Bruce Springsteen (vocals, acoustic guitar, harmonica), Marc Anthony Thompson (acoustic guitar, backing vocals), Patti Scialfa (backing vocals, acoustic guitar), Frank Bruno (acoustic guitar, backing vocals, washboard), Soozie Tyrell (violin, backing vocals), Sam Bardfeld (violin), Greg Liszt (banjo), Marty Rifkin (pedal steel guitar), Charles Giordano (piano, organ, accordion), Jeremy Chatzky (upright bass, electric bass), Larry Eagle (drums), Lisa Lowell (backing vocals), Curtis King Jr. (backing vocals), Cindy Mizelle (backing vocals), Art Baron (tuba, trombone), Eddie Manion (saxophone), Mark Pender (trumpet), Curt Ramm (trumpet), Richie "La Bamba" Rosenberg (trombone), and Clark Gayton (trombone).

2007

In February Springsteen wins two Grammy Awards, for Best Traditional Folk Album (*We Shall Overcome: The Seeger Sessions*) and Best Long Form Music Video (*Wings for Wheels: The Making of Born to Run*).

Also in February *We All Love Ennio Morricone* is published, a tribute album in honor of the great maestro on the occasion of the Oscar awarded to him for his many contributions throughout his career.

Studio sessions begin in Atlanta for a new album with the E Street Band, with producer Brendan O'Brien. A five-day "rehearsal and basic tracks" recording session takes place at Southern Tracks from March 7–11 with E Street Band members Tallent, Weinberg, and Bittan. This subgroup continues scattered recording sessions during March. Van Zandt, Lofgren, Federici, Clemons, Scialfa, and Soozie Tyrell appear to have traveled to Atlanta to add specific overdubs during the latter (late March to early May) stages of the sessions.

Meanwhile, on April 5, Springsteen makes an unadvertised guest appearance at a benefit/tribute show held in his honor at Carnegie Hall, called "Celebrating the Music of Bruce Springsteen: Music for Youth Benefit." Among the twenty artists honoring him we find Steve Earle ("Nebraska"), Patti Smith ("Because the Night"), Badly Drawn Boy ("Thunder Road"), Pete Yorn ("Dancing in the Dark"), Jesse Malin with Ronnie Spector ("Hungry Heart"), and Odetta ("57 Channels"). Springsteen gets onstage last, playing "The Promised Land" and "Rosalita," first in solo acoustic versions, and then "Rosalita" again together with the other artists.

On May 12, at the fifth annual benefit for the Count Basie Theatre Foundation, Springsteen guests on "Barbara Ann" and "Love and Mercy" during the show of the legendary Beach Boys' leader, Brian Wilson.

With the individual ESB members' roles completed by early May, Springsteen and O'Brien spend the rest of the month and part of June putting the final touches on the album.

On June 5, Columbia releases *Bruce Springsteen with the Sessions Band: Live in Dublin*, a two-CD album and home video that captures concert performances recorded in November 2006 at the Point Theatre in Dublin.

On July 30, Terry Magovern, Springsteen's personal assistant and close friend, dies. Two days later, at Magovern's memorial service in Red Bank, Bruce performs a new song called "Terry's Song," which will be later added as an unlisted bonus track on the *Magic* album.

Magic, the fifteenth studio album by Bruce Springsteen, is released on September 25, debuting at #1 on the *Billboard* 200 chart. Three days later, Bruce Springsteen and the E Street Band perform "The Promised Land," "Radio Nowhere," "Livin' in the Future," "My Hometown," and "Night" live at Rockefeller Plaza in New York City for NBC-TV's *Today* show.

The Magic Tour kicks off from Hartford, Connecticut, on October 2. Twelve days later, during the concert in Ottawa, Ontario, Springsteen performs "State Trooper" and "Keep the Car Running" with with Win Butler and Régine Chassagne of Arcade Fire. On Halloween night at the Los Angeles Sports Arena, Bruce emerges from a coffin to open the show, echoing his prior Halloween night performances at this venue in 1980 and 1984. The last show of the first American leg is scheduled on November 19 at the Boston Garden. Nobody yet knows that this will prove to be Danny Federici's last complete show. Two days later, it is announced that he will take a leave of absence from the tour to pursue treatment for melanoma. Springsteen states: "Danny is one of the pillars of our sound and has played beside me as a great friend for more than forty years. We all eagerly await his healthy and speedy return." For the European leg that kicks off from Madrid on November 25, Charles Giordano from the Sessions Band takes his place.

2008

In February Springsteen wins three Grammy Awards: Best Rock Song ("Radio Nowhere"), Best Male Rock Vocal Performance ("Radio Nowhere"), and Best Rock Instrumental Performance ("Once Upon a Time in the West"). In the meantime, senator Barack Obama, interviewed during a TV show, answers the question "Who would you most like to meet?" by saying, "Without doubt Bruce Springsteen."

On March 17, during a concert in Milwaukee, Wisconsin, jazz bassist Richard Davis, who performed on the original album version, guests on a rare "Meeting Across the River," played by sign request. Three days later, at the Conseco Fieldhouse in Indianapolis, Indiana, after eleven songs Charlie Giordano leaves his place behind the keyboards to its rightful owner, Danny Federici, for "The Promised Land" and "Spirit in the Night." Federici then takes up his accordion and steps forward. "Before we went on, I asked him what he wanted to play," Springsteen would recall few weeks later. "He said, 'Sandy.' He wanted to strap on the accordion and revisit the boardwalk of our youth during the summer nights when we'd walk along the boards with all the time in the world . . . He wanted to play once more the song that is of course about the end of something wonderful and the beginning of something unknown and new." Federici plays the organ on the encores ("Backstreets," "Kitty's Back," "Born to Run," "Dancing in the Dark," and "American Land"). The band all knew that they wouldn't see Danny onstage again.

The Magic Tour continues in the U.S. On April 7, at the Honda Center in Anaheim, California, Springsteen offers a new rock arrangement of "The Ghost of Tom Joad" with searing guitar solos from guest Tom Morello of Rage Against the Machine. On April 13, Jon Bon Jovi guests on "Glory Days" at the American Airlines Center in Dallas. The night after that, in Houston, "Terry's Song" is played live for the first time, dedicated to Terry Cox, a sixteen-year-old who died in a swimming accident, on what would have been Terry Magovern's sixty-eighth birthday. Bruce is joined onstage by Alejandro Escovedo for "Always a Friend" and by Joe Ely for "All Just to Get to You."

Danny Federici dies on April 17, at the Memorial Sloan-Kettering Cancer Center in New York City, at the age of fifty-eight. Three shows of the Magic Tour are rescheduled due to his passing. On April 21, Springsteen delivers a eulogy during the funeral service in Red Bank. The next night, the concert in Tampa opens—as will all the others on the rest of this leg of the tour—with a film montage in tribute to Federici set to "Blood Brothers."

On April 23, Roger McGuinn of the Byrds guests on "Turn! Turn! Turn!" and "Mr. Tambourine Man." During those days, Springsteen's endorsement for Obama's candidature in the presidential elections in November finally comes through.

On May 4, Bruce Springsteen is inducted into the New Jersey Hall of Fame, together with other local heroes such as Frank Sinatra, Toni Morrison, Albert Einstein, and Meryl Streep. *Time* magazine puts him in their list of the one hundred most influential people in the world, together with Putin, the Dalai Lama, Barack Obama, Steve Jobs, George Clooney, the Cohen brothers, Oprah Winfrey, Hillary Clinton, Radiohead, Brad Pitt, and Angelina Jolie. On May 2, meanwhile, after twenty-seven dates, the second American leg of the Magic Tour concludes. Five days later, Bruce Springsteen and the E Street Band play at the Count Basie Theatre in Red Bank. In a show that will be long remembered, Bruce and the band run through the entire *Darkness on the Edge of Town* and *Born to Run* albums in order, as close to the original recordings as possible. Mark Pender guests on trumpet for "Meeting Across the River," and a full horn section joins the band on "Tenth Avenue Freeze-Out" and the encores. A test run, perhaps, for what would become a regular occurrence towards the end of the Working on a Dream Tour.

On May 22, the European stadium leg of the Magic Tour kicks off from Dublin, closing with a two-night stand at Camp Nou in Barcelona, where 143,000 fans gather to see Bruce Springsteen and the E Street Band. On the last night, members of the Springsteen family (including Bruce's son Evan) are onstage dancing along to "American Land."

On July 15, Columbia releases the *Magic Tour Highlights* EP only for digital download. It consists of four live audio tracks and their accompanying videos, recorded during 2008: "Always a Friend" featuring Alejandro Escovedo, "The Ghost of Tom Joad" featuring Tom Morello, "Turn! Turn! Turn!" featuring Roger McGuinn, and "4th of July, Asbury Park (Sandy)," with Danny Federici's last performance with the E Street Band. The proceeds from the sales will support the Danny Federici Melanoma Fund.

On July 27, the last leg of the Magic Tour begins with a three-night stand at Giants Stadium, ending on August 30 in Milwaukee, Wisconsin, where Springsteen and the band are the featured entertainment at the Harley Davidson 105th Anniversary Festival. In total, Springsteen holds a hundred concerts in seventy cities around the world, selling around 2.6 million tickets and grossing more than $235 million.

In September, the film *The Wrestler*, directed by Darren Aronofsky, wins the Golden Lion for best film at the Venice Film Festival. On the credits a new Springsteen song is heard, with the same title as the film.

On October 4, 5, and 6, Springsteen make a three-city solo mini-tour (Philadelphia, Columbus, and Ypsilanti) in support of Barack Obama's presidential bid, and plays the "Change Rocks" benefit show held at the Hammerstein Ballroom in New York City for Obama's campaign, backed by Roy Bittan, Patti Scialfa, and Billy Joel with his band. John Legend and India Arie join on "The Rising" and "People Get Ready," and Barack Obama himself joins on the finale, "Signed, Sealed, Delivered, I'm Yours."

On November 11, Springsteen performs at a "Change We Need" rally in Cleveland in support of Barack Obama's presidential campaign, playing a new song titled "Working on a Dream." Two days later, Barack Obama is elected as the forty-fourth president of the United States and and holds a historic speech in Chicago, at the end of which "The Rising" resounds in the air.

2009

On January 11, Springsteen picks up the Golden Globe Award for Best Original Song in a Motion Picture for "The Wrestler." Two days later, Columbia releases *Bruce Springsteen & the E Street Band Greatest Hits*, a compilation album released as a limited edition first in the U.S., Canada, and Australia exclusively through Wal-Mart retailers.

On January 18, over 500,000 people meet up in front of the Lincoln Memorial in Washington for the ceremony opening the three days in which the United States celebrate their new president, Barack Obama. At the show called "We Are One," Tom Hanks, Denzel Washington, Samuel L. Jackson, Marisa Tomei, and Tiger Woods are guest stars, among others, and the president-elect speaks in interludes between performances by Mary J. Blige, Stevie Wonder with Usher and Shakira, John Mellencamp, James Taylor with John Legend, Garth Brooks, Sheryl Crow with Herbie Hancock, Bon Jovi, U2, and Bruce Springsteen, who opens the event performing "The Rising" backed by a large gospel choir and gets back onstage after Obama's speech to sing "This Land Is Your Land" together with the eighty-nine-year-old Pete Seeger.

Working on a Dream—the sixteenth studio album by Bruce Springsteen—is released on January 27, debuting at #1 on the *Billboard* 200 chart and reaching #1 in seventeen other countries around the world. Critical reception ranges widely.

Rolling Stone gives it a five-star rating, but *Los Angeles Times* writer Ann Powers says, "The best thing that can be said about *Working on a Dream* is that it's boisterously scatterbrained, exhilaratingly bad."[17]

On February 1, at the Raymond James Stadium in Tampa, Springsteen closes what has probably been the busiest month of his life performing the halftime show at Super Bowl XLIII. Bruce and the band, joined by a horn section, play "Tenth Avenue Freeze-Out," "Born to Run," "Working on a Dream," and "Glory Days," with all songs being shortened to fit into the twelve-minute time slot of the show. More than 100,000,000 Americans watch the live TV broadcast.

The Working on a Dream Tour kicks off from San Jose, California, on April 1. The longtime members of the E Street Band (Bittan, Van Zandt, Lofgren, Tallent, Scialfa, Clemons, and Weinberg) are backed up by Charlie Giordano (keyboards), Soozie Tyrell (violin), Curtis King Jr. and Cindy Mizelle (backing vocals). Max Weinberg's eighteen-year-old son, Jay, becomes his replacement for parts of the shows, due to Max's bandleader obligations to *The Tonight Show with Conan O'Brien*. On this tour—the first to include the E Street Band without Danny Federici—the "stump the band" routine becomes established: Springsteen collects request signs from the pit audience as an extended introduction to "Raise Your Hand" is played. Once that song is completed, Springsteen selects two or three numbers to play from the requests: rare Springsteen songs or decades-past oldies, like "Wild Thing," "96 Tears," "Mony Mony," "Jailhouse Rock," "My Generation," "Like a Rolling Stone," "I Wanna Be Sedated," and "London Calling." The activity leads to impromptu arrangements being worked out onstage: Springsteen has been known to taunt the audience afterwards with declarations that the E Street Band cannot be stumped: "This is the greatest bar band in the land!"

In late spring, the Tour goes to Europe, where Bruce Springsteen and the E Street Band are also billed in various rock festivals, such as PinkPop in the Netherlands, Glastonbury and Hard Rock Calling in England, and the Festival des Vielles Charreus in France. On July 19, at Stadio Olimpico in Rome, Springsteen walks on stage to the notes of Morricone's "Once Upon a Time in the West." "We are so glad to play in the most beautiful city in the world," he says. Then he asks for some silence. "We don't play this one often," he says. "We want to dedicate this song to the people of L'Aquila." And he delivers a stunning "My City of Ruins." The day before the show, I was on the radio with Steve Van Zandt, and I gave him a letter for Bruce that I received from "Vittorio and the fans from L'Aquila." The letter said,

> Dear Bruce, for long time I have dreamed to have a chance to ask you to sing
> a song that is special to me. Today I want to ask you to sing a song that has

unfortunately acquired a new and stronger meaning to me and many of my friends since last April 6. That day, our area was struck by a terrible earthquake. About 300 people died, thousands were injured, tens of thousands are now homeless and they do not know when they will be able to have their homes rebuilt. Most of the people are still living in tents; factories, offices, schools, the university, everything is gone now, and it is difficult to think about tomorrow. Our city is in ruins, Bruce, so some days ago I found myself thinking that I would love to listen to "My City of Ruins" in the show in Rome, and so would my friends from L'Aquila and all the area, as many of us will be there for you.

Back in the U.S.A., Bruce Springsteen and the E Street Band open their five-night stand at Giants Stadium with a new song that Bruce has written in honor of the soon-to-be-demolished venue. "Join us tonight to shut the old lady down!" he says before performing "Wrecking Ball." During the five nights in New Jersey, in front of almost 300,000 people, Springsteen plays in sequence these entire albums: *Born to Run* (on the first and fourth nights), *Darkness on the Edge of Town* (on the second night), and *Born in the U.S.A.* (on the third and fifth nights).

In October, Johnny Cash's daughter, Rosanne, releases her new album, *The List*, also containing a duet with Springsteen on "Sea of Heartbreak."

On October 29 and 30, the Rock & Roll Hall of Fame celebrates its twenty-fifth anniversary with two concerts destined to make history, with performances by Jerry Lee Lewis, U2, Patti Smith, Simon & Garfunkel, Metallica, James Taylor, Bonnie Raitt, Mick Jagger, Lou Reed, Ray Davies, Ozzy Osbourne, Paul Simon, Jeff Beck, Buddy Guy, Aretha Franklin, Stevie Wonder, Sting, Little Anthony and the Imperials, and Crosby, Stills and Nash. The first night runs almost six hours with Bruce Springsteen and the E Street Band closing the concert with special guests John Fogerty, Darlene Love, Tom Morello, Sam Moore, Jackson Browne, Peter Wolf, and Billy Joel.

On November 7 and 8, Springsteen returns to Madison Square Garden with two concerts of his Working on a Dream Tour featuring *The Wild, the Innocent & the E Street Shuffle* and *The River* in their entirety. The tour ends in Buffalo, on November 22, with the longest show of the year (thirty-four songs and nearly three and a half hours), with Bruce performing his first album, *Greetings from Asbury Park, NJ*, in its entirety, dedicated to Mike Appel.

On December 5, President Obama gives Springsteen the Kennedy Center Honors—the nation's highest award for those who have defined American culture through the arts. Also honored are Robert De Niro, Mel Brooks, Dave Brubeck, and Grace Bumbry. Jon Stewart opens the tribute to Springsteen, and performers including John Mellencamp, Melissa Etheridge, Eddie Vedder, Jennifer Nettles, Ben Harper, and Sting cover Bruce's songs as he watches from the presidential box with Michelle and Barack Obama. Before the performance, the president said, "Bruce has been a great friend over the last year, and when I watched him on the steps of the Lincoln Memorial when he rocked the National Mall before my inauguration, I thought it captured as well as anything the spirit of what America *should* be about. On a day like that, and today, I remember I'm the President, but he's the Boss . . ."

2010

In January, Clarence Clemons undergoes back surgery in New York. In a statement to the Associated Press, he says that he's "in great spirits" and "looking forward to a brighter future and playing more music!"

On January 20, the Sundance Channel and UK Channel 4-TV broadcast *Spectacle: Elvis Costello with . . . Bruce Springsteen*, taped on September 25, 2009, at the Apollo Theater in New York City. Over the course of a nearly four-hour taping, Springsteen and Costello discussed everything from their Catholic upbringings to fatherhood to the role of the songwriter in a democratic society. And the music . . . Costello and the Imposters open the show with a cover of "Point Blank," while Bruce opens with "Wild Billy's Circus Story," for which he is joined onstage by an acoustic Nils Lofgren and Roy Bittan on accordion. "American Skin (41 Shots)" is Bruce solo. "Galveston Bay" is Bruce and Roy. Elvis Costello sings "Black Ladder" and "Brilliant Disguise" with Bruce and Nils backing. "I Can't Stand Up for Falling Down," "Seeds," and the Radio medley ("Radio Silence"—"Radio Nowhere"—"Radio Radio") are full band: Bruce, Roy, and Nils, plus Elvis Costello & the Imposters.

On January 22, Bruce performs for Hope for Haiti Now, a benefit for the victims of the Haiti earthquake, playing "We Shall Overcome." The track will be subsequently available for sale on iTunes and Amazon.

In February, Springsteen is honored at the 52nd Grammy Awards for Best Solo Rock Vocal Performance for "Working on a Dream," up against Bob Dylan, John Fogerty, Prince, and Neil Young.

On April 24, Springsteen and Steve Van Zandt join the Rascals on stage at the annual Kristen Ann Carr Fund benefit in New York City and play "Good Lovin.'"

On May 6, Springsteen and poet Robert Pinsky, along with John Wesley Harding, appear at "Jersey Rain: Robert Pinsky and Bruce Springsteen in Conversation and Performance with John Wesley Harding," a part of the 2010 WAMFEST

Words and Music Festival. For two hours, the artists discuss and perform their work for a packed auditorium of 400 students. David Porter reports for the *Associated Press*: "The two men, joined at times by Harding, performed their works separately and together. Pinsky's poem 'Shirt' segued into Springsteen's 'The River,' and Springsteen read Pinsky's 'Samurai Song' as a prelude to his own 'Darkness on the Edge of Town,' played on 12-string guitar. Springsteen also performed 'The Promised Land,' 'Nebraska,' and 'Born to Run,' and he joked that 'you have to be careful if you're a songwriter reading poetry, because the temptation to steal is ever present.' Springsteen also remarked, 'What I've been trying to write about for 40 years, Robert gets into a single poem.'"

Less than a year after the June 28, 2009, Hard Rock Calling festival in London, Bruce Springsteen and the E Street Band's performance there is released as *London Calling: Live in Hyde Park* two-DVD set.

After a long wait, the Holy Grail for any Springsteen fan is finally released on November 16. *The Promise: The Darkness on the Edge of Town Story* is a six-disc set including three CDs and three DVDs containing a remastered version of the *Darkness on the Edge of Town* album; a new two-CD album, *The Promise*, containing twenty-one previously unreleased outtakes from the *Darkness* sessions; a documentary titled *The Promise: The Making of Darkness on the Edge of Town*; and two DVDs of live performances: Bruce and the E Street Band's intimate and complete album performance of *Darkness* shot in 2009; about an hour's worth of previously unseen archival footage from the Thrill Hill Vault, including complete song performances taken from private band rehearsals, studio sessions, and live concerts during the *Darkness* era; and the previously unreleased complete concert performance from December 8, 1978, at the Summit in Houston, Texas, toward the end of the Darkness Tour. The deluxe box set contains an 80–page spiral-bound reproduction of Springsteen's original notebooks documenting the recording sessions for the album, containing alternate lyrics, song ideas, recording details, and personal notes. The documentary already received its première on September 14, at the Toronto International Film Festival. *The Promise* is also released as a two-CD album, and in that format enters the UK Albums Chart at #7.

The same day of the box set release, Springsteen guests on *Late Night with Jimmy Fallon* and plays a song titled "Whip My Hair," featuring Jimmy Fallon disguised as Neil Young, and Bruce as himself, circa 1975. For "Because the Night" and "Save My Love" Bruce is backed by Steve Van Zandt, Roy Bittan, and the in-house band the Roots.

On December 7, at the Carousel House in Asbury Park, Bruce Springsteen and the E Street Band in front of a small crowd of around sixty are videotaped for a future webcast and official video release. The Band is comprised of the original 1978 performers only, with Charlie Giordano substituting for Danny.

2011

In January, Springsteen starts to work with producer Ron Aniello on new songs that Bruce has written in the previous months: "We Take Care of Our Own," "Shacked and Drawn," "Rocky Ground," and others were coming "along for almost a gospel album package I was thinking about," Springsteen later explained. Other songs were written as a solo material: "Just me and a guitar singing these songs," as he put it. The subjects of these songs were greed, corruption, and the current state of America. Soon the focus moved away from a solo album. "Then Ron brought a large library of sound that allowed me to explore—like maybe a hip-hop drum loop or country-blues stomp loop. The actual drums came later. There was no preconceived set of instruments that needed to be used; I could go anywhere, do anything, use anything. It was very wide open."

At the 26th Annual Rock & Roll Hall of Fame Induction Ceremony, Springsteen joins inductee Darlene Love on stage for three songs. Bette Midler is also on stage for "He's a Rebel."

A new Dropkick Murphys album, *Going Out in Style*, is released in March. Springsteen guests, trading lead vocals with Ken Casey on "Peg o' My Heart." A few days later, *Rolling Stone* polls readers on their favorite live act of all time. The winner—"without a close second anywhere in sight"—is Bruce Springsteen and the E Street Band. The Rolling Stones are #2 and the Who #3. Ray Davies's new album *See My Friends*, a collection of Davies and friends' new takes on Kinks classics, leads off with his duet with Springsteen on the Kinks' "Better Things."

In April, Springsteen makes his debut appearance on Steve Van Zandt's *Little Steven's Underground Garage* radio show. The interview is broadcast in three parts on April 1, 8, and 15 on over 200 terrestrial FM radio stations across the United States. It is more an informal, spontaneous chat between friends than an interview: topics included in the show are wide-ranging, but primarily cover Bruce and Steve's musical influences (Elvis Presley, the Beatles, the Animals, the Kinks, the Yardbirds, Bob Dylan, the Rolling Stones, the Who, and Them).

Recording sessions for a new album continue. Unlike the previous two albums that were recorded with the E Street Band, this new one features an extensive list of guest musicians. In fact, there will be only three songs that feature the E Street Band—"Wrecking Ball," "Land of Hope and Dreams," and the bonus track "American Land." The rest see Springsteen and Aniello accompanied by Sessions

Band members, choirs, strings, and horns. Roy Bittan and Garry Tallent do not appear at all, and Steve Van Zandt only lends vocals to two tracks.

In May, Lady Gaga releases her *Born This Way* album. Clarence Clemons blows his saxophone on two tracks, "The Edge of Glory" and "Hair." On June 12, news has it that Clarence Clemons has suffered a massive stroke. After two subsequent brain surgeries at a Florida hospital, he is reported to be "currently responsive and in stable condition." The next day, Springsteen writes from his website: "By now, many of you have heard that our beloved comrade and sax player Clarence Clemons has suffered a serious stroke. While all initial signs are encouraging, Clarence will need much care and support to achieve his potential once again. He has his wonderfully supportive wife, Victoria, excellent doctors and health care professionals, and is surrounded by friends and family. I thank you all for your prayers and positive energy and concern. This is a time for us all to share in a hopeful spirit that can ultimately inspire Clarence to greater heights." On June 18, Clarence Clemons dies. Springsteen writes: "Clarence lived a wonderful life. He carried within him a love of people that made them love him. He created a wondrous and extended family. He loved the saxophone, loved our fans and gave everything he had every night he stepped on stage. His loss is immeasurable and we are honored and thankful to have known him and had the opportunity to stand beside him for nearly forty years. He was my great friend, my partner, and with Clarence at my side, my band and I were able to tell a story far deeper than those simply contained in our music. His life, his memory, and his love will live on in that story and in our band."

On June 21, Springsteen takes part in a private memorial service for Clarence Clemons in Palm Beach, Florida, playing a solo acoustic guitar "Tenth Avenue Freeze-Out." The ceremony closes with "You're a Friend of Mine" performed by Springsteen, Jackson Browne, and the E Street Band. Bruce also delivers a eulogy. A month later, he attends a U2 show with his son Evan at the New Meadowlands Stadium in East Rutherford, New Jersey, where U2 pays tribute to Clarence Clemons in the intro to "Moment of Surrender" and finishes the song reading out the lyrics to the final verse of "Jungleland."

On October 1, Springsteen participates in a charity concert at the Beacon Theatre in New York City marking Sting's sixtieth birthday, and plays "I Hung My Head" with Sting's band before embarking on a solo acoustic "Fields of Gold." Sting joins Bruce for "Can't Stand Losing You" before the grand finale with "Every Breath You Take" and "Happy Birthday" with all the night's artists on stage, including Lady Gaga, Stevie Wonder, Branford Marsalis, will.i.am, Mary J. Blige, Rufus Wainwright, and Billy Joel.

Talking with *Spin* magazine about the new Coldplay album *Mylo Xyloto*, singer Chris Martin names Bruce as an inspiration for its third-person perspective: "You can sometimes get your own feelings across more strongly if you pretend that you're singing it from someone else's angle. But it's always from me. It's just a new way of framing it. That's definitely from listening to so much Springsteen."

On December 19, Vincent Manniello, who laid down the beat for Bruce's early band the Castiles, passed away. In 1966, Vinny "Skibotts" Manniello replaced drummer Bart Haynes, who shipped out to Vietnam and was later killed in action. Manniello was part of the lineup that recorded the "Baby I" single in May of '66, Springsteen's first record.

2012

On January 19, "We Take Care of Our Own," the first single from Springsteen's new album, is digitally released. On February 2, at Los Angeles' Staples Center, Bruce Springsteen and the E Street Band, accompanied by a fourteen-piece string section, open the 54th Annual Grammy Awards with the live premiere of "We Take Care of Our Own."

During the final week of February, Jimmy Fallon dedicates an entire week of his *Late Night with Jimmy Fallon* show to Springsteen's music.

Wrecking Ball—the seventeenth studio album by Bruce Springsteen, is released March 5. Produced by Ron Aniello, the album contains thirteen songs (included two additional tracks) all written in 2011 with the exception of "Jack of All Trades" (written in 2009 and previously unreleased), "Wrecking Ball" (written in 2009 for the demolition of Giants Stadium), "American Land" (written during the 2006 Seeger Sessions but never released before in a studio version), and "Land of Hope and Dreams" (first performed on the 1999 Reunion Tour but never released before in a studio version). The album includes tracks that feature Clarence Clemons, who died in June 2011: the Big Man performs the saxophone solos on "Land of Hope and Dreams" and backing saxophone rhythms on the title track. The album—named best album of 2012 by *Rolling Stone*—debuted at #1 in sixteen different countries including both the U.S. and UK charts. *Wrecking Ball* became Springsteen's tenth #1 album in the United States, tying him with Elvis Presley for third most #1 albums of all time. Only the Beatles (at nineteen) and Jay-Z (at twelve) have more #1 albums.

On March 9, Bruce Springsteen and the E Street Band play the Apollo Theater to celebrate the tenth anniversary of SiriusXM Radio, the satellite network that also broadcasts E Street Radio.

On March 15, Springsteen delivers the keynote speech at the South by Southwest music festival in Austin, Texas. Arriving on stage thirty-five minutes later than the scheduled twelve p.m., he begins by saying, "Good morning. Why are we up so fucking early? How important can this speech be if we're giving it at noon, when every decent musician in town is asleep?" He speaks about his musical influences during his hour-long speech before leaving the stage to a standing ovation. Following the keynote speech, Bruce performs an intimate concert at Moody Theater, featuring a twenty-four-song set with plenty of special guests. Jimmy Cliff shares the stage with Bruce and the E Street Band for "Many Rivers to Cross," "Time Will Tell," and "The Harder They Come." The Animals' Eric Burdon performs with Springsteen for the first time in an appearance that was arranged following Bruce's passionate speech about The Animals' influence on his music: the two share the microphone on "We Gotta Get Out of This Place." "This Land Is Your Land" closes the set with the accompaniment of Joe Ely, Alejandro Escovedo, Tom Morello, Garland Jeffreys, Arcade Fire, and the Low Anthem.

The Wrecking Ball Tour kicks off from Atlanta, Georgia, on March 18. Clarence Clemons's nephew, Jake, takes his place on the saxophone, backed by a horn section formed by Clark Gayton (trombone), Curt Ramm (trumpet), Barry Danielian (trumpet), and Eddie Manion (saxophone). Cindy Mizelle, Curtis King, and Michelle Moore provide backing vocals. Tom Morello guests on guitar in multiple shows. "Tenth Avenue Freeze-Out" is always performed during the encores as a tribute song to Clarence Clemons. Shows are longer than on recent tours, culminating in Helsinki on July 31, with the longest performance of Springsteen's career to date at four hours and six minutes.

On July 14, Bruce and band return to the Hard Rock Festival in Hyde Park with a fantastic concert opened by "Thunder Road," sung with just the accompaniment of Roy Bittan on piano. Morello guests on several numbers, and John Fogerty joins for "The Promised Land." The final guest for the evening is Sir Paul McCartney, and together they play "I Saw Her Standing There" followed by a raucous "Twist and Shout." Unfortunately, only a few minutes past the ten-thirty curfew, the concert organizers choose to cut the sound at the conclusion of "Twist and Shout." Springsteen is unable to play a final song, nor is he able to say his farewells to the crowd. Instead he sings a brief a cappella, unamplified "Goodnight Irene," and leaves the stage. Steve takes to Twitter following the show to express his disappointment and anger, while Bruce comments, "I wasn't aware the plug had been pulled, and people couldn't hear what I was singing. Afterwards I said to Paul, 'I can understand them pulling the plug on me, but you? Aren't you a knight?'" Paul McCartney remembers, "Bruce, sort of, got in touch and said, 'Do you wanna get up? We'd like you to get up.' I said, 'Well, I don't know, I'll just come along to the show,' so we're in the side of the show in the wings, and he says, 'Are you gonna get up, man?' I said, 'I don't know, maybe.' Then his roadie says, 'I've got a bass for you, I've got a guitar, it's all tuned, it's ready to go.' I go, 'Oh, you're *really* ready!' So they're all really ready to go, so, what have they rehearsed? He said 'Twist and Shout' and 'I Saw Her Standing There.' So at last minute, I sort of have to say, 'Yeah, I'll do it,' so I go on, and it's great, they really have rehearsed it, and I'm the only one who sort of doesn't know it, even though I wrote the bloody thing. So then they go to 'Twist and Shout,' and I'm singing it, and someone had whispered, 'We haven't got any time, we can't do it,' but it was so nice, Bruce is going, 'Yeah, come on, man.' Bruce is, you know, he's a do-er, a go-getter, so I was happy. 'Yeah!' We're rocking away, all our monitors stayed on, so we weren't really aware that the plug had been pulled on the audience, that you see on the YouTube later, it's all gone dead. And he is singing, he's gonna then go back and sing 'Good Night Irene,' which I think was all dead, but we had a laugh again. You've gotta have a laugh, it would just be so terrifying if you didn't, so we just had a laugh afterwards, I was just apologetic, like, 'I'm sorry, man, only in Britain!' It's the only place . . . You can't imagine in New York somewhere like that, them pulling the plug. And it got everyone, of course, so that was the big story. Everyone in America was going to me, 'Is it true, man? They pulled the plug on you and Springsteen?!' and I'm saying, 'Yeah, well, you know, just some guy. Some bloody jobsworth . . .'"

The tour returns to the United States in August and focuses on baseball and football stadiums. The tour's third (and final) show at MetLife Stadium in East Rutherford, is delayed for two hours due to a strong thunderstorm. The show finally gets underway around ten thirty p.m., prompting fans to sing "Happy Birthday" to Springsteen at midnight to celebrate his sixty-third birthday. At the end of the show, Springsteen is presented with a guitar-shaped birthday cake onstage. On October 29, the New Jersey area is hit hard by Hurricane Sandy. Springsteen's show in Rochester, New York, the following day must be postponed until October 31. That night, Springsteen dedicates his performance to those affected by the storm and those helping with the recovery. Springsteen and the E Street Band perform "Land of Hope and Dreams" during a one-hour televised telethon called *Hurricane Sandy: Coming Together* on November 2. He will later participate in the *12-12-12: The Concert for Sandy Relief* at Madison Square Garden.

2013

On February 8, at the Los Angeles Convention Center, Springsteen is honored as the 2013 MusiCares Person of the Year "in recognition of his extraordinary creative accomplishments as well as his significant charitable work, which has included an impressive range of philanthropic activities over the years." The gala includes a reception, silent auction, dinner, award presentation, and star-studded tribute concert. The guest performances include "Adam Raised a Cain" by Alabama Shakes, "Dancing in the Dark" by John Legend, "Because the Night" by Patti Smith, "I'm on Fire" by Mumford & Sons, "American Skin (41 Shots)" by Jackson Browne and Tom Morello, "Streets of Philadelphia" by Elton John, "Lonesome Day" by Sting, and "Born in the U.S.A." by Neil Young and the Crazy Horse.

In March, Bruce Springsteen and the E Street Band perform in Australia for the first time in a decade. Tom Morello is standing in for Steve Van Zandt, who is filming his successful TV show *Lilyhammer*. "Miami" Steve returns for the 2013 European leg of the tour, whose climax is reached in Milan, where Springsteen appears for the fifth time in his career at the famous San Siro Stadium, greeted by the crowd on the bleachers forming a gigantic "OUR LOVE IS REAL" sign with the colors of the Italian banner on the notes of Morricone's *Once Upon a Time in the West* theme, and in Rome, where Bruce follows "Kitty's Back" with the complete side two of *The Wild, the Innocent & the E Street Shuffle*, until "New York City Serenade," only played ten times since 1999, and only in the U.S. This stunning, long-awaited European debut is enriched by the Roma Sinfonietta, a string section directed by Leandro Piccioni, a group of musicians whose collaborations range from Michael Nyman to Quincy Jones, and from Roger Waters to, last but not least, Ennio Morricone.

In September, Springsteen plays four shows in South America (Chile, Argentina, and Brazil). The Wrecking Ball Tour ends in Rio de Janeiro at the Rock in Rio Festival.

The Wrecking Ball Tour featured over 215 different songs, grossing $400 million from 134 shows.

2014

High Hopes—the eighteenth studio album by Bruce Springsteen—is released on January 14, becoming his eleventh #1 in the U.S., and his tenth #1 in the UK. The album is a collection of cover songs, outtakes, and reimagined versions of tracks from past albums, Eps, and tours.

The High Hopes Tour kicks off from Cape Town on January 26. Bruce Springsteen and the E Street Band open their first show in South Africa playing the Specials' "Free Nelson Mandela," and dedicating "We Are Alive" to Mandela. After the African and Oceanic legs, the High Hopes Tour ends with sixteen gigs in North America.

On April 10, fifteen years after Springsteen's entry, the E Street Band are finally inducted into the Rock & Roll Hall of Fame. Bruce himself inducts the band, followed by acceptance speeches by David Sancious; Vini Lopez; Jason Federici for his father, Danny; Nils Lofgren; Victoria Clemons for her husband, Clarence; Patti Scialfa; Garry Tallent; Roy Bittan; Max Weinberg; and Steve Van Zandt. Three songs follow, with a unique lineup of two drummers and David Sancious on the organ for the first time in many years.

On April 19, Columbia releases *American Beauty*, a four-song EP with outtakes from Springsteen's 2014 album *High Hopes*.

On May 29, Springsteen joins the Rolling Stones on stage at the Rock in Rio Festival in Lisbon, Portugal, performing "Tumbling Dice" together.

In November, Simon & Schuster publishes *Outlaw Pete*, a storybook with artwork by Frank Caruso, based on the song of the same name from Springsteen's *Working on a Dream* album. *Outlaw Pete* is about a bank-robbing baby whose exploits become a meditation on sin, fate, and free will.

On December 1, following Bono's recent bike accident in Central Park, Springsteen and other artists step in to save U2's surprise World AIDS Day performance in Times Square. Adam Clayton, the Edge, and Larry Mullen Jr. are joined by Springsteen and Coldplay's Chris Martin, each of whom will take a turn as front man on the U2 songs. Bruce sings "Where the Streets Have No Name" and "I Still Haven't Found What I'm Looking For" at the conclusion of the hour-long concert.

2015

On January 17, Springsteen makes a surprise appearance at the 2015 Light of Day charity concert. The Light of Day organization funds research into possible cures, improved treatments, and support for persons suffering from Parkinson's disease and related illnesses. Bruce guests with Willie Nile and La Bamba's Big Band before a solo acoustic "Janey Don't You Lose Heart" and a fifteen-song set with Joe Grushecky and the Houserockers.

On February 6, he performs at the 25th MusiCares Person of the Year gala to honor Bob Dylan, playing "Knockin' on Heaven's Door."

In April, WikiLeaks reveals a new Springsteen contract, with release plans. The document goes into a lot of economical details (higher royalty rates, a $31 million advance, a contract extension until June 2027, etc.), including details of the benefits the 2005 contract brought to Columbia ($73 million on top of the $101 million paid to Springsteen). Most interesting for Springsteen fans are the details of the release plans for the next twelve years, which include thirteen projects (besides the current Archival Series): four new studio albums (delivered at least twelve months apart;) one anniversary box set, with three CDs, for the *Born in the U.S.A.* album;

one anniversary box set, with three CDs, for *The River* album; one anniversary box set, with two CDs, for the *Nebraska* album; one box set with three or four discs of unreleased songs (the second volume of *Tracks*); and five complete live-concert albums (the box sets and live albums will be released at least six months apart). One of the clauses specifies that Springsteen "will have the right to sell downloads of his live concerts directly or through third parties." The new contract also specifies that Springsteen has total control over the production of all recordings and their contents. With the new deal Springsteen will stay at Columbia at least until June 30, 2027 (if he has delivered all thirteen products by then), or for two years after delivering the last of the products. In the emails between the Sony execs they admit, "It's obviously a rich deal given his stature," but "this is not an artist we can afford to lose."

On July 1, Bruce joins Brian Wilson and his band on stage for two songs during the encore of Wilson's set at the PNC Bank Arts Center in Holmdel. Apparently keen to remain in the background and keep the focus on Brian Wilson, Springsteen sings harmonies on "Barbara Ann" before picking up a guitar and playing backup on "Surfin' U.S.A." On July 31, he makes a surprise appearance at the final night of U2's eight-night stand at Madison Square Garden. After hinting at what is to come by singing a few lines of "Hungry Heart" at the end of "Beautiful Day," Bono speaks about Springsteen's profound influence on the band before introducing Bruce, who plays guitar and shares vocals on "I Still Haven't Found What I'm Looking For" after letting the crowd sing the opening verse. They then transition into an impromptu "Stand by Me."

On December 4, Columbia celebrates the thirty-fifth anniversary of *The River* by releasing a box set titled *The Ties that Bind: The River Collection*. The set contains fifty-two tracks on four CDs along with four hours of video on three DVDs. The first two CDs feature the remastered version of *The River* and the third CD contains the previously unreleased *The River: Single Album*, originally to be titled *The Ties that Bind*. The fourth CD, *The River: Outtakes*, spans all of the River sessions in 1979 and 1980 and contains eleven previously unreleased outtakes. The fifth DVD disc contains a sixty-minute documentary, *The Ties that Bind*, which features an interview with Springsteen as he reflects on writing and recording *The River*. The remaining discs feature *Bruce Springsteen and the E Street Band: The River Tour, Tempe 1980*, a new film produced from footage professionally filmed in 1980 from Springsteen's November 5, 1980, concert at Arizona State University in Tempe, Arizona. Also included is twenty minutes of footage from the late September 1980 River Tour rehearsals held in Lititz, Pennsylvania. The boxed set also includes a 148-page coffee table book featuring 200 rare or previously unseen photos and memorabilia.

2016

The River 2016 World Tour kicks off on January 16 from the Consol Energy Center in Pittsburgh. The E Street Band is backing Springsteen: Roy Bittan, Nils Lofgren, Patti Scialfa, Garry Tallent, Steve Van Zandt, and Max Weinberg with Soozie Tyrell, Charles Giordano, and Jake Clemons. Each show on the opening U.S. leg will feature a complete performance of *The River*, in sequence. The encores open with "Rebel Rebel," in tribute to David Bowie, who died on January 10, at the age of 69.

The European leg starts from the Camp Nou in Barcelona, Spain, and continues throughout the first part of the summer with amazing concerts that often reach four hours playing time. On July 16, the tour premiere of "New York City Serenade" opens Springsteen's set at the ancient Circus Maximus in Rome, with the Roma Sinfonietta Orchestra providing strings.

Springsteen and the E Street Band kick off the second North American leg of the tour on August 23, 2016, at the MetLife Stadium in East Rutherford. On September 7, at Citizens Bank Park in Philadelphia, Springsteen again breaks his longest show record, clocking in at four hours and four minutes, which now stands as his longest show in the United States and second longest ever.

On September 27, Simon & Schuster releases *Born to Run*, the long-awaited Bruce Springsteen autobiography, with its companion piece, *Chapter and Verse*, a career-spanning album featuring songs from all stages of his career. On the date of the book's release, Springsteen embarks on a nine-date book tour in the United States. The book has received critical acclaim.

On Bruce Springsteen

"They call him the Boss. Well that's a bunch of crap. He's not the boss. He works *for* us. More than a boss, he's the owner, because more than anyone else, Bruce Springsteen owns America's heart."

—Bono (U2)[18]

"The performers who changed my life were individuals, They didn't conform to any sense of reality but their own. The last performer who stood up to be counted as an original is Bruce Springsteen, I think. Individuals move me, not mobs. People with originality, whether it's Hector, Achilles, Ted Turner or Jerry Lee Lewis or Hank Williams."

—Bob Dylan[19]

"For most of us nine jillion Bruce Springsteen fans who've stood through years of his barn-burning, bombs-dropping, ceiling-cracking, ozone-splitting three-hour mega-extravaganza concerts, in all manner of nasty weather and good, who've bought and rebought album after album, who've pored over lyrics, mused over his complex musical and band life, as well as his privacy-shrouded marital, familial and psychic forays, and who've demarked sovereign occasions in our own lives with the strains of 'No Surrender' running through our hectic brains—for all of us in his global audience—the perpetual fascination of *Bruce* (I've never, I give you my word, shouted that out at a performance) is simply: How the hell do you get from Freehold, N.J., to *this* in only 50 short years? It's reminiscent of the old Maine farmer who, when asked directions to the next town over the hill, allows that you can't get there from here. Really, in Springsteen's or anybody's life, you *can't* get there from here. But, well . . . here he is. Are we not all present to testify?"

—Richard Ford[20]

"They say that if you only ever read one book you should make it Steinbeck's *Grapes of Wrath*. I say that if you had to listen to only one rock record you could do no worse than . . . *Born to Run*, the one that captivates me to this day."

—Jim Kerr (Simple Minds)[21]

"Springsteen had such an influence on our home. My father gave me, I believe it was for Christmas, a Bruce Springsteen songbook for the piano and on it was 'Thunder Road,' which is my favorite Bruce Springsteen song. My dad said, 'If you learn how to play this song we will take out a loan for a grand piano, a baby grand.' So I remember it was the hardest thing for me. I was playing these huge classical pieces, like 15 pages long . . . and then there was this Bruce Springsteen song. I opened up the book and there was like chords, guitar chords. I was so confused. I didn't understand it, so I just started to read it and eventually, eventually I got it down."

—Lady Gaga[22]

"Me and the Boss met for the first time years ago at a local restaurant when a cute teen girl—like a girl out of a Springsteen song—approached our table. Bruce gave the lass a huge smile, and even reached into his pocket for a pen. But she said, 'Aren't you Stephen King?' It was one of the best moments of my young life!"

—Stephen King[23]

"Bruce Springsteen's 'Hungry Heart,' which I think is a great record, to me is the same kind of period sound of 'Starting Over': the Fifties. [. . .] God help Bruce Springsteen when they decide he's no longer God. I haven't seen him, but I've heard such good things about him. Right now his fans are happy. He's told them about being drunk and chasing girls and cars and everything, and that's about the level they enjoy. But when he gets down to facing his own success and growing older and having to produce it again and again, they'll turn on him, and I hope he survives it."

—John Lennon (The Beatles)[24]

"In my opinion, the greatest artist in history is Bruce Springsteen."

—Chris Martin (Coldplay)[25]

"Springsteen's very wise. He's a very down-to-Earth guy. He's a very self-analytical and self-demanding person who wants to be a real human being and work on what it means to be a human being."

—Edward Norton[26]

"In contemporary American music, Springsteen is its most enduring and robust giver . . . You always get a sense of personal truth, humility and passion. A sense of humor, a sense of rock 'n' roll and a raconteurism once solely the domain of tribal chiefs. But *chief* comes from *chieftain*. And that's just not an American word. *Boss?* Now that comes from *boss man*, and if this guy ain't the boss . . . man, nobody is."

—Sean Penn[27]

"One of my favorite bandleaders is Bruce Springsteen. I've watched him many years. I was backstage one night, and I saw him turn around and give a cue, and the band switched on a dime. I used to see James Brown do that a lot, too—you learn from the best."

—Prince[28]

"There's an epic vision at the heart of Bruce Springsteen's music. . . . And that epic vision is there in the amazing range of emotions in his songs—exhilaration, tragedy, desire, sorrow, hope, resignation, anger, betrayal, longing . . . Simply put, Bruce Springsteen is a major American artist."

—Martin Scorsese[29]

"When Springsteen sings . . . that's not about *fun*. That's fucking triumph, man."

—Pete Townshend (The Who)[30]

"God, I love his songs, I wish I had written 'Meeting Across the River.' His early songs are like little black-and-white films. Things like 'Wild Billy's Circus Story' were real well crafted. He's got a great visual sense, a great balance."

—Tom Waits[31]

"With Bruce, we are on similar paths, writing and singing out own kind of songs around the world, along with Bob [Dylan] and a few other singer/songwriters. It is a silent fraternity of sorts, occupying this space in people's souls with our music."

—Neil Young[32]

---

1. Scott Hisler, "David Bowie Opens Up a Little," *Musician*, August 1987.

2. Greil Marcus, "Springsteen's Thousand and One American Nights."

3. Lester Bangs, "Hot Rod Rumble in the Promised Land," *CREEM*, November 1975.

4. Dave Marsh. *Born to Run*.

5. William Borroughs, quoted in Christopher Sandford, *Springsteen: Point Blank*.

6. Robert Hilburn, *Springsteen* (Atlanta: Rolling Stone Press, 1985).

7. Paul Nelson, "Let Us Now Praise Famous Men."

8. Paolo Hewitt, "Bruce Springsteen: 'The River,'" *Melody Maker*, October 11, 1980.

9. Bruce Springsteen, quoted in Dave Marsh, *Glory Days*.

10. Bruce Springsteen, quoted in David Kamp, "The Book of Bruce Springsteen," *Vanity Fair*, October 2016.

11. Bruce Springsteen. *Born to Run*.

12. Steve Pond, "Bruce's Hard Look at Love," *Rolling Stone*, December 3, 1987.

13. Steven Hyden, "Overrated, Underrated, or Properly Rated: Bruce Springsteen," *Grantland*, January 7, 2014.

14. Clarence Clemons and Don Reo, *Big Man*.

15. Thom Jurek, "The Rising—Bruce Springsteen," AllMusic.com. Retrieved May 17, 2014.

16. "Album of the Month: 'The Rising,'" *Uncut*, September 2002.

17. Ann Powers, "Album review: Bruce Springsteen and the E Street Band's 'Working on a Dream," *Los Angeles Times*, January 24, 2009.

18. Bono. Bruce Springsteen's Rock & Roll Hall of Fame Induction Speech (The Waldorf Astoria, New York, March 15, 1999).

19. Bob Dylan, quoted in Edna Gundersen. "Dylan's Art Is Forever A-Changing." *USA Today*, August 28, 2006.

20. Richard Ford. "Richard Ford Reviews Bruce Springsteen's Memoir." *The New York Times*, September 22, 2016.

21. Jim Kerr. "Springsteen? Oh My God!" www.simpleminds.com, February 3, 2009.

22. Lady Gaga, quoted in Phil Gallo. "Lady Gaga Reflects on Spriingsteen Influence for 'Inside the Outside' Doc." *Billboard*, May 18, 2011.

23. Stephen King, quoted in Ian Mohr. "Stephen King's Epic First Meeting with Bruce Springsteen." *Page Six*, June 8, 2016.

24. John Lennon, quoted in Jonathan Cott. "John Lennon: The Last Interview." *Rolling Stone*, December 23, 2010.

25. Chris Martin, during a Coldplay concert at MetLife Stadium, East Rutherford, NJ, July 16, 2016.

26. Edward Norton, quoted in Kaleem Aftab. "Edward Norton Interview: Fight Club Actor Talks Bruce Springsteen Relationship Advice, American History X, Socialism and President Obama." *The Independent*, August 14, 2015.

27. Sean Penn. "Bruce Springsteen." *Time*, May 12, 2008.

28. Prince interviewed on ABC's *The View* TV talk show, January 17, 2012.

29. Martin Scorsese. Foreword to *Racing in the Street*.

30. Pete Townshend, quoted in Dave Marsh. *Two Hearts*.

31. Tom Waits, quoted in Patrick Humphries. *The Many Lives of Tom Waits*. London: Omnibus Press, 2009.

32. Neil Young. *Waging Heavy Peace: A Hippie Dream*. New York: Plume, 2013.

Works

Albums

Greetings from Asbury Park, NJ

(Single studio album—Columbia 01/05/1973)

BLINDED BY THE LIGHT / GROWIN' UP / MARY QUEEN OF ARKANSAS / DOES THIS BUS STOP AT 82ND STREET? / LOST IN THE FLOOD / THE ANGEL / FOR YOU / SPIRIT IN THE NIGHT / IT'S HARD TO BE A SAINT IN THE CITY

All songs written by Bruce Springsteen ◆ Produced by Mike Appel and Jim Cretecos ◆ Recorded June–October 1972 at 914 Sound Studios, Blauvelt, NY ◆ Recording engineer: Louis Lahav

Bruce Springsteen: lead vocals, acoustic guitar, electric guitar, harmonica, bass, piano, keyboards, handclaps ◆ David Sancious: piano, organ, keyboards ◆ Garry Tallent: bass ◆ Vini "Mad Dog" Lopez: drums, backing vocals, handclaps ◆ Clarence Clemons: saxophone, backing vocals, handclaps on "Blinded by the Light" and "Spirit in the Night" ◆ Harold Wheeler: piano on "Blinded by the Light" and "Spirit in the Night" ◆ Richard Davis: upright double bass on "The Angel" ◆ Steve Van Zandt: sound effects on "Lost in the Flood"

Peak position on US charts: #60
Peak position on UK charts: —

The Wild, the Innocent & the E Street Shuffle

(Single studio album—Columbia 11/05/1973)

THE E STREET SHUFFLE / 4TH OF JULY, ASBURY PARK (SANDY) / KITTY'S BACK / WILD BILLY'S CIRCUS STORY / INCIDENT ON 57TH STREET / ROSALITA (COME OUT TONIGHT) / NEW YORK CITY SERENADE

All songs written by Bruce Springsteen ◆ Produced by Mike Appel and Jim Cretecos ◆ Recorded May–September 1973 at 914 Sound Studios, Blauvelt, NY ◆ Recording engineer: Louis Lahav

Bruce Springsteen: lead vocals, acoustic guitar, electric guitar, harmonica, mandolin, maracas ◆ David Sancious: piano, organ, electric piano, clavinet, soprano saxophone on "The E Street Shuffle," string arrangement on "New York City Serenade" ♦ Danny Federici: accordion, backing vocals, 2nd piano on "Incident on 57th Street," organ on "Kitty's Back" ♦ Garry Tallent: bass, tuba, backing vocals ♦ Clarence Clemons: saxophone, backing vocals ♦ Vini "Mad Dog" Lopez: drums, backing vocals, cornet on "The E Street Shuffle" ♦ Richard Blackwell: conga, percussion ♦ Albany "Al" Tellone: baritone saxophone on "The E Street Shuffle" ♦ Suki Lahav: backing vocals on "4th of July, Asbury Park (Sandy)" and "Incident on 57th Street"

Peak position on US charts: #47
Peak position on UK charts: —

Born to Run

(Single studio album—Columbia—09/01/1975)

THUNDER ROAD / TENTH AVENUE FREEZE-OUT / NIGHT / BACKSTREETS / BORN TO RUN / SHE'S THE ONE / MEETING ACROSS THE RIVER / JUNGLELAND

All songs written by Bruce Springsteen ♦ Produced by Bruce Springsteen, Jon Landau and Mike Appel ♦ Recorded May 1974–July 1975 at The Record Plant, New York, NY, and 914 Sound Studios, Blauvelt, NY ♦ Recording engineers: Jimmy Iovine and Louis Lahav

Bruce Springsteen: lead vocals, producer, lead and rhythm guitars, harmonica, percussion ♦ Roy Bittan: piano, Fender Rhodes, organ, harpsichord, glockenspiel, background vocals on all tracks except "Born to Run" ♦ Garry W. Tallent: bass ♦ Clarence Clemons: saxophone, tambourine, background vocals ♦ Max Weinberg: drums on all tracks except "Born to Run" ♦ Danny Federici; organ and glockenspiel on "Born to Run" ♦ David Sancious: piano, organ on "Born to Run" ♦ Ernest "Boom" Carter: drums on "Born to Run" ♦ Steve Van Zandt: guitar and background vocals on "Thunder Road," horn arrangements on "Tenth Avenue Freeze-Out" ♦ Suki Lahav: violin on "Jungleland" ♦ Randy Brecker: trumpet on "Meeting Across the River" and "Tenth Avenue Freeze-Out" ♦ Michael Brecker: tenor saxophone on "Tenth Avenue Freeze-Out" ♦ Wayne Andre: trombone on "Tenth Avenue Freeze-Out" ♦ David Sanborn: baritone saxophone on "Tenth Avenue Freeze-Out" ♦ Richard Davis: double bass on "Meeting Across the River" ♦ Mike Appel: background vocals on "Thunder Road" ♦ Charles Calello: conductor, string arrangements on "Jungleland"

Peak position on US charts: #3
Peak position on UK charts: #16

Darkness on the Edge of Town
(Single studio album—Columbia 06/02/1978)

BADLANDS / ADAM RAISED A CAIN / SOMETHING IN THE NIGHT / CANDY'S ROOM / RACING IN THE STREET / THE PROMISED LAND / FACTORY / STREETS OF FIRE / PROVE IT ALL NIGHT / DARKNESS ON THE EDGE OF TOWN

All songs written by Bruce Springsteen ◆ Produced by Bruce Springsteen and Jon Landau ◆ Recorded at Atlantic Studios, New York, NY (June–August 1977) and The Record Plant, New York, NY (July 1977–March 1978) ◆ Recording engineer: Jimmy Iovine

Bruce Springsteen: lead vocals, lead guitar, harmonica ◆ Roy Bittan: piano, backing vocals ◆ Clarence Clemons: saxophone, backing vocals ◆ Danny Federici: organ, glockenspiel ◆ Garry Tallent: bass ◆ Steve Van Zandt: rhythm guitar, backing vocals ◆ Max Weinberg: drums

Peak position on US charts: #5
Peak position on UK charts: #16

The River
(Double studio album—Columbia 10/17/1980)

THE TIES THAT BIND / SHERRY DARLING / JACKSON CAGE / TWO HEARTS / INDEPENDENCE DAY / HUNGRY HEART / OUT IN THE STREET / CRUSH ON YOU / YOU CAN LOOK (BUT YOU BETTER NOT TOUCH) / I WANNA MARRY YOU / THE RIVER / POINT BLANK / CADILLAC RANCH / I'M A ROCKER / FADE AWAY / STOLEN CAR / RAMROD / THE PRICE YOU PAY / DRIVE ALL NIGHT / WRECK ON THE HIGHWAY

All songs written by Bruce Springsteen ◆ Produced by Bruce Springsteen, Jon Landau and Steve Van Zandt ◆ Recorded May 1979–August 1980 at Power Station Studios, New York, NY ◆ Recording engineer: Neil Dorfsman, except "The Ties that Bind" by Bob Clearmountain, and "Drive All Night" by Jimmy Iovine

Bruce Springsteen: lead vocals, electric and acoustic guitars, 12-string electric guitar, harmonica, percussion, piano on "Drive All Night" ◆ Roy Bittan: piano, organ on "I'm a Rocker" and "Drive All Night," background vocals ✦ Clarence Clemons: tenor saxophone, baritone saxophone, percussion, background vocals ✦ Danny Federici: organ, glockenspiel ✦ Garry Tallent: bass ✦ Steve Van Zandt: rhythm guitar, acoustic guitar, lead guitar on "Crush on You," harmony vocals, background vocals ✦ Max Weinberg: drums, percussion ✦ Howard Kaylan: harmony vocals ✦ Mark Volman: harmony vocals ✦ Flo & Eddie: backing vocals on "Hungry Heart"

Peak position on US charts: #1
Peak position on UK charts: #2

Nebraska
(Single studio album—Columbia 09/20/1982)

NEBRASKA / ATLANTIC CITY / MANSION ON THE HILL / JOHNNY 99 / HIGHWAY PATROLMAN / STATE TROOPER / USED CARS / OPEN ALL NIGHT / MY FATHER'S HOUSE / REASON TO BELIEVE

All songs written by Bruce Springsteen ✦ Produced by Bruce Springsteen. Recorded January 1982 at Thrill Hill East, Colts Neck, NJ ✦ Recording engineer: Toby Scott

Bruce Springsteen: vocals, guitar, harmonica, mandolin, glockenspiel, tambourine, organ, synthesizer

Peak position on US charts: #3
Peak position on UK charts: #3

Born in the U.S.A.
(Single studio album—Columbia 04/06/1984)

BORN IN THE U.S.A. / COVER ME / DARLINGTON COUNTY / WORKING ON THE HIGHWAY / DOWNBOUND TRAIN / I'M ON FIRE / NO SURRENDER / BOBBY JEAN / I'M GOIN' DOWN / GLORY DAYS / DANCING IN THE DARK / MY HOMETOWN

All songs written by Bruce Springsteen ✦ Produced by Bruce Springsteen, Jon Landau, Chuck Plotkin, and Steve Van Zandt ✦ Recorded January 1982– March 1984 at The Power Station, NY; The Hit Factory, NY; and Thrill Hill West, LA ✦ Recording engineers: Toby Scott (Hit Factory/Power Station) and Mike Batlan (Thrill Hill West)

Bruce Springsteen: lead vocals, electric guitar, acoustic guitar ✦ Roy Bittan: piano, synthesizer, background vocals ✦ Clarence Clemons: saxophone, percussion, background vocals ✦ Danny Federici: organ, glockenspiel, piano on "Born in the U.S.A." ✦ Garry Tallent: bass guitar, background vocals ✦ Steve Van Zandt: acoustic guitar, mandolin, harmony vocals ✦ Max Weinberg: drums, background vocals ✦ Richie "La Bamba" Rosenberg: background vocals on "Cover Me" and "No Surrender" ✦ Ruth Davis: background vocals on "My Hometown"

Peak position on US charts: #1
Peak position on UK charts: #1

Bruce Springsteen & the E Street Band Live/1975–85
(Quintuple live album—Columbia 11/10/1986)

THUNDER ROAD / ADAM RAISED A CAIN / SPIRIT IN THE NIGHT / 4TH OF JULY, ASBURY PARK (SANDY) / PARADISE BY THE "C" / FIRE / GROWIN' UP / IT'S HARD TO BE A SAINT IN THE CITY /BACKSTREETS / ROSALITA (COME OUT TONIGHT) / RAISE YOUR HAND / HUNGRY HEART / TWO HEARTS / CADLLAC RANCH / YOU CAN LOOK (BUT YOU BETTER NOT TOUCH) / INDEPENDENCE DAY / BADLANDS / BECAUSE THE NIGHT / CANDY'S ROOM / DARKNESS ON THE EDGE OF TOWN / RACING IN THE STREET / THIS LAND IS YOUR LAND / NEBRASKA / JOHNNY 99 / REASON TO BELIEVE / BORN IN THE U.S.A. / SEEDS / THE RIVER / WAR / DARLINGTON COUNTY / WORKING ON THE HIGHWAY / THE PROMISED LAND / COVER ME / I'M ON FIRE / BOBBY JEAN / MY HOMETOWN / BORN TO RUN / NO SURRENDER / TENTH AVENUE FREEZE-OUT / JERSEY GIRL

All songs written by Bruce Springsteen, except "Raise Your Hand" (Cropper, Floyd, Isbell), "Because the Night (Springsteen, Smith), "This Land Is Your Land (Guthrie), "War" (Strong, Whitfield), "Jersey Girl" (Waits) ✦ Produced by Bruce Springsteen, Jon Landau, and Chuck Plotkin ✦ Recorded live 1975–85 ✦ Recording engineers: Toby Scott and Bruce Jackson

Bruce Springsteen: vocals, electric guitar, harmonica, acoustic guitar ✦ Roy Bittan: piano, synthesizer, backing vocals ✦ Clarence Clemons: saxophone, percussion, backing vocals ✦ Danny Federici: organ, accordion, glockenspiel, piano, synthesizer, backing vocals ✦ Nils Lofgren (1984–85): electric and acoustic guitar, backing vocals ✦ Patti Scialfa (1984–85): backing vocals, synthesizer ✦ Garry Tallent: bass, backing vocals ✦ Steve Van Zandt (1975–81): electric guitar, acoustic guitar, backing vocals ✦ Max Weinberg: drums ✦ Flo & Eddie: backing vocals on "Hungry Heart" ✦ The Miami Horns (Stan Harrison, Eddie Manion, Mark Pender, Richie "La Bamba" Rosenberg): horns on "Tenth Avenue Freeze-Out"

Peak position on US charts: #1
Peak position on UK charts: #4

Tunnel of Love
(Single studio album—Columbia 10/06/1987)

AIN'T GOT YOU / TOUGHER THAN THE REST / ALL THAT HEAVEN WILL ALLOW / SPARE PARTS / CAUTIOUS MAN / WALK LIKE A MAN / TUNNEL OF LOVE / TWO FACES / BRIL-LIANT DISGUISE / ONE STEP UP / WHEN YOU'RE ALONE / VALENTINE'S DAY

All songs written by Bruce Springsteen ✦ Produced by Bruce Springsteen, Jon Landau, and Chuck Plotkin ✦ Recorded January–July 1987 at Thrill Hill East, Colts Neck, NJ. Additional recording at The Hit Factory, New York, NY; A&M Studios, Los Angeles, CA; and Kren Studio, Los Angeles, CA ✦ Recording engineer: Toby Scott

Bruce Springsteen: lead vocals, backing vocals, guitar, mandolin, bass guitar, keyboards, harmonica, percussion, drum machines ✦ Roy Bittan: piano on "Brilliant Disguise," synthesizers on "Tunnel of Love" ✦ Clarence Clemons: backing vocals on "When You're Alone" ✦ Danny Federici: organ on "Tougher than the Rest," "Spare Parts," "Two Faces," and "Brilliant Disguise" ✦ Nils Lofgren: guitar on "Tunnel of Love," backing vocals on "When You're Alone" ✦ Patti Scialfa: backing vocals on "Tunnel of Love," "One Step Up," and "When You're Alone" ✦ Garry Tallent: bass guitar on "Spare Parts" ✦ Max Weinberg: drums on "All That Heaven Will Allow," "Two Faces," and "When You're Alone;" percussion on "Tougher than the Rest," "Spare Parts," "Walk Like a Man," "Tunnel of Love," and "Brilliant Disguise" ✦ James Wood: harmonica on "Spare Parts"

Peak position on US charts: #1
Peak position on UK charts: #1

Human Touch

(Single studio album—Columbia 03/31/1992)

HUMAN TOUCH / SOUL DRIVER / 57 CHANNELS (AND NOTHIN' ON) / CROSS MY HEART / GLORIA'S EYES / WITH EVERY WISH / ROLL OF THE DICE / REAL WORLD / ALL OR NOTHIN' AT ALL / MAN'S JOB / I WISH I WERE BLIND / LONG GOODBYE / REAL MAN / PONY BOY

All songs written by Bruce Springsteen, except "Cross My Heart" (Springsteen, Williamson), "Roll of the Dice" and "Real World" (Springsteen, Bittan), and "Pony Boy" (traditional) • Produced by Bruce Springsteen, Jon Landau, Chuck Plotkin, and Roy Bittan • Recorded September 1989–March 1991 at A&M Studios, Soundworks West, Oceanway Studios, One On One Studio, The Record Plant, Westlake Studios, and Thrill Hill West, Los Angeles, CA • Recording engineer: Toby Scott

Bruce Springsteen: guitar and lead vocals, bass on "57 Channels (And Nothin' On)" • Randy Jackson: bass • Jeff Porcaro: drums, percussion • Roy Bittan: keyboards • Sam Moore: backing vocals on "Soul Driver," "Roll of the Dice," "Real World," and "Man's Job" • Patti Scialfa: harmony vocals on "Human Touch" and "Pony Boy" • David Sancious: Hammond organ on "Soul Driver" and "Real Man" • Bobby King: backing vocals on "Roll of the Dice" and "Man's Job" • Tim Pierce: guitar on "Soul Driver" and "Roll of the Dice" • Michael Fisher: percussion on "Soul Driver" • Bobby Hatfield: harmony vocals on "I Wish I Were Blind" • Mark Isham: trumpet on "With Every Wish"

Peak position on US charts: #2
Peak position on UK charts: #1

Lucky Town

(Single studio album—Columbia 03/31/1992)

BETTER DAYS / LUCKY TOWN / LOCAL HERO / IF I SHOULD FALL BEHIND / LEAP OF FAITH / THE BIG MUDDY / LIVING PROOF / BOOK OF DREAMS / SOULS OF THE DEPARTED / MY BEAUTIFUL REWARD

All songs written by Bruce Springsteen • Produced by Bruce Springsteen, Jon Landau and Chuck Plotkin • Recorded September 1991–January 1992 at Thrill Hill West and A&M Studios, Los Angeles, CA • Recording engineer: Toby Scott

Bruce Springsteen: guitar, lead vocals, keyboards, bass guitar, harmonica, percussion ✦ Gary Mallaber: drums ✦ Roy Bittan: keyboards on "Leap of Faith," "The Big Muddy," and "Living Proof" ✦ Patti Scialfa: backing vocals on "Better Days," "Local Hero," and "Leap of Faith" ✦ Soozie Tyrell: backing vocals on "Better Days," "Local Hero," and "Leap of Faith" ✦ Lisa Lowell: backing vocals on "Better Days," "Local Hero," and "Leap of Faith" ✦ Randy Jackson: bass guitar on "Better Days" ✦ Ian McLagan: organ on "My Beautiful Reward"

Peak position on US charts: #3
Peak position on UK charts: #2

In Concert/MTV Plugged
(Single live album—Columbia 04/12/1993)

RED-HEADED WOMAN / BETTER DAYS / ATLANTIC CITY / DARKNESS ON THE EDGE OF TOWN / MAN'S JOB / HUMAN TOUCH / LUCKY TOWN / I WISH I WAS BLIND / THUNDER ROAD / LIGHT OF DAY / IF I SHOULD FALL BEHIND / LIVING PROOF / MY BEAUTIFUL REWARD

All songs written by Bruce Springsteen ✦ Produced by Bruce Springsteen ✦ Recorded live on September 22, 1992, at the Warner Hollywood Studios, Los Angeles, CA ✦ Recording engineer: Toby Scott

Bruce Springsteen: lead vocals, lead and rhythm guitar, harmonica ✦ Zachary Alford: drums ✦ Roy Bittan: keyboards ✦ Shane Fontayne: lead and rhythm guitar ✦ Tommy Sims: bass ✦ Crystal Taliefero: acoustic guitar, percussion, background vocals ✦ Gia Ciambotti: background vocals ✦ Carol Dennis: background vocals ✦ Cleopatra Kennedy: background vocals ✦ Bobby King: background vocals ✦ Angel Rogers: background vocals ✦ Patti Scialfa: acoustic guitar, harmony vocals on "Human Touch"

Peak position on US charts: #189
Peak position on UK charts: #4

Greatest Hits
(Single collection album—02/28/1995)

BORN TO RUN / THUNDER ROAD / BADLANDS / THE RIVER / HUNGRY HEART / ATLANTIC CITY / DANCING IN THE DARK / BORN IN THE U.S.A. / MY HOMETOWN / GLORY DAYS /

BRILLIANT DISGUISE / HUMAN TOUCH / BETTER DAYS / STREETS OF PHILADELPHIA* / SECRET GARDEN** / MURDER INCORPORATED / BLOOD BROTHERS** / THIS HARD LAND**

All songs written by Bruce Springsteen ✦ Produced by Bruce Springsteen, Jon Landau, Mike Appel, Chuck Plotkin, Steve Van Zandt, and Roy Bittan ✦ Recorded 1975–1992 in various locations; (*) August 1993 at Thrill Hill West, Los Angeles, CA; (**) January 1995 at the Hit Factory, New York, NY ✦ Recording engineer: Toby Scott

Various musicians on already released songs. (**) Bruce Springsteen: lead vocals, guitar, harmonica ✦ Roy Bittan: piano, synthesizer ✦ Clarence Clemons: saxophone, percussion ✦ Danny Federici: organ, synthesizer, accordion ✦ Nils Lofgren: guitar ✦ Patti Scialfa: vocals on "Secret Garden" ✦ Garry Tallent: bass ✦ Steve Van Zandt: mandolin on "This Hard Land" ✦ Max Weinberg—drums ✦ Frank Pagano: percussion on "Blood Brothers" and "This Hard Land"

Peak position on US charts: #1
Peak position on UK charts: #1

The Ghost of Tom Joad
(Single studio album—11/21/1995)

THE GHOST OF TOM JOAD / STRAIGHT TIME / HIGHWAY 29 / YOUNGSTOWN / SINALOA COWBOYS / THE LINE / BALBOA PARK / DRY LIGHTNING / THE NEW TIMER / ACROSS THE BORDER / GALVESTON BAY / MY BEST WAS NEVER GOOD ENOUGH

All songs written by Bruce Springsteen ✦ Produced by Bruce Springsteen and Chuck Plotkin ✦ Recorded March–September 1995 at Thrill Hill West, Los Angeles, CA ✦ Recording engineer: Toby Scott

Bruce Springsteen: lead vocals, guitar, keyboards, harmonica ✦ Danny Federici: accordion, keyboards ✦ Gary Mallaber: drums ✦ Garry Tallent: bass ✦ Jim Hanson: bass ✦ Marty Rifkin: pedal steel guitar ✦ Soozie Tyrell: violin, background vocals ✦ Lisa Lowell: background vocals ✦ Patti Scialfa: background vocals ✦ Jennifer Condos: bass in "Across the Border" ✦ Jim Hanson: bass in "Youngstown" ✦ Chuck Plotkin: keyboards on "Youngstown"

Peak position on US charts: #11
Peak position on UK charts: #16

Tracks

(Quatruple collection album—11/10/1998)

MARY QUEEN OF ARKANSAS (demo version) / IT'S HARD TO BE A
SAINT IN THE CITY (demo version) / GROWIN' UP (demo version) /
DOES THIS BUS STOP AT 82ND STREET? (demo version) / BISHOP
DANCED / SEASIDE BAR SONG / ZERO AND BLIND TERRY /
LINDA LET ME BE THE ONE / THUNDERCRACK / RENDEZVOUS
(live) / GIVE THE GIRL A KISS / ICEMAN / BRING ON THE NIGHT
/ SO YOUNG AND IN LOVE / HEARTS OF STONE / DON'T
LOOK BACK / RESTLESS NIGHTS / A GOOD MAN IS HARD TO
FIND (PITTSBURGH) / ROULETTE / DOLLHOUSE / WHERE THE
BANDS ARE / LOOSE ENDS / LIVING ON THE EDGE OF THE
WORLD / WAGES OF SIN / TAKE 'EM AS THEY COME / BE TRUE
/ RICKY WANTS A MAN OF HER OWN / I WANNA BE WITH YOU
/ MARY LOU / STOLEN CAR (alternate version) / BORN IN THE U.S.A.
(demo version) / JOHNNY BYE-BYE / SHUT OUT THE LIGHT /
CYNTHIA / MY LOVE WILL NEVER LET YOU DOWN / THIS
HARD LAND / FRANKIE / TV MOVIE / STAND ON IT (demo version)
/ LION'S DEN / CAR WASH / ROCKAWAY THE DAYS / BROTHERS
UNDER THE BRIDGES '83 / MAN AT THE TOP / PINK CADILLAC
/ TWO FOR THE ROAD / JANEY DON'T LOSE YOUR HEART /
WHEN YOU NEED ME / THE WISH / THE HONEYMOONERS /
LUCKY MAN / LEAVIN' TRAIN / SEVEN ANGELS / GAVE IT A
NAME* / SAD EYES / MY LOVER MAN / OVER THE RISE /
WHEN THE LIGHTS GO OUT / LOOSE CHANGE / TROUBLE IN
PARADISE / HAPPY / PART MAN, PART MONKEY / GOIN' CALI /
BACK IN YOUR ARMS / BROTHERS UNDER THE BRIDGE '95

All songs written by Bruce Springsteen, except "Johnny Bye-Bye" (Springsteen,
Berry), and "Trouble in Paradise" (Springsteen, Bittan) ◆ Produced (1998) by
Bruce Springsteen and Chuck Plotkin ◆ Recorded 1972–1998 in various locations. (*) Recorded August 1998 at Thrill Hill East, Rumson, NJ ◆ Recording
engineer (1998): Toby Scott

Various musicians. (*) Bruce Springsteen: lead vocal, electric guitar, tambourine
◆ Roy Bittan: keyboards

Peak position on US charts: #27
Peak position on UK charts: #20

18 Tracks
(Single collection album—Columbia 04/03/1999)

GROWIN' UP (demo version) / SEASIDE BAR SONG / RENDEZVOUS / HEART OF STONE / WHERE THE BANDS ARE / LOOSE ENDS / I WANNA BE WITH YOU / BORN IN THE U.S.A. (demo version) / MY LOVE WILL NOT LET YOU DOWN / LION'S DEN / PINK CADILLAC / JANEY DON'T YOU LOSE HEART / SAD EYES / PART MAN, PART MONKEY / TROUBLE RIVER / BROTHERS UNDER THE BRIDGE / THE FEVER / THE PROMISE*

All songs written by Bruce Springsteen ✦ (*) Produced by Bruce Springsteen and Chuck Plotkin ✦ Recorded 1972–1998 in various locations. (*) Recorded on February 12, 1999 at Thrill Hill East, Rumson, NJ ✦ (*) Recording engineer: Toby Scott

Various musicians. (*) Bruce Springsteen: lead vocal, piano

Peak position on US charts: #64
Peak position on UK charts: #23

Live in New York City
(Double live album—Columbia 03/27/2001)

MY LOVE WILL NOT LET YOU DOWN / PROVE IT ALL NIGHT / TWO HEARTS / ATLANTIC CITY / MANSION ON THE HILL / THE RIVER / YOUNGSTOWN / MURDER INCORPORATED / BADLANDS / OUT IN THE STREET / BORN TO RUN / TENTH AVENUE FREEZE-OUT / LAND OF HOPE AND DREAMS / AMERICAN SKIN (41 SHOTS) / LOST IN THE FLOOD / BORN IN THE U.S.A. / DON'T LOOK BACK / JUNGLELAND / RAMROD / IF I SHOULD FALL BEHIND

All songs written by Bruce Springsteen ✦ Produced by Bruce Springsteen, Jon Landau, and Chuck Plotkin ✦ Recorded live on June 29 and July 1, 2000, at Madison Square Garden, New York, NY ✦ Recording engineer: Toby Scott

Bruce Springsteen: lead vocal, guitars, harmonica ✦ Roy Bittan: piano ✦ Clarence Clemons: saxophone, percussion, backing vocals ✦ Danny Federici: organ, keyboards, accordion ✦ Nils Lofgren: guitar, backing vocals ✦ Patti Scialfa:

guitar, backing vocals ◆ Garry Tallent: bass ◆ Steve Van Zandt: guitar, mandolin, backing vocals ◆ Max Weinberg: drums

Peak position on US charts: #5
Peak position on UK charts: #11

The Rising
(Single studio album—Columbia 07/30/2002)

LONESOME DAY / INTO THE FIRE / WAITIN' ON A SUNNY DAY / NOTHING MAN / COUNTIN' ON A MIRACLE / EMPTY SKY / WORLDS APART / LET'S BE FRIENDS (SKIN TO SKIN) / FURTHER ON (UP THE ROAD) / THE FUSE / MARY'S PLACE / YOU'RE MISSING / THE RISING / PARADISE / MY CITY OF RUINS

All songs written by Bruce Springsteen ◆ Produced by Brendan O'Brien ◆ Recorded January–March 2002 at Southern Tracks Studio, Atlanta, GA ◆ Recording engineer: Nick DiDia

Bruce Springsteen: lead guitar, vocals, acoustic guitar, baritone guitar, harmonica ◆ Roy Bittan: keyboards, piano, Mellotron, Kurzweil, pump organ, Korg M1, Crumar ◆ Clarence Clemons: saxophone, background vocals ◆ Danny Federici: Hammond B3, Vox Continental, Farfisa ◆ Nils Lofgren: electric guitar, dobro, slide guitar, banjo, background vocals ◆ Patti Scialfa: vocals ◆ Garry Tallent: bass ◆ Steve Van Zandt: electric guitar, background vocals, mandolin ◆ Max Weinberg: drums ◆ Soozie Tyrell: violin, background vocals ◆ Brendan O'Brien: hurdy-gurdy, glockenspiel, orchestra bells on "Into the Fire," "Waitin' on a Sunny Day," and "Empty Sky" ◆ Larry Lemaster and Jere Flint: cello on "Lonesome Day" and "You're Missing ◆ Jane Scarpantoni: cello on "Into the Fire," "Mary's Place," "The Rising," and "My City of Ruins" ◆ Asid Ali Khan and Group: voices on "Worlds Apart" ◆ Nashville String Machine: strings on "Countin' on a Miracle" and "You're Missing," arranged and conducted by Ricky Keller ◆ Alliance Singers: backing vocals on "Let's Be Friends (Skin to Skin)" and "Mary's Place" ◆ Mark Pender and Mike Spengler: trumpet on "Mary's Place" ◆ Rich Rosenberg: trombone on "Mary's Place" ◆ Jerry Vivino: tenor saxophone on "Mary's Place" ◆ Ed Manion: baritone saxophone on "Mary's Place"

Peak position on US charts: #1
Peak position on UK charts: #1

The Essential

(Triple collection album—Columbia 11/11/2003)

BLINDED BY THE LIGHT / FOR YOU / SPIRIT IN THE NIGHT / 4TH OF JULY, ASBURY PARK (SANDY) / ROSALITA (COME OUT TONIGHT) / THUNDER ROAD / BORN TO RUN / JUNGLELAND / BADLANDS / DARKNESS ON THE EDGE OF TOWN / THE PROMISED LAND / THE RIVER / HUNGRY HEART / NEBRASKA / ATLANTIC CITY / BORN IN THE U.S.A. / GLORY DAYS / DANCING IN THE DARK / TUNNEL OF LOVE / BRILLIANT DISGUISE / HUMAN TOUCH / LIVING PROOF / LUCKY TOWN / STREETS OF PHILADELPHIA / THE GHOST OF TOM JOAD / THE RISING / MARY'S PLACE / LONESOME DAY / AMERICAN SKIN (41 SHOTS) (live) / LAND OF HOPE AND DREAMS (live) / FROM SMALL THINGS (BIG THINGS ONE DAY COME) / THE BIG PAYBACK / HELD UP WITHOUT A GUN (live) / TRAPPED (live) / NONE BUT THE BRAVE / MISSING / LIFT ME UP / VIVA LAS VEGAS / COUNTY FAIR / CODE OF SILENCE (live) / DEAD MAN WALKIN' / COUNTIN' ON A MIRACLE (acoustic)

All songs written by Bruce Springsteen, except "Trapped" (Cliff), "Viva Las Vegas" (Pomus, Shuman), and "Code of Silence" (Springsteen, Grushecky) • Produced by Bruce Springsteen and Jon Landau • Recorded 1972–2002 in various locations • Recording engineers: various

Various musicians

Peak position on US charts: #14
Peak position on UK charts: #15

Devils & Dust

(Single studio album—Columbia 04/26/2005)

DEVILS & DUST / ALL THE WAY HOME* / RENO / LONG TIME COMIN'* / BLACK COWBOYS / MARIA'S BED / SILVER PALOMINO / JESUS WAS AN ONLY SON / LEAH / THE HITTER / ALL I'M THINKIN' ABOUT / MATAMOROS BANKS

All songs written by Bruce Springsteen • Produced by Brendan O'Brien • (*) Produced by Brendan O'Brien, Bruce Springsteen, and Chuck Plotkin • Recorded 1996–2004 at Thrill Hill East, Colts Neck, NJ, and Thrill Hill West,

Los Angeles, CA; horns and instrument overdubbing recorded 2004 at Southern Tracks Studios, Atlanta, GA; strings recorded 2004 at Masterphonics Studio, Nashville, TN ✦ Recording engineers: Toby Scott (Thrill Hill East, Thrill Hill West and Southern Tracks) and Nick Didia (Southern Tracks and Masterphonics).

Bruce Springsteen: vocals, guitar, keyboards, bass, drums, harmonica, tambourine, percussion ✦ Brendan O'Brien—hurdy-gurdy, sarangi, sitar, bass guitar, tambura ✦ Steve Jordan: drums ✦ Soozie Tyrell: violin on "Long Time Comin'" and "Maria's Bed," backing vocals on "Long Time Comin'," "Maria's Bed," "Jesus Was an Only Son," and "All I'm Thinking About" ✦ Chuck Plotkin: piano on "All the Way Home" ✦ Susan Welty and Thomas Witte: horns on "Devils & Dust" and "Black Cowboys" ✦ Marty Rifkin: steel guitar on "All the Way Home" and "Long Time Comin'" ✦ Danny Federici: organ on "Long Time Comin'" ✦ Nashville String Machine: strings on "Black Cowboys," "Silver Palomino," and "Matamoros Banks" ✦ Mark Pender: trumpet on "Leah" ✦ Patti Scialfa and Lisa Lowell: backing vocals on "Long Time Comin'," "Maria's Bed," "Jesus Was an Only Son," and "All I'm Thinking About."

Peak position on US charts: #1
Peak position on UK charts: #1

Hammersmith Odeon London '75
(Double live album—Columbia 02/28/2006)

THUNDER ROAD / TENTH AVENUE FREEZE-OUT / SPIRIT IN THE NIGHT / LOST IN THE FLOOD / SHE'S THE ONE / BORN TO RUN / THE E STREET SHUFFLE-HAVING A PARTY / IT'S HARD TO BE A SAINT IN THE CITY / BACKSTREETS / KITTY'S BACK / JUNGLELAND / ROSALITA (COME OUT TONIGHT) / 4TH OF JULY ASBURY PARK (SANDY) / DETROIT MEDLEY / FOR YOU / QUARTER TO THREE

All songs written by Bruce Springsteen, except "Having a Party (Cooke), "Detroit Medley" ("Devil with a Blue Dress": Stevenson, Long; "See See Rider": Rainey, Arant; "Good Golly Miss Molly": Blackwell, Marascalco; "Jenny Take a Ride": Crewe, Johnson, Penniman) and "Quarter to Three" (Barge, Guida, Royster, Anderson) ✦ Produced by Bruce Springsteen, Jon Landau, Barbara Carr, and Thom Zimny ✦ Recorded live on November 18, 1975, at Hammersmith Odeon, London, UK

Bruce Springsteen: guitar, vocals, harmonica, piano on "For You" ✦ Roy Bittan: piano, backing vocals ✦ Clarence Clemons: saxophone, percussion, backing vocals ✦ Danny Federici: keyboards ✦ Garry Tallent: bass ✦ Steve Van Zandt: guitar, slide guitar, backing vocals ✦ Max Weinberg: drums

Peak position on US charts: #18
Peak position on UK charts: #33

We Shall Overcome: The Seeger Sessions
(Single studio album—Columbia 04/24/2006)

OLD DAN TUCKER / JESSE JAMES / MRS. MCGRATH / O MARY DON'T YOU WEEP / JOHN HENRY / ERIE CANAL / JACOB'S LADDER / MY OKLAHOMA HOME / EYES ON THE PRIZE / SHENANDOAH / PAY ME MY MONEY DOWN / WE SHALL OVERCOME / FROGGIE WENT A-COURTIN'

All songs: Traditional, except "Jesse James" (Gashade), "Erie Canal" (Allen), "My Oklahoma Home" (Cunningham, Cunningham), "We Shall Overcome" (Tindley) ✦ Produced by Bruce Springsteen ✦ Recorded in November 1997, March 2005, and January 2006 at Thrill Hill East, Colts Neck, NJ ✦ Recording engineer: Toby Scott

Bruce Springsteen: lead vocals, guitar, harmonica, B-3 organ, and percussion ✦ Sam Bardfeld: violin ✦ Art Baron: tuba ✦ Frank Bruno: guitar ✦ Jeremy Chatzky: upright bass ✦ Mark Clifford: banjo ✦ Larry Eagle: drums and percussion ✦ Charles Giordano: B-3 organ, piano, and accordion ✦ Ed Manion: saxophone ✦ Mark Pender: trumpet, backing vocals ✦ Richie "La Bamba" Rosenberg: trombone, backing vocals ✦ Patti Scialfa: backing vocals ✦ Soozie Tyrell: violin, backing vocals

Peak position on US charts: #3
Peak position on UK charts: #3

We Shall Overcome: The Seeger Sessions—American Land Edition
(Single studio album—10/03/2006)

OLD DAN TUCKER / JESSE JAMES / MRS. MCGRATH / O MARY DON'T YOU WEEP / JOHN HENRY / ERIE CANAL / JACOB'S LADDER / MY OKLAHOMA HOME / EYES ON THE PRIZE /

SHENANDOAH / PAY ME MY MONEY DOWN / WE SHALL OVERCOME / FROGGIE WENT A-COURTIN' / BUFFALO GALS / HOW CAN I KEEP FROM SINGING / HOW CAN A POOR MAN STAND SUCH TIMES AND LIVE (live) * / BRING 'EM HOME / AMERICAN LAND (live) **

All songs: Traditional, except "Jesse James" (Gashade), "Erie Canal" (Allen), "My Oklahoma Home" (Cunningham, Cunningham), "We Shall Overcome" (Tindley), "How Can I Keep from Singing?" (Lowry, Plenn), "How Can a Poor Man Stand Such Times and Live" (Reed, Springsteen), "Bring 'Em Home" (Seeger, Musselman), "American Land" (Springsteen) ◆ Produced by Bruce Springsteen ◆ Recorded in November 1997, March 2005, and January 2006 at Thrill Hill East, Colts Neck, NJ (*) Recorded live on April 13, 2006 at the Convention Hall, Asbury Park, NJ (**) Recorded live on June 22, 2006 at Madison Square Garden, New York, NY ◆ Recording engineer: Toby Scott

Bruce Springsteen: lead vocals, guitar, harmonica, B-3 organ, and percussion ◆ Sam Bardfeld: violin ◆ Art Baron: tuba ◆ Frank Bruno: guitar ◆ Jeremy Chatzky: upright bass ◆ Mark Clifford: banjo ◆ Larry Eagle: drums and percussion ◆ Charles Giordano: B-3 organ, piano, and accordion ◆ Ed Manion: saxophone ◆ Mark Pender: trumpet, backing vocals ◆ Richie "La Bamba" Rosenberg: trombone, backing vocals ◆ Patti Scialfa: backing vocals ◆ Soozie Tyrell: violin, backing vocals

Peak position on US charts: —
Peak position on UK charts: —

Live in Dublin

(Double live album—Columbia 06/05/2007)

ATLANTIC CITY / OLD DAN TUCKER / EYES ON THE PRIZE / JESSE JAMES / FURTHER ON (UP THE ROAD) / O MARY DON'T YOU WEEP / ERIE CANAL / IF I SHOULD FALL BEHIND / MY OKLAHOMA HOME / HIGHWAY PATROLMAN / MRS. MCGRATH / HOW CAN A POOR MAN STAND SUCH TIMES AND LIVE / JACOB'S LADDER / LONG TIME COMIN' / OPEN ALL NIGHT / PAY ME MY MONEY DOWN / GROWIN' UP / WHEN THE SAINTS GO MARCHIN' IN / THIS LITTLE LIGHT OF MINE / AMERICAN LAND / BLINDED BY THE LIGHT / LOVE OF THE COMMON PEOPLE / WE SHALL OVERCOME

All songs written by Bruce Springsteen, except "Jesse James" (Gashade), "Erie Canal" (Allen), "My Oklahoma Home" (Cunningham, Cunningham), "We Shall Overcome" (Tindley), "How Can a Poor Man Stand Such Times and Live" (Reed, Springsteen), "This Little Light of Mine" (Loes), "Love of the Common People" (Hurley, Wilkins), "Old Dan Tucker," "Eyes on the Prize," "O Mary Don't You Weep," "Mrs. McGrath," "Jacob's Ladder," "Pay Me My Money Down," "When the Saints Go Marchin' In" (Traditional) ✦ Produced by George Travis ✦ Recorded live on November 17 and 19, 2006, at the Point Theatre, Dublin, IRL ✦ Recording engineer: Toby Scott

Bruce Springsteen: lead vocal, guitar, harmonica ✦ Sam Bardfeld: violin, vocals ✦ Art Baron: sousaphone, trombone, mandolin, penny whistle, euphonium ✦ Frank Bruno: acoustic guitar, vocals, field drum ✦ Jeremy Chatzky: bass, double bass ✦ Larry Eagle: drums, percussion ✦ Clark Gayton: trombone, vocals, percussion ✦ Charles Giordano: accordion, piano, Hammond organ, vocals ✦ Curtis King Jr.: vocals, percussion ✦ Greg Lizst: banjo, vocals ✦ Lisa Lowell: vocals, percussion ✦ Ed Manion: tenor and baritone saxophones, vocals, percussion ✦ Cindy Mizelle: vocals, percussion ✦ Curt Ramm: trumpet, vocals, percussion ✦ Marty Rifkin: steel guitar, dobro, mandolin ✦ Patti Scialfa: acoustic guitar, vocals ✦ Marc Anthony Thompson: acoustic guitar, vocals ✦ Soozie Tyrell: violin, vocals

Peak position on US charts: —
Peak position on UK charts: —

Magic

(Single studio album—Columbia 09/25/2007)

RADIO NOWHERE / YOU'LL BE COMIN' DOWN / LIVIN' IN THE FUTURE / YOUR OWN WORST ENEMY / GYPSY BIKER / GIRLS IN THEIR SUMMER CLOTHES / I'LL WORK FOR YOUR LOVE / MAGIC / LAST TO DIE / LONG WALK HOME / DEVIL'S ARCADE / TERRY'S SONG

All songs written by Bruce Springsteen ✦ Produced by: Brendan O'Brien ✦ Recorded March–May 2007 at Southern Tracks Studios, Atlanta, GA ✦ Recording Engineer: Nick Didia

Bruce Springsteen: lead and backing vocals, guitars, pump organ, harmonica, synthesizer, glockenspiel, percussion ✦ Roy Bittan: piano, organ ✦ Clarence Clemons: saxophone, backing vocals ✦ Danny Federici: organ, keyboards

• Nils Lofgren: guitars, backing vocals • Patti Scialfa: backing vocals • Garry Tallent: bass • Steve Van Zandt: guitars, mandolin, backing vocals • Max Weinberg: drums • Soozie Tyrell: violin on "Livin' in the Future," "I'll Work for Your Love," "Magic," and "Last to Die" • Jeremy Chatzky: upright bass on "Magic" • Daniel Laufer: cello on "Devil's Arcade" • Patrick Warren: Chamberlin, tack piano on "Your Own Worst Enemy," "Girls in Their Summer Clothes," "Magic," "Long Walk Home," and "Devil's Arcade" • String section on "Your Own Worst Enemy" and "Girls in Their Summer Clothes": Kenn Wagner, Jay Christy, Justin Bruns, William Pu, Cristopher Pulgram, John Meisner, Olga Shpitko, Sheela Lyengar (violins), Tania Maxwell Clements, Amy Chang, Lachlan McBane (viola), Karen Freer, Daniel Laufer, Charae Kruege (cello)

Peak position on US charts: #1
Peak position on UK charts: #1

Bruce Springsteen & the E Street Band Greatest Hits
(American Edition)
(Single collection album—Columbia 01/13/2009)

ROSALITA (COME OUT TONIGHT) / BORN TO RUN / THUNDER ROAD / DARKNESS ON THE EDGE OF TOWN / BADLANDS / HUNGRY HEART / GLORY DAYS / DANCING IN THE DARK / BORN IN THE U.S.A. / THE RISING / LONESOME DAY / RADIO NOWHERE

All songs written by Bruce Springsteen • Various producers • Recorded 1973–2007 in various locations

Various musicians

Peak position on US charts: #43
Peak position on UK charts: —

Bruce Springsteen & The E Street Band Greatest Hits
(European Edition)
(Single collection album—Columbia 06/01/2009)

BLINDED BY THE LIGHT / ROSALITA (COME OUT TONIGHT) / BORN TO RUN / THUNDER ROAD / BADLANDS / DARKNESS ON THE EDGE OF TOWN / HUNGRY HEART / THE RIVER / BORN IN THE U.S.A. / I'M ON FIRE / GLORY DAYS / DANCING IN

THE DARK / THE RISING / LONESOME DAY / RADIO NOWHERE / LONG WALK HOME / BECAUSE THE NIGHT (live) / FIRE (live)

All songs written by Bruce Springsteen, except "Because the Night" (Springsteen, Smith) ◆ Various producers ◆ Recorded 1972–2007 in various locations

Various musicians

Peak position on US charts: —
Peak position on UK charts: #3

Working on a Dream

(Single studio album—Columbia 01/27/2009)

OUTLAW PETE / MY LUCKY DAY / WORKING ON A DREAM / QUEEN OF THE SUPERMARKET / WHAT LOVE CAN DO / THIS LIFE / GOOD EYE / TOMORROW NEVER KNOWS / LIFE ITSELF / KINGDOM OF DAYS / SURPRISE, SURPRISE / THE LAST CARNIVAL / THE WRESTLER

All songs written by Bruce Springsteen ◆ Produced by Brendan O'Brien ◆ Recorded at Southern Tracks Studios, Atlanta, GA; Avatar Studios and Clinton Recording Studios, New York, NY; Henson Recording Studios, Hollywood, CA; and Thrill Hill East, Colts Neck, NJ ◆ Recording engineer: Nick DiDia

Bruce Springsteen: lead vocals, guitars, harmonica, keyboards, percussion, glockenspiel ◆ Roy Bittan: piano, organ, accordion ◆ Clarence Clemons: saxophone, vocals ◆ Danny Federici: organ ◆ Nils Lofgren: guitars, vocals ◆ Patti Scialfa: vocals ◆ Garry Tallent: bass ◆ Steven Van Zandt: guitars, vocals ◆ Max Weinberg: drums ◆ Soozie Tyrell: violin, vocals ◆ Patrick Warren: organ, piano, keyboards on "Outlaw Pete," "This Life," "Tomorrow Never Knows" ◆ Jason Federici: accordion on "The Last Carnival" ◆ Eddie Horst: string and horn arrangements on "Outlaw Pete," "Tomorrow Never Knows," "Surprise Surprise," "Kingdom of Days"

Peak position on US charts: #1
Peak position on UK charts: #1

The Promise

(Double collection album—Columbia 11/16/2010)

RACING IN THE STREET ('78) / GOTTA GET THAT FEELING / OUTSIDE LOOKING IN / SOMEDAY (WE'LL BE TOGETHER) / ONE WAY STREET / BECAUSE THE NIGHT / WRONG SIDE OF THE

STREET / THE BROKENHEARTED / RENDEZVOUS / CANDY'S BOY / SAVE MY LOVE / AIN'T GOOD ENOUGH FOR YOU / FIRE / SPANISH EYES / IT'S A SHAME / COME ON (LET'S GO TONIGHT) / TALK TO ME / THE LITTLE THINGS (MY BABY DOES) / BEAKAWAY / THE PROMISE / CITY OF NIGHT / THE WAY

All songs written by Bruce Springsteen, except "Because the Night" (Springsteen, Smith) ✦ Produced by Bruce Springsteen and Jon Landau ✦ Recorded 1977–1978 at The Record Plant, New York, NY, and 2010 at Thrill Hill East, Colts Neck, NJ ✦ Recording engineers: Jimmy Iovine (Record Plant) and Toby Scott (Thrill Hill East)

Bruce Springsteen: lead vocals, lead guitar, harmonica ✦ Roy Bittan: piano, vocals ✦ Clarence Clemons: saxophone, vocals ✦ Danny Federici: organ, glockenspiel ✦ Garry Tallent: bass ✦ Steve Van Zandt: rhythm guitar, vocals ✦ Max Weinberg: drums ✦ Tiffany Andrews: backing vocals on "Someday (We'll Be Together)" and "Breakaway" ✦ Corinda Crawford: backing vocals on "Someday (We'll Be Together)" and "Breakaway" ✦ Barry Danielian: trumpet on "The Brokenhearted," "It's a Shame," and "Breakaway" ✦ Rick Gazda: trumpet on "Talk to Me" ✦ Stan Harrison: tenor saxophone on "The Brokenhearted," "It's a Shame," "Talk to Me" and "Breakaway" ✦ Dan Levine: trombone on "The Brokenhearted," "It's a Shame," and "Breakaway" ✦ David Lindley: violin on "Racing in the Street ('78)" ✦ Ed Manion: baritone saxophone on "The Brokenhearted," "It's a Shame," "Talk to Me," and "Breakaway" ✦ Michelle Moore: backing vocals on "Someday (We'll Be Together)" and "Breakaway" ✦ Bob Muckin: trumpet on "Talk to Me" ✦ Curt Ramm: trumpet on "The Brokenhearted," "It's a Shame," and "Breakaway" ✦ Richie "La Bamba" Rosenberg: trombone on "Talk to Me" ✦ Antionette Savage: backing vocals on "Someday (We'll Be Together)" and "Breakaway" ✦ Patti Scialfa: backing vocals on "Someday (We'll Be Together)" and "Breakaway" ✦ Soozie Tyrell: backing vocals on "Someday (We'll Be Together)" and "Breakaway"

Peak position on US charts: #16
Peak position on UK charts: #7

Wrecking Ball

(Single studio album—Single collection album—Columbia 03/05/2012)

WE TAKE CARE OF OUR OWN / EASY MONEY / SHACKLED AND DRAWN / JACK OF ALL TRADES / DEATH TO MY HOME-TOWN / THIS DEPRESSION / WRECKING BALL / YOU'VE GOT

IT / ROCKY GROUND / LAND OF HOPE AND DREAMS / WE ARE ALIVE / SWALLOWED UP (IN THE BELLY OF THE WHALE) / AMERICAN LAND

All songs written by Bruce Springsteen ✦ Produced by Ron Aniello and Bruce Springsteen ✦ Recorded 2009–2011 at Thrill Hill East, Colts Neck, NJ ✦ Recording engineers: Ross Peterson, Ron Aniello, Rob Lebret, Clif Norrell, and Toby Scott

Bruce Springsteen: vocals, guitars, banjo, piano, organ, drums, percussion, loops ✦ Ron Aniello: guitar, bass, keyboards, piano, drums, loops ✦ Max Weinberg: drums on "Wrecking Ball," "We Are Alive," and "American Land" ✦ Matt Chamberlain: drums on "Shackled and Drawn," "Death to My Hometown," "You've Got It," and "Land of Hope and Dreams" ✦ Charlie Giordano: accordion, piano, organ, synth, celeste on "Shackled and Drawn," "Death to My Hometown," "Wrecking Ball," "Rocky Ground," "Land of Hope and Dreams," "Swallowed Up (In the Belly of the Whale)" ✦ Soozie Tyrell: violin on "Easy Money," "Wrecking Ball," "land of Hope and Dreams," and "We Are Alive" ✦ Clarence Clemons: saxophone on "Wrecking Ball" and "Land of Hope and Dreams" ✦ Tom Morello: electric guitar on "Jack of All Trades" and "This Depression" ✦ Greg Leisz: banjo, mandocello on "We Are Alive," lap steel guitar on "You've Got It" ✦ Marc Muller: pedal steel on "You've Got It") ✦ Steve Van Zandt: mandolin on "Land of Hope and Dreams" and "American Land," backing vocals on "Wrecking Ball," "Land of Hope and Dreams," and "American Land" ✦ Horn Section (Curt Ramm, Clark Gayton, Stan Harrison, Ed Manion, Dan Levine, Art Baron) on "Shackled and Drawn," "Jack of All Trades," "Wrecking Ball," and "Land of Hope and Dreams" ✦ Darrel Leonard: trumpet solo on "We Are Alive" ✦ Kevin Buell: marching drum on "Death to My Hometown" ✦ Rob Lebret: electric guitar on "Wrecking Ball" ✦ Clif Norrell: tuba on "Shackled and Drawn" ✦ Steve Jordan: tambourine on "Easy Money" ✦ Backing vocals arranged by Patti Scialfa (Lisa Lowell, Soozie Tyrell) on "We Take Care of Our Own," "Shackled and Drawn," "This Depression," "Wrecking Ball," "Land of Hope and Dreams," and "We Are Alive" ✦ Michelle Moore: vocals on "Rocky Ground" and "Land of Hope and Dreams" ✦ Cindy Mizelle: outro vocal on "Shackled and Drawn" ✦ Ron Aniello: backing vocals on "We Take Care of Our Own" and "Swallowed Up (In the Belly of the Whale)" ✦ Kevin Buell: backing vocals on "Death to My Hometown" ✦ Victorious Gospel Choir: choir on "Rocky Ground" and "Land of Hope and Dreams" directed by Lilly "Crawford" Brown

Peak position on US charts: #1
Peak position on UK charts: #1

Collection 1973–2012

(Australia and Europe)
(Single collection album—Columbia 03/08/2013)

ROSALITA (COME OUT TONIGHT) / THUNDER ROAD / BORN TO RUN / BADLANDS / THE PROMISED LAND / HUNGRY HEART / ATLANTIC CITY / BORN IN THE U.S.A. / DANCING IN THE DARK / BRILLIANT DISGUISE / HUMAN TOUCH / STREETS OF PHILADELPHIA / THE GHOST OF TOM JOAD / THE RISING / RADIO NOWHERE / WORKING ON A DREAM / WE TAKE CARE OF OUR OWN / WRECKING BALL

All songs written by Bruce Springsteen • Various producers • Recorded 1972–2012 in various locations

Various musicians

Peak position on US charts: —
Peak position on UK charts: —

High Hopes

(Single studio album—Columbia 01/14/2014)

HIGH HOPES / HARRY'S PLACE / AMERICAN SKIN (41 SHOTS) / JUST LIKE FIRE WOULD / DOWN IN THE HOLE / HEAVEN'S WALL / FRANKIE FELL IN LOVE / THIS IS YOUR SWORD / HUNTER OF INVISIBLE GAME / THE GHOST OF TOM JOAD / THE WALL / DREAM BABY DREAM

All songs written by Bruce Springsteen, except "High Hopes" (McConnell), "Just Like Fire Would" (Bailey), and "Dream Baby Dream" (Rev, Vega) • Produced by Bruce Springsteen, Brendan O'Brien, and Ron Aniello • Recorded 2002–2013 at Thrill Hill East and Stone Hill Studio, Colts Neck, NJ; Renegade Studio, Electric Lady Studios, Avatar Studios, and Sear Sound, New York, NY; Southern Tracks, Atlanta, GA; Very Loud House, Veritas Studio, East West Studios, NRG Studios, Village Studios, Record Plant, Los Angeles, CA; Berkeley Street Studio, Santa Monica, CA; Studios 301, Byron Bay and Sydney, Australia • Recording engineers: Nick DiDia, Ross Petersen, and Toby Scott

Bruce Springsteen: lead vocals, guitar, percussion, bass, organ, synthesizers, piano, banjo, mandolin, vibraphone, drums, harmonium ✦ Roy Bittan: piano, organ on "This Is Your Sword" ✦ Clarence Clemons: saxophone on "Harry's Place" and "Down in the Hole" ✦ Danny Federici: organ on "Down in the Hole" and "The Wall" ✦ Nils Lofgren: guitar on "High Hopes," "Harry's Place," "Just Like Fire Would," and "The Wall," backing vocals on "American Skin (41 Shots)" ✦ Patti Scialfa: background vocals ✦ Garry Tallent: bass ✦ Steve Van Zandt: guitar on "American Skin (41 Shots)," backing vocals ✦ Max Weinberg: drums ✦ Ron Aniello: drum loops, percussion loops, bass, synthesizers, guitar, 12-string guitar, Farfisa organ, accordion, vibraphone ✦ Tom Morello: guitar, lead vocals on "The Ghost of Tom Joad" ✦ Jake Clemons: saxophone on "American Skin (41 Shots)" and "Just Like Fire Would" ✦ Charles Giordano: organ on "American Skin (41 Shots)" and "Just Like Fire Would," accordion on "The Ghost of Tom Joad" ✦ Ed Manion: saxophone on "High Hopes," "American Skin (41 Shots)," "Just Like Fire Would," and "Dream Baby Dream" ✦ Soozie Tyrell: violin on "Down in the Hole" "Hunter of Invisible Game," and "The Ghost of Tom Joad," background vocals ✦ Sam Bardfeld: violin: on "Heaven's Wall," "Frankie Fell in Love," and "This Is Your Sword" ✦ Everett Bradley: backing vocals on "High Hopes" and "Just Like Fire Would," percussion on "High Hopes," "Just Like Fire Would," and "Heaven's Wall" ✦ Barry Danielian: trumpet saxophone on "High Hopes," "American Skin (41 Shots)," "Just Like Fire Would," and "Dream Baby Dream" ✦ Josh Freese: drums on "This Is Your Sword" ✦ Clark Gayton: trombone, tuba, saxophone on "High Hopes," "American Skin (41 Shots)," "Just Like Fire Would," and "Dream Baby Dream" ✦ Stan Harrison: saxophone on "High Hopes," "American Skin (41 Shots)," and "Dream Baby Dream" ✦ Curtis King: backing vocals on "High Hopes," "American Skin (41 Shots)," "Just Like Fire Would," and "Heaven's Wall" ✦ Cindy Mizelle: backing vocals on background vocals on "High Hopes," "American Skin (41 Shots)," "Just Like Fire Would," and "Heaven's Wall" ✦ Michelle Moore: backing vocals on background vocals on "High Hopes" and "Just Like Fire Would" ✦ Curt Ramm: trumpet and saxophone on "High Hopes," "American Skin (41 Shots)," "Just Like Fire Would," and "Dream Baby Dream," cornet on "The Wall" ✦ Evan, Jessica, and Samuel Springsteen: backing vocals on "Down in the Hole" ✦ Cillian Vallely: uilleann pipes, low whistle, tin whistle on "This Is Your Sword"

Peak position on US charts: #1
Peak position on UK charts: #1

The Essential (2015 Edition)

(Triple collection album—Columbia 10/23/2015)

GROWIN' UP / BLINDED BY THE LIGHT / FOR YOU / SPIRIT IN THE NIGHT / 4TH OF JULY, ASBURY PARK (SANDY) / ROSALITA (COME OUT TONIGHT) / THUNDER ROAD / BORN TO RUN / TENTH AVENUE FREEZE-OUT / BADLANDS / THE PROMISED LAND / PROVE IT ALL NIGHT / THE RIVER / HUNGRY HEART / THE TIES THAT BIND / OUT IN THE STREET / ATLANTIC CITY / JOHNNY 99 / BORN IN THE U.S.A. / GLORY DAYS / DANCING IN THE DARK / TOUGHER THAN THE REST / BRILLIANT DISGUISE / ONE STEP UP / HUMAN TOUCH / BETTER DAYS / IF I SHOULD FALL BEHIND / STREETS OF PHILADELPHIA / MURDER INCORPORATED / THE GHOST OF TOM JOAD / THE RISING / LONESOME DAY / DEVILS & DUST / LONG TIME COMIN' / RADIO NOWHERE / WORKING ON A DREAM / MY LUCKY DAY / THE WRESTLER / WE TAKE CARE OF OUR OWN / HUNTER OF INVISIBLE GAME

All songs written by Bruce Springsteen ◆ Produced by Bruce Springsteen and Jon Landau ◆ Recorded 1972–2014 in various locations ◆ Recording engineers: various

Various musicians

Peak position on US charts: —
Peak position on UK charts: —

Chapter and Verse

(Single collection album—Columbia 09/23/2016)

BABY I / YOU CAN'T JUDGE A BOOK BY THE COVER / HE'S GUILTY (THE JUDGE SONG) / BALLAD OF JESSE JAMES / HENRY BOY / GROWIN' UP / 4TH OF JULY, ASBURY PARK (SANDY) / BORN TO RUN / BADLANDS / THE RIVER / MY FATHER'S HOUSE / BORN IN THE U.S.A. / BRILLIANT DISGUISE / LIVING PROOF / THE GHOST OF TOM JOAD / THE RISING / LONG TIME COMIN' / WRECKING BALL

All songs written by Bruce Springsteen, except "Baby I" (Springsteen, Theiss) and "You Can't Judge a Book by the Cover" (Dixon) ◆ Produced by Bruce

Springsteen ✦ Recorded 1966–2012 in various locations ✦ Recording engineers: various

Various musicians

Peak position on US charts: #5
Peak position on UK charts: #2

Extended Plays

Chimes of Freedom
(Live EP—Columbia 10/12/1988)

TOUGHER THAN THE REST / BE TRUE / CHIMES OF FREE-DOM / BORN TO RUN (acoustic)

All songs written by Bruce Springsteen, except "Chimes of Freedom (Dylan) ✦ Produced by Bruce Springsteen, Jon Landau, and Chuck Plotkin ✦ Recorded live March–July 1988 ✦ Recording engineer: Toby Scott

Bruce Springsteen: lead vocals, guitar, harmonica ✦ Roy Bittan: synthesizer, piano ✦ Clarence Clemons: saxophone, percussion ✦ Danny Federici: organ ✦ Nils Lofgren: guitar ✦ Patti Scialfa: vocals, guitar ✦ Garry Tallent: bass ✦ Max Weinberg: drums ✦ Mario Cruz: saxophone ✦ Eddie Manion: saxophone ✦ Mark Pender: trumpet ✦ Richie "La Bamba" Rosenberg: trombone ✦ Mike Spengler: trumpet

Peak position on US charts: —
Peak position on UK charts: #13

Blood Brothers
(Studio EP—Columbia 11/19/1996)

BLOOD BROTHERS (alternate rock version) / HIGH HOPES / MURDER INCORPORATED (live)* / SECRET GARDEN (string version) / WITHOUT YOU

All songs written by Bruce Springsteen, except "High Hopes" (McConnell) ✦ Produced by Bruce Springsteen, Jon Landau, and Chuck Plotkin ✦ Recorded January–February 1995 at The Hit Factory, New York, NY (*) Recorded live on February 21, 1995 at Tramps, New York, NY ✦ Recording engineer: Toby Scott

Bruce Springsteen: lead vocals, guitar, harmonica ✦ Roy Bittan: piano, synthe-sizer ✦ Clarence Clemons: saxophone, backing vocals, percussion ✦ Danny Federici: organ, synthesizer, backing vocals ✦ Nils Lofgren: guitar, backing vocals ✦ Patti Scialfa: acoustic guitar, backing vocals ✦ Garry Tallent: bass, backing vocals ✦ Steve Van Zandt: guitar, backing vocals ✦ Max Weinberg: drums, backing vocals ✦ David Kahne: string arrangement and string synthesizer on "Secret Garden" ✦ Lisa Lowell: backing vocals on "High Hopes" ✦ Frank Pagano: percussion on "High Hopes," backing vocals on "Without You" ✦ Chuck Plotkin: backing vocals on "Without You" ✦ Soozie Tyrell: backing vocals on "Without You"

Peak position on US charts: —
Peak position on UK charts: —

American Beauty
(Studio EP—Columbia 04/19/2014)

AMERICAN BEAUTY / MARY MARY / HURRY UP SUNDOWN / HEY BLUE EYES

All songs written by Bruce Springsteen ✦ Produced by Brendan O'Brien and Ron Aniello ✦ Recorded 2007 and 2014 at Southern Tracks, Atlanta, GA, and Thrill Hill East, Colts Neck, NJ ✦ Recording engineers: Nick DiDia, Ross Petersen, and Toby Scott

Bruce Springsteen: lead vocals, 6- and 12-string acoustic guitar, electric guitar, slide guitar, keyboards, synth, bass, percussion, pump organ, and tambourine ✦ Charles Giordano: organ, Farfisa ✦ Patti Scialfa: backing vocals ✦ Ron Ani-ello: bass, piano, synth ✦ Josh Freese: drums, timpani on "American Beauty" ✦ Songa Lee: violin on "Mary Mary" and "Hurry Up Sundown" ✦ Steve Rich-ards: cello on "Mary Mary" and "Hurry Up Sundown" ✦ Toby Scott: drum programming on on "Mary Mary" and "Hurry Up Sundown" ✦ Scott Tibbs: string arrangement and conductor on on "Mary Mary" and "Hurry Up Sun-down" ✦ Max Weinberg: drums on "Hey Blue Eyes" ✦ Garry Tallent: bass on "Hey Blue Eyes" ✦ Roy Bittan: piano on "Hey Blue Eyes" ✦ Nils Lofgren: guitar, pedal steel on "Hey Blue Eyes" ✦ Patrick Warren: keyboards on "Hey Blue Eyes"

Peak position on US charts: —
Peak position on UK charts: #83

Singles

Title	Country	Release Date	US Chart	UK Chart
BLINDED BY THE LIGHT / THE ANGEL	US	Feb–73	143	–
SPIRIT IN THE NIGHT / FOR YOU	US	May–73	–	–
4TH OF JULY ASBURY PARK (SANDY) / THE E STREET SHUFFLE	Europe	Feb–75	–	–
BORN TO RUN / MEETING ACROSS THE RIVER	World	Sep–75	23	–
TENTH AVENUE FREEZE-OUT / SHE'S THE ONE	World	Dec–75	83	–
BORN TO RUN / SPIRIT IN THE NIGHT	UK	Nov–76	–	–
PROVE IT ALL NIGHT / FACTORY	World	Jun–78	33	–
BADLANDS / SOMETHING IN THE NIGHT	World	Jul–78	42	–
BADLANDS / STREETS OF FIRE	World	Aug–78	–	–
THE PROMISED LAND / STREETS OF FIRE	UK	Oct–78	–	–
ROSALITA (COME OUT TONIGHT) / NIGHT	Europe	Apr–79	–	–
HUNGRY HEART / HELD UP WITHOUT A GUN	World	Oct–80	5	44
FADE AWAY / BE TRUE	US	Dec–80	20	–
SHERRY DARLING / BE TRUE	Europe	Jan–81	–	–
SHERRY DARLING / INDEPENDENCE DAY	UK	Jan–81	–	–
CADILLAC RANCH / WRECK ON THE HIGHWAY	UK	Feb–81	–	–
THE RIVER / INDEPENDENCE DAY	Europe	May–81	–	35
THE RIVER / BORN TO RUN / ROSALITA (COME OUT TONIGHT)	UK	Jul–81	–	'
ATLANTIC CITY / MANSION ON THE HILL	UK	Sep–82	–	15
OPEN ALL NIGHT / THE BIG PAYBACK	Europe	Oct–82	–	'
DANCING IN THE DARK / PINK CADILLAC	World	May–84	2	4

DANCING IN THE DARK (Blaster Mix) / DANCING IN THE DARK (Radio) / DANCING IN THE DARK (Dub)	World	Jun–84	–	–
COVER ME / JERSEY GIRL (live)	World	Jul–84	7	16
COVER ME (Undercover Mix) / COVER ME (Dub 1) / COVER ME (Radio) / COVER ME (Dub 2)	US	Jul–84	–	–
COVER ME (Dub 1) / JERSEY GIRL (live) / DANCING IN THE DARK (Dub)	UK	Jul–84	–	–
BORN IN THE U.S.A. / SHUT OUT THE LIGHT	World	Oct–84	9	10
BORN IN THE U.S.A. (Freedom Mix) / BORN IN THE U.S.A. (Dub) /BORN IN THE U.S.A. (Radio)	World	Oct–84	–	–
I'M ON FIRE / JOHNNY BYE BYE	World	Feb–85	6	-
I'M ON FIRE / BORN IN THE U.S.A.	UK	Apr–85	–	5
I'M ON FIRE / ROSALITA / BORN IN THE U.S.A. (Freedom Mix) / JOHNNY BYE BYE	UK	Apr–85	–	–
GLORY DAYS / STAND ON IT	World	May–85	5	17
GLORY DAYS / STAND ON IT / SHERRY DARLING / RACING IN THE STREET	UK	Jun–85	–	–
I'M GOING DOWN / JANEY DON'T YOU LOSE HEART	World	Aug–85	9	15
MY HOMETOWN / SANTA CLAUS IS COMING TO TOWN (live)	World	Dec–85	6	9
SANTA CLAUS IS COMING TO TOWN (live) /MY HOMETOWN	USA, UK	Dec–85	16	9
WAR (live) / MERRY CHRISTMAS BABY (live)	World	Nov–86	8	18
WAR (live) /MERRY CHRISTMAS BABY (live) / INCIDENT ON 57TH STREET (live)	Europe	Nov–86	–	–
FIRE (live) / INCIDENT ON 57TH STREET (live)	US	Jan–87	46	–
FIRE (live) / FOR YOU (live)	Europe	Jan–87	–	54
FIRE (live) / FOR YOU (live) / BORN TO RUN (live) / NO SURRENDER (live) / TENTH AVENUE FREEZE-OUT	Europe	Jan–87	–	–

BORN TO RUN (live) / JOHNNY 99 (live) / SEEDS (live)	Europe	Feb–87	–	16
BRILLIANT DISGUISE / LUCKY MAN	World	Sep–87	5	20
TUNNEL OF LOVE / TWO FOR THE ROAD	World	Nov–87	9	45
TUNNEL OF LOVE / SANTA CLAUS IS COMING TO TOWN (live) / TWO FOR THE ROAD	Europe	Nov–87	–	–
ONE STEP UP / ROULETTE	World	Jan–88	13	–
TOUGHER THAN THE REST/ TOUGHER THAN THE REST (live)	World	May–88	12	–
TOUGHER THAN THE REST / TOUGHER THAN THE REST (live) /BE TRUE (live)/ BORN TO RUN (live)	Europe	Jun–88	–	13
SPARE PARTS / SPARE PARTS (live)	Europe	Sep–88	–	32
SPARE PARTS / PINK CADILLAC / SPARE PARTS (live) / CHIMES OF FREEDOM (live)	Europe	Sep–88	–	–
HUMAN TOUCH / BETTER DAYS	World	Mar–92	16	–
HUMAN TOUCH / SOULS OF THE DEPARTED	Europe	Mar–92	–	11
HUMAN TOUCH / SOULS OF THE DEPARTED / THE LONG GOODBYE	Europe	Mar–92	–	–
BETTER DAYS / TOUGHER THAN THE REST (live)	Europe	Mar–92	–	34
BETTER DAYS / TOUGHER THAN THE REST (live) / PART MAN, PART MONKEY	UK	Mar–92	–	–
57 CHANNELS (AND NOTHIN' ON) / PART MAN, PART MONKEY	USA	May–92	68	–
57 CHANNELS (AND NOTHIN' ON) / 57 CHANNELS (AND NOTHIN' ON) (Little Steven Version 1 Edit)	Europe	May–92	–	32
57 CHANNELS (AND NOTHIN' ON) (Little Steven Mix Version 1) / 57 CHANNELS (AND NOTHIN' ON) (Little Steven Mix Version 2) /57 CHANNELS (AND NOTHIN' ON) (There's a Riot Goin' On)	World	May–92	–	–

57 CHANNELS (AND NOTHIN' ON) / STAND ON IT / JANEY DON'T YOU LOSE HEART	Europe	Jun–92	–	–
LEAP OF FAITH / LEAP OF FAITH (live) / 30 DAYS OUT	Europe	Sep–92	–	46
LEAP OF FAITH / THE BIG PAYBACK / SHUT OUT THE LIGHT	Europe	Sep–92	–	–
LUCKY TOWN (live) / LEAP OF FAITH (live)	UK	Nov–92	–	48
IF I SHOULD FALL BEHIND / IF I SHOULD FALL BEHIND (live) /ONE STEP UP / MEETING ACROSS THE RIVER	Europe	Jan–93	–	51
LUCKY TOWN (live) /LEAP OF FAITH (live) / 30 DAYS OUT	Europe	Jan–93	–	48
LUCKY TOWN (live) / LUCKY TOWN	UK	Feb–93	–	–
STREETS OF PHILADELPHIA / IF I SHOULD FALL BEHIND (live)	World	Jan–94	–	–
STREETS OF PHILADELPHIA / IF I SHOULD FALL BEHIND (live) / GROWIN' UP (live) / THE BIG MUDDY (live)	World	Jan–94	9	2
STREETS OF PHILADELPHIA / IF I SHOULD FALL BEHIND (live) / GROWIN' UP (live) / LIGHT OF DAY (live)	US	Feb–94	–	–
MURDER INCORPORATED / BECAUSE THE NIGHT (live) / PINK CADILLAC / 4TH OF JULY, ASBURY PARK (SANDY)	Europe	Feb–95	–	–
SECRET GARDEN / THUNDER ROAD (live)	USA	Apr–95	63	–
SECRET GARDEN / SECRET GARDEN (string version) / MURDER INCORPORATED (live) / THUNDER ROAD (live)	Europe	Apr–95	–	44
HUNGRY HEART / THUNDER ROAD / HUNGRY HEART '95 (live) / THUNDER ROAD '95 (live)	World	Nov–95	32	28
THE GHOST OF TOM JOAD / STRAIGHT TIME (live) / SINALOA COWBOYS (live) / DARKNESS ON THE EDGE OF TOWN (live)	Europe	Feb–96	–	26

THE GHOST OF TOM JOAD / MEETING ACROSS THE RIVER / ONE STEP UP / NEBRASKA	Europe	Mar–96	–	–
DEAD MAN WALKIN' / THIS HARD LAND (live)	Europe	Nov–96	–	–
DEAD MAN WALKIN' / HIGHWAY 29 / THIS HARD LAND LIVE / DOES THIS BUS STOP AT 82ND STREET? LIVE	Europe	Nov–96	–	–
MISSING / DARKNESS ON THE EDGE OF TOWN (live)	Europe	Nov–96	–	–
MISSING / DARKNESS ON THE EDGE OF TOWN (live) / BORN IN THE U.S.A. (live) / SPARE PARTS (live)	Europe	Nov–96	–	–
SECRET GARDEN / MISSING	World	Feb–97	19	17
SECRET GARDEN (string version / BLOOD BROTHERS (alternate version) / STREETS OF PHILADELPHIA / HIGHWAY 29	UK	Feb–97	–	–
SAD EYES / MISSING / MAN AT THE TOP / TAKE 'EM AS THEY COME	Europe	Nov–98	–	–
SAD EYES / I WANNA BE WITH YOU	USA	Apr–99	–	–
I WANNA BE WITH YOU / WHERE THE BANDS ARE / BORN IN THE U.S.A. (acoustic) / BACK IN YOUR ARMS	Europe	Jun–99	–	–
THE RISING / LAND OF HOPES AND DREAMS (live)	World	Jul–02	52	94
LONESOME DAY / LAND OF HOPES AND DREAMS (live)	World	Nov–02	–	–
LONESOME DAY / SPIRIT IN THE NIGHT (live) / THE RISING (live) / LONESOME DAY (video)	World	Nov–02	74	39
WAITIN' ON A SUNNY DAY / BORN TO RUN (live) / DARKNESS ON THE EDGE OF TOWN (live) / THUNDER ROAD (live)	World	Feb–03	83	–
DEVILS & DUST	US	Apr–05	72	–
ALL THE WAY HOME	Europe	Apr–05	–	–
ALL I'M THINKIN' ABOUT	World	May–05	–	–
PAY ME MY MONEY DOWN / JACOB'S LADDER / WE SHALL OVERCOME	World	May–06		

RADIO NOWHERE	World	Aug–07	–	96
LONG WALK HOME	Europe	Nov-07	–	57
SANTA CLAUS IS COMIN' TO TOWN (live)	Europe	Dec–07	–	60
GIRLS IN THEIR SUMMER CLOTHES (winter mix) / GIRLS IN THEIR SUMMER CLOTHES (live) / GIRLS IN THEIR SUMMER CLOTHES (video)	World	Jan–08	95	–
DREAM BABY DREAM / The Suicide: "Dream Baby Dream" / Mr. Ray: "Beat the Devil"	World	Jun–08	–	–
WORKING ON A DREAM	World	Nov–08	95	133
MY LUCKY DAY	US	Nov–08	–	–
THE WRESTLER	World	Dec–08	–	93
WHAT LOVE CAN DO / A NIGHT WITH THE JERESY DEVIL	US	Apr–09	–	–
BORN TO RUN	Europe	Jul–09	–	93
WRECKING BALL (live)	World	Sep–09	–	–
SAVE MY LOVE / BECAUSE THE NIGHT	US	Nov–10	-	–
GOTTA GET THIS FEELING / RACING IN THE STREET ('78)	Europe	Apr–11	–	–
WE TAKE CARE OF OUR OWN	World	Jan–12	106	111
ROCKY GROUND / THE PROMISE (live)	Europe	Apr–12	–	–
DEATH TO MY HOMETOWN	World	May–12	–	–
HIGH HOPES	World	Nov–13	–	167

Video

Video Anthology 1978–1988

(Home video—Columbia 01/31/1989)

ROSALITA (COME OUT TONIGHT) (live) / THE RIVER (live) / THUNDER ROAD (live) / ATLANTIC CITY / DANCING IN THE DARK / BORN IN THE U.S.A. / I'M ON FIRE / GLORY DAYS / MY HOMETOWN / WAR (live) / FIRE (live) / BORN TO RUN (live) / BRILLIANT DISGUISE / TUNNEL OF LOVE / ONE STEP UP /

TOUGHER THAN THE REST (live) / SPARE PARTS (live) / BORN TO RUN (live acoustic)

All songs written by Bruce Springsteen, except "War" (Barrett, Strong) • Produced by Thrill Hill Productions • Directed by various directors • All Springsteen's music videos

Bruce Springsteen and the E Street Band

In Concert/MTV Plugged
(Home video—Columbia 12/15/1992)

RED-HEADED WOMAN / BETTER DAYS / LOCAL HERO / ATLANTIC CITY / DARKNESS ON THE EDGE OF TOWN / MAN'S JOB / GROWIN' UP / HUMAN TOUCH / LUCKY TOWN / I WISH I WAS BLIND / THUNDER ROAD / LIGHT OF DAY / THE BIG MUDDY / 57 CHANNELS (AND NOTHIN' ON) / MY BEAUTIFUL REWARD / GLORY DAYS / LIVING PROOF / IF I SHOULD FALL BEHIND / ROLL OF THE DICE

All songs written by Bruce Springsteen, except "Roll of the Dice" (Springsteen, Bittan) • Produced by Alex Coletti and Joe Gallen • Directed by Larry Jordan • Filmed live on September 22, 1992 at Warner Hollywood Studios, Los Angeles, CA

Bruce Springsteen: lead vocals, lead and rhythm guitar, harmonica • Zachary Alford: drums • Roy Bittan: keyboards • Shane Fontayne: lead and rhythm guitar • Tommy Sims: bass • Crystal Taliefero: acoustic guitar, percussion, background vocals • Gia Ciambotti: background vocals • Carol Dennis: background vocals • Cleopatra Kennedy: background vocals • Bobby King: background vocals • Angel Rogers: background vocals • Patti Scialfa: acoustic guitar, harmony vocals on "Human Touch"

Blood Brothers
(Documentary film—Columbia—03/03/1996)

BLOOD BROTHERS / HIGH HOPES / SECRET GARDEN #2 / MURDER INCORPORATED LIVE* / BACK IN YOUR ARMS / THIS HARD LAND / WITHOUT YOU

All songs written by Bruce Springsteen, except "High Hopes" (McConnell) • Produced by Jon Landau, Barbara Carr, Jack Gulick, Ernie Fritz and Lee

Rolontz ✦ Directed by Ernie Fritz ✦ Filmed January 9–16, 1995 at the Hit Factory, New York (*) Filmed live on February 21, 1995 at Tramps, New York, NY

Bruce Springsteen: lead vocals, guitar, harmonica ✦ Roy Bittan: piano, synthesizer ✦ Clarence Clemons: saxophone, backing vocals, percussion ✦ Danny Federici: organ, synthesizer, backing vocals ✦ Nils Lofgren: guitar, backing vocals ✦ Patti Scialfa: acoustic guitar, backing vocals ✦ Garry Tallent: bass, backing vocals ✦ Steve Van Zandt: guitar, backing vocals ✦ Max Weinberg: drums, backing vocals ✦ David Kahne: string arrangement and string synthesizer on "Secret Garden" ✦ Lisa Lowell: backing vocals on "High Hopes" ✦ Frank Pagano: percussion on "High Hopes," backing vocals on "Without You" ✦ Chuck Plotkin: backing vocals on "Without You" ✦ Soozie Tyrell: backing vocals on "Without You"

The Complete Video Anthology 1978–2000
(Home video—Columbia 01/16/2001)

ROSALITA (COME OUT TONIGHT) (live) / THE RIVER (live) / THUNDER ROAD (live) / ATLANTIC CITY / DANCING IN THE DARK / BORN IN THE U.S.A. / I'M ON FIRE / GLORY DAYS / MY HOMETOWN / WAR (live) / FIRE (live) / BORN TO RUN (live) / BRILLIANT DISGUISE / TUNNEL OF LOVE / ONE STEP UP / TOUGHER THAN THE REST (live) / SPARE PARTS (live) / BORN TO RUN (live acoustic) / HUMAN TOUCH / BETTER DAYS / 57 CHANNELS (AND NOTHIN' ON) / LEAP OF FAITH (live) / STREETS OF PHILADELPHIA / MURDER INCORPORATED (live) / SECRET GARDEN / HUNGRY HEART '95 (live) / DEAD MAN WALKING / THE GHOST OF TOM JOAD / THE GHOST OF TOM JOAD (live) / HIGHWAY PATROLMAN / IF I SHOULD FALL BEHIND (live) / BORN IN THE U.S.A. (live acoustic) / SECRET GARDEN #2

All songs written by Bruce Springsteen ✦ Produced by Thrill Hill Productions ✦ Directed by various directors ✦ All Springsteen's music videos

Bruce Springsteen and various musicians

Live in New York City
(Home video—Columbia 11/06/2001)

MY LOVE WILL NOT LET YOU DOWN / PROVE IT ALL NIGHT / TWO HEARTS / ATLANTIC CITY / MANSION ON THE HILL /

THE RIVER / YOUNGSTOWN / MURDER INCORPORATED / BADLANDS / OUT IN THE STREET / TENTH AVENUE FREEZE-OUT / BORN TO RUN / LAND OF HOPES AND DREAMS / AMERICAN SKIN (41 SHOTS) / BACKSTREETS / DON'T LOOK BACK / DARKNESS ON THE EDGE OF TOWN / LOST IN THE FLOOD / BORN IN THE U.S.A. / JUNGLELAND / LIGHT OF DAY / THE PROMISE / THUNDER ROAD / RAMROD / IF I SHOULD FALL BEHIND

All songs written by Bruce Springsteen ◆ Produced by Jon Landau, George Travis, and Bruce Springsteen ◆ Directed by Chris Hilson ◆ Filmed live on June 29 and July 1, 2000, at Madison Square Garden, New York, NY

Bruce Springsteen: lead vocal, guitars, harmonica ◆ Roy Bittan: piano ◆ Clarence Clemons: saxophone, percussion, backing vocals ◆ Danny Federici: organ, keyboards, accordion ◆ Nils Lofgren: guitar, backing vocals ◆ Patti Scialfa: guitar, backing vocals ◆ Garry Tallent: bass ◆ Steve Van Zandt: guitar, mandolin, backing vocals ◆ Max Weinberg: drums

Live in Barcelona

(Home video—Columbia 11/18/2003)

THE RISING / LONESOME DAY / PROVE IT ALL NIGHT / DARKNESS ON THE EDGE OF TOWN / EMPTY SKY / YOU'RE MISSING / WAITIN' ON A SUNNY DAY / THE PROMISED LAND / WORLDS APART / BADLANDS / SHE'S THE ONE / MARY'S PLACE / DANCING IN THE DARK / COUNTIN' ON A MIRACLE / SPIRIT IN THE NIGHT / INCIDENT ON 57TH STREET / INTO THE FIRE / NIGHT / RAMROD / BORN TO RUN / MY CITY OF RUINS / BORN IN THE U.S.A. / LAND OF HOPE AND DREAMS / THUNDER ROAD / *DROP THE NEEDLE AND PRAY* (documentary)

All songs written by Bruce Springsteen ◆ Produced by Jon Landau, Barbara Carr, and George Travis ◆ Directed by Chris Hilson ◆ Filmed live at Palau San Jordi, Barcelona, October 16, 2002

Bruce Springsteen: vocals, guitars, harmonica, piano on "Into the Fire" and "Spirit in the Night" ◆ Roy Bittan: piano, keyboards ◆ Danny Federici: organ, keyboards ◆ Nils Lofgren: electric guitar, backing vocals ◆ Steve Van Zandt: electric and acoustic guitars, mandolin, backing vocals ◆ Garry Tallent: bass ◆ Clarence Clemons: saxophone, percussion, backing vocals ◆ Patti Scialfa:

acoustic guitar, percussion, backing vocals ✦ Max Weinberg: drums ✦ Soozie Tyrell: violin, backing vocals

Devils & Dust—Bonus DVD
(Home video—Columbia 04/25/2005)

DEVILS & DUST / LONG TIME COMIN' / RENO / ALL I'M THINKIN' ABOUT / MATAMOROS BANKS

All songs written by Bruce Springsteen ✦ Produced by Chuck Plotkin ✦ Directed by Danny Clinch ✦ Filmed on March 2005

Bruce Springsteen: vocals, acoustic guitar, harmonica

VH1 Storytellers: Bruce Springsteen
(Home video—Columbia 09/06/2005)

DEVILS & DUST / BLINDED BY THE LIGHT / BRILLIANT DISGUISE / NEBRASKA / JESUS WAS AN ONLY SON / WAITIN' ON A SUNNY DAY / THE RISING / THUNDER ROAD

All songs written by Bruce Springsteen ✦ Produced by Jon Landau, Barbara Carr, George Travis, Bill Flanningan and Lee Rolontz ✦ Directed by Dave Diomedi ✦ Filmed live on April 4, 2005 at Two River Theater, Red Bank, NJ

Bruce Springsteen: vocals, guitars, piano, harmonica

We Shall Overcome—Bonus DVD
(Home video—Columbia 04/25/2006)

JOHN HENRY / PAY ME MY MONEY DOWN / BUFFALO GALS / ERIE CANAL / O MARY DON'T YOU WEEP / SHENANDOAH

All songs: Traditional ✦ Produced by Thom Zimny ✦ Directed by Thom Zimny ✦ Filmed in 2006

Bruce Springsteen: lead vocals, guitar, harmonica, B-3 organ, and percussion ✦ Sam Bardfeld: violin ✦ Art Baron: tuba ✦ Frank Bruno: guitar ✦ Jeremy Chatzky: upright bass ✦ Mark Clifford: banjo ✦ Larry Eagle: drums and percussion ✦ Charles Giordano: B-3 organ, piano, and accordion ✦ Ed Manion: saxophone ✦ Mark Pender: trumpet, backing vocals ✦ Richie "La Bamba" Rosenberg: trombone, backing vocals ✦ Patti Scialfa: backing vocals ✦ Soozie Tyrell: violin, backing vocals

We Shall Overcome American Land Edition—Bonus DVD
(Home video—Columbia 10/03/2006)

HOW CAN A POOR MAN STAND SUCH TIMES AND LIVE / BRING 'EM HOME / AMERICAN LAND / PAY ME MY MONEY DOWN

All songs: Traditional, except "How Can a Poor Man Stand Such Times and Live" (Reed, Springsteen), "Bring 'Em Home" (Seeger, Musselman), "American Land" (Springsteen) ◆ Produced by Thom Zimny ◆ Directed by Thom Zimny and Chris Hilson ◆ Filmed in 2006

Bruce Springsteen: lead vocals, guitar, harmonica, B-3 organ, and percussion ◆ Sam Bardfeld: violin ◆ Art Baron: tuba ◆ Frank Bruno: guitar ◆ Jeremy Chatzky: upright bass ◆ Mark Clifford: banjo ◆ Larry Eagle: drums and percussion ◆ Charles Giordano: B-3 organ, piano, and accordion ◆ Ed Manion: saxophone ◆ Mark Pender: trumpet, backing vocals ◆ Richie "La Bamba" Rosenberg: trombone, backing vocals ◆ Patti Scialfa: backing vocals ◆ Soozie Tyrell: violin, backing vocals

Live in Dublin
(Home video—Columbia 06/05/2007)

ATLANTIC CITY / OLD DAN TUCKER / EYES ON THE PRIZE / JESSE JAMES / FURTHER ON UP THE ROAD / O MARY DON'T YOU WEEP / ERIE CANAL / IF I SHOULD FALL BEHIND / MY OKLAHOMA HOME / HIGHWAY PATROLMAN / MRS. MCGRATH / HOW CAN A POOR MAN STAND SUCH TIMES AND LIVE / JACOB'S LADDER / LONG TIME COMIN' / OPEN ALL NIGHT / PAY ME MY MONEY DOWN / GROWIN' UP / WHEN THE SAINTS GO MARCHIN' IN / THIS LITTLE LIGHT OF MINE / AMERICAN LAND / BLINDED BY THE LIGHT / LOVE OF THE COMMON PEOPLE / WE SHALL OVERCOME

All songs written by Bruce Springsteen, except "Jesse James" (Gashade), "Erie Canal" (Allen), "My Oklahoma Home" (Cunningham, Cunningham), "We Shall Overcome" (Tindley), "How Can a Poor Man Stand Such Times and Live" (Reed, Springsteen), "This Little Light of Mine" (Loes), "Love of the Common People" (Hurley, Wilkins), "Old Dan Tucker," "Eyes on the Prize," "O Mary Don't You Weep," "Mrs. McGrath," "Jacob's Ladder," "Pay Me My Money

Down," "When the Saints Go Marchin' In" (Traditional) ✦ Produced by Jon Landau, Barbara Carr, and George Travis ✦ Directed by Thom Zimny ✦ Filmed live on November 17 and 19, 2006, at the Point Theatre, Dublin, IRL

Bruce Springsteen: lead vocal, guitar, harmonica ✦ Sam Bardfeld: violin, vocals ✦ Art Baron: sousaphone, trombone, mandolin, penny whistle, euphonium ✦ Frank Bruno: acoustic guitar, vocals, field drum ✦ Jeremy Chatzky: bass, double bass ✦ Larry Eagle: drums, percussion ✦ Clark Gayton: trombone, vocals, percussion ✦ Charles Giordano: accordion, piano, Hammond organ, vocals ✦ Curtis King Jr.: vocals, percussion ✦ Greg Lizst: banjo, vocals ✦ Lisa Lowell: vocals, percussion ✦ Ed Manion: tenor and baritone saxophones, vocals, percussion ✦ Cindy Mizelle: vocals, percussion ✦ Curt Ramm: trumpet, vocals, percussion ✦ Marty Rifkin: steel guitar, dobro, mandolin ✦ Patti Scialfa: acoustic guitar, vocals ✦ Marc Anthony Thompson: acoustic guitar, vocals ✦ Soozie Tyrell: violin, vocals

London Calling: Live in Hyde Park

(Home video—Columbia 06/22/2010)

LONDON CALLING / BADLANDS / NIGHT / SHE'S THE ONE / OUTLAW PETE / OUT IN THE STREET / WORKING ON A DREAM / SEEDS / JOHNNY 99 / YOUNGSTOWN / GOOD LOVIN' / BOBBY JEAN / TRAPPED / NO SURRENDER / WAITING ON A SUNNY DAY / THE PROMISED LAND / RACING IN THE STREET / RADIO NOWHERE / LONESOME DAY / THE RISING / BORN TO RUN / ROSALITA (COME OUT TONIGHT) / HARD TIMES (COME AGAIN NO MORE) / JUNGLELAND / AMERICAN LAND / GLORY DAYS / DANCING IN THE DARK

All songs written by Bruce Springsteen, except "London Calling" (Strummer, Jones), "Good Lovin'" (Clark, Resnick), "Trapped" (Cliff), and "Hard Times (Come Again No More" (Foster) ✦ Produced by Thom Zimny ✦ Directed by Chris Hilson ✦ Filmed live on June 22, 2010, at Hyde Park, London, UK

Bruce Springsteen: lead vocals, guitar, harmonica ✦ Roy Bittan: piano, keyboards, accordion ✦ Charlie Giordano: organ, piano, accordion, backing vocals ✦ Steve Van Zandt: guitar, madolin, backing vocals ✦ Nils Lofgren: guitar, vocals ✦ Garry Tallent: bass ✦ Clarence Clemons: saxophone, percussion, backing vocals ✦ Soozie Tyrell: violin, guitar, mandolin, percussion, backing vocals ✦ Max Weinberg: drums ✦ Curtis King Jr.: backing vocals, percussion ✦ Cindy Mizelle: backing vocals, percussion ✦ Curt Ramm: trumpet on "Wrecking Ball" ✦ Brian Fallon: vocals on "No Surrender"

Springsteen & I

(Documentary film—Black Dog Films 07/22/2013)

DOCUMENTARY / THUNDER ROAD * / BECAUSE THE NIGHT * / SHACKLED AND DRAWN * / WE ARE ALIVE * / TWIST AND SHOUT (with Paul McCartney) * / I SAW HER STANDING THERE (with Paul McCartney) *

All songs written by Bruce Springsteen except "Because the Night" (Springsteen, Smith), "Twist and Shout" (Medley, Berns), and "I Saw Her Standing There" (Lennon, McCartney) ✦ Produced by Baillie Walsh, Ridley Scott Associates, Black Dog Films, and Scott Free Productions ✦ Directed by Ander Jon Petersen and Oliver Nice ✦ Filmed 2012 in various locations (*) Filmed live on July 14, 2017 at Hyde Park, London, UK

Bruce Springsteen: lead vocals, guitar, harmonica ✦ Roy Bittan: piano, keyboards ✦ Charlie Giordano: organ, backing vocals ✦ Steve Van Zandt: guitar, backing vocals ✦ Nils Lofgren: guitar, vocals ✦ Garry Tallent: bass ✦ Jake Clemons: saxophone ✦ Soozie Tyrell: violin, guitar, percussion, backing vocals ✦ Max Weinberg: drums ✦ Curtis King Jr.: backing vocals, percussion ✦ Cindy Mizelle: backing vocals, percussion ✦ Michelle Moore: backing vocals ✦ Everett Bradley: percussion, backing vocals ✦ Curt Ramm: trumpet, percussion ✦ Barry Danielian: trumpet, percussion ✦ Clark Gayton: trombone, tuba, percussion ✦ Eddie Manion: saxophone, percussion

Born in the U.S.A. Live: London 2013

(Home video—Columbia 01/14/2014)

BORN IN THE U.S.A. / COVER ME / DARLINGTON COUNTY / WORKING ON THE HIGHWAY / DOWNBOUND TRAIN / I'M ON FIRE / NO SURRENDER / BOBBY JEAN / I'M GOIN' DOWN / GLORY DAYS / DANCING IN THE DARK / MY HOMETOWN

All songs written by Bruce Springsteen ✦ Produced by Thom Zimny ✦ Directed by Chris Hilson ✦ Filmed live on June 30, 2013, at Queen Elizabeth Olympic Park, London, UK

Bruce Springsteen: lead vocals, guitar, harmonica ✦ Roy Bittan: piano, keyboards ✦ Charlie Giordano: organ, backing vocals ✦ Steve Van Zandt: guitar, backing vocals ✦ Nils Lofgren: guitar, vocals ✦ Garry Tallent: bass ✦ Jake Clemons: saxophone ✦ Soozie Tyrell: violin, guitar, percussion, backing vocals ✦ Max Weinberg: drums ✦ Curtis King Jr.: backing vocals, percussion ✦ Cindy Mizelle: backing vocals, percussion ✦ Michelle Moore: backing vocals, rapping on "Rocky Ground" ✦ Everett Bradley: percussion, backing vocals ✦ Curt Ramm: trumpet, percussion ✦ Barry Danielian: trumpet, percussion ✦ Clark Gayton: trombone, tuba, percussion ✦ Eddie Manion: saxophone, percussion

A MusiCares Tribute to Bruce Springsteen
(Home video—Columbia 03/25/2014)

ADAM RAISED A CAIN (performed by Alabama Shakes) / BECAUSE THE NIGHT (performed by Patti Smith) / ATLANTIC CITY (performed by Natalie Maines, Ben Harper, and Charlie Musselwhite) / AMERICAN LAND (performed by Ken Casey) / MY CITY OF RUINS (performed by Mavis Staples and Zac Brown) / AMERICAN SKIN (41 SHOTS) (performed by Jackson Browne and Tom Morello) / MY HOMETOWN (performed by Emmylou Harris) / ONE STEP UP (performed by Kenny Chesney) / STREETS OF PHILADELPHIA (performed by Elton John) / HUNGRY HEART (performed by Juanes) / TOUGHER THAN THE REST (performed by Tim McGraw and Faith Hill) / THE GHOST OF TOM JOAD (performed by Jim James and Tom Morello) / DANCING IN THE DARK (performed by John Legend) / LONESOME DAY (performed by Sting) / BORN IN THE U.S.A. (performed by Neil Young and the Crazy Horse) / WE TAKE CARE OF OUR OWN (performed by Bruce Springsteen and the E Street Band) / (performed by Bruce Springsteen and the E Street Band) / THUNDER ROAD (performed by Bruce Springsteen and the E Street Band) / BORN TO RUN (performed by Bruce Springsteen and the E Street Band) / GLORY DAYS (performed by Bruce Springsteen and the E Street Band)

All songs written by Bruce Springsteen, except "Because the Night" (Springsteen, Smith) ✦ Produced by Dana Tomarken, Tom Swift, and Kristi Foely ✦ Directed by Leon Knoles ✦ Filmed on February 28, 2013, at the Convention Center, Los Angeles, CA

Bruce Springsteen: lead vocals, guitar, harmonica ✦ Roy Bittan: piano, keyboards ✦ Charlie Giordano: organ, backing vocals ✦ Steve Van Zandt: guitar, backing vocals ✦ Nils Lofgren: guitar, vocals ✦ Garry Tallent: bass ✦ Jake Clemons: saxophone ✦ Soozie Tyrell: violin, guitar, percussion, backing vocals ✦ Max Weinberg:

drums ✦ Curtis King Jr.: backing vocals, percussion ✦ Cindy Mizelle: backing vocals, percussion ✦ Everett Bradley: percussion, backing vocals ✦ Curt Ramm: trumpet, percussion ✦ Barry Danielian: trumpet, percussion ✦ Clark Gayton: trombone, tuba, percussion ✦ Eddie Manion: saxophone, percussion ✦ other musicians listed above

Combo Box Sets

Born to Run—30th Anniversary Edition
(Studio and live box set—Columbia 11/14/2005)

Born to Run
(Remastered single studio album)

THUNDER ROAD / TENTH AVENUE FREEZE-OUT / NIGHT / BACKSTREETS / BORN TO RUN / SHE'S THE ONE / MEETING ACROSS THE RIVER / JUNGLELAND

All songs written by Bruce Springsteen ✦ Produced by Bruce Springsteen, Jon Landau, and Mike Appel ✦ Recorded May 1974 – July 1975 at The Record Plant, New York, NY, and 914 Sound Studios, Blauvelt, NY ✦ Recording engineers: Jimmy Iovine and Louis Lahav

Bruce Springsteen: lead vocals, producer, lead and rhythm guitars, harmonica, percussion ✦ Roy Bittan: piano, Fender Rhodes, organ, harpsichord, glockenspiel, background vocals on all tracks except "Born to Run" ✦ Garry W. Tallent: bass ✦ Clarence Clemons: saxophone, tambourine, background vocals ✦ Max Weinberg: drums on all tracks except "Born to Run" ✦ Danny Federici; organ and glockenspiel on "Born to Run" ✦ David Sancious: piano, organ on "Born to Run" ✦ Ernest "Boom" Carter: drums on "Born to Run" ✦ Steve Van Zandt: guitar and background vocals on "Thunder Road," horn arrangements on "Tenth Avenue Freeze-Out" ✦ Suki Lahav: violin on "Jungleland" ✦ Randy Brecker: trumpet on "Meeting Across the River" and "Tenth Avenue Freeze-Out" ✦ Michael Brecker: tenor saxophone on "Tenth Avenue Freeze-Out" ✦ Wayne Andre: trombone on "Tenth Avenue Freeze-Out" ✦ David Sanborn: baritone saxophone on "Tenth Avenue Freeze-Out" ✦ Richard Davis: double bass on "Meeting Across the River" ✦ Mike Appel: background vocals on "Thunder Road" ✦ Charles Calello: conductor, string arrangements on "Jungleland"

Wings for Wheels: The Making of Born to Run
(Home video)

THE MAKING OF BORN TO RUN (documentary)* / SPIRIT IN THE NIGHT** / WILD BILLY'S CIRCUS SONG** / THUNDER-CRACK**

All songs written by Bruce Springsteen ♦ Produced by Thom Zimmy, Bruce Springsteen, Jon Landau, and Barbara Carr ♦ Directed by Tom Zimny ♦ * Documentary filmed in 2005 (with 1974–75 footage filmed by Barry Rebo) ** Filmed live on May 1, 1973, at the Ahmanson Theater in Los Angeles, CA

Bruce Springsteen: lead vocals, guitar, harmonica ♦ David Sancious: piano ♦ Danny Federici: organ ♦ Garry Tallent: bass ♦ Vini Lopez: drums

Hammersmith Odeon, London '75
(Home video)

THUNDER ROAD / TENTH AVENUE FREEZE-OUT / SPIRIT IN THE NIGHT / LOST IN THE FLOOD / SHE'S THE ONE / BORN TO RUN / THE E STREET SHUFFLE-HAVING A PARTY / IT'S HARD TO BE A SAINT IN THE CITY / BACK-STREETS / KITTY'S BACK / JUNGLELAND / ROSALITA (COME OUT TONIGHT) / 4TH OF JULY ASBURY PARK (SANDY) / DETROIT MEDLEY / FOR YOU / QUARTER TO THREE

All songs written by Bruce Springsteen, except "Having a Party (Cooke), "Detroit Medley" ("Devil with a Blue Dress": Stevenson, Long; "See See Rider": Rainey, Arant; "Good Golly Miss Molly": Blackwell, Marascalco; "Jenny Take a Ride": Crewe, Johnson, Penniman) and "Quarter to Three" (Barge, Guida, Royster, Anderson) ♦ Produced by Bruce Springsteen, Jon Landau, Barbara Carr, and Thom Zimny. ♦ Recorded live on November 18, 1975, at Hammersmith Odeon, London, UK

Bruce Springsteen: guitar, vocals, harmonica, piano on "For You" ♦ Roy Bittan: piano, backing vocals ♦ Clarence Clemons: saxophone, percussion, backing vocals ♦ Danny Federici: keyboards ♦ Garry Tallent: bass ♦ Steve Van Zandt: guitar, slide guitar, backing vocals ♦ Max Weinberg: drums

The Promise: The Darkness on the Edge of Town Story
(Studio and live box set—Columbia 11/16/2010)

The Promise: The Making of Darkness on the Edge of Town
(Documentary)

Produced by Jon Landau and Barbara Carr ◆ Directed by Thom Zimny ◆ Filmed in 2010

Darkness on the Edge of Town—Paramount Theatre, Asbury Park, NJ, 2009
(Home video)

BADLANDS / ADAM RAISED A CAIN / SOMETHING IN THE NIGHT / CANDY'S ROOM / RACING IN THE STREET / THE PROMISED LAND / FACTORY / STREETS OF FIRE / PROVE IT ALL NIGHT / DARKNESS ON THE EDGE OF TOWN

All songs written by Bruce Springsteen ◆ Produced by Jon Landau, Barbara Carr, and George Travis ◆ Directed by Thom Zimny ◆ Filmed on December 13, 2009, at the Paramount Theatre, Asbury Park, NJ

Bruce Springsteen: lead vocals, lead guitar, harmonica ◆ Roy Bittan: piano, backing vocals ◆ Clarence Clemons: saxophone, backing vocals ◆ Charlie Giordano: organ, glockenspiel ◆ Garry Tallent: bass ◆ Steve Van Zandt: rhythm guitar, backing vocals ◆ Max Weinberg: drums

Thrill Hill Vault (1976–1978)
(Home video)

SAVE MY LOVE * / CANDY'S BOY * / SOMETHING IN THE NIGHT ** / DON'T LOOK BACK *** / AIN'T GOOD ENOUGH FOR YOU *** / THE PROMISE *** / CANDY'S ROOM (demo) *** / BADLANDS **** / THE PROMISED LAND **** / PROVE IT ALL NIGHT **** / BORN TO RUN **** / ROSALITA (COME OUT TONIGHT) ****

All songs written by Bruce Springsteen ◆ Produced by Thom Zimny ◆ Directed by Barry Rebo and Arnold Levine ◆ * Filmed at Springsteen residence, Holmdel, NJ, 1976 ** Filmed live on August 5, 1976, at Monmouth Arts Center, Red Bank, NJ *** Filmed at the Record Plant Studios, New York, NY, 1978 ****Filmed live on July 8, 1978, at Arizona Veterans Memorial Coliseum, Phoenix, AZ

Bruce Springsteen: lead vocals, lead guitar, harmonica • Roy Bittan: piano, backing vocals • Clarence Clemons: saxophone, backing vocals • Danny Federici: organ, glockenspiel • Garry Tallent: bass • Steve Van Zandt: rhythm guitar, backing vocals • Max Weinberg: drums

Houston '78 Bootleg: House Cut
(Home video)

BADLANDS / STREETS OF FIRE / IT'S HARD TO BE A SAINT IN THE CITY / DARKNESS ON THE EDGE OF TOWN / SPIRIT IN THE NIGHT / INDEPENDENCE DAY / THE PROMISED LAND / PROVE IT ALL NIGHT / RACING IN THE STREET / THUNDER ROAD / JUNGLELAND / THE TIES THAT BIND / SANTA CLAUS IS COMING TO TOWN / THE FEVER / FIRE / CANDY'S ROOM / BECAUSE THE NIGHT / POINT BLANK / SHE'S THE ONE / BACKSTREETS / ROSALITA (COME OUT TONIGHT) / BORN TO RUN / DETROIT MEDLEY / TENTH AVENUE FREEZE-OUT / YOU CAN'T SIT DOWN / QUARTER TO THREE

All songs written by Bruce Springsteen, except "Santa Claus Is Coming to Town" (Gillespie, Coots), "Because the Night" (Springsteen, Smith), "Detroit Medley" ("Devil with a Blue Dress": Stevenson, Long; "See See Rider": Rainey, Arant; "Good Golly Miss Molly": Blackwell, Marascalco; "Jenny Take a Ride": Crewe, Johnson, Penniman), "You Can't Sit Down" (Clark, Cornell, Muldrow), and "Quarter to Three" (Barge, Guida, Royster, Anderson) • Produced by Thom Zimny • Directed by Thom Zimny • Filmed live on December 8, 1978, at The Summit, Houston, TX

Bruce Springsteen: lead vocals, lead guitar, harmonica • Roy Bittan: piano, backing vocals • Clarence Clemons: saxophone, backing vocals • Danny Federici: organ, glockenspiel • Garry Tallent: bass • Steve Van Zandt: rhythm guitar, backing vocals • Max Weinberg: drums

Darkness on the Edge of Town
(Remastered single studio album)

BADLANDS / ADAM RAISED A CAIN / SOMETHING IN THE NIGHT / CANDY'S ROOM / RACING IN THE STREET / THE PROMISED LAND / FACTORY / STREETS OF FIRE / PROVE IT ALL NIGHT / DARKNESS ON THE EDGE OF TOWN

All songs written by Bruce Springsteen • Produced by Bruce Springsteen and Jon Landau • Recorded at Atlantic Studios, New York, NY (June–August 1977) and The Record Plant, New York, NY (July 1977–March 1978) • Recording engineer: Jimmy Iovine

Bruce Springsteen: lead vocals, lead guitar, harmonica • Roy Bittan: piano, backing vocals • Clarence Clemons: saxophone, backing vocals • Danny Federici: organ, glockenspiel • Garry Tallent: bass • Steve Van Zandt: rhythm guitar, backing vocals • Max Weinberg: drums

The Promise
(Double collection album)

RACING IN THE STREET ('78) / GOTTA GET THAT FEELING / OUTSIDE LOOKING IN / SOMEDAY (WE'LL BE TOGETHER) / ONE WAY STREET / BECAUSE THE NIGHT / WRONG SIDE OF THE STREET / THE BROKENHEARTED / RENDEZVOUS / CANDY'S BOY / SAVE MY LOVE / AIN'T GOOD ENOUGH FOR YOU / FIRE / SPANISH EYES / IT'S A SHAME / COME ON (LET'S GO TONIGHT) / TALK TO ME / THE LITTLE THINGS (MY BABY DOES) / BREAKAWAY / THE PROMISE / CITY OF NIGHT / THE WAY

All songs written by Bruce Springsteen, except "Because the Night" (Springsteen, Smith) • Produced by Bruce Springsteen and Jon Landau • Recorded 1977–1978 at The Record Plant, New York, NY, and 2010 at Thrill Hill East, Colts Neck, NJ • Recording engineers: Jimmy Iovine (Record Plant) and Toby Scott (Thrill Hill East)

Bruce Springsteen: lead vocals, lead guitar, harmonica • Roy Bittan: piano, vocals • Clarence Clemons: saxophone, vocals • Danny Federici: organ, glockenspiel • Garry Tallent: bass • Steve Van Zandt: rhythm guitar, vocals • Max Weinberg: drums • Tiffany Andrews: backing vocals on "Someday (We'll Be Together)" and "Breakaway" • Corinda Crawford: backing vocals on "Someday (We'll Be Together)" and "Breakaway" • Barry Danielian: trumpet on "The Brokenhearted," "It's a Shame," and "Breakaway" • Rick Gazda: trumpet on "Talk to Me" • Stan Harrison: tenor saxophone on "The Brokenhearted," "It's a Shame," "Talk to Me" and "Breakaway" • Dan Levine: trombone on "The Brokenhearted," "It's a Shame," and "Breakaway" • David Lindley: violin on "Racing in the Street ('78)" • Ed Manion: baritone saxophone on "The Brokenhearted," "It's a Shame," "Talk to Me" and "Breakaway" ♦ Michelle Moore: backing vocals on "Someday (We'll Be Together)" and "Breakaway" ♦ Bob Muckin: trumpet on "Talk to Me" ♦ Curt Ramm: trumpet on "The Brokenhearted," "It's a Shame," and "Breakaway" ♦ Richie "La Bamba" Rosenberg: trombone on "Talk to Me" ♦ Antionette Savage: backing vocals on "Someday (We'll Be Together)" and "Breakaway" ♦ Patti Scialfa: backing vocals on "Someday (We'll Be Together)" and "Breakaway" ♦ Soozie Tyrell: backing vocals on "Someday (We'll Be Together)" and "Breakaway"

The Ties that Bind: The River Collection
(Studio and live box set—Columbia 12/04/2015)

The River
(Remastered double studio album)

THE TIES THAT BIND / SHERRY DARLING / JACKSON CAGE / TWO HEARTS / INDEPENDENCE DAY / HUNGRY HEART / OUT IN THE STREET / CRUSH ON YOU / YOU CAN LOOK / I WANNA MARRY YOU / THE RIVER / POINT BLANK / CADILLAC RANCH / I'M A ROCKER / FADE AWAY / STOLEN CAR / RAMROD / THE PRICE YOU PAY / DRIVE ALL NIGHT / WRECK ON THE HIGHWAY

All songs written by Bruce Springsteen ♦ Produced by Bruce Springsteen, Jon Landau, and Steve Van Zandt ♦ Recorded May 1979 – August 1980 at Power Station Studios, New York, NY ♦ Recording engineer: Neil Dorfsman, except "The Ties that Bind" by Bob Clearmountain, and "Drive All Night" by Jimmy Iovine

Bruce Springsteen: lead vocals, electric and acoustic guitars, 12-string electric guitar, harmonica, percussion, piano on "Drive All Night" ♦ Roy Bittan: piano, organ on "I'm a Rocker" and "Drive All Night," background vocals ♦ Clarence Clemons: tenor saxophone, baritone saxophone, percussion, background vocals ♦ Danny Federici: organ, glockenspiel ♦ Garry Tallent: bass ♦ Steve Van Zandt: rhythm guitar, acoustic guitar, lead guitar on "Crush on You," harmony vocals, background vocals ♦ Max Weinberg: drums, percussion ♦ Howard Kaylan: harmony vocals ♦ Mark Volman: harmony vocals ♦ Flo & Eddie: backing vocals on "Hungry Heart"

The River: Single Album

(Remastered single collection album)

THE TIES THAT BIND / CINDY / HUNGRY HEART / STOLEN CAR / BE TRUE / THE RIVER / YOU CAN LOOK (BUT YOU BETTER NOT TOUCH) / THE PRICE YOU PAY / I WANNA MARRY YOU / LOOSE ENDS

All songs written by Bruce Springsteen ◆ Produced by Bruce Springsteen, Jon Landau, and Steve Van Zandt ◆ Recorded May 1979 – August 1980 at Power Station Studios, New York, NY ◆ Recording engineer: Neil Dorfsman, except "The Ties that Bind" by Bob Clearmountain

Bruce Springsteen: lead vocals, electric and acoustic guitars, 12-string electric guitar, harmonica, percussion ◆ Roy Bittan: piano, background vocals ◆ Clarence Clemons: tenor saxophone, baritone saxophone, percussion, background vocals ◆ Danny Federici: organ, glockenspiel ◆ Garry Tallent: bass ◆ Steve Van Zandt: rhythm guitar, acoustic guitar, harmony vocals, background vocals ◆ Max Weinberg: drums, percussion ◆ Howard Kaylan: harmony vocals ◆ Mark Volman: harmony vocals ◆ Flo & Eddie: backing vocals on "Hungry Heart"

The River: Outtakes

(Remastered single collection album)

MEET ME IN THE CITY / THE MAN WHO GOT AWAY / LITTLE WHITE LIES / THE TIME THAT NEVER WAS / NIGHT FIRE / WHITETOWN / CHAIN LIGHTNING / PARTY LIGHTS / PARADISE BY THE "C" / STRAY BULLET / MR. OUTSIDE / ROULETTE / RESTLESS NIGHTS / WHERE THE BANDS ARE / DOLLHOUSE / LIVING ON THE EDGE OF THE WORLD / TAKE 'EM AS THEY COME / RICKY WANTS A MAN OF HER OWN / I WANNA BE WITH YOU / MARY LOU / HELD UP WITHOUT A GUN / FROM SMALL THINGS (BIG THINGS ONE DAY COME)

All songs written by Bruce Springsteen ◆ Produced by Bruce Springsteen, Jon Landau and Steve Van Zandt ◆ Recorded May 1979 – August 1980 at Power Station Studios, New York, NY ◆ Recording engineer: Neil Dorfsman, except "The Ties that Bind" by Bob Clearmountain

Bruce Springsteen: lead vocals, electric and acoustic guitars, 12-string electric guitar, harmonica, percussion ◆ Roy Bittan: piano, background vocals ◆ Clarence Clemons: tenor saxophone, baritone saxophone, percussion, background vocals ◆ Danny Federici: organ, glockenspiel ◆ Garry Tallent: bass ◆ Steve Van Zandt: rhythm guitar, acoustic guitar, harmony vocals, background vocals ◆ Max Weinberg: drums, percussion ◆ Howard Kaylan: harmony vocals ◆ Mark Volman: harmony vocals

The Ties that Bind
(documentary)

Produced by Thom Zimny ◆ Directed by Thom Zimny ◆ Filmed in 2015

Bruce Springsteen and the E Street Band: The River Tour, Tempe 1980
(Home video)

BORN TO RUN / PROVE IT ALL NIGHT / TENTH AVENUE FREEZE-OUT / JACKSON CAGE / TWO HEARTS / THE PROMISED LAND / OUT IN THE STREET / THE RIVER / BADLANDS / THUNDER ROAD / NO MONEY DOWN / CADILLAC RANCH / HUNGRY HEART / FIRE / SHERRY DARLING / I WANNA MARRY YOU / CRUSH ON YOU / RAMROD / YOU CAN LOOK (BUT YOU BETTER NOT TOUCH) / DRIVE ALL NIGHT / ROSALITA (COME OUT TONIGHT) / I'M A ROCKER / JUNGLELAND / DETROIT MEDLEY / RAMROD * / CADILLAC RANCH * / FIRE * / CRUSH ON YOU * / SHERRY DARLING

All songs written by Bruce Springsteen, except "No Money Down" (Berry) and "Detroit Medley" ("Devil with a Blue Dress": Stevenson, Long; "See See Rider": Rainey, Arant; "Good Golly Miss Molly": Blackwell, Marascalco; "Jenny Take a Ride": Crewe, Johnson, Penniman) ◆ Produced by Bruce Springsteen and Jon Landau ◆ Filmed live on November 5, 1980, at Arizona State University Activity Center, Tempe, AZ

Bruce Springsteen: lead vocals, guitar, harmonica ◆ Roy Bittan: piano ◆ Clarence Clemons: saxophone, percussion, backing vocals ◆ Danny Federici: organ ◆ Garry Tallent: bass ◆ Steve Van Zandt: guitar, backing vocals ◆ Max Weinberg: drums

Songs in VV.AA. Compilation Releases

STAY (live with Jackson Browne) on *No Nukes—The M.U.S.E. Concerts for a Non-Nuclear Future* (1979)

DEVIL WITH THE BLUE DRESS MEDLEY (live) on *No Nukes—The M.U.S.E. Concerts for a Non-Nuclear Future* (1979)

SANTA CLAUS IS COMING TO TOWN (live) on *In Harmony 2* (1981)

TRAPPED (live) on *U.S.A. for Africa: We Are the World* (1985)

REMEMBER WHEN THE MUSIC on *Harry Chapin Tribute* (1987)

MERRY CHRISTMAS BABY (live) on *A Very Special Christmas* (1987)

AIN'T GOT NO HOME on *Folkways: A Vision Shared—A Tribute to Woody Guthrie and Leadbelly* (1988)

VIGILANTE MAN on *Folkways: A Vision Shared—A Tribute to Woody Guthrie and Leadbelly* (1988)

VIVA LAS VEGAS on *The Last Temptation of Elvis* (1990)

CHICKEN LIPS AND LIZARD HIPS on *For Our Children* (1991)

GYPSY WOMAN on *A Tribute to Curtis Mayfield—All Men Are Brothers* (1994)

SHAKE, RATTLE AND ROLL (live with Jerry Lee Lewis) on *The Concert for the Rock and Roll Hall of Fame* (1996)

GREAT BALLS OF FIRE (live with Jerry Lee Lewis) on *The Concert for the Rock and Roll Hall of Fame* (1996)

WHOLE LOTTA SHAKIN' GOIN' ON (live with Jerry Lee Lewis) on *The Concert for the Rock and Roll Hall of Fame* (1996)

RIDING MY CAR (live) on *'Til We Outnumber 'Em—A Tribute to Woody Guthrie* (2000)

PLANE WRECK AT LOS GATOS (DEPORTEE) (live) on *'Til We Outnumber 'Em—A Tribute to Woody Guthrie* (2000)

MY CITY OF RUINS (live) on *America: A Tribute to Heroes* (2001)

GIVE MY LOVE TO ROSE on *Kindred Spirtis—A Tribute to the Music of Johnny Cash* (2002)

MY RIDE'S HERE on *Enjoy Every Sandwich: The Songs of Warren Zevon* (2004)

ONCE UPON A TIME IN THE WEST on *We All Love Ennio Morricone* (2007)

THE RISING (live) on *We Are One: The Obama Inaugural Celebration* (2009)

THIS LAND IS YOUR LAND (live with Pete Seeger) on *We Are One: The Obama Inaugural Celebration* (2009)

THE GHOST OF TOM JOAD (live with Tom Morello) on *The 25th Anniversary Rock & Roll Hall of Fame Concerts* (2010)

FORTUNATE SON (live with John Fogerty) on *The 25th Anniversary Rock & Roll Hall of Fame Concerts* (2010)

OH, PRETTY WOMAN (live with John Fogerty) on *The 25th Anniversary Rock & Roll Hall of Fame Concerts* (2010)

JUNGLELAND (live) on *The 25th Anniversary Rock & Roll Hall of Fame Concerts* (2010)

A FINE FINE BOY (live with Darlene Love) on *The 25th Anniversary Rock & Roll Hall of Fame Concerts* (2010)

NEW YORK STATE OF MIND (live with Billy Joel) on *The 25th Anniversary Rock & Roll Hall of Fame Concerts* (2010)

BORN TO RUN (live with Billy Joel) on *The 25th Anniversary Rock & Roll Hall of Fame Concerts* (2010)

(YOUR LOVE KEEPS LIFTING ME) HIGHER AND HIGHER (live with Darlene Love, John Fogerty, Sam Moor, Billy Joel, and Tom Morello) on *The 25th Anniversary Rock & Roll Hall of Fame Concerts* (2010)

BECAUSE THE NIGHT (live with U2 and Patti Smith) on *The 25th Anniversary Rock & Roll Hall of Fame Concerts* (2010)

I STILL HAVEN'T FOUND WHAT I'M LOOKING FOR (live with U2) on *The 25th Anniversary Rock & Roll Hall of Fame Concerts* (2010)

WE SHALL OVERCOME (live) on *Hope for Haiti Now* (2010)

EVERY BREATH YOU TAKE (live with Sting) on *¡Released!—1988: Human Rights Now!* (2013)

BORN IN THE U.S.A. (live) on *¡Released!—1988: Human Rights Now!* (2013)

I'M ON FIRE (live) on *¡Released!—1988: Human Rights Now!* (2013)

THE RIVER (live with Sting) on *¡Released!—1988: Human Rights Now!* (2013)

RAISE YOUR HAND (live) on *¡Released!—1988: Human Rights Now!* (2013)

TWIST AND SHOUT / LA BAMBA (live) on *¡Released!—1988: Human Rights Now!* (2013)

CHIMES OF FREEDOM (live with Sting, Peter Gabriel, Tracy Chapman, and Youssou N'Dour)

GET UP, STAND UP (live with Sting, Peter Gabriel, Tracy Chapman, and Youssou N'Dour)

LINDA PALOMA (live) on *Looking into You: A Tribute to Jackson Browne* (2014)

Guest Appearances

FIRE (pianoforte) on Robert Gordon, *Fresh Fish Special* (1977)

SAY GOODBYE TO HOLLYWOOD (guitar) on Ronnie Spector and the E Street Band, "Say Goodbye to Hollywood" / "Baby, Please Don't Go" (1977)

BABY, PLEASE DON'T GO (guitar) on Ronnie Spector and the E Street Band, "Say Goodbye to Hollywood" / "Baby Please Don't Go" (1977)

HEARTS OF STONE (guitar, backing vocal) on Southside Johnny and the Asbury Jukes, *Hearts of Stone* (1978)

TRAPPED AGAIN (backing vocal) on Southside Johnny and the Asbury Jukes, *Hearts of Stone* (1978)

FASTER AND LOUDER (vocals) on The Dictators, *Bloodbrothers* (1978)

STREET HASSLE (vocals) on Lou Reed, *Street Hassle* (1978)

ENDLESS NIGHT (background vocals) on Graham Parker, *The Up Escalator* (1980)

PARALYZED (background vocals) on Graham Parker, *The Up Escalator* (1980)

JOLE BLON (vocals, guitar) on Gary "U.S." Bonds, *Dedication* (1981)

THIS LITTLE GIRL (background vocals) on Gary "U.S." Bonds, *Dedication* (1981)

YOUR LOVE (vocals) on Gary "U.S." Bonds, *Dedication* (1981)

DEDICATION (guitar, background vocals) on Gary "U.S." Bonds, *Dedication* (1981)

OUT OF WORK (guitar) on Gary "U.S." Bonds, *On the Line* (1982)

ANGELYNE (guitar) on Gary "U.S." Bonds, *On the Line* (1982)

UNTIL THE GOOD IS GONE (background vocals) on Little Steven & the Disciples of Soul, *Men Without Women* (1982)

ANGEL EYES (background vocals) on Little Steven & the Disciples of Soul, *Men Without Women* (1982)

MEN WITHOUT WOMEN (background vocals) on Little Steven & the Disciples of Soul, *Men Without Women* (1982)

PROTECTION (guitar, backing vocals) on Donna Summer, *Donna Summer* (1982)

SAVIN' UP (guitar) on Clarence Clemons & the Red Bank Rockers, *Rescue* (1983)

WE ARE THE WORD (shared vocal) on VV.AA., *U.S.A. for Africa: We Are the World* (1985)

SUN CITY (shared vocals) on Artists United Against Apartheid, *Sun City* (1985)

WE'VE GOT THE LOVE (guitar) on Jersey Artists for Mankind, "We've Got the Love" / "Save Love, Save Life" (1986)

NATIVE AMERICAN (vocals) on Little Steven, *Freedom—No Compromise* (1987)

DREAM BABY (guitar, backing vocals) on Roy Orbison, *A Black & White Night Live* (1989)

OOBY DOOBY (guitar, backing vocals) on Roy Orbison, *A Black & White Night Live* (1989)

UPTOWN (guitar, backing vocals) on Roy Orbison, *A Black & White Night Live* (1989)

DOWN THE LINE (guitar, backing vocals) on Roy Orbison, *A Black & White Night Live* (1989)

OH, PRETTY WOMAN (guitar, backing vocals) on Roy Orbison, *A Black & White Night Live* (1989)

UP TO YOU (harmonica) on The Epidemics, *Eye Catcher* (1989)

VALENTINE (backing vocals) on Nils Lofgren, *Silver Lining* (1991)

TAKE A LOOK AT MY HEART (backing vocals) on John Prine, *The Missing Years* (1991)

IT'S BEEN A LONG TIME (vocals) on Southside Johnny and the Asbury Jukes, *Better Days* (1992)

ALL THE WAY HOME (guitar, keyboards, backing vocals) on Southside Johnny and the Asbury Jukes, *Better Days* (1992)

BIG BLACK HEAVEN (guitar) on Patti Scialfa, *Rumble Doll* (1993)

TALK TO ME LIKE THE RAIN (guitar, keyboards) on Patti Scialfa, *Rumble Doll* (1993)

ALL JUST TO GET YOU (backing vocals) on Joe Ely, *Letter to Laredo* (1995)

I'M A THOUSAND MILES FROM HOME (backing vocals) on Joe Ely, *Letter to Laredo* (1995)

DARK AND BLOODY GROUND (guitar, backing vocals) on Joe Grushecky, *American Babylon* (1995)

CHAIN SMOKIN' (guitar, mandolin, keyboards) on Joe Grushecky, *American Babylon* (1995)

NEVER BE ENOUGH TIME (guitar) on Joe Grushecky, *American Babylon* (1995)

LABOR OF LOVE (guitar, mandolin) on Joe Grushecky, *American Babylon* (1995)

WHAT DID YOU DO IN THE WAR (guitar, harmonica) on Joe Grushecky, *American Babylon* (1995)

HOMESTEAD (guitar, mandolin, backing vocals) on Joe Grushecky, *American Babylon* (1995)

ONLY LOVERS LEFT ALIVE (guitar) on Joe Grushecky, *American Babylon* (1995)

BILLY'S WALZ (mandolin) on Joe Grushecky, *American Babylon* (1995)

EVERYTHING I DO (vocals) on Elliot Murphy, *Selling the Gold* (1995)

PUMPING IRON (guitar) on Joe Grushecky, *Labour Of Love* (1996)

TALKING TO THE KING (guitar) on Joe Grushecky, *Labour Of Love* (1996)

GIMME SHELTER (guitar) on Joe Grushecky, *Labour Of Love* (1996)

MISERY LOVES COMPANY (guitar, backing vocals) on Mike Ness, *Cheating at Solitaire* (1999)

DOWN THE ROAD APIECE (vocals, guitar) on Joe Grushecky and the Houserockers, *Down the Road Apiece—Live* (1999)

TRAGEDY (backing vocals) on Emmylou Harris, *Red Dirt Girl* (2000)

WRECK ON THE HIGHWAY (vocals, guitar) on John Wesley Harding, *Awake* (2001)

FLOAT AWAY (guitar, backing vocals) on Marah, *Float Away with the Friday Night Gods* (2002)

WHITE LINES (guitar) on Soozie Tyrell, *White Lines* (2003)

STE. GENEVIEVE (backing vocals) on Soozie Tyrell, *White Lines* (2003)

DISORDER IN THE HOUSE (vocals, guitar) on Warren Zevon, *The Wind* (2003)

PRISON GROVE (backing vocals) on Warren Zevon, *The Wind* (2003)

RAISE YOUR HAND (vocals, guitar) on Clarence Clemons Temple of Soul, *Live in Asbury Park Vol. II* (2004)

CAN'T TEACH AN OLD DOG NEW TRICKS (guitar, backing vocals) on Gary "U.S." Bonds, *Back in 20* (2004)

YOU CAN'T GO BACK (guitar, keyboards) on Patti Scialfa, *23rd Street Lullaby* (2004)

ROSE (guitar, keyboards) on Patti Scialfa. *23rd Street Lullaby* (2004)

LOVE (STAND UP) (guitar, keyboards) on Patti Scialfa. *23rd Street Lullaby* (2004)

AS LONG AS I (CAN BE WITH YOU) (guitar) on Patti Scialfa, *23rd Street Lullaby* (2004)

WENDY (guitar, backing vocals) on Patti Scialfa, *23rd Street Lullaby* (2004)

BETTER TO HAVE AND NOT NEED (backing vocals) in Sam Moore, *Overnight Sensational* (2006)

AIN'T NO LOVE (vocals) on Sam Moore, *Overnight Sensational* (2006)

PINK CADILLAC (backing vocals) on Jerry Lee Lewis, *Last Man Standing* (2006)

BROKEN RADIO (vocals) on Jesse Malin, *Glitter in the Gutter* (2007)

LOOKING FOR ELVIS (guitar, harmonica) on Patti Scialfa, *Play It as It Lays* (2007)

TOWN CALLED HEARTBREAK (guitar) on Patti Scialfa, *Play It as It Lays* (2007)

PLAY AROUND (B3 organ) on Patti Scialfa, *Play It as It Lays* (2007)

RAINY DAY MAN (guitar) on Patti Scialfa, *Play It as It Lays* (2007)

PLAY IT AS IT LAYS (B3 organ, guitar) on Patti Scialfa, *Play It as It Lays* (2007)

GLORY DAYS (vocals, guitar) on Bernie Williams, *Moving Forward* (2009)

SEA OF HEARTBREAK (vocals) on Rosanne Cash, *The List* (2009)

WHEN WILL I BE LOVED (vocals) on John Fogerty, *The Blue Ridge Rangers Rides Again* (2009)

BETTER THINGS (vocals) on Ray Davies, *See My Friends* (2010)

FAITH (vocals) on Alejandro Escovedo, *Street Songs of Love* (2010)

PEG O' MY HEART (vocals) on Dropkick Murphys, *Going Out in Style* (2011)

GOD'S COUNTING ON ME . . . GOD'S COUNTING ON YOU (vocals) on Pete Seeger & Lorre Wyatt, *A More Perfect Union* (2012)

WHIP MY HAIR (vocals) on Jimmy Fallon, *Blow Your Pants Off* (2012)

ROSE TATTOO (vocals) on Dropkick Murphys, *Rose Tattoo: For Boston Charity EP* (2013)

Prizes and Awards

Academy Awards (Oscars)

1994	Best Original Song	"Streets of Philadelphia"	winner
1996	Best Original Song	"Dead Man Walkin'"	nominated

American Music Awards

1985	Pop/Rock Male Artist	Bruce Springsteen	winner
1985	Pop/Rock Male Video Artist	Bruce Springsteen	nominated
1986	Pop/Rock Male Artist	Bruce Springsteen	winner
1986	Pop/Rock Album	*Born in the U.S.A.*	winner
1986	Pop/Rock Male Video Artist	Bruce Springsteen	winner

ASCAP Film & Television Music Awards

1995	Song of the Year	"Streets of Philadelphia"	winner

Brit Awards

1986	International Male Artist	Bruce Springsteen	winner
2002	International Male Artist	Bruce Springsteen	nominated

Golden Globe

1994	Best Original Song	"Streets of Philadelphia"	winner
2009	Best Original Song	"The Wrestler"	winner

Grammy Awards

1981	Best Rock Vocal Performance, Male	"Detroit Medley"	nominated
1982	Best Rock Vocal Performance, Male	"The River"	nominated
1985	Best Rock Vocal Performance, Male	"Dancing in the Dark"	winner
1985	Album of the Year	*Born in the U.S.A.*	nominated
1986	Record of the Year	*Born in the U.S.A.*	nominated
1988	Best Rock Vocal Solo Performance	"Tunnel of Love"	winner
1988	Best Rock Vocal Performance, Male	"Brilliant Disguise"	nominated
1988	Best Rock Instrumental Performance	"Paradise by the "C""	nominated
1993	Best Rock Song	"Human Touch"	nominated

1993	Best Rock Vocal Performance, Male	"Human Touch"	nominated
1995	Song of the Year	"Streets of Philadelphia"	winner
1995	Best Rock Song	"Streets of Philadelphia"	winner
1995	Best Rock Vocal Performance, Male	"Streets of Philadelphia"	winner
1995	Best Song for a Motion picture	"Streets of Philadelphia"	winner
1995	Record of the Year	"Streets of Philadelphia"	nominated
1997	Best Contemporary Folk Album	*The Ghost of Tom Joad*	winner
1997	Best Rock Vocal Performance, Male	"Dead Man Walkin'"	nominated
1997	Best Music Video, Long Form	*Blood Brothers*	nominated
1998	Best Rock Vocal Performance, Male	"Thunder Road"	nominated
2000	Best Rock Song	"The Promise"	nominated
2000	Best Rock Vocal Performance, Male	"The Promise"	nominated
2003	Album of the Year	*The Rising*	nominated
2003	Best rock Album	*The Rising*	winner
2003	Song of the Year	"The Rising"	nominated
2003	Best Rock Song	"The Rising"	winner
2003	Best Rock Vocal Performance, Male	"The Rising"	winner
2004	Best Rock Performance by Duo/Group	"Disorder in the House"	winner
2005	Best Rock Vocal Performance, Male	"Code of Silence"	winner
2006	Best Contemporary Folk Album	*Devils & Dust*	nominated
2006	Best Music Video, Long Form	*Devils & Dust*	nominated
2006	Song of the Year	"Devils & Dust"	nominated
2006	Best Rock Song	"Devils & Dust"	nominated
2006	Best Rock Vocal Performance, Male	"Devils & Dust"	winner
2007	Best traditional Folk Album	*We Shall Overcome*	winner
2007	Best Music Video, Long Form	*Wings for Wheels*	winner
2008	Best Rock Album	*Magic*	nominated
2008	Best Rock Song	"Radio Nowhere"	winner
2008	Best Solo Rock Vocal Performance	"Radio Nowhere"	winner
2008	Best Rock Instrumental Performance	"Once Upon a Time in the West"	winner
2009	Best Rock Song	"Girls in Their Summer Clothes"	winner
2009	Best Solo Rock Vocal Performance	"Girls in Their Summer Clothes"	nominated
2010	Best Song for a Motion Picture	"The Wrestler"	nominated
2010	Best Pop Collaboration with Vocals	"Sea of Heartbreak"	nominated

2010	Best Rock Song	"Working on a Dream"	nominated
2010	Best Solo Rock Vocal Performance	"Working on a Dream"	winner
2013	Best Rock Album	*Wrecking Ball*	nominated
2013	Best Rock Song	"We Take Care of Our Own"	nominated
2013	Best Rock Performance	"We Take Care of our Own"	nominated

MTV Music Awards

1985	Best Male Video	"I'm on Fire"	winner
1985	Best Stage Performance in a Video	"Dancing in the Dark"	winner
1985	Best Overall Performance in a Video	"Dancing in the Dark"	winner
1986	Best Male Video	"Glory Days"	nominated
1986	Best Overall Performance in a Video	"Glory Days"	nominated
1987	Best Overall Performance in a Video	"Born to Run"	nominated
1987	Best Overall Performance in a Video	"War"	nominated
1988	Video of the Year	"Tunnel of Love"	nominated
1988	Best Male Video	"Tunnel of Love"	nominated
1988	Best Art Direction in a Video	"Tunnel of Love"	nominated
1988	Best Editing in a Video	"Tunnel of Love"	nominated
1992	Best Male Video	"Human Touch"	nominated
1994	Best Video from a Film	"Streets of Philadelphia"	winner
1994	Best Male Video	"Streets of Philadelphia"	nominated
1997	Best Video from a Film	"Secret Garden"	nominated
2000	Best Cameo	*High Fidelity*	nominated

Other Prizes and Awards

1997	Polar Music Prize recipient
1999	Inducted into the Rock & Roll Hall of Fame
1999	Inducted into the Songwriters Hall of Fame
2000	Rock & Roll Hall of Fame's 500 Songs That Shaped Rock & Roll: "Born to Run," "Dancing in the Dark," "Rosalita (Come Out Tonight)"
2001	The minor planet 23990, discovered September 4, 1999, by I. P. Griffin at Auckland, New Zealand, is named in his honor
2003	*Rolling Stone*'s 500 Greatest Albums of All Time: *Born to Run* (#18), *Born in the U.S.A.* (#85), *The Wild, the Innocent & the E Street Shuffle* (#132), *Darkness on the Edge of Town* (#151), *Nebraska* (#224), *The River* (#250), *Greetings from Asbury Park, NJ* (#379), *Tunnel of Love* (#475)

2003   Zagat Survey Music Guide: *Born to Run* (#1 Most Popular Album of All Time)

2004   *Rolling Stone's* 500 Greatest Songs of All Time: "Born to Run (#21), "Thunder Road" (#86), "Born in the U.S.A." (#275)

2004   *Rolling Stone's* 100 Greatest Artists of All Time: Bruce Springsteen (#23)

2008   *Time's* 100 Most Influential People of the Year: Bruce Springsteen

2009   *Forbes'* Celebrity 100: Bruce Springsteen (#6)

2009   Kennedy Center Honors recipient

2013   Named MusiCares Person of the Year

2016   Presidential Medal of Freedom recipient

Bruce Springsteen Live

Tour	# Shows	Attendance	Revenue (US$)
Greetings Tour	118	255,103	1,275,515
The Wild Tour	153	119,989	599,945
Born to Run Tour	210	517,189	3,620,323
Darkness Tour	117	813,315	6,506,520
The River World Tour	141	1,888,595	15,108,760
Born in the U.S.A. Tour	158	4,796,683	86,340,294
Tunnel of Love Express Tour	68	2,080,973	47,862,379
"Human Rights Now!" Tour	20	1,276,000	31,900,000
World Tour	102	1,986,273	57,601,917
The Ghost of Tom Joad Tour	129	393,192	22,018,752
Reunion Tour	132	2,627,810	170,807,650
The Rising Tour	120	4,075,657	221,789,424
Vote for Change Tour	7	127,219	10,177,520
Devils & Dust Tour	73	816,345	72,654,705
The Seeger Sessions Tour	56	898,706	79,984,834
Magic Tour	100	2,505,971	242,809,266
Working on a Dream Tour	83	2,169,970	194,520,402
Wrecking Ball Tour	134	3,958,629	399,068,832
High Hopes Tour	34	594,236	67,929,714
The River World Tour	89	2,486,048	293,703,964
Total	2,044	34,387,903	2,026,280,716

Highest-Grossing Concert Tours of All Time

	Artist	Tour Name	Year	Gross (US$)
1.	U2	360° Tour	2009–11	736,421,584
2.	The Rolling Stones	A Bigger Bang Tour	2005–07	558,255,524
3.	Roger Waters	The Wall Live	2010–13	458,673,798
4.	AC/DC	Black Ice World Tour	2008–10	441,121,000
5.	Madonna	Sticky & Sweet Tour	2008–09	408,000,000
6.	Bruce Springsteen	Wrecking Ball Tour	2012–13	399,068,832
7.	U2	Vertigo Tour	2005–06	389,047,636
8.	The Police	Reunion Tour	2007–08	362,000,000
9.	The Rolling Stones	Voodoo Lounge Tour	1994–95	320,000,000
10.	The Rolling Stones	Licks Tour	2002–03	311,000,000

Tours with Highest Attendance of All Time

	Artist	Tour Name	Year	Attendance
1.	U2	360° Tour	2009–11	7,272,046
2.	The Rolling Stones	Voodoo Lounge Tour	1994–95	6,336,776
3.	Pink Floyd	The Division Bell Tour	1994	5,987,345
4.	Garth Brooks	World Tour	1996–98	5,437,320
5.	U2	Zoo TV Tour	1992–93	5,350,554
6.	Bruce Springsteen	Born in the U.S.A. Tour	1984–85	4,796,683
7.	AC/DC	Black Ice World Tour	2008–10	4,486,965
8.	The Rolling Stones	A Bigger Bang Tour	2005–07	4,680,000
9.	U2	Vertigo Tour	2005–06	4,619,021
10.	Michael Jackson	HIStory World Tour	1996–97	4,543,456

Sales

Springsteen Albums Overall Sales

(Figures in Sales columns represent millions of records sold.)

Title	Diamond Discs	Platinum Discs	Golden Discs	US Sales	RoW Sales	Total Sales
Born in the U.S.A.	1	15	2	15.9	15.2	31.1
Live/1975–85	1	13	1	13.2	6.9	20.1
Greatest Hits	0	4	1	4.8	8.8	13.6
Born to Run	0	6	1	6.8	3.2	10
The River	0	5	1	5.4	4	9.4
Tunnel of Love	0	3	1	3.8	3.8	7.6
Darkness on the Edge of Town	0	3	1	3.7	2.1	5.8
The Rising	0	2	1	2.4	2.8	5.2
The Essential	0	2	1	2.2	1.8	4.0
Human Touch	0	1	1	1.5	2.4	3.9
The Wild, the In nocent & the E Street Shuffle	0	2	1	2.6	0.9	3.5
Greetings from Asbury Park	0	2	1	2.5	0.9	3.4
Lucky Town	0	1	1	1.3	2.0	3.3
Nebraska	0	1	1	1.8	1.5	3.3
Live in New York City	0	1	1	1.6	1.6	3.2
Magic	0	1	1	1.1	1.7	2.8
Tracks	0	1	1	1.4	1.2	2.6
The Ghost of Tom Joad	0	0	1	0.8	1.6	2.4
Working on a Dream	0	0	1	0.7	1.2	1.9
We Shall Overcome: The Seeger Sessions	0	0	1	0.7	1.2	1.9
Devils & Dust	0	0	1	0.7	1.1	1.8
Wrecking Ball	0	0	1	0.5	1.1	1.6
The Promise	0	0	1	0.6	0.9	1.5
In Concert /MTV Plugged	0	0	0	0.4	0.8	1.2
18 Tracks	0	0	0	0.4	0.6	1.0
High Hopes	0	0	0	0.2	0.7	0.9
Bruce Springsteen & The ESB Greatest Hits	0	0	0	0.2	0.5	0.7

Chapter and Verse	0	0	0	0.3	0.4	0.7
Live in Dublin	0	0	0	0.2	0.4	0.6
Hammersmith Odeon, London 75	0	0	0	0.2	0.2	0.4
Collection 1973-2012	0	0	0	0.0	0.2	0.2
Total	2	63	24	77.9	71.7	149.6

Springsteen Singles Overall Sales

(Figures in Sales columns represent millions of records sold.)

Title	Diamond Discs	Platinum Discs	Golden Discs	US Sales	RoW Sales	Total Sales
Dancing in the Dark	0	1	1	1.9	1.8	3.7
Streets of Philadelphia	0	0	1	0.9	1.4	2.3
Santa Claus Is Coming to Town	0	0	1	0.8	0.7	1.5
Cover Me	0	0	1	0.8	0.5	1.3
My Hometown	0	0	1	0.6	0.7	1.3
Born in the U.S.A.	0	0	1	0.7	0.6	1.3
I'm on Fire	0	0	0	0.4	0.6	1.0
Glory Days	0	0	0	0.4	0.4	0.8
Brilliant Disguise	0	0	0	0.4	0.4	0.8
I'm Goin' Down	0	0	0	0.4	0.3	0.7
War	0	0	0	0.4	0.3	0.7
Hungry Heart	0	0	0	0.4	0.2	0.6
Born to Run	0	0	0	0.1	0.5	0.6
Tunnel of Love	0	0	0	0.3	0.3	0.6
Tougher than the Rest	0	0	0	0.3	0.2	0.5
Human Touch	0	0	0	0.2	0.3	0.5
One Step Up	0	0	0	0.2	0.2	0.4
Secret Garden	0	0	0	0.2	0.2	0.4
Lonesome Day	0	0	0	0.2	0.1	0.3
Fade Away	0	0	0	0.2	0.1	0.3
Atlantic City	0	0	0	0.0	0.2	0.2
The Ghost of Tom Joad	0	0	0	0.1	0.1	0.2
Others	0	0	0	1.1	0.9	2.0
Total	0	1	6	11.0	11.0	22.0

Springsteen Videos Overall Sales
(Figures in Sales columns represent millions of units sold.)

Title	Diamond Discs	Platinum Discs	Golden Discs	US Sales	RoW Sales	Total Sales
Live in Barcelona	0	4	1	0.40	0.60	1.00
Video Anthology	0	3	1	0.30	0.20	0.50
Live in New York City	0	3	1	0.30	0.40	0.70
In Concert/MTV Plugged	0	0	1	0.07	0.10	0.17
Blood Brothers	0	0	1	0.05	0.08	0.13
Live in Dublin	0	0	1	0.06	0.10	0.16
VH1 Storytellers	0	0	1	0.06	0.05	0.11
London Calling: Live in Hyde Park	0	0	0	0.04	0.08	0.12
Total	0	10	7	1.28	1.61	2.89

List of Best-Selling Music Artists of All Time

1.	The Beatles	610		14.	Mariah Carey	171
2.	Elvis Presley	590		15.	AC/DC	170
3.	Michael Jackson	350		16.	Queen	162
4.	Elton John	300		17.	Taylor Swift	160
5.	Led Zeppelin	290		18.	Garth Brooks	158
6.	Madonna	275		19.	U2	155
7.	Pink Floyd	255		20.	Eagles	150
8.	Rihanna	230		21.	Eminem	145
9.	The Rolling Stones	200		22.	Billy Joel	140
10.	ABBA	190		23.	Frank Sinatra	136
11.	Whitney Houston	185		24.	Barbra Streisand	133
12,	Celine Dion	180		25.	Phil Collins	130
13.	Bruce Springsteen	172				

The artists in the above table are listed with figures that consider both their claimed sales figure along with their total of certified units. All artists included on this list who have begun charting on official albums or singles charts have their available claimed figures supported by at least 20 percent in certified units. The certified units are sourced from available online databases of local music industry associations. The figures refer to "records" (singles, albums, videos).

List of Best-Selling Albums of All Time

1.	Michael Jackson	*Thriller*	65
2.	AC/DC	*Back in Black*	50
3.	Pink Floyd	*The Dark Side of the Moon*	45
4.	VV.AA. (W. Houston)	*The Bodyguard—Soundtrack*	44
5.	Eagles	*Their Greatest Hits (1971–1975)*	43
6.	Meat Loaf	*Bat Out of Hell*	42
7.	VV.AA. (Bee Gees)	*Saturday Night Fever—Soundtrack*	39
8.	Fleetwood Mac	*Rumours*	40
9.	Shania Twain	*Come On Over*	39
10.	Led Zeppelin	*Led Zeppelin IV*	37
11.	Michael Jackson	*Bad*	35
12.	Alanis Morissette	*Jagged Little Pills*	33
13.	The Beatles	*Sgt. Pepper's Lonely Hearts Club Band*	32
14.	Bruce Springsteen	*Born in the U.S.A.*	31
15.	The Beatles	*1*	30
16.	The Beatles	*Abbey Road*	30
17.	Adele	*21*	30
18.	Celine Dion	*Falling into You*	30
19.	Nirvana	*Nevermind*	30
20.	VV.AA.	*Dirty Dancing*	30

Recording Industry Association of America (RIAA)

This is the list of the top 100 highest-certified music artists in the United States based on album certifications by RIAA. Since 2016, the RIAA album certification has also included on-demand audio/video streams (1,500 streams = 1 album unit) and track sale equivalent (10 track sales = 1 album unit).

1.	The Beatles	178.0	11.	Bruce Springsteen	71.0
2.	Garth Brooks	148.0	12.	George Strait	69.0
3.	Elvis Presley	136.0	13.	Barbra Streisand	68.5
4.	Led Zeppelin	111.5	14.	The Rolling Stones	66.5
5.	The Eagles	101.0	15.	Aerosmith	66.0
6.	Billy Joel	82.5	16.	Madonna	64.5
7.	Michael Jackson	81.0	17.	Mariah Carey	64.0
8.	Elton John	77.0	18.	Metallica	62.0
9.	Pink Floyd	75.0	19.	Whitney Houston	57.0
10.	AC/DC	72.0	20.	Van Halen	56.5

BIBLIOGRAPHY

✦ Books on Springsteen quoted in this volume

Bruce Springsteen and Philosophy: Darkness on the Edge of Truth. Popular Culture and Philosophy, Vol. 32. Edited by Randall E. Auxier and Doug Anderson. Chicago: Open Court, 2008.

Bruce Springsteen—The Rolling Stone Files: The Ultimate Compendium of Interviews, Articles, Facts and Opinions from the Files of Rolling Stone. New York: Hyperion Press, 1996.

Racing in the Street: The Bruce Springsteen Reader. Edited by June Skinner Sawyers. New York: Penguin, 2004.

Springsteen dalla A alla Z. Edited by Ermanno Labianca e Massimo Cotto. Roma: Arcana, 1999.

Talk About a Dream. The Essential Interview of Bruce Springsteen. Edited by Christopher Phillips and Louis P. Masur. New York: Bloomsbury Press, 2013.

The Ties that Bind: Bruce Springsteen A to E to Z. Edited by Gary Graff. Canton: Visible Ink Press, 2005.

Beviglia, Jim. *Counting Down Bruce Springsteen: His 100 Finest Songs.* Lanham: Rowman & Littlefield, 2014.

Carlin, Peter Ames. *Bruce.* New York: Touchstone, 2012.

Clemons, Clarence, and Don Reo. *Big Man: Real Life & Tall Tales.* New York: Grand Central Publishing, 2009.

Coles, Robert. *Bruce Springsteen's America: The People Listening, a Poet Singing.* New York: Random House, 2004.

Crane, Bob. *A Place to Stand: A Guide to Bruce Springsteen's Sense of Place.* Baltimore: Palace Books, 2002.

Cullen, Jim. *Born in the U.S.A.: Bruce Springsteen and the American Tradition.* Middletown: Wesleyan University Press, 2005.

D'Amore, Antonella. *Mia città di rovine. L'America di Bruce Springsteen.* Roma: Manifestolibri, 2002.

Dolan, Marc. *Bruce Springsteen and the Promise of Rock 'n' Roll.* New York: W.W. Norton and Company, 2012.

Gambaccini, Peter. *Bruce Springsteen.* London: Omnibus Press, 1981.

Garman, Bryan K. *A Race of Singers: Whitman's Working-Class Hero from Guthrie to Springsteen.* Chapel Hill: University of North Carolina Press, 2000.

Heylin, Clinton. *Springsteen Song by Song: A Critical Look.* New York: Viking Books, 2012.

—. *E Street Shuffle: The Glory Days of Bruce Springsteen and the E Street Band.* London: Constable, 2012.

Hilburn, Robert. *Springsteen.* Atlanta: Rolling Stone Press, 1985.

Humphries, Patrick, and Chris Hunt. *Bruce Springsteen: Blinded by the Light.* London: Plexus, 1985.

Humphries, Patrick. *The Complete Guide to the Music of Bruce Springsteen.* New York: Omnibus Press, 1996.

Kamp, David. "The Book of Bruce Springsteen." *Vanity Fair*, October 2016.

Kirkpatrick, Rob. *The Words and Music of Bruce Springsteen*. Westport: Greenwood, 2007.

Labianca, Ermanno. *American Skin. Vita e musica di Bruce Springsteen*. Firenze: Giunti, 2000.

— and Giovanni Canitano. *Real World. Sulle strade di Bruce Springsteen*. Roma: Fazi, 2005.

Marsh, Dave. *Born to Run: The Bruce Springsteen Story*. New York: Doubleday, 1979.

—. *Glory Days: Bruce Springsteen in the 1980s*. New York: Pantheon Books, 1987.

—. *Two Hearts: The Definitive Biography, 1972–2003*. New York: Routledge, 2003.

—. *Bruce Springsteen on Tour: 1968–2005*. New York: Bloomsbury, 2006.

Masciotra, David. *Working on a Dream: The Progressive Political Vision of Bruce Springsteen*. New York: Continuum, 2010.

Masur, Louis P. *Runaway Dream. "Born to Run" and Bruce Springsteen's American Vision*. New York: Bloomsbury Press, 2010.

Portelli, Alessandro. *Badlands. Springsteen e l'America: il lavoro e i sogni*. Roma: Donzelli, 2015.

Sandford, Christopher. *Springsteen: Point Blank*. London: Omnibus Press, 2004.

Skinner Sawyers, June. *Tougher than the Rest: 100 Best Bruce Springsteen Songs*. New York: Omnibus Press, 2006.

Springsteen, Bruce. *Songs*. New York: HarperEntertainment, 2003.

—. *Born to Run*. London: Simon & Schuster, 2016.

Wiersema, Robert. *Walk Like a Man: Coming of Age with the Music of Bruce Springsteen*. Vancouver: Greystone Books, 2011.

Wolff, Daniel. *4th of July, Asbury Park: A History of the Promised Land*. New York: Bloomsbury, 2006.

♦ Articles on Springsteen quoted in this volume

"100 Greatest Bruce Springsteen Songs of All Time." *Rolling Stone*, January 16, 2014.

"Album of the Month:'The Rising.'" *Uncut*, September 2002.

"Bruce Springsteen: By the Book." *The New York Times*, November 2, 2014.

"Bruce Springsteen's 40 Greatest Songs." *Uncut*, February 17, 2015.

"Bruce Springsteen:'I Cried When I Heard Clarence Clemons on "Wrecking Ball."'" *New Musical Express*, March 14, 2012.

"The Lost Interviews. 1975." excerpted in *Backstreets* #57, Winter 1997, and *Backstreets* #58, Spring 1998.

Appelo, Tim. "Bruce Springsteen's New Album Is His'Angriest' Yet." *Hollywood Reporter*, January 13, 2012.

Bangs, Lester. "Hot Rumble in the Promised Land." *CREEM*, November 1975.

Beviglia, Jim. "The 10 Best Bruce Springsteen Songs of All Time: Bowing Out as an HBO Documentary Beckons." Posted August 8, 2010, http://houston.culturemap.com/

—. "Bruce Springsteen:'Wrecking Ball.'" *American Songwriter*, March 5, 2012.

—. "Counting Down Bruce Springsteen: #48,'The Last Carnival.'" *American Songwriter*, June 30, 2014.

—. "Counting Down Bruce Springsteen: #94,'Valentine's Day.'" *American Songwriter*, June 30, 2014.

Binelli, Mark. "Bruce Springsteen's American Gospel." *Rolling Stone*, August 22, 2002.

Bonca, Cornel. "Save Me Somebody: Bruce Springsteen's Rock 'n' Roll Covenant." *Killing the Buddha*, July 29, 2001.

Bottazzi, Blue. "Bruce Springsteen: 'Nebraska.'" *Il Mucchio Selvaggio*, November 1982.

Bull, Debby. "Bruce Springsteen Gives the Little Guy Something to Cheer About." *Rolling Stone*, July 19–August 2, 1984.

Carithers, David. "'Come On and Rise Up': Springsteen's Experiential Art After 9/11." *Nebula*, September 2005.

Castaldo, Gino. "Provaci ancora Bruce." *La Repubblica*, April 1, 1999.

Chianca, Peter. "Tired Fans to Bruce Springsteen: Cut It Out!" Posted August 29, 2016, http://www.wickedlocal.com/

Cilia, Eddy. "Nebraska." *Velvet Gallery*, June 1990.

Cocks, Jay. "Rock's New Sensation: The Backstreets Phantom of Rock." *Time Magazine*, October 27, 1975.

Coleman, Ray. "Springsteen Crazy." *Melody Maker*, November 1975.

Cott, Roger, and Patrick Humphries. "American Heartbeat: The Bruce Springsteen Interview." *Hot Press*, November 2, 1984.

Cotto, Massimo. "Born to Run." *Velvet Gallery*, June 1990.

Coyne, Kevin. "Story Behind the Glory." *Cape Cod Times*, July 10, 2011.

Cross, Charles R. "Interview with Mike Appel." *Backstreets* #34/35, Fall 1990 / Winter 1991.

Dawidoff, Nicholas. "The Pop Populist." *The New York Time Magazine*, January 26, 1997.

DiMartino, Dave. "Bruce Springsteen Takes It to the River: So Don't Call Him Boss, OK?" *Creem*, January 1981.

Earls, John. "David Bowie Abandoned Covering Bruce Springsteen After Meeting Him." *New Musical Express*, August 19, 2016.

Emerson, Ken. "Springsteen Goes Gritty and Serious. 'The Wild, the Innocent & the E Street Shuffle' Album Review." *Rolling Stone*, January 31, 1974.

Everett-Green, Robert. "Springsteen Is No Less than Storyteller-in-Chief for His Generation." *Toronto Globe and Mail*, July 16, 2005.

Flannigan, Erik, and Christopher Phillips. "'Tracks': The Backstreets Liner Notes." *Backstreets* #61, Winter 1998.

Flannigan, Erik. "Trust None of What You Hear." *Backstreets* #87, Spring 2008.

Ford, Richard. "Richard Ford Reviews Bruce Springsteen's Memoir." *The New York Times*, September 22, 2016.

Fricke, David. "Tunnel of Love." *Rolling Stone*, December 17, 1987.

—. "Bruce Springsteen: Magic." *Rolling Stone*, October 18, 2007.

Gardner, Elysa. "Illustrator Draws on the Boss for 'Outlaw Pete' Book." *USA Today*, November 3, 2014.

Garman, Bryan K. "The Ghost of History: Bruce Springsteen, Woody Guthrie and the Hurt Song." *Popular Music and Society*, Summer 1996.

Gilbert, Jerry. "Bruce: Under the Boardwalk." *Sounds*, March 16, 1974.

Gilmore, Mikal. "Bruce Springsteen: What Does it Mean, Springsteen Asked, to Be an American?" *Rolling Stone*, November 15, 1980.

—. "The Ghost of Tom Joad." *Rolling Stone*, December 17, 1995.

Graydon, Samuel. "America Needs Bruce Springsteen." *The Times Literary Supplement*, October 26, 2016.

Greene, Andy. "Bruce Springsteen, Billy Joel Form Supergroup for Obama in NYC." *Rolling Stone*, October 17, 2008.

—. "Max Weinberg on His Future with Conan and Bruce." *Rolling Stone*, June 2010.

—. "Bruce Springsteen Producer Breaks Down 'High Hopes': Exclusive." *Rolling Stone*, December 30, 2013.

Greenman, Ben. "American Sounds." *The New Yorker*, October 1, 2007.

Hagen, Mark. "The Midnight Cowboy." *Mojo*, January 1999.

—. "Meet the New Boss." *The Observer*, January 1, 2009.

Harris, Keith. "Lift Every Voice." *The Village Voice*, August 6, 2002.

Hart, Benjamin. "Bruce Springsteen Talks Occupy Movement, New Album." *The Huffington Post*, February 18, 2012.

Hausler, Philip. "Wheels of Fire." *Backstreets* #75, Fall 2002.

Henke, James. "Interview with Bruce Springsteen." *Rolling Stone*, August 6, 1992.

—. "The Magician's Tool." *Backstreets* #89, Summer 2010.

Hewitt, Paolo. "Bruce Springsteen: 'The River.'" *Melody Maker*, October 11, 1980.

Hiatt, Bryan. "Springsteen Goes Back to Basics." *Rolling Stone*, April 21, 2005.

—. "Bruce's Dream. An Intimate Visit." *Rolling Stone*, January 23, 2009.

—. "Bruce Springsteen on Making 'Born to Run': 'We Went to Extremes.'" *Rolling Stone*, August 25, 2015.

Hilburn, Robert. "Out in the Streets." *Los Angeles Times*, October 15, 1980.

Horovitz, David. "Bruce Springsteen's Kibbutz Violinist." *The Jerusalem Post*, October 22, 2007.

Humphries, Patrick. "Springsteen." *Record Collector*, February 1999.

Hyden, Steven. "Overrated, Underrated, or Properly Rated: Bruce Springsteen." *Grantland*, January 7, 2014.

Jurek, Thom. "The Rising—Bruce Springsteen." AllMusic.com. Retrieved May 17, 2014.

Kamp, David. "The Book of Bruce Springsteen." *Vanity Fair*, October 2016.

Karlsberg, Jesse P., and John Plunkett. "Bruce Springsteen's Sacred Harp Sample." Posted March 28, 2012, http://originalsacredharp.com/

Kerr, Jim. "Springsteen? Oh My God!" www.simpleminds.com, February 3, 2009.

Knobler, Peter. "I Was the Girl in the Song." *More*, April 2008.

Landau, Jon. "Growing Young with Rock and Roll." *The Real Paper*, May 22, 1974.

Levy, Joe. "Bruce Springsteen's Restless Heart: The Rolling Stone Interview." *Rolling Stone*, October 17, 2007.

—. "The E Street Band Chief Talks About Making His Most Romantic Record Since 'Born to Run.'" *Rolling Stone*, November 1, 2007.

Light, Alan. "The Missing." *The New Yorker*, August 5, 2002.

Lombardi, John. "St. Boss—The Sanctification of Bruce Springsteen and the Rise of Mass Hip." *Esquire*, December 1988.

Mangione, Lorraine. "Spirit in the Night to Mary's Place: Loss, Death, and the Transformative Power of Relationships." *The Psychology of Aesthetics, Creativity & the Arts*, July 2008.

Manzoor, Sarfraz. "My Favourite Album: 'Tunnel of Love' by Bruce Springsteen." *The Guardian*, August 31, 2011.

Marchese, David. "The Boss Finally Gets What He Wants, but What About Us?" *Spin*, January 22, 2009.

Marcus, Greil. "Springsteen's Thousand and One American Nights. 'Born to Run' Album Review." *Rolling Stone*, October 9, 1975.

Marsh, Dave. "Bruce Springsteen: A Rock Star Is Born." *Rolling Stone*, September 25, 1975.

—. "Bruce Springsteen Raises Cain." *Rolling Stone*, August 24, 1978.

—. "Springsteen." *Musician*, February 1981.

Massimino, Andrew E. "And the Next Day . . ." *Backstreets* #83/84, Winter 2005/2006.

Massimino, Andrew E., and Christopher Phillips. "Beyond the Songs." *Backstreets* #75, Fall 2002.

Masur, Louis P. "Tramps Like Us. The Birth of 'Born to Run.'" *Slate*, September 22, 2009.

McConnell, Frank. "A Rock Poet: From Fitzgerald to Springsteen." *Commonweal*, August 12, 1983.

Milazzo, Melissa. "Bruce Springsteen: Reason to Believe." Posted May 10, 2010, http://melissamilazzo. wordpress.com/

Mohr, Ian. "Stephen King's Epic First Meeting with Bruce Springsteen." *Page Six*, June 8, 2016.

Mörke, Torsten. "Interview with David Hazlett." Posted November 2000, http://www.castiles. net/

Morris, Marya. "Geography and Place. From 'My Hometown' to 'This Hard Land': Bruce Springsteen's Use of Geography, Landscapes, and Places to Depict the American Experience." *Interdisciplinary Literary Studies*, Vol. 9, No. 1, Glory Days: A Bruce Springsteen Celebration, Penn State University Press, Fall 2007.

Nelson, Paul. "Let Us Now Praise Famous Men." *Rolling Stone*, December 1980.

—. "Bruce Springsteen: 'Nebraska.'" *Musician*, November 1982.

Orth, Maureen, Janet Huck and Peter S. Greenberg. "The Making of a Rock Star." *Newsweek*, October 27, 1975.

Pareles, Jon. "Springsteen Looks at Love." *The New York Times*, October 4, 1987.

—. "Springsteen: An Old-Fashioned Rocker in a New Era." *The New York Times*, March 29, 1992.

—. "Music; His Kind of Heroes, His Kind of Songs." *The New York Times*, July 14, 2002.

— "Bruce Almighty." *The New York Times*, April 24, 2005.

Peay, Pythia. "Soul Searching." *Washingtonian*, January–February 2001.

Penn, Sean. "Bruce Springsteen." *Time*, May 12, 2008.

Percy, Will. "Rock and Read: Will Percy Interviews Bruce Springsteen." *Double Take*, Spring 1998.

Petridis, Alexis. "CD of the Week: Bruce Springsteen and the E Street Band." *The Guardian*. July 25, 2002.

Phillips, Christopher. "Seachin' Through the Dust." *Backstreets* #75, Fall 2002.

—. "The Real World." *Backstreets* #79, Spring 2004.

—. "Citizen Bruce." *Backstreets* #95, Summer/Fall 2004.

—. "The Devil's in the Details." *Backstreets* double issue #83/84, Winter 2005/2006.

—. "With These Hands." *Backstreets* #83/84, Winter 2005/2006.

—. "The Devil's in the Details." *Backstreets* #83/84, Winter 2005/2006.

—. "Heck of a Job, Brucie." *Backstreets* #91, Fall/Winter 2013.

Pistolini, Stefano. "Separare le carriere della politica e del rock." *IL*, Ocotber 2012.

Pitts, Leonard, Jr. "Springsteen Captures the State of America." *Chicago Tribune*, March 21, 2012.

Pond, Steve. "Bruce's Hard Look at Love." *Rolling Stone*, December 3, 1987.

Powers, Ann. "Album Review: Bruce Springsteen and the E Street Band's 'Working on a Dream.'" *Los Angeles Times*, January 24, 2009.

Raimondo, Luca. "Soundcheck: 'Nebraska.'" *Follow That Dream*, June 1991.

Remnick, David. "We Are Alive." *The New Yorker*, July 30, 2012.

Rodgers, Larry. "Bruce Springsteen, Born in the U.S.A., 25 Years Old Today." *The Arizona Republic*, June 4, 2009.

Roland, Tom. "Bruce Springsteen's Enduring Effect on the Country Charts Influences Two Top 10 Singles." *Billboard*, May 8, 2012.

Rose, Caryn. "Somerville Nights." *Backstreets* #76, Winter/Spring 2003.

—. "10 of the Best: Bruce Springsteen." *The Guardian*, March 19, 2014.

Russell, Bob. "Bruce Springsteen: 'Wrecking Ball.'" *Pop Culture Ponderings*, April 9, 2012.

Scott, Anthony O. "The Poet Laureate of 9/11. Apocalypse and Salvation on Springsteen's New Album." *Slate*, August 6, 2002.

Sennett, Sean. "Bruce Springsteen Q&A: On Top Down Under." *Rolling Stone*, March 11, 2014.

Shruers, Fred. "Bruce Springsteen and the Secret of the World." *Rolling Stone*, February 5, 1981.

Strauss, Neil. "Springsteen Looks Back but Keeps Walking On." *The New York Times*, May 7, 1995.

—. "Human Touch." *Guitar World*, October 1995.

Sutcliffe, Phil. "You Talking to Me?" *Mojo*, January 2006.

Sweeting, Adam. "Into the Fire." *Uncut*, September 2002.

Tyrangiel, Josh. "Born to Stump." *Time*, October 10, 2004.

Tziampiris, Aristotle. "Why Springsteen Could Have Been President." *The Huffington Post*, August 30, 2016.

Vulliamy, Ed. "Bruce Springsteen: Last of the Protest Singers." *The Observer*, June 10, 2012.

Wieseltier, Leon. "A Saint in the City." *The New Republic*, August 1, 2012.

Zambellini, Mauro. "All Those Years of Human Touch." *Il Mucchio Selvaggio*, April 1992.

—. "Born to Run." *Il Mucchio Selvaggio*, June 1992.

‣ Other books quoted in this volume

Chambers's Encyclopaedia, Vol. 2. London: George Newnes, 1961.

Conversations on the Craft of Poetry with Robert Frost, John Crowe Ransom, Robert Lowell, Theodore Roethke. Edited by Cleanth Brooks and Robert Penn Warren. New York: Holt, Rinehart and Winston, 1961.

Inner Voices, Inner View: Conversations with Southern Writers. Norwalk: Enolam Group, 2005.

Music for Pleasure: Essays in the Sociology of Pop. New York: Routledge, 1988.

Stranded: Rock and Roll for a Desert Island. Edited by Greil Marcus. New York: Da Capo Press, 1996.

Studies in Art and Religious Interpretation, 2. New York: Mellen, 1982.

Sweet Nothings: An Anthology of Rock and Roll. Bloomington: Indiana University Press, 1994.

The EmBodyment of American Culture, Edited by Heinz Tschachler, Maureen Devine, Michael Draxlbauer. Münster: LIT Verlag, 2003.

The Norton Anthology of Poetry. New York: W. W. Norton & Company, 1983.

Baudelaire, Charles. *Journaux intimes*. Paris: Les Éditions G. Crés et Cie, 1920.

—. *Œuvres completes*. Paris, Gallimard, 1975–1976.

Blesh, Rudi, and Janis Blesh. *They All Played Ragtime*. New York: Alfred A. Knopf, 1950.

Bloom, Harold. *The Western Canon: The Books and Schools of the Age*. New York: Harcourt, 1994.

Booth, Wayne C. *The Rhetoric of Fiction*. Chicago: University of Chicago Press, 1961.

Boyle, T.C. *Greasy Lake and Other Stories*. New York: Viking Penguin, 1985.

Campbell, Joseph. *The Hero with a Thousand Faces*. New York: Pantheon Books, 1948.

Carver, Raymond. *Where Water Comes Together with Other Water*. New York: Vintage, 1986.

—. *Where I'm Calling From: Selected Stories*. New York: Vintage, 1988.

Cioran, Emil. *Syllogismes de l'amertume*. Paris: Gallimard, 1952.

Clarke Keogh, Pamela. *Elvis Presley: The Man. The Life. The Legend*. New York: Atria Books, 2004.

Conan Doyle, Arthur. *Songs of the Road*. London: Smith, Elder & Co., 1911.

Croce, Benedetto. *Estetica come scienza dell'espressione e linguistica generale. Teoria e storia*. Milano: Adelphi, 1990.

Dees, Morris. *A Season for Justice*. New York: Charles Scribner's Sons, 1991.

De Simone, Mariano. *"Doo-dah! Doo-dah!" Musica e musicisti nell'America dell'Ottocento*. Roma: Arcana, 2003.

Dickinson, Emily. *The Poems of Emily Dickinson*. Edited by Thomas H. Johnson. Boston: Belknap Press of Harvard University Press, 1955.

Dylan, Bob. *Chronicles. Volume One*. London: Simon & Schuster, 2004.

Eliot, Thomas Stearns. *Selected Essays 1917–1932*. London: Faber & Faber, 1951.

—. *Four Quartets*. New York: Harcourt, Brace & World, 1962.

Epstein, Dena J. *Sinful Tunes and Spirituals: Black Folk Music to the Civil War*. Chicago: University of Illinois Press, 1977.

Farber, David G. *Sloan Rules: Alfred P. Sloan and the Triumph of General Motors*. Chicago: University of Chicago Press, 2012.

Faulkner, William. *The Sound and the Fury*. London: Jonathan Cape and Harrison Smith, 1929.

Flanagan, Bill. *Written in My Soul: Conversations with Rock's Great Songwriters*. Chicago: Contemporary Books, 1987.

Franklin, Benjamin. *The Autobiography: 1706–1757*. Bedford: Applewood Books, 2008.

Friedrich, Hugo. *The Structure of Modern Poetry: From the Mid-nineteenth to the Mid-twentieth Century*. Evanston, Northwestern University Press, 1974.

Gilmore, Mikal. *Night Beat: A Shadow History of Rock & Roll*. New York: Anchor, 1998.

Ginsberg, Allen. *Howl and Other Poems*. San Francisco: City Lights, 1956.

Graves, Robert. *The White Goddess*. London: Faber & Faber, 1948.

Guagliardo, Huey. *Perspectives on Richard Ford: Redeemed by Affection*. Jackson: University Press of Mississippi, 2000.

Gundersen, Edna. "Dylan's Art Is Forever A-Changing." *USA Today*, August 28, 2006.

Heaney, Seamus. *The Government of the Tongue*. London: Faber, 1988.

Hedin, Benjamin. *Studio A: The Bob Dylan Reader*. New York: W. W. Norton & Company, 2004.

Hemingway, Ernest. *Men Without Women*. New York: Charles Scribner's Sons, 1927.

—. *A Farewell to Arms*. New York: Charles Scribner's Sons, 1929.

—. *Death in the Afternoon*. New York: Charles Scribner's Sons, 1932.

Hornby, Nick. *Songbook*. San Francisco: McSweeney's, 2002.

Humphries, Patrick. *The Many Lives of Tom Waits*. London: Omnibus Press, 2009.

Jordan, Terry G. *North American Cattle Ranching Frontiers: Origins, Diffusion, and Differentiation*. Albuquerque: University of New Mexico Press, 1993.

Kazin, Alfred. *Bright Book of Life. American Novelists and Storytellers from Hemingway to Mailer*. London: Secker & Walburg, 1974.

Kerouac, Jack. *On the Road*. New York: Viking Press, 1957.

—. *Romanzi*. Milano: Mondadori, 2001.

Le Corbusier. *When Cathedrals Were White*. Columbus: McGraw-Hill, 1964.

Lomax, Alan. *Land Where the Blues Began*. New York: New Press, 2002.

Lomax, John A. *American Ballads and Folk Songs*. New York: Macmillan Company, 1934.

Lowell, Robert. *Lord Weary's Castle*. San Diego: Harcourt Brace, 1946.

—. *Life Studies*. New York: Farrar, Straus & Giroux, 1959.

Maharidge, Dale. *Journey to Nowhere—The Saga of the New Underclass*, photography by Michael Williamson. New York: Hyperion Books, 1986.

Marcus, Greil. *In the Fascist Bathroom: Punk in Pop Music, 1977–1992*. Cambridge: Harvard University Press, 1999.

Mason, Bobby Ann. *In Country*. New York: Harper & Row, 1985.

Masters, Edgar Lee. *Spoon River Anthology*. New York: MacMillan, 1916.

Melville, Herman. *Moby-Dick; or, The Whale*. New York: Harper & Brothers, 1851.

Monda, Antonio. *La magnifica illusione. Un viaggio nel cinema americano*. Roma: Fazi, 2007.

Morris, Timothy. *Becoming Canonical in American Poetry*. Chicago: University of Illinois Press, 1995.

O'Connor, Flannery. *A Good Man Is Hard to Find*. San Diego: Harcourt, Brace and Company, 1955.

—. *Mystery & Manners: Occasional Prose*. Selected and edited by Sally and Robert Fitzgerald. New York: Farrar, Straus & Giroux, 1961.

—. *The Complete Stories*. New York: Farrar, Straus and Giroux, 1989.

Ott, Christine. *Montale e la parola riflessa*. Milano: Franco Angeli, 2006.

Owen, Wilfred. *Poems*. London: Chatto & Windus, 1920.

Percy, Walker. *The Moviegoer*. New York: Knopf, 1961.

Perone, James E. *The Album: A Guide to Pop Music's Most Provocative, Influential, and Important Creations*, Volume 1. Santa Barbara: Praeger, 2012.

Pound, Ezra. *ABC of Reading*. Cambridge: New Directions, 1934.

Rahv, Philip. *Essays on Literature and Politics 1932–1972*. Boston: Houghton Mifflin, 1978.

Raimondi, Giorgio. *La scrittura sincopata. Jazz e letteratura nel Novecento italiano*. Milano: Bruno Mondadori, 1999.

Sabin, Roger. *Punk Rock: So What?: The Cultural Legacy of Punk*. London: Routledge, 1999.

Savage, Jon. *Teenage: The Creation of Youth Culture*. New York: Viking, 2007.

Shakespeare, William. *Macbeth*. London: Penguin, 2007.

Smith, John. *The Generall Historie of Virginia, New-England, and the Summer Isles*. London: Michael Sparkes, 1624.

Stedman, Edmund Clarence, and Ellen Mackay Hutchinson. *A Library of American Literature*, Vol. 1. New York: Charles Webster, 1889.

Steinbeck, John. *The Grapes of Wrath*. New York: The Viking Press-James Lloyd, 1939.

Tocqueville, Alexis de. *Selected Letters on Politics and Society*. Edited by Roger Boesche. Berkley: University of California Press, 1985.

Twain, Mark. *Roughing It*. Chicago: American Publishing Company, 1872.

Vogler, Christopher. *The Writer's Journey: Mythic Structure for Writers*. Los Angeles: Michael Wiese Productions, 2007.

Whitehead, Colson. *John Henry Days*. New York: Doubleday, 1991.

Whitfield, James M. *America and Other Poems*. Buffalo: James S. Leavitt, 1853.

Whitman, Walt. *Leaves of Grass*. Philadelphia: David McKay, 1900.

—. *Foglie d'erba*. Milano: Rizzoli, 2004.

Wyatt, David. *Out of the Sixties. Storytelling and the Vietnam Generation*. Cambridge: Cambridge University Press, 1993.

Young, Neil. *Waging Heavy Peace: A Hippie Dream*. New York: Plume, 2013.

Zollo, Paul. *Songwriters on Songwriting*. New York: Da Capo Press, 2005.

♦ Other articles quoted in this volume

"Aronowsky Quizzed Springsteen over One-legged Dog Line." *IMDb*, November 26, 2010.

"George Bush Meet Woodrow Wilson." *New York Times*, November 20, 1990.

"Irvine Welsh Slams Nobel Prize Award for Bob Dylan." *The Scotsman*, October 13, 2016.

Aftab, Kaleem. "Edward Norton Interview: Fight Club Actor Talks Bruce Springsteen Relationship Advice, American History X, Socialism and President Obama." *The Independent*, August 14, 2015.

Arax, Mark, and Tom Gordo. "California's Illicit Farm Belt Export." *Los Angeles Times*, March 19, 1995.

Barth, John. "The Literature of Exhaustion." *The Atlantic Monthly*, August 1967.

Buford, Bill. "Dirty Realism." *Granta*, Summer 1983.

Bussey, John. "The Eye of the Storm: One Man's Journey Through Desperation and Chaos." *The Wall Street Journal*, September 12, 2001.

Christgau, Robert. "Review of 'Please Kill Me: The Uncensored Oral History of Punk.'" *New York Times Book Review*, 1996.

Cott, Jonathan. "The Lost Lennon Tapes." *Rolling Stone*, December 8, 2010.

—. "John Lennon: The Last Interview." *Rolling Stone*, December 23, 2010.

Crane, Stephen. "Parades and Entertainments." *The New York Tribune*, August 21, 1892.

Davis, Stephen. "Van Morrison. The Interview." *New Age*, August 1985.

DeLillo, Don. "In the Ruins of the Future: Reflections on Terror and Loss in the Shadow of September." *Harper's*, December 2001.

Douglas, Edward. "Mickey Rourke Piledrives 'The Wrestler.'" *Coming Soon*, December 17, 2008.

Gallo, Phil. "Lady Gaga Reflects on Springsteen Influence for 'Inside the Outside' Doc." *Billboard*, May 18, 2011.

Hansen, Chadwick. "The Character of Jim and the Ending of 'Huckleberry Finn.'" *The Massachussetts Review*. Vol. 5, No. 1, Autumn 1963.

Hisler, Scott. "David Bowie Opens Up a Little." *Musician*, August 1987.

Mailer, Norman. "The Hip and the Square." *Village Voice*, April 25, 1956.

Phipps, Keith. "The Restless Dreams and Lonely Highways of Two-Lane Blacktop." *The Dissolve*, May 26, 2015.

Poe, Edgar Allan. "Marginalia." *Democratic Review*, November, 1844.

Pynchon, Thomas. "The Deadly Sins. Sloth: Nearer, My Couch, to Thee." *The New York Times*, June 6, 1993.

Ramone, Tommy. "Fight Club." *Uncut*, January, 2007.

Reeves, Jay. "Case Closed; Cherry Guilty." *Times Daily*, May 23, 2002.

Ronner, Abby. "Giddy Out: Will New York's Federation of Black Cowboys Be Sent Packing?" *The Village Voice*, April 20, 2016.

Rotella, Sebastian. "Children of the Border." *Los Angeles Times*, April 3, 1993.

♦ Books on Springsteen not quoted but consulted for this volume

Bruce Springsteen and the American Soul: Essays on the Songs and Influence of a Cultural Icon. Edited by David Garrett Izzo. Jefferson: McFarland, 2011.

Brucetellers. Pistoia: Nuove Esperienze, 2011.

Our Love Is Real. Edited by Henry Ruggeri. Roma: Arcana, 2013.

Reading the Boss: Interdisciplinary Approaches to the Works of Bruce Springsteen. Edited by Roxanne Harde and Irwin Streight. Lanham, Lexington Books, 2010.

Barco, Stefano, and Alberto Neri. *Bruce Springsteen Anthology*. Padova: Arcana, 1999.

Cavicchi, Daniel. *Tramps Like Us: Music and Meaning Among Springsteen Fans*. New York: Oxford Univeristy Press, 1998.

De Rossi, Patrizia. *She's the One: Bruce Springsteen e le donne*. Reggio Emilia: Imprimatur, 2014.

Dolan, Mark. *Bruce Springsteen and the Promise of Rock 'n' Roll*. New York: W.W. Norton & Company, 2013.

Duffy, John W. *Bruce Springsteen Talking*. London: Omnibus Press, 2004.

Goddard, Peter. *Springsteen Live*. Toronto: Stoddart Publishing, 1984.

Goldsmith, Lynn. *Springsteen: Access All Areas*. New York, Universe Publishing, 2000.

Heylin, Clinton, and Simon Gee. *The E Street Shuffle: Springsteen & the E Street Band in Performance 1972–1988*. Cheshire: Labour of Love Productions, 1989.

Hilburn, Robert. *Springsteen*. New York: Rolling Stone Press, 1985.

Himes, Geoffrey. *Bruce Springsteen*. Milano: No Reply, 2008.

Jones, Tennessee. *Deliver Me from Nowhere*. Brooklyn: Soft Skull Press, 2005.

Linch, Kate. *Springsteen: No Surrender*. New York: Proteus, 1984.

Kirsh Lawrence. *The Light in Darkness*. Montreal: Kirsh Communications, 2009.

Mårtensson, Anders, and Jorgen Johannsson. *Local Heroes. The Asbury Park Music Scene.* Chapel Hill: Rutgers Univerity Press, 2008.

Meola, Erica. *Born to Run: The Unseen Photos.* San Rafael: InSight Editions, 2006.

Petrillo, Marina. *Nativo americano. La voce folk di Bruce Springsteen.* Milano: Feltrinelli, 2010.

Primeau, Patrick. *The Moral Passion of Bruce Springsteen.* Bethesda: International Scholars Publications, 1996.

Rosen, Steven. *Bruce Springsteen.* Chessington: Castle Communications, 1995.

Santelli, Robert. *Greetings from E Street: The Story of Bruce Springsteen and the E Street Band.* San Francisco: Chronicle Books, 2006.

Stefanko, Frank. *Days of Hope and Dreams: An Intimate Portrait of Bruce Springsteen.* San Rafael: InSight Editions, 2003.

Symynkywicz, Jeffrey B. *The Gospel According to Bruce Springsteen.* Louisville, Westminister John Knox Press, 2008.

⬧ Articles on Springsteen not quoted but consulted for this volume

Bangs, Lester. "Hot Rod Rumble in the Promised Land." *Creem*, November 1975.

Barol, Bill. "He's on Fire." *Newsweek*, August 5,1985.

Barry, Dave. "Glory Days." *Miami Herald*, July 10, 1994.

Bird, Elizabeth. "'Is That Me Baby?' Image, Authenticity, and the Career of Bruce Springsteen." *American Studies*, 35, No. 2, 1994.

Brooks, David. "The Other Education." *The New York Times*, November 26, 2009.

Carlin, Peter Ames. "The Secret Life of Bruce Springsteen, aged 13¾." *The Word*, December 2010.

Coyne, Kevin. "The Faulkner of Freehold." *Asbury Park Press*, March 14, 1999.

Costas, Bob. "Bruce Springsteen Talks About His Music and His Career." *Today*, December 7, 1998.

Douglas, Ann. "Bruce Springsteen and Narrative Rock: The Art of Extended Urgency." *Dissent*, Fall 1985.

Filippo, Chet. "Bruce Springsteen: A Rock 'n' Roll Evangelist for Our Times Crusades for Patriotism and Puritanism of a Different Stripe." *Musician*, November 1984.

Fricke, David. "Review of 'Magic.'" *Rolling Stone*, October 18, 2007.

Fusilli, Jim. "The Heart of Darkness." *The Wall Street Journal*, October 10, 2010.

Gavin, Martin. "Hey Joad, Don't Make It Sad." *New Musical Express*, March 9, 1996.

Griffin, John. "Springsteen Has Winner in River." *The Gazette*, October 16, 1980.

Hilburn, Robert. "Springsteen Off and Running." *The Los Angeles Times*, September 28, 1975.

Holden, Stephen. "Bruce Springsteen: Of Time and 'The River.'" *The Village Voice*, October 28, 1980.

Knobler, Peter, and Greg Mitchell. "Who Is Bruce Springsteen and Why Are We Saying All These Wonderful Things About Him?" *Crawdaddy*, March 1973.

Knopper, Steve. "Influencing the Boss: Springsteen Mines Many Sources for Inspiration." *Milwaukee Journal Sentinel*, September 27, 2002.

Morse, Steve. "Bruce Looks Back: Springsteen Talks About Life, Changes, and His New Boxed Set." *Boston Globe*, November 20, 1998.

Rockwell, John. "New Dylan from New Jersey? It Might as Well Be Springsteen." *Rolling Stone*, October 9, 1975.

Rufford, Nick. "Bruce Springsteen: Just a Regular Millionaire." *Sunday Times Magazine*, November 23, 2010.

Tucker, Ken. "Springsteen: The Interview." *Entertainment Weekly*, February 28, 2003.

Wolcott, James. "The Hagiography of Bruce Springsteen." *Vanity Fair*, December 1985.

♦ Other books and articles not quoted but consulted for this volume

Altschuler, Glenn C. *All Shook Up: How Rock 'n' Roll Changed America*. New York: Oxford University Press, 2003.

Berendt, Joachim-Ernst. *The Jazz Book: From Ragtime to Fusion and Beyond*. New York: Lawrence Hill & Co, 1975.

Campbell, Michael. *Popular Music in America. And the Beat Goes On*. Tempe: Engage Learning, 2008.

Coleman, Rick. *Blue Monday: Fats Domino and the Lost Dawn of Rock 'n' Roll*. New York: Da Capo Press, 2007.

Davis, Miles, and Quincy Troupe. *Miles, The Autobiography*. New York: Simon & Schuster, 1989.

Ferlinghetti, Lawrence. *Berlin*, Naples: Golden Mountain Press, 1961.

Gambaccini Paul. *Masters of Rock*. London: Omnibus Press, 1982.

Garst, John. "Chasing John Henry in Alabama and Mississippi: A Personal Memoir of Work in Progress." *Journal of the Alabama Folklife Association* #5, 2002.

Gilmore, Mikal. *Night Beat. Collected Writing on Rock & Roll Culture and Other Disruptions*. New York: Bantam Doubleday Dell, 1997.

Greenway, John. *American Folksongs of Protest*. Philadelphia: University of Pennsylvania Press, 1953.

Guthrie, Woody. *Pastures of Plenty: A Self-Portrait*. Edited by Dave Marsh and H. Leventhal. New York: HarperCollins, 1990.

Hammond, John, and Irving Townsend. *John Hammond on Record*. New York: Penguin Books, 1977.

Johnson, Nunnally. *The Grapes of Wrath* (Screenplay). Hollywood: Script City, 1940.

Kerouac, Jack. *241st Chorus, Mexico City Blues: 242 Choruses*. New York: Grove/Evergreen, 1959.

Klein, Joe. *Woody Guthrie: A Life*. New York: Knopf, 1980.

Marling Karal, Ann. *Graceland: Going Home with Elvis*. Cambridge: Harvard University Press, 1997.

Matthiessen, Francis Otto. *American Renaissance: Art and Expression in the Age of Emerson and Whitman*. Oxford: Oxford University Press, 1941.

Moriarty, Frank. *Seventies Rock. The Decade of Creative Chaos*. Lanham: Taylor Trade Publishing, 2003.

Percy, Walker. *The Message in the Bottle: How Queer Man Is, How Queer Language Is, and What One Has to Do with the Other*. New York: Picador/Farrar, Strauss and Giroux, 2000.

Reiken, Frederick. *The Lost Legends of New Jersey*. Harvest Books, New York, 2001.

Riggan, William. *Pícaros, Madmen, Naïfs, and Clowns: The Unreliable First-Person Narrator*. Norman: University of Oklahoma Press, 1981.

Samway, Patrick S.J. *Walker Percy: A Life*. Chicago: Loyola Press, 1999.

Scaduto, Anthony. *Bob Dylan*. New York: New American Library, 1979.

Stokes, Niall. *Into the Heart: The Story Behind Every U2 Song*. Australia: HarperCollins, 1996.

Thompson Jim. *The Killer Inside Me*. New York: Vintage Books, 1991.

Weinberg, Max, and Robert Santelli. *The Big Beat*. Chicago: Contemporary Books, 1984.

♦ Speeches, Radio & TV Interviews

Bono. "Bruce Springsteen's Rock & Roll Hall of Fame Induction Speech." Waldorf Astoria, New York, March 15, 1999.

Springsteen, Bruce. Interview for the *Wings for Wheels* home video (2005).

Springsteen, Bruce. "Springsteen Discusses His Latest Release, Part 1." Interview with Renée Montagne. National Public Radio's *Morning Edition*, April 26, 2005.

Borick, Christopher, and David Rosenwasser. "Springsteen's Right Side: A Liberal Icon's Conservatism." Paper at the Bruce Springsteen Symposium, West Long Branch, NJ, September 26, 2009.

Dylan, Bob. "Banquet Speech." Paper presented by the U.S. Ambassador to Sweden Azita Raji at the Nobel Banquet in Stockholm, December 10, 2016. Copyright ©2016 The Nobel Foundation.

Hamburger, Susan. "'Bruce, We Need You Now': Bruce Springsteen's Response to 9/11 with 'The Rising." Paper read at the South Atlantic Modern Language Association meeting, Durham, NC, November 9, 2012.

Springsteen, Bruce. "Jackson Browne's Rock & Roll Hall of Fame Induction Speech." Waldorf Astoria, New York, March 15, 2004.

Springsteen, Bruce. International press conference. Théâtre Marigny, Paris, France, February 16, 2012.

Springsteen, Bruce. "Keynote Speech." Paper presented at the South by Southwest Conference, Austin, TX, March 15, 2012.

Springsteen, Bruce. Speech at Barak Obama presidential rally. Madison, WI, November 5, 2012.

Springsteen, Bruce. Interview during Dave Marsh's *Live From E Street Nation* show on Sirius XM's E Street Radio channel, December 19, 2013. The interview premiered on January 10, 2014.

♦ Websites

brucebase.wikispaces.com

brucetapes.com

friendsofthespringsteencollection.nexxtblog.com

northofboston.wickedlocal.com/springsteen

springsteenlyrics.com

www.backstreets.com
www.blogitallnight.com
www.brucespringsteen.it
www.brucespringsteen.net
www.greasylake.org
www.lostintheflood.priv.at

ACKNOWLEDGMENTS

I have seen Bruce Springsteen in concert so many times I've lost track of the number. The first was on June 21, 1985, at the Meazza Stadium, with two of my friends with whom the previous summer I had listened to a cassette tape with *Nebraska* on the A-side, and *Born to Run* on side B. During those days radio and TV channels had been playing "Dancing in the Dark," which at the time did not seem like such a great song to me. But when *Nebraska* came out of the speakers, I was floored: it was totally different from all the music I had loved up until then. We listened to the album in silence. Then we flipped sides. How could it be that the author of "Reason to Believe" was the same as for "Thunder Road"?

This book cannot be concluded without my heartfelt thanks going to Niccolò Borella and Bernardino Sassoli, the two friends with whom I discovered Springsteen and first saw him live; and the many others I met up with on the way, sharing the same passion for Springsteen's music (how could I forget Pierluigi De Palma?).

Sincere thanks must be given to Giulio Mozzi and Massimiliano Bianchini, who ten years ago published the first edition of this book in Italy for Sironi Publishing. And to John Cerullo, Bernadette Malavarca, and Ilaria Narici, who made the publishing of the English edition possible, with the precious contribution of my agent, Carmen Prestia, and of Mona Okada (Grubman, Indursky & Schindler).

Ennio Morricone honored me with his preface to the book, as did Dave Marsh, who acted (and continues to be) like a "maestro," guide, counselor, and friend to me.

The English edition of *Like a Killer in the Sun* would never have been possible without the approval and encouragement of Bruce Springsteen and of Jon Landau Management (my heartfelt gratitude to you, Barbara Carr!), not forgetting my great friend Susan Duncan Smith, who has been helping Bruce for years in all his Italian activities.

On August 11, 1999, I attended a Bruce Springsteen show at the Meadowlands Arena in East Rutherford, New Jersey. My friend Kevin Cleary gave me the tickets (in the second row!). Two years later, on September 11, 2001, Kevin died in his office on the eighty-fourth floor of the north tower of the World Trade Center. This book is dedicated to his memory.

Francesca Bolza has worked on the present edition with enthusiasm, professionalism and talent, transforming my highfalutin Italian into English—*grazie mille*!

My deepest apologies go to my beloved wife, Gaia, for my escapes to arenas and stadiums worldwide trailing behind Springsteen's tracks, with my thanks for having stood by me raising Margherita and Matteo with the sacred cult for the Jersey Devil—guys, sing with me: "These are better days, baby . . . yeah, better days shining through."

PERMISSIONS

Lyrics

"4th of July, Asbury Park (Sandy)" (Springsteen) Copyright © 1973 Bruce Springsteen GMR

"57 Channels (An Nothin' On)" (Springsteen) Copyright © 1992 Bruce Springsteen GMR

"Across the Border" (Springsteen) Copyright © 1995 Bruce Springsteen GMR

"Adam Raised a Cain" (Springsteen) Copyright © 1978 Bruce Springsteen GMR

"American Land" (Springsteen) Copyright © 2006 Bruce Springsteen GMR

"Atlantic City" (Springsteen) Copyright © 1982 Bruce Springsteen GMR

"Backstreets" (Springsteen) Copyright © 1975 Bruce Springsteen GMR

"Badlands" (Springsteen) Copyright © 1978 Bruce Springsteen GMR

"Balboa Park" (Springsteen) Copyright © 1995 Bruce Springsteen GMR

"Because the Night" (Springsteen, Smith) Copyright © 1978 Bruce Springsteen GMR, Patti Smith ASCAP

"Better Days" (Springsteen) Copyright ©1992 Bruce Springsteen GMR

"Black Cowboys" (Springsteen) Copyright © 2005 Bruce Springsteen GMR

"Blinded by the Light" (Springsteen) Copyright © 1972 Bruce Springsteen GMR

"Blood Brothers" (Springsteen) Copyright © 1995 Bruce Springsteen GMR

"Bobby Jean" (Springsteen) Copyright © 1984 Bruce Springsteen GMR

"Born in the U.S.A." (Springsteen) Copyright © 1984 Bruce Springsteen GMR

"Born to Run" (Springsteen) Copyright © 1975 Bruce Springsteen GMR

"Brilliant Disguise" (Springsteen) Copyright © 1987 Bruce Springsteen GMR

"Candy's Room" (Springsteen) Copyright © 1978 Bruce Springsteen GMR

"Car Wash" (Springsteen) Copyright ©1998 Bruce Springsteen GMR

"Cautious Man" (Springsteen) Copyright © 1987 Bruce Springsteen GMR

"Come On (Let's Go Tonight)" (Springsteen) Copyright © 2010 Bruce Springsteen GMR

"Dancing in the Dark" (Springsteen) Copyright © 1984 Bruce Springsteen GMR

"Darkness on the Edge of Town" (Springsteen) Copyright © 1978 Bruce Springsteen GMR

"Death to My Hometown" (Springsteen) Copyright © 2012 Bruce Springsteen GMR

"Devil's Arcade" (Springsteen) Copyright © 2007 Bruce Springsteen GMR

"Devils & Dust" (Springsteen) Copyright © 2005 Bruce Springsteen GMR

"Downbound Train" (Springsteen) Copyright © 1984 Bruce Springsteen GMR

"Easy Money" (Springsteen) Copyright © 2012 Bruce Springsteen GMR

"Empty Sky" (Springsteen) Copyright © 2002 Bruce Springsteen GMR

Text